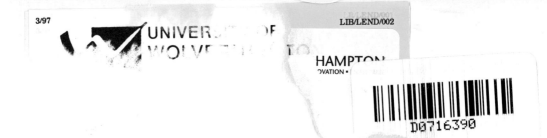

Apley's

SYSTEM OF ORTHOPAEDICS AND FRACTURES

8th Edition

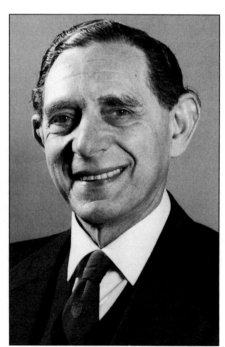

Alan Graham Apley 1914–1996
Inspired teacher, wise mentor and
joyful friend

Apley's

SYSTEM OF ORTHOPAEDICS AND FRACTURES

8th Edition

Louis Solomon
MB, ChB, MD, FRCS, FRCSEd
Emeritus Professor of Orthopaedic Surgery, University of Bristol

David Warwick
MD, BM, DIMC, FRCS, FRCS(Orth)
Consultant Orthopaedic Surgeon, Southampton University Hospitals
Formerly: Lecturer in Orthopaedic Surgery, University of Bristol

Selvadurai Nayagam
MB, ChB, MCh(Orth), FRCS(Orth)Ed
Consultant Orthopaedic Surgeon, Royal Liverpool Children's Hospital and
Royal Liverpool University Hospital

Foreword by

Henry J. Mankin
MD, FRCS(Hon)
Former Chief of the Orthopaedic Service, Massachusetts General Hospital,
Edith M. Ashley Professor of Orthopaedics, Harvard Medical School, Boston, USA

ARNOLD

A member of the Hodder Headline Group
LONDON
Co-published in the USA by
Oxford University Press Inc., New York

First published in Great Britain in 2001
by Arnold, a member of the Hodder Headline Group,
338 Euston Road, London NW1 3BH

http://www.arnoldpublishers.com

Co-published in the USA by Oxford University Press Inc.,
198 Madison Avenue, New York, NY10016

British Library Cataloguing-in-Publication Data
A catalogue record for this book is available from the British Library

Library of Congress Cataloging-in-Publication Data
A catalog record for this book is available from the Library of Congress

ISBN 0 340 76372 8 (hb)
ISBN 0 340 76373 6 (pb, International Students Edition)

1 2 3 4 5 6 7 8 9 10

Design and illustration by Inperspective Ltd

Printed and bound in India by Ajanta Offset, New Delhi

What do you think about this book? Or any other Arnold title?
Please send your comments to feedback.arnold@hodder.co.uk

Contents

FOREWORD   vii
PREFACE   ix
ACKNOWLEDGEMENTS   xi

PART 1 – GENERAL ORTHOPAEDICS

1. ORTHOPAEDIC DIAGNOSIS   3

2. INFECTION   27

3. RHEUMATIC DISORDERS   51

4. CRYSTAL DEPOSITION DISORDERS   69

5. OSTEOARTHRITIS   77

6. OSTEONECROSIS AND RELATED DISORDERS   91

7. METABOLIC AND ENDOCRINE DISORDERS   105

8. GENETIC DISORDERS, SKELETAL DYSPLASIAS
    AND MALFORMATIONS   133

9. TUMOURS   167

10. NEUROMUSCULAR DISORDERS   201

11. PERIPHERAL NERVE INJURIES   229

12. ORTHOPAEDIC OPERATIONS   255

PART 2 – REGIONAL ORTHOPAEDICS

13. THE SHOULDER AND PECTORAL GIRDLE   277

14. THE ELBOW   303

15. THE WRIST   315

16. THE HAND   333

17. THE NECK   357

18. THE BACK   371

19. THE HIP   405

20. THE KNEE   449

21. THE ANKLE AND FOOT   485

PART 3 – FRACTURES AND JOINT INJURIES

22. THE MANAGEMENT OF MAJOR INJURIES   521

23. PRINCIPLES OF FRACTURES   539

24. INJURIES OF THE SHOULDER, UPPER ARM
    AND ELBOW   583

25. INJURIES OF THE FOREARM AND WRIST   611

26. HAND INJURIES   629

27. INJURIES OF THE SPINE   643

28. INJURIES OF THE PELVIS   667

29. INJURIES OF THE HIP AND FEMUR   681

30. INJURIES OF THE KNEE AND LEG   705

31. INJURIES OF THE ANKLE AND FOOT   733

INDEX   761

Foreword

In the Preface to the 6th edition of *Apley's System of Orthopaedics and Fractures*, the authors pointed out that the first outline for this great educational book was in 1954, and that over the decades since then, the question as to whether a general textbook of orthopaedics was still a worthwhile endeavour was constantly raised. The answer was self-evident. The magnificent text which they published in 1993 as the 7th edition proved to be a superb addition to our educational tools in orthopaedics; as in the past, it was concise, clear and easily readable.

It is with deep regret that we record the passing of Alan Graham Apley at the age of 82 in December of 1996. In a sense this Foreword is a posthumous salute to a great educator, talented clinician and wonderful author who not only contributed hugely to our life in orthopaedics but was a friend to many of us. It should be noted however that this Foreword has another purpose, which is an endorsement and admiration for Mr Apley's co-author in the 6th and 7th editions and now the principal author of the 8th edition, Professor Louis Solomon. No better choice of successor to Alan Apley could be made and the new volume not only lives up to our expectations, based on the previous seven, but exceeds them. The text has been extended and modernized, without losing any of its former clarity, and the 8th edition emerges as a testimony to the combined educational skills of Alan Apley, Louis Solomon and the two new contributors, David Warwick and Selvadurai Nayagam, who have joined the authorial team.

In the Foreword to the 7th edition I made the statement that it was enough in our 'salad days' to be able to describe a disease, define its differential diagnosis and give some idea of the management regimens which were in use. That was sufficient for the time, but not for today. Not for our patients, not for ourselves as musculoskeletal scientists and, fortunately for the readers, not for the authors of this new edition of the reigning classic. We now read not only of the diagnostic features and principles of care, but for many of the entities we find discussions in clear and precise language about the pathophysiology, the biology, the molecular genetics, the modern diagnostic tools and the technical details of management of the common (and sometimes not so common) disorders. The authors – including including Alan Apley, who I believe still to be a contributor to the book! – are to be praised for their ability to cover all these areas and still maintain the readability of the book and keep the volume down to size. This is the ultimate test of a good textbook: to be able to put enough into each chapter to impart significant, valid, up-to-date information and to engage the attention of the serious student without exhausting the interest of the casual browser. This is the gift that separates the present volume from a host of multi-volume, multi-authored textbooks that are used only as references and are often left to gather dust on library shelves.

Returning to the question posed in the opening paragraph of this foreword: Why another edition of an old textbook? What does it give us that is not already available in other treatises? Who will benefit? The answer is that, notwithstanding the burgeoning growth of hi-tech information systems, this and some other key textbooks still form the standard educational resource for our discipline, providing our students and ourselves with easy and inexpensive access to truths and lines of logical thought in the broad field of orthopaedic surgery. Anyone who has lived with prior editions, as well as new readers discovering the book for the first time, will know after a few sentences why this book has become a treasure, a dependable friend who can be trusted to tell the truth, to counsel and to guide the way in a very special and graceful manner.

Henry J. Mankin MD, FRCS (Hon)
Former Chief of the Orthopaedic Service
Chief of Orthopaedic Oncology
Massachusetts General Hospital
Edith M. Ashley Professor of Orthopaedics
Harvard Medical School
Boston, Massachusetts, USA

It was almost 50 years ago that Alan Apley wrote the first outline of his *System of Orthopaedics and Fractures*. In the years that followed, hundreds of young surgeons were taught by him and the Apley Course became a legend. This most inspiring of teachers is no longer alive but his spirit still pervades the book which has now reached its 8th edition.

When I first joined Alan as a co-author in 1980, I gave no thought to the day when I, too, would have to share this work with others. But all things change, and no change is more welcome than an infusion of new blood into a well-worn body. David Warwick and Durai Nayagam have joined me in the preparation of this volume. We hope that what emerges from our particular special interests has the ring of a single authorial voice.

As before, the book is divided into three major sections: General Orthopaedics, which comprises the main categories of musculoskeletal disorders such as infection, arthritis, metabolic bone disease, developmental abnormalities, tumours and neuromuscular conditions; then Regional Orthopaedics, which is an overview of conditions affecting individual joints; and thirdly Fractures and Joint Injuries, covering the principles of skeletal trauma and the fracture patterns encountered in each region. This leads inevitably to some repetition, but we make no apology for this. Understanding comes from constant cross-referral between the general and the particular.

The new edition is again bigger than its predecessors. This is necessitated by the ever-increasing volume of research and technical development which has made its way from reports and reviews to established practice. What was true yesterday may no longer be true today; the speculative ideas of the past are filtered by long and rigorous critical appraisal to become the new orthodoxy. In these pages we have strived to find the right balance between dogma and creative innovation, so that we do not leave the reader with a range of 'options' that ultimately falls short of true guidance. Some readers will disagree with the amount of coverage or the degree of emphasis we give to one subject or another. "Why write six pages on tuberculosis and four on poliomyelitis when these conditions are no longer seen in our hospitals?" asked one commentator of the 7th edition. Or "Why go on telling people that a plaster cast is a good alternative to internal fixation for this or that fracture?". The answer is that the world is our arena and there are millions of people somewhere on the map who still suffer from diseases that have all but disappeared in more privileged communities, and thousands of doctors who have neither the training nor the expensive facilities to treat fractures in the 'modern' way.

Many of the older illustrations have been replaced, and many more added. For the first time we are using full colour, wherever appropriate, throughout the book. The page design has been modernised but the illustrations (over 2500 of them) again appear as 'composites' – groups or sequential series of pictures that tell a story rather than merely illustrate a particular appearance. This has been a feature of the book since the earliest editions, and in the past many readers have used the pictures and their captions for rapid revision when preparing for examinations.

When the *System of Orthopaedics and Fractures* first appeared in print, it was aimed primarily at registrars preparing for their general surgical examinations. Orthopaedic trainees today are expected to know a great deal more than their predecessors; the new *System* has set out firmly to meet this need, yet without pretending to be an exhaustive reference work. Thus, the main appeal of the book will be to senior trainees and practising orthopaedic surgeons. However, the principles that underpin our subject are presented in a way which should be helpful to anyone who is interested in musculoskeletal disorders and trauma; as with the previous edition, the book also serves as a parallel resource for those who are more comfortable with the companion volume – the *Concise System* – and only occasionally need to pursue a particular problem in greater detail.

Operations are described only in outline, with the emphasis on indications, pitfalls, complications and outcome. Here and there descriptions are replaced by simple line drawings. No-one should expect to use the book as an instruction manual in the operating theatre; such details are better sought in reference works on operative surgery, titles of which appear at the end of Chapter 12.

We have also pondered the value of adding long lists of journal references at the end of each chapter, and have decided to limit these citations to papers and texts which present a new, or particularly useful, approach to any subject. In doing so we intend no disrespect to those giants of our profession who were either the first to report a new idea or the most influential in promoting it. Their place in history is secure.

We hope that those readers who have grown up with *Apley's System* will recognise an old companion in the new work, and that those who come to it for the first time will find it a fitting introduction to the orthopaedics of the new millennium.

L. S.

Acknowledgements

We are deeply indebted to the many colleagues who were kind enough to offer constructive criticisms of the previous edition of this book and in so doing help us in the preparation of the present edition. Equally valuable were the casual remarks that enriched innumerable conversations during the past few years, many of which found their way into the manuscript without our even knowing that we were quoting others. And then there were those who most generously took on the task of reading through entire chapters and giving us the benefit of their expert commentary. In particular we wish to thank Mr Stephen Eisenstein, Director of the Department for Spinal Disorders in the Robert Jones and Agnes Hunt Orthopaedic Hospital, Oswestry; Mr Peter Burge and Mr Andrew Carr, Consultant Orthopaedic Surgeons at the Nuffield Orthopaedic Centre, Oxford; Mr John Dixon, Consultant Orthopaedic Surgeon at the Avon Orthopaedic Centre, Bristol; Ms Lisa Sacks, Consultant Plastic Surgeon at Frenchay Hospital, Bristol; Mr Martin Gargan and Mr Peter Witherow, Consultant Orthopaedic Surgeons at the Royal Hospital for Sick Children, Bristol.

Many of the pictures in the previous edition were provided by colleagues in Britain and abroad. These were duly acknowledged in that volume. New pictures or x-rays for the present edition have been generously supplied by local colleagues: Mr John Albert, Mr John Dorgan, Mr Stephen Eisenstein, Mr Neeraj Garg, Mr Martin Gargan, Mr Mike Manning, Mr Ian Nelson, Mr Alistair Ross, Mr Evert Smith and Dr John Wakeley. Dr Kjeld Søballe, Aarhus University Hospital, Denmark, provided pictures of the Ganz triple osteotomy of the pelvis and Mr H.K. Wong, National University Hospital, Singapore, allowed us to use his pictures showing ossification of the posterior longitudinal ligament of the cervical spine, a condition seldom seen in Britain. Professor Sidney Biddulph, Johannesburg, generously suppled us with the pictures for the section on hand infections. We are deeply grateful to them for this assistance.

New drawings were prepared by Mr Peter Cox of Creative Design and many new photographs by the Department of Medical Illustration at the Bristol Royal Infirmary.

The manuscript was typed by Ms Carol Marks, a model of patience, efficiency and willing attention.

We wish to express our admiration and gratitude to Paul Wilkinson, Lee Smith and Ian Spick of Inperspective, London, for their painstaking work on the design and setting of the System in its present style.

We are deeply grateful also to Joan Solomon, whose aesthetic instinct and artistic expertise contributed immensely to the general presentation of this work.

We take this opportunity to thank Dr Geoffrey Smaldon, our patient Editor who, for many years, coddled and encouraged us during the preparation of each new edition of the System.

Other contributors are more difficult to identify. We owe a deep debt of gratitude to the many patients who have allowed us to intrude upon their suffering and use their case histories, x-rays and photographs as illustrations. We cannot name them, for reasons of confidentiality, but we do thank them most sincerely.

Finally, we acknowledge – often with humility – the students and trainees whose healthy scepticism and persistent, unselfconscious questions motivated us in the long journey to complete this work.

L. S.
D.W.
S. N.

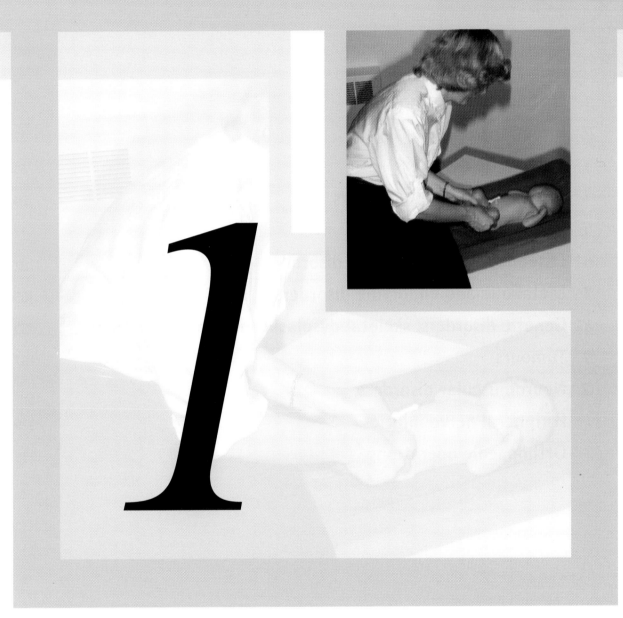

General Orthopaedics

In This Section

1 **Orthopaedic diagnosis** 3

2 **Infection** 27

3 **Rheumatic disorders** 51

4 **Crystal deposition disorders** 69

5 **Osteoarthritis** 77

6 **Osteonecrosis and related disorders** 91

7 **Metabolic and endocrine disorders** 105

8 **Genetic disorders, skeletal dysplasias and malformations** 133

9 **Tumours** 167

10 **Neuromuscular disorders** 201

11 **Peripheral nerve injuries** 229

12 **Orthopaedic operations** 255

1

Orthopaedic diagnosis

Information consists of differences that make a difference.
Gregory Bateson

Orthopaedics is concerned with bones, joints, muscles, tendons and nerves – the skeletal system and all that makes it move. Conditions that affect these structures fall into seven easily remembered pairs:

1. Congenital and developmental abnormalities
2. Infection and inflammation
3. Arthritis and rheumatic disorders
4. Metabolic and endocrine disorders
5. Tumours and lesions that mimic them
6. Sensory disturbance and muscle weakness
7. Injury and mechanical derangement

Diagnosis in orthopaedics, as in all of medicine, is the identification of disease. It begins from the very first encounter with the patient and is gradually modified and fine-tuned until we have a picture, not only of a *pathological process* but also of the *functional loss* and the *disability* that goes with it. Understanding evolves from the systematic gathering of information from the history, the physical examination, tissue and organ imaging and special investigations. Systematic, but never mechanical; behind the enquiring head there should also be what D. H. Lawrence has called the intelligent heart. It must never be forgotten that the patient is also a person, with a mind and a personality, a job and hobbies, a family and a home; all have a bearing upon – and are in turn affected by – the disorder and its treatment.

HISTORY

'Taking a history' is a misnomer. The patient tells a story; it is we the listeners who construct a history. The story may be maddeningly disorganized; the history has to be systematic. Carefully and patiently compiled, it can be every bit as informative as examination or laboratory tests.

As we record it, certain key words will inevitably stand out: *injury, pain, stiffness, swelling, deformity, instability, weakness, altered sensibility* and *loss of function*. Each symptom is pursued for more detail: we need to know when it began, whether suddenly or gradually, spontaneously or after some specific event; how it has changed or progressed; what makes it worse; what makes it better.

While listening, we consider if the story fits some pattern that we recognize – for we are already thinking of a diagnosis. Every piece of information should be thought of as part of a larger picture which gradually unfolds in our understanding. 'Disease reveals itself in casual parentheses', is the way Trotter described it.

SYMPTOMS

Pain

Pain is the most common symptom in orthopaedics. It is described in terms that range from the most boring and bland to the impossibly dramatic and bizarre. The metaphors used tell us more about the patient's psyche than about the pathology; yet there are clearly differences between the throbbing pain of an abscess and the aching pain of chronic arthritis, between the 'burning pain' of neuralgia and the 'stabbing pain' of a ruptured tendon.

Severity is even more subjective. High and low thresholds undoubtedly exist, but to the patient pain is as bad as it feels, and any system of 'pain grading' must take this into account. The main value of estimating severity is in assessing the progress of the disorder or the response to treatment. The following is a simple and useful system:

- *Grade I (mild)* Pain that can easily be ignored.
- *Grade II (moderate)* Pain that cannot be ignored, interferes with function and needs treatment from time to time.
- *Grade III (severe)* Pain that is present most of the time, demanding constant attention.
- *Grade IV (excruciating)* Totally incapacitating pain.

Patients are often vague about the site of pain. Yet its precise location is important, and in orthopaedics it is particularly useful to ask the patient to point to where it hurts; not merely to tell us, but actually to point. But don't assume that the site of pain is always the site of pathology; 'referred' pain and 'autonomic' pain can be very deceptive.

Referred pain Pain arising in or near the skin is usually localized accurately. Pain arising in deep structures is more diffuse and is sometimes of unexpected distribution; thus, hip disease may manifest with pain in the knee (so might an obturator hernia). This is not because sensory nerves connect the two sites; it is due to inability of the cerebral cortex to distinguish between sensory

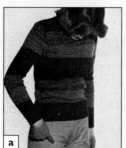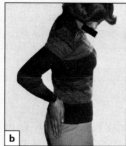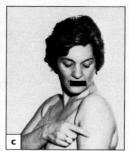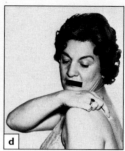

1.1 'Point to where it hurts' In (**a**) and (**b**) the complaint would be of hip pain; in (**c**) and (**d**) of shoulder pain. Only in (**a**) is the patient's assumption likely to be correct; the other pictures show typical sites of referred pain for (**b**) a lumbar spine problem, (**c**) supraspinatus tendinitis and (**d**) cervical spondylosis.

messages from embryologically related sites. Further examples are shown in Fig. 1.1.

Autonomic pain We are so accustomed to matching pain with some discrete anatomical structure and its known sensory nerve supply that we are apt to dismiss any pain that does not fit the usual pattern as 'atypical' or 'inappropriate'. However, pain can also arise in the autonomic nerves that accompany the peripheral blood vessels. This 'autonomic pain' (e.g. after operation) is much more vague, often widespread and accompanied by vasomotor and trophic abnormalities. It is poorly understood, often doubted, but none the less real.

Stiffness

Stiffness may be *generalized* (typically in systemic disorders such as rheumatoid arthritis and ankylosing spondylitis) or *localized* to a particular joint. Patients often have difficulty in distinguishing localized stiffness from painful movement; limitation of movement should not be assumed until verified by examination.

Ask when it occurs: regular early morning stiffness of many joints is one of the cardinal symptoms of rheumatoid arthritis, whereas transient stiffness of one or two joints after periods of inactivity is typical of osteoarthritis.

Locking, a special variety of stiffness, is the sudden inability to complete one particular movement; it suggests a mechanical block – for example, due to a loose body or a torn meniscus becoming trapped between the articular surfaces. Unfortunately, patients use the term for any painful limitation of movement; much more reliable is a history of sudden 'unlocking' when the offending body slips out of the way.

Swelling

Swelling may be in the soft tissues, the joint or the bone; to the patient they are all the same. It is important to

establish whether the swelling followed an injury, whether it appeared rapidly (probably a haematoma or a haemarthrosis) or slowly (soft tissue inflammation, a joint effusion or a tumour), whether it is painful (acute inflammation, infection – or a tumour), whether it is constant or comes and goes, and whether it is continuing to enlarge.

Deformity

The common deformities are well described in terms such as round shoulders, spinal curvature, knock knees, bow legs, pigeon toes and flat feet. Deformity of a single bone or joint is less easily described and the patient may simply declare that the limb is 'crooked'.

Some 'deformities' are merely variations of the normal (e.g. short stature or wide hips); others disappear spontaneously with growth (e.g. flat feet or bandy legs in an infant). However, if the deformity is *progressive* it may be serious.

Weakness

Generalized weakness is a feature of all chronic illness. However, true muscular weakness – especially if it is confined to one limb or to a single muscle group – is much more specific and suggests some neurological or muscle disorder. Patients sometimes say that the limb is 'dead' when it is actually weak, and this can be a source of confusion. Questions should be framed to discover precisely which movements are affected, for this may give important clues, if not to the exact diagnosis at least to the site of the lesion.

Instability

The patient may complain of a joint 'giving way'. This may be due to muscle weakness or to ligamentous deficiency from laxity or rupture. If there is a history of injury its precise nature is important.

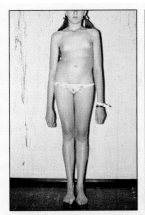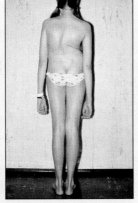

1.2 Deformity This young girl complained of a prominent right hip; the real deformity was scoliosis.

development of ankylosing spondylitis or osteoporosis. Similarly, rheumatic disorders may be suggested by a history of eye, skin or urogenital disease. Patients should also be asked about previous medication; many drugs, and especially corticosteroids, have long-term effects on bone. Alcohol and drug abuse are important, and we must not be afraid to ask about them.

FAMILY HISTORY

Patients often wonder (and worry) about inheriting a disease or passing it on to their children. To the doctor, information about musculoskeletal disorders in the patient's family may help with both diagnosis and counselling.

SOCIAL BACKGROUND

No history is complete without enquiry about the patient's background: details about work, travel, recreation, home circumstances and the level of support from family and friends. These always impinge on the assessment of disability; occasionally a particular activity (at work, on the sports field or in the kitchen) is responsible for the entire condition.

Change in sensibility

Tingling or numbness signifies interference with nerve function – pressure from a neighbouring structure (e.g. a prolapsed intervertebral disc), local ischaemia (e.g. nerve entrapment in a fibro-osseous tunnel) or a peripheral neuropathy. It is important to establish its exact distribution; from this we can tell whether the fault lies in a peripheral nerve or in a nerve root. We should also ask what makes it worse or better; a change in posture might be the trigger, thus focusing attention on a particular site.

Loss of function

Functional disability is more than the sum of individual symptoms and its expression depends upon the needs of the patient. The patient may say 'I can't sit for long' rather than 'I have backache', or 'I can't put my socks on' rather than 'my hip is stiff. Moreover, what to one patient is merely inconvenient may, to another, be incapacitating. Thus a lawyer or a teacher may readily tolerate a stiff knee provided it is painless and does not impair walking; but to a plumber or a parson the same disorder might spell economic or spiritual disaster. One question should elicit the important information: *'What can't you do that you used to be able to do?'*

PAST HISTORY

Patients often forget to mention previous illnesses or accidents, or they may simply not appreciate their relevance to the present complaint. They should be asked specifically about childhood disorders, periods of incapacity and old injuries. A 'twisted ankle' many years ago may be the clue to the onset of osteoarthritis in what is otherwise an unusual site for this condition. Gastrointestinal disease, which in the patient's mind 'has nothing to do with bones', may be important in the later

EXAMINATION

In *A Case of Identity* Sherlock Holmes has the following conversation with Dr Watson.

Watson: You appeared to read a good deal upon [your client] which was quite invisible to me.
Holmes: Not invisible but unnoticed, Watson.

Some disorders can be diagnosed at a glance: who would mistake the facies of acromegaly or the hand deformities of rheumatoid arthritis for anything else? Nevertheless, even in these cases a systematic approach is rewarding; it keeps reinforcing the habit and the patients feel that they have been properly attended to.

The examination actually begins from the moment we set eyes on the patient. We observe his or her general appearance, posture and gait. Are they walking freely or do they use a stick? Are they in pain? Do their movements look natural? Can you spot any distinctive features immediately: A characteristic facies? A spinal curvature? A short limb? Any type of asymmetry? They may have a tell-tale gait suggesting a painful hip, an unstable knee or a foot-drop. The clues are endless and the game is played by everyone (qualified or lay) at each new encounter throughout life. In the clinical setting the assessment needs to be more focused.

When we proceed to the structured examination, the patient must be suitably undressed; no mere rolling up of a trouser leg is sufficient. If one limb is affected, both must be exposed so that they can be compared.

We examine the good limb, then the bad. There is a great temptation to rush in with both hands – a temptation that must be resisted. Only by proceeding in a purposeful, orderly way can we avoid missing important signs. The system we use is simple but comprehensive:

First we LOOK
Then we FEEL
Then we MOVE

Of course, we recognize that some flexibility is desirable. Sometimes we need to look while we move (e.g. a spinal deformity may become apparent only when the patient bends forwards); or we may have to move a joint (especially one that is swollen) before we can feel exactly where it is! Our purpose in emphasizing the discipline – LOOK, FEEL, MOVE – is to encourage the habit of systematic thought which alone ensures that no important detail will be neglected or forgotten.

LOOK

Skin We look first at the skin, especially for scars and colour changes. Scars are a record of the past – surgical archaeology so to speak. Colour reflects pigmentation or vascular status – for example, the blueness of cyanosis or bruising and the redness of inflammation. Abnormal creases, unless due to fibrosis, suggest underlying deformity which is not always obvious; shiny skin with no creases suggests oedema or trophic change.

Shape Next we look at the shape. Is there swelling, or wasting (one often enhances the appearance of the other)? Or is there a definite lump? And is a normally straight bone bent?

Position A joint is three dimensional and it is important to look for deformity in three planes. In many joint disorders and in most nerve lesions the limb assumes a characteristic posture.

FEEL

Feeling is exploring, not groping aimlessly. Know your anatomy and you will know where to feel for the landmarks; find the landmarks and you can trace a diagnostic map in your mind's eye.

The skin Is it warm or cold; moist or dry; and is sensation normal?

The soft tissues Is there a lump; if so, what are its characteristics? Are the pulses normal?

The bones and joints Are the outlines normal? Is the synovium thickened? Is there excessive joint fluid?

Tenderness When feeling for tenderness keep your eyes on the patient's face; a grimace will tell you more than a grunt. Try to localize any tenderness to a particular structure; knowing *where* it is will often tell you *what* it is.

MOVE

'Movement' comprises several different activities: active movement, passive movement, abnormal or unstable movement, and provocative movement.

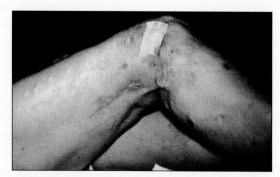

1.3 Look for scars Scars are a map of the past. The faded scar on this patient's thigh tells of an old operation – internal fixation of a femoral fracture. The scar behind this is where the postoperative infection was drained. Chronic osteomyelitis has also left the scars of sinuses, one of them still draining

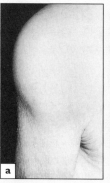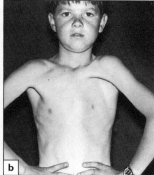

1.4 Shape (a) This large swelling of the shoulder appeared slowly. Is it in the muscle, the bone or the joint? (b) This is no mere wasting of muscle; the boy has a congenitally absent pectoralis major on the left.

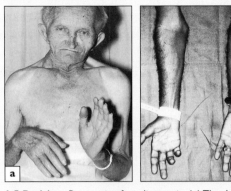

1.5 Position Posture is often diagnostic. (**a**) The drop wrist of a radial nerve palsy due to carcinomatous infiltration of the supraclavicular lymph nodes on the right. (**b**) A typical ulnar claw hand, in this case due to valgus deformity of the right elbow causing tension on the ulnar nerve.

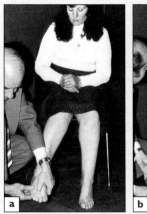
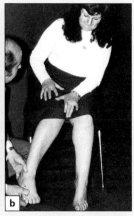

1.6 Feeling for tenderness (**a**) How not to do it. It is better to watch the patient's face (**b**), and to stop the moment she feels pain.

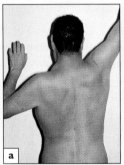
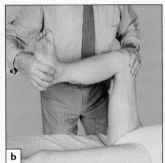
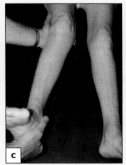
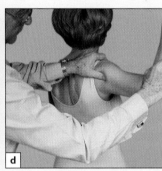

1.7 Move (**a**) Active movement – the patient moves the joint. The right shoulder is normal; the left has restricted active movement. (**b**) Passive movement – the examiner moves the joint. (**c**) Unstable movement – the joint can be moved across the normal planes of action, in this case demonstrating valgus instability of the right knee. (**d**) Provocative movement – the examiner moves (or manipulates) the joint so as to provoke the symptoms of impending pain or dislocation. Here he is reproducing the position in which an unstable shoulder is likely to dislocate.

Active movement Ask the patient to move without your assistance. This will give you an idea of the degree of mobility and whether it is painful or not. Active movement is also used to assess muscle power.

Passive movement Here it is the examiner who moves the joint in each anatomical plane. Note whether there is any difference between the range of active and passive movement.

The range of movement is recorded in degrees, starting from zero which, by convention, is the neutral or anatomical position of the joint. For accuracy you can use a goniometer (Fig. 1.8e), but with practice you will learn to estimate the angles by eye. What is important is to compare the symptomatic with the asymptomatic or normal side.

Describing the range of movement is often made to seem difficult. Words such as 'full', 'good', 'limited' and 'poor' are misleading. *Always cite the range or span,*

from start to finish, in degrees. For example, 'knee flexion 0–140°' means that the range of flexion is from zero (the knee absolutely straight) through an arc of 140 degrees (the leg making an acute angle with the thigh). Similarly, 'knee flexion 20–90°' means that flexion begins at 20 degrees (i.e. the joint cannot extend fully to the anatomical zero position) and movement continues only to 90 degrees.

While testing movement, feel for *crepitus*. Joint crepitus is usually coarse and fairly diffuse; tendon crepitus is fine and precisely localized to the affected tendon sheath.

Unstable movement This is movement which is inherently unphysiological. You may be able to shift or angulate a joint out of its normal plane of movement, thus demonstrating that the joint is unstable. Such abnormal movement may be obvious (e.g. a wobbly knee); often, though, you have to use special manoeuvres to pick up minor degrees of instability.

Provocative movement One of the most telling clues to diagnosis is reproducing the patient's symptoms by applying a specific, provocative movement. Shoulder pain due to impingement of the subacromial structures may be 'provoked' by moving the joint in a way that is calculated to produce such impingement; the patient recognizes the similarity between this pain and his or her daily symptoms. Likewise, a patient who has had a previous dislocation or subluxation can be vividly reminded of that event by stressing the joint in such a way that it again threatens to dislocate; indeed, merely starting the movement may be so distressing that the patient goes rigid with anxiety at the anticipated result – this is aptly called the *apprehension test.*

The terminology of movement

Flexion/extension These are movements in the sagittal plane; for example, at the knee, elbow, ankle and the joints of the fingers and toes.

Adduction/abduction These are movements in the coronal plane, towards or away from the midline.

External rotation/internal rotation These are rotational movements around a longitudinal axis. Strictly speaking they should be called lateral and medial rotation.

Pronation/supination These, too, are rotatory movements, but the terms are applied only to movements of the forearm and the foot.

Circumduction This is a composite movement made up of a rhythmic sequence of all the other movements. It is possible only for ball-and-socket joints (hip, shoulder).

Specialized movements Certain movements, such as opposition of the thumb, lateral flexion and rotation of the spine, and inversion or eversion of the foot, are described under the relevant regions.

Joint stiffness

The term 'stiffness' covers a variety of limitations. We consider three types of stiffness in particular: (1) all movements absent; (2) all movements limited; (3) one or two movements limited.

All movements absent Surprisingly, although movement is completely blocked, the patient may retain such good function that the restriction goes unnoticed until the joint is examined. Surgical fusion is called 'arthrodesis'; pathological fusion is called 'ankylosis'. Acute suppurative arthritis typically ends in bony ankylosis; tuberculous arthritis heals by fibrosis and causes *fibrous ankylosis* – not strictly a 'fusion' because there may still be a small jog of movement.

All movements limited After severe injury, movement may be limited as a result of oedema and bruising. Later, adhesions and loss of muscle extensibility may perpetuate the stiffness.

With active inflammation all movements are restricted and painful and the joint is said to be 'irritable'. In acute arthritis spasm may prevent all but a few degrees of movement.

In osteoarthritis the capsule fibroses and movements become increasingly restricted, but pain occurs only at the extremes of motion.

Some movements limited When one particular movement is blocked the cause is usually mechanical. Thus a torn

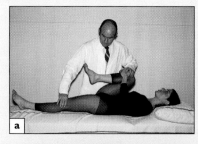
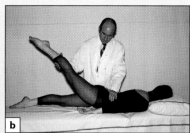
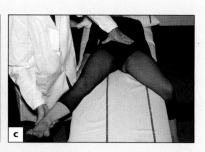
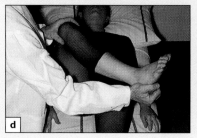
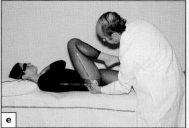

1.8 Planes of movement (a) Flexion, (b) extension, (c) abduction and (d) rotation of the hip. The range of movement can be estimated by eye or measured accurately using a goniometer (e).

and displaced meniscus may prevent full extension of the knee but not flexion.

Bone deformity may alter the arc of movement, such that it is limited in one direction (loss of abduction in coxa vara is an example) but movement in the opposite direction is full or even increased.

These are all examples of *'fixed deformity'*.

Joint laxity

Children's joints are much more mobile than those of adults; their greater flexibility allows children to adopt postures that would be impossible for their parents. An unusual degree of mobility can, of course, be attained in dancers and athletes, but when the exercises are stopped mobility soon reverts to the normal range.

Persistent generalized joint hypermobility This occurs in about 5% of normal people and is inherited as a simple mendelian dominant. The knees and elbows can be hyperextended, and the hands and feet can attain unusual positions. Such hypermobile joints are not necessarily unstable – as witness the controlled performances of acrobats – but they do have a tendency to recurrent dislocation (e.g. of the shoulder or patella). They also have a tendency to unexplained joint pains (arthralgia). There is, however, no convincing evidence that hypermobility by itself predisposes to degenerative arthritis; only if the joint becomes unstable is this likely to develop.

Generalized hypermobility is not usually associated with any obvious disease; but severe laxity is a feature of certain rare connective tissue disorders such as Marfan's syndrome, Ehlers–Danlos syndrome, Larsen's disease and osteogenesis imperfecta.

DEFORMITY

The word 'deformity' may be applied to a person, a bone or a joint. Shortness of stature is a kind of defor-

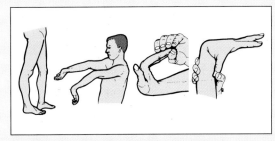

1.9 Tests for joint hypermobility Hyperextension of knees and elbows; metacarpophalangeal joints extending to 90 degrees; thumb able to touch forearm.

mity; it may be due to shortness of the limbs or of the trunk, or both. An individual bone also may be abnormally short; this is rarely important in the upper limbs, but it is in the lower.

If a limb appears to be crooked, it is important to establish whether the deformity is in the bone or in the joint.

A joint may be held in an unnatural position either because of faulty alignment or because it lacks full movement. The more common deformities are designated by special terms.

Varus and valgus It seems pedantic to replace 'bow legs' and 'knock knees' with 'genu varum' and 'genu valgum'. But comparable colloquialisms are not available for deformities of the elbow, hip or big toe; and, besides, the formality is justified by the need for clarity and consistency. *Varus* means that the part distal to the joint is displaced towards the midline, *valgus* away from it.

Kyphosis and lordosis Seen from the side, the spine has a series of curves – convex posteriorly in the dorsal region (kyphosis), and convex anteriorly in the cervical and lumbar regions (lordosis). Excessive curvature constitutes kyphotic or lordotic deformity (also sometimes referred to as hyperkyphosis and hyperlordosis).

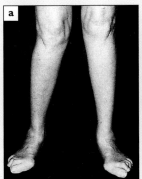 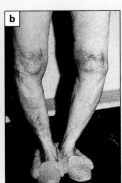 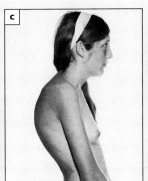 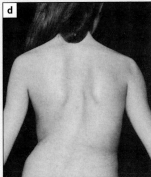

1.10 Common deformities (a) Valgus knees (and great toes); (b) varus knees; (c) kyphosis; (d) scoliosis.

Scoliosis Seen from behind, the normal spine is straight. Any curvature in the coronal plane is called a scoliosis.

Postural deformity A postural deformity is one which the patient can, if he chooses, correct by voluntary effort; for example, a postural kyphosis due to slumped shoulders, or a sciatic 'scoliosis' due to spasm of the paravertebral muscles.

Structural deformity A deformity which results from a permanent change in anatomical structure cannot be voluntarily corrected. It is important to distinguish postural scoliosis from structural (fixed) scoliosis. The former is non-progressive, benign and needs no treatment in itself; the latter is usually progressive and may require treatment.

'Fixed deformity' This term is ambiguous. It seems to mean that a joint is deformed and immobile. Not so – it means that one particular movement cannot be completed. Thus, if a knee can flex fully but cannot extend fully it is said to have a 'fixed flexion deformity'.

Joint deformity

There are four basic causes of joint deformity:
1. *Contracture of the overlying soft tissues* This is seen typically when there is severe scarring across the flexor aspect of a joint (e.g. after a burn) or after muscle fibrosis and contracture.
2. *Muscle imbalance* Unbalanced muscle weakness or spasticity will result in joint deformity which will eventually become fixed. This is seen most typically in poliomyelitis and cerebral palsy. Tendon rupture, likewise, may cause deformity.
3. *Dislocation* If a joint is disarticulated it cannot assume its normal position.
4. *Joint destruction* Trauma, infection or arthritis may destroy the joint and lead to severe deformity.

Bone deformity

Bone deformity in a child may be the result of distorted growth due to a genetic abnormality, injury or disease. Examples are achondroplasia (genetic), physeal fractures (trauma) and rickets (vitamin D deficiency).

In adults the more likely causes are malunion of a fracture, Paget's disease and bone tumours.

BONY LUMPS

A bony lump may be due to faulty development, injury, inflammation or a tumour. Although x-ray examination is essential, the clinical features can be highly informative.

Size A large lump attached to bone, or a lump that is getting bigger, is nearly always a tumour.

Site A lump near a joint is most likely to be a tumour (benign or malignant); a lump in the shaft may be fracture callus, inflammatory new bone or a tumour.

Margin A benign tumour has a well-defined margin; malignant tumours, inflammatory lumps and callus have a vague edge.

Consistency A benign tumour feels bony hard; malignant tumours often give the impression that they can be indented.

Tenderness Lumps due to active inflammation, recent callus or a rapidly growing sarcoma are tender.

Multiplicity Multiple bony lumps are uncommon: they occur in hereditary multiple exostosis and in Ollier's disease.

NEUROLOGICAL EXAMINATION

If the symptoms include weakness or incoordination or a change in sensibility, or if they point to any disorder of the neck or back, a complete neurological examination of the related part is mandatory.

Once again we follow a systematic routine, first looking at the *general appearance,* then assessing *motor function* (muscle tone, power and reflexes) and finally testing for *sensory function* (both skin sensibility and deep sensibility).

Appearance

Some neurological disorders result in postures that are so characteristic as to be diagnostic at a glance: the claw hand of an ulnar nerve lesion; drop wrist following radial nerve palsy; or the 'waiter's tip' deformity of the arm in brachial plexus injury. Usually, however, it is when the patient moves that we can best appre-

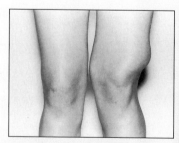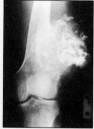

1.11 Bony lumps The lump above the left knee is hard, well-defined and not increasing in size. The clinical diagnosis of cartilage-capped exostosis (osteochondroma) is confirmed by the x-rays.

ciate the type and extent of motor disorder: the dangling arm following a brachial plexus injury; the flail lower limb of poliomyelitis; the symmetrical paralysis of spinal cord lesions; the characteristic drop-foot gait following sciatic or peroneal nerve damage; and the jerky, 'spastic' movements of cerebral palsy.

Concentrating on the affected part, we look for trophic changes that signify loss of sensibility: the smooth, hairless skin that seems to be stretched too tight; atrophy of the fingertips and the nails; scars that tell of accidental burns; and ulcers that refuse to heal. Muscle wasting is important; if localized and asymmetrical, it may suggest dysfunction of a specific motor nerve.

Tone and power

Tone in individual muscle groups is tested by moving the nearby joint to stretch the muscle. Increased tone (spasticity) is characteristic of upper motor neuron disorders such as cerebral palsy and stroke. It must not be confused with rigidity (the 'lead-pipe' or 'cogwheel' effect) which is seen in Parkinson's disease. Decreased tone (flaccidity) is found in lower motor neuron lesions; for example, poliomyelitis. Muscle power is diminished in all three states; it is important to recognize that a 'spastic' muscle may still be weak.

Testing for power is not as easy as it sounds; few patients have studied anatomy, and we must make ourselves understood. The easiest way is shown in Fig. 1.13. The sequence is important: you place the limb – he holds it – you try to force movement, asking him to resist while you feel the muscle. The normal limb is examined first, then the affected limb and the two are compared. Finer muscle actions, such as those of the thumb and fingers, may be reproduced by first demonstrating the movement yourself, then testing it in the unaffected limb and then in the affected one. We may learn even more about composite movements by asking the patient to perform specific tasks, such as holding a pen or gripping a rod.

Muscle power is usually graded on the Medical Research Council scale:

Grade 0 – no movement
Grade 1 – only a flicker of movement
Grade 2 – movement with gravity eliminated
Grade 3 – movement against gravity
Grade 4 – movement against resistance
Grade 5 – normal power

It is important to recognize that muscle weakness may be due to muscle disease rather than nerve disease. In muscle disorders the weakness is usually symmetrical and sensation is normal.

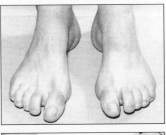
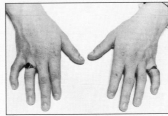

1.12 Neurological examination This young man presented with pes cavus and claw toes. He also has mild clawing of the fingers. Diagnosis: hereditary motor and sensory neuropathy (peroneal muscular atrophy).

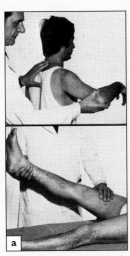
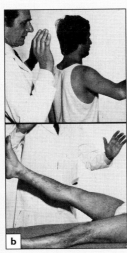
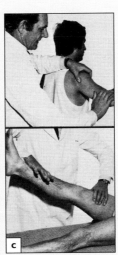

1.13 Testing muscle power The sequence is always the same, no matter whether the deltoid, quadriceps or any other muscle is being examined. (**a**) 'Let me lift it'. (**b**) 'Hold it there'. (**c**) 'Keep it there'.

Tendon reflexes

A deep tendon reflex is elicited by rapidly stretching the tendon near its insertion. A sharp tap with the tendon hammer does this well; but all too often this is performed with a flourish and with such force that the finer gradations of response are missed. It is better to employ a series of taps, starting with the most forceful and reducing the force with each successive tap until there is no response. Comparing the two sides in this way, we can pick up fine differences showing that a reflex is 'diminished' rather than 'absent'. In the upper limb we test biceps, triceps and brachioradialis; and in the lower limb the patellar and Achilles tendons.

The tendon reflexes are monosynaptic segmental reflexes; that is, the reflex pathway takes a 'short cut' through the spinal cord at the segmental level. Depression or absence of the reflex signifies interruption of the pathway at the posterior nerve root, the anterior horn cell, the motor nerve root or the peripheral nerve. It is a reliable pointer to the segmental level of dysfunction: thus, a depressed biceps jerk suggests pressure on the fifth or sixth cervical (C5 or 6) nerve roots while a depressed ankle jerk signifies a similar abnormality at the first sacral level (S1). An unusually brisk reflex, on the other hand, is characteristic of an upper motor neuron disorder (e.g. cerebral palsy, a stroke or injury to the spinal cord); the lower motor neuron is released from the normal central inhibition and there is an exaggerated response to tendon stimulation. This may manifest as *ankle clonus*: a sharp upward jerk on the foot (dorsiflexion) causes a repetitive, 'clonic' movement of the foot; similarly, a sharp downward push on the patella may elicit patellar clonus.

Superficial reflexes

The superficial reflexes are elicited by stroking the skin at various sites to produce a specific muscle contraction; the best known are the abdominal (T7–T12), cremasteric (L1, 2) and anal (S4, 5) reflexes. These are corticospinal (upper motor neuron) reflexes. Absence of the reflex indicates an upper motor neuron lesion (usually in the spinal cord) above that level.

The plantar reflex

Forceful stroking of the sole normally produces flexion of the toes (or no response at all). An extensor response (the big toe extends while the others remain in flexion) is characteristic of upper motor neuron disorders. This is the Babinski sign – a type of withdrawal reflex which is present in young infants and normally disappears after the age of 18 months.

Sensibility

Sensibility to touch and to pinprick may be increased (*hyperaesthesia*) in certain irritative nerve lesions. More often, though, it is diminished (*hypoaesthesia*) or absent (*anaesthesia*), signifying pressure on or interruption of a peripheral nerve, a nerve root or the sensory pathways in the spinal cord. The area of sensory change can be mapped out on the skin and compared with the known segmental or dermatomal pattern of innervation. If the abnormality is well defined it is an easy matter to establish the level of the lesion, even if the precise cause remains unknown.

Brisk percussion along the course of an injured nerve may elicit a tingling sensation in the distal distribution of the nerve (*Tinel's sign*). The point of hypersensitivity marks the site of abnormal nerve sprouting: if it progresses distally at successive visits this signifies regeneration; if it remains unchanged this suggests a local neuroma.

Tests for *temperature recognition* and *two-point discrimination* (the ability to recognize two touch-points a few millimetres apart) are sometimes used in the assessment of peripheral nerve injuries.

Deep sensibility can be examined in several ways. In the *vibration test* a sounded tuning-fork is placed over a peripheral bony point (e.g. the medial malleolus or the head of the ulna); the patient is asked if he or she can feel the vibrations and to say when they disappear. By comparing the two sides, differences can be noted. *Position sense* is tested by asking the patient to find certain points on the body with the eyes closed – for example, touching the tip of the nose with the forefinger. *The sense of joint posture* is tested by grasping the big toe and placing it in different positions of flexion and extension. The patient is asked to say whether it is 'up' or 'down'. *Stereognosis*, the ability to recognize shape and texture by feel alone, is tested by giving the patient (whose eyes are closed) a variety of familiar objects to hold and asking him or her to name each object.

The pathways for deep sensibility run in the posterior columns of the spinal cord. Disturbances are, therefore, found in peripheral neuropathies and in spinal cord lesions such as posterior column injuries or tabes dorsalis. The sense of balance is also carried in the posterior columns. This can be tested by asking the patient to stand upright with his or her eyes closed; excessive body sway is abnormal (Romberg's sign).

Cortical and cerebellar function

A staggering gait may imply an unstable knee – or a disorder of the spinal cord or cerebellum. If there is no musculoskeletal abnormality to account for the sign, a full examination of the central nervous system will be necessary.

EXAMINATION IN SPECIAL SITUATIONS

The methods described here should be regarded as a guide, not a set of laws engraved on tablets of stone. The sequence may sometimes have to be changed because a patient is in pain or very severely disabled. Some special tests are applicable only to certain sites; these are described under the relevant sections.

The entire approach may need to be modified when examining patients with acute injuries. Obviously you would not try to 'move' a limb with a suspected fracture when an x-ray can provide the answer. Moreover, resuscitation will always take priority and in severely injured patients the detailed local examination may have to be curtailed or deferred.

Paediatric practice requires special skills. You may have no first-hand account of the symptoms; a baby screaming with pain will tell you very little, and overanxious parents will probably tell you too much. When examining the child, you should be flexible. If he or she is moving a particular joint, take your opportunity to examine movement then and there. You will learn much more by adopting methods of play than by applying a rigid system of examination. And leave any test for tenderness until last!

DIAGNOSTIC IMAGING

The map is not the territory.
Alfred Korzybski

PLAIN FILM RADIOGRAPHY

Plain film x-ray examination is over 100 years old. Notwithstanding the extraordinary technical advances of the past few decades, it remains the most useful method of diagnostic imaging. Whereas other methods may define an inaccessible anatomical structure more accurately, or may reveal some localized tissue change, the plain film provides information simultaneously on the size, shape, tissue 'density' and bone architecture – characteristics which, taken together, usually suggest a diagnosis, or at least a range of possible diagnoses.

The radiographic image

Radiographic images are produced by the attenuation of x-rays as they pass through intervening tissues before striking an appropriately sensitized plate or film. The more dense and impenetrable the tissue, the greater the attenuation and therefore the more blank, or white, the image in the film. Thus, a metal implant appears intensely white, bone less so and soft tissues in varying shades of grey depending on their 'density'. Cartilage, which causes little attenuation, appears as a dark area between adjacent bone ends; this 'gap' is usually called the joint space, though of course it isn't a space at all, it is merely a 'radiolucent' zone filled with cartilage (Fig. 1.18). Other 'radiolucent' areas are produced by very osteoporotic bone or by fluid-filled cysts in bone.

One bone overlying another (e.g. the femoral head inside the acetabular socket) produces superimposed images; any abnormality seen in the resulting combined image could be in either bone, so it is important to obtain several images from different projections in order to separate the anatomical outlines. Similarly, the bright image of a metallic foreign body superimposed upon that of, say, the femoral condyles could mean that the foreign body is in front of, inside or behind the bone. A second projection, at right angles to the first, will give the answer.

How to read an x-ray

The term 'x-ray' has become entrenched by usage. 'Radiograph' is more correct, and 'roetgenogram' has its adherents. Everyone knows that an 'x-ray' is the film which the doctor puts up on an 'x-ray viewing box'. So we eschew pedantry and stick with 'x-ray'. In most cases at least two projections of each part will be needed.

The process of interpretation should be as methodical as clinical examination. It is seductively easy to be led astray by some flagrant anomaly; systematic study is the only safeguard. A convenient sequence for examination is: *patient – soft tissues – bone – joint – diagnostic associations*.

The patient

Make sure that the name on the film is that of your patient; mistaken identity is a potent source of error. The clinical details are important; it is surprising how much more you can see on the x-ray when you know the background. Similarly, when requesting an x-ray examination, give the radiologist enough information to indicate your line of thinking.

The soft tissues

Unless examined early, these are liable to be forgotten. Look for variations in shape and variations of density.

Shape Muscle planes are often visible and may reveal wasting or swelling. Bulging outlines around a hip, for example, may suggest a joint effusion; and soft-tissue swelling around interphalangeal joints may be the first radiographic sign of rheumatoid arthritis.

Density Increased density in the soft tissues follows calcification in a tendon, a blood vessel, a haematoma or an abscess; often the shape and site suggest which is involved. The radiographic density of a metallic foreign body is usually unmistakable; but even wood or glass may show in suitable films. The precise localization of foreign bodies necessitates multiple views.

Decreased density of soft tissues is due either to fat (the most radiolucent tissue) or to gas.

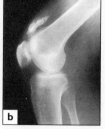

1.14 X-ray signs in soft tissues (**a**) Calcification of the supraspinatus tendon. (**b**) Heterotopic ossification in the quadriceps tendon.

The bones

Again, think in terms of shape and density.

Shape Look at the overall shape of the bones and how they fit together. Identify the anatomical structures and study each one carefully. For example, for the spine, look at the overall vertebral alignment, then at the disc spaces, and then at each vertebra separately, moving from the body to the pedicles, the facet joints and finally to the spinous appendages. For the pelvis, see if the shape is symmetrical with the bones in their normal positions, then look at the sacrum, the two innominate bones, the pubic rami and the ischial tuberosities, then the femoral heads and the upper ends of the femora, always comparing the two sides.

The bone as a whole may be bent, or it may be unduly wide – as in Paget's disease. A localized deformity or swelling may be due to bulging from within (a cyst or other radiolucent lesion) or to excessive new bone formation (perhaps a tumour). Examine carefully *the periosteal surface* (periosteal new bone is characteristic of infection, fracture or malignancy), the *cortex* (for evidence of destruction or fracture) and the *endosteum* (is it sharp and clear, or is it excavated?).

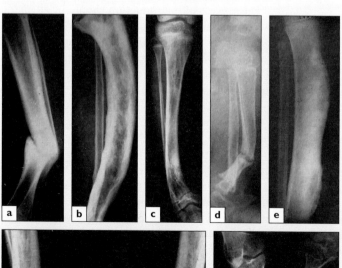

1.15 Bent tibiae
Unilateral: (**a**) malunited fracture; (**b**) Paget's disease; (**c**) dyshondroplasia; (**d**) congenital pseudarthrosis; (**e**) syphilitic sabre tibia.

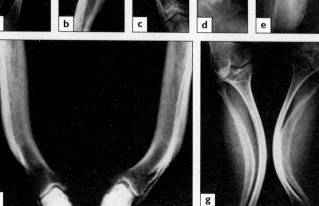

Bilateral: (**f**) old rickets; (**g**) osteogenesis imperfecta.

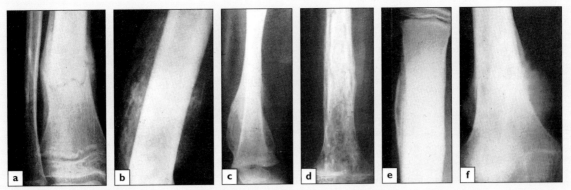

1.16 'Visible periosteum' Ossification just outside the cortex is seen when periosteum has been lifted away from the bone. It may have been lifted by blood, as in (**a**) callus, (**b**) myositis ossificans and (**c**) scurvy; or by inflammatory material, as in (**d**) chronic osteomyelitis and (**e**) syphilitic periostitis; or by tumour material, as in (**f**) osteosarcoma.

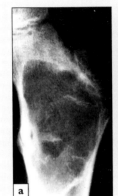
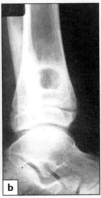
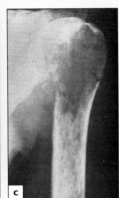

1.17 Rare areas in bone (**a**) This may represent a true cyst, but any radiolucent lesion can look 'cystic' – as with the abscess in (**b**) and the metastatic tumour in (**c**).

Density Note whether the 'density' is increased (sclerosis) or diminished (osteoporosis or replacement by abnormal tissue). The trabecular structure is usually visible: Is it regular? Is it disarranged, or even absent? Now look carefully for 'vacant areas'. Focal defects with sharp margins are usually benign; defects with fuzzy margins may signify infection or a malignant lesion; and those with a 'moth-eaten' appearance are almost certainly malignant. Remember that a 'vacant area' in the image is not necessarily vacant in reality; any tissue that is radiolucent looks dark, so a fibrous tumour may look very much like a cyst! The site of the lesion is important. Bone cysts usually occur in the metaphyses; giant cell tumours always at the very ends of the bone.

The joint

The radiographic 'joint' consists of the articulating bones and the 'space' between them. The 'joint space' is, of course, illusory; it is occupied by a film of synovial fluid plus radiolucent articular cartilage which varies in thickness from 1 mm or less (the carpal joints) to 6 mm (the knee). It looks much wider in children than in adults because much of the epiphysis is still cartilaginous and therefore radiolucent.

Shape Note the general orientation of the joint and the congruity of the bone ends (the subarticular bone plates), if necessary comparing the abnormal with the normal opposite side. Then look for narrowing or asymmetry of the joint 'space', which could signify loss of articular cartilage thickness – a classic sign of arthritis. Further stages of joint destruction are revealed by interruption of the subarticular bone plates and radiolucent bone cysts or periarticular erosions. Bony outgrowths from the joint margins (osteophytes) are typical of osteoarthritis.

Density Lines of increased density within the articular space may be due to calcification of the cartilage or menisci (chondrocalcinosis). Loose bodies, if they are radio-opaque, appear as rounded or irregular patches overlying the normal structures.

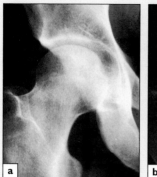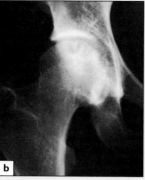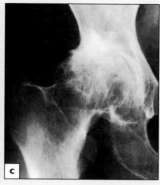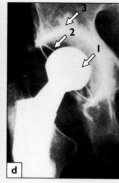

1.18 Plain x-rays of the hip Stages in the development of osteoarthritis (OA). **(a)** Normal hip: anatomical shape and position, with joint 'space' (articular cartilage) fully preserved. **(b)** Early OA, showing joint space slightly decreased and a subarticular cyst in the femoral head. **(c)** Advanced OA: joint space markedly decreased; osteophytes at the joint margin. **(d)** Hip replacement: the cup is radiolucent but its position is shown by a circumferential wire marker. Note the differing image 'densities': **(1)** the metal femoral implant; **(2)** the polyethylene cup (radiolucent); **(3)** acrylic cement impacted into the adjacent bone.

Diagnostic associations

However carefully the individual x-ray features are observed, the diagnosis will not leap ready-made off the x-ray plate. Even a fracture is not always obvious. It is the pattern of abnormalities that counts: if you see one feature that is suggestive, look for others that are commonly associated.

- Narrowing of the joint space + subarticular cysts + osteophytes = osteoarthritis.
- Narrowing of the joint space + osteoporosis + periarticular erosions = inflammatory arthritis.
- Bone destruction + periosteal new-bone formation = infection or malignancy until proven otherwise.

The search for associated abnormalities, or clarification of some poorly observed feature in the plain film, may call for further examination by one of the other imaging techniques.

X-RAYS USING CONTRAST MEDIA

Substances that alter x-ray attenuation characteristics can be used to produce images which contrast with those of the normal tissues. The contrast media used in orthopaedics are mostly iodine-based liquids which can be injected into sinuses, joint cavities or the spinal theca. Air or gas also can be injected into joints to produce a 'negative image' outlining the joint cavity.

Oily iodides are not absorbed and maintain maximum concentration after injection. However, because they are non-miscible, they do not penetrate well into all the nooks and crannies. They are also tissue irritants, especially if used intrathecally. Ionic, water-soluble iodides permit much more detailed imaging and, although also somewhat irritant and neurotoxic, are rapidly absorbed and excreted. Metrizamide, a non-ionic iodide, is the least toxic and least irritant.

Sinography

Sinography is the simplest form of contrast radiography. The medium (usually one of the ionic water-soluble compounds) is injected into an open sinus; the film shows the track and whether or not it leads to the underlying bone or joint.

Arthrography

Arthrography is a particularly useful form of contrast radiography. Intra-articular loose bodies will produce filling defects in the opaque contrast medium. In the knee, torn menisci, ligament tears and capsular ruptures can be shown. In children's hips, arthrography is a useful method of outlining the cartilaginous (and therefore radiolucent) femoral head. In adults with avascular necrosis of the femoral head, arthrography may show up torn flaps of cartilage. After hip replacement, loosening of a prosthesis may be revealed by seepage of the contrast medium into the cement/bone interface. In the ankle, wrist and shoulder, extrusion of the injected contrast medium may disclose tears in the capsular structures. In the spine, contrast radiography can be used to diagnose disc degeneration (discography) and abnormalities of the small facet joints (facetography).

Myelography

Myelography was used extensively in the past for the diagnosis of disc prolapse and other spinal canal lesions. It has been largely replaced by non-invasive methods such

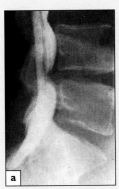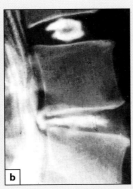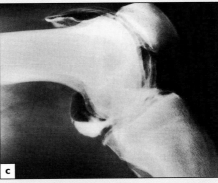

1.19 Contrast radiography (a) Myelography shows the outline of the spinal theca. Where facilities are available, myelography has been largely replaced by CT and MRI. (b) Discography is sometimes useful: note the difference between a normal intervertebral disc (upper level) and a degenerate disc (lower level). (c) Contrast arthrography of the knee shows a small popliteal herniation.

as computed tomography (CT) and magnetic resonance imaging (MRI). However, it is still indicated for the investigation of cervical nerve root lesions and as an adjunct to other methods in patients with back pain.

The oily media are no longer used, and even with the ionic water-soluble iodides there is a considerable incidence of complications, such as low-pressure headache (due to the lumbar puncture), muscular spasms or convulsions (due to neurotoxicity, especially if the chemical is allowed to flow above the mid-dorsal region) and arachnoiditis (which is attributed to the hyperosmolality of these compounds in relation to cerebrospinal fluid). Precautions, such as keeping the patient sitting upright after myelography, must be strictly observed.

Metrizamide has low neurotoxicity and at working concentrations it is more or less isotonic with cerebrospinal fluid. It can therefore be used throughout the length of the spinal canal; the nerve roots are also well delineated (radiculography). A bulging disc, an intrathecal tumour or narrowing of the bony canal will produce characteristic distortions of the opaque column in the myelogram.

TOMOGRAPHY

Tomography provides an image 'focused' on a selected plane. By moving the tube and the x-ray film in opposite directions on an imaginary pivot during the exposure, images on either side of the pivotal plane are deliberately blurred out. When several 'cuts' are studied, lesions obscured in conventional x-rays may be revealed. The method is useful for diagnosing segmental bone necrosis and depressed fractures in cancellous bone (e.g. of the vertebral body or the tibial plateau); these defects are often obscured in the plain x-ray by the surrounding intact mass of bone. Small radiolucent lesions, such as osteoid osteomas and bone abscesses, can also be revealed.

A good standby in former years, conventional tomography has been largely supplanted by CT and MRI.

COMPUTED TOMOGRAPHY

Like simple tomography, CT produces 'cutting' images through selected tissue planes – but with much greater resolution. A further advance over conventional tomography is that the images are transaxial (like transverse anatomical sections), thus exposing anatomical planes that are never viewed in plain film x-rays. A general (or 'localization') view is obtained, the region of interest is selected and a series of cross-sectional images is produced. Slices through the larger joints or tissue masses may be 5–10 mm apart; those through the small joints or intervertebral discs have to be much thinner.

Since it achieves such excellent contrast resolution, CT is able to display the size and shape of bone and soft-tissue masses in transverse planes. This makes it particularly useful in the assessment of tumour size and spread, even if it is unable to characterize the tumour type. Other common applications are in the diagnosis of spinal disorders (especially intervertebral disc prolapse), joint abnormalities and pelvic lesions. It is invaluable – sometimes indispensable – in the assessment of complex fractures, or indeed of any fractures in sites not normally accessible to plain x-rays (e.g. vertebral bodies, tibial condyles, tarsal and carpal bones, and the sacroiliac joints), and the detection of intra-articular bone fragments.

The value of CT can be extended in several ways. Intravascular, intra-articular or intrathecal contrast media can be used to highlight blood vessels or cavity outlines and show their relationship to adjacent masses. CT-guided procedures (e.g. tumour biopsy) are also helpful. With suitable equipment transaxial images can be reconstructed to give sagittal or coronal images, or even three-dimensional images of

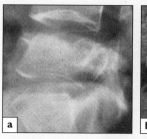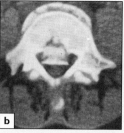

1.20 Computed tomography (CT) The plain x-ray (**a**) shows a fracture of the vertebral body, but one cannot tell precisely how the bone fragments are displaced. The CT scan (**b**) shows clearly that they are dangerously close to the cauda equina.

bones with complicated shapes, like the vertebrae or the hip. With appropriate computer software the images may be 'taken apart' to allow inspection of a particular site (for example the interior of the acetabulum without the femoral head); or bones may be 'reconstructed' by editing out certain parts and putting the pieces of the image together again in a new shape. This is sometimes helpful in planning operations. Computer-linked CT is also used to design customized implants, e.g. for complicated joint replacements.

One disadvantage of CT is the relatively high radiation exposure. It should, therefore, be used with discretion.

MAGNETIC RESONANCE IMAGING

Unlike x-ray imaging, MRI relies upon radiofrequency emissions from atoms and molecules in tissues exposed to a static magnetic field. The images produced by these signals are similar to those of CT scans, but with even better contrast resolution and more refined differentiation of tissues. Moreover, the sectional images can be obtained in almost any plane, and can be reconstituted to give a three-dimensional picture, thus adding even further to the information available.

All atomic nuclei with an odd number of protons possess the property of magnetic resonance, but, because it is so abundant in human tissues and so easily detectable, the hydrogen nucleus is the one currently employed for MR imaging. The intensity of the MR signal depends partly on the density of hydrogen nuclei in the tissue scanned and partly on the spin characteristics and relaxation rates following proton excitation. This phenomenon of relaxation is defined by two independent time constants, T_1 and T_2, thus giving rise to two simultaneous signals.

Tissues containing abundant hydrogen (fat, cancellous bone and marrow) emit high-intensity signals and produce the brightest images; those containing little hydrogen (cortical bone, ligament, tendon and air) appear black; intermediate in the grey scale are cartilage, spinal canal and muscle. In producing the images, either the T_1 or the T_2 characteristics of the tissue may be enhanced, or 'weighted', to give complementary information. The T_1-weighted images show greater definition and provide almost 'anatomical' pictures; the T_2-weighted images tell more about the physiological characteristics of the tissue. Other pulse sequences often used are proton density and short tau inversion recovery (STIR), which suppresses the signal from fat and increases the contrast for water-containing tissues.

By selecting the most appropriate anatomical plane, coil type, slice thickness, magnification and pulse sequence, different tissues and organs can be displayed with extraordinary clarity. Bone tumours can be shown in their transverse and longitudinal extent, and extraosseous spread can be accurately assessed. Moreover, there is the potential for characterizing the actual tissue, thus allowing a pathological as well as an anatomical diagnosis.

Other areas of usefulness are in the early diagnosis of bone ischaemia and necrosis, the investigation of backache and spinal disorders, and the elucidation of cartilage and ligament injuries. In the knee, especially, MRI is as accurate as arthroscopy in diagnosing meniscal tears and cruciate ligament injuries; furthermore, it can detect osteochondral lesions which are not visible

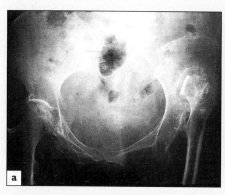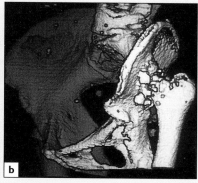

1.21 Reconstructed CT images (**a**) The plain x-ray shows an old untreated congenital dislocation on the left. (**b**) The three-dimensional image reveals just how far the femoral head is from the anatomical socket, information that is important in planning hip surgery.

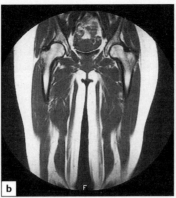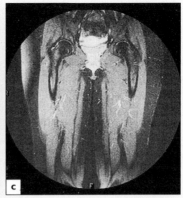

1.22 Magnetic resonance imaging (MRI) (**a**, **b**) T_1-weighted and (**c**) STIR (short tau inversion recovery) sequences of the torso and thigh areas, showing the contrasting definition and brightness of the various structures and tissues.

on arthroscopy. MRI is now proving equally useful in diagnosing rotator cuff tears and labral injuries in the shoulder and ligament injuries around the ankle.

As MRI is so versatile, and free of the risks of ionizing radiation, it is tempting to overindulge its use. It is well to remember that it is still only one diagnostic method among many.

DIAGNOSTIC ULTRASOUND

High-frequency sound waves, generated by a transducer, can penetrate several centimetres into the soft tissues; as they pass through the tissue interfaces some of these waves are reflected back (like echoes) to the transducer, where they are registered as electrical signals and displayed as images on a screen or plate. With modern equipment, tissues of varying density can be 'imaged' in gradations of grey that allow reasonable definition of the anatomy. Real-time display on a moni-

tor gives a dynamic image, which is more useful than the usual static images on transparent plates. One big advantage of this technique is that the equipment is simple and portable and can be used almost anywhere. Another is that it produces no harmful side effects.

Depending on their structure, different tissues are referred to as highly echogenic, mildly echogenic or echo-free. Fluid-filled cysts are echo-free; fat is highly echogenic; and semi-solid organs manifest varying degrees of 'echo-genicity' which permits their spatial identification.

As a result of the marked echogenic contrast between cystic and solid masses, ultrasonography is particularly useful for identifying hidden 'cystic' lesions such as haematomas, abscesses, popliteal cysts and arterial aneurysms. It is also capable of detecting intra-articular fluid and may be used to diagnose a synovial effusion or to monitor the progress of an 'irritable hip'. More recently it has

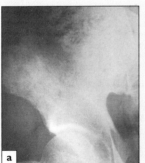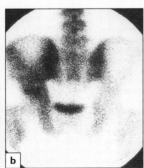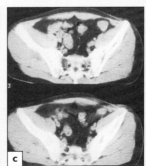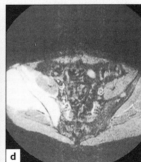

1.23 Imaging (**a**) Plain x-rays of this 40-year-old man showed only non-specific destructive changes in the right innominate bone. (**b**) The radioisotope scan revealed diffuse activity throughout the ilium and also in the ischium. (**c**) CT studies added further information: there is increased bulk in the glutei and the iliacus. (**d**) The MRI (STIR sequence) shows the full extent of the lesion – a large tumour involving the whole of the iliac blade with soft-tissue masses in the glutei and iliacus. Note also the matastatic deposit in the opposite iliac blade. Biopsy revealed a non-Hodgkin's lymphoma.

come into its own as a means of screening newborn babies for congenital dislocation (or dysplasia) of the hip; the cartilaginous femoral head and the acetabular labrum can be clearly identified, and their relationship to each other shows whether the hip is normal or abnormal. Ultrasound has also been used to diagnose rotator cuff tears of the shoulder, though the interpretation of these images can be difficult.

RADIONUCLIDE IMAGING

Photon emission by radionuclides taken up in specific tissues can be recorded by either a simple rectilinear scanner or a gamma camera, to produce an image which reflects current activity in that tissue or organ. The ideal isotope for this purpose is technetium-99m (^{99m}Tc): it has the appropriate energy characteristics for gamma-camera imaging, it has a relatively short half-life (6 hours) and it is rapidly excreted. The low background activity means that any site of increased uptake is readily visible. When ^{99m}Tc is linked to a bone-seeking phosphate compound, it is selectively concentrated in skeletal tissues.

Bone-seeking isotopes

Technetium-labelled hydroxymethylene diphosphophonate (^{99m}Tc-HDP) is injected intravenously and its activity is recorded at two stages: (1) shortly after injection, while it is still in the blood stream or the perivascular space (the *perfusion* or *bloodpool phase*), and (2) 3 hours later when the isotope has been taken up in bone *(the bone phase)*. Normally, in the early perfusion phase the vascular soft tissues around the joints produce the darkest (most active) image; 3 hours later this activity has faded and the bone outlines are shown more clearly, the greatest activity appearing in the cancellous tissue at the ends of the long bones.

Changes in radioactivity are most significant when they are sharply localized or asymmetrical. Four types of abnormality are seen, described below.

Increased activity in the perfusion phase This is due to increased soft-tissue blood flow – one of the cardinal features of inflammation (e.g. acute or chronic synovitis).

Decreased activity in the perfusion phase This is much less common and signifies local vascular insufficiency.

Increased activity in the bone phase This could be due either to excessive isotope uptake in the osseous extracellular fluid or to more avid incorporation into newly forming bone tissue; either would be likely in a fracture, infection, a local tumour or healing after necrosis, and nothing in the bone scan itself distinguishes between these conditions.

Diminished activity in the bone phase This is due to an absent blood supply (e.g. in the femoral head after a fracture of the femoral neck) or to replacement of bone by pathological tissue.

The clinical applications are manifold and include: (1) the diagnosis of stress fractures (or other undisplaced fractures) that do not appear on the plain x-ray; (2) the detection of a small bone abscess, or an osteoid osteoma; (3) the investigation of loosening or infection around prostheses; (4) the diagnosis of femoral head ischaemia in Perthes' disease or avascular necrosis in adults; (5) the early detection of bone metastases. The scintigraphic appearances in these conditions are described in the relevant chapters. In most cases the isotope scan serves chiefly to pinpoint the site of abnormality and it should always be read in conjunction with other modes of imaging.

Other radionuclide compounds

Technetium-labelled sulphur colloid (^{99m}Tc-S$_c$) is taken up by phagocytes in the reticuloendothelial system and is therefore a better indicator of marrow vascularity than the bone-seeking compounds. Its use may permit early diagnosis of femoral head ischaemia, but the method is not sensitive enough to justify its routine use in hip fractures or suspected femoral head necrosis.

Gallium-67 (^{67}Ga) concentrates in inflammatory cells and has been used to identify sites of hidden infection; for example, in the investigation of prosthetic

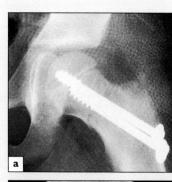

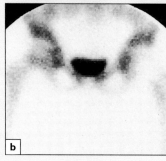

1.24 Radionuclide imaging (a) This fractured femoral neck in a child has resulted in loss of the blood supply, as shown by **(b)** the 'void' in the left hip on the technetium scan.

loosening after joint replacement. However, it is arguable whether it gives any more reliable information than the ^{99m}Tc bone scan.

Indium-111-labelled leucocytes can also be used as markers for infection. Leucocytes from the patient's own blood are labelled with ^{111}In and then re-injected into the blood stream. Areas of increased activity show where they are concentrated.

BLOOD TESTS

Non-specific blood tests

Non-specific blood abnormalities are common in bone and joint disorders; their interpretation hinges on the clinical and x-ray findings.

Hypochromic anaemia is usual in rheumatoid arthritis; but it may also be a consequence of gastrointestinal bleeding due to the anti-inflammatory drugs.

Leucocytosis is generally associated with infection; but a mild leucocytosis is not uncommon in rheumatoid arthritis and during an attack of gout.

The erythrocyte sedimentation rate (ESR) is usually increased in acute and chronic inflammatory disorders and after tissue injury. However, patients with low-grade infection may have a normal ESR and this should not be taken as a reassuring sign. The ESR is strongly affected by the presence of monoclonal immunoglobulins; a high ESR is almost mandatory in the diagnosis of myelomatosis.

C-reactive protein (and other acute phase proteins) may be abnormally increased in chronic inflammatory arthritis and (temporarily) after injury. The test is often used to monitor the progress and activity of rheumatoid arthritis and chronic infection.

Plasma gamma-globulins can be measured by protein electrophoresis. Their precise characterization is helpful in the assessment of certain rheumatic disorders, and more particularly in the diagnosis of myelomatosis.

Rheumatoid factor tests

Rheumatoid factor is an autoantibody (or antiglobulin) which is often present in patients with rheumatoid arthritis. However, it is not diagnostic and some patients remain 'seronegative'. Rheumatoid factor is also absent in patients with ankylosing spondylitis,

Reiter's disease or psoriatic arthritis; these disorders have been grouped together as the 'seronegative spondarthritides'.

Tissue typing

HLA antigens can be detected in white blood cells and they are used to characterize individual tissue types. The seronegative spondarthritides are closely associated with the presence of HLA-B27 on chromosome 6; this is frequently used as a confirmatory test in patients suspected of having ankylosing spondylitis or Reiter's disease, but it should not be regarded as a specific test because it is positive in about 8% of normal Caucasians.

Biochemistry

Biochemical tests are essential in monitoring patients after any serious injury. They are also used routinely in the investigation of rheumatic disorders and abnormalities of bone metabolism. Their significance is discussed under the relevant conditions.

SYNOVIAL FLUID ANALYSIS

Arthrocentesis is a much-neglected diagnostic procedure; given the correct indications it can yield valuable information. It should be considered in the following conditions (see Table 1.1).

Acute joint swelling after injury The distinction between synovitis and bleeding may not be obvious; aspiration will settle the question immediately.

Suspected infection Careful examination and laboratory investigations may provide the answer, but they take time. Joint aspiration is essential for early diagnosis.

Acute synovitis in adults Synovial fluid analysis may be the only way to distinguish between infection, gout and pseudogout.

Chronic synovitis Here joint aspiration is less urgent, and is only one of many diagnostic procedures in the investigation of suspected tuberculosis or atypical rheumatic disorders.

Technique

The joint should be aspirated under strict aseptic conditions. Even a small quantity of fluid (less than 0.5 ml) is enough for diagnostic analysis.

Table 1.1 Examination of synovial fluid

Suspected condition	Appearance	Viscosity	White cells	Crystals	Biochemislry	Bacteriology
Normal	Clear yellow	High	Few	–	As for plasma	–
Septic arthritis	Purulent	Low	+	–	Glucose low	+
Tuberculous arthritis	Turbid	Low	+	–	Glucose low	+
Rheumatoid arthritis	Cloudy	Low	++	–	–	–
Gout	Cloudy	Normal	++	urate	–	–
Pseudogout	Cloudy	Normal	+	pyrophosphate	–	–
Osteoarthritis	Clear yellow	High	Few	Often +	–	–

Gross examination

The volume of fluid and its appearance are immediately noted. Normal synovial fluid is clear and slightly yellow. A cloudy or turbid fluid is due to the presence of cells, usually a sign of inflammation. Blood-stained fluid may be found after injury, but is also seen in acute inflammatory disorders and in pigmented villonodular synovitis.

Microscopic examination

A single drop of fresh synovial fluid is placed on a glass slide and examined through the microscope. Blood cells are easily identified; abundant leucocytes may suggest infection. Crystals may be seen, though this usually requires a careful search; they are better characterized by polarized light microscopy (see Fig. 4.3).

Dry smears are prepared with heparinized fluid; more concentrated specimens can be obtained if the fluid is centrifuged. After suitable staining (Wright's and Gram's), the smear is examined for pus cells and organisms. Remember, though, *that negative findings do not exclude infection.*

Laboratory tests

If enough fluid is available, it is sent for full laboratory investigation (cells, biochemistry and bacteriological culture). A simultaneous blood specimen allows comparison of synovial and blood glucose concentration; a marked reduction of synovial glucose suggests infection.

A high white cell count (more than 100,000/mm³) is usually indicative of infection, but a moderate leucocytosis is also seen in gout and other types of inflammatory arthritis.

Bacteriological culture and tests for antibiotic sensitivity are essential in any case of suspected infection.

BONE BIOPSY

Bone biopsy is often the crucial means of making a diagnosis or distinguishing between local conditions that closely resemble one another. Confusion is most likely to occur when the x-ray or MRI discloses an area of bone destruction that could be due to a compression fracture, a bone tumour or infection (e.g. a collapsed vertebral body). In other cases it is obvious that the lesion is a tumour – but what type of tumour? Benign or malignant? Primary or metastatic? Radical surgery should never be undertaken for a suspected neoplasm without first confirming the diagnosis histologically – no matter how 'typical' or 'obvious' the x-ray appearances may be.

In bone infection, the biopsy permits not only histological proof of acute inflammation but also bacteriological typing of the organism and tests for antibiotic sensitivity.

The investigation of metabolic bone disease is, likewise, seldom complete without a biopsy to show (1) the type of abnormality (osteoporosis, osteomalacia, hyperparathyroidism) and (2) the severity of the disorder.

Open or closed?

Open biopsy, with exposure of the lesion and excision of a sizeable portion of the bone, seems preferable, but it has several drawbacks. (1) It requires an operation, with the attendant risks of anaesthesia and infection. (2) New tissue planes are opened up, predisposing to spread of infection or tumour. (3) The biopsy incision may jeopardize subsequent wide excision of the lesion. (4) The more inaccessible lesions (e.g. a tumour of the acetabular floor) can be reached only by dissecting widely through healthy tissue.

A carefully performed 'closed' biopsy, using a needle or trephine of appropriate size to ensure the removal of an adequate sample of tissue, is the procedure of choice except when the lesion cannot be accurately localized or when the tissue consistency is such that a sufficient sample cannot be obtained. Solid or semi-solid tissue is removed intact by the cutting needle or trephine; fluid material can be aspirated through the biopsy needle.

Precautions

The appropriate size of biopsy needle or cutting trephine should be selected. A soft tumour, or focus of infection, can be sampled with a comparatively thin needle (1–2 mm diameter); an iliac crest biopsy for histomorphometry in metabolic bone disease requires a trephine at least 5 mm in diameter.

The biopsy site and approach should be carefully planned with the aid of x-rays or other imaging techniques. If there is any possibility of the lesion being malignant, the approach should be sited so that the wound and biopsy track can be excised if later radical surgery proves to be necessary.

The procedure is carried out in an operating theatre, under anaesthesia (local or general) and with full aseptic techniques. For deep-seated lesions, fluoroscopic control of the needle insertion is essential. Even then, very small lesions may be difficult to find; however, if it is a bone-forming tumour (e.g. an osteoid osteoma) it can be labelled by giving an intravenous injection of ^{99m}Tc-HDP 3 hours beforehand and then located with a sterilized radiation probe during open operation

It goes without saying that a knowledge of the local anatomy and of the likely consistency of the lesion, is important. Large blood vessels and nerves must be avoided; potentially vascular tumours may bleed profusely and the means to control haemorrhage should be readily to hand. More than one surgeon has plunged a wide-bore needle into an aneurysm which was mistaken for a soft-tissue tumour or an abscess!

Finally, the tissue obtained at the biopsy should be suitably processed. If infection is suspected, the material should go into a culture tube and be sent to the laboratory as soon as possible. A smear may also be useful. Whole tissue is transferred to a jar containing formalin, without damaging the specimen or losing any material. Aspirated blood should be allowed to clot and can then be preserved in formalin for later paraffin embedding and sectioning. Tissue thought to contain crystals should not be placed in formalin as this may destroy the crystals; it should either be kept unaltered for immediate examination or stored in saline.

No matter how careful the biopsy, there is always the risk that the tissue will be too scanty or too unrepresentative for accurate diagnosis. Close consultation with the radiologist and pathologist beforehand will minimize this possibility. In the best hands, needle biopsy has an accuracy rate of over 95%.

ARTHROSCOPY

Arthroscopy is performed for both diagnostic and therapeutic reasons. Almost any joint can be reached but the procedure is most usefully employed in the knee, shoulder, wrist, ankle and hip. If the suspect lesion is amenable to surgery, it can often be dealt with at the same sitting without the need for an open operation. However, arthroscopy is an invasive procedure and its mastery requires skill and practice; it should not be used simply as an alternative to clinical examination and imaging.

Technique

The instrument is basically a rigid telescope fitted with fibreoptic illumination. Tube diameter ranges from about 2 mm (for small joints) to 4–5 mm (for the knee). It carries a lens system that gives a magnified image. The eyepiece allows direct viewing by the arthroscopist, but it is far more convenient to fit a small, sterilizable solid-state television camera which produces a picture of the joint interior on a television monitor.

The procedure is best carried out under general anaesthesia; this gives good muscle relaxation and permits manipulation and opening of the joint compartments. The joint is distended with fluid and the arthroscope is introduced percutaneously. Various instruments (probes, curettes and forceps) can be inserted through other skin portals; they are used to help expose the less accessible parts of the joint, or to obtain biopsies for further examination. Guided by the image on the monitor, the arthroscopist explores the joint in a systematic fashion, manipulating the arthroscope with one hand and the probe or forceps with the other. At the end of the procedure the joint is washed out and the small skin wounds are sutured. The patient is usually able to return home later the same day.

Diagnosis

The *knee* is the most accessible joint. The appearances of the synovium and the articular surfaces usually allow differentiation between inflammatory and non-inflammatory, destructive and non-destructive lesions. Meniscal tears can be diagnosed and treated immediately by repair or removal of partially detached segments. Cruciate ligament deficiency, osteocartilaginous fractures, cartilaginous loose bodies and synovial 'tumours' are also readily visualized.

Arthroscopy of the *shoulder* is more difficult, but the articular surfaces and glenoid labrum can be adequately explored. Rotator cuff lesions can often be diagnosed and treated at the same time.

Arthroscopy of the *wrist* is useful for diagnosing torn triangular fibrocartilage and interosseous ligament ruptures.

Arthroscopy of the *hip* is less widely used, but it is proving to be useful in the diagnosis of unexplained hip pain. Labral tears, synovial lesions, loose bodies and articular cartilage damage (all of which are difficult to detect by conventional imaging techniques) have been diagnosed with a reported accuracy rate of about 50%.

Complications

Diagnostic arthroscopy is safe but not entirely free of complications, the commonest of which are haemarthosis, thrombophlebitis, infection and joint stiffness. There is also a significant incidence of algodystrophy (complex regional pain syndrome) following arthroscopy.

ELECTRODIAGNOSIS

Nerve and muscle function can be studied by various electrical methods. This information on physiological activity is invaluable in the diagnosis of neuromuscular disorders, but it must be used to supplement – not replace – the systematic clinical examination. Two types of investigation are employed: nerve conduction studies and electromyography.

Motor nerve conduction

Electrical stimulation of a motor nerve normally produces contraction of the muscles supplied by that nerve. The stimulus is applied to the skin over the

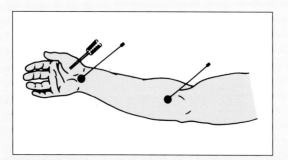

1.25 Electrodiagnosis Electrodes at different levels are used to stimulate the median nerve and one in the thenar muscle records contraction. If the distance between the electrodes is measured and the time interval (from stimulation to muscle contraction) is recorded, conduction velocity can be calculated.

nerve, and the motor unit response is measured by a concentric needle electrode inserted into the muscle; the electrical discharge, *or motor action potential (MAP)*, is amplified and displayed on an oscilloscope.

The time interval between stimulation of the nerve and the appearance of the MAP is the *latency*. If the test is repeated at two points a measured distance apart along the nerve, and the latency values obtained are subtracted from one another, the conduction velocity between those two points can be determined. Normal values are about 50–60m/s.

Conduction velocity is slowed in peripheral nerve damage or compression, and the site of the lesion can be established by taking measurements in different segments of the nerve (e.g. in the diagnosis of nerve entrapment syndromes). With more severe demyelination, the amplitude of the MAP is also diminished. If the nerve is completely divided, from the 14th day after injury there is no response to either faradic or galvanic stimulation of the nerve, and there is an abnormal response from galvanic stimulation of the muscle (the 'reaction of degeneration'). By plotting the strength of current against the duration of stimulus necessary to produce contraction, a strength/duration curve can be obtained, which reflects the degree of denervation and progressive changes in nerve function over time. Other lower motor neuron disorders produce characteristic changes in latency and motor action potentials.

Sensory nerve conduction

If a sensory nerve is stimulated distally, the *sensory nerve action potential (SNAP)* can be recorded at a proximal site. Here again, by measuring the distance between stimulating and recording electrodes, and the time lapse between stimulus and response, the sensory nerve conduction velocity can be calculated. In compression or entrapment of a mixed nerve, sensory conduction is often affected before motor conduction, so it is useful to measure both. The amplitude of the SNAP gives an indication of the proportion of functioning nerve fibres.

A special application of this test is in the recording of *somatosensory evoked potentials (SEPs)*. Percutaneous electrical stimulation of a peripheral nerve (for convenience usually the median nerve at the wrist or the posterior tibial nerve at the ankle) produces a response that can be recorded by electrodes placed on the spinal cord, on the skin over one of the vertebrae or on the scalp over the cerebral cortex. This is useful in monitoring the integrity of the spinal cord during operative correction of severe spinal deformities and other potentially dangerous procedures. A significant fall in signal amplitude or an increase in latency is regarded as a sign of danger, and tension on the cord can be released before irreversible damage occurs.

The same principle is used in the diagnosis of sensory neuropathies such as Friedreich's ataxia, and in the investigation of brachial plexus injuries where the anatomy makes it impossible to carry out the more usual nerve conduction studies.

Electromyography

Electromyography (EMG) does not involve electrical nerve stimulation. Instead, a concentric needle in the muscle is used to record motor unit activity at rest and when attempts are made to contract the muscle.

Normally there is no electrical activity at rest. However, spontaneous discharges may occur after partial or complete denervation, with pressure on spinal nerve roots, with anterior horn cell degeneration (e.g. in progressive muscular atrophy) and in various muscle disorders. This is thought to be due to increased sensitivity of the denervated (or abnormal) muscle fibres to circulating acetylcholine.

On voluntary muscle contraction, characteristic oscilloscope patterns appear. The number, shape, amplitude and duration of these action potentials make up a pattern that can distinguish between neuropathic and myopathic disorders. In myopathies the action potentials are smaller; in neuropathies they are abnormally large and extended. Mapping denervation activity in peripheral muscles can give important information on the exact levels of nerve and spinal cord lesions.

Interpretation and diagnosis

Electromyography is not a print-out of disease; it should always be considered in conjunction with clinical findings, x-ray, biochemical tests, nerve conduction studies and – if necessary – muscle biopsy before a diagnosis is reached. It is also important to remember, when using EMG in the diagnosis of *nerve injuries*, that it takes 3 weeks for denervation discharges to appear; therefore one cannot distinguish between temporary damage and permanent damage until 'recovery potentials' appear in the former.

With the development of computer-assisted analysis, electrodiagnosis will have considerably wider application in the future.

REFERENCES AND FURTHER READING

Apley AG, Solomon L (1997) *Physical Examination in Orthopaedics*. Butterworth Heinemann, Oxford

Kimura J (1983) *Electrodiagnosis in Diseases of Nerve and Muscle: Principles and Practice*. F A Davis, Philadelphia

Murphy WA, Destouet JM, Gilula LA (1981) Percutaneous skeletal biopsy: a procedure for radiologists – results, review and recommendations. *Radiology* 139, 545–549

Resnick D, Niwayama G (1988) *Diagnosis of Bone and Joint Disorders*, vol 1, Diagnostic Techniques, 2nd edn. W B Saunders, Philadelphia

Watt I (1988) Musculoskeletal system. In: *Nuclear Medicine: Applications to Surgery* (eds ER Davies, WEG Thomas). Castle House Publ, Tunbridge Wells, 219–253

Micro-organisms may reach the bones and joints either *directly* through a break in the skin (a pinprick, a stab wound, a laceration, an open fracture or an operation) or *indirectly via the blood stream* from a distant site such as the nose or mouth, the respiratory tract, the bowel or the genito-urinary tract. Depending on the type of invader, the site of infection and the host response, the result may be a *pyogenic osteomyelitis or arthritis*, a chronic *granulomatous reaction* (classically seen in tuberculosis), or an indolent response to an *unusual organism* (e.g. a fungal infection). *Parasitic lesions* such as hydatid disease also are considered in this chapter, although these are infestations rather than infections.

GENERAL ASPECTS OF INFECTION

Infection – as distinct from mere residence of micro-organisms – is a condition in which pathogenic organisms multiply and spread within the body tissues. This usually gives rise to an acute or chronic inflammatory reaction, which is the body's way of combating the invaders and destroying them, or at least immobilizing them and confining them to a single area. The signs of inflammation are recounted in the classical mantra: redness, swelling, heat, pain and loss of function.

Acute pyogenic infections are characterized by the formation of pus – a concentrate of defunct leucocytes, dead and dying bacteria and tissue debris – which is often localized in an abscess. Pressure builds up within the abscess and infection may then extend directly along the tissue planes. It may also spread further afield via lymphatics (causing lymphangitis and lymphadenopathy) or via the bloodstream (bacteraemia and septicaemia). The accompanying systemic reaction varies from a vague feeling of lassitude with mild pyrexia to severe illness, fever, toxaemia and shock. The generalized effects are due to the release of bacterial enzymes and endotoxins as well as cellular breakdown products from the host tissues.

Chronic infection may follow on acute or, depending on the type of organism and the host reaction, it may be 'chronic' from the start. It usually involves the formation of granulation tissue (a combination of fibroblastic and vascular proliferation) leading to fibrosis. Some organisms provoke a non-pyogenic reaction involving the formation of cellular granulomas which consist largely of lymphocytes, modified macrophages and multinucleated giant cells; this is seen most typically in tuberculosis. Systemic effects are less acute but may ultimately be very debilitating, with lymphadenopathy, splenomegaly and tissue wasting.

The host response is crucial in determining the course of the disease. Resistance is likely to be depressed in the very young and the very old, in states of malnutrition or immuno-suppression, and in certain diseases such as diabetes.

Local factors also are important. Damaged muscle is a favourable substrate for certain organisms, and the presence of foreign material may interfere with the phagocytic response to invading bacteria. Bone, which consists of a collection of rigid compartments, is more susceptible than soft tissues to vascular damage and cell death from the build-up of pressure in acute inflammation; unless it is rapidly controlled, bone infection will inevitably lead to necrosis. Bone structure – a honeycomb of inaccessible spaces – also makes it very difficult to eradicate infection once it is established.

The principles of treatment are: (1) to provide analgesia and general supportive measures; (2) to rest the affected part; (3) effective antibiotic or chemotherapy; and (4) surgical eradication of infected and necrotic tissue. Special laboratory investigations may be needed to identify the infecting microbe and test for the most effective microbicide. For acute infections, the timing of surgery is all-important: in the early stages, antibiotics should be given a chance and the clinical condition carefully monitored to detect signs of improvement or deterioration; if there is pus, it must be let out and the sooner the better. For chronic infection, the choice between conservative and surgical treatment is much more difficult and each case must be decided on its merits.

ACUTE HAEMATOGENOUS OSTEOMYELITIS

Acute osteomyelitis is almost invariably a disease of children. When adults are affected it may be because their resistance is lowered by debility, disease or drugs. An association with diabetes has long been recognized, whilst immunosuppression, either acquired or induced, is increasingly encountered as a predisposing factor. Trauma may determine the site of infection, possibly by causing a small haematoma or fluid collection in a bone.

The causal organism is usually *Staphylococcus aureus*, less often one of the other Gram-positive cocci, such as *Streptococcus pyogenes* or *S. pneumoniae*. In children under 4 years of age the Gram-negative *Haemophilus influenzae* is a fairly common pathogen, the quoted incidence varying from 5 to 50%. Other Gram-negative organisms (e.g. *Escherichia coli, Pseudomonas aeruginosa, Proteus mirabilis* and the anaerobic *Bacteroides fragilis*) occasionally cause acute bone infection. Other anaerobic organisms (particularly *Peptococcus magnus*) have been found in patients with osteomyelitis – usually as part of a mixed infection. Unusual organisms are more likely to be found in heroin addicts and as opportunistic pathogens in patients with compromised immune defence mechanisms. Curiously, patients with sickle-cell disease are prone to infection by *Salmonella*.

The blood stream is invaded, perhaps from a minor skin abrasion, a boil, a septic tooth or – in the newborn – from an infected umbilical cord. In adults the source of infection may be a urethral catheter, an indwelling arterial line or a dirty needle and syringe.

Organisms usually settle in the metaphysis, most often in the proximal tibia or in the distal and proximal ends of the femur. This predilection for the metaphysis has been attributed to the peculiar arrangement of the blood vessels in that area: the non-anastomosing terminal branches of the nutrient artery twist back in hairpin loops before entering the large network of sinusoidal veins; the relative vascular stasis favours bacterial colonization. In young infants, in whom there is still a free anastomosis between metaphyseal and epiphyseal blood vessels, infection can just as easily lodge in the epiphysis. In adults, haematogenous infection is more common in the vertebrae than in the long bones.

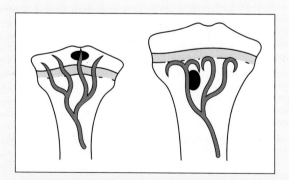

2.1 Acute osteomyelitis (1) In babies infection may settle near the very end of the bone; joint infection and growth disturbance easily follow. In children, metaphyseal infection is usual; the growth disc acts as a barrier to spread.

Pathology

The pathological picture varies considerably, depending on the patient's age, the site of infection, the virulence of the organism and the host response. However, underlying the variations there is a characteristic pattern marked by *inflammation, suppuration, necrosis, reactive new bone formation* and, ultimately, *resolution and healing*.

INFLAMMATION The earliest change is an acute inflammatory reaction with vascular congestion, exudation of fluid and infiltration by polymorphonuclear leucocytes. The intraosseous pressure rises rapidly, causing intense pain, obstruction to blood flow and intravascular thrombosis. Even at an early stage the tissues are threatened by impending ischaemia.

SUPPURATION By the second or third day, pus forms within the bone and forces its way along the Volkmann canals to the surface where it produces a subperiosteal abscess. From there the pus spreads along the shaft, to re-enter the bone at another level or burst into the surrounding soft tissues. In infants, infection often extends through the physis into the epiphysis and thence into the joint. In older children the physis is a barrier to direct spread but where the metaphysis is partly intracapsular (e.g. at the hip, shoulder or elbow) pus may discharge through the periosteum into the joint. In adults the abscess is more likely to spread within the medullary cavity. Vertebral infection may spread through the end-plate and the intervertebral disc into the adjacent vertebral body.

NECROSIS The rising intraosseous pressure, vascular stasis, infective thrombosis and periosteal stripping increasingly compromise the blood supply; by the end of a week there is usually microscopic evidence of bone death. Bacterial toxins and leucocytic enzymes also may play their part in the advancing tissue destruction. In infants the growth disc is often irreparably damaged and the epiphysis may undergo avascular necrosis. With the gradual ingrowth of granulation tissue the boundary between dead and living bone becomes defined. Pieces of dead bone separate as sequestra varying in size from mere spicules to large necrotic segments. Macrophages and lymphocytes arrive in increasing numbers and the debris is slowly removed by a combination of phagocytosis and osteoclastic resorption. However, the larger sequestra remain entombed in cavities of bone, inaccessible to either final destruction or repair.

NEW BONE FORMATION New bone forms from the deep layers of the stripped periosteum. This is typical of pyogenic infection and is usually obvious by the end of the second week. With time the new bone thickens to form an involucrum enclosing the infected tissue

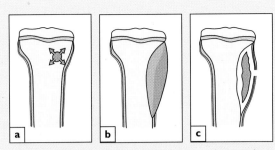

2.2 Acute osteomyelitis (2) (a) Infection in the metaphysis may spread towards the surface, to form a subperiosteal abscess (b). Some of the bone may die, and is encased in periosteal new bone as a sequestrum (c). The encasing involucrum is sometimes perforated by sinuses.

and sequestra. If the infection persists, pus and tiny sequestrated spicules of bone may continue to discharge through perforations (cloacae) in the involucrum and track by sinuses to the skin surfaces; the condition is now established as a chronic osteomyelitis.

RESOLUTION Once common, chronic osteomyelitis following on acute is nowadays seldom seen. If infection is controlled and intraosseous pressure released at an early stage, this dire progress can be aborted. The bone around the zone of infection is at first osteoporotic (probably due to hyperaemia). With healing, there is fibrosis and appositional new bone formation; this, together with the periosteal reaction, results in sclerosis and thickening of the bone. In some cases, remodelling may restore the normal contours; in others, though healing is sound, the bone is left permanently deformed.

Clinical features

The patient, *usually a child*, presents with severe pain, malaise and a fever; in neglected cases, toxaemia may be marked. The parents will have noticed that the child refuses to use one limb or to allow it to be handled or even touched. There may be a recent history of infection – a septic toe, a boil, a sore throat or a discharge from the ear.

Typically the child looks ill and feverish; the pulse rate is likely to be over 100 and the temperature is raised. The limb is held still and there is acute tenderness near one of the larger joints (e.g. above or below the knee, in the popliteal fossa or in the groin). Even the gentlest manipulation is painful and joint movement is restricted. Local redness, swelling, warmth and oedema are later signs and signify that pus has escaped from the interior of the bone. Lymphadenopathy is common but non-specific. It is important to remember

that all these features may be attenuated if antibiotics have been administered.

In infants, and especially in the newborn, the constitutional disturbance can be misleadingly mild; the baby simply fails to thrive and is drowsy but irritable. Suspicion should be aroused by a history of birth difficulties, umbilical artery catheterization or a site of infection (however mild) such as an inflamed intravenous infusion point. Metaphyseal tenderness and resistance to joint movement can signify either osteomyelitis or septic arthritis; indeed, both may be present, so the distinction hardly matters. Look for other sites – multiple infection is not uncommon.

In adults the commonest site of infection is the thoracolumbar spine. There may be a history of some urological procedure followed by a mild fever and backache. Local tenderness is not very marked and it may take weeks before x-ray signs appear; when they do appear the diagnosis may still need to be confirmed by fine-needle aspiration and bacteriological culture.

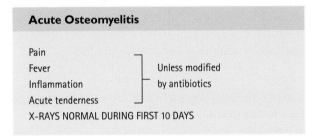

Other bones are occasionally involved, especially if there is a background of diabetes, malnutrition, drug addiction, leukaemia, immunosuppressive therapy or debility. In the very elderly, and in those with immune deficiency, systemic features are mild and the diagnosis is easily missed.

Diagnostic imaging

During the first few days the *plain x-ray* shows no abnormality of the bone. Displacement of the fat planes signifies soft-tissue swelling, but this could as well be due to a haematoma or soft-tissue infection. By the end of the second week there may be a faint extra-cortical outline due to periosteal new bone formation. This is the classic x-ray sign of pyogenic osteomyelitis, but treatment should not be delayed while waiting for it to appear. Later the periosteal thickening becomes more obvious and there is patchy rarefaction of the metaphysis; later still the ragged features of bone destruction appear.

An important late sign is the combination of regional osteoporosis with a localized segment of apparently increased density (e.g. in the femoral head). Osteoporosis

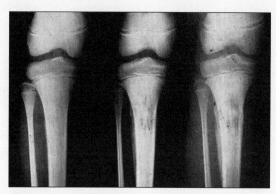

2.3 Acute osteomyelitis (3) The first x-ray, 2 days after symptoms began, is normal – it always is; metaphyseal mottling and periosteal changes were not obvious until the second film, taken 14 days later; eventually much of the shaft was involved.

is a feature of metabolically active, and thus living, bone; the segment that fails to become osteoporotic is metabolically inactive and possibly dead.

Ultrasound may detect a subperiosteal collection of fluid in the early stages of osteomyelitis, but it cannot distinguish between a haematoma and pus.

Radioscintigraphy with ^{99m}Tc-HDP reveals increased activity in both the perfusion phase and the bone phase. This is a highly sensitive investigation, even in the very early stages, but it has relatively low specificity and other inflammatory lesions can show similar changes. In doubtful cases, scanning with ^{67}Ga-citrate or ^{111}In labelled leucocytes may be more revealing.

MRI is extremely sensitive, even in the early phase of bone infection, and can therefore help to differentiate between soft-tissue infection and osteomyelitis. The most typical feature is a reduced intensity signal in T_1-weighted images.

Investigations

The most certain way to confirm the clinical diagnosis is to aspirate pus from the metaphyseal subperiosteal abscess or the adjacent joint. Even if no pus is found, a smear of the aspirate is examined immediately for cells and organisms; a simple Gram stain may help to identify the type of infection and assist with the initial choice of antibiotic. A sample is also sent for detailed bacteriological examination and tests for sensitivity to antibiotics.

The white cell count and C-reactive protein values are usually high and the haemoglobin concentration diminished; the ESR also rises but it may take several days to do so and it often remains elevated even after the infection subsides. In the very young and the very old these tests are less reliable and may show values within the range of normal.

Blood culture is positive in only about half the cases of proven infection.

Antistaphylococcal antibody titres may be raised. This test is most useful in atypical cases where the diagnosis is in doubt.

Osteomyelitis in an unusual site or with an unusual organism should alert one to the possibility of heroin addiction, deficient host defence mechanisms or sickle-cell disease. *Salmonella* may be cultured from the faeces.

Differential diagnosis

CELLULITIS This is often mistaken for osteomyelitis. There is widespread superficial redness and lymphangitis. The source of skin infection may not be obvious and should be searched for (e.g. on the sole or between the toes). The organism is usually staphylococcus or streptococcus. Mild cases will respond to an oral penicillinase-resistant penicillin; severe cases need intravenous antibiotics.

STREPTOCOCCAL NECROTIZING MYOSITIS Group A β-haemolytic streptococci (the same organisms which are responsible for the common 'sore throat') occasionally invade muscles and cause an acute myositis which, in its early stages, may be mistaken for cellulitis or osteomyelitis. Although the condition is rare, it should be kept well to the foreground in the differential diagnosis because it may rapidly spiral out of control towards muscle necrosis, septicaemia and death. Intense pain and board-like swelling of the limb in a patient with fever and a general feeling of illness are warning signs of a medical emergency. MRI will reveal muscle swelling and possibly signs of tissue breakdown. Immediate treatment with intravenous antibiotics is essential. Surgical debridement of necrotic tissue – and sometimes even amputation – may be needed to save a life.

ACUTE SUPPURATIVE ARTHRITIS Tenderness is diffuse, and all movement at the joint is abolished by muscle spasm. In infants the distinction between osteomyelitis and septic arthritis is somewhat theoretical, as both usually coexist. A progressive rise in C-reactive protein values over 24–48 hours is suggestive of concurrent septic arthritis (Unkila-Kallis *et al.*, 1994).

ACUTE RHEUMATISM The pain is less severe and it tends to flit from one joint to another, and there may be carditis, rheumatic nodules or erythema marginatum.

SICKLE-CELL CRISIS The patient may present with features indistinguishable from those of acute osteomyelitis. In areas where *Salmonella* is endemic it would be wise to treat such patients with suitable antibiotics until infection is definitely excluded.

GAUCHER'S DISEASE Pseudo-osteitis may occur with features closely resembling those of osteomyelitis. The diagnosis is made by finding other stigmata of the disease, especially enlargement of the spleen and liver.

Treatment

If osteomyelitis is suspected on clinical grounds, blood and fluid samples should be taken and then treatment started immediately without waiting for final confirmation of the diagnosis.

There are four important aspects to the management of the patient: (1) supportive treatment for pain and dehydration; (2) splintage of the affected part; (3) antibiotic therapy; and (4) surgical drainage.

GENERAL SUPPORTIVE TREATMENT The distressed child needs to be comforted and treated for pain. Analgesics should be given at repeated intervals without waiting for the patient to ask for them. Septicaemia and fever can cause severe dehydration and it may be necessary to give fluid intravenously.

SPLINTAGE Some type of splintage is desirable, partly for comfort but also to prevent joint contractures. Simple skin traction may suffice and, if the hip is involved, this also helps to prevent dislocation. At other sites a plaster slab or half-cylinder may be used but it should not obscure the affected area.

ANTIBIOTICS Blood and aspiration material are sent immediately for examination and culture, but the prompt administration of antibiotics is so vital that treatment should not await the result. Initially the choice of antibiotics is based on the findings from direct examination of the pus smear and a 'best guess' at the most likely pathogen; a more appropriate drug can be substituted, if necessary, once the organism is identified and its antibiotic sensitivity is known. Factors such as the patient's age, general state of resistance, renal function, degree of toxaemia and previous history of allergy must be taken into account. The following recommendations are offered as a guide rather than a specific policy.

Older children and previously fit adults, who probably have a staphylococcal infection, are started on intravenous flucloxacillin and fusidic acid, which are administered continuously until the condition begins to improve and the C-reactive protein values return to normal levels – usually after 1 or 2 weeks. Thereafter, antibiotics are given orally for another 3–6 weeks; during that period it is wise to track the serum antibiotic levels in order to ensure that the minimal inhibitory concentration is maintained. Fusidic acid is preferred to benzylpenicillin (a) because of the increasing prevalence of penicillin-resistant staphylococci and (b) because it is well concentrated in bone. However, for a streptococcal infection benzylpenicillin is probably better.

In children under 4 years (who have a high incidence of haemophilus infection) and in any case in which *Gram-negative organisms* are seen in the smear, it is advisable to start with one of the cephalosporins (cefuroxime or cefotaxime). This is effective against both staphylococci and Gram-negative bacteria; it can be given intravenously or orally and reaches high concentrations in bone. A good alternative is the combination of amoxycillin and clavulanic acid (co-amoxiclav, a β-lactamase inhibitor).

Patients with sickle-cell disease are prone to bone infection and in most cases this is due to salmonellae and/or other Gram negative organisms (Ebong, 1986). The recommended treatment is with chloramphenicol or co-trimoxazole or combined amoxycillin and clavulanic acid.

Heroin addicts and immunocompromised patients often have unusual infections (e.g. pseudomonas, proteus or bacteroides). When the background is known, it is wise to start with one of the newer cephalosporins or with gentamicin and flucloxacillin.

DRAINAGE If antibiotics are given early, drainage is often unnecessary. However, if the clinical features do not improve within 36 hours of starting treatment, or even before that if there are signs of deep pus (swelling, oedema, fluctuation), and most certainly if pus is aspirated, the abscess should be drained by open operation under general anaesthesia. If pus is found – and released – there is little to be gained by drilling into the medullary cavity. If there is no obvious abscess, it is reasonable to drill a few holes into the bone in various directions. There is no evidence that widespread drilling has any advantage and it may do more harm than good; if there is an extensive intramedullary abscess, drainage can be better achieved by cutting a small window in the cortex. The wound is closed without a drain and the splint (or traction) is reapplied. At present about one-third of patients with confirmed osteomyelitis are likely to need an operation; adults with vertebral infection seldom do.

Once the signs of infection subside, movements are encouraged and the child is allowed to walk with the aid of crutches. Full weightbearing is usually possible after 3–4 weeks.

Complications

A lethal outcome from septicaemia is nowadays extremely rare; with antibiotics the child nearly always recovers and the bone may return to normal.

But morbidity is common, especially if treatment is delayed or the organism is insensitive to the chosen antibiotic.

METASTATIC INFECTION This is sometimes seen – generally in infants – and may involve other bones, joints, serous cavities, the brain or lung. In some cases the infection may be multifocal from the outset. It is easy to miss secondary sites of infection when attention is focused on one particular area; it is important to be alert to this complication and to examine the child all over and repeatedly.

SUPPURATIVE ARTHRITIS This may occur: (1) in very young children, in whom the growth disc is not an impenetrable barrier; (2) where the metaphysis is intracapsular, as in the upper femur; or (3) from metastatic infection. In infants it is so common as almost to be taken for granted, especially with osteomyelitis of the femoral neck. Ultrasound will help to demonstrate an effusion, but the definitive diagnosis is given by joint aspiration.

ALTERED BONE GROWTH In infants, physeal damage may lead to arrest of growth and shortening of the bone. In older children, however, the bone occasionally grows too long because metaphyseal hyperaemia has stimulated the growth disc.

CHRONIC OSTEOMYELITIS Despite improved methods of diagnosis and treatment, acute osteomyelitis sometimes fails to resolve and the patient is left with a chronic infection and a draining sinus. This may be due to neglect but is also seen in debilitated patients and in those with compromised defence mechanisms.

SUBACUTE HAEMATOGENOUS OSTEOMYELITIS

This condition is no longer rare, and in some countries the incidence is almost equal to that of acute osteomyelitis. Its relative mildness is presumably due to the organism being less virulent or the patient more resistant (or both). It is more variable in skeletal distribution than acute osteomyelitis, but the distal femur and the proximal and distal tibia are the favourite sites.

Pathology

Typically there is a well-defined cavity in cancellous bone, containing glairy seropurulent fluid (rarely pus). The cavity is lined by granulation tissue containing a mixture of acute and chronic inflammatory cells. The surrounding bone trabeculae are often thickened.

Clinical features

The patient is usually a child or adolescent who has had pain near one of the larger joints for several weeks or even months. He may have a limp and often there is slight swelling, muscle wasting and local tenderness. The temperature is usually normal and there is little to suggest an infection. The white cell count may be normal but the ESR is often raised.

Imaging

The typical radiographic lesion is a circumscribed, round or oval 'cavity' 1–2 cm in diameter; most often it is seen in the tibial or femoral metaphysis, but it may occur in the epiphysis or in one of the cuboidal bones (e.g. the calcaneum). Sometimes the 'cavity' is surrounded by a halo of sclerosis (the classic *Brodie's abscess*); occasionally it is less well defined, extending into the diaphysis. Metaphyseal lesions cause little or no periosteal reaction; diaphyseal lesions may be associated with periosteal new bone formation and marked cortical thickening.

The radioisotope scan shows markedly increased activity.

Diagnosis

The clinical and x-ray appearances may resemble those of an osteoid osteoma; occasionally they mimic a malignant bone tumour. The diagnosis often remains in doubt until a biopsy is performed. If fluid is encountered, it should be sent for bacteriological culture; this is positive in about half the cases and the organism is almost always *Staph. aureus*.

Treatment

Treatment may be conservative if the diagnosis is not in doubt; immobilization and antibiotics (flucloxacillin and fusidic acid) for 6 weeks usually result in healing, though this may take another 6–12 months. If the diagnosis is in doubt, an open biopsy is needed and the lesion may be curetted at the same time. Curettage is also indicated if the x-ray shows that there is no healing after conservative treatment; this is always followed by a further course of antibiotics.

GARRÉ'S SCLEROSING OSTEOMYELITIS

Garré, in 1893, described a rare form of non-suppurative osteomyelitis which is characterized by marked sclerosis and cortical thickening. There is no abscess, only a diffuse

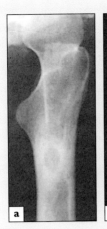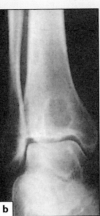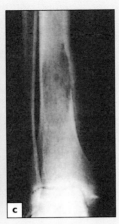

2.4 Subacute osteomyelitis (**a**, **b**) The classic Brodie's abscess looks like a small walled-off cavity in the bone with little or no periosteal reaction; (**c**) sometimes rarefaction is more diffuse and there may be cortical erosion and periosteal reaction.

enlargement of the bone at the affected site – usually the diaphysis of one of the tubular bones or the mandible. The patient is typically an adolescent or young adult with a long history of aching and slight swelling over the bone. Occasionally there are recurrent attacks of more acute pain accompanied by malaise and slight fever.

X-rays show increased bone density and cortical thickening; in some cases the marrow cavity is completely obliterated. There is no abscess cavity.

Diagnosis can be difficult. If a small segment of bone is involved, it may be mistaken for an osteoid osteoma. If there is marked periosteal layering of new bone, the lesion resembles a Ewing's sarcoma. The biopsy will disclose a low-grade inflammatory lesion with reactive bone formation. Microorganisms are seldom cultured but the condition is usually ascribed to a staphylococcal infection.

Treatment is by operation: the abnormal area is excised and the exposed surface thoroughly curetted. Bone grafts, bone transport or free bone transfer may be needed.

MULTIFOCAL NON-SUPPURATIVE OSTEOMYELITIS

This obscure disorder – it is not even certain that it is an infection – was first described in isolated cases in the 1960s and 1970s, and later in a more comprehensive report on 20 patients of mixed age and sex (Björkstén and Boquist, 1980). It is now recognized that (1) it is not as rare as initially suggested; (2) it comprises several different syndromes which have certain features in common; and (3) there is an association with chronic skin infection, especially pustular lesions of the palms and soles (palmo-plantar pustulosis) and pustular psoriasis.

In children the condition usually takes the form of multifocal (often symmetrical), recurrent lesions in the long-bone metaphyses, clavicles and anterior rib-cage; in adults the changes appear predominantly in the sterno-costo-clavicular complex and the vertebrae. In

recent years the various syndromes have been drawn together under the convenient acronym SAPHO – standing for synovitis, acne, pustulosis, hyperostosis and osteitis (Boutin and Resnick, 1998).

Early osteolytic lesions show histological features suggesting a subacute inflammatory condition; in long-standing cases there may be bone thickening and round cell infiltration. The aetiology is unknown. Despite the local and systemic signs of inflammation, there is no purulent discharge and microorganisms have seldom been isolated.

The two most characteristic clinical syndromes are described here (see also page 297 and Fig. 13.28).

SUBACUTE RECURRENT MULTIFOCAL OSTEOMYELITIS

This appears as an inflammatory bone disorder affecting mainly children and adolescents. Patients develop recurrent attacks of pain, swelling and tenderness around one or other of the long-bone metaphyses (usually the distal femur or the proximal or distal tibia), the medial ends of the clavicles or a vertebral segment. Over the course of several years multiple sites are affected, sometimes symmetrically and sometimes simultaneously; with each exacerbation the child is slightly feverish and may have a raised ESR (Carr *et al.*, 1993).

X-ray changes are characteristic. There are small lytic lesions in the metaphysis, usually closely adjacent to the physis. Some of these 'cavities' are surrounded by sclerosis, others show varying stages of healing. The clavicle may become markedly thickened. If the spine is affected, it may lead to collapse of a vertebral body. *Radioscintigraphy* shows increased activity around the lesions.

Biopsy of the lytic focus is likely to show the typical histological features of acute or subacute inflammation. In long-standing lesions there is a chronic inflammatory reaction with lymphocyte infiltration. Bacteriological cultures are almost invariably negative.

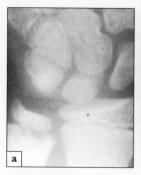
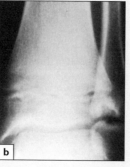

2.5 Multifocal osteomyelitis The small lesions at the junction of metaphysis and physis in (**a**) the ulna and (**b**) the fibula are typical of multifocal osteomyelitis.

Treatment is entirely palliative; antibiotics have no effect on the disease. Although the condition may run a protracted course, the prognosis is good and the lesions eventually heal without complications.

STERNO–COSTO–CLAVICULAR HYPEROSTOSIS

Patients are usually in their forties or fifties and men are affected more often than women. Clinical and radiological changes are usually confined to the sternum and adjacent bones and the vertebral column. As with recurrent multifocal osteomyelitis, there is a curious association with cutaneous pustulosis. The usual complaint is of pain, swelling and tenderness around the sternoclavicular joints; sometimes there is also a slight fever and the ESR may be elevated. Patients with vertebral column involvement may develop back pain and stiffness.

X-rays show hyperostosis of the medial ends of the clavicles, the adjacent sternum and the anterior ends of the upper ribs, as well as ossification of the sternoclavicular and costoclavicular ligaments. Vertebral changes include sclerosis of individual vertebral bodies, ossification of the anterior longitudinal ligament, anterior intervertebral bridging, end-plate erosions, disc space narrowing and vertebral collapse.

Radioscintigraphy shows increased activity around the sternoclavicular joints and affected vertebrae.

The condition usually runs a protracted course with recurrent 'flares'. There is no effective treatment but in the long-term symptoms tend to diminish or disappear; however, the patient may be left with ankylosis of the affected joints.

INFANTILE CORTICAL HYPEROSTOSIS (CAFFEY'S DISEASE)

Infantile cortical hyperostosis is a rare disease of infants and young children. It usually starts during the first few months of life with painful swelling over the tubular bones and/or the mandible. The child may be feverish and irritable, refusing to move the affected limb. Infection may be suspected but, apart from the swelling, there are no local signs of inflammation. The ESR, though, is usually elevated.

X-rays characteristically show periosteal new-bone formation resulting in thickening of the affected bone.

After a few months the local features may resolve spontaneously, only to reappear somewhere else. Flat bones, such as the scapula and cranial vault, may also be affected.

Other causes of hyperostosis (osteomyelitis, scurvy) must be excluded. The cause of Caffey's disease is unknown but a virus infection has been suggested. Antibiotics are sometimes employed; it is doubtful whether they have any effect.

POST-TRAUMATIC OSTEOMYELITIS

Open fractures are always contaminated and are therefore prone to infection. The combination of tissue injury, vascular damage, oedema, haematoma, dead

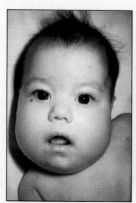
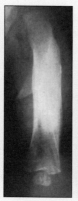
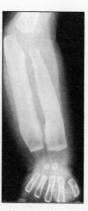

2.6 Caffey's disease This infant with Caffey's disease develped marked thickening of the mandible and long bones. The lesions gradually cleared up, leaving little or no trace of their former ominous appearance.

bone fragments and an open pathway to the atmosphere must invite bacterial invasion even if the wound is not contaminated with particulate dirt. This is the most common cause of osteomyelitis in adults.

Staph. aureus is the usual pathogen, but other organisms such as *E. coli*, *Proteus* and *Pseudomonas*. are sometimes involved. Occasionally, anaerobic organisms (*Clostridia*, anaerobic *Streptococci* or *Bacteroides*) appear in contaminated wounds.

Clinical features

The patient becomes feverish and develops pain and swelling over the fracture site; the wound is inflamed and there may be a seropurulent discharge. Blood tests reveal a leucocytosis and an increased ESR. A wound swab should be examined and cultured for organisms.

Treatment

The essence of treatment is prophylaxis: thorough cleansing and debridement of open fractures, the provision of drainage by leaving the wound open, immobilization of the fracture and antibiotics. In most cases a combination of benzylpenicillin and flucloxacillin, given 6-hourly for 48–72 hours, will suffice. Better still is a broad-spectrum cephalosporin. If the wound is clearly contaminated, it is wise also to give metronidazole for 4 or 5 days to control both aerobic and anaerobic organisms. Wound closure is delayed until the infection has settled.

Pyogenic wound infection, once it has taken root, is difficult to eradicate. The presence of necrotic soft tissue and dead bone, together with a mixed bacterial flora, conspire against effective antibiotic control. Treatment calls for regular wound dressing and repeated excision of all dead and infected tissue. Loose or ineffectual implants should be removed; stable implants are left undisturbed until the fracture has united. If the fracture is unfixed, or if it becomes unstable, an external fixator can be applied.

If these measures fail, the management is essentially that of chronic osteomyelitis.

POSTOPERATIVE OSTEOMYELITIS

Osteomyelitis can occur after any operation on bone, but especially after operating on open fractures and after procedures involving the use of foreign implants. The reported incidence of infection after orthopaedic operations on a broad cross-section of patients varies from 0.2% to over 10%. Much depends on the criteria for diagnosing 'postoperative' infection. Do the figures include superficial wound infection? And very late

infection? The true incidence is probably around 5% and the risk is considerably greater in the elderly, the obese, those with diabetes or other chronic diseases, patients with sickle-cell disease, Gaucher's disease or leukaemia, patients on corticosteroid or immunosuppressive therapy, and patients who have had multiple previous operations at the same site.

Organisms may be introduced directly into the wound from the atmosphere, the instruments, the patient or the surgeon; or indirectly by haematogenous spread from a distant focus.

The resulting infection is sometimes obvious within days, but it may not occur until months or even years later. A practical classification is suggested in the Box. Its value lies in the recognition that the different 'types' of infection call for different approaches to treatment.

Classification of postoperative infection

A. Early infection
1. Superficial
2. Deep
3. Superficial and deep

B. Late infection
1. Following early infection
2. Covert infection appearing later
3. Following a long period of normality

The organisms in postoperative osteomyelitis are usually a mixture of pathogenic bacteria (*Staph. aureus*, *Proteus*, *E. coli*, *Pseudomonas*) and others that are not normally pathogenic (e.g. *Staph. epidermidis*) but may become so in the presence of a foreign implant.

Local factors that favour bacterial invasion are: (1) soft-tissue damage; (2) haematoma formation; and (3) bone death.

Whatever the 'cause' of the infection, and whether 'early' or 'late', the *foreign implant* is both a predisposing factor and an important element in its persistence. Bacteria as well as human tissue cells have an affinity for molecules on the surface of the implant. Both compete for occupancy of the same surface – the tissue cells by adaptation and integration, the bacteria by adhesion and colonization. This contest has been aptly called 'the race for the surface' (Gristina, 1988). If the tissue cells win, the implant is incorporated as an 'inert' biomaterial. If the bacteria win, the resulting infection usually persists until the implant is removed.

Clinical features

Early postoperative infection (within 1 month) is usually fairly obvious. With a purely superficial infection the symptoms are minimal, but if the infection is deep, the patient complains of persistent pain and may have a fever. The skin over the implant is inflamed, and there may be a purulent discharge from the wound. Often there is tenderness and pain on moving the limb. The ESR and white cell count are elevated, and blood culture may be positive. Bacteriological examination of the wound discharge will help to identify the organism and establish the antibiotic sensitivity.

Initially the infection usually appears to be superficial. This is no cause for optimism, for the bone may be involved from the outset. Plain x-rays and MRI are unlikely to be helpful, as they cannot distinguish between the tissue changes due to the operation and those associated with infection.

Rarely (e.g. in patients on immunosuppressive therapy) there may be a fulminant postoperative infection with septicaemia and toxaemia.

Intermediate postoperative infection is seen between 1 month and 1 year after the operation. Often there is a history of 'wound problems' in the early postoperative period, followed by a long quiescent period during which both the surgeon and the patient may be falsely reassured while the organisms lurk in hidden corners, waiting to proliferate and spread when local conditions favour their emergence.

Late postoperative infection is much more difficult to diagnose. Several years may have elapsed since the operation, during which the patient was completely asymptomatic. Pain usually starts insidiously and may never become acute. Often there is no more than a low-grade inflammatory reaction, little different from that due to aseptic loosening of the implant; this is especially true of cemented joint prostheses. Local examination, x-ray signs of bone resorption and increased activity on radionuclide scanning may equally fail to distinguish between aseptic loosening and infection. However, if there is marked periosteal new bone formation and cortical destruction, with increased scintigraphic activity in both the perfusion phase and the bone phase, the likelihood of infection is greatly increased. The MRI may show a localized area of high signal activity due to pus.

Blood investigations are sometimes helpful. The ESR is always elevated after joint replacement but it should return to normal by 6 months.

Confirmation of the diagnosis is obtained by aspirating purulent material from the area, or by culturing the organism in washings taken after attempted aspiration.

Prevention

'Prevention is better than cure.' This adage applies with particular force to postoperative infection. The risk of implant-mediated infection can be reduced by: (1) avoiding operations on immune-depressed patients;

(2) eliminating any focus of infection before operating; (3) insisting on optimal operative sterility; (4) giving prophylactic antibiotics; (5) handling tissues gently; (6) using high-quality implant materials; (7) ensuring close fit and secure fixation of the implant; and (8) preventing or counteracting later intercurrent infection.

ANTIBIOTICS AND CLEAN AIR The introduction by Charnley of the ultra-clean air operating enclosure and special operating suits with body exhausts brought a substantial reduction in his incidence of wound infection (especially 'early' infection) after hip replacement. Significant reductions have also been achieved with prophylactic antibiotics (e.g. one of the cephalosporins, given intravenously shortly before and then 8-hourly for two further doses after operation). Wearing impervious operative clothing also is of value. Using all methods combined, the sepsis rate for total hip replacement can be reduced to below 0.2% (Lidwell, 1986).

Treatment

OPERATIONS WITHOUT IMPLANTS Postoperative infection in these cases is similar to post-traumatic infection – with the advantage of less tissue damage. Treatment follows the same lines.

INFECTION AFTER INTERNAL FIXATION OF FRACTURES Appropriate antibiotics, given intravenously and in large doses, are the first line of defence. If there is an abscess, it should be drained and the wound left open until it is clean. These measures alone may suffice. If they fail, excision of infected and necrotic material followed by intermittent antibiotic irrigation and suction drainage may yet control the infection and prevent it from becoming an intractable chronic osteomyelitis. If at all possible the fixation device should be retained until the fracture has united; even worse than a septic fracture is a septic unstable fracture! If the implant has to be removed in order to achieve adequate debridement, the fracture should be held securely with an external fixator.

INFECTION FOLLOWING JOINT REPLACEMENT *Early postoperative infection* is treated as above, by antibiotics and local drainage with excision of dead and avascular tissue. However, even if the wound heals, there remains the risk of recurrent late infection.

The variability of presentation of *late infection* calls for a flexible strategy. As a general rule, unless there is pus which needs drainage, it is the stability of the prosthesis rather than the presence of bacteria that dictates treatment. If the prosthesis is secure and the patient not in pain, there is no absolute indication for operation.

If the prosthesis is loose, or painful, or if there is a copiously draining sinus, the choice of treatment is determined by the patient's general condition. Those who are unfit for the very extensive operation that will be necessary are better treated with long-term antibiotics and restriction of activities. Those who are fit can be offered a 'revision arthroplasty' – i.e. meticulous removal of the infected prosthesis, acrylic cement and infected bone, followed by the insertion of a new prosthesis. If a frank abscess is encountered, the revision is done in two stages, with a period of 4–6 weeks of intermittent irrigation and suction of the entire infected field between removal of the old and insertion of the new implant. If there is no abscess, a one-stage revision is carried out, using either antibiotic-impregnated acrylic cement or no cement at all.

The alternative (especially with infected hip replacements) is simply to remove the implant and acrylic cement, leaving an unstable joint. The infection may heal but function is not very satisfactory.

CHRONIC OSTEOMYELITIS

This used to be the dreaded sequel to acute haematogenous osteomyelitis; nowadays it more frequently follows an open fracture or operation.

The usual organisms (and with time there is always a mixed infection) are *Staph. aureus, E. coli, S. pyogenes, Proteus* and *Pseudomonas*; in the presence of foreign implants *Staph. epidermidis*, which is normally non-pathogenic, is the commonest of all.

Pathology

Bone is destroyed or devitalized in a discrete area at the focus of infection or more diffusely along the surface of a foreign implant. Cavities containing pus and pieces of dead bone (sequestra) are surrounded by

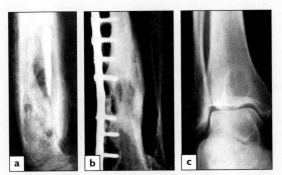

2.7 Chronic osteomyelitis Chronic bone infection, with a persistent sequestrum, may be a sequel to acute osteomyelitis (**a**). More often it follows an open fracture or operation (**b**). Occasionally it presents as a Brodie's abscess (**c**).

vascular tissue, and beyond that by areas of sclerosis – the result of chronic reactive new bone formation. The sequestra act as substrates for bacterial adhesion in much the same way as foreign implants, ensuring the persistence of infection until they are removed or discharged through draining sinuses. Sinuses may seal off for weeks or even months, giving the appearance of healing, only to reopen (or appear somewhere else) when the tissue tension rises. Bone destruction, and the increasingly brittle sclerosis, may occasionally result in a pathological fracture. The histological picture is one of chronic inflammatory cell infiltration around areas of acellular bone or microscopic sequestra.

Clinical features

The patient presents because pain, pyrexia, redness and tenderness have recurred (a 'flare'), or with a discharging sinus. In long-standing cases the tissues are thickened and often puckered or folded in where a scar or sinus is attached to the underlying bone. There may be a sero-purulent discharge and excoriation of the surrounding skin. In post-traumatic osteomyelitis the bone may be deformed or non-united.

Imaging

X-ray examination will usually show bone resorption – either as a patchy loss of density or as frank excavation around an implant – with thickening and sclerosis of the surrounding bone. However, there are marked variations: there may be no more than localized loss of trabeculation, or an area of osteoporosis, or periosteal thickening; sequestra show up as unnaturally dense fragments, in contrast to the surrounding vascularized bone; sometimes the bone is crudely thickened and misshapen, resembling a bone tumour. A *sinogram* may help to localize the site.

Radioisotope scintigraphy is sensitive but not specific. ^{99m}Tc-HDP scans show increased activity in both the perfusion phase and the bone phase. Scanning with ^{67}Ga-citrate or ^{111}In-labelled leucocytes is said to be more specific for osteomyelitis; such scans are useful for showing up hidden foci of infection.

CT and MRI are invaluable in planning operative treatment: together they will show the extent of bone destruction and reactive oedema, hidden abscesses and sequestra.

Investigations

During acute flares the ESR and blood white cell count may be increased; these non-specific signs are helpful in assessing the progress of bone infection but they are not diagnostic.

Antistaphylococcal antibody titres may be elevated – a valuable sign in the diagnosis of hidden infections and in tracking progress to recovery.

Organisms cultured from discharging sinuses should be tested repeatedly for antibiotic sensitivity; with time, they often change their characteristics and become resistant to treatment.

Treatment

ANTIBIOTICS Chronic infection is seldom eradicated by antibiotics alone. Yet bactericidal drugs are important (a) to stop the spread of infection to healthy bone and (b) to control acute flares. The choice of antibiotic depends on bacteriological studies, but the drug must be capable of penetrating sclerotic bone and should be non-toxic with long-term use. Fusidic acid, clindamycin and the cephalosporins are good examples.

LOCAL TREATMENT A sinus may be painless and need dressing simply to protect the clothing. Colostomy paste can be used to stop excoriation of the skin. An acute abscess may need urgent incision and drainage, but this is only a temporary measure.

OPERATION A waiting policy, punctuated by spells of bed rest and antibiotics to control flares, may have to be patiently endured until there is a clear indication for radical surgery, i.e. significant symptoms, combined with the clear evidence of a sequestrum or dead bone.

Under antibiotic cover all infected soft tissue and all dead or devitalized bone must be excised; dead material can be identified by the preoperative injection of sulphan blue which stains all living tissues green, leaving dead material unstained; the patient and his or her visitors should be warned that the skin will (temporarily) look green. Double-lumen tubes are laid in the resulting cavity and the tissues are closed with the tubes emerging through separate stab wounds. An appropriate antibiotic solution is instilled 4-hourly and cleared shortly before the next instillation by low-pressure suction. (This is more tidy than continuous irrigation, which normally fails after a few days due to leakage from the wound.) Cavity injection and drainage should be continued until the effluent is sterile (usually 3–6 weeks); the tubes are then gradually withdrawn as the cavity diminishes in size. The method needs meticulous care and supervision.

As an alternative, porous gentamicin-impregnated beads may be used to 'sterilize' the cavity. This is easier, but less successful; moreover, if the beads are not taken out by 2–3 weeks they are extremely difficult to remove.

Another way of preventing recurrent infection and encouraging healing is to fill completely the dead space left after excision of necrotic tissue with living – or potentially living – material. The best-tried methods are the *Papineau technique* and muscle flap transfer. With the Papineau technique the cavity is packed with small cancellous bone grafts (preferably autogenous) mixed with an antibiotic and a fibrin sealant. Where possible, the area is covered by adjacent muscle and the skin wound is sutured without tension. With *muscle flap transfer*, in suitable sites a large wad of muscle, with its blood supply intact, can be mobilized and laid into the cavity; the surface is later covered with a split-skin graft. In areas with too little adjacent muscle (e.g. the distal part of the leg), the same thing can be achieved by transferring a myocutaneous island flap on a long vascular pedicle.

In refractory cases it may be possible to excise the infected and/or devitalized segment of bone and then close the gap by the *Ilizarov method* of 'transporting' a viable segment from the remaining diaphysis. This is especially useful if infection is associated with an ununited fracture (see page 263).

AFTERCARE Success is difficult to measure; a minute focus of infection might escape the therapeutic onslaught, only to flare into full-blown osteomyelitis many years later. Prognosis should always be guarded; local trauma must be avoided and any recurrence of symptoms, however slight, should be taken seriously and investigated. The watchword is 'cautious optimism' – a 'probable cure' is better than no cure at all.

2.8 Chronic osteomyelitis – treatment The surest way of delivering antibiotics to the site of infection is by one or more double-lumen tubes. A narrow catheter is threaded (like an intravenous line) into the wider suction tube; antibiotic solution is run in through the catheter and sucked out through the drainage tube. (Courtesy of Mr C. Lautenbach, Johannesburg General Hospital.)

ACUTE SUPPURATIVE ARTHRITIS

A joint can become infected (1) by direct invasion through a penetrating wound, intra-articular injection or arthroscopy; (2) by direct spread from an adjacent bone abscess; or (3) by blood spread from a distant site. In infants it is often difficult to tell whether the infection started in the bone and spread to the joint or vice versa. In practice it hardly matters and in advanced cases it should be assumed that the entire joint and the adjacent bone ends are involved.

The causal organism is usually *Staph. aureus*; however, in infants *Haemophilus influenzae* is an important pathogen. Occasionally other organisms, such as *Streptococcus, E. coli* and *Proteus*, are encountered.

Predisposing conditions are rheumatoid arthritis, chronic debilitating disorders, intravenous drug abuse, immunosuppressive drug therapy and acquired immunodeficiency syndrome (AIDS).

Pathology

The usual trigger is a haematogenous infection which settles in the synovial membrane; there is an acute inflammatory reaction with a serous or seropurulent exudate and an increase in synovial fluid. As pus appears in the joint, articular cartilage is eroded and destroyed, partly by bacterial enzymes and partly by enzymes released from synovium, inflammatory cells and pus. In infants the entire epiphysis, which is still largely cartilaginous, may be severely damaged; in older children, vascular occlusion may lead to necrosis of the epiphyseal bone. In adults the effects are usually confined to the articular cartilage, but in late cases there may be extensive erosion due to synovial proliferation and ingrowth.

If the infection goes untreated, it will spread to the underlying bone or burst out of the joint to form abscesses and sinuses.

With healing there may be: (1) complete resolution and a return to normal; (2) partial loss of articular cartilage and fibrosis of the joint; (3) loss of articular cartilage and bony ankylosis; or (4) bone destruction and permanent deformity of the joint.

Clinical features

The clinical features differ somewhat according to the age of the patient.

In newborn infants the emphasis is on septicaemia rather than joint pain. The baby is irritable and refuses to feed; there is a rapid pulse and sometimes a fever. Infection is usually suspected, but it could be anywhere! The joints should be carefully felt and moved to elicit the local signs of warmth, tenderness and resistance to movement. The umbilical cord should be examined for a source of infection. An inflamed intravenous infusion site should always excite suspicion.

In children the usual features are acute pain in a single large joint (commonly the hip) and reluctance to move the limb ('pseudoparesis'). The child is ill, with a rapid pulse and a swinging fever. The overlying skin looks red and in a superficial joint swelling may be obvious. There is local warmth and marked tenderness. All movements are restricted, and often completely abolished, by pain and spasm. It is essential to look for a source of infection – a septic toe, a boil or a discharge from the ear.

In adults it is often a superficial joint (knee, wrist or ankle) that is painful, swollen and inflamed. There is warmth and marked local tenderness, and movements are restricted. The patient should be questioned and examined for evidence of gonococcal infection or drug abuse. Patients with rheumatoid arthritis, and especially those on corticosteroid treatment, may develop a 'silent' joint infection. Suspicion may be aroused by an unexplained deterioration in the patient's general condition; every joint should be carefully examined.

Imaging

Early on the *x-ray* is usually normal but *ultrasound* shows a joint effusion. In children the joint 'space' may

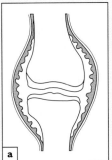 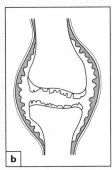 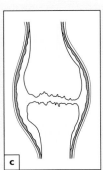 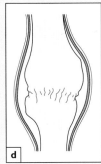

2.9 Acute suppurative arthritis In the early stage **(a)** there is an acute synovitis with a purulent joint effusion. **(b)** Soon the articular cartilage is attacked by bacterial and cellular enzymes. If the infection is not arrested, the cartilage may be completely destroyed **(c)**; healing then leads to bony ankylosis **(d)**.

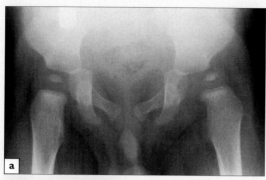

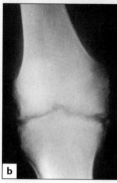

2.10 Suppurative arthritis (a)
In a child: the left hip is subluxated and the soft tissues are swollen. **(b)** *In an adult*: marked erosion of the articular surfaces of the knee.

injury does not exclude infection. Diagnosis may remain in doubt until the joint is aspirated.

IRRITABLE JOINT At the onset the joint is painful and lacks some movement. But the child is not really ill and there are no signs of infection.

HAEMOPHILIC BLEED An acute haemarthrosis closely resembles septic arthritis. The history is usually conclusive, but aspiration will resolve any doubt.

RHEUMATIC FEVER Typically the pain flits from joint to joint, but at the onset one joint may be misleadingly inflamed. However, there are no signs of septicaemia.

GOUT AND PSEUDOGOUT In adults, acute crystal-induced synovitis may closely resemble infection. On aspiration the joint fluid is often turbid, with a high white cell count; however, microscopic examination by polarized light will show the characteristic crystals.

GAUCHER'S DISEASE In this rare condition acute joint pain and fever can occur without any organism being found ('pseudo-osteitis'). Because of the predisposition to true infection, antibiotics should be given.

seem to be widened (because of fluid in the joint) and there may be slight subluxation of the joint. With *E. coli* infections there is sometimes gas in the joint. Narrowing or irregularity of the joint space are late features.

Investigations

The white cell count and ESR are raised and blood culture may be positive. However, special investigations take time and it is much quicker (and usually more reliable) to aspirate the joint and examine the fluid. It may be frankly purulent – but beware! – in early cases the fluid may look clear. A white cell count and Gram stain should be carried out immediately: the normal synovial fluid leucocyte count is under 300 per ml; it may be over 10,000 per ml in non-infective inflammatory disorders, but counts of over 50,000 per ml are highly suggestive of sepsis. Gram-positive cocci are probably *Staph. aureus*; Gram-negative cocci are either *H. influenzae* (in children) or *Gonococcus* (in adults). Samples of fluid are also sent for full bacteriological examination and tests for antibiotic sensitivity.

Differential diagnosis

ACUTE OSTEOMYLEITIS In young children, osteomyelitis may be indistinguishable from septic arthritis; often one must assume that both are present.

TRAUMA Traumatic synovitis or haemarthrosis may be associated with acute pain and swelling. A history of

Treatment

The first priority is to aspirate the joint and examine the fluid. Treatment is then started without further delay and follows the same lines as for acute osteomyelitis. Once the blood and tissue samples have been obtained, there is no need to wait for detailed results before giving antibiotics.

GENERAL SUPPORTIVE CARE Analgesics are given for pain and intravenous fluids for dehydration.

SPLINTAGE The joint must be rested either on a splint or in a widely split plaster. With hip infection, the joint should be held abducted and 30 degrees flexed, on traction to prevent dislocation.

ANTIBIOTICS The initial choice of antibiotics is based on judgement of the most likely pathogens; a more appropriate drug can be substituted after full bacteriological investigation.
   Older children and adults are given flucloxacillin and fusidic acid, intravenously for 2–7 days and then orally for another 3 weeks.
   Children under 4 years, in whom there is a high incidence of haemophilus infection, should be treated with ampicillin or one of the newer cephalosporins from the outset.

DRAINAGE Under anaesthesia the joint is opened through a small incision, drained and washed out with physiological saline. A small catheter is left in place and the wound is closed; suction-irrigation is continued for another 2 or 3 days. This is the safest policy and is certainly advisable (1) in very young infants, (2) when the hip is involved and (3) if the aspirated pus is very thick. For the knee, arthroscopic debridement and copious irrigation may be equally effective. Older children with early septic arthritis (symptoms for less than 3 days) involving any joint except the hip can often be treated successfully by repeated closed aspiration of the joint; however, if there is no improvement within 48 hours, open drainage will be necessary.

AFTERCARE Once the patient's general condition is satisfactory and the joint is no longer painful or warm, further damage is unlikely. If articular cartilage has been preserved, gentle and gradually increasing active movements are encouraged. If articular cartilage has been destroyed the aim is to keep the joint immobile while ankylosis is awaited. Splintage in the optimum position is therefore continuously maintained, usually by plaster, until ankylosis is sound.

Complications

BONE DESTRUCTION and, at the hips, dislocation of the joint are serious threats if infection is not rapidly controlled. The x-ray sometimes gives a misleadingly pessimistic picture: the femoral head may seem to have disappeared, but as the condition resolves and the bone recalcifies the true state of affairs becomes apparent.

CARTILAGE DESTRUCTION may lead to either fibrous or bony ankylosis. In adults, partial destruction of the joint will result in secondary osteoarthritis.

GROWTH DISTURBANCE may occur, presenting either as a localized deformity or as shortening of the bone.

GONOCOCCAL ARTHRITIS

Neisseria gonorrhoea is the commonest cause of septic arthritis in adults. The condition should always be suspected in the older age group and patients should be examined for other signs of genito-urinary infection (e.g. a urethral discharge). Joint aspiration may reveal the typical Gram-negative organisms, but bacteriological investigations are often disappointing.

Treatment is similar to that of pyogenic arthritis. Patients will usually respond fairly quickly to cephalosporin given intravenously or intramuscularly. If the organism is sensitive to penicillin (and the patient is not allergic!), treatment with ampicillin or amoxycillin and clavulanic acid is equally effective.

SEPTIC ARTHRITIS AND HIV-1 INFECTION

Septic arthritis has been encountered quite frequently in HIV-positive intravenous drug users, HIV-positive haemophiliacs and other patients with AIDS. The usual organisms are *Staph. aureus* and *Streptococcus*; however, opportunistic infection by unusual organisms is not uncommon.

The patient may present with an acutely painful, inflamed joint and marked systemic features of bacteraemia or septicaemia. In some cases the infection is confined to a single, unusual site such as the sacroiliac joint; in others several joints may be affected simultaneously. Opportunistic infection by unusual organisms may produce a more indolent clinical picture.

Treatment follows the general principles outlined before. Patients with staphylococcal and streptococcal infections usually respond well to antibiotic treatment and joint drainage; opportunistic infections may be more difficult to control.

SPIROCHAETAL INFECTION

Although rarely seen in many countries, spirochaetal bone infection is still quite common in some parts of the world.

EARLY CONGENITAL SYPHILIS

Treponema pallidum can cross the placental barrier and infect the fetus during the latter half of pregnancy. However, bone changes do not usually appear until several weeks after birth (Rasool and Govender, 1989).

The infant is sick and irritable. The commonest clinical features are hepatosplenomegaly. Serological tests are usually positive in both mother and child.

The first signs of skeletal involvement may be joint swelling and 'pseudoparalysis' – the child refuses to move a painful limb. Several sites may be involved, often symmetrically, with slight swelling and tenderness at the ends or along the shafts of the tubular bones.

X-rays The characteristic changes are of two kinds: (1) 'periostitis' – diffuse periosteal new-bone formation along the diaphysis, usually of mild degree but sometimes producing an 'onion-peel' effect; and (2) 'metaphysitis' – trabecular erosion in the juxtaepiphyseal region, showing first as a lucent band near the physis and later as frank bone destruction.

Diagnosis The condition must be distinguished from scurvy (rare in the first 6 months of life), multifocal osteomyelitis, the battered baby syndrome and Caffey's disease (see page 34).

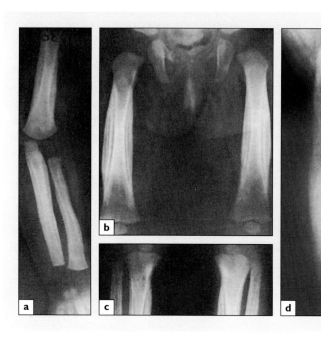

2.11 Syphilis (a, b, c) Congenital syphilis, with diffuse periostitis of many bones. (d) Acquired syphilitic periostitis of the tibia.

LATE CONGENITAL AND ACQUIRED SYPHILIS

Bone lesions in older children and adults are usually manifestations of tertiary disease, the result of gumma formation and endarteritis. Gummata appear either as discrete, punched-out radiolucent areas in the medulla or as more extensive destructive lesions in the cortex. The surrounding bone is thick and sclerotic. Sometimes the dense endosteal and periosteal new-bone formation is the predominant feature, affecting almost the entire bone (the classic 'sabre tibia').

TREATMENT Antibiotics are ineffectual in tertiary syphilis. An operation is occasionally needed if the gumma breaks down or if there is a pathological fracture.

YAWS

Yaws is a non-venereal spirochaetal infection caused by *Treponema pertenue*. It is seen mainly in the tropics, and usually in children, presenting with features resembling those of syphilis. The characteristic bone changes are periosteal new-bone formation and cortical rarefaction or destruction. Sclerosis is less marked than in syphilis. Active infection is treated with penicillin.

TUBERCULOSIS

Once common throughout the world, tuberculosis showed a steady decline in its prevalence in developed countries during the 1960s and 1970s, no doubt due to the effectiveness of public health programmes and advances in chemotherapy. In the past two decades, however, the annual incidence (particularly of extra-pulmonary tuberculosis) has risen again, a phenomenon which has been attributed variously to changes in population movements, the spread of intravenous drug abuse and the emergence of AIDS.

The skeletal manifestations of the disease are seen chiefly in the large joints and the spine, but the infection may appear in any bone. Predisposing conditions include chronic debilitating disorders, drug abuse, prolonged corticosteroid medication, AIDS and other disorders resulting in reduced defence mechanisms.

Pathology

Mycobacterium tuberculosis (usually human, sometimes bovine) enters the body via the lung (droplet infection) or the gut (swallowing infected milk products) or, rarely, through the skin. In contrast to pyogenic infection, it causes a granulomatous reaction which is associated with tissue necrosis and caseation.

PRIMARY COMPLEX The initial lesion in lung, pharynx or gut is a small one with lymphatic spread to regional lymph nodes; this combination is the primary complex. Usually the bacilli are fixed in the nodes and no clinical illness results, but occasionally the response is excessive, with enlargement of glands in the neck or abdomen.

Even though there is usually no clinical illness, the initial infection has two important sequels: (1) within nodes which are apparently healed or even calcified, bacilli may survive for many years, so that a reservoir exists; (2) the body has been sensitized to the toxin (a positive Heaf test being an index of sensitization) and,

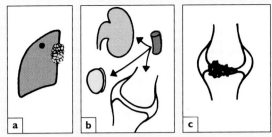

2.12 The tuberculous process The primary infection is usually arrested in the local lymph glands (**a**); secondary spread is by the blood stream (**b**); the term 'tertiary' can be used for the local destructive lesion (**c**).

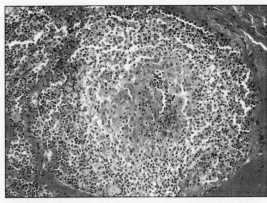

2.13 Tuberculosis – histology A typical tuberculous granuloma, with central necrosis and scattered giant cells surrounded by lymphocytes and histiocytes.

should reinfection occur, the response is quite different, the lesion being a destructive one which spreads by contiguity.

SECONDARY SPREAD If resistance to the original infection is low, widespread dissemination via the blood stream may occur, giving rise to miliary tuberculosis or meningitis. More often, blood spread occurs months or years later and bacilli are deposited in extrapulmonary tissues. Some of these foci develop into destructive lesions to which the term 'tertiary' may be applied.

TERTIARY LESION Bones or joints are affected in about 5% of patients with tuberculosis. There is a predilection for the vertebral bodies and the large synovial joints. Multiple lesions occur in about one-third of patients. In established cases it is difficult to tell whether the infection started in the joint and then spread to the adjacent bone or vice versa; synovial membrane and subchondral bone have a common blood supply and they may, of course, be infected simultaneously.

Once the bacilli have gained a foothold, they elicit a chronic inflammatory reaction. The characteristic microscopic lesion is the tuberculous granuloma – a collection of epithelioid and multinucleated giant cells surrounding an area of necrosis, with round cells (mainly lymphocytes) around the periphery.

Within the affected area, small patches of caseous necrosis appear. These may coalesce into a larger yellowish mass, or the centre may break down to form an abscess containing pus and fragments of necrotic bone.

Bone lesions tend to spread quite rapidly. Epiphyseal cartilage is no barrier to invasion and soon the infection reaches the joint. Only in the vertebral bodies, and more rarely in the greater trochanter of the femur or the small bones of the hands or feet, does the infection persist as a pure chronic osteomyelitis.

If the synovium is involved, it becomes thick and oedematous, giving rise to a marked effusion. A pannus of granulation tissue may extend across the joint and articular cartilage is slowly destroyed, though the rapid and complete destruction elicited by pyogenic organisms does not occur in the absence of secondary infection. At the edges of the joint, along the synovial reflections, there may be active bone erosion. In addition, the increased vascularity causes local osteoporosis.

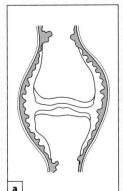
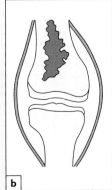
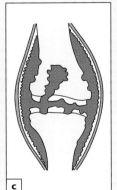
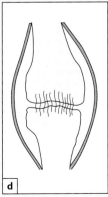

2.14 Tuberculous arthritis The disease may begin as synovitis (**a**) or osteomyelitis (**b**), both of which can resolve. From either it may extend to become a true arthritis (**c**); not all the cartilage is destroyed, and healing is usually by fibrous ankylosis (**d**).

If unchecked, caseation and infection extend into the surrounding soft tissues to produce a 'cold' abscess ('cold' only in comparison to a pyogenic abscess). This may burst through the skin, forming a sinus, or it may track along the tissue planes to point at some distant site. Secondary infection by pyogenic organisms is common. If the disease is arrested at an early stage, healing may be by resolution to apparent normality. If articular cartilage has been damaged, healing is by fibrosis and incomplete ankylosis, with progressive joint deformity. Within the fibrocaseous mass, mycobacteria may remain imprisoned, retaining the potential to flare up into active disease many years later.

Clinical features

There may be a history of previous infection or recent contact with tuberculosis. The patient, usually a child or young adult, complains of pain and (in a superficial joint) swelling. In advanced cases there may be attacks of fever or lassitude and loss of weight. Relatives tell of 'night cries': the joint, splinted by muscle spasm during the day, relaxes with sleep and the damaged tissues are stretched or compressed, causing sudden episodes of intense pain. Muscle wasting is characteristic and synovial thickening is often striking. Movements are limited in all directions. As articular erosion progresses the joint becomes stiff and deformed.

In tuberculosis of the spine, pain may be deceptively slight – often no more than an ache when the spine is jarred. Consequently the patient may not present until there is a visible abscess (usually in the groin or the lumbar region to one side of the midline) or until collapse causes a localized kyphosis. Occasionally the presenting feature is weakness or loss of sensibility in the lower limbs.

Multiple foci of infection are sometimes found, with bone and joint lesions at different stages of development. This is more likely in people with lowered resistance.

X-ray

Soft-tissue swelling and periarticular osteoporosis are characteristic. The bone ends take on a 'washed-out' appearance and the articular space is narrowed. In children the epiphyses may be enlarged, probably the result of long-continued hyperaemia. Later on there is erosion of the subarticular bone; characteristically this is seen on *both sides of the joint*, indicating an inflammatory process starting in the synovium. Cystic lesions may appear in the adjacent bone ends but there is little or no periosteal reaction. In the spine the characteristic appearance is one of bone erosion and collapse around an intervertebral disc space; the soft-tissue shadows may define a paravertebral abscess.

Investigations

The ESR is increased and there may be a relative lymphocytosis. The Mantoux or Heaf test will be positive: these are sensitive but not specific tests; i.e. a negative Mantoux virtually excludes the diagnosis, but a positive test merely indicates tuberculous infection, now or at some time in the past.

If synovial fluid is aspirated, it may be cloudy, the protein concentration is increased and the white cell count is elevated.

Acid-fast bacilli are identified in synovial fluid in 10–20% of cases, and cultures are positive in over half. A synovial biopsy is more reliable; sections will show the characteristic histological features, and acid-fast bacilli may be identified; cultures are positive in over 80% of cases.

Diagnosis

Except in areas where tuberculosis is common, diagnosis is often delayed simply because the disease is not suspected. Features that should trigger more active investigation are:

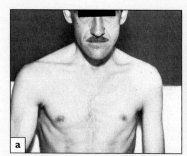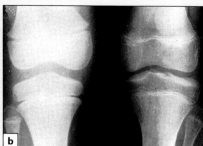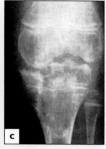

22.15 Tuberculosis A characteristic feature of tuberculosis is wasting of muscle (**a**). The knees in (**b**) show osteoporosis on the left, due to synovitis. This often resolves with treatment but, if cartilage and bone are destroyed (**c**), healing is by fibrosis.

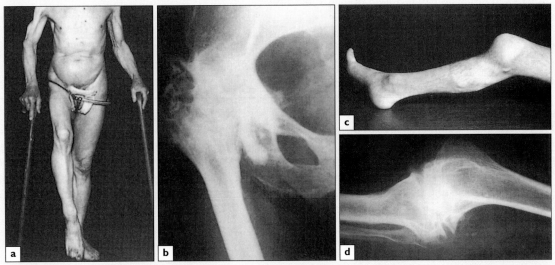

2.16 The aftermath of tuberculous arthritis Joint destruction and deformity: flexion and adduction at the hip (**a, b**); flexion, lateral rotation and backward subluxation at the knee (**c, d**).

- A long history
- Involvement of only one joint
- Marked synovial thickening
- Marked muscle wasting
- Periarticular osteoporosis
- A positive Mantoux test

Synovial biopsy for histological examination and culture is often necessary.

Joint tuberculosis must be differentiated from the following.

TRANSIENT SYNOVITIS This is fairly common in children. At first it seems no different from any other low-grade inflammatory arthritis; however, it always settles down after a few weeks' rest in bed. If the synovitis recurs, further investigation (even a biopsy) may be necessary.

MONARTICULAR RHEUMATOID ARTHRITIS Occasionally rheumatoid arthritis starts in a single large joint. This is clinically indistinguishable from tuberculosis and the diagnosis may have to await the results of synovial biopsy.

SUBACUTE ARTHRITIS Diseases such as amoebic dysentery or brucellosis are sometimes complicated by arthritis. The history, clinical features and pathological investigations usually enable a diagnosis to be made.

HAEMORRHAGIC ARTHRITIS The physical signs of blood in a joint may resemble those of tuberculous arthritis. If the bleeding has followed a single recent injury, the history and absence of marked wasting are diagnostic. Following repeated bleeding, as in haemophilia, the clinical resemblance to tuberculosis is closer, but there is also a history of bleeding elsewhere.

PYOGENIC ARTHRITIS In long-standing cases it may be difficult to exclude an old septic arthritis.

Treatment

REST Hugh Owen Thomas long ago urged that tuberculosis should be treated by rest – which had to be 'prolonged, uninterrupted, rigid and enforced'. This often involved splintage of the joint and traction to overcome muscle spasm and prevent collapse of the articular surfaces. With modern chemotherapy this is no longer mandatory; rest and splintage are varied according to the needs of the individual patient. Those who are diagnosed and treated early are kept in bed only until symptoms subside, and thereafter are allowed restricted activity until the joint changes resolve (usually 6 months to a year). Those with progressive joint destruction may need a longer period of rest and splintage to prevent ankylosis in a bad position; however, as soon as symptoms permit, movements are again encouraged.

CHEMOTHERAPY The most effective treatment is a combination of antituberculous drugs, which should always include rifampicin and isoniazid. During the past decade the incidence of drug resistance has increased and this has led to the addition of various 'potentiating' drugs to the list. A recommended regimen is rifampicin, isoniazid and ethambutol (or pyrazinamide) for 8 weeks, and thereafter rifampicin and isoniazid for a further 6–12 months. Streptomycin and ethambutol are more toxic and should not be used for long-term treatment. A full review of treatment protocols can be found in the paper by Perez-Stable and Hopewell (1989).

OPERATION Operative drainage or clearance of a tuberculous focus is seldom necessary nowadays. However, a cold abscess may need immediate draining.

Once the condition is controlled and arthritis has completely subsided, normal activity can be resumed, though the patient must report any renewed symptoms. If, however, the joint is painful and the articular surface is destroyed, arthrodesis or replacement arthroplasty may be considered. The longer the period of inactivity, the less the risk of reactivation of the disease; there is always some risk and it is essential to give chemotherapy before and after the operation.

BRUCELLOSIS

Brucellosis is an unusual but none the less important cause of subacute or chronic granulomatous infection in bones and joints. Three species of organism are seen in humans: *Brucella melitensis, B. abortus* (from cattle) and *B. suis* (from pigs). Infection usually occurs from drinking unpasteurized milk or from coming into contact with infected meat (e.g. among farmers and meat packers). In the past it has been more common in countries around the Mediterranean and in certain parts of Africa and India. About 50% of patients with chronic brucellosis develop arthritis.

Pathology

The organism enters the body with infected milk products or, occasionally, directly through the skin or mucosal surfaces. It is taken up by the lymphatics and then carried by the blood stream to distant sites. Foci of infection may occur in bones (usually the vertebral bodies) or in the synovium of the larger joints. The characteristic lesion is a chronic inflammatory granuloma with round-cell infiltration and giant cells. There may be central necrosis and caseation leading to abscess formation and invasion of the surrounding tissues.

Clinical features

The patient usually presents with fever, headache and generalized weakness, followed by joint pains and backache. The initial illness may be acute and alarming; more often it begins insidiously and progresses until the symptoms localize in a single large joint (usually the hip or knee) or in the spine. The joint becomes painful, swollen and tender; movements are restricted in all directions. If the spine is affected, there is usually local tenderness and back movements are restricted.

The systemic illness follows a fluctuating course, with alternating periods of fever and apparent improvement (hence the older term 'undulant fever'). Diagnosis is often long delayed and may not be resolved until destructive changes are advanced.

X-rays The picture is that of a subacute arthritis, with loss of articular space, slowly progressive bone erosion and periarticular osteoporosis. In the spine there may be destruction and collapse of adjacent vertebral bodies with obliteration of the disc.

Investigations A positive agglutination test (titre above 1/80) is diagnostic. Joint aspiration or biopsy may allow the organism to be cultured and identified.

Diagnosis

Diagnosis is usually delayed while other types of subacute arthritis are excluded.

Tuberculosis and brucellosis have similar clinical and radiological features. The distinction is often difficult and may have to await the results of agglutination tests, synovial biopsy and bacteriological investigation.

Reiter's disease and other forms of reactive arthritis often follow an initial systemic illness. However, fever is not so marked and joint erosion is usually late and mild.

Treatment

ANTIBIOTICS The infection usually responds to a combined onslaught with tetracycline and streptomycin for 3–4 weeks. Alternative drugs, which are equally effective and which may be used as 'combination therapy', are rifampicin and the newer cephalosporins.

OPERATION An abscess will need drainage, and necrotic bone and cartilage should be meticulously excised. If the joint is destroyed, arthrodesis or arthroplasty may be necessary once the infection is completely controlled.

MYCOTIC INFECTIONS

Mycotic or fungal infection causes an indolent granulomatous reaction, often leading to abscess formation, tissue destruction and ulceration. When the musculoskeletal system is involved, it is usually by direct spread from the adjacent soft tissues. Occasionally, however, a bone or joint may be infected by haematogenous spread from a distant site.

These disorders are conveniently divided into 'superficial' and 'deep' infections.

SUPERFICIAL MYCOSES These are primarily infections of the skin or mucous surfaces, which spread into the adjacent soft tissues and bone. The more common examples are the *maduromycoses* (a group consisting of several species), *Sporothrix* and various species of *Candida*.

The *actinomycoses* are usually included with the superficial fungal infections. The causal organisms, of which *Actinomyces israelii* is the commonest in humans, are not really fungi but anaerobic bacilli with fungus-like appearance and behaviour.

DEEP MYCOSES This group comprises infections by *Blastomyces, Histoplasma, Coccidioides, Cryptococcus, Aspergillus* and other rare fungi species. The organisms, which occur in rotting vegetation and bird droppings, gain entry through the lungs and, in humans, may cause an influenza-like illness. Bone or joint infection is uncommon except in patients with compromised host defences.

MADUROMYCOSIS

This chronic fungal infection is seen mainly in northern Africa and the Indian subcontinent. The organisms usually enter through a cut in the foot; from there they spread through the subcutaneous tissues and along the tendon sheaths. The bones and joints are infected by direct invasion; local abscesses form and break through the skin as multiple sinuses. The patient may present at an early stage with a tender subcutaneous nodule (when the diagnosis is seldom entertained); more often he or she is seen when the foot is swollen and indurated, with discharging sinuses and ulcers. X-rays may show multiple bone cavities or progressive bone destruction. The organism can be identified in the sinus discharge or in tissue biopsies.

Treatment is unsatisfactory as there is no really effective chemotherapy. Intravenous amphotericin B is advocated, but it is fairly toxic and causes side effects such as headaches, vomiting and fever. Necrotic tissue should be widely excised. Even then it is sometimes difficult to stop further invasion, and amputation is sometimes necessary.

CANDIDIASIS

Candida albicans is a normal commensal in humans and it often causes superficial infection of the skin or mucous membranes. Deep and systemic infections are rare except under conditions of immunosuppression.

Candida osteomyelitis and arthritis may follow direct contamination during surgery or other invasive

procedures such as joint aspiration or arthroscopy. The diagnosis is usually made only after tissue sampling and culture.

Treatment consists of thorough joint irrigation and curettage of discrete bone lesions, together with intravenous amphotericin B.

ACTINOMYCOSIS

Infection is usually by *A. israelii*, an anaerobic Gram-positive bacillus. Although rare, it is important that it should be diagnosed because the organism is sensitive to antibiotics.

The most common site of infection is the mandible (from the mouth and pharynx), but bone lesions are also seen in the vertebrae (spreading from the lung or gut) and the pelvis (spreading from the caecum or colon). Peripheral lesions may occur by direct infection of the soft tissues and later extension to the bones. There may be a firm, tender swelling in the soft tissues, going on to form an abscess and one or more chronic discharging sinuses. X-rays may show cyst-like areas of bone destruction. The organism can be readily identified in the sinus discharge, but only on anaerobic culture.

Treatment, by large doses of penicillin G, tetracycline or erythromycin, has to be continued for several months.

THE DEEP MYCOSES

Histoplasmosis, blastomycosis and coccidioidomycosis are rare causes of bone and joint infection, but they

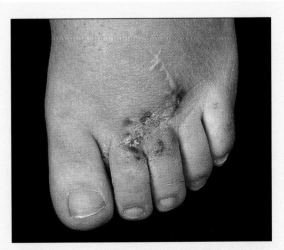

2.17 Maduromycosis This Mediterranean market-worker was perpetually troubled by tiny abscesses and weeping sinuses in her foot. X-rays showed that bone destruction had already spread to the tarsal bones, and after 2 years of futile treatment the foot had to be amputated.

should always be considered in patients on immuno-suppressive therapy who develop arthritis of one of the large joints or osteomyelitis in an unusual site. Diagnosis is usually delayed and often involves specialized micro-biological investigations to identify the organism.

Treatment with intravenous amphotericin B is moderately effective. Operation may be necessary to drain an abscess or to remove necrotic tissue.

HYDATID DISEASE

Hydatid disease is caused by the tapeworm *Echinococcus*. Parasitic infestation is common among sheep farmers, but bone lesions are rare.

The organism, a cestode worm, has a complicated life-cycle. The definitive host is the dog or some other carni-vore that carries the tapeworm in its bowel. Segments of worm and ova pass out in the faeces and are later ingested by one of the intermediate hosts – usually sheep or cattle or man. Here the larvae are carried via the portal circulation to the liver, and occasionally beyond to other organs, where they produce cysts containing numerous scolices. Infested meat is then eaten by dogs (or humans), giving rise to a new generation of tapeworm.

Scolices carried in the blood stream occasionally settle in bone and produce hydatid cysts that slowly enlarge with little respect for cortical or epiphyseal boundaries. The bones most commonly affected are the vertebrae, pelvis, femur and ribs.

Clinical features

The patient may complain of pain and swelling, or may present for the first time with a pathological fracture or compression of the spinal cord. The diagnosis is more likely if the patient comes from a sheep-farming district.

X-rays These show solitary or multiloculated bone cysts, but only moderate expansion of the cortices. In the spine, hydatid disease may involve adjacent verte-brae, with large cysts extending into the paraverte-bral soft tissues; these features are best seen on *CT and MRI*.

Investigations Casoni's (complement fixation) test may be positive. The diagnosis can be confirmed by carrying out a needle biopsy.

Treatment Hydatid disease is extremely difficult to erad-icate, and the location and size of the cysts often make surgical excision impractical or impossible (e.g. hydatid of the spine).

The anthelminthic drug albendazole is moderately effective in destroying the parasite. It has to be given in repeated courses (at least six) of 4 weeks each and it is said to be more effective when combined with praz-iquantel (Bonifacino *et al.*, 1997). However, the bone cysts do not heal and may require curettage and bone grafting to lessen the risk of pathological fracture. At operation the cavity can be further 'sterilized' with copious amounts of hypertonic saline to lessen the risk of recurrence.

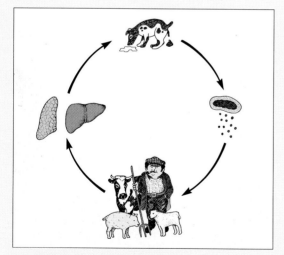

2.18 Hydatid disease The life-cycle of the tapeworm which causes hydatid disease.

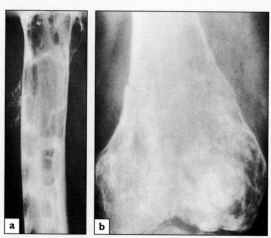

2.19 Hydatid disease of bone Two examples of hydatid involvement of bone: there is no expansion of the cortex in **(a)** and very little in **(b)**.

REFERENCES AND FURTHER READING

Björkstén B, Boquist L (1980) Histopathological aspects of chronic recurrent multifocal osteomyelitis. *Journal of Bone and Joint Surgery* **62B**, 276–380

Bonifacino R, Dogliani E, Craig PS (1997) Albendazole treatment and serological follow-up in hydatid disease of bone. *International Orthopaedics* 2, 127–132

Boutin RD, Resnick D (1998) The SAPHO syndrome: an evolving concept for unifying several idiopathic disorders of bone and skin. *American Journal of Roentgenology* **170**, 585–591

Carr AJ, Cole WG, Robertson DM, Chow CW (1993) Chronic multifocal osteomyelitis. *Journal of Bone and Joint Surgery* **75B**, 582–591

Ebong WW (1986) Acute osteomyelitis in Nigerians with sickle-cell disease. *Annals of Rheumatic Diseases* **45**, 911

Gristina AG (1988) Biomaterial-centred infection: microbial adhesion versus tissue integration. *Science* **237**, 437–451

Lidwell OM (1986) Clean air at operation and subsequent sepsis in the joint. *Clinical Orthopaedics and Related Research* 211, 91–102

Perez-Stable EJ, Hopewell PC (1989) Current tuberculosis treatment regimens: choosing the right one for your patient. *Clinics of Chest Medicine* 10, 323

Rasool MN, Govender S (1989) The skeletal manifestations of congenital syphilis. *Journal of Bone and Joint Surgery* **71B**, 752–755

Unkila-Kallis L, Kallis MJT, Peltola H (1994) The usefulness of C-reactive protein levels in the identification of concurrent septic arthritis in children who have acute haematogenous osteomyelitis. *Journal of Bone and Joint Surgery* **76A**, 848–853

Rheumatic disorders

The term 'rheumatic disorders' covers a number of diseases that cause chronic pain, stiffness and swelling around joints and tendons. Many common conditions, such as influenza, are associated with painful muscles and joints, but the rheumatic disorders are distinguished by (1) their chronicity and (2) the appearance of local and systemic features of inflammation. Many – perhaps all – result from a faulty immune reaction to an antigenic stimulus, against a background of genetic predisposition.

RHEUMATOID ARTHRITIS

Rheumatoid arthritis (RA) is the commonest cause of chronic inflammatory joint disease. The most typical features are a symmetrical polyarthritis and tenosynovitis, morning stiffness, elevation of the erythrocyte sedimentation rate (ESR) and the appearance of anti-IgG globulins (rheumatoid factors) in the serum. However, changes can be widespread in the tissues of the body and the condition should really be called rheumatoid *disease.*

The reported prevalence of RA is 1–3%, with a peak incidence in the fourth or fifth decade. Women are affected 3 or 4 times as commonly as men. Both the prevalence and the clinical expression vary between populations; the disease is more common (and generally more severe) in the urban communities of Europe and North America than in the rural populations of Africa (Solomon *et al.,* 1975).

Cause

The cause of RA is still incompletely worked out. However, a great deal is now known about the circumstances in which it develops and hypotheses about its etiology and pathogenesis have been narrowed down to manageable lines of discussion. The following is a very simplified account; for more detailed information the reader is referred to one of the larger reference works (Kelley *et al.,* 1997).

Important factors in the evolution of RA are (1) genetic susceptibility; (2) an immunological reaction, possibly involving a foreign antigen, preferentially focused on synovial tissue; (3) an inflammatory reaction in joints and tendon sheaths; (4) the appearance of anti-IgG antibodies ('rheumatoid factors') in the blood and synovium; (5) perpetuation of the inflammatory process; and (6) articular cartilage destruction.

Genetic susceptibility A genetic association is suggested by the fact that RA is more common in first-degree relatives of patients than in the population at large; furthermore twin studies have revealed a concordance rate of around 30% if one of the pair is affected.

Immunological processes The human leukocyte antigen (HLA) DR4 occurs in about 70% of people with RA, compared to a frequency of less than 30% in normal controls. HLA-DR4 is encoded in the major histocompatibility complex (MHC) region on chromosome 6. In common with other HLA Class II molecules, it appears as a surface antigen on cells of the immune system (B lymphocytes, macrophages, dendritic cells) which can act as antigen-presenting cells (APCs). In some T-cell immune reactions, the process is initiated only when the antigenic peptide is presented in association with a specific HLA allele. It has been suggested that this is the case in people who develop RA; the idea is even more attractive if one posits that the putative antigen has a special affinity for synovial tissue. So far no such antigen has been discovered, but the conditions surrounding the early development of RA suggest that it might be an arthrotropic virus or retrovirus.

The inflammatory reaction Once the APC/T-cell interaction is initiated, various local factors come into play and lead to a progressive enhancement of the immune response. There is a marked proliferation of cells in the synovium, with the appearance of cytokines, which are important in mediating intercellular communication and activating macrophages and B-cells. Local factors also have a role in stimulating vascular proliferation. The resulting synovitis, both in joints and in tendon sheath linings, is the hallmark of early RA.

Rheumatoid factor B cell activation leads to the production of anti-IgG auto-antibodies, which are detected in the blood as 'rheumatoid factor' (RF). This finding is so characteristic that it was once regarded as diagnostic (even pathognomonic) of RA. It is now known not to be so, but patients with a positive RF test tend to be more severely affected than those with a negative test. A current theory is that the RF antiglobulins play an important role in perpetuating the chronic inflammatory process.

Chronic synovitis and joint destruction Chronic rheumatoid synovitis is associated with the production of proteolytic enzymes, tissue factors such as prostaglandins and interleukin-1 (IL-1), and possibly also anti-collagen antibodies. Immune complexes are deposited in the synovium and on the articular cartilage, where they appear to augment the inflammatory process. This combination of factors leads to depletion of the cartilage matrix and, eventually, damage to the chondrocytes. Vascular proliferation and osteoclastic activity, most marked at the edges of the articular surface, may contribute further to cartilage destruction and periarticular bone erosion.

Pathology

The condition is widespread, but the brunt of the attack falls on synovium. The constant and characteristic feature is a chronic inflammation; an inconstant but pathognomonic lesion is the rheumatoid nodule.

JOINTS AND TENDONS

The pathological changes, if unchecked, proceed in three stages.

Stage 1 – synovitis Early changes are vascular congestion, proliferation of synoviocytes and infiltration of the subsynovial layers by polymorphs, lymphocytes and plasma cells. There is thickening of the capsular structures, villous formation of the synovium and a cell-rich effusion into the joints and tendon sheaths. Though painful, swollen and tender, these structures are still intact and mobile, and the disorder is potentially reversible.

Stage 2 – destruction Persistent synovitis causes joint and tendon destruction. Articular cartilage is eroded, partly by proteolytic enzymes, partly by vascular tissue in the folds of the synovial reflections and partly due to direct invasion of the cartilage by a pannus of granulation tissue creeping over the articular surface. At the margins of the joint, bone is eroded by granulation tissue invasion and osteoclastic resorption. Recent evidence suggests that bone erosions are the result of synovial hyperplasia rather than inflammation (Kirwan, 1997).

Similar changes occur in tendon sheaths, causing tenosynovitis, invasion of the collagen bundles and, eventually, partial or complete rupture of tendons.

A synovial effusion, often containing copious amounts of fibrinoid material, produces swelling of the joints, tendons and bursae.

Stage 3 – deformity The combination of articular destruction, capsular stretching and tendon rupture leads to progressive instability and deformity of the joints. By this time the inflammatory process may have subsided; the emphasis is now on the mechanical and functional effects of joint and tendon disruption.

EXTRA-ARTICULAR TISSUES

The rheumatoid nodule is a small granulomatous lesion consisting of a central necrotic zone surrounded by a radially disposed palisade of local histiocytes, and beyond that by inflammatory granulation tissue. Nodules occur under the skin (especially over bony prominences), in the synovium, on tendons, in the sclera and in many of the viscera.

Lymphadenopathy can affect not only the nodes draining inflamed joints, but also those at a distance such as the mediastinal nodes. This, as well as a mild *splenomegaly*, is due to hyperactivity of the reticuloendothelial system. *Vasculitis,* more usually associated with disseminated lupus, may be fairly widespread.

Muscle weakness is common. It may be due to a generalized *myopathy* or *neuropathy*, but it is important to exclude spinal cord disease or cord compression due to vertebral displacement. Sensory changes may be part of a neuropathy, but localized sensory and motor symptoms can also result from *nerve compression* by thickened synovium.

Visceral disease can occur in the lungs, heart, kidneys, gastrointestinal tract and brain.

Clinical features

The onset of RA is usually insidious, with symptoms emerging over a period of months. Occasionally the disease starts quite suddenly.

In the early stages the picture is mainly that of a polysynovitis, with soft-tissue swelling and stiffness. Typically, a woman of 30–40 years complains of pain, swelling and loss of mobility in the proximal joints of the fingers. There may be a previous history of 'muscle pain', tiredness, loss of weight and a general lack of well-being. As time passes the symptoms 'spread' to other joints – the wrists, feet, knees and shoulders in order of frequency. Another classic feature is generalized stiffness after periods of inactivity, and especially after rising from bed in the early morning.

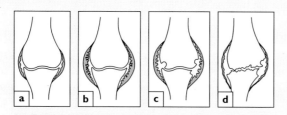

3.1 Pathology of rheumatoid arthritis (a) The normal joint. **(b)** Stage 1 – synovitis and joint swelling. **(c)** Stage 2 – early joint destruction with periarticular erosions. **(d)** Stage 3 – advanced joint destruction and deformity.

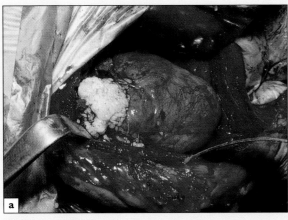
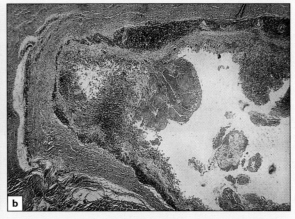

3.2 Rheumatoid synovitis (**a**) The macroscopic appearance of rheumatoid synovitis with fibrinoid material oozing through a rent in the capsule. (**b**) Histology shows proliferating synovium with round-cell infiltration and fibrinoid particles in the joint cavity (×120).

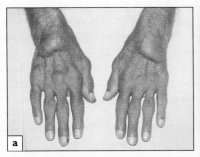
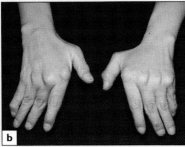
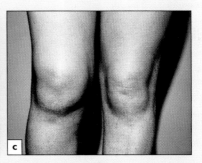

3.3 Rheumatoid arthritis – clinical features (**a**) Early – spindling of the fingers and synovitis of the wrists. (**b**) The classic hand deformities of established RA. (**c**) Occasionally RA starts with synovitis of a single large joint (in this case the right knee).

Physical signs may be slight, but usually there is symmetrically distributed swelling and tenderness of the metacarpophalangeal joints, the proximal interphalangeal joints and the wrists. Tenosynovitis is common in the extensor compartments of the wrist and the flexor sheaths of the fingers; it is diagnosed by feeling thickening, tenderness and crepitation over the back of the wrist or the palm while passively moving the fingers. If the larger joints are involved, local warmth, synovial hypertrophy and intra-articular effusion may be more obvious. Movements are often limited but the joints are still stable and deformity is unusual.

In the later stages joint deformity becomes increasingly apparent and the acute pain of synovitis is replaced by the more constant ache of progressive joint destruction. The combination of joint instability and tendon rupture produces the typical 'rheumatoid' deformities: ulnar deviation of the fingers, radial and volar displacement of the wrists, valgus knees, valgus feet and clawed toes.

Joint movements are restricted and often very painful. About a third of all patients develop pain and stiffness in the cervical spine. Function is increasingly disturbed and patients may need help with grooming, dressing and eating.

EXTRA-ARTICULAR FEATURES are often seen in patients with severe disease. The most characteristic is the appearance of *nodules*. They are usually found as small subcutaneous lumps, rubbery in consistency, at the back of the elbows, but they also develop in tendons (where they may cause 'triggering' or rupture), in the viscera and the eye. They are pathognomonic of RA, but occur in only 25% of patients.

Less specific features include *muscle wasting, lymphadenopathy, scleritis, nerve entrapment syndromes, skin atrophy or ulceration* and *peripheral sensory neuropathy*. Marked visceral disease, such as pulmonary fibrosis, is rare. Vasculitis of some degree is almost ubiquitous and may account for many of the features listed here.

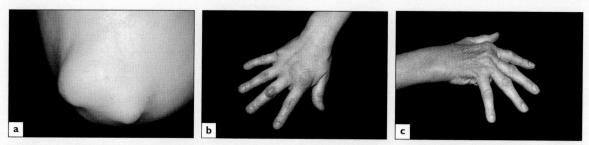

3.4 Extra-articular features (**a,b**) Subcutaneous nodules occur typically on the extensor aspects of the elbow and the hand. They are pathognomonic of RA. (**c**) Tendon rupture is common; the 'drop fingers' in this patient are due to rupture of the extensor tendons at the wrist.

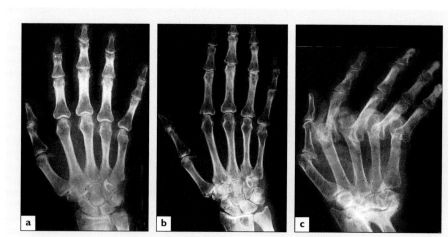

3.5 Rheumatoid arthritis – sequence of changes The progress of disease is well shown in this patient's x-rays. (**a**) First there was only soft-tissue swelling and periarticular osteoporosis; (**b**) later juxta-articular erosions appeared; (**c**) ultimately the joints became unstable and deformed, with four of the metacarpophalangeal joints dislocated.

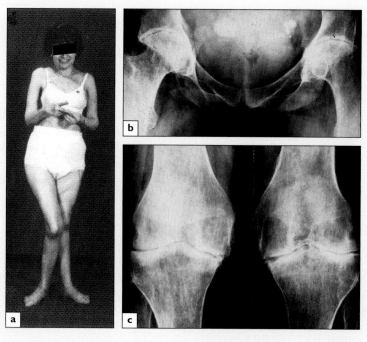

3.6 Rheumatoid arthritis – aftermath The acute phase is over, but the patient is left with secondary osteoarthritis of (**a, b**) the hips and (**a, c**) knees.

X-rays

Early on, x-rays show only the features of synovitis: soft-tissue swelling and periarticular osteoporosis. The later stages are marked by the appearance of marginal bony erosions and narrowing of the articular space, especially in the proximal joints of the hands and feet.

In advanced disease, articular destruction and joint deformity are obvious. Flexion and extension views of the cervical spine often show subluxation at the atlanto-axial or mid-cervical levels; surprisingly, this causes few symptoms in the majority of cases.

Blood investigations

Normocytic, hypochromic anaemia is common and is a reflection of abnormal erythropoiesis due to disease activity. It may be aggravated by chronic gastro-intestinal blood loss caused by anti-inflammatory drugs.

In active phases the ESR is raised, C-reactive protein may be present and mucoprotein levels are high.

Serological tests for RF are positive in about 80% of patients and antinuclear factors are present in 30%. Neither of these tests is specific and neither is required for a diagnosis of RA.

Synovial biopsy

Synovial tissue may be obtained by needle biopsy, via the arthroscope, or by open operation. Unfortunately, most of the histological features of RA are non-specific and the report is more likely to read 'consistent with' rather than 'diagnostic of'.

Diagnosis

The usual criteria for diagnosing rheumatoid disease are the presence of a bilateral, symmetrical polyarthritis involving the proximal joints of the hands or feet, and persisting for at least 6 weeks. If there are subcutaneous nodules or x-ray signs of periarticular erosions, the diagnosis is certain. *A positive test for RF in the absence of the above features is not sufficient evidence of RA, nor does a negative test exclude the diagnosis if the other features are all present.* The chief value of the RF tests is in the assessment of prognosis: persistently high titres herald more serious disease.

Atypical forms of presentation are not uncommon. The early stages may be punctuated by long spells of quiescence, during which the diagnosis is doubted, but sooner or later the more characteristic features appear. Occasionally, in older people, the onset is explosive, with the rapid appearance of severe joint pain and stiffness; paradoxically these patients have a relatively good prognosis. Now and then (more so in young women) the disease starts with chronic pain and swelling of a single large joint and it may take months or years before other joints are involved.

In the differential diagnosis of polyarthritis several disorders must be considered.

SERONEGATIVE INFLAMMATORY POLYARTHRITIS Polyarthritis is a feature of a number of conditions vaguely related to RA: psoriatic arthritis, juvenile chronic arthritis (JCA; Still's disease), systemic lupus erythematosus (SLE) and other connective-tissue diseases. These are considered in later sections.

ANKYLOSING SPONDYLITIS This is primarily a disease of the sacroiliac and intervertebral joints, causing back pain and progressive stiffness; however, it may also involve the peripheral joints.

REITER'S DISEASE The larger joints and the lumbosacral spine are the main targets. There is usually a history of urethritis or colitis and often also conjunctivitis.

POLYARTICULAR GOUT Tophaceous gout affecting multiple joints can, at first sight, be mistaken for RA. On x-ray the erosions are quite different from those

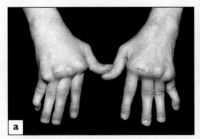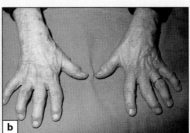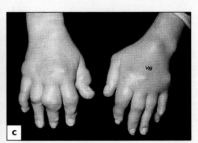

3.7 Rheumatoid arthritis – differential diagnosis These three patients all presented with painful swollen finger joints. (**a**) The proximal joints are enlarged and deformed (rheumatoid arthritis); (**b**) the distal joints are the worst (Heberden's osteoarthritis); (**c**) the asymmetrical nodules are actually gouty tophi.

of RA; the diagnosis is clinched by identifying the typical birefringent crystals in the joint fluid or a nodular tophus.

It is a curious fact that, although both gout and RA are fairly common, the two conditions are rarely seen in the same patient. The reason for this is unknown.

CALCIUM PYROPHOSPHATE DEPOSITION DISEASE This condition is usually seen in older people. Typically it affects large joints, but it may occur in the wrist and metacarpophalangeal joints as well. X-ray signs are fairly characteristic and crystals may be identified in synovial fluid or synovium.

OSTEOARTHRITIS Polyarticular osteoarthritis (OA), which typically involves the finger joints, is often mistaken for RA. A moment's reflection will usually dispel any doubt: OA always involves the *distal* interphalangeal joints and causes a nodular arthritis with radiologically obvious osteophytes, whereas RA affects the *proximal* joints of the hand and causes predominantly erosive features.

Some confusion may arise from the fact that RA, in its later stages, is associated with loss of articular cartilage and *secondary OA*. Enquiry into the early history will usually untangle the diagnosis. Sometimes, however, RA atypically affects only a few of the larger joints and it is then very difficult to distinguish from OA; x-ray features such as loss of articular cartilage throughout the entire joint and lack of hypertrophic bone changes (sclerosis and osteophytes) should suggest an inflammatory arthritis.

SARCOIDOSIS Sarcoid disease sometimes presents with a symmetrical small-joint polyarthritis and no bone involvement; erythema nodosum and hilar lymphadenopathy are clues to the diagnosis. The condition usually subsides spontaneously within 6 months. Another form of the disease, with chronic granulomatous infiltration of bone, synovium and other organs, is more common in black Africans and descendants. In addition to polyarthritis and tenosynovitis, x-rays show punched-out 'cysts' and cortical erosions in the bones of the hands and feet. The ESR is raised and the Kveim test may be positive. Treatment with non-steroidal anti-inflammatory drugs (NSAIDs) may be adequate but in more intractable cases corticosteroids are necessary

POLYMYALGIA RHEUMATICA This condition, which is seen mainly in middle-aged or elderly women, is characterized by aching discomfort around the pectoral and pelvic girdles, post-inactivity stiffness and muscular weakness. The joints are not tender but the muscles are. The ESR is almost always remarkably high. This is a form of giant-cell arteritis and carries the risk of temporal arteritis resulting in blindness. Corticosteroids (as little as 10mg a day) provide rapid and dramatic relief of all symptoms, and this response is often used as a diagnostic test.

Treatment

There is no cure for RA. This must be explained to the patient, who also needs to be reassured that it is not necessarily a crippling disease, that much can be done to alleviate symptoms and delay progression and that there is every chance of a useful and active life despite some functional limitations.

Management is guided by five injunctions: *(1) stop the synovitis; (2) keep the joints moving; (3) prevent deformity; (4) reconstruct; (5) rehabilitate.*

A multidisciplinary approach is needed from the beginning: ideally the therapeutic team should include a rheumatologist, orthopaedic surgeon, physiotherapist, occupational therapist, orthotist and social worker. Their deployment and priorities will vary according to the stage of the disease. The following scheme should meet the needs of the 'average' patient.

At the onset of the disease both the patient and the doctor will be uncertain about the likely rate of progress. Treatment is mainly palliative and supportive: the control of pain and stiffness with NSAIDs, maintaining muscle tone and joint mobility by a balanced programme of exercise and general advice on coping with the activities of daily living.

During the early phase of established RA (the first 6–12 months) the main problem is the control of synovitis. NSAIDs may have to be stepped up and, if the pain, swelling, stiffness and joint tenderness are not alleviated, may need to be supplemented by the introduction of low-dosage corticosteroids (5–7.5mg prednisolone daily) and 'second-line' drugs such as gold or penicillamine.

Systemic corticosteroids, once feared because of their side-effects, have been shown to be effective at low dosage in delaying the onset of articular erosion and slowing disease progression (Kirwan *et al.*, 1995; Kirwin, 1997). It is recommended that they be used in the early active phase of RA for up to 2 years. During that time, the 'second-line' drugs, which take a long time to start acting, can be introduced and then continued (if necessary) when corticosteroid treatment is tailed off.

Additional measures include the injection of long-acting corticosteroid preparations into inflamed joints and tendon sheaths. It is sometimes feared that such injections may themselves cause damage to articular cartilage or tendons. However, there is little evidence that they are harmful, provided they are used sparingly and with full precautions against infection.

Physiotherapy is still important. But so is rest – one of the oldest methods of treating inflammation. During an acute flare-up, the patient may benefit from a few weeks' rest in bed; gentle active and passive exercises are kept up and care should be taken to prevent

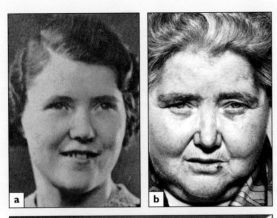

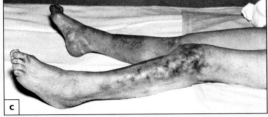

3.8 Treatment of rheumatoid arthritis – side-effects of systemic corticosteroids. Anti-inflammatory drugs are necessary – but can be harmful. (**a, b**) This young woman on corticosteroids became severely cushingoid. (**c**) This patient had multiple ecchymoses which, combined with tissue-paper skin, add to the risks of limb surgery.

gold, penicillamine or methotrexate. However, these drugs cannot restore what has already been destroyed, and local counteractive measures become increasingly important. Preventive splintage and orthotic devices may delay the march of events. If these fail to restore and maintain function, operative treatment is indicated. At first this consists mainly of soft-tissue procedures (synovectomy, tendon repair or replacement and joint stabilization); in some cases osteotomy may be more appropriate.

In late rheumatoid disease (5–20 years), severe joint destruction, fixed deformity and loss of function are clear indications for reconstructive surgery. Arthrodesis, osteotomy and arthroplasty all have their place and are considered in the appropriate chapters. However, it should be recognized that patients who are no longer suffering the pain of active synovitis and who are content with a limited pattern of life may not want or need heroic surgery merely to improve their anatomy. Careful assessment for occupational therapy, the provision of mechanical aids and adjustments to their home environment may be much more useful.

NOTE: The various drugs employed in the treatment of RA, and the indications for using them, are reviewed in a 'guidelines' paper published by the American College of Rheumatology (1996).

postural deformities. Sometimes a week or two of continuous splintage (e.g. for the knees or wrists) is effective; night splints can be used intermittently at any stage of the disease.

During the phase of progressive erosive arthritis (1–5 years), the combination of muscle weakness, joint instability and tendon rupture may lead to progressive deformity. By now the patient will probably be on long-term treatment with one of the 'second-line' drugs such as

Complications

FIXED DEFORMITIES The perils of RA are often the commonplace ones resulting from ignorance and neglect. Early assessment and planning should prevent postural deformities, which will result in joint contractures.

MUSCLE WEAKNESS Even mild degrees of myopathy or neuropathy, when combined with prolonged inactivity, may lead to profound muscle wasting and weakness. This

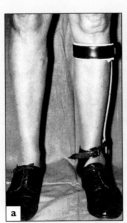

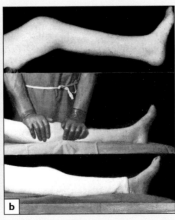

3.9 Treatment of rheumatoid arthritis – prevent deformity (**a**) Splintage to rest inflamed joints may, if started early, halt the progress of deformity. (**b**) An early fixed deformity of the knee can be corrected by gentle manipulation and temporary plaster splintage.

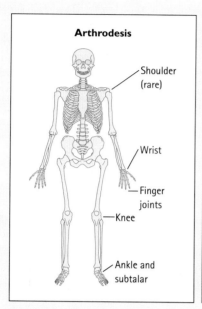

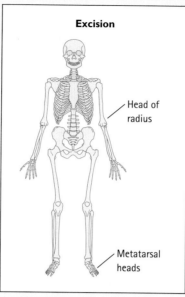

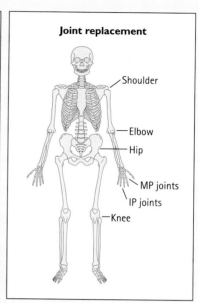

3.10 Surgical treatment of rheumatoid arthritis Sites where reconstructive operations may be useful.

should be prevented by physiotherapy and pain control, if possible; if not, the surgeon must be forewarned of the difficulty of postoperative rehabilitation.

JOINT RUPTURE Occasionally the joint lining ruptures and synovial contents spill into the soft tissues. Treatment is directed at the underlying synovitis – i.e. splintage and injection of the joint, with synovectomy as a second resort.

INFECTION Patients with RA – and even more so those on corticosteroid therapy – are susceptible to infection. Sudden clinical deterioration, or increased pain in a single joint, should alert one to the possibility of septic arthritis and the need for joint aspiration.

SPINAL CORD COMPRESSION This is a rare complication of cervical spine instability. The onset of weakness and upper motor neuron signs in the lower limbs is suspicious. If they occur, immobilization of the neck is essential and spinal fusion should be carried out as soon as possible.

SYSTEMIC VASCULITIS Vasculitis is a rare but potentially serious complication. High doses of corticosteroids and intravenous plasma volume expanders may be called for.

AMYLOIDOSIS This is another rare but potentially lethal complication of long-standing rheumatoid disease. The patient presents with proteinuria and progressive renal failure. The diagnosis is made by finding amyloid in a rectal or renal biopsy. There is no specific treatment.

Prognosis

RA runs a variable course. When the patient is first seen it is difficult to predict the outcome, but high titres of RF, periarticular erosions, rheumatoid nodules, severe muscle wasting, joint contractures and evidence of vasculitis are poor prognostic signs. Women, on the whole, fare somewhat worse than men. About 10% of patients improve steadily after the first attack of active synovitis; 60% have intermittent phases of disease activity and remission, but with a slow downhill course over many years; 20% have severe joint erosion, which is usually evident within the first 5 years; and 10% end up completely disabled.

ANKYLOSING SPONDYLITIS

Like RA, ankylosing spondylitis (AS) is a generalized chronic inflammatory disease – but its effects are seen mainly in the spine and sacroiliac joints. It is characterized by pain and stiffness of the back, with variable involvement of the hips and shoulders and (more rarely) the peripheral joints. Its reported prevalence is 0.0%–0.2% in western Europe and North America, but is much lower in Japanese and black African peoples. Males are affected more frequently than females (estimates vary from 2:1 to 10:1) and the usual age at onset is between 15 and 25 years. There is a strong tendency to familial aggregation and association with the genetic marker HLA-B27.

Cause

The cause of AS is similar to that of RA. There is considerable evidence for regarding it as a genetically determined immunopathological disorder. The disease is much more common in family members than in the general population; HLA-B27 is present in over 90% of Caucasian patients and in half of their first-degree relatives (as compared with 8% of the general population); and racial groups with an unusually low prevalence of AS also show a very low prevalence of HLA-B27 (e.g. less than 1% in Japanese people). There are various theories about the 'triggering factor' that initiates the abnormal immune response. It may be a bacterial antigen which closely resembles HLA-B27 that induces an antibody response which targets also the HLA-B27 positive cells; or, as in the case of RA, the HLA-B27 molecule may be involved in the presentation of a specific antigen to the T-cells which then react with the antigen-presenting cells. Since classic AS is sometimes associated with genitourinary or bowel infection, and disorders such as Reiter's disease and ulcerative colitis cause vertebral and sacroiliac changes indistinguishable from those of AS, it is thought that the putative organism may be carried to the spine by local lymphatic drainage.

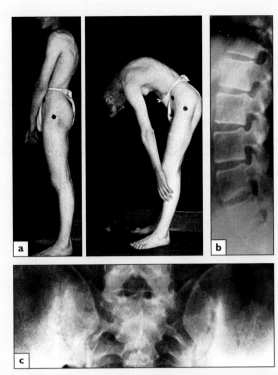

3.11 Ankylosing spondylitis – early The early features are (**a**) a stiff spine, (**b**) 'squaring' of the lumbar vertebrae and (**c**) bilateral sacroiliac erosion.

Pathology

There are two basic lesions: synovitis of diarthrodial joints and inflammation at the fibro-osseous junctions of syndesmotic joints and tendons. The preferential involvement of the insertion of tendons and ligaments (the entheses) has spawned the unwieldy term *enthesopathy*.

Synovitis of the sacroiliac and vertebral facet joints causes destruction of articular cartilage and periarticular bone. The costovertebral joints also are frequently involved, leading to diminished respiratory excursion. When peripheral joints are affected the same changes occur.

Inflammation of the fibro-osseous junctions affects the intervertebral discs, sacroiliac ligaments, symphysis pubis, manubrium sterni and the bony insertions of large tendons. Pathological changes proceed in three stages: (1) an inflammatory reaction with round-cell infiltration, granulation tissue formation and erosion of adjacent bone; (2) replacement of the granulation tissue by fibrous tissue; and (3) ossification of the fibrous tissue, leading to ankylosis of the joint.

Ossification across the surface of the disc gives rise to small bony bridges or syndesmophytes linking adjacent vertebral bodies. If many vertebrae are involved the spine may become absolutely rigid.

Clinical features

The disease starts insidiously: a teenager or young adult complains of backache and stiffness recurring at intervals over a number of years. This is often diagnosed as 'back strain', but (unlike back strain) the symptoms are worse in the early morning and after inactivity. Referred pain in the buttocks and thighs may appear as 'sciatica' and some patients are mistakenly treated for intervertebral disc prolapse. Gradually pain and stiffness become continuous and other symptoms begin to appear: general fatigue, pain and swelling of joints, tenderness at the insertion of the tendo Achillis, 'foot strain', or intercostal pain and tenderness.

Occasionally the disease starts with pain and slight swelling in a peripheral joint such as the ankle, or pain and stiffness of the hip. Sooner of later, though, backache will come to the fore.

Early on there is little to see apart from slight flattening of the lower back and limitation of extension in the lumbar spine. There may be diffuse tenderness over the spine and sacroiliac joints, or (occasionally) swelling and tenderness of a single large joint.

In established cases the posture is typical: loss of the normal lumbar lordosis, increased thoracic kyphosis and a forward thrust of the neck; upright posture and balance are maintained by standing with the hips and knees slightly flexed, and in late cases these may become fixed deformities. Spinal movements are diminished in all directions, but loss of extension is always the earliest and the most severe disability. It is revealed dramatically by the 'wall test': the patient is asked to stand with his or her back to the wall; heels, buttocks, scapulae and occiput should all be able to touch the wall simultaneously. If extension is seriously diminished the patient will find this impossible. In the most advanced stage the spine may be completely ankylosed from occiput to sacrum, sometimes in positions of grotesque deformity. Marked loss of cervical extension may restrict the line of vision to a few paces.

Chest expansion, which should be at least 7cm in young men, is often markedly decreased. In old people, who may have pulmonary disease, this test is unreliable.

Peripheral joints (usually shoulders, hips and knees) are involved in over a third of the patients; they show the features of inflammatory arthritis – swelling, tenderness, effusion and loss of mobility. There may also be tenderness of the ligament and tendon insertions close to a large joint or under the heel.

EXTRASKELETAL MANIFESTATIONS General fatigue and loss of weight are common. Acute anterior uveitis occurs in about 25% of patients; it usually responds well to treatment but, if neglected, may lead to glaucoma. Other extraskeletal disorders, such as aortic valve disease, carditis and pulmonary fibrosis, are rare and occur very late in the disease.

X-rays

The cardinal sign – and often the earliest – is erosion and fuzziness of the sacroiliac joints. Later there may be periarticular sclerosis, especially on the iliac side of the joint, and finally bony ankylosis.

The earliest vertebral change is flattening of the normal anterior concavity of the vertebral body ('squaring'). Later, ossification of the ligaments around the intervertebral discs produces delicate bridges (syndesmophytes) between adjacent vertebrae. Bridging at several levels gives the appearance of a 'bamboo spine'.

Osteoporosis is common in long-standing cases and there may be hyperkyphosis of the thoracic spine due to wedging of the vertebral bodies.

Peripheral joints may show erosive arthritis or progressive bony ankylosis.

Special investigations

The ESR is usually elevated during active phases of the disease. HLA-B27 is present in 90% of cases. Serological tests for RF are negative.

Diagnosis

Diagnosis is easy in patients with spinal rigidity and typical deformities, but it is often missed in those with early disease or unusual forms of presentation. In over 10% of cases the disease starts with an asymmetrical inflammatory arthritis – usually of the hip, knee or ankle – and it may be several years before back pain appears. Atypical onset is more common in women, who may show less obvious changes in the sacroiliac joints. A history of AS in a close relative is strongly suggestive.

MECHANICAL DISORDERS Low back pain in young adults is usually attributed to one of the more common disorders such as muscular strain, facet joint dysfunction or

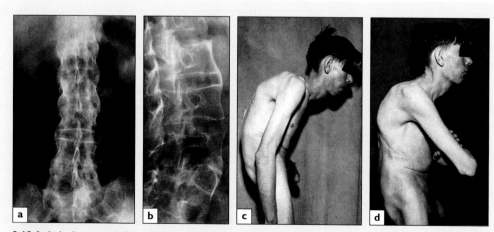

3.12 Ankylosing spondylitis – late (**a, b**) Bony bridges (syndesmophytes) between the vertebral bodies convert the spine into a rigid column ('bamboo spine'); note that the sacroiliac joints have fused. Spinal osteotomy may be necessary at this stage: (**c**) before operation this man could see only a few paces ahead; (**d**) after osteotomy his back is still rigid, but his posture, function and outlook are vastly improved.

spondylolisthesis. These conditions differ from AS in several ways: the onset of pain is related to specific physical activities, stiffness is less pronounced and symptoms are eased rather than aggravated by inactivity. Tenderness is also more localized and the peripheral joints are normal.

ANKYLOSING HYPEROSTOSIS (FORESTIER'S DISEASE) This is a fairly common disorder, predominantly of older men, characterized by widespread ossification of ligaments and tendon insertions. X-rays show pronounced but asymmetrical intervertebral spur formation and bridging throughout the dorsolumbar spine. Although it bears a superficial resemblance to AS, it is not an inflammatory disease, spinal pain and stiffness are seldom severe, the sacroiliac joints are not eroded and the ESR is normal.

THE SERONEGATIVE SPONDARTHRITIDES A number of disorders are associated with vertebral and sacroiliac lesions indistinguishable from those of AS. They are *Reiter's disease, psoriatic arthritis, ulcerative colitis, Crohn's disease, Whipple's disease and Behçet's syndrome.* In each there are certain characteristic features: the rash or nail changes of psoriasis, intestinal ulceration in enterocolitis, genitourinary and ocular inflammation in Reiter's disease, buccal and genital ulceration in Behçet's syndrome. Yet there is considerable overlap between them; all show some familial aggregation and all are associated with the histocompatibility antigen, HLA-B27. Patients with one of these disorders (including AS) often have close relatives with another, or with a positive HLA-B27.

Treatment

The disease is not nearly as damaging as RA and most patients continue to lead an active life. In the absence of a specific agent, treatment consists of (1) general measures to maintain satisfactory posture and preserve movement, (2) anti-inflammatory drugs to counteract pain and stiffness and (3) operations to correct deformity or restore mobility.

GENERAL MEASURES Patients are encouraged to remain active and follow their normal pursuits as far as possible. They should be taught how to maintain satisfactory posture and urged to perform spinal extension exercises every day. Swimming, dancing and gymnastics are ideal forms of recreation. Rest and immobilization, effective in other inflammatory joint diseases, are contraindicated because they tend to increase the general feeling of stiffness.

NON-STEROIDAL ANTI-INFLAMMATORY DRUGS It is doubtful whether these drugs prevent or retard the progress to ankylosis, but they do control pain and counteract

soft-tissue stiffness, thus making it possible to benefit from exercise and activity. Indomethacin is often used but other, less powerful, drugs may be adequate; they usually have to be continued for many years.

OPERATION Stiffness of the hips can be treated by joint replacement, though this seldom provides more than moderate mobility. Moreover, the incidence of infection is higher than usual and patients may need prolonged rehabilitation.

Deformity of the spine may be severe enough to warrant lumbar or cervical osteotomy. These are difficult and potentially hazardous procedures; fortunately, with improved activity and exercise programmes, they are seldom needed. If spinal deformity is combined with hip stiffness, hip replacements (permitting full extension) often suffice.

Complications

SPINAL FRACTURES The spine is often both rigid and osteoporotic; fractures may be caused by comparatively mild injuries. The commonest site is C5–7, but it is prudent to x-ray the entire spine in accident victims who have AS. Treatment in these cases is directed at preventing further deformity.

HYPERKYPHOSIS In long-standing cases the spine may become severely kyphotic, so much so that the patient has difficulty lifting his head to see in front of his feet.

SPINAL CORD COMPRESSION This is uncommon, but it should be thought of in patients who develop long-tract symptoms and signs. It may be caused by atlanto-axial subluxation or by ossification of the posterior longitudinal ligament.

LUMBOSACRAL NERVE ROOT COMPRESSION Patients may occasionally develop root symptoms, including lower limb weakness and paraesthesia, in addition to their 'usual' pelvic girdle symptoms.

REITER'S SYNDROME AND REACTIVE ARTHRITIS

The syndrome described by Hans Reiter in 1916 (and 100 years before that by Benjamin Brodie) is a clinical triad of *urethritis, arthritis* and *conjunctivitis* occurring some weeks after either *dysentery* or *venereal infection.* It is now recognized that this is one of the classic forms of reactive arthritis, i.e. an aseptic inflammatory arthritis associated with non-specific urogenital or bowel infection.

Its prevalence is difficult to assess, but it is probably the commonest type of large-joint polyarthritis in young men. It is thought to occur in 1–3% of all people who develop either non-specific urogenital infection or *Shigella* dysentery, but its incidence may be as high as 25% in those who are HLA-B27 positive. Men are affected more often than women (the ratio is about 10:1), but this may simply reflect the difficulty of diagnosing the venereal infection in women. The usual age at onset is between 20 and 40 years, but children are affected too – perhaps after an episode of diarrhoea.

Cause

Familial aggregation, overlap with other forms of seronegative spondarthritis in first-degree relatives and a close association with HLA-B27 point to a genetic predisposition, the bowel or urogenital infection acting as a trigger. Dysenteric organisms include *Shigella flexneri*, *Salmonella*, *Campylobacter* species and *Yersinia enterocolitica*. *Lymphogranuloma venereum* and *Chlamydia trachomatis* have been implicated as sexually transmitted infections. All these bacteria can survive in human cells; assuming that either the bacterium or a peptide bacterial fragment acts as the antigen, the pathogenesis could be the same as that suggested for AS.

Pathology

The pathological changes are essentially the same as those in AS, with the emphasis first on subacute large-joint synovitis and later tending towards sacroiliitis and spondylitis.

Clinical features

The acute phase of the disease is marked by an asymmetrical inflammatory arthritis of the lower limb joints – usually the knee and ankle but often the tarsal and toe joints as well. The joint may be acutely painful, hot and swollen with a tense effusion, suggesting gout or infection. Tendo Achillis tenderness and plantar fasciitis (evidence of enthesopathy) are common, and the patient may complain of backache even in the early stage. Conjunctivitis, urethritis and bowel infections are often mild and easily missed; the patient should be carefully questioned about symptoms during the previous few weeks. Cystitis and cervicitis may occur in women.

Less frequent, but equally characteristic, features are a vesicular or pustular dermatitis of the feet (keratoderma blennorrhagicum), balanitis and mild buccal ulceration.

The acute disorder usually lasts for a few weeks or months and then subsides, but most patients have either recurrent attacks of arthritis or other features of chronic disease.

The chronic phase is more characteristic of a spondarthropathy. Over half of the patients with Reiter's disease complain of mild, recurrent episodes of polyarthritis (including upper limb joints). About half of those again develop sacroiliitis and spondylitis with features resembling those of AS. Uveitis is also fairly common and may give rise to posterior synechiae and glaucoma.

X-RAYS Sacroiliac and vertebral changes are similar to those of AS. If peripheral joints are involved, they may show features of erosive arthritis.

SPECIAL INVESTIGATIONS Tests for HLA-B27 are positive in 75% of patients with sacroiliitis. The ESR may be high in the active phase of the disease. The causative organism can sometimes be isolated from urethral fluids or faeces, and tests for antibodies may be positive.

Diagnosis

The diagnosis should be considered in any young adult who presents with an acute or subacute arthritis in the lower limbs. It is more likely to be missed in women, in

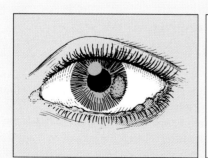 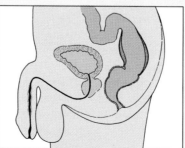 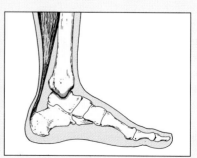

3.13 Reiter's syndrome – the classic triad The classic triad of Reiter's syndrome – conjunctivitis, urethritis (sometimes colitis) and arthritis. Tenderness of the tendo Achillis and the plantar fascia is also common.

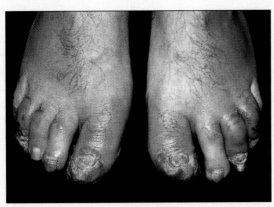

3.14 Reiter's disease – other features The characteristic pustular dermatitis of the feet – keratoderma blenorrhagicum.

children and in those with very mild (and often forgotten) episodes of urogenital or bowel infection. Some patients never develop the full syndrome and one should be alert to the *forme fruste* with large-joint arthritis alone.

GOUT AND INFECTIVE ARTHRITIS Reiter's disease, gout and infection should all be considered in the differential diagnosis of inflammation in a large peripheral joint. Examination of synovial fluid for organisms and crystals may provide important clues.

GONOCOCCAL ARTHRITIS Gonococcal arthritis takes two forms: (1) bacterial infection of the joint, and (2) a reactive arthritis with sterile joint fluid. A history of venereal infection further complicates the distinction from Reiter's disease, and diagnosis may depend on identifying the organism or gonococcal antibodies.

ENTEROPATHIC ARTHRITIS Ulcerative colitis and Crohn's disease may be associated with subacute synovitis, causing pain and swelling of one or more of the peripheral joints. These subside when the intestinal disease is controlled.

Treatment

There is no specific treatment for Reiter's disease; even if the triggering infection is identified, treating it will have no effect on the reactive arthritis. However, there is some evidence that treatment of *Chlamydia* infection with tetracycline for periods of up to 3 months can reduce the risk of recurrent joint disease (Bardin *et al.*, 1992).

Acute arthritis or tendinitis may benefit from local injection of corticosteroids and a period of splintage. Topical corticosteroids are also used for severe uveitis.

For the rest, treatment is palliative and supportive. Patients may need long-term non-steroidal anti-inflammatory and analgesic therapy. If spinal and sacroiliac changes are marked, treatment is the same as for AS.

PSORIATIC ARTHRITIS

Polyarthritis and psoriasis are often seen together. Usually this is simply a chance concurrence of two fairly common disorders. In some cases, however, the patient has a true psoriatic arthritis – a distinct entity characterized by seronegative polysynovitis, erosive (sometimes very destructive) arthritis and a significant incidence of sacroiliitis and spondylitis. The prevalence of psoriasis is 1–2%; only about 5% of those affected will develop psoriatic arthritis. The sex ratio is reported as 1:1 and the usual age at onset 30–50 years (much later than the skin lesions).

Cause

As with the other seronegative spondarthritides, there is a strong genetic component: patients often give a family history of psoriasis; there is a significantly increased incidence of other spondarthritides in close relatives; and 60% of those with psoriatic spondylitis or sacroiliitis have HLA-B27.

Psoriatic skin lesions may well be a reactive phenomenon, and the joint lesions a form of 'reactive arthritis'. However, no specific trigger agent has thus far been identified.

Pathology

The joint changes are similar to those in RA – chronic synovitis with round-cell infiltration and exudate, going on to fibrosis. Cartilage and bone destruction may be unusually severe ('arthritis mutilans'). However, rheumatoid nodules are not seen.

Sacroiliac and spine changes, which occur in about 30% of patients, are similar to those in AS.

Clinical features

The patient usually presents with a comparatively mild, asymmetrical oligoarthritis or polyarthritis affecting some of the interphalangeal joints of the fingers or toes. The condition progresses slowly and may become quiescent. Sometimes (particularly in women) joint involvement is more symmetrical, and in these cases the condition may be indistinguishable from seronegative RA. Asymmetrical swelling of two or three fingers may be due to a combination of interphalangeal arthritis and tenosynovitis. Occasionally a patient may present with an isolated ensethopathy or dactylitis (Salvarini *et al.*, 1997)

Sacroiliitis and spondylitis are seen in about one-third of patients, and occasionally this is the predominant change with a clinical picture resembling AS. As

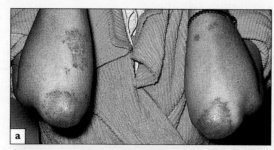

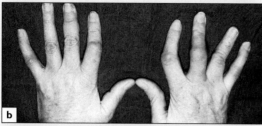

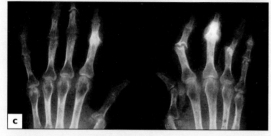

3.15 Psoriatic arthritis (1) **(a)** Psoriasis of the elbows and forearms; **(b)** typical finger deformities, and **(c)** x-rays show distal joint involvement – clearly the disease is not simply rheumatoid arthritis in a patient with psoriasis.

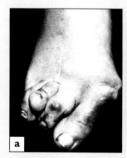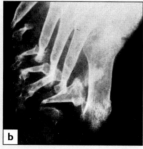

3.16 Psoriatic arthritis (2) The feet and toes are often involved. In this case the patient developed a severely destructive form of the disease (arthritis mutilans).

in the other spondarthritides, heel pain (enthesitis) is not uncommon.

In the worst cases both the spine and the peripheral joints may be involved. Fingers and toes are severely deformed due to erosion and instability of the interphalangeal joints (arthritis mutilans). Psoriasis of the skin or nails usually precedes the arthritis, but hidden lesions (in the natal cleft or umbilicus) are easily overlooked.

Ocular inflammation occurs in about 30% of patients.

X-RAYS There may be severe destruction of the interphalangeal joints of the hands and feet; changes in the large joints are similar to those of rheumatoid disease. Sacroiliac erosion is fairly common; if the spine is involved the appearances are identical to those of AS.

SPECIAL INVESTIGATIONS Tests for RF are almost always negative. HLA-B27 occurs in 50–60% of cases, especially in those with overt sacroiliitis.

Diagnosis

The main difficulty is to distinguish 'psoriatic arthritis' from 'psoriasis with seronegative RA'. The important distinguishing features of psoriatic arthritis are: (1) asymmetrical joint distribution; (2) involvement of distal finger joints; (3) the presence of sacroiliitis or spondylitis; and (4) the absence of rheumatoid nodules.

Treatment

Although joint erosion usually progresses, psoriatic arthritis is usually milder than RA. Most patients require no more than topical preparations to control the skin disease and NSAIDs for the arthritis. In resistant forms of arthritis, low-dosage immunosuppressive agents (azathioprine, cyclosporin and methotrexate) have proved effective, but should not be used if there is renal impairment (Pitzalis and Pipitone, 2000).

Local treatment, when necessary, consists of judicious splintage to avoid undue deformity, and surgery for unstable joints. Arthrodesis of the distal interphalangeal joints may greatly improve function.

ENTEROPATHIC ARTHRITIS

Both Crohn's disease and ulcerative colitis may be associated with either peripheral arthritis or sacroiliitis and spondylitis.

Peripheral arthritis is fairly common, occurring in about 15% of patients with inflammatory bowel disease. Typically one or perhaps a few of the larger joints are involved. Pain and swelling appear quite suddenly and may last for 2–3 months before subsiding. Synovitis is usually the only feature and joint erosion is rare. Men and women are affected with equal frequency and there is no particular association with HLA-B27. Treatment is directed at the underlying disorder: attacks of arthritis are triggered by a flare-up of bowel disease, and when the latter is brought under control the arthritis disappears. Anti-inflammatory drugs are useful if synovitis is marked; they have not been shown to have any deleterious effect on the bowel disease.

Sacroiliitis and spondylitis are seen in about 10% of patients with inflammatory bowel disease, and in half of these patients the clinical picture closely resembles that of AS. HLA-B27 is positive in 60% of cases and there is an increased incidence of AS in close relatives. Unlike the peripheral arthritis, sacroiliitis shows no temporal relationship to gastrointestinal inflammation and its course is unaffected by treatment of the bowel disease. Management is the same as that of AS.

Complications

In addition to spondarthritis, there are several unusual but important complications of inflammatory bowel disease that may confuse the clinical picture.

SEPTIC ARTHRITIS OF THE HIP Infection may spread directly from the bowel. The patient presents with a fever and pain in the groin. Hip movements are limited and there may be swelling due to an abscess. Treatment is by antibiotics and operative drainage.

PSOAS ABSCESS In Crohn's disease a posterior fistula may track into the psoas sheath. The patient complains of back pain and may develop a typical psoas abscess with pain in the hip, limitation of movement and a tender mass in the groin. Treatment is by operative drainage of the abscess.

OSTEOPENIA Patients with chronic bowel disease often develop osteoporosis and osteomalacia – partly due to malabsorption and partly as a consequence of treatment with corticosteroids. Compression fractures of the spine may cause severe back pain. Treatment is futile if the patient has to remain on cortisone.

JUVENILE CHRONIC ARTHRITIS

Juvenile chronic arthritis (JCA) is the preferred term for non-infective inflammatory joint disease of more than 3 months' duration in children under 16 years of age. It embraces a group of disorders in all of which pain, swelling and stiffness of the joints are common features. The prevalence is about 1 per 1000 children, and boys and girls are affected with equal frequency.

The cause is similar to that of rheumatoid disease: an abnormal immune response to some antigen in children with a particular genetic predisposition. However, RF is usually absent.

The pathology, too, is like that of RA: primarily a synovial inflammation leading to fibrosis and ankylosis. Stiffening tends to occur in whatever position the joint is allowed to assume; thus flexion deformities are a common and characteristic feature. Chronic inflammation and alterations in the local blood supply may affect the epiphyseal growth plates, leading to both local bone deformities and an overall retardation of growth. However, cartilage erosion is less marked than in RA and severe joint instability is uncommon.

Clinical features

Children with JCA present in several characteristic ways. About 15% have a *systemic illness*, and arthritis only develops somewhat later; the majority (60–70%) have a *pauciarticular arthritis* affecting a few of the larger joints; about 10% present with *polyarticular arthritis*, sometimes closely resembling RA; the remaining 5–10% develop a *seronegative spondarthritis*.

SYSTEMIC JCA This, the classic *Still's disease*, is usually seen below the age of 3 years and affects boys and girls equally. It starts with intermittent fever, rashes and malaise; during these episodes, which occur almost daily, the child appears to be quite ill but after a few hours the clinical condition improves again. Less constant features are lymphadenopathy, splenomegaly and hepatomegaly. Joint swelling occurs some weeks or months after the onset; fortunately, it usually resolves when the systemic illness subsides but it may go on to progressive seronegative polyarthritis, leading to permanent deformity of the larger joints and fusion of the cervical apophyseal joints. By puberty there may be stunting of growth, often abetted by the earlier use of corticosteroids.

PAUCIARTICULAR JCA This is by far the commonest form of JCA. It usually occurs below the age of 6 years and is much more common in girls; occasionally older children are affected. Only a few joints are involved and there is no systemic illness. The child presents with pain and swelling of medium-sized joints (knees, ankles, elbows and wrists); sometimes only one joint is affected. RF tests are negative. A serious complication is chronic iridocyclitis, which occurs in about 50% of cases. The arthritis often goes into remission after a few years, but by then the child is left with asymmetrical deformities and growth defects that may be permanent.

POLYARTICULAR JCA Polyarticular arthritis, typically with involvement of the temporomandibular joints and the cervical spine, is usually seen in older children, mainly girls. The hands and wrists are often affected, but the classic deformities of RA are uncommon and RF is usually absent. In some cases, however, the condition is

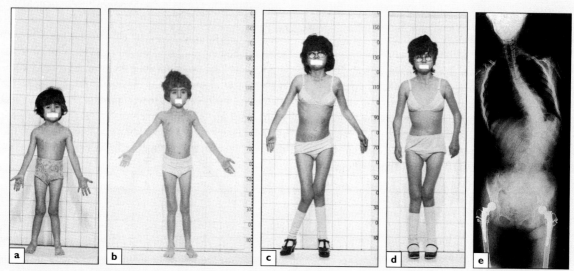

3.17 Juvenile chronic arthritis (a–d) This young girl developed JCA when she was 5 years old. Here we see her at 6, 9 and 14 years of age. The arthritis has become inactive, leaving her with a knee deformity which was treated by osteotomy. Her eyes, too, were affected by iridocyclitis. (Courtesy of Mr Malcolm Swann and Dr Barbara Ansell). **(e)** X-ray of another young girl who required hip replacements at the age of 14 years and, later, surgical correction of her scoliosis.

indistinguishable from adult RA, with a positive RF test; these probably warrant the designation 'juvenile RA'.

SERONEGATIVE SPONDARTHRITIS In older children – usually boys – the condition may take the form of sacroiliitis and spondylitis; hips and knees are sometimes involved as well. Tests for HLA-B27 are often positive and this should probably be regarded as 'juvenile AS'.

X-rays

In early disease non-specific changes such as soft-tissue swelling may be seen, but x-ray is mainly useful to exclude other painful disorders. Later there may be signs of progressive joint erosion and deformity.

Investigations

The white cell count and ESR are markedly raised in systemic JCA, less so in the other forms. RF tests are positive only in juvenile RA. Joint aspiration and synovial fluid examination may be essential to exclude infection or haemarthrosis.

Diagnosis

In the early stages, before chronic arthritis is fully established, diagnosis may be difficult. Systemic JCA may start with an illness resembling a viral infection. Pauciarticular JCA, especially if only one joint is involved, is indistinguishable from *Reiter's disease* or *septic arthritis* (if the signs are acute) or *tuberculous synovitis* (if they are more subdued).

Other conditions that need to be excluded are *rheumatic fever*, one of *the bleeding disorders* and *leukaemia*.

In most cases the problem is resolved once the full pattern of joint involvement is established, but blood investigations, joint aspiration and synovial biopsy may be required to clinch the diagnosis.

Treatment

GENERAL TREATMENT Systemic treatment is similar to that of RA, including the use of second-line drugs such as hydroxychloroquine, sulfasalazine or low-dose methotrexate for those with seropositive juvenile RA. Corticosteroids should be used only for severe systemic disease and for chronic iridocyclitis unresponsive to topical therapy.

Children and parents alike need sympathetic counselling to help them cope with the difficulties of social adjustments, education and training.

LOCAL TREATMENT The priorities are to prevent stiffness and deformity. Night splints are useful for the wrists, hands, knees and ankles; prone lying for some period of each day may prevent flexion contracture of the hips. Between periods of splinting, active exercises are encouraged; these are started by the physiotherapist but the parents must be taught how to continue the programme.

Fixed deformities may need correction by serial plasters or by a spell in hospital on a CPM machine; when progress is no longer being made, joint capsulotomy may help. For painful eroded joints, useful procedures include custom-designed arthroplasties of the hip and knee (even in children), and arthrodesis of the wrist or ankle.

Complications

ANKYLOSIS Whilst most patients recover good function, some loss of movement is common. Hips, knees and elbows may be unable to extend fully, and in the spondylitic form of JCA the spine, hips and knees may be almost rigid. Temporomandibular ankylosis and stiffness of the cervical spine can make general anaesthesia difficult and dangerous.

GROWTH DEFECTS There is a general retardation of growth, aggravated by prolonged corticosteroid therapy. In addition, epiphyseal disturbances lead to characteristic deformities: external torsion of the tibia, dysplasia of the distal ulna, underdevelopment of the mandible, shortness of the neck and scoliosis.

FRACTURES Children aged under 5 years with chronic joint disease may suffer osteoporosis and they are prone to fractures.

IRIDOCYCLITIS This is most common in pauciarticular disease; untreated it may lead to blindness.

AMYLOIDOSIS In children with long-standing active disease there is a serious risk of amyloidosis, which may be fatal.

Prognosis

Fortunately, most children with JCA recover from the arthritis and are left with only moderate deformity and limitation of function. However, 5–10% (and especially those with juvenile RA) are severely crippled and require treatment throughout life.

A significant number of children with JCA (about 3%) still die – usually as a result of renal failure due to amyloidosis, or following overwhelming infection.

THE SYSTEMIC CONNECTIVE TISSUE DISEASES

This term is applied to a group of closely related conditions that have features which overlap with those of rheumatoid disease. Like RA, these are 'autoimmune disorders', probably triggered by viral infection in genetically predisposed individuals.

SYSTEMIC LUPUS ERYTEMATOSUS

Systemic lupus occurs mainly in young females and may be difficult to differentiate from RA. Although joint pain is usual, it is often overshadowed by systemic symptoms such as malaise, anorexia, weight loss and fever. Characteristic clinical features are skin rashes (especially the 'butterfly rash' of the face), Raynaud's phenomenon, peripheral vasculitis, splenomegaly, and disorders of the kidney, heart, lung, eye and central nervous system. Anaemia, leucopenia and elevation of the ESR are common. Tests for antinuclear factor are always positive.

Treatment Corticosteroids are indicated for severe systemic disease and may have to be continued for life. Progressive joint deformity is unusual and the arthritis can almost always be controlled by anti-inflammatory drugs, physiotherapy and intermittent splintage.

Complications A curious complication of SLE is avascular necrosis (usually of the femoral head). This may be due in part to the corticosteroid treatment, but the disease itself seems to predispose to bone ischaemia, possibly as a manifestation of the antiphospholipid syndrome which sometimes accompanies SLE (see Chapter 6).

REFERENCES AND FURTHER READING

American College of Rheumatology and Ad Hoc Committee on Clinical Guidelines (1996) Guidelines for monitoring drug therapy in rheumatoid arthritis. *Arthritis and Rheumatism* 39, 723–731

Bardin T, Enel C, Cornelis F *et al.* (1992) Antibiotic treatment of venereal disease and Reiter's syndrome in a Greenland population. *Arthritis and Rheumatism* 350, 190

Kelley WN, Harris ED, Ruddy S, Sledge CB (1997) *Textbook of Rheumatology*, 5th edn. WB Saunders Co, Philadelphia

Kirwin JR and the Arthritis and Rheumatism Council Low-dosage Glucocorticoid Study Group (1995) The effect of glucocorticoids on joint destruction in rheumatoid arthritis. *New England Journal of Medicine* 333, 142–146

Kirwin JR (1997) The relationship between synovitis and erosions in rheumatoid arthritis. *British Journal of Rheumatology* 36, 225–228

Pitzalis C, Pipitone N (2000) Psoriatic arthritis. *Journal of the Royal Society of Medicine* 93, 412–415

Salvarini C, Cantini F, Olivieri I *et al.* (1997) Isolated peripheral enthesitis and for dactylitis: a subset of psoriatic arthritis. *Journal of Rheumatology* 24, 1106–1110

Solomon L, Beighton P, Valkenburg HA *et al.* (1975) Rheumatic disorders in the South African Negro. *South African Medical Journal* 49, 1292–1296

4 Crystal deposition disorders

The crystal deposition disorders are a group of conditions characterized by the presence of crystals in and around joints, bursae and tendons. Although many different crystals are found, three clinical conditions in particular are associated with this phenomenon:

- gout
- calcium pyrophosphate dihydrate (CPPD) deposition disease
- calcium hydroxyapatite (HA) deposition disorders

Characteristically, in each of the three conditions, crystal deposition has three distinct consequences: (1) it may be totally *inert and asymptomatic*; (2) it may induce *an acute inflammatory reaction*; or (3) it may result in *slow destruction* of the affected tissues.

GOUT

This is a disorder of purine metabolism characterized by hyperuricaemia, deposition of monosodium urate monohydrate crystals in joints and per-articular tissues and recurrent attacks of acute synovitis. Late changes include cartilage degeneration, renal dysfunction and uric acid urolithiasis.

The clinical disorder was known to Hippocrates and its association with hyperiuricaemia was recognized well over 100 years ago. The prevalence of symptomatic gout varies from 1 to over 10 per thousand, depending on the race, sex and age of the population studied. It is much commoner in Caucasian than in black African peoples; it is more widespread in men than in women (the ratio may be as high as 20:1) and it is rarely seen before the menopause in females.

Although the risk of developing clinical features of gout increases with increasing levels of serum uric acid, only a fraction of those with hyperuricaemia develop symptoms. However, 'hyperuricaemia' and 'gout' are generally regarded as part and parcel of the same disorder.

Pathology

HYPERURICAEMIA Nucleic acid and purine metabolism normally proceeds, through complex pathways, to the production of hypoxanthine and xanthine; the final breakdown to uric acid is catalysed by the enzyme xanthine oxidase. Monosodium urate appears in ionic form in all the body fluids; about 70% is derived from endogenous purine metabolism and 30% from purine-rich foods in the diet. It is excreted (as uric acid) mainly by the kidneys and partly in the gut.

Urate is poorly soluble, with a plasma saturation value of only 7mg/dl (0.42mmol/l). This concentration is commonly exceeded in normal individuals and epidemiological studies have identified entire populations (for example the Maoris of New Zealand) who have unusually high levels of serum uric acid. The term 'hyperuricaemia' is therefore generally reserved for individuals with a serum urate concentration which is significantly higher than that of the population to which they belong (more than two standard deviations above the mean); this is about 0.42mmol/l for men and 0.35mmol/l for women in Western Caucasian peoples. By this definition, about 5% of men and less than 1% of women have hyperuricaemia; the majority suffer no pathological consequences and they remain asymptomatic throughout life.

GOUT Urate crystals are deposited in minute clumps in connective tissue, including articular cartilage; the commonest sites are the small joints of the hands and feet. For months, perhaps years, they remain inert. Then, possibly as a result of local trauma, the needle-like crystals are dispersed into the joint and the surrounding tissues where they excite an acute inflammatory reaction. Individual crystals may be phagocytosed by synovial cells and polymorphs or may float free in the synovial fluid.

With the passage of time, urate deposits may build up in joints, periarticular tissues, tendons and bursae; common sites are around the metatarsophalangeal joints of the big toes, the Achilles tendons, the olecranon bursae and the pinnae of the ears. These clumps of chalky material, or tophi (L. *tophus* = porous stone), vary in size from less than 1mm to several centimetres in diameter. They may ulcerate through the skin or destroy cartilage and periarticular bone.

Classification

Gout is often classified into 'primary' and 'secondary' forms. *Primary gout* (95%) occurs in the absence of any obvious cause and may be due to constitutional under-excretion (the vast majority) or overproduction of urate.

Secondary gout (5%) results from prolonged hyperuricaemia due to acquired disorders such as myeloproliferative diseases, administration of diuretics or renal failure.

This division is somewhat artificial; people with an initial tendency to 'primary' hyperuricaemia may develop gout only when secondary factors are introduced – for example obesity and alcohol abuse, or treatment with diuretics or salicylates which increase tubular reabsorption of uric acid.

Clinical features

Patients are usually men over the age of 30 years; women are seldom affected until after the menopause. Often there is a family history of gout.

The gouty stereotype is obese, rubicund, hypertensive and fond of alcohol. However, many patients have none of these attributes and some are nudged into an attack by the uncontrolled administration of diuretics or aspirin.

THE ACUTE ATTACK The sudden onset of severe joint pain that lasts for a week or two before resolving completely is typical of acute gout. The attack usually comes out of the blue, but may be precipitated by minor trauma, operation, intercurrent illness, unaccustomed exercise or alcohol. The commonest sites are the metatarsophalangeal joint of the big toe, the ankle and finger joints, and the olecranon bursa. Occasionally, more than one site is involved. The skin looks red and shiny and there is considerable swelling. The joint feels hot and extremely tender, suggesting a cellulitis or septic arthritis. Sometimes the only feature is acute pain and tenderness in the heel or the sole. Hyperuricaemia is present at some stage, though not necessarily during an acute attack. However, whilst a low serum uric acid makes gout unlikely, hyperuricaemia is not 'diagnostic' and is often seen in normal middle-aged men.

The true diagnosis can be established beyond doubt by finding the characteristic negatively birefringent urate crystals in the synovial fluid. A drop of fluid on a glass slide is examined by polarizing microscopy. Crystals may be sparse but if the fluid specimen is centrifuged a concentrated pellet may be obtained for examination.

CHRONIC GOUT Recurrent acute attacks may eventually merge into polyarticular gout. Joint erosion causes chronic pain, stiffness and deformity; if the finger joints are affected, this may be mistaken for rheumatoid arthritis (RA). Tophi may appear around joints, over the olecranon, in the pinna of the ear and – less frequently – in almost any other tissue. A large tophus can ulcerate through the skin and discharge its chalky material. Renal lesions include calculi, due to uric acid precipitation in the urine, and parenchy-mal disease due to deposition of monosodium urate from the blood.

X-rays

During the acute attack x-rays show only soft-tissue swelling. Chronic gout may result in joint space narrowing and secondary osteoarthritis. Tophi appear as characteristic punched-out 'cysts' or deep erosions in the para-articular bone ends; these excavations are larger and slightly further from the joint margin than the typical rheumatoid erosions. Occasionally, bone destruction is more marked and may resemble neoplastic disease (see Fig. 9.2).

Differential diagnosis

INFECTION Cellulitis, septic bursitis, an infected bunion or septic arthritis must all be excluded, if necessary by immediate joint aspiration. Remember that crystals and sepsis may coexist, so always send fluid for both culture and crystal analysis.

REITER'S DISEASE This may present with acute pain and swelling of a knee or ankle, but the history is more protracted and the response to anti-inflammatory drugs less dramatic.

PSEUDOGOUT Pyrophosphate crystal deposition may cause an acute arthritis indistinguishable from gout – except that it tends to affect large rather than small joints and is somewhat more common in women than in men. Articular calcification may show on x-ray. Demonstrating the crystals in synovial fluid establishes the diagnosis.

RHEUMATOID ARTHRITIS Polyarticular gout affecting the fingers may be mistaken for RA, and elbow tophi for rheumatoid nodules. In difficult cases biopsy will establish the diagnosis. RA and gout seldom occur together.

Treatment

The acute attack should be treated by resting the joint and giving large doses of one of the non-steroidal anti-inflammatory drugs. Colchicine is less effective and may cause diarrhoea, nausea and vomiting. A tense joint effusion may require aspiration and local injection of hydrocortisone.

Between attacks, attention should be given to simple measures such as losing weight, cutting out alcohol and eliminating diuretics. Interval therapy is indicated if acute attacks recur at frequent intervals, if there are tophi or if renal function is impaired. Asymptomatic hyperuricaemia does not call for treatment. Uricosuric

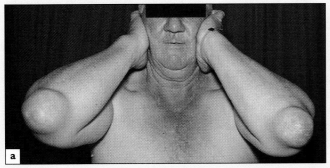

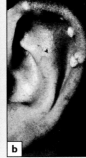

4.1 Gout (1) This man with chronic gout declares his diagnosis at a glance, with his rubicund face, bulging olecranan bursae and tophi.

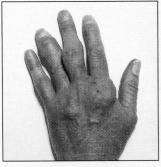

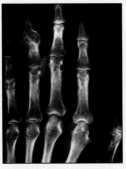

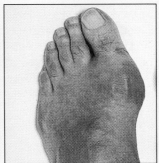

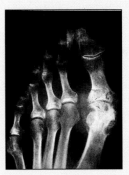

4.2 Gout (2) In both the hand and the foot, joints are asymmetrically swollen; x-rays show large periarticular excavations, which are filled with uric acid deposits. The joints are curiously 'pulpy'.

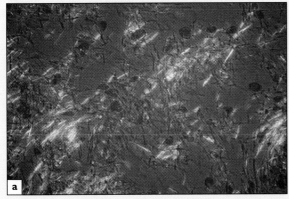

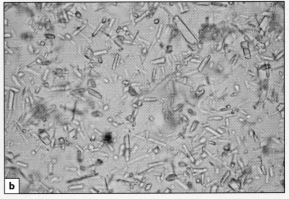

4.3 Crystals In polarized light, crystals appear bright on a dark background. If a compensator is added to the optical system, the background appears in shades of mauve and the birefringent crystals as yellow or blue, depending on their spatial orientation. In these two specimens (obtained from crystal deposits in cartilage) there are differences in shape, size and type of birefringence of the crystals. **(a)** Urate crystals are needle-like, 5–20cm long and exhibit strong negative birefringence. **(b)** Pyrophosphate crystals are rhomboid-shaped, slightly smaller than urate crystals and show weak positive birefringence. (Courtesy of Professor PA Dieppe.)

drugs (probenecid or sulfinpyrazone) can be used if renal function is normal. Allopurinol, a xanthine oxidase inhibitor, is usually preferred. *These drugs should never be started during an acute attack, and they should always be covered by an anti-inflammatory preparation or colchicine*; otherwise they may actually precipitate an acute attack. In chronic tophaceous gout, and in all patients with renal complications, allopurinol is the drug of choice. With prolonged administration, adjusted to maintain a normal serum uric acid level (less than 0.4mmol/l), tophi may gradually dissolve. Ulcerating tophi that fail to heal with conservative treatment can be evacuated by curettage; the wound is left open and dressings are applied until it heals.

CALCIUM PYROPHOSPHATE DIHYDRATE DEPOSITION

'CPPD deposition' encompasses three overlapping conditions: (1) *chondrocalcinosis* – the appearance of calcific material in articular cartilage and menisci; (2) *pseudo-gout* – a crystal-induced synovitis; and (3) *chronic pyrophosphate arthropathy* – a type of degenerative joint disease. Any one of these conditions may occur on its own or in any combination with the others (Dieppe *et al.*, 1982). In contrast to classic gout, serum biochemistry shows no consistent abnormality.

CPPD crystal deposition is known to occur in certain metabolic disorders (e.g. hyperparathyroidism and haemochromatosis) that cause a critical change in ionic calcium and pyrophosphate equilibrium in cartilage. The rare familial forms of chondrocalcinosis are probably due to a similar biochemical defect. However, in the vast majority of cases chondrocalcinosis follows some local change in the cartilage due to ageing, degeneration, enzymatic degradation or trauma.

Pathology

Pyrophosphate is probably generated in abnormal cartilage by enzyme activity at chondrocyte surfaces; it combines with calcium ions in the matrix where crystal nucleation occurs on collagen fibres. The crystals grow into microscopic 'tophi', which appear as nests of amorphous material in the cartilage matrix. Chondrocalcinosis is most pronounced in fibrocartilaginous structures (e.g. the menisci of the knee, triangular ligament of the wrist, pubic symphysis and intervertebral discs), but may also occur in hyaline articular cartilage, tendons and periarticular soft tissues.

From time to time CPPD crystals are extruded into the joint where they excite an inflammatory reaction similar to gout. The long-standing presence of CPPD crystals also seems to influence the development of osteoarthritis in joints not usually prone to this condition (e.g. elbows and ankles). Characteristically, there is a hypertrophic reaction with marked osteophyte formation but sometimes, for reasons that are poorly understood, the joint shows severe destructive changes.

Clinical features

The clinical disorder takes several forms, all of them appearing with increasing frequency in relation to age. Most of the patients are women over the age of 60 years.

ASYMPTOMATIC CHONDROCALCINOSIS Calcification of the menisci is common in elderly people and is usually asymptomatic. When it is seen in association with osteoarthritis, this does not necessarily imply cause and effect. Both are common in elderly people and they are bound to be seen together in some patients; x-rays may reveal chondrocalcinosis in other, asymptomatic, joints. Chondrocalcinosis in patients under 50 years of age should suggest the possibility of an underlying metabolic disease or a familial disorder.

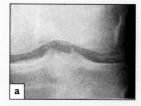
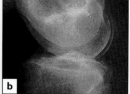

4.4 Chondrocalcinosis Calcium pyrophosphate crystals may be deposited in cartilage, causing (**a**) calcification of menisci and (**b**) a thin, dense line within the articular cartilage. Usually no specific cause is found, but chondrocalcinosis may be associated with metabolic disorders such as hyperparathyroidism and haemochromatosis.

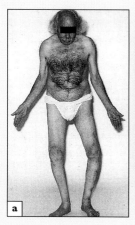
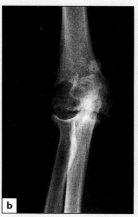
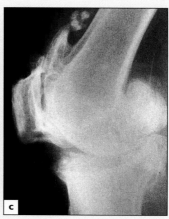

4.5 Pyrosphate arthropathy (**a, b**) A middle-aged man who presented with osteoarthritis in several of the larger joints, including unusual sites such as the elbow and ankle. (**c**) The left knee was the worst and x-ray showed the characteristic features of articular calcification, loose bodies in the joint and large trailing osteophytes around the patellofemoral joint.

ACUTE SYNOVITIS (PSEUDOGOUT) The patient, typically a middle-aged woman, complains of acute pain and swelling in one of the larger joints – usually the knee. Sometimes the attack is precipitated by a minor illness or operation. The joint is tense and inflamed, though usually not as acutely as in gout. Untreated the condition lasts for a few weeks and then subsides spontaneously. *X-rays* may show signs of chondrocalcinosis, and the diagnosis can be confirmed by finding *positively birefringent crystals* in the synovial fluid.

CHRONIC PYROPHOSPHATE ARTHROPATHY The patient, usually an elderly woman, presents with polyarticular 'osteoarthritis' affecting the larger joints (hips, knees) and – more helpfully – unusual joints, such as the ankles, shoulders, elbows and wrists where osteoarthritis is seldom seen. There are the usual features of pain, stiffness, swelling, joint crepitus and loss of movement. It is often diagnosed, simply, as 'generalized osteoarthritis', but the x-ray features are distinctive. Sometimes alternating bouts of acute synovitis and chronic arthritis may mimic rheumatoid disease. Occasionally joint destruction is so marked as to suggest neuropathic joint disease.

X-rays

The characteristic x-ray features arise from a combination of (1) intra-articular and periarticular calcification, and (2) degenerative arthritis in distinctive sites (Resnick and Resnick, 1983).

Calcification is usually seen in and around the knees, wrists, shoulders, hips, pubic symphysis and intervertebral discs; it is often bilateral and symmetrical. In articular cartilage it appears as a thin line parallel to the joint. In the fibrocartilaginous menisci and discs it produces cloudy, irregular opacities. Less common sites are the joint synovium, capsule, ligaments, tendons and bursae.

Degenerative changes are similar to those of straightforward osteoarthritis but notably involving unusual sites such as the non-weightbearing joints, the isolated patellofemoral compartment in the knee and the talonavicular joint in the foot. In advanced cases joint destruction may be marked, with the formation of loose bodies.

Diagnosis

THE ACUTE ATTACK
'Pseudogout' must be distinguished from other acute inflammatory disorders.

Acute gout usually occurs in men, and typically in smaller joints or in the olecranon bursa. The final word often lies with joint aspiration and identification of the characteristic crystals.

Post-traumatic haemarthrosis can be misleading; pseudogout is often precipitated by trauma. A clear history and aspiration of blood-stained fluid will solve the problem.

Septic arthritis must not be missed; a delay of 24 hours can mean the difference between successful and unsuccessful treatment. Systemic features are more evident, but blood tests and joint aspiration are essential to clinch the diagnosis; joint fluid should be submitted with a request for both crystal analysis and bacteriological culture.

Reiter's disease can start in a single large joint; always enquire about (and look for) signs of conjunctivitis, urethritis and colitis.

CHRONIC CPPD ARTHROPATHY
Chronic pyrophosphate arthropathy usually affects multiple joints and it has to be distinguished from other types of polyarticular arthritis.

Osteoarthritis and joint calcification are both common in older people; the two together do not necessarily make it a CPPD arthropathy. The distinctive x-ray features, and especially the involvement of unusual joints (the elbow, wrist and ankle), point to a CPPD disorder, rather than a simple concurrence of two common conditions.

Inflammatory polyarthritis usually involves the smaller joints as well, and systemic features of inflammation are more marked.

Metabolic disorders such as *hyperparathyroidism, haemochromatosis* and *alkaptonuria* may be associated with calcification of articular cartilage and fibrocartilage as well as joint symptoms. It is important to exclude such generalized disorders before labelling a patient as 'just another case of chondrocalcinosis'.

Haemochromatosis is an uncommon disorder of middle-aged people (usually men), resulting from chronic iron overload. The clinical features are those of cirrhosis and diabetes, with a typical bronze pigmentation of the skin. About half of the patients develop

Table 4.1 Gout and pseudogout	
Gout	**Pseudogout**
Smaller joints	Large joints
Pain intense	Pain moderate
Joint inflamed	Joint swollen
Hyperuricaemia	Chondrocalcinosis
Uric acid crystals	Ca pyrophosphate crystals

joint symptoms (particularly in the hands and fingers); some also have chronic backache. X-rays reveal chondrocalcinosis and a destructive arthropathy, typically in the metacarpophalangeal joints. The plasma iron and iron-binding capacity are raised.

Alkaptonuria is a rare, heritable metabolic disorder characterized by the appearance of homogentisic acid in the urine, dark pigmentation of the connective tissues (*ochronosis*) and calcification of hyaline and fibrocartilage. The inborn error is an absence of homogentisic acid oxidase in the liver and kidney. Those affected usually remain asymptomatic until the third or fourth decade when they present with pain and stiffness of the spine and (later) larger joints. There may also be dark pigmentation of the ear cartilage and the sclerae, and clothes may become stained by homogentisic acid in the sweat. X-rays reveal narrowing and calcification of the intervertebral discs at multiple levels, and spinal osteoporosis. At a later stage the large peripheral joints may show chondrocalcinosis and severe osteoarthritis. The feature which gives the condition its name is that the urine turns dark brown when it is alkalinized or if it is left to stand for some hours.

Hyperparathyroidism is described on page 123.

Treatment

The treatment of *pseudogout* is the same as that of acute gout: rest and high-dosage anti-inflammatory therapy. In elderly patients joint aspiration and intra-articular corticosteroid injection is the treatment of choice as these patients are more vulnerable to the side effects of non-steroidal anti-inflammatory drugs.

Chronic chondrocalcinosis appears to be irreversible. Fortunately it usually causes few symptoms and little disability. When it is associated *with progressive joint degeneration* the treatment is essentially that of advanced osteoarthritis.

CALCIUM HYDROXYAPATITE DEPOSITION DISORDERS

Crystalline calcium HA is a normal component of bone mineral. It also occurs abnormally in dead or damaged tissue. Minute deposits in joints and periarticular tissues can give rise to either an acute reaction (synovitis or tendinitis) or a chronic, destructive arthropathy.

Prolonged hypercalcaemia or hyperphosphataemia, of whatever cause, may result in widespread metastatic calcification. However, by far the most common cause of HA crystal deposition in and around joints is local tissue damage – torn ligaments, tendon attrition and cartilage damage or degeneration.

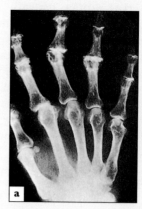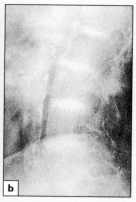

4.6 Haemochromatosis and alkaptonuria
(a) *Haemochromatosis*: the degenerative arthritis of the proximal finger joints is typical. (b) *Alkaptonuria*: the intervertebral discs are calcified – this man has backache.

Pathology

The minute (less than 1μm) HA crystals are deposited around chondrocytes in articular cartilage and in relatively avascular or damaged parts of tendons and ligaments – most notably around the shoulder and knee. The deposits grow by crystal accretion and eventually may be detectable by x-ray in the periarticular tendons or ligaments. Calcification of the posterior longitudinal ligament of the cervical spine may also be associated with HA crystal deposition.

Sometimes the calcific deposit has a creamy consistency but in long-standing cases it is more like chalk. The mini-tophus may be completely inert; but in symptomatic cases it is surrounded by an acute vascular reaction and inflammation. Crystal shedding into joints may give rise to synovitis. More rarely this is complicated by the development of a rapidly destructive, erosive arthritis.

Clinical features

Two clinical syndromes are associated with HA crystal deposition: (1) an acute or subacute periarthritis, and (2) a chronic destructive arthritis.

ACUTE OR SUBACUTE PERIARTHRITIS
This is by far the commonest form of HA crystal deposition disorder affecting joints. The patient, usually an adult between 30 and 50 years, complains of pain close to one of the larger joints – most commonly the shoulder or the knee. Symptoms may start suddenly, perhaps after minor trauma, and rise to a crescendo during which the tissues around the joint are swollen, warm and exquisitely tender – but tender *near* the joint in relation to a tendon or ligament, rather than *in* the joint. At other times the onset is more gradual and it is

easier to localize the area of tenderness to one of the periarticular structures. Both forms of the condition are seen most commonly in the rotator cuff lesions of the shoulder. Symptoms usually subside after a few weeks or months; sometimes they are aborted only when the calcific deposit is removed or the surrounding tissues are decompressed. In acute cases, operation may disclose a tense globule of creamy material oozing from between the frayed fibres of tendon or ligament.

CHRONIC DESTRUCTIVE ARTHRITIS

HA crystals are sometimes found in association with a chronic erosive arthritis; whether they cause the arthritis or modify a pre-existing disorder remains uncertain.

A more dramatic type of rapidly destructive arthritis of the shoulder is occasionally seen in elderly patients with rotator cuff lesions. This was described in 1981 by McCarty and his colleagues from Milwaukee and has acquired the sobriquet 'Milwaukee shoulder'. Similar conditions affect the hip and knee. They have been attributed to HA crystal (or mixed HA and CPPD crystal) shedding, but there remains some doubt about the true association with crystal deposition.

X–rays

With periarthritis, calcification may be seen in tendons or ligaments close to the joint, most commonly in the rotator cuff around the shoulder.

Articular cartilage and fibrocartilaginous menisci and discs never show the type of calcification seen in CPPD deposition disease, but 'loose bodies' may be seen in synovial joints. Erosive arthritis causes loss of the articular space, with little or no sclerosis or osteophyte formation. In destructive arthritis, subchondral bone is severely eroded or excavated.

Investigations

There is little help from special investigations. Serum biochemistry is usually normal, except in those patients

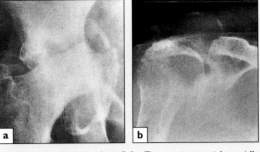

4.7 Rapidly destructive OA Two patients with rapidly destructive OA of a large joint, (**a**) the hip in one and (**b**) the shoulder in the other. Common features are rapid progression to joint disruption, crumbling of the sub-articular bone and peri-articular ossification.

with hypercalcaemia or hyperphosphataemia. Synovial fluid examination may reveal high counts of polymorphonuclear leucocytes, but this hardly serves to distinguish the condition from other types of subacute synovitis. HA crystals can be identified only by electron probe or transmission electron microscopy.

Treatment

Acute periarthritis should be treated by rest and non-steroidal anti-inflammatory drugs. Resistant cases may respond to local injection of corticosteroids; they should be used only to weather the acute storm – repeated injections for lesser pain may dampen the repair process in damaged tendons or ligaments and thus predispose to recurrent attacks. Persistent pain and tenderness may call for operative removal of the calcific deposit or 'decompression' of the affected tendon or ligament.

Erosive arthritis is treated like osteoarthritis. However, rapidly progressive bone destruction calls for early operation: in the case of the shoulder, synovectomy and soft-tissue repair; for the hip, usually total joint replacement.

REFERENCES AND FURTHER READING

Dieppe PA, Alexander GJM, Jones HE *et al.* (1982) Pyrophosphate arthropathy: a clinical and radiological study of 105 cases. *Annals of the Rheumatic Diseases* 41, 371-376

McCarty DJ, Halverson PB, Carrera GF *et al.* (1981) 'Milwaukee shoulder' – association of microspheroids containing hydroxyapatite crystals, active collagenase and neutral protease with rotator cuff defects. *Arthritis and Rheumatism* 24, 464-473

Resnick CS, Resnick D (1983) Crystal deposition disease. *Seminars in Arthritis and Rheumatism* 12, 390-403

5 Osteoarthritis

ARTICULAR CARTILAGE

Hyaline cartilage, the pearly gristle which covers the bone ends in every diarthrodeal joint, is supremely adapted to transmit load and movement from one skeletal segment to another. It increases the area of the articular surfaces and helps to improve their adaptability and stability; it changes its shape under load and distributes compressive forces widely to the subarticular bone; and, covered by a film of synovial fluid, it is more slippery than any man-made material, offering very little frictional resistance to movement and surface gliding.

This specialized connective tissue has a gel-like matrix consisting of a proteoglycan ground substance in which are embedded an architecturally structured collagen network and a relatively sparse scattering of specialized cells, the chondrocytes, which are responsible for producing all the structural components of the tissue. It has a high water content (60–80%), most of which is exchangeable with the synovial fluid.

The proteoglycans exist mainly in the form of aggregan, a large aggregating molecule with a protein core along which are arranged up to 100 chondroitin sulphate and keratan sulphate glycosaminoglycans (GAGs), rather like the bristles on a bottlebrush. Hundreds of aggregan molecules are linked, in turn, to a long, unbranched hyalurinate chain (hyaluronan), to form an even larger molecule with a molecular weight of over 100 million Daltons. These negatively charged macromolecules are responsible for the stiffness and springiness of articular cartilage.

The fibrillar component of articular cartilage is mainly type II collagen. The collagen bundles are arranged in structured patterns, parallel to the articular surface in the superficial zones and perpendicular to the surface in the deeper layers where they anchor the articular cartilage to the subchondral bone.

There is considerable interaction between the molecules of each component and between the molecules of the different components of cartilage: if these links are degraded or broken, the cartilage will tend to unravel. This happens to some degree with ageing, but much more so in pathological states leading to osteoarthritis.

Proteoglycans have a strong affinity for water, resulting in the collagen network being subjected to considerable tensile stresses. With loading, the cartilage deforms and water is slowly squeezed onto the surface where it helps to form a lubricating film. When loading ceases, the surface fluid seeps back into the cartilage up to the joint where the swelling pressure in the cartilage is balanced by the tensile force of the collagen network. As long as the network holds and the proteoglycans remain intact, cartilage retains its compressibility and elasticity. If the collagen network is disrupted, the matrix becomes waterlogged and soft; this, in turn, is followed by loss of proteoglycans, cellular damage and splitting ('fibrillation') of the articular cartilage. Trouble mounts up further as the damaged chondrocytes begin to release matrix-degrading enzymes.

OSTEOARTHRITIS

Osteoarthritis (OA) is a chronic joint disorder in which there is progressive softening and disintegration of articular cartilage accompanied by new growth of cartilage and bone at the joint margins (osteophytes) and capsular fibrosis. It differs from simple wear and tear in several ways: it is asymmetrically distributed and often localized to only one part of a joint; and it is related to abnormal loading rather than frictional wear. In its most common form, it is unaccompanied by any systemic illness and, although there are sometimes local signs of inflammation, it is not primarily an inflammatory disorder.

It is also not a purely degenerative disorder, and the term 'degenerative arthritis' – which is often used as a synonym for OA – is a misnomer. OA is a dynamic phenomenon; it shows features of both destruction and repair. Cartilage softening and disintegration are accompanied from the very outset by hyperactive new bone formation, osteophytosis and remodelling. The final picture is determined by the relative vigour of these opposing processes. In addition, there are various secondary factors which influence the progress of the disorder: the appearance of calcium-containing crystals in the joint; ischaemic changes (especially in elderly people) which result in areas of osteonecrosis in the subchondral bone; the appearance of joint instability; and the effects of prolonged anti-inflammatory medication.

Etiology

The most obvious thing about OA is that it increases in frequency with age. This does not mean that OA is simply an expression of senescence. Cartilage does 'age', showing diminished cellularity, reduced proteoglycan

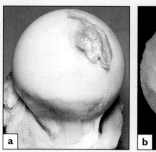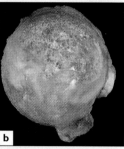

5.1 Osteoarthritis: non-progressive and progressive (a)
Non-progressive OA changes are common in older people; here
we see them along the inferomedial edge of the femoral head,
while the articular cartilage over the rest of the head looks perfect. **(b)** Progressive OA changes are seen characteristically in
the maximal load-bearing area; in the hip this is the superior part
of the joint. Articular cartilage has been destroyed, leaving a bald
patch on the dome of the femoral head.

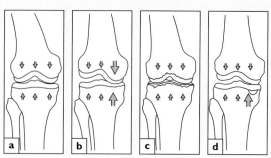

5.2 Osteoarthritis – causal factors In the normal joint **(a)**
the forces are evenly distributed. The remaining diagrams show
the three ways in which cartilage may be damaged: **(b)** deformity increases the stress in a localized area by concentrating the
load at this point; **(c)** cartilage which has been weakened by some
preceding disorder is unable to bear even normal loads; **(d)** if the
subarticular bone is abnormal it may be unable to support the
cartilage adequately.

concentration, loss of elasticity and a decrease in breaking strength with advancing years. These factors may
well predispose to OA, but it is significant that the
progressive changes which are associated with clinical and
radiological deterioration are restricted to certain joints,
and to specific areas of those joints, while other areas
show little or no progression with age (Byers *et al.*, 1970).

Primary changes in cartilage matrix might (theoretically) weaken its structure and thus predispose to cartilage breakdown; crystal deposition disease and
ochronosis are well-known examples, and genetic
defects in type II collagen have been demonstrated in
some cases (Palotie *et al.*, 1989; Knowlton *et al.*, 1990).
However, it is unlikely that factors such as these are the
sole determinants of OA.

Articular cartilage may be damaged by previous
inflammatory disorders. Enzymes released by synovial
cells and leucocytes can cause leaching of proteoglycans
from the matrix, and synovial-derived interleukin-1 (IL-
1) may suppress proteoglycan synthesis. This may
explain the appearance of secondary OA in patients with
rheumatoid diseases; whether similar processes operate
in 'idiopathic' or 'primary' OA is unknown.

In the majority of cases the precipitating cause of OA
is increased mechanical stress in some part of the articular surface. This may be due to increased load (e.g. in
deformities that affect the lever system around a joint) or
to a reduction of the articular contact area (e.g. with joint
incongruity or instability). Both factors operate in varus
deformity of the knee and in acetabular dysplasia –
common precursors of OA. Changes in the subchondral
bone may also increase stress concentration in the overlying cartilage, either by altering the shape of the articular surface or by an increase in bone density (e.g.
following fracture healing) which reduces the shock-
absorbing effect of the supporting cancellous bone.

From the foregoing outline it should be apparent
that the division of OA into 'primary' (when there is no
obvious antecedent factor) and 'secondary' (when it
follows a demonstrable abnormality) is somewhat artificial. This is borne out in clinical practice: patients
with 'secondary' OA of the knee following meniscectomy have been found also to have a higher than usual
incidence of 'primary' OA in other joints (Doherty *et
al.*, 1986). Perhaps primary, generalized factors (genetic,
metabolic or endocrine) alter the physical properties of
cartilage and thereby determine who is likely to develop
OA, while secondary factors such as anatomical defects
or trauma specify when and where it will occur. OA is,
ultimately, more process than disease, occurring in any
condition which causes a disparity between the
mechanical stress to which articular cartilage is
exposed and the ability of the cartilage to withstand
that stress.

Pathogenesis

The initial stages of OA have been studied in animal
models with induced joint instability and may not be
representative of all types of OA.

The earliest changes, while the cartilage is still
morphologically intact, are an increase in water content
of the cartilage and easier extractability of the matrix
proteoglycans; similar findings in human cartilage have
been ascribed to failure of the internal collagen
network that normally restrains the matrix gel. At a
slightly later stage there is loss of proteoglycans and
defects appear in the cartilage. As the cartilage becomes
less stiff, secondary damage to chondrocytes may cause
release of cell enzymes and further matrix breakdown.
Cartilage deformation may also add to the stress on the

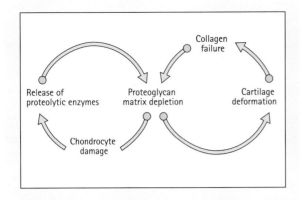

Pathology

The cardinal features are: (1) progressive cartilage destruction; (2) subarticular cyst formation, with (3) sclerosis of the surrounding bone; (4) osteophyte formation; and (5) capsular fibrosis.

Initially the cartilaginous and bony changes are confined to one part of the joint – the most heavily loaded part. There is softening and fraying, or fibrillation, of the normally smooth and glistening cartilage. The term 'chondromalacia' (Gr = cartilage softening) seems apt for this stage of the disease, but it is used only of the patellar articular surfaces where it features as one of the causes of anterior knee pain in young people.

With progressive disintegration of cartilage, the underlying bone becomes exposed and some areas may be polished, or burnished, to ivory-like smoothness (eburnation). Sometimes small tufts of fibrocartilage may be seen growing out of the bony surface. At a distance from the damaged area the articular cartilage looks relatively normal, but at the edges of the joint there is remodelling and growth of osteophytes covered by thin, bluish cartilage.

Beneath the damaged cartilage the bone is dense and sclerotic. Often within this area of subchondral sclerosis, and immediately subjacent to the surface, are one or more cysts containing thick, gelatinous material.

The joint capsule usually shows thickening and fibrosis, sometimes of extraordinary degree. The synovial lining, as a rule, looks only mildly inflamed; sometimes, however, it is thick and red and covered by villi.

The *histological appearances* vary considerably, according to the degree of destruction. Early on, the cartilage shows small irregularities or splits in the

collagen network, thus amplifying the changes in a cycle that leads to tissue breakdown.

Articular cartilage has an important role in distributing and dissipating the forces associated with joint loading. When it loses its integrity these forces are increasingly concentrated in the subchondral bone. The result: focal trabecular degeneration and cyst formation, as well as increased vascularity and reactive sclerosis in the zone of maximal loading.

What cartilage remains is still capable of regeneration, repair and remodelling. As the articular surfaces become increasingly malapposed and the joint unstable, cartilage at the edges of the joint reverts to the more youthful activities of growth and endochondral ossification, giving rise to the bony excrescences, or osteophytes, that so clearly distinguish OA (once called 'hypertrophic arthritis') from 'atrophic' disorders such as rheumatoid disease.

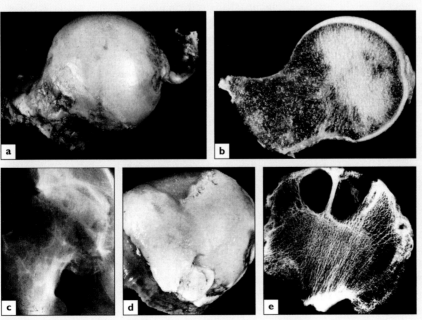

5.3 Osteoarthitis – pathology (a) Normal ageing causes slight degeneration of the articular surface, but the coronal section (**b**) shows that the cartilage thickness is well preserved even in old age. By contrast, in progressive osteoarthritis (lower row) the weight-bearing area is severely damaged: the x-ray (**c**) shows cartilage loss at the superior pole and cysts in the underlying bone; the specimen (**d**) shows that the top of the femoral head was completely denuded of cartilage; and a fine-detail x-ray of the specimen (**e**) shows that the subchondral bone plate has been perforated.

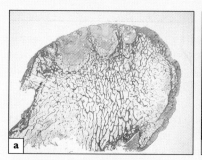 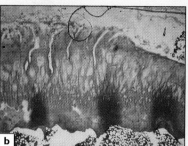 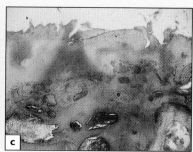

5.4 Osteoarthritis – histology (**a**) Destructive changes (loss of articular cartilage and cyst formation) are most marked where stress is greatest; reparative changes are represented by sclerosis around the cysts and new bone formation (osteophytes) in less stressed areas. (**b**) In this high-power view, the articular cartilage shows loss of metachromasia and deep clefts in the surface (fibrillation). Attempts at repair result in (**c**) subarticular sclerosis and buds of fibrocartilage mushrooming where the articular surface is destroyed.

surface, while in the deeper layers there is patchy loss of metachromasia (obviously corresponding to the depletion of matrix proteoglycans). Most striking, however, is the increased cellularity, and the appearance of clusters, or clones, of chondrocytes – 20 or more to a batch. In later stages, the clefts become more extensive and in some areas cartilage is lost to the point where the underlying bone is completely denuded. The biochemcial abnormalities corresponding to these changes were described by Mankin *et al.* (1971).

The subchondral bone shows marked osteoblastic activity, especially on the deep aspect of any cyst. The cyst itself contains amorphous material; its origin is mysterious – it could arise from stress disintegration of small trabeculae, from local areas of osteonecrosis or from the forceful pumping of synovial fluid through cracks in the subchondral bone plate. As in all types of arthritis, small areas of osteonecrosis are quite common.

The osteophytes appear to arise from cartilage hyperplasia and ossification at the edge of the articular surface.

The capsule and synovium are often thickened but cellular activity is slight; however, sometimes there is marked inflammation or fibrosis of the capsular tissues.

A feature of OA, which is difficult to appreciate from the morbid anatomy, is the marked vascularity and venous congestion of the subchondral bone. This can be shown by angiographic studies and the demonstration of increased intraosseous pressure. It is also apparent from the intense activity around osteoarthritic joints shown on radionuclide scanning.

Prevalence

OA is the commonest of all joint diseases. It is a truly universal disorder, affecting both sexes and all races; everyone who lives long enough will have it somewhere, in some degree. However, there are significant differences in its rate of occurrence in different ethnic groups, in the different sexes within any group and in the different joints.

Reports of prevalence rates vary, depending on the method of evaluation. Autopsy studies show OA changes in everyone over the age of 65 years. Radiographic surveys suggest that the prevalence rises from 1% below the age of 30 years to over 50% in people above the age of 60 years. OA of the finger joints is particularly common in elderly women, affecting more than 70% of those over 70 years.

Men and women are equally likely to develop OA, but more joints are affected in women than in men.

OA is much more common in some joints (the fingers, hip, knee and spine) than in others (the elbow, wrist and ankle). This may simply reflect the fact that some joints are more prone to predisposing abnormalities than others.

A similar explanation may account for certain geographic and ethnic differences in prevalence. For example, the female-to-male ratio for OA of the hip is about 1:1 in northern Europe but it is nearer 2:1 in southern Europe where there is a high incidence of acetabular dysplasia in girls. Even more striking is the virtual absence of hip OA in southern Chinese and African blacks (Hoagland *et al.*, 1973; Solomon *et al.*, 1976); this may simply be because predisposing disorders such as developmental displacement of the hip, Perthes' disease and slipped femoral epiphysis are uncommon in these populations. That they have no inherent resistance to OA is shown by the fact that they often develop the condition in other joints, for example the knee.

Risk factors

Joint dysplasia Disorders such as congenital acetabular dysplasia and Perthes' disease presage a greater than normal risk of OA in later life. However, OA is by no means inevitable and one should not be in any hurry to undertake 'prophylactic' surgery in a child with asymptomatic dysplasia.

Trauma Fractures involving the articular surface are obvious precursors of secondary OA. So, too, are lesser injuries which result in joint instability. What is less certain is whether malunion of a long-bone fracture predisposes to OA by causing segmental overload in a joint above or below the healed fracture (for example, in the knee or ankle after a tibial fracture). Contrary to popular belief, research has shown that moderate angular deformities of the tibia (up to 15°) are not associated with an increased risk of OA (Merchant and Dietz, 1989). This applies to mid-shaft fractures; malunion close to a joint may well predispose to secondary OA.

Occupation There is good evidence of an association between OA and certain occupations which cause repetitive stress; for example OA of the knees in workers engaged in knee-bending activities (Felson *et al.*, 1987), OA in the upper limbs in people working with heavy vibrating tools (Schumacher *et al.*, 1972) and OA of the hands in cotton mill workers (Lawrence, 1961). More controversial is the relationship of OA to sporting activity. Boxers are certainly prone to developing OA of the hands but this may be due to trauma. The same applies to footballers with OA of the knees and baseball pitchers with OA of the shoulder. More convincing evidence of a causative relationship comes from studies which have shown a significant increase in the risk of hip and knee OA in athletes (Harris *et al.*, 1994; Kulkala *et al.*, 1994).

Bone density It has long been known that women with femoral neck fractures seldom have OA of the hip. This negative association between OA and osteoporosis is reflected in studies which have demonstrated a significant increase in bone mineral density in people with OA compared to those without (Hannan *et al.*, 1992; Hart *et al.*, 1994). However, this may not be simple cause and effect: bone density is determined by a variety of genetic, hormonal and metabolic factors which may also influence cartilage metabolism independently of any effect due to bone density.

Obesity The simple idea that obesity causes increased joint loading and therefore predisposes to OA may be correct, at least for OA of the knees. However, the association is closer in women than in men and therefore (as with bone density) it may reflect other endocrine or metabolic factors in the pathogenesis of OA.

Family history Women with generalized OA are likely to see the same condition developing in their daughters. The particular trait which is responsible for this is not known.

Clinical features

Patients usually present after middle age. Joint involvement follows several different patterns: symptoms centre either on one or two of the weightbearing joints (hip or knee), on the interphalangeal joints (especially in women) or on any joint that has suffered a previous affliction (e.g. congenital dysplasia, osteonecrosis or intra-articular fracture). A family history is common in patients with polyarticular OA.

Pain is the usual presenting symptom. It is often quite widespread, or it may be referred to a distant site – for example, pain in the knee from OA of the hip. It starts insidiously and increases slowly over months or years. It is aggravated by exertion and relieved by rest, although with time relief is less and less complete. In the late stage the patient may have pain in bed at night. There are several possible causes of pain: capsular fibrosis, with pain on stretching the shrunken capsule; muscular fatigue; and, perhaps most important of all, bone pressure due to vascular congestion and intraosseous hypertension.

Stiffness is common; characteristically it occurs after periods of inactivity, but with time it becomes constant and progressive.

Swelling may be intermittent (suggesting an effusion) or continuos (with capsular thickening or large osteophytes).

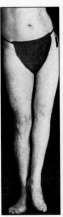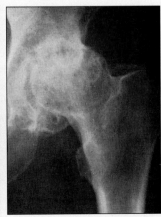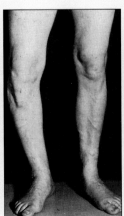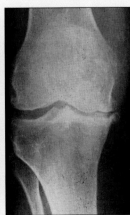

5.5 Osteoarthritis – clinical and x-rays Deformity and loss of articular 'space' at the hip and the knee.

Deformity may result from capsular contracture or joint instability; but beware, it may have preceded and contributed to the onset of OA.

Loss of function, though not the most dramatic, is often the most distressing symptom. A limp, difficulty in climbing stairs, restriction of walking distance or progressive inability to perform everyday tasks or enjoy recreation may eventually drive the patient to seek help.

Typically, the symptoms of OA follow an intermittent course, with periods of remission sometimes lasting for months.

Although the patient complains of only one or two joints, examination may show that others are affected in varying degrees. Swelling and deformity may be obvious in peripheral joints; at the hip, deformity is usually masked by postural adjustments of the pelvis and spine. In long-standing cases there is muscle wasting. Tell-tale scars denote previous abnormalities. Local tenderness is common, and in superficial joints fluid, synovial thickening or osteophytes may be felt.

Movement is always restricted, but is often painless within the permitted range; it may be accompanied by crepitus. Some movements are more curtailed than others; thus, at the hip extension, abduction and internal rotation are usually the most severely limited.

In the late stages joint instability may occur for any of three reasons: loss of cartilage and bone; asymmetrical capsular contracture; and muscle weakness.

Imaging

X-rays are so characteristic that other forms of imaging are seldom necessary. The four cardinal signs are asymmetric loss of cartilage (narrowing of the 'joint space'), sclerosis of the subchondral bone under the area of cartilage loss, cysts close to the articular surface and osteophytes at the margins of the joint. In addition there may be evidence of previous disorders (congenital defects, old fractures, rheumatoid arthritis, chondrocalcinosis).

In the late stage, displacement of the joint is common and bone destruction may be severe.

Radionuclide scanning with ^{99m}Tc-HDP shows increased activity during the bone phase in the subchondral regions of affected joints. This is due to increased vascularity and new bone formation.

Arthroscopy

Arthroscopy may show cartilage damage long before x-ray changes appear. The problem is that it reveals too much, and the patient's symptoms may be ascribed to OA when they are, in fact, due to some other disorder.

Natural history

OA usually evolves as a slowly progressive disorder. However, symptoms may wax and wane in intensity, sometimes disappearing for several months.

The x-rays show no such fluctuation. However, there is considerable variation between cases in the relative degrees of destruction and repair. Most of the men and half of the women have a *hypertrophic* reaction, with marked sclerosis and large osteophytes. In about 20% of cases – most of them women – reactive changes are more subdued, inviting descriptions such as *atrophic*

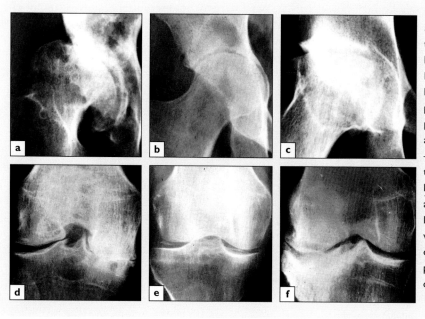

5.6 Osteoarthritis – x-rays The three types of osteoarthritis are shown in the hip (**a, b, c**) and the knee (**d, e, f**). In type I mechanical overload has damaged a localized area of cartilage – the upper pole in this hip (**a**) and the medial compartment in this knee (**d**). In type II the articular cartilage was already abnormal – following an inflammatory arthritis of the hip (**b**) and chondrocalcinosis of the knee (**e**), so that even normal loads damaged the surfaces. In type III the underlying bone was defective – either too weak as in osteonecrosis of the hip (**c**) or too sclerotic, as in this old tibial plateau fracture (**f**) causing breakdown of the covering cartilage.

or *osteopenic* OA. Occasionally OA takes the form of a *rapidly progressive* disorder.

Complications

Capsular herniation OA of the knee is sometimes associated with a marked effusion and herniation of the posterior capsule (Baker's cyst).

Loose bodies Cartilage and bone fragments may give rise to loose bodies, resulting in episodes of locking.

Rotator cuff dysfunction OA of the acromioclavicular joint may cause rotator cuff impingement, tendinitis or cuff rupture.

Spinal stenosis Long-standing hypertrophic OA of the lumbar apophyseal joints may give rise to acquired spinal stenosis. The abnormality is best demonstrated by computed tomography (CT).

Spondylolisthesis In patients over 60 years of age, destructive OA of the apophyseal joints may result in severe segmental instability and spondylolisthesis (so-called 'degenerative' spondylolisthesis, which almost always occurs at L4/5).

Clinical variants

Although the features of OA in any particular joint are fairly consistent, the overall clinical picture shows variations which define a number of sub-groups.

MONARTICULAR AND PAUCIARTICULAR OA
In its 'classic' form, OA presents with pain and dysfunction in one or two of the large weightbearing joints. There may be an obvious underlying abnormality; acetabular dysplasia, old Perthes' disease or slipped epiphysis, a previous fracture or damage to ligaments or menisci. In the majority of cases, however, the abnormality is more subtle and one may question whether its discovery will influence subsequent treatment.

POLYARTICULAR (GENERALIZED) OA
This is far and away the most common form of OA, though most of the patients never consult an orthopaedic surgeon. The patient is usually a middle-aged woman who presents with pain, swelling and stiffness of the finger joints. The first carpometacarpal and the big toe metatarsophalangeal joints, or the knees and lumbar facet joints, may be affected as well.

The changes are most obvious in the hands. The interphalangeal joints become swollen and tender, and in the early stages they often appear to be inflamed. Over a period of years osteophytes and soft-tissue swelling produce a characteristic knobbly appearance of the distal

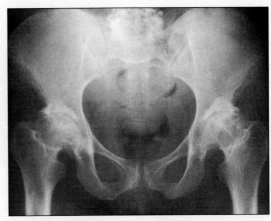

5.7 Secondary OA The flattened femoral head and shortened femoral necks are tell-tale signs of multiple epiphyseal dysplasia in this patient with secondary OA.

interphalangeal joints (Herberden's nodes) and, less often, the proximal interphalangeal joints (Bouchard's nodes); pain may disappear but stiffness and deformity can be disturbing. Some patients present with painful knees or backache and the knobbly fingers are noticed only in passing. There is a strong association with carpal tunnel syndrome and isolated tenovaginitis.

X-rays show the characteristic features of OA, usually maximal in the distal interphalangeal joints of the fingers.

OA IN UNUSUAL SITES
OA is uncommon in the shoulder, elbow, wrist and ankle. If any of these joints is affected one should suspect a previous abnormality – congenital or traumatic – or an associated generalized disease such as a crystal arthropathy.

ENDEMIC OA
OA occasionally occurs as an endemic disorder affecting entire communities. It may due either to some environmental factor peculiar to that region or to an underlying generalized dysplasia in a genetically isolated community.

Kashin–Beck disease is seen in the north-eastern parts of Russia and China; in some areas it is thought to affect over 8% of the population (Sokoloff, 1985). It usually manifests as a generalized OA of the finger joints, elbows, knees and ankles. Shortness of stature is common, suggesting that the condition starts in childhood. It remains uncertain whether the widespread bone deformity and cartilage degeneration are due to a genetic disorder, an unusually dietary deficiency or the ingestion of mycotoxins in spoiled wheat.

Mseleni joint disease is a polyarticular arthritis that is seen among the Tsonga people around the village of Mseleni

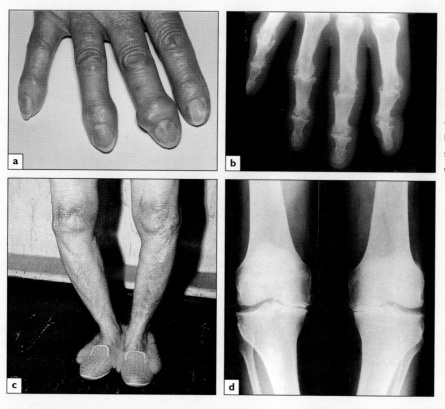

5.8 Polyarticular (generalized) OA (**a, b**) An almost invariable feature of polyarticular OA is involvement of the terminal finger joints – Heberden's nodes. The thumb carpometacarpal joint also may be affected. (**c, d**) There is a strong association with OA of the knees.

on the eastern seaboard of Southern Africa. OA of the hips is common but numerous other joints are affected as well, leading to crippling deformities in older adults. X-rays show features of secondary OA associated with two distinct underlying disorders – multiple epiphyseal dysplasia, which affects men and women in equal proportions, and protrusio acetabuli, which occurs almost exclusively in women (Solomon *et al.*, 1986).

It is important to recognize endemic disorders of this kind as it may be possible to reduce the prevalence of OA by appropriate public health measures and genetic counselling.

RAPIDLY DESTRUCTIVE OA (see also page 75)

Every so often a patient with apparently straightforward OA shows rapid and startling progression of bone destruction. The condition was at one time thought to be due to the dampening of pain impulses by powerful anti-inflammatory drugs – a notional type of analgesic arthropathy. It is now recognized that it occurs mainly in elderly women and that it is often associated with calcium crystal deposition (Doherty *et al.*, 1986). Usually it is the hip that is affected, but similar changes may be seen in other joints.

NEUROPATHIC JOINT DISEASE (CHARCOT'S DISEASE)

The most destructive arthropathy is that associated with lack of pain sensibility and position sense. This condition is discussed under a separate heading at the end of the chapter.

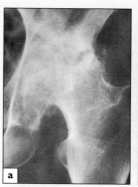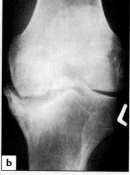

5.9 Rapidly destructive OA (**a**) This looked, at first, like 'ordinary' OA of the hip. At the next visit, 6 months later, x-ray showed severe crumbling of the joint surfaces. (**b**) Similar changes are seen (though less often) in other joints.

Differential diagnosis of OA

A number of conditions may mimic OA, some presenting as a monarthritis and some as a polyarthritis affecting the finger joints.

AVASCULAR NECROSIS 'Idiopathic' necrosis causes joint pain and local effusion. Early on the diagnosis is made by MRI. Once bone destruction occurs the x-ray changes can be mistaken for those of OA; *the cardinal*

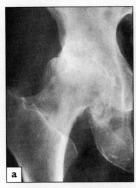
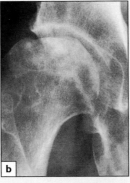

5.10 Differential diagnosis – osteoarthritis and osteonecrosis (a) OA with marked subarticular bone collapse is sometimes mistaken for osteonecrosis. The clue to the diagnosis is that in OA the articular 'space' (cartilage) is progressively reduced before bone collapse occurs, whereas in primary osteonecrosis **(b)** articular cartilage is preserved even while the underlying bone crumbles.

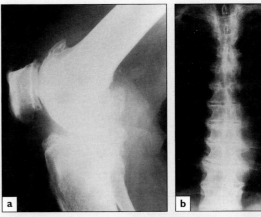

5.11 Diffuse idiopathic skeletal hyperostosis – DISH
(a) The large bony outgrowths around the knee suggest something more than the usual OA. X-rays of the spine **(b)** show the typical features of DISH.

distinguishing feature is that in osteonecrosis the 'joint space' (articular cartilage) is preserved in the face of progressive bone collapse and deformity.

INFLAMMATORY ARTHROPATHIES Rheumatoid arthritis, ankylosing spondylitis and Reiter's disease may start in one or two large joints. The history is short and there are local signs of inflammation. X-rays show a predominantly atrophic or erosive arthritis. Sooner or later other joints are affected and systemic features appear.

POLYARTHRITIS OF THE FINGERS Polyarticular OA may be confused with other disorders which affect the finger joints (see Fig. 3.7). Close observation shows several distinguishing features. *Nodal OA* affects predominantly the distal joints, *rheumatoid arthritis* the proximal joints. *Psoriatic arthritis* is a purely destructive arthropathy and there are no interphalangeal 'nodes'. *Tophaceous gout* may cause knobbly fingers, but the knobs are tophi, not osteophytes. X-rays will show the difference.

DIFFUSE IDIOPATHIC SKELETAL HYPEROSTOSIS (DISH) This is a fairly common disorder of middle-aged people, characterized by bone proliferation at the ligament and tendon insertions around peripheral joints and the intervertebral discs (Resnick *et al.*, 1975). On x-ray examination the large bony spurs are easily mistaken for osteophytes. DISH and OA often appear together, but DISH is not OA: the bone spurs are symmetrically distributed, especially along the pelvic apophyses and throughout the vertebral column. When DISH occurs by itself it is usually asymptomatic.

MULTIPLE DIAGNOSIS OA is so common after middle age that it is often found in patients with other conditions that cause pain in or around a joint. Before jumping to the conclusion that the symptoms are due to the OA

features seen on x-ray, be sure to exclude periarticular disorders as well as more distant abnormalities giving rise to referred pain.

Management

The management of OA depends on the joint (or joints) involved, the stage of the disorder, the severity of the symptoms, the age of the patient and his or her functional needs. Three observations should be borne in mind: (1) symptoms characteristically wax and wane, and pain may subside spontaneously for long periods; (2) some forms of OA actually become less painful with the passage of time and the patient may need no more than reassurance and a prescription for pain killers; (3) at the other extreme, the recognition (from serial x-rays) that the patient has a rapidly progressive type of OA may warrant an early move to reconstructive surgery before bone loss compromises the outcome of any operation.

EARLY TREATMENT
There is, as yet, no drug that can modify the effects of OA. Treatment is, therefore, symptomatic. The principles are: (1) maintain movement and muscle strength; (2) protect the joint from 'overload'; (3) relieve pain; and (4) modify daily activities.

Physiotherapy The mainstay of treatment in the early case is physiotherapy, which should be directed at maintaining joint mobility and improving muscle strength. The programme can include aerobic exercise, but care should be taken to avoid activities which increase impact loading. Other measures, such as massage and the application of warmth, may reduce pain but improvement is short-lived and the treatment has to be repeated.

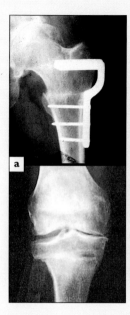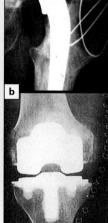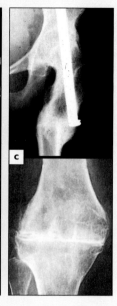

5.12 Operative treatment The three basic operations: **(a)** osteotomy, **(b)** arthroplasty, **(c)** athrodesis – at the hip.

– at the knee

Load reduction Protecting the joint from excessive load may slow down the rate of cartilage loss. It is also effective in relieving pain. Common sense measures such as weight reduction for obese patients, wearing shock-absorbing shoes, avoiding activities like climbing stairs, and using a walking stick will pay excellent dividends.

Analgesic medication Pain relief is important, but not all patients require drug therapy and those who do may not need it all the time. If other measures do not provide symptomatic improvement, patients may respond to a simple analgesic such as paracetamol. If this fails to control pain, a non-steroidal anti-inflammatory preparation may be better.

INTERMEDIATE TREATMENT
Joint debridement (removal of interfering osteophytes, cartilage tags and loose bodies) may give some improvement. This technique, previously all but abandoned, has gained acceptance again in the form of arthroscopic surgery for OA of the knee.

Localized cartilage defects can be 'grafted' with autologous chondrocytes. However, the use of cartilage transplants to obtain resurfacing of an osteoarthritic joint is still in the realm of experimental surgery.

If symptoms and signs increase, then at some joints (chiefly the hip and knee) realignment osteotomy should be considered. It must be done while the joint is still stable and mobile and x-rays show that a major part of the articular surface (the radiographic 'joint space') is preserved. Pain relief is often dramatic and is ascribed to (1) vascular decompression of the subchondral bone, and (2) redistribution of loading forces towards less damaged parts of the joint. After load redistribution, fibrocartilage may grow to cover exposed bone.

LATE TREATMENT
Progressive joint destruction, with increasing pain, instability and deformity (particularly of one of the weightbearing joints), usually requires reconstructive surgery. Arthrodesis is indicated if the stiffness is acceptable and neighbouring joints are not likely to be prejudiced. With arthroplasty, timing is essential. Too early, and the odds against a durable result lengthen in proportion to the demands of strenuous activity and time; too late, and bone destruction, deformity, stiffness and muscle atrophy make the operation more difficult and the results more unpredictable.

For OA of the hip and knee, total joint replacement has transformed the lives of millions of patients. Similar operations for the shoulder, elbow and ankle are less successful but techniques are improving year by year.

HAEMOPHILIC ARTHROPATHY

Recurrent intra-articular bleeding may lead to chronic synovitis and progressive articular destruction. Clinically, this is seen only in classic haemophilia, in which there is a deficiency of clotting factor VIII, and Christmas disease, due to deficiency of factor IX. Both are X-linked recessive disorders manifesting in males but carried by females. Their incidence is about 1 per 10,000 male births. Plasma-clotting factor levels above 40% of the normal are compatible with normal control of haemorrhage. Patients with clotting factor levels above 5% ('mild haemophilia') may have prolonged bleeding after injury or operation; those with levels below 1% ('severe haemophilia') have frequent spontaneous joint and muscle haemorrhages.

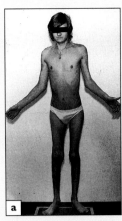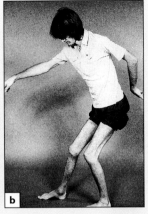

5.13 Haemophilic arthropathy – clinical features
(a) Recurrent haemarthrosis and chronic synovitis led to contractures of the elbow joints and deformities of the knees and ankles. (b) This man, with contractures of the knees and ankles, had difficulty staying upright, let alone walking, without support.

Pathology

Haemorrhage into the joint causes synovial irritation, inflammation and subsynovial fibrosis. Haemosiderin appears in the synovial cells and macrophages and after repeated bleeds the synovium becomes thick and heavily pigmented. A vascular pannus creeps over the articular surface and the cartilage is gradually eroded. The subchondral bone may be exposed and penetrated, and occasionally large cysts develop at the bone ends. These changes are attributed to cartilage-degrading enzymes released by the proliferative synovities and by cells that have accumulated iron, but an additional factor may be the interference with normal cartilage nutrition due to prolonged or repeated joint immobilization.

Bleeding into muscles is less common but equally harmful. Increased tension may lead to muscle necrosis, reactive fibrosis and joint contractures. Sometimes nerves are compressed, causing a neurapraxia; temporary weakness may contribute further to the development of joint deformity.

Cysts and pseudotumours are rare phenomena. A large soft-tissue haematoma may become encapsulated before it is absorbed, and may then draw in more fluid by osmosis to produce a slowly expanding 'cyst'. A subperiosteal haematoma occasionally stimulates cystic resorption of bone resembling a tumour.

Clinical features

Only males are affected and in severe haemophilia joint bleeds usually begin when the child starts to walk. The clinical picture depends on the severity of the disorder, the site of bleeding and the efficacy of long-term treatment. The commonest features are acute bleeding into joints or muscles, chronic arthritis and joint contractures. The sites most frequently involved are the knees, ankles, elbow, shoulders and hips.

ACUTE BLEEDING INTO A JOINT, MUSCLE OR NERVE With trivial injury a joint (usually the knee, elbow or ankle) may rapidly fill with blood. Pain, warmth, boggy swelling, tenderness and limited movement are the outstanding features. The resemblance to a low-grade inflammatory joint is striking, but the history is diagnostic.

Acute bleeding into muscles (especially the forearm, calf or thigh) is less common. A painful swelling appears and movement of the related joint is resisted. The distinction from a haemarthosis may be difficult (e.g. with groin pain due to iliopsoas haemorrhage); usually only those movements that stretch the affected muscles are painful, whereas in haemarthrosis all movements are painful.

Bleeding into a peripheral nerve causes intense pain followed by a variable degree of sensory change and muscle weakness. Nerve function usually recovers after several months.

Neurological symptoms and signs may also be caused by a large soft-tissue haematoma. Following effective treatment, the haematoma is usually resorbed within 10–14 days but full movement may take longer to return.

Bleeding into the forearm or leg may give rise to a classic compartment syndrome. The tell-tale signs of acute pain and tissue tension should be heeded before sensory and motor impairment are obvious.

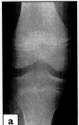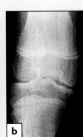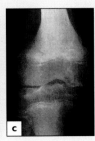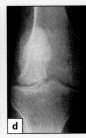

5.14 Haemophilic arthritis (a) At first there is blood in the joint but the surfaces are intact; (b) later the cartilage is attacked and the joint 'space' narrows; (c) bony erosions appear and eventually the joint becomes deformed and unstable; in (d) early subluxation is obvious.

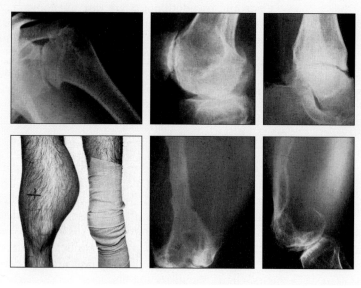

5.15 Haemophilia Top row: degeneration in several joints after repeated bleeding. Bottom row: since it threatened the integrity of the femur, this large pseudotumour was extirpated; at the same time massive bone grafts were inserted – no light undertaking in a haemophilic.

JOINT DEGENERATION This, the sequel to repeated bleeding, usually begins before the age of 15 years. Chronic synovitis is followed by cartilage degeneration. An affected joint shows wasting, limitation of movement and fixed deformity not unlike a tuberculous or rheumatoid joint. In long-standing cases, articular destruction may lead to instability.

X-ray changes vary according to the stage of the disorder. A useful classification is that of Arnold and Hilgartner (1977): *Stage I* – soft-tissue swelling; *Stage II* – osteoporosis and epiphyseal overgrowth; *Stage III* – slight narrowing of the articular space and squaring of the bone ends; *Stage IV* – marked narrowing of the articular space; and *Stage V* – joint disintegration.

Cysts and pseudotumours are rare complications (see above).

Treatment

The most important aspect of treatment is to provide the patient with the means to counteract the haemorrhage as soon as it occurs. Patients are taught to recognize the early symptoms of bleeding and to administer the appropriate clotting factor concentrate themselves.

It is important to establish the precise diagnosis; factor VIII or IX is effective only for the specific disorder. Frozen cryoprecipitate is sometimes used instead, but is much less effective. Fresh-frozen plasma is no longer used.

THE ACUTE BLEED Bleeding into the tissues is treated by immediate factor replacement. Analgesics are given for pain and the limb is immobilized in a splint – but not for more than a day or two. Once the acute episode has passed, movement is encouraged, under continuing cover with factor concentrate. Joint aspiration is avoided unless distension is severe or there is a strong suspicion of infection. Nerve palsy may require intermittent splintage and physiotherapy until the neurapraxia recovers, and during this time the skin must be protected from injury.

CHRONIC ARTHROPATHY The aim is to prevent the development of joint contractures, stiffness and progressive muscle weakness. Under cover of factor infusions the patient is given physiotherapy, and impending contractures are managed by intermittent splintage and, if necessary, traction or passive correction by an inflatable splint.

Operative treatment has become safer since the introduction of clotting factor concentrates. However, patients who develop antifactor antibodies are unsuitable for any form of surgery. It is also important to screen patients for hepatitis B virus and HIV antibodies, as their presence demands special precautions during the operation.

The clotting factor concentration should be raised to above 25% for factor VIII and above 15% for factor IX, and it should be kept at those levels throughout the postoperative period. It goes without saying that operative treatment should be carried out in a hospital with the appropriate multidisciplinary expertise on site.

Useful procedures are tendon lengthening (to correct contractures), osteotomy (for established deformity) and arthrodesis of the knee or ankle (for painful joint destruction). Synovectomy is sometimes performed but the benefits are dubious. Total hip replacement is technically feasible, but tissue dissection should be kept to a minimum and meticulous haemostatis is needed. Not surprisingly, the complication rate is higher than for hip replacement in non-bleeders (Nelson *et al.*, 1992).

NEUROPATHIC JOINT DISEASE (CHARCOT'S DISEASE)

Charcot, in 1868, described a type of destructive arthropathy associated with disease of the central nervous system. Almost all his patients had tabes dorsalis, but the name 'Charcot joint disease' came to be applied to any destructive arthropathy arising from loss of pain sensibility and position sense. The most common causes are neurosyphilis (affecting mainly the lower limb joints), syringomyelia (upper and lower limbs), multiple sclerosis, myelomeningocele, spinal cord compression, peripheral neuritis (usually diabetic), leprosy and congenital indifference to pain. The term is also applied (less accurately) to rapidly destructive forms of OA where there is no neurological lesion.

Pathogenesis and pathology

Neuropathic joints lack the normal reflex safeguards against abnormal stress or injury and the subchondral bone disintegrates with alarming speed. Unlike OA, this is a mainly destructive condition and there are few signs of repair. Some cases show increased vascularity and osteoclastic activity in the subchondral bone; in others, capsular and ligamentous laxity and joint instability go hand in hand with articular disintegration.

The early changes are similar to those of OA. However, it soon becomes apparent that this is a rapidly destructive process; the articular surface breaks up, fragments of bone and cartilage appear in the joint or embedded in the synovium and there is thickening of the synovial membrane and marked joint effusion. In the late stages, there is complete loss of articular cartilage, fragmentation of the subchondral bone and joint subluxation.

Clinical featues

The patient complains of weakness, instability, swelling, laxity and progressive deformity of the joint (usually the knee or ankle). The joint is neither warm nor particularly tender, but swelling is marked, fluid is greatly increased and in the late stages bits of bone may be felt everywhere. There is always some instability and in the worst cases the joint is flail. The appearances suggest that movement would be agonizing and yet it is often painless. The paradox is diagnostic. General examination may reveal features of the underlying neurological disorder.

X-rays The radiogaphic changes may at first be mistaken for those of OA. However, thinning of the articular space is unusually rapid and there is little in the way of osteophyte formation. Joint swelling and the appearance of intra-articular 'calcification' are further clues. Ultimately, there is gross erosion of the articular surfaces and displacement of the joint.

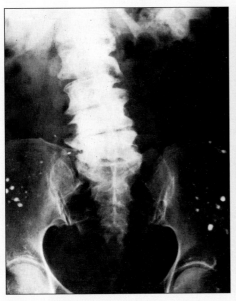
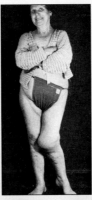
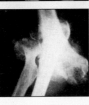
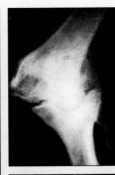
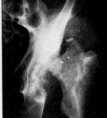

5.16 Charcot's disease
The vertebrae are distorted and dense, the buttocks show the radio-opaque remains of former injections; the knee, elbow and hip joints look grotesque. Moral: 'If it's bizarre, do a WR'. Note also the happy smile (though not all Charcot joints are tabetic, nor are they always painless).

Treatment

There is no way of halting or slowing the destructive process. Treatment is usually conservative and consists of splintage of the unstable joint. Despite the bizarre appearances, patients often seem to manage well. Some patients complain of pain and may need analgesic medication.

Weightbearing joints are sometimes so unstable that splintage is useless. Arthrodesis may be attempted, but the patient should be warned that there is only a small chance of success.

REFERENCES AND FURTHER READING

Arnold WD, Hilgartner MW (1977) Hemophilic arthopathy. *Journal of Bone and Joint Surgery* 59A, 287-305

Byers PD, Contepomi CA, Farkas TA (1970) A post mortem study of the hip joint including the prevalence of features on the right side. *Annals of the Rheumatic Diseases* 29, 15-31

Doherty M, Holt M, MacMillan P *et al.* (1986) A reappraisal of 'analgesic hip'. *Annals of the Rheumatic Diseases* 45, 272-276

Felson DT, Anderson JJ, Namack A *et al.* (1987) Obesity and symptomatic knee osteoarthritis. *Arthritis and Rheumatism* 30, S130

Hannan MT, Zhang Y, Anderson JJ *et al.* (1992) Bone mineral density and knee osteoarthritis in elderly men and women: The Framingham Study. *Arthritis and Rheumatism* 35, S1 (S40)

Harris PA, Hart DJ, Jawad S *et al.* (1994) Risk of osteoarthritis (OA) associated with running: A radiological survey. *Arthritis and Rheumatism* 37, S369

Hart DJ, Mootoosamy I, Doyle DV *et al.* (1994) The relationship between osteoarthritis and osteoporosis in the general population: The Chingford Study. *Annals of the Rheumatic Diseases* 53, 158

Hoaglund FT, Yau ACMC, Wong WL (1973) Osteoarthritis of the hip and other joints in Southern Chinese in Hong Kong. *Journal of Bone and Joint Surgery* 55A, 545-557

Knowlton RG, Katzenstein PL, Moskowitz RW *et al.* (1990) Genetic linkage of a polymorphism in the type II procollagen gene (COL2A1) to primary osteoarthritis associated with mild chondrodysplasia. *New England Journal of Medicine* 322, 526

Kulkala UM, Kaprio J, Sarno S (1994) Osteoarthritis of weight bearing joints of lower limbs in former elite male athletes. *British Medical Journal* 308, 231

Lawrence JS (1961) Rheumatism in cotton operatives. *British Journal of Industrial Medicine* 18, 270-276

Mankin HJ, Dorfman DD, Lippiello L, Zarins A (1971) Biochemical and metabolic abnormalities in articular cartilage from osteoarthritic human hips. II. Correlation of morphology with metabolic data. *Journal of Bone and Joint Surgery* 53A, 523-537

Merchant TC, Dietz FR (1989) Long-term follow-up after fractures of the tibial and fibular shafts. *Journal of Bone and Joint Surgery* 71A, 599-606

Nelson IW, Sivamerugan S, Latham PD *et al.* (1992) Total hip arthroplasties for haemophilic arthropathies. *Clinical Orthopaedics and Related Research* 276, 210-213

Palotie A, Vaisanen P, Ott J *et al.* (1989) Predisposition to familial osteoarthrosis linked to type II colagen gene. *Lancet* 2, 924

Resnick D, Shaul SR, Robins JM (1975) Diffuse idiopathic skeletal hyperostosis (DISH): Forestier's disease with extraspinal manifestations. *Radiology* 115, 513-524

Schumacher HR, Agudelo C, Labowitz R (1972) Jackhammer arthropathy. *Journal of Occupational Medicine* 14, 563

Sokoloff L (1985) Endemic forms of osteoarthitis. *Clinics in Rheumatic Diseases* 11, 187-202

Solomon L (1976) Patterns of osteoarthritis of the hip. *Journal of Bone and Joint Surgery* 58B, 176-183

Solomon L, McLaren P, Irwig L *et al.* (1986) Distinct types of hip disorder in Mselini joint disease. *South African Medical Journal* 69, 15-17

6

Osteonecrosis and related disorders

Avascular necrosis has long been recognized as a complication of femoral head fractures, the simplistic explanation being traumatic severance of the blood supply to the femoral head. Segmental osteonecrosis also appears as a distinctive feature in a number of non-traumatic disorders: joint infection, Perthes' disease, caisson disease, Gaucher's disease, systemic lupus erythematosus (SLE), high-dosage corticosteroid administration and alcohol abuse, to mention only the more common ones.

Whatever the cause, the condition, once establshed, may come to dominate the clinical picture, demanding attention in its own right.

Aetiology and pathogenesis

Sites which are peculiarly vulnerable to ischaemic necrosis are the femoral head, the femoral condyles, the head of the humerus, the capitulum and the proximal parts of the scaphoid and talus. These subarticular regions lie at the most distant parts of the bone's vascular territory, and they are largely enclosed by cartilage, giving restricted access to local blood vessels. The subchondral trabeculae are further compromised in that they are sustained largely by a system of endarterioles with limited collateral connections.

Another factor which needs to be taken into account is that the vascular sinusoids which nourish the marrow and bone cells, unlike arterial capillaries, have no adventitial layer and their patency is determined by the volume and pressure of the surrounding marrow tissue, which itself is encased in unyielding bone. The system functions essentially as a closed compartment within which one element can expand only at the expense of the others. Local changes such as decreased blood-flow, haemorrhage or marrow swelling can, therefore, rapidly spiral to a vicious cycle of ischaemia, reactive oedema or inflammation, marrow swelling, increased intraosseous pressure and further ischaemia.

The process described above can be initiated in at least four different ways: (1) severance of the local blood supply; (2) venous stasis and retrograde arteriolar stoppage; (3) intravascular thrombosis; and (4) compression of capillaries and sinusoids by marrow swelling. *Ischaemia, in the majority of cases, is due to a combination of several of these factors.*

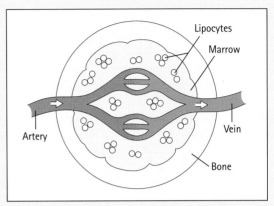

6.1 Avascular necrosis – pathogenesis The medullary cavity of bone is virtually a closed compartment containing myeloid tissue, marrow fat and capillary blood vessels. Any increase in fat cell volume will reduce capillary circulation and may result in bone ischaemia.

Table 6.1 Main conditions associated with non-traumatic osteonecrosis

Infection
    Osteomyelitis
    Septic arthritis
Haemoglobinopathy
    Sickle cell disease
Storage disorders
    Gaucher's disease
Caisson disease
    Dysbaric osteonecrosis
Coagulation disorders
    Familial thrombophilia
    Hypofibrinolysis
    Hypolipoproteinaemia
    Thrombocytopenic purpura
Other
    Perthes' disease
    Cortisone administration
    Alcohol abuse
    SLE (? increase in antiphospholipid antibodies)
    Pregnancy (? decreased fibrinolysis; ? fatty liver)
    Anaphylactic shock
    Ionizing radiation

TRAUMATIC OSTEONECROSIS

In traumatic osteonecrosis the vascular anatomy is particularly important. In fractures and dislocations of the hip the retinacular vessels supplying the femoral head are easily torn. If, in addition, there is damage to or thrombosis of the ligamentum teres, osteonecrosis is inevitable. Little wonder that displaced fractures of the femoral neck are complicated by osteonecrosis in over 20% of cases. Undisplaced fractures, or lesser injuries, also sometimes result in subchondral necrosis; this may be due to thrombosis of intraosseous capillaries or sinusoidal occlusion due to marrow oedema.

Other injuries which are prone to osteonecrosis are fractures of the scaphoid and talus. Significantly, it is always the proximal fragment which suffers. This is because the principal vessels enter the bones near their distal ends and take an intra-osseous course from distal to proximal.

Impact injuries and osteoarticular fractures at any of the convex articular surfaces behave in the same way and often develop localized ischaemic changes. These small lesions are usually referred to as 'osteochondroses' and many of them have acquired eponyms which are firmly embedded in orthopaedic history.

NON-TRAUMATIC OSTEONECROSIS

The mechanisms here are more complex and may involve several pathways to intravascular stasis or thrombosis, as well as extravascular swelling and capillary compression.

Intravascular thrombosis Various mechanisms leading to capillary thrombosis have been demonstrated in patients with non-traumatic osteonecrosis. Over 80% of cases are associated with high-dosage corticosteroid medication or alcohol abuse (or both, acting cumulatively). These conditions give rise to hyperlipidaemia and fatty degeneration of the liver. Jones (1994) has favoured the idea that fat embolism plays a part, giving rise to capillary endothelial damage, platelet aggregation and thrombosis.

Glueck *et al.* (1996; 1997a) have suggested that thrombophilia and hypofibrinolysis are important aetiological factors in both adult osteonecrosis and Perthes' disease. Recent studies, however, have failed to confirm this association (Liesner, 1999). Other coagulopathies have been implicated – e.g. antiphospholipid deficiency in SLE (Asherson *et al.*, 1993) and enhanced coagulability in sickle-cell disease (Francis, 1991), and it now seems likely that coagulation abnormalities of one sort or another play at least a contributory role in most of the disorders associated with non-traumatic osteonecrosis.

Extravascular marrow swelling High dosage corticosteroid administration and alcohol overuse cause fat cell swelling in the marrow, a feature which is very obvious in bone specimens obtained during joint replacement. There is a demonstrable rise in intra-osseous pressure and contrast venography shows slowing of venous blood-flow from the bone. Ficat and Arlet (1980) posited that the increase in marrow fat volume in the femoral head caused sinusoidal compression, venous stasis and retrograde ischaemia leading to trabecular bone death; in other words, the establishment of a compartment syndrome.

Whichever of these mechanisms offers the primary pathway to non-traumatic bone ischaemia, it is almost certain that both come into play at a fairly early stage and each enhances the effect of the other.

Pathology and natural history

Bone cells die after 12–48 hours of anoxia, yet for days or even weeks the gross appearance of the affected segment remains unaltered. During this time the most striking histological changes are seen in the marrow: loss of fat cell outlines, inflammatory cell infiltration, marrow oedema, the appearance of tissue histiocytes, and eventual replacement of necrotic marrow by undifferentiated mesenchymal tissue.

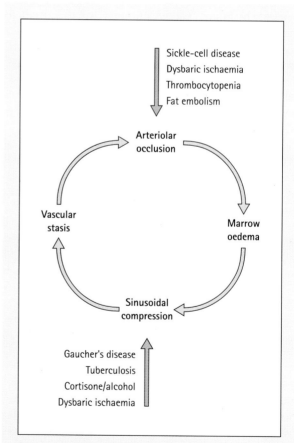

6.2 Avascular necrosis Algorithm showing how various disorders may enter the vicious cycle of capillary stasis and marrow engorgement.

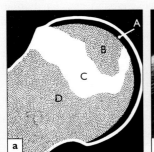
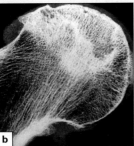
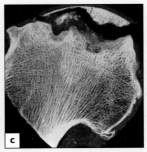
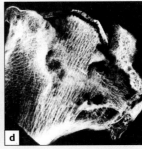

6.3 Avascular necrosis of bone – pathology These fine-detail x-rays of necrotic femoral heads show the progress of osteonecrosis. The articular cartilage (A) remains intact for a long time. The necrotic segment (B) has a texture similar to that of normal bone, but it may develop fine cracks. New bone surrounds the dead trabeculae and causes marked sclerosis (C). Beyond this the bone remains unchanged (D). In the later stages the necrotic bone breaks up and finally the joint surface is destroyed.

A characteristic feature of ischaemic segmental necrosis is the tendency to bone repair, and within a few weeks one may see new blood vessels and osteoblastic proliferation at the interface between ischaemic and live bone. As the necrotic sector becomes demarcated, vascular granulation tissue advances from the surviving trabeculae and new bone is laid down upon the dead; it is this increase in mineral mass that later produces the radiographic appearance of increased density or 'sclerosis'.

Reparative new bone formation proceeds slowly and probably does not advance for more than 8–10mm into the necrotic zone. With time, structural failure begins to occur in the most heavily stressed part of the necrotic segment. Usually this takes the form of a linear tangential fracture close to the articular surface, possibly due to shearing stress. The crack may break through the articular cartilage and at operation it may be possible to lift the 'lid' off the necrotic segment like the cracked shell of a hard-boiled egg. However, until very late the articular cartilage retains its thickness and viability. In the final stages, fragmentation of the necrotic bone leads to progressive deformity and destruction of the joint surface.

In the past, when diagnosis was based entirely on x-ray changes, it was thought that osteonecrosis always progressed to bone collapse. Now that it is possible to detect the earliest signs by magnetic resonance imaging (MRI), it has become apparent that this is not the case.

The size of the necrotic segment, as defined by a hypointense band in the T_1-weighted MRI, is usually established at the time of the initiating ischaemic event, and from then on it rarely increases; indeed, there is evidence that non-traumatic lesions sometimes diminish in size and occasionally they even disappear (Sakamoto *et al.*, 1997). In persistent lesions, the rate of bone collapse depends largely on the site and extent of the necrotic segment: lesions which lie outside the normal stress trajectories may remain structurally intact while those that involve large segments of the loadbearing surface usually collapse within 3 years (see under Staging the Lesion).

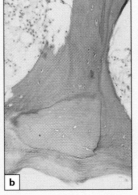

6.4 Avascular necrosis – histology (a) Section across the junction between articular cartilage and bone shows living cartilage cells but necrotic subchondral marrow and bone. (b) A high power view shows islands of dead bone with empty osteocytic lacunae enfolded by new, living bone.

Clinical features

The earliest stage of bone death is asymptomatic; by the time the patient presents, the lesion is usually well advanced. Pain is a common complaint. It is felt in or near a joint, and perhaps only with certain movements. Some patients complain of a 'click' in the joint, probably due to snapping or catching of a loose articular fragment. In the later stages the joint becomes stiff and deformed. Local tenderness may be present and, if a superficial bone is affected, there may be some swelling. Movements – or perhaps one particular movement – may be restricted; in advanced cases there may be fixed deformities.

Imaging

X-RAY The early signs of ischaemia are confined to the bone marrow and cannot be detected by plain x-ray examination. X-ray changes, when they appear (seldom before 3 months after the onset of ischaemia), are due to (a) reactive new bone formation at the boundary of the ischaemic area and (b) trabecular failure in the necrotic segment. An area of increased radiographic density appears in the subchondral bone; soon afterwards, suitable views may show a thin tangential fracture line just below the articular surface – the 'crescent sign'. In the late stages there is distortion of the articular surface and more intense 'sclerosis', now partly due to bone compression in a collapsed segment. Occasionally the necrotic portion separates from the parent bone as a discrete fragment. With all these changes (and this is the cardinal feature distinguishing primary avascular necrosis from the sclerotic and destructive forms of osteoarthritis, the 'joint space' retains its normal width because the articular cartilage is not destroyed until very late.

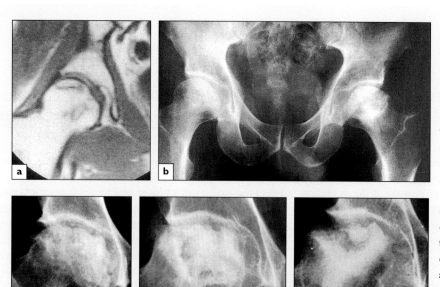

6.5 Avascular necrosis – imaging (a) The earliest changes are seen in the MRI: a hypo-intensive band in the T_1-weighted image. (b) X-ray of the same patient shows only a hint of sclerosis in the right femoral head but well-marked changes on the left.

(c–e) In long-standing cases the details may differ but the major features are constant: increased bone density and distortion of the bone architecture, but an intact joint space. Sometimes the necrotic segment separates ('dissects') as a discrete fragment (e).

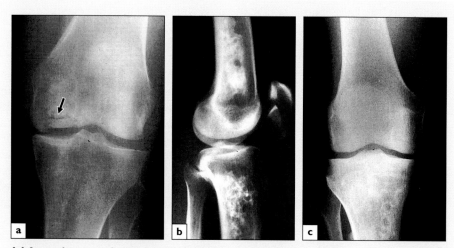

6.6 Avascular necrosis – x-rays (a) Osteonecrosis of the femoral condyle always affects the highest point of the articular surface, thus distinguishing it from osteochondritis dissecans which occurs adjacent to the intercondylar notch. (b) Medullary sclerosis, like dense puffs of smoke inside the bone away from the articular surface, is typical of bone infarction; this patient was x-rayed only because he fractured his patella. (c) A less common type of bone infarction appearing as rings of increased density in the metaphysis.

RADIOSCINTIGRAPHY Radionuclide scanning with ^{99m}Tc-sulphur colloid, which is taken up in myeloid tissue, may reveal an avascular segment. This is most likely in traumatic avascular necrosis, where a large segment of bone is involved, or in sickle-cell disease where a 'cold' area contrasts significantly with the generally high nuclide uptake due to increased erythroblastic activity. ^{99m}Tc-HDP scans (in the bone phase) may also show a 'cold' area, particularly if a large segment of bone is avascular (e.g. after fracture of the femoral neck). More often, however, the picture is dominated by *increased* activity, reflecting hyperaemia and new bone formation in the area around the infarct.

MRI This is the most reliable way of diagnosing marrow changes and bone ischaemia at a comparatively early stage. The first sign is a band-like low-intensity signal on the T_1-weighted SE image (and a similar but high-intensity signal on the STIR image), corresponding to the interface between ischaemic and normal bone. The site and size of the demarcated necrotic zone have been used to predict the progress of the lesions (see page 439).

COMPUTED TOMOGRAPHY CT involves considerable radiation exposure and it is not very useful for diagnosing osteonecrosis. However, it does show the area of bone destruction very clearly and it may be useful in planning surgery.

Tests for haemodynamic function

During the early stage of ischaemic necrosis the intramedullary pressure is often markedly raised. This phenomenon is most easily demonstrated in the femoral head. A cannula introduced into the metaphysis enables measurements to be taken (1) at rest and (2) after rapid injection of saline. The normal resting pressure is 10–20mmHg, rising by about 15mmHg after saline injection; in early osteonecrosis both the intramedullary pressure and the response to saline injection may be increased three- or fourfold. Venous stasis can also be demonstrated by venography after injection of radio-opaque medium into the bone.

Similar findings have been recorded in OA, but the change is not nearly as marked as in osteonecrosis.

Staging the lesion

Ficat and Arlet (1980) introduced the concept of *radiographic staging* for osteonecrosis of the hip to distinguish between early (pre-symptomatic) signs and later features of progressive demarcation and collapse of the necrotic segment in the femoral head. Their classification has since been slightly modified and applied also to other sites. *Stage 1* showed no x-ray change and the

diagnosis was based on measurement of intra-osseous pressure and bone biopsy. In *Stage 2* the femoral head contour was still normal but there were early signs of reactive change in the subchondral area. *Stage 3* was defined by clearcut x-ray signs of osteonecrosis with evidence of structural damage and distortion of the bone outline. In *Stage 4* there was collapse of the articular surface and signs of secondary OA. There are worries about the reproducibility and reliability of this system (Smith *et al.*, 1996); moreover, it cannot be used to predict the progress of early lesions.

Recent modifications involving assessment of both *the extent* and *the location* of the early changes on plain x-ray and MRI have proved to be more reliable as predictors of outcome, at least in relation to femoral head necosis (Shimizu *et al.*, 1994; Steinberg *et al.*, 1995). The location and size of the necrotic segment in Ficat stages 1–3 are defined by the hypo-intense band on the T_1-weighted MRI. Two general observations can be made: (1) The size of the ischaemic segment is determined at a very early stage and it rarely increases after that. (2) Small lesions which do not involve the maximally loaded zone of the articular surface tend not to collapse, whereas large lesions extending under the maximally loaded articular surface break down in over 60% of cases.

Shimizu's classification is particularly useful in planning treatment for osteonecrosis of the femoral head. This is discussed in Chapter 19.

Diagnosis of the underlying disorder

In many cases of osteonecrosis an underlying disorder will be obvious from the history: a known episode of trauma, an occupation such as deep-sea diving or working under compressed air, a family background of Gaucher's disease or sickle-cell disease.

There may be a record of high-dosage corticosteroid administration; for example, after renal transplantation where the drug is used for immunosuppression. However, smaller doses (e.g. as short-term treatment for asthma or as an adjunct in neurosurgical emergencies) and even topical corticosteroid preparations can also be dangerous in patients with other risk factors (Solomon and Pearse, 1994). Combinations of drugs (e.g. corticosteroids and azathioprine, or corticosteroids after a period of alcohol abuse) also can be potent causes of osteonecrosis; occasionally corticosteroids have been given without the patient's knowledge.

Alcohol abuse is often difficult to determine because patients tend to hide the information. There is no biochemical marker that is specific for high alcohol intake, but elevation of three or four of the following is highly suggestive: aspartate transaminase, γ-glutamyl transpeptidase (γ-GT), serum urate, serum triglyceride and mean red cell volume (Whitehead, *et al.*, 1978).

It has been suggested that patients with very early non-traumatic osteonecrosis, and children with early Perthes' disease, should undergo laboratory tests for coagulopathies; this has been justified by reports of cases in which the condition has been halted or reversed by treatment with antithrombotic preparations such as warfarin and stanozolol (Glueck *et al.*, 1997b). Unfortunately the tests are very expensive and there is understandable resistance to adopting this approach in routine management, especially since the hypothesis on which it is based is highly controversial (Liesner, 1999).

In cases of suspected SLE, antiphospholipid antibodies may be measured.

Prevention

The risk of developing osteonecrosis can be reduced by attention to certain measures: a policy of using corticosteroids only when essential and in minimal effective dosage; being aware of the cumulative effect of even moderate doses of corticosteroids in patients with a history of alcohol abuse; rigorous application of decompression procedures for divers and compressed-air workers; care in preventing anoxia in patients with haemoglobinopathies. Whether it is worth aspirating post-traumatic hip effusions or haemarthrosis to prevent capsular tamponade is still uncertain.

Studies now in progress will show whether it is justifiable to offer prophylactic treatment to relatives of patients with familial coagulopathies and osteonecrosis.

Treatment

In planning treatment, all the factors that influence the natural course of the condition must be taken into account: the general medical background, the type of ischaemic necrosis, the site and extent of the necrotic segment, its stage of development, the patient's age and capacity for bone repair, the persistence or otherwise of the aetiological agent and its effect on bone turnover.

Only general principles will be discussed here; the treatment of osteonecrosis in specific sites is dealt with in the appropriate chapters on regional orthopaedics.

EARLY OSTEONECROSIS

While the bone contour is intact there is always the hope that structural failure can be prevented. Some lesions heal spontaneously or, at any rate, do not progress to bone collapse; this is seen especially in areas which are not severely stressed: the non-weight-bearing joints, the superomedial part of the femoral head and the non-weightbearing surfaces of the femoral condyles and talus. Here one can afford to pursue a waiting policy. Antithrombotic medication is theoretically feasible in those cases shown to be associated with thrombophilia and hypofibrinolysis.

Heavily loaded lesions in weightbearing joints have a poor prognosis and will probably end in structural failure if left untreated. If the bone contour is still intact, an 'unloading' osteotomy will help to preserve the anatomy while remodelling proceeds. This approach is applicable especially to the hip and knee.

Medullary decompression and bone grafting may have a place in Ficat stage 1 and 2 osteonecrosis of the femoral head (page 439).

INTERMEDIATE STAGE OSTEONECROSIS

Once there is structural damage and distortion of the articular surface, conservative operations are inappropriate. However, the joint may still be salvageable and in this situation realignment osteotomy – either alone

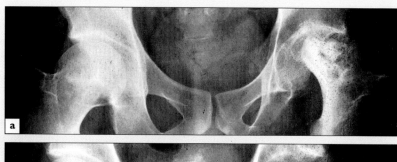
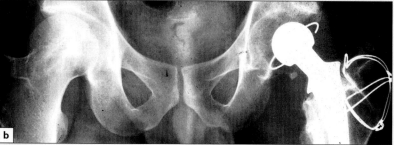

6.7 Osteonecrosis – treatment (a) Alcohol abuse has led to bilateral femoral head necrosis, advanced on the left but detectable only by MRI on the right. (b) The left hip had to be replaced; at the same time the right side was treated by drilling of the femoral neck (medullary decompression). This x-ray was taken 8 years later.

or combined with curettage and bone grafting of the necrotic segment – has a useful role.

If mobility can be sacrificed without severe loss of function (e.g. in the ankle or wrist), arthrodesis will relieve pain and restore stability.

LATE STAGE OSTEONECROSIS

Destruction of the articular surface may be give rise to pain and severe loss of function. Three options are available: (1) Non-operative management, concentrating on pain control, modification of daily activities and, where appropriate, splintage of the joint. (2) Arthrodesis of the joint, e.g. the ankle or wrist. Or (3) partial or total joint replacement, the preferred option for the shoulder, hip and knee.

SYSTEMIC DISORDERS ASSOCIATED WITH OSTEONECROSIS

DRUG-INDUCED NECROSIS

Alcohol, corticosteroids, immunosuppressives and cytotoxic drugs, either singly or in combination, are the commonest causes of non-traumatic osteonecrosis. 'At risk' doses for these drugs have not been established; the threshold depends not only on the total intake but also on the time over which the intake is spread and the presence or absence of associated disorders which themselves may predispose to osteonecrosis. A cumulative dose of 2000mg of prednisone equivalent administered over several years (for example in the treatment of rheumatoid arthritis) is less likely to cause osteonecrosis than the same dose given over a period of months (e.g. after organ transplantation). It is important to bear in mind that multiple causative agents have an additive effect; thus, osteonecrosis has been encountered after comparatively short courses and low doses of corticosteroids (totals of 800mg or less), but in these cases an additive factor can almost always be identified (Solomon and Pearse, 1994).

The threshold dose for alcohol is equally vague. However, based on the known dose relationship of alcohol-induced fatty degeneration of the liver, we would set it at around 150mg of ethanol per day for men and considerably less for women. Asking patients 'How much do you drink?' is unlikely to elicit an accurate response. However, the presence of raised serum triglyceride and γ-GT levels, together with an increased mean corpuscular volume (MCV), is highly suggestive of excessive alcohol intake.

SICKLE-CELL DISEASE

Sickle-cell disease is a genetic disorder in which the red cells contain abnormal haemoglobin (HbS). In deoxygenated blood there is increased aggregation of the haemoglobin molecules and distortion of the red cells, which become somewhat sickle-shaped. At first this is reversible and the cells reacquire their normal shape when the blood is oxygenated. Eventually, however, the red cell membrane becomes damaged and the cells are permanently deformed.

The sickle cell trait, which originated in West and Central Africa centuries ago, is an example of natural selection for survival in areas where malaria was endemic. From there the gene was carried to countries along the Mediterranean, the Persian Gulf, parts of India and across the Atlantic where it appears in people of Afro-American descent. In recent years it has spread more widely in Europe but it is rarely encountered south of the equator.

Sickle-cell disease is most likely in homozygous offspring (those with HbS genes from both mother and father), but it may also occur in heterozygous children with HbS/C haemoglobinopathy and HbS/thalassaemia. Inheritance of one HbS gene and one normal β-globin gene confers the (heterozygous) *sickle-cell trait*; HbS concentration is low and sickling occurs only under conditions of hypoxia (e.g. under inefficient anaesthesia, in extreme cold, at very high altitudes and when flying in unpressurized aircraft).

In the established disorder, the main clinical features are due to a combination of chronic haemolytic anaemia and a tendency to clumping of the sickle-shaped cells which results in diminished capillary flow and recurrent episodes of intracapillary thrombosis. Secondary changes such as trabecular coarsening, infarctions of the marrow, periostitis and osteonecrosis are common. Complications include hyperuricaemia (due to increased red cell turnover) and an increased susceptibility to bacterial infection.

CLINICAL FEATURES Children during the first 2 years of life may present with swelling of the hands and feet. X-rays at first seem normal, but later there may be suggestive features such as marrow densities and periosteal new bone formation ('dactylitis'). These changes are usually transient, but treatment is required for pain.

In older children a typical feature is recurrent episodes of severe pain, sometimes associated with fever. These 'crises', which may affect almost any part of the body, are thought to be due to infarcts.

Osteonecrosis of the femoral head is common, both in children (when it is sometimes mistaken for Perthes' disease) and in young adults, in whom other causes of non-traumatic osteonecrosis have to be excluded (Iwegbu and Fleming, 1985). Males and females are affected with almost equal frequency. The child develops a painful limp and movements are restricted. X-rays may show no more than a diffuse increase in density of the epiphysis; however, in most cases the changes are very similar to those of Perthes' disease, usually going on to flattening of the epiphysis. In

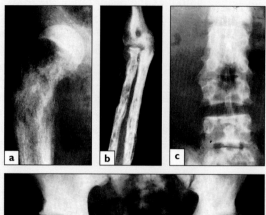

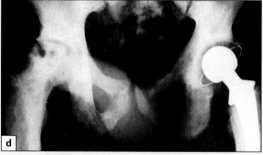

6.8 Sickle-cell disease (a) Typical changes in the femur due to marrow hyperplasia, with bone infarction and necrosis of the femoral head. (b) In severe cases infarctions of tubular bones may resemble osteomyelitis, with sequestra and a marked periosteal reaction (sometimes a true salmonella infection supervenes). (c) The spine also may be involved. (d) In adults osteoporosis is followed by endosteal sclerosis, seen clearly in the right femur; the left hip has already been replaced following femoral head necrosis.

young adults there are both destructive lesions and diffuse sclerosis of the femoral head.

The head of the humerus and the femoral condyles may be similarly affected.

Other bone changes are due to a combination of marrow hyperplasia and medullary infarctions. Trabecular coarsening and thickening of the cortices may be mistaken for signs of infection.

Bacterial osteomyelitis and *septic arthritis*, sometimes involving multiple sites, are serious complications, particularly in children. In over 50% of cases the organism is *Salmonella*.

TREATMENT A follow-up study of untreated children with femoral head necrosis due to sickle-cell disease showed that 80% of them had permanently damaged hips with severe loss of function (Hernigou *et al.*, 1991). This may be due to recurrent infarction and inflammatory changes in the joint.

Hypoxic conditions favouring the occurrence of crises should be avoided. If episodes of bone pain are frequent, transfusions may be necessary to reduce the concentration of HbS. During a crisis the patient should be given adequate analgesia and should be kept fully oxygenated. Infections should be guarded against, or treated promptly with the appropriate antibiotics.

Femoral head necrosis in children should be treated in the same way as Perthes' disease (see page 425). Adults are treated along the lines described on page 439. The emphasis in all cases should be on conservatism. Anaesthesia carries definite risks; failure to maintain adequate oxygenation may precipitate vascular occlusion in the central nervous system, lungs or kidneys. Prophylactic antibiotics are advisable as the risk of postoperative infection is high.

CAISSON DISEASE AND DYSBARIC OSTEONECROSIS

Decompression sickness (caisson disease) and osteonecrosis are important causes of disability in deep-sea divers and compressed-air workers building tunnels or underwater structures. Under increased air pressure the blood and other tissues (especially fat) become supersaturated with nitrogen; if decompression is too rapid the gas is released as bubbles, which cause local tissue damage, generalized embolic phenomena and intracapillary coagulation. Prolonged compression may also cause swelling of marrow fat cells and decreased intramedullary blood flow, possibly due to oxygen toxicity (Pooley and Walder, 1984).

The symptoms of decompression sickness, which may develop within minutes, are pain near the joints ('the bends'), breathing difficulty and vertigo ('the staggers'). In the most acute cases there can be circulatory and respiratory collapse, severe neurological changes, coma and death. Only 10% of patients with bone necrosis give a history of decompression sickness.

Radiological bone lesions have been found in 17% of compressed-air workers in Britain; almost half the lesions are juxta-articular – mainly in the humeral head and femoral head – but microscopic bone death is much more widespread than x-rays suggest.

Clinical and x-ray features The necrosis may cause pain and loss of joint movement, but many lesions remain 'silent' and are found only on routine x-ray examination. Medullary infarcts cause mottled calcification or areas of dense sclerosis. Juxta-articular changes are similar to those in other forms of osteonecrosis.

Management The aim is prevention; the incidence of osteonecrosis is proportional to the working pressure, the length of exposure, the rate of decompression and the number of exposures. Strict enforcement of suitable working schedules has reduced the risks considerably. The treatment of established lesions follows the principles already outlined.

GAUCHER'S DISEASE (see also page 158)

In this familial disorder lack of a specific enzyme results in the abnormal storage of glucocerebroside in the macrophages of the reticuloendothelial system. The effects are seen chiefly in the liver, spleen and bone marrow, where the large polyhedral 'Gaucher cells' accumulate. Bone complications are common and osteonecrosis is among the worst of them. The hip is most frequently affected, but lesions also appear in the distal femur, the talus and the head of the humerus. Bone ischaemia is usually attributed to the increase in medullary cell volume and sinusoidal compression, but it is likely that other effects (abnormal cell emboli and increased blood viscosity) are equally important.

Clinical features Bone necrosis may occur at any age and causes pain around one of the larger joints (usually the hip). In long-standing cases movements are restricted. There is a tendency for the Gaucher deposits to become infected and the patient may present with septicaemia. Blood tests reveal anaemia, leucopenia and thrombocytopenia. A diagnostic, though inconstant, finding is a raised serum acid phosphatase level.

X-ray The appearances resemble those in other types of osteonecrosis, and 'silent' lesions may be found in a number of bones. A special feature (due to replacement of myeloid tissue by Gaucher cells) is expansion of the tubular bones, especially the distal femur, producing the Erlenmeyer flask appearance. Cortical thinning and osteoporosis may lead to pathological fracture.

Treatment The condition can now be treated by replacement of the missing enzyme and there is evidence that this will reduce the incidence of bone complications.

The management of established osteonecrosis follows the principles outlined earlier. However, there is a greater risk of infection following operation and suitable precautions should be taken. For adults, total joint replacement is probably preferable to other procedures.

RADIATION NECROSIS

Ionizing radiation, if sufficiently intense or prolonged, may cause bone death. This is due to the combined effects of damage to small blood vessels, marrow cells and bone cells. Such changes, which are dose-related, often occurred in the past when low-energy radiation was in use. Nowadays, with megavoltage apparatus and more sophisticated planning techniques, long-term bone damage is much less likely; patients who present with osteonecrosis are usually those who were treated some years ago. Areas affected are mainly the shoulder and ribs (after external irradiation for breast cancer), the sacrum, pelvis and hip (after irradiation of pelvic lesions) and the jaws (after treatment of tumours around the head and neck).

Pathology Unlike the common forms of ischaemic necrosis, which always involve subchondral bone, radiation necrosis is more diffuse and the effects more variable. Marrow and bone cells die, but for months or even years there may be no structural change in the bone. Gradually, however, stress fractures appear and may result in widespread bone destruction. A striking feature is the absence of repair and remodelling. The surrounding bone is usually osteoporotic; in the jaw, infection may follow tooth extraction.

Clinical features The patient usually presents with pain around the shoulder, the hip, the sacrum or the pubic symphysis. There will always be a history of previous treatment by ionizing radiation, though this may not come to light unless appropriate questions are asked.

There may be local signs of irradiation, such as skin pigmentation, and the area is usually tender. Movements in the nearby joint are restricted. General examination may reveal scars or other evidence of the

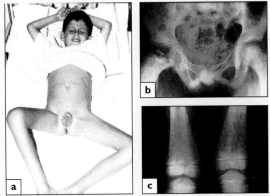

6.9 Gaucher's disease This young boy, whose sister also had Gaucher's disease, developed pain in the right hip; abduction was limited and painful. X-rays show necrosis of the right femoral head and widening of the femoral shafts (the Erlenmeyer flask appearance).

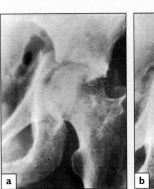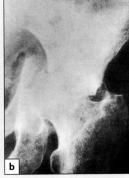

6.10 Radiation necrosis – x-rays This patient received radiation therapy for carcinoma of the bladder. One year later he developed pain in the left hip and x-ray showed (**a**) a fracture of the acetabulum. Diagnosis of radiation necrosis was confirmed when (**b**) the fracture failed to heal and the joint crumbled.

original lesion. X-rays show areas of bone destruction and patchy sclerosis; in the hip there may be an unsuspected fracture of the acetabulum or femoral neck, or collapse of the femoral head.

Treatment Treatment depends on the site of osteonecrosis, the quality of the surrounding bone and the life expectancy of the patient. If a large joint is involved (e.g. the hip), replacement arthroplasty may be considered; however, bone quality is often poor and there is a high risk of early implant loosening. Nevertheless, if pain cannot be adequately controlled, and if the patient has a reasonable life expectancy, joint replacement is justified.

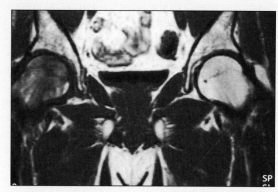

6.11 Bone marrow oedema MRI showing the typical diffuse area of low signal intensity in the right femoral head in the T$_1$-weighted image.

BONE MARROW OEDEMA SYNDROME

In 1959 Curtiss and Kincaid described an uncommon clinical syndrome characterized by pain and *transient osteoporosis* of one or both hips affecting women in the last trimester of pregnancy. It is now recognized that the condition can occur in patients of either sex and at all ages from late adolescence onwards. Although quite distressing at its onset, the condition typically lasts for only 6–12 months, after which the symptoms subside and radiographic bone density is restored. Sometimes successive joints are affected ('*regional migratory osteoporosis*'), with similar symptoms occurring at each site.

The aetiology of the condition is obscure. The intense activity shown on radionuclide scanning suggests a neurovascular abnormality akin to that of reflex sympathetic dystrophy (RSD). However, there are no trophic changes in the soft tissues and no long-term effects, such as one sees in RSD. The demonstration of diffuse changes on MRI – low signal intensity on T$_1$-weighted images and matching high signal intensity on

T$_2$-weighted images – corresponding to the areas of increased scintigraphic activity are characteristic of bone marrow oedema (Wilson *et al.*, 1988), and this is now thought to be an important aspect of transient osteoporosis. What causes it is still unknown.

Similar 'marrow oedema changes' are sometimes seen in areas around typical lesions of osteonecrosis and it has been suggested that transient osteoporosis is due to a sublethal, reversible episode of ischaemia associated with reactive hyperaemia in the surrounding bone (Hofmann *et al.*, 1993). Many would disagree with this hypothesis; the most significant differences between the two conditions are listed in Table 6.2. Furthermore, histological examination has failed to demonstrate necrosis in either bone or marrow in patients with typical transient osteoporosis (Yamamoto *et al.*, 1999). The issue is important because transient osteoporosis is a reversible disorder which requires only symptomatic treatment while osteonecrosis often calls for operative intervention.

Table 6.2 Differences between transient bone-marrow oedema and osteonecrosis

	Bone marrow oedma	Osteonecrosis
Sex distribution (M:F)	1:3	1:1
Predisposing factors	Pregnancy	Systemic disorders
		Corticosteroids
Onset	Acute	Gradual
Clinical progress	Self-limiting	Progressive
X-ray	Osteopenia	Sclerosis
Scintigraphy	Increased activity	Reduced activity
MRI	Diffuse changes	Focal changes
Histology	Marrow oedema	Marrow necrosis
	Minimal bone death	Bone necrosis

(See Guerra and Steinberg, 1995)

OSTEOCHONDRITIS (OSTEOCHONDROSIS)

The terms 'osteochondritis', or 'osteochondrosis', has for many years been applied to a group of conditions in which there is compression, fragmentation or separation of a small segment of articular cartilage and bone. The affected area shows many of the features of ischaemic necrosis, including death of bone cells in the osteoarticular fragment and reactive vascularity and osteogenesis in the surrounding bone. The disorder occurs mainly in adolescents and young adults, often during phases of increased physical activity, and may be initiated by trauma or repetitive stress. However, there must be other predisposing factors, for the condition is sometimes multifocal and sometimes runs in families. Recent observations suggest that some children are unusually predisposed to bone ischaemia because of an underlying vascular coagulopathy. Despite the name, there are no signs of inflammation.

Impact injuries may cause bleeding or oedema in the subarticular bone, resulting in capillary compression or thrombosis and localized ischaemia. Osteoarticular fractures can cause severance of the local blood supply and separation of a necrotic osteochondral fragment. And traction injuries may similarly damage the blood supply to an apophysis. These mechanisms are reflected in the somewhat simplistic subdivision into 'crushing', 'splitting' and 'pulling' osteochondritis.

CRUSHING OSTEOCHONDRITIS

This is usually seen in late adolescence, but adults also are sometimes affected. It is characterized by apparently spontaneous necrosis of the ossific nucleus in a long-bone epiphysis or one of the cuboidal bones of the wrist or foot. Local anatomical features (e.g. a metatarsal bone that is longer than usual, or disproportion in the lengths of radius and ulna) which could result in undue compressive stress being applied to the bone, can sometimes be identified.

The pathological changes are the same as those in other forms of osteonecrosis: bone death, fragmentation or distortion of the necrotic segment, and reactive new bone formation around the ischaemic trabeculae.

Pain and limitation of joint movement are the usual complaints. Tenderness is sharply localized to the affected bone. X-rays show the characteristic increased density, accompanied in the later stages by distortion and collapse of the necrotic segment.

The common examples of crushing osteochondritis have, by long tradition, acquired eponymous labels: *Freiberg's disease* of the metatarsal; *Köhler's disease* of the navicular; *Kienböck's disease* of the carpal lunate; and *Panner's disease* of the capitulum.

Vertebral osteochondritis (*Scheuermann's disease*) is similar in kind but without clear evidence of bone death. Compression and fragmentation of the vertebral epiphyseal plates lead to distorted growth of the vertebral bodies. The condition occurs during adolescence and may cause back pain and dorsal kyphosis. X-rays show irregularity or fragmentation of the vertebral endplates; in the thoracic spine the affected vertebrae may end up slightly wedge-shaped (hence the kyphosis).

SPLITTING OSTEOCHONDRITIS (OSTEOCHONDRITIS DISSECANS)

A small segment of articular cartilage and the subjacent bone may separate (dissect) as an avascular fragment. This occurs typically in young adults, usually men, and affects particular sites: the lateral surface of the medial femoral condyle in the knee, the anteromedial corner of the talus in the ankle, the superomedial part of the femoral head, the humeral capitulum and the first metatarsal head.

The cause is almost certainly repeated minor trauma resulting in osteochondral fracture of a convex surface; the fragment loses its blood supply.

The knee is much the commonest joint to be affected. The patient presents with intermittent pain, swelling and joint effusion. If the necrotic fragment

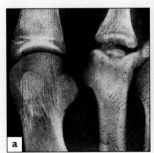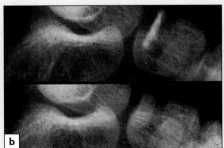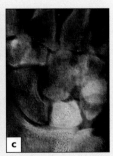

6.12 Crushing osteochondritis (a) Freiberg's disease of the second metatarsal; (b) Köhler's disease of the navicular, compared with the normal side below; (c) Kienbock's disease of the lunate.

becomes completely detached, it may cause locking of the joint or unexpected episodes of giving way. Less frequently, similar episodes occur in the hip or ankle.

X-rays must be taken with the joint in the appropriate position to show the affected part of the articular surface in tangential projection. The dissecting fragment is defined by a radiolucent line of demarcation. When it separates, the resulting 'crater' may be obvious.

The early changes (i.e. before demarcation of the dissecting fragment) are better shown by MRI: there is decreased signal intensity in the area around the affected osteochondral segment. Radionuclide scanning with ^{99m}Tc-HDP shows markedly increased activity in the same area.

Treatment in the early stage consists of load reduction and restriction of activity. In children, complete healing may occur, though it takes up to 2 years; in adults, it is doubtful whether the future course of events can be significantly influenced. However, it is generally recommended that partially detached fragments are pinned back in position after roughening of the base, while completely detached fragments should be pinned back only if they are fairly large and completely preserved. In the knee, these procedures may be carried out by arthroscopy. If the fragment becomes detached and causes symptoms, it should be fixed back in position or else completely removed.

PULLING OSTEOCHONDRITIS (TRACTION APOPHYSITIS)

Localized pain and increased radiographic density in an unfused apophysis may result from tensile stress on the physeal junction. This is seen at two sites: the tibial tuberosity (*Osgood–Schlatter's disease*) and the calcaneal apophysis (*Sever's disease*); both are subject to unusual traction forces from powerful tendons which insert into the apophysis. The bone changes may be a reaction to repetitive local trauma but this never leads to true necrosis.

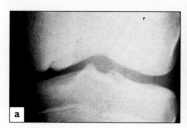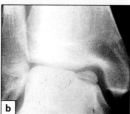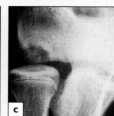

6.13 Splitting osteochondritis The osteochondral fragment usually remains in place at the articular surface. The most common sites are (**a**) the medial femoral condyle, (**b**) the talus and (**c**) the capitulum.

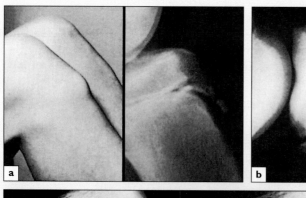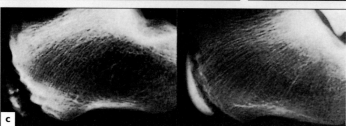

6.14 Pulling osteochondritis These are merely traction lesions, dignified by eponyms: (**a**) Osgood–Schlatter's disease involves the apophysis into which the knee extensor mechanism is inserted; (**b**) in Johannson–Larsen's disease the calcification is a sequel to the patellar ligament partially pulling away from the bone; (**c**) Sever's disease, compared with the normal side.

REFERENCES AND FURTHER READING

Asherson RA, Lioté F, Page B *et al.* (1993) Avascular necrosis of bone and antiphospholipid antibodies in systemic lupus erythematosus. *Journal of Rheumatology* **20**, 284-288

Curtiss PH, Kincaid WE (1959) Transitory demineralization of the hip in pregnancy: a report of three cases. *Journal of Bone and Joint Surgery* **41**A, 1327-1333

Ficat RP (1985) Idiopathic bone necrosis of the femoral head: early diagnosis and treatment. *Journal of Bone and Joint Surgery* **67**B, 3-9

Ficat RP, Arlet J (1980) *Ischemia and Necroses of Bone* (edited and adapted by DS Hungerford). Williams & Wilkins, Baltimore

Francis RB Jr (1991) Platelets, coagulation and fibrinolysis in sickle-cell disease: Their possible role in vascular occlusion. *Blood Coagulation and Fibrinolysis* **2**, 341-353

Glueck CJ, Crawford A, Roy D *et al.* (1996) Association of antithrombotic factor deficiencies and hypofibrinolysis with Legg-Perthes' disease. *Journal of Bone and Joint Surgery* **78**A, 3-13

Glueck CJ, Freiberg R, Tracy T *et al.* (1997a) Thrombophilia and hypofibrinolysis: Pathophysiologies of osteonecrosis. *Clinical Orthopaedics* **334**, 43-56

Glueck CJ, Crawford A, Roy D *et al.* (1997b) Correspondence. *Journal of Bone and Joint Surgery* **79**A, 1114-5

Guerra JJ, Steinberg ME (1995) Distinguishing transient osteoporosis from avascular necrosis of the hip. *Journal of Bone and Joint Surgery* **77**A, 616-624

Hernigou P, Galacteros F, Bachir D *et al.* (1991) Deformities of the hip in adults who have sickle-cell disease and had avascular necrosis in childhood. *Journal of Bone and Joint Surgery* **73**A, 81-92

Hofmann S, Engel A, Neuhold A *et al.* (1993) Bone-marrow oedema syndrome and transient osteoporosis of the hip. *Journal of Bone and Joint Surgery* **75**B, 210-216

Iwegbu CF, Fleming AF (1985) Avascular necrosis of the femoral head in sickle-cell disease. *Journal of Bone and Joint Surgery* **67**B, 29-32

Jones JP Jr (1994) Concepts of etiology and early pathogenesis of osteonecrosis. In: Schafer IM (ed), *Instructional Course Lectures.* American Academy of Orthopaedic Surgeons **43**, 499-512

Liesner RJ (1999) Editorial. Does thrombophilia cause Perthes' disease in children? *Journal of Bone and Joint Surgery* **81**B, 565–566

Pooley J, Walder DN (1984) The effect of compressed air on bone marrow blood flow and its relationship to caisson disease of bone. In: *Bone Circulation* (eds J Arlet, RP Ficat and DS Hungerford). Williams & Wilkins, Baltimore, 53-67

Sakamoto M, Shimizu K, Iida S *et al.* (1997) Osteonecrosis of the femoral head: A prospective study with MRI. *Journal of Bone and Joint Surgery* **79**B, 213-219

Shimizu K, Moriya H, Akita T (1994) Prediction of collapse with magnetic resonance imaging of avascular necrosis of the femoral head. *Journal of Bone and Joint Surgery* **76**A, 215-223

Smith SW, Meyer RA, Connor PM *et al.* (1996) Interobserver reliability and intraobserver reproducibility of the modified Ficat classification system of osteonecrosis of the femoral head. *Journal of Bone and Joint Surgery* **78**A, 1702-1706

Solomon L, Pearse MF (1994) Osteonecrosis following low-dose short-course corticosteroids, *Journal of Orthopaedic Rheumatology* **7**, 203-205

Steinberg ME, Hayken GD, Steinberg DR (1995) A quantitative system for staging avascular necrosis. *Journal of Bone and Joint Surgery* **77**B, 34-41

Whitehead TP, Clarke CA, Whitfield AGW (1978) Biochemical and haematological markers of alcohol intake. *Lancet* **1**, 978-981

Wilson ΛJ, Murphy WΛ, Hardy DC *et al.* (1988) Transient osteoporosis: transient bone marrow oedema? *Radiology* **167**, 757-760

Yamamoto T, Kubo T, Hirasawa Y *et al.* (1999) A cliniocopathologic study of transient osteoporosis of the hip. *Skeletal Radiology* **28**, 621-627

Metabolic and endocrine disorders

Bones have obvious mechanical functions: they support and protect the soft tissues, transmit load and muscular force from one part of the body to another and mediate movement and locomotion.

Bone as a tissue has an equally important role as a mineral reservoir which helps to regulate the composition – and in particular the calcium ion concentration – of the extracellular fluid. For all its solidity, bone is in a continuous state of flux, its internal shape and structure changing from moment to moment in concert with the normal variations in mechanical function and mineral exchange. All modulations in bone structure and composition are brought about by cellular activity, which is regulated by hormones and local factors; these agents, in turn, are controlled by alterations in mineral ion concentrations. The metabolic bone disorders are conditions in which generalized skeletal abnormalities result from disruption of this complex interactive system.

BONE AND BONES

BONE COMPOSITION

Bone consists of a largely collagenous matrix which is impregnated with mineral salts and populated by cells.

The matrix

The matrix is composed of *type I collagen* lying in a *mucopolysaccharide* ground substance. There are also small amounts of non-collagenous protein, mainly in the form of *proteoglycans* and the bone-specific proteins *osteonectin,* which appears to be involved in bone mineralization, and osteocalcin – or Gla protein – whose function is unknown. Gla protein is produced only by osteoblasts and its concentration in the blood is, to some extent, a measure of osteoblastic activity. The unmineralized matrix is known as osteoid; normally it is seen only as a thin layer on surfaces where active new bone formation is taking place, but the proportion of osteoid to mineralized bone increases significantly in rickets and osteomalacia.

Bone mineral

Almost half the bone volume is mineral matter – mainly *calcium* and *phosphate* in the form of *crystalline hydroxyapatite* which is laid down in osteoid at the calcification front. The interface between bone and osteoid can be labelled by administering tetracycline, which is taken up avidly in newly mineralized bone and shows as a fluorescent band on ultraviolet light microscopy. In mature bone the proportions of calcium and phosphate are constant and the molecule is firmly bound to collagen; 'demineralization' occurs only by resorption of the entire matrix.

Bone cells

There are of three types of bone cell: osteoblasts, osteocytes and osteoclasts.

Osteoblasts are concerned with bone formation; they are derived from local mesenchymal precursors and form rows of small (20μm) cuboidal cells along the free surfaces of trabeculae and haversian systems where new bone is laid down. They are rich in alkaline phosphatase and are responsible for the production of type I collagen as well as the non-collagenous bone proteins and for the mineralization of bone matrix (Peck and Woods, 1988). They may also be involved in the initiation and control of osteoclastic activity. At the end of a bone remodelling cycle the osteoblast either remains on the newly formed surface as a quiescent lining cell or becomes enveloped in the matrix as a resting osteocyte.

Osteocytes can therefore be regarded as spent osteoblasts. Lying in their bony lacunae, they communicate with each other and with the surface lining cells by slender cytoplasmic processes. Their function is obscure: they may, under the influence of parathyroid hormone, participate in bone resorption ('osteocytic osteolysis') and calcium ion transport (Peck and Woods, 1988). It has also been suggested that they are sensitive to mechanical stimuli and communicate information and changes in stress and strain to the active osteoblasts (Skerry *et al.,* 1989).

Osteoclasts are the principal mediators of bone resorption. These large multinucleated cells are derived from monocytic precursors in the marrow and, under appropriate conditions, they are attracted by chemotactic stimuli to bone surfaces which have been 'prepared' in some way by the lining osteoblasts. A specific region on the cell surface the – so-called ruffled border – has been identified as the zone of attachment to bone. Once activated, osteoclastic bone resorption is carried out by lysozomal enzymes. With resorption of the organic matrix, the osteoclasts are left in shallow excavations along the surface – Howship's lacunae. By identifying these excavations one can distinguish 'resorption surfaces' from the smooth 'formation surfaces' or 'resting surfaces' in histological sections.

BONE STRUCTURE

Bone in its immature state is called *woven bone*; the collagen fibres are arranged haphazardly and the cells have no specific orientation. Typically it is found in the early stages of fracture healing, where it acts as a temporary weld before being replaced by mature bone. The mature tissue is *lamellar bone*, in which the collagen fibres are arranged parallel to each other to form multiple layers (or laminae) with the osteocytes lying between the lamellae. Unlike woven bone, which is laid down in fibrous tissue, lamellar bone forms only on existing bone surfaces.

Lamellar bone exists in two structurally different forms, *compact (cortical) bone* and *cancellous (trabecular) bone*.

Compact bone

Compact (cortical) bone is dense to the naked eye. It is found where support matters most: the outer walls of all bones but especially the shafts of tubular bones, and the subchondral plates supporting articular cartilage. It is made up of compact units – haversian systems or osteons – each of which consists of a central canal (the haversian canal) containing blood vessels, lymphatics and nerves and enclosed by closely packed, more or less concentric lamellae of bone. Between the lamellae lie osteocytes, bedded in lacunae which appear to be discrete but which are in fact connected by a network of fine canaliculae. The haversian canal offers a free surface lined by bone cells; its size varies, depending on whether the osteon is in a phase of resorption or formation. During resorption osteoclasts eat into the surrounding lamellae and the canal widens out; during formation osteoblasts lay down new lamellae on the inner surface and the canal closes down again.

Cancellous bone

Cancellous (trabecular) bone has a honeycomb appearance; it makes up the interior meshwork of all bones and is particularly well developed in the ends of the tubular

bones and the vertebral bodies. The structural units of trabecular bone are flattened sheets or spars that can be thought of as unfolded osteons. Three-dimensionally the trabecular sheets are interconnected (like a honeycomb) and arranged according to the mechanical needs of the structure, the thickest and strongest along trajectories of compressive stress and the thinnest in the planes of tensile stress. The interconnectedness of this meshwork lends added strength to cancellous bone beyond the simple effect of tissue mass. The spaces between trabeculae – the 'opened out' vascular spaces – contain the marrow and the fine sinusoidal vessels that course through the tissue, nourishing both marrow and bone.

Trabecular bone is obviously more porous than cortical bone. Though it makes up only one-quarter of the total skeletal mass, it provides two-thirds of the total bone surface. Add to this the fact that it is covered with marrow and it is easy to understand why the effects of metabolic disorders are usually seen first in trabecular bone.

Haversian system

Bones vary greatly in size and shape. At the most basic level, however, they are similar: compact on the outside and spongy on the inside. Their outer surfaces (except at the articular ends) are covered by a tough *periosteal membrane*, the deepest layer of which consists of potentially bone-forming cells. The inner, endosteal, surfaces are irregular and lined by a fine *endosteal membrane* in close contact with the marrow spaces.

The osteonal pattern in the cortex is usually depicted from two-dimensional histological sections. A three-dimensional reconstruction would show that the *haversian canals* are long branching channels running in the longitudinal axis of the bone and connecting extensively with each other and with the endosteal and periosteal surfaces by smaller channels (*Volkmann canals*). In this way the vessels in the haversian canals form a rich anastomotic network between the medullary and periosteal blood supply. Blood flow in this capillary network is normally centrifugal – from the medullary cavity outwards – and it has long been held that the cortex is supplied entirely from this source. However, it seems likely that at least the outermost layers of the cortex are normally also supplied by periosteal vessels, and if the medullary vessels are blocked or destroyed the periosteal circulation can take over entirely and the direction of blood flow is reversed.

BONE MODELLING AND REMODELLING

New bone growth occurs in two different ways: (1) by ossification of proliferating cartilage (*endochondral ossification*), typically at the epiphyseal growth plate (physis) or during bone repair; and (2) by direct ossification in

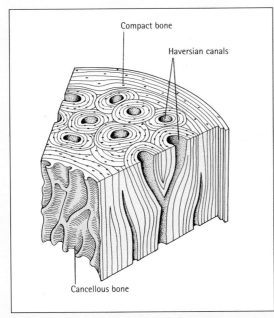

7.1 Bone structure A slice of cortex shows the basic elements of compact bone: outer laminae of subperiosteal bone, densely packed osteons each made up of concentric layers of bone and osteocytes around a central haversian canal which contains the vessels, and the inner surface (endosteum) which merges into a lattice of cancellous bone.

connective tissue (*membranous ossification*), as seen in the formation of subperiosteal new bone.

During growth the most newly formed bone has continuously to be 'sculpted' into the normal shape of that particular region. How else can a long bone retain its shape as the flared ends are carried further and further from the midshaft during growth? This 'sculpting', properly known as *modelling*, proceeds by co-ordinated phases of osteoclastic resorption and osteoblastic formation of bone. At the same time the internal trabecular pattern is fashioned according to the functional needs of the bone: trabeculae that lie along lines of compressive stress end up thicker than those lying in planes of tensile stress (see Wolff's Law, page 111).

The same process continues throughout adult life, except now it is directed not at the modelling of a particular shape but at the constant *remodelling* of existing bone. This serves a crucial purpose in the preservation of skeletal structure: 'old bone' is continually replaced by 'new bone' and in this way the skeleton is protected from exposure to excessive loading frequencies and stress failure. Besides, the maintenance of calcium homeostasis requires a constant turnover of the mineral deposits which would otherwise stay locked in bone.

At each *remodelling site* work proceeds in an orderly and unvarying sequence: osteoclasts gather on a free bone surface and excavate a cavity; they disappear and, after a period of quiescence, are replaced by osteoblasts which proceed to fill in the excavation with new bone. Each cycle of bone turnover – which takes from 4 to 6 months – is conducted by groups of cells that appear to work in concert; together they make a *bone remodelling unit*. The annual rate of turnover has been estimated as 4% for cortical bone and 25% for trabecular bone (Parfitt, 1988). The rate of bone turnover may be increased or decreased either by alterations in the number of remodelling units at work or by changes in the remodelling time.

Resorption starts when osteoclasts are activated and attracted by chemotaxis to a mineralized surface. The organic matrix and mineral are removed together; on a trabecular plate this produces a simple excavation, but in cortical bone the cells either enlarge an existing haversian canal or else burrow into the compact bone to create *a cutting cone* – like miners sinking a new shaft. After 2–3 weeks resorption ceases and the osteoclasts disappear. A week or two later the cavity surface is covered with osteoblasts and for the next 3 months bone *formation and mineralization* slowly restore the lost tissue.

During bone remodelling, resorption and formation are *coupled*, the one ineluctably following the other.

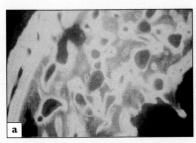 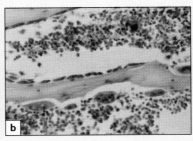 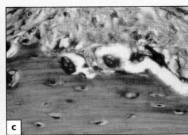

7.2 Bone turnover (**a**) Bone can be 'labelled' by administering tetracycline which appears in newly mineralized bone as a fluorescent band. Actively forming osteons are easily identified. (**b**) The cells that govern bone turnover are the osteoclasts (along the scalloped surface of this trabeculum) and the more populous osteoblasts (lining the opposite, bone-forming surface). (**c**) High-power of osteoclasts in Howship's lacunae.

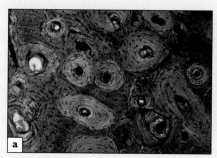
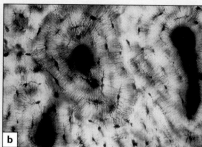

7.3 Histology (a) Low-power and (b) high-power views showing the osteons in various stages of formation and resorption.

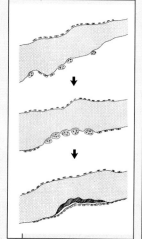
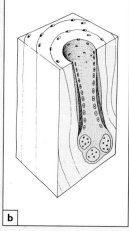

7.4 Bone remodelling Bone is remodelled by a regular, almost invariable sequence of cellular activities. (a) Open surfaces are first excavated by osteoclasts and then lined and filled in again by a following train of osteoblasts. (b) In compact bone the osteoclasts burrow deeply to produce a cutting cone, with the osteoblasts appearing behind them to reline the cavity with new bone.

REGULATION OF BONE TURNOVER AND MINERAL EXCHANGE

Over 98% of the body's calcium and 85% of its phosphorus are tightly packed in bone and capable of only very slow exchange. A small amount of mineral is in a rapidly exchangeable form, either in partially formed crystals or in the extracellular fluid where calcium and phosphate concentrations depend mainly on intestinal absorption and renal excretion; transient alterations in serum levels are accommodated quickly by changes in renal tubular absorption.

The control of calcium is much more critical than that of phosphate; thus, in persistent calcium deficiency the extracellular calcium ion concentration is maintained by drawing on bone, whereas phosphate deficiency simply leads to lowered serum phosphate concentration. The regulation of calcium exchange is therefore linked inescapably to that of bone formation and bone resorption. The complex balance between calcium absorption, renal tubular excretion, extracellular circulation and calcium turnover in bone is controlled by an array of systemic and local factors.

Calcium

Calcium is essential for normal cell function and physiological processes such as nerve conduction and muscle contraction. An uncompensated fall in extracellular calcium concentration may cause tetany; an excessive rise can lead to depressed neuromuscular transmission.

The normal calcium concentration in plasma and extracellular fluid is 2.2–2.6mmol/l (8.8–10.4mg/dl). Much of this is bound to protein; about half is ionized and effective in cell metabolism and the regulation of calcium homoeostasis.

The recommended daily intake of calcium is 800–1000mg (20–25mmol), and ideally this should be increased to 1500mg during pregnancy and lactation. However, it is well known that many people in underdeveloped countries manage on half these amounts. About 50% of the dietary calcium is absorbed (mainly

This ensures that, at least over the short term, a balance is maintained, though at any moment and at any particular site one or other process may predominate.

In the long term, change is inevitable. During the first half of life, formation slightly exceeds resorption and bone mass increases; in later years resorption exceeds formation and bone mass steadily diminishes. Rapid bone loss leading to osteoporosis is usually due to excessive resorption rather than diminished formation.

Tilting the balance in the remodelling cycle towards bone loss is relatively easy: any number of disorders – and even minor physiological deviations like lack of exercise – may lead to osteoporosis. To regain lost bone, on the other hand, is extremely difficult. Remodelling follows a simple slogan: *No gain without prior loss!* Under normal circumstances bone formation occurs only after a preceding cycle of resorption. Any attempt to shift the emphasis away from resorption and towards formation must take account of this paradox.

in the upper gut) but much of that is secreted back into the bowel and only about 200mg (5mmol) enters the circulation.

Calcium absorption is mediated by vitamin D metabolites and requires a suitable calcium/phosphate ratio. Absorption is inhibited by excessive intake of phosphates (common in soft drinks), oxalates (found in tea and coffee), phytates (chapatti flour) and fats, by the administration of certain drugs (including corticosteroids) and in malabsorption disorders of the bowel.

Urinary excretion varies between 2.5 and 5mmol (100–200mg) per 24 hours; if calcium intake is reduced, urinary excretion is adjusted by increasing tubular reabsorption. If calcium concentration is persistently reduced, calcium is drawn from the skeleton by increased bone resorption. These compensatory shifts in intestinal absorption, renal excretion and bone remodelling are regulated by parathyroid hormone (PTH) and vitamin D metabolites.

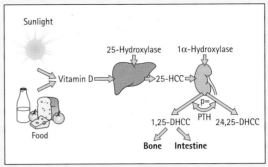

7.5 Vitamin D metabolism Cholecalciferol is derived either from the diet or by conversion of precursors when the skin is exposed to sunlight. This inactive 'vitamin' is hydroxylated, first in the liver and then in the kidney, to form the active metabolite 1,25-dihydroxycholecalciferol (DHCC).

Phosphorus

Phosphorus is needed for many important metabolic processes. Plasma concentration – almost entirely in the form of ionized inorganic phosphates – is 0.9–1.3mmol/l (2.8–4.0mg/dl). It is abundantly available in the diet and is absorbed in the small intestine, more or less in proportion to the amount ingested; however, absorption is reduced in the presence of antacids such as aluminium hydroxide, which binds phosphorus in the gut.

Phosphate excretion is extremely efficient, but 90% is reabsorbed in the proximal tubules. Tubular reabsorption is decreased (and overall excretion increased) by PTH.

While PTH undoubtedly plays a part in phosphate homeostasis, its main role is to regulate calcium concentration, with phosphate taking second place. Recently, however, evidence has accumulated which points to the existence of another hormone, phosphatonin, which also decreases tubular reabsorption of phosphate independently of PTH and which therefore has an important role in regulating phosphate concentration. Where it is secreted is uncertain, but the most likely source is thought to be the liver (Nesbitt and Drezner, 1996).

Magnesium

Magnesium plays a small but important part in mineral homeostasis. The cations are distributed in the cellular and extracellular compartments of the body and appear in high concentration in bone. Magnesium is necessary for the efficient secretion and peripheral action of PTH. Thus, if hypocalcaemia is accompanied by hypomagnesaemia it cannot be fully corrected until normal magnesium concentration is restored.

Vitamin D

Vitamin D, through its active metabolites, is principally concerned with calcium absorption and transport and (acting together with PTH) bone remodelling. Target organs are the small intestine and bone.

Naturally occurring vitamin D_3 (cholecalciferol) is derived from two sources: directly from the diet and indirectly by the action of ultraviolet light on the precursor 7-dihydrocholesterol in the skin. The normal requirement is about 400IU per day. In most countries this is obtained mainly from exposure to sunlight; those who lack such exposure are likely to suffer from vitamin D deficiency. Vitamin D itself is inactive. Conversion to active metabolites (which function as hormones) takes place first in the liver by 25-hydroxylation to form 25-hydroxycholecalciferol (25-HCC), and then in the kidneys by further hydroxylation (mediated by PTH) to 1,25-dihydroxycholecalciferol (1,25-DHCC). The concentration of these metabolites can be measured in serum samples.

The terminal metabolite, 1,25-DHCC (calcitriol), is the most active form. Acting on the *lining cells of the small intestine*, it increases the absorption of calcium and phosphate. *In bone* it acts together with PTH to promote osteoclastic resorption; it also enhances calcium transport across the cell membrane and indirectly assists with osteoid mineralization.

Other, less active, vitamin D metabolites are formed by the kidney. Indeed, 24,25-DHCC is normally present in far greater quantity than 1,25-DHCC, but during negative calcium balance production switches to 1,25-DHCC in response to PTH secretion (see below); the increased 1,25-DHCC then helps to maintain the serum calcium concentration by promoting intestinal absorption of calcium.

Parathyroid hormone

PTH is the fine regulator of calcium exchange. It maintains the extracellular calcium concentration between very narrow limits; production and release are stimulated by a fall and suppressed (up to a point) by a rise in plasma ionized calcium. Target organs are the kidney, bone and (indirectly) the gut. The active terminal fragment of the PTH molecule can be readily estimated in blood samples.

Acting on the *renal tubules*, PTH increases phosphate excretion by restricting its reabsorption, and conserves calcium by increasing its reabsorption. These responses rapidly compensate for any change in plasma ionized calcium. Acting on *the kidney parenchyma*, it controls hydroxylation of the vitamin D metabolite, 25-HCC.

In *bone* PTH promotes osteoclastic resorption and the release of calcium and phosphate into the blood. This it does, not by direct action on osteoclasts but by stimulating the osteoblasts to prepare the bone surface for resorption and to initiate osteoclast chemotaxis; the net effect is a prolonged rise in plasma calcium. There may also be a rapid stimulation of osteocytic osteolysis.

In the *intestine* PTH has an indirect action; it stimulates calcium absorption by promoting the conversion of vitamin D to its active metabolite in the kidney.

Calcitonin

Calcitonin, which is secreted by the C cells of the thyroid, does more or less the opposite of PTH: it suppresses osteoclastic bone resorption and increases renal calcium excretion. This occurs especially when bone turnover is high, as in Paget's disease. Its secretion is stimulated by a rise in serum calcium concentration above 2.25mmol/l (9mg/dl).

Other hormones

A number of hormones that influence epiphyseal growth, bone formation and bone resorption play a secondary role in calcium balance.

Oestrogen is thought to stimulate calcium absorption and to protect bone from the unrestrained action of PTH. Its withdrawal leads to bone depletion and, in some cases, frank osteoporosis. This occurs naturally at the menopause, but a similar effect is seen in amenorrhoeic young women who may actually lose bone at a time when their peers are building up to peak bone mass.

Adrenal corticosteroids in excess cause a pernicious type of osteoporosis due to a combination of increased bone resorption, diminished bone formation, decreased intestinal calcium absorption and increased calcium excretion; collagen synthesis may also be defective.

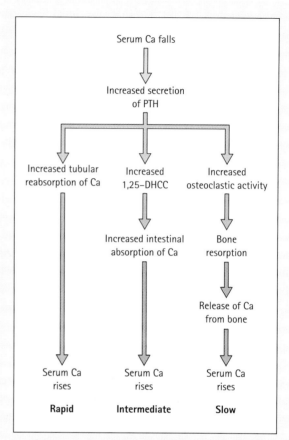

7.6 Homoeostatic loop Effect of a fall in serum calcium.

Thyroxine increases both formation and resorption, but more so the latter; hyperthyroidism is associated with high bone turnover and osteoporosis.

Local factors

Systemic hormones have a large-scale effect on bone turnover; they translate the shifts in calcium and phosphate balance to the work-front where bone remodelling takes place. But the intimate processes of signalling between osteoblasts and osteoclasts, cell recruitment and activation, spatial organization and mineral transport are mediated by local factors derived from bone cells, matrix components and cells of the immune system. Some serve as messengers between systemic and local agents; others behave as autocrines and paracrines. *Insulin-like growth factor I (somatomedin C)* is produced mainly in the liver but probably also by osteoblasts under the influence of growth hormone. It stimulates osteoblast proliferation and osteoblastic activity in bone formation. *Transforming growth factors* produced during bone resorption can stimulate osteoblastic activity; this may account for the coupling of resorption and formation. *Interleukin-1 (IL-1)* and *osteoclast-activating factor (OAF)*, cytokines derived from monocytes and lymphocytes, are powerful activators of bone resorption; they are thought to be responsible

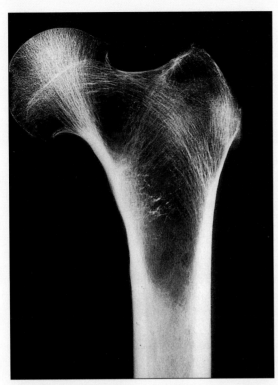

7.7 Wolff's law The elegant trabecular pattern of the upper femur shows how well the anatomical structure conforms to the imposed forces; the thickest trabeculae lie in the lines of the greatest stress.

for osteoporosis in inflammatory disorders, multiple myeloma and other malignant tumours. *Prostaglandins* are produced by bone cells and regulate both osteoclastic and osteoblastic activity. They are important in promoting bone resorption in inflammatory disorders and fractures and may also account for the bone destruction and hypercalcaemia in metastatic bone disease.

There is considerable interaction between cytokines and some of the hormones which control bone turnover. For example, oestrogen deficiency leads to activation of cytokines which, in turn, stimulate osteoclastic activity (Horowitz, 1993).

Bone morphogenetic protein (BMP), which can be extracted from bone matrix, induces chondrogenesis and bone formation. This process – known as bone induction – may be important in fracture healing and bone graft replacement.

Mechanical stress

It is well known that the direction and thickness of trabeculae in cancellous bone are related to regional stress trajectories. This is recognized in Wolff's law (1896), which says that the architecture and mass of the skeleton are adjusted to withstand the prevailing forces imposed by functional need or deformity. Physiological stress is supplied by gravity, load-bearing, muscle action and vascular pulsation. If a continuous bending force is applied, more bone will form on the concave surfaces (where there is compression) and bone will thin down on the convex surfaces (which are under tension). Weightlessness, prolonged bed rest, lack of exercise, muscular weakness and limb immobilization are all associated with osteoporosis. How physical signals are transmitted to bone cells is not known, but they almost certainly operate through local growth factors.

Electrical stimulation

When bone is loaded or deformed, small electrical potentials are generated - negative on compressed surfaces and positive on surfaces under tension (Brighton and McCluskey, 1986). This observation led to the idea that stress-generated changes in bone mass may be mediated by electrical signals; from this it was a logical step to suggest that induced electrical potentials can affect bone formation and resorption. How, precisely, this is mediated remains unknown. Electromagnetic field potentials have been used for the treatment of delayed fracture union and regional osteoporosis, so far with inconclusive results.

Other environmental factors

Moderate rises in temperature or oxygen tension have been shown experimentally to increase bone formation. *Acid–base balance* affects bone resorption, which is increased in chronic acidosis and decreased in alkalosis.

Increased dietary phosphates or pyrophosphates tend to inhibit bone resorption. Pyrophosphate analogues (*bisphosphonates*) are used in the treatment of osteoporosis, where they appear to inhibit both resorption and formation.

Fluoride has complex effects on bone, the most important being direct stimulation of osteoblastic activity, the formation of fluoroapatite crystals (which are resistant to osteoclastic resorption) and an apparent increase in mineral density without a concomitant gain in strength; there is also evidence of calcium retention and secondary hyperparathyroidism. *Fluorosis* occurs as an endemic disorder in India and some other parts of the world due to an excess of fluoride in the drinking water.

AGE-RELATED CHANGES IN BONE

Bone turnover or remodelling goes on throughout life. It varies in rate, extent and distribution according to the demands of growth, endocrine activity, mechanical stress and biochemical exchange. During

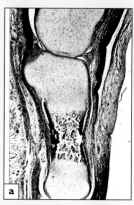 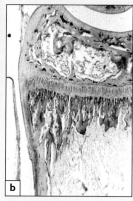 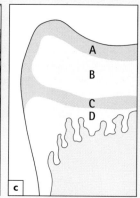

7.8 Bone growth (a) A foetal phalanx, with bone forming in its cartilage model.

(b, c) During childhood the bone shows the familiar separation into
(A) articular cartilage
(B) epiphysis
(C) cartilaginous growth plate (physis)
(D) newly formed juxtaepiphyseal bone.

growth the entire bone increases in size and changes somewhat in shape. At the epiphyseal growth plate (physis), new bone is added by endochondral ossification; on the surface, bone is formed directly by subperiosteal appositional ossification; the medullary cavity is expanded by endosteal bone resorption; bulbous bone ends are re-formed and sculpted continuously by co-ordinated formation and resorption. Although during childhood each bone gets longer and wider, the bone tissue of which it is made remains quite light and porous.

Between puberty and 30 years of age the haversian canals and intertrabecular spaces are to some extent filled in and the cortices increase in overall thickness; i.e. the bones become heavier and stronger. Bone mass increases at the rate of about 3% per year and during the third decade each individual attains a state of peak bone mass, the level of which is determined by genetic, hormonal, dietary and environmental factors. The greater the peak bone mass, the less marked will be the effects of the inevitable depletion which occurs in later life.

From 30 years onwards there is a slow but inexorable loss of bone; haversian spaces enlarge, trabeculae become thinner, the endosteal surface is resorbed and the medullary space expands – i.e. year by year the bones become slightly more porous. The diminution in bone mass proceeds at a rate of about 0.3% per year in men and 0.5% per year in women up to the menopause.

From the onset of the menopause and for the next 10 years the rate of bone loss in women accelerates to about 3% per year, occurring predominantly in trabecular bone. This steady depletion is due mainly to excessive resorption – osteoclastic activity seeming to be released from the restraining influence of gonadal hormone. (Similar changes are seen in younger women about 5 years after oophorectomy.) About 30% of white women will lose bone to the extent of developing postmenopausal osteoporosis. For reasons that are not fully understood, the degree of bone depletion is much less marked in blacks than in whites.

From the age of 65 or 70 years the rate of bone loss gradually tails off and by the age of 75 years it is about 0.5% per year. This later phase of depletion is due mainly to diminishing osteoblastic activity (Parfitt, 1988).

Men are affected in a similar manner, but the phase of rapid bone loss occurs 15 or 20 years later than in women, at the climacteric.

Bone mass and bone strength

It is important to recognize that throughout life, and regardless of whether *bone mass* increases or decreases, the degree of *mineralization* in normal people varies very little from age to age or from one person to another. With advancing years the loss of bone mass is accompanied by a *disproportionate loss of bone strength*, which is explained in a number of ways. (1) The absolute diminution in bone mass is the most important, but not the only, factor. (2) With increased postmenopausal bone resorption, gaps appear in the plates of trabecular bone; not all these defects are repaired and the loss of structural connectivity further reduces the overall strength of the bone. (3) In old age the decrease in bone cell activity makes for a slow remodelling rate; old bone takes longer to be replaced and microtrauma to be repaired, thus increasing the likelihood of stress failure.

METABOLIC DISORDERS

The common metabolic bone disorders are associated, in varying degree, with depletion of bone tissue or bone mineral and (in some cases) with systemic features of altered mineral metabolism. The most common conditions fall into three groups: (1) *osteoporosis*, in which the quantity of bone (bone mass) is abnormally low; (2) *osteomalacia*, in which the osseous connective tissue (osteoid) is present but insufficiently mineralized; and (3) *osteitis fibrosa*, in which PTH overproduction leads to bone resorption and replacement by fibrous tissue.

CLINICAL ASSESSMENT

The clinical features of metabolic bone disease are essentially those of *skeletal failure* (bone pain, fractures and deformity), *hypercalcaemia* (anorexia, abdominal pain, depression, renal stone or metastatic calcification) or some *underlying endocrine disorder*.

X-rays may show *stress fractures, vertebral compression, cortical thinning, loss of trabecular structure* or merely an ill-defined loss of radiographic density – *osteopenia* – which can signify either osteomalacia or osteoporosis.

These appearances are so common in old people that they seldom generate a call for detailed investigation. However, in patients under the age of 50 years, those with repeated fractures or bone deformities and those with associated systemic features, a full *clinical, radiological and biochemical evaluation* is essential.

History

The duration of symptoms and their relationship to previous disease, drug therapy or operations are important.

Other causal associations are retarded growth, malnutrition, dietary fads, intestinal malabsorption, alcohol abuse and cigarette smoking.

Examination

The patient's appearance may be suggestive of an endocrine or metabolic disorder: the moon face and cushingoid build of hypercortisonism; the smooth, hairless skin of testicular atrophy; physical underdevelopment in rickets. Thoracic kyphosis is a non-specific feature of spinal osteoporosis.

X-rays

Decreased skeletal radiodensity is a late and unreliable sign of bone loss; it becomes apparent only after a 30% reduction in mineral or skeletal mass.

One of the earliest signs of osteoporosis is loss of the horizontal trabeculae in the vertebral bodies; the remaining vertical trabeculae seem, by contrast, to be more conspicuous and the vertebral cortices are sharply etched around the faded interiors. There may be obvious fractures – new and old – especially in the spine, ribs, pubic rami or corticocancellous junctions of the long bones. Small stress fractures are more difficult to detect: they may be found in the proximal parts of the femur or tibia. The vertebral bodies may show compression fractures, minor wedging at multiple levels or biconcave distortion of the end-plates due to bulging of intact intervertebral discs.

In addition to these general signs of reduced bone mass or defective mineralization, there may be specific features of bone disorders such as rickets, hyperparathyroidism, metastatic bone disease or myelomatosis.

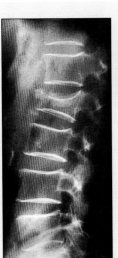
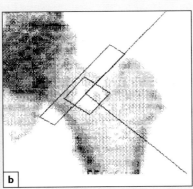
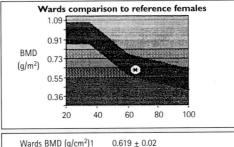

Wards comparison to reference females

Wards BMD (g/cm²)1	0.619 ± 0.02
Wards % young females	68 ± 3
Wards % age matched	95 ± 3

7.9 Osteoporosis - x-ray and bone density scan (a) This x-ray shows a compression fracture of a single vertebra - L2. Other characteristic signs are loss of vertebral 'density', with relative accentuation of the vertebral end-plates and the remaining vertical trabeculae. (b) Bone mass is best measured by dual-energy x-ray absorptiometry scan. In this case the value fell towards the lower limit of normal for the relevant age group.

Measurement of bone mass

The investigation of bone-losing disorders has been greatly advanced by the development of methods for measuring bone mineral density (BMD) and bone mass. Measurement is based on the principle that a beam of energy is attenuated as it passes through bone, and the degree of attenuation is related to the mass and mineral content of the bone. BMD is expressed in grams per unit area (or unit volume in the case of computed tomography, CT) and is recorded in comparison to the sex- and age-specific distribution of these values in the general population. The measurements are specific for each location (lumbar spine, femoral neck, distal radius, etc).

Radiographic absorptiometry Density is measured using standard radiographs and comparing the values against those of an aluminium reference wedge. The method is applicable only to appendicular sites such as the hand or calcaneum. However, it is simple and cheap and can be used as a crude screening procedure in general practice.

Single-energy x-ray absorptiometry This measures the attenuation of a collimated photon beam as it passes through bone. The method is simple and not very expensive. However, it is applicable only to the appendicular skeleton, and measuring the BMD at the wrist (for example) does not accurately reflect bone density in the spine or femoral neck.

Quantitative computed tomography Quantitative CT permits measurement of mineral content per unit volume of bone, which is a true expression of bone density. It also provides separate values for cortical and cancellous bone. Its main drawback is the high radiation exposure, and it is no more accurate than dual-energy x-ray absorptiometry (DEXA).

Dual-energy x-ray absorptiometry This is now the method of choice. Precision and accuracy are excellent, x-ray exposure is not excessive and measurements can be obtained anywhere in the skeleton (Mirsky and Einhorn, 1998). It should, however, be noted that the presence of spinal osteophytes and bone bridges will make vertebral density measurements unreliable. Some investigators have reported good correlation between measurements in the appendicular and axial skeleton. However, the risk of fracture at any particular site is best gauged by measuring bone density at the target site.

INDICATIONS
The main indications for using bone densitometry are: (a) to assess the degree and progress of bone loss in patients with clinically diagnosed metabolic bone disease or conditions such as hyperparathyroidism, corticosteroid-induced osteoporosis, gonadal deficiency or other endocrine disorders; (b) as a screening procedure for perimenopausal women with multiple risk factors for osteoporotic fractures; and (c) to monitor the effect of treatment for osteoporosis.

Biochemical tests

Serum calcium and phosphate concentrations should be measured in the fasting state, and it is the ionized calcium fraction that is important.

Serum alkaline phosphatase concentration is an index of osteoblastic activity; it is raised in osteomalacia and in disorders associated with high bone turnover (hyperparathyroidism, Paget's disease, bone metastases).

Osteocalcin (Gla protein) is a more specific marker of bone formation; elevated serum levels suggest increased bone turnover.

Parathyroid hormone activity can be estimated from serum assays of the COOH terminal fragment. However, in renal failure the test is unreliable because there is reduced clearance of the COOH fragment.

Vitamin D activity is assessed by measuring the serum 25-HCC concentration. Serum 1,25-DHCC levels do not necessarily reflect vitamin uptake but are reduced in advanced renal disease.

Urinary calcium and phosphate excretion can be measured. Significant alterations are found in malabsorption disorders, hyperparathyroidism and other conditions associated with hypercalcaemia.

Urinary hydroxyproline excretion is a measure of bone resorption. It may be increased in high-turnover conditions such as Paget's disease but it is not sensitive enough to reflect lesser increases in bone resorption.

Excretion of pyridinium compounds and telopeptides derived from bone collagen cross-links is a much more sensitive index of bone resorption (Rosen *et al.*, 1994). This may be useful in monitoring the progress of hyperparathyroidism and other types of osteoporosis. However, excretion is also increased in chronic arthritis associated with bone destruction.

NB: Laboratory reports should always state the normal range for each test, which may be different for infants, children and adults.

Bone biopsy

Standardized bone samples are easily obtained from the iliac crest and can be examined (without prior decalcification) for histological bone volume, osteoid formation and the relative distribution of formation and resorption surfaces. The rate of bone remodelling can also be gauged by labelling the bone with tetracycline on two occasions (2 weeks apart) before obtaining the biopsy. Tetracycline is taken up in new bone and produces a fluorescent strip on ultraviolet light microscopy. By measuring the distance between the two labels, the rate of new bone formation can be calculated. Characteristically in osteomalacia there is a decrease in the rate of bone turnover and an increase in the amount of uncalcified osteoid.

OSTEOPOROSIS

Osteoporosis, in the broadest sense, describes a state in which bone is fully mineralized but its structure is abnormally porous and its strength is less than normal for a person of that age and sex. Stated more pedantically: there is a significant decrease in bone mass per unit volume of bone tissue and this is accompanied by increased fragility of the bone.

Bone depletion may be brought about by predominant bone resorption, decreased bone formation or a combination of the two. It seems self-evident that the main reason for the loss of bone strength is the reduction in bone mass; however, in the trabecular bone that is still present there may also be a loss of structural connectivity, and this so alters the mechanical properties that the loss of strength is out of proportion to the diminution in bone mass. As a consequence, the bone – particularly around the diaphyseo-metaphyseal junctions in tubular bones and in the mainly cancellous vertebral bodies – eventually reach a state in which a comparatively minor strain causes a fracture.

The defining radiographic features of osteoporosis are loss of trabecular definition and thinning of the cortices. The term '*osteopenia*' is sometimes used to describe bone which appears to be less dense than normal on x-ray, without defining whether the loss of density is due to osteoporosis or to osteomalacia, or indeed whether it is sufficiently marked to be regarded as at all pathological. In an attempt to avoid confusion, osteoporosis is sometimes defined in terms of BMD as measured by DEXA of the spine and hips, using the lower value of the two. For example, anything more than 2.5 standard deviation (SD) below the average for premenopausal women in the relevant population group may be defined as osteoporosis. While this provides a useful statistical index for calculating the risk of skeletal failure, it ignores the importance of other risk factors in determining whether or not a particular person will suffer an insufficiency fracture.

Osteoporosis may be confined to a particular bone or group of bones – *regional osteoporosis* – (for example due to disuse) – or it may appear as *generalized osteoporosis*. It is also conveniently classified as *primary*, in which no specific cause can be found but which is usually related to ageing processes and decreased gonadal activity, and *secondary* (due to a variety of endocrine, metabolic and neoplastic disorders).

PRIMARY OSTEOPOROSIS

Primary osteoporosis usually manifests as an exaggerated form of the 'physiological' bone depletion that normally accompanies ageing and loss of gonadal activity (see page 111). Two overlapping patterns are described: an early postmenopausal syndrome characterized by rapid bone loss due predominantly to increased osteoclastic resorption (type I or high turnover osteoporosis), and a less well-defined syndrome which emerges in very elderly people and is due to a gradual slow-down in osteoblastic activity and the increasing appearance of dietary insufficiencies and chronic ill health (type II or low turnover osteoporosis).

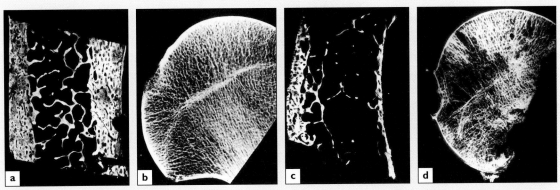

7.10 Osteoporosis Fine detail x-rays of iliac crest biopsies and femoral head slices, showing the contrast between trabecular density in a healthy 40-year old woman (**a, b**) and one of 70 years with post-menopausal osteoporosis (**c, d**).

Postmenopausal osteoporosis

Women at the menopause, and for the next 10 years, lose bone at an accelerated rate – about 3% per year compared with 0.3% during the preceding decade. This is due mainly to increased bone resorption, the withdrawal of oestrogen having removed one of the normal restraints on osteoclastic activity. In some cases this process is exaggerated and results in osteoporosis and skeletal failure.

RISK FACTORS   A number of risk factors for this group have been identified: Caucasoid (white) or Asiatic ethnicity; a family history of osteoporosis; a history of anorexia nervosa and/or amenorrhoea; low peak bone mass in early adulthood; early onset of menopause; early hysterectomy; skinny or emaciated build; dietary insufficiency; alcohol abuse; cigarette smoking; and chronic lack of exercise. The question of low calcium intake as a risk factor is controversial, with conflicting evidence both for and against.

CLINICAL FEATURES   A woman at or near the menopause develops back pain and increased thoracic kyphosis; she, or someone in the family, may have noticed that her height has diminished. X-rays may show wedging or compression of one or more vertebral bodies. This is the typical picture, but sometimes the first clinical event is a low-energy fracture of the distal radius or one of the other bone ends.

DEXA scans may show significantly reduced bone density in the vertebral bodies or femoral neck.

The rate of bone turnover is either normal or slightly increased; measurement of excreted collagen cross-link products and telopeptides may suggest a high-turnover type of bone loss.

Once the general diagnosis has been established, screening tests should be performed to rule out causes of secondary osteoporosis (see page 118).

PREVENTION AND TREATMENT   Bone densitometry can be used to identify women who are at more than usual risk of suffering a fracture at the menopause, and prophylactic treatment of this group would seem sensible. However, routine DEXA screening (even in countries where it is available) is still a controversial issue; for practical purposes, it is usually reserved for women with multiple risk factors and particularly those with suspected oestrogen deficiency (premature or surgically induced menopause) or some other bone-losing disorder, and those who have suffered previous low-energy fractures at the menopause.

Women approaching the menopause should be advised to maintain adequate levels of dietary calcium and vitamin D, to keep up a high level of physical activity and to avoid smoking and excessive consumption of alcohol. If necessary, the recommended daily requirements should be met by taking calcium and vitamin D supplements; these measures have been shown to reduce the risk of low-energy fractures in elderly women (Chapuy *et al.*, 1994).

Oestrogen medication (hormone replacement therapy, or HRT) is the most effective way of maintaining bone density and reducing the risk of fracture after the menopause; when treatment is stopped, bone loss proceeds at the usual rate. However, there are drawbacks to HRT, notably the risk of recurrent bleeding after the menopause and fears about an increase in the incidence of breast and uterine cancer after long-term treatment, and this has inhibited its more general acceptance. For practical purposes, HRT is encouraged for women with positive risk factors and low BMD on

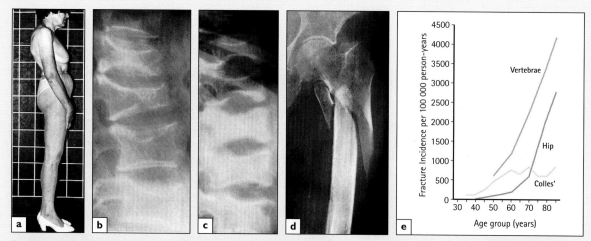

7.11 Osteoporosis (a) This woman noticed that she was becoming more and more round-shouldered; she also had chronic backache and her x-rays **(b)** show compression of vertebral bodies. **(c)** The spine of a similar patient who, 6 years after this film was taken, fell in her kitchen and sustained the fracture shown in **(d)**. The fracture incidence in women rises steeply after the menopause **(e)**.

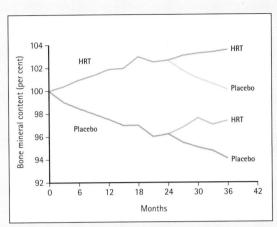

7.12 Postmenopausal osteoporosis – treatment Controlled trials have shown that hormone replacement therapy can prevent the otherwise inevitable bone loss that occurs after the menopause. When HRT is replaced by placebo (cross-over trials), there is a significant drop in bone mineral content (after Lindsay, *et al.*, 1984).

DEXA scanning– especially if there are other reasons for wanting to prescribe this medication – and is contraindicated if risk factors for breast cancer are identified. In women who have not had a hysterectomy, the risk of uterine cancer can be eliminated by administering a combination of oestrogen and progestin.

Bisphosphonates offer a useful alternative to HRT. The newer preparations (especially alendronate) have been shown to prevent bone loss and to reduce the risk of vertebral and hip fractures (Liberman *et al.*, 1995; Black *et al.*, 1996). Gastrointestinal side effects are a bother and suitable precautions should be taken.

Calcitonin has also been used with moderately good effect and is available in the form of a nasal spray.

Fluoride is one of the few drugs which directly stimulate osteoblastic activity. As originally used, in the form of sodium fluoride, it produced an increase in vertebral bone density but bone quality was, if anything, adversely affected and long-term studies failed to show a reduction in fracture rates. More recently, slow-release fluoride in low dosage together with calcium supplements has given better results (Pak *et al.*, 1995).

Osteoporosis of old age
(involutional or 'senile' osteoporosis)

Fifteen years after the menopause in women, and at the same age (the seventh or eight decade) in men, there is still a steady loss of bone mass – about 0.5% per year. This is so universal as to be regarded as a physiological manifestation of ageing. However, in some people (and much more often in women) bone loss reaches the point where fractures occur after comparatively minor trauma. This is most likely to happen in women who have already shown signs of poor bone mass around the menopause; significantly, the incidence of vertebral fracture rises steadily from the age of 50 years onwards, and by 70 years almost a third of white women will have at least one vertebral fracture. Worse still, after 65 years there is a rising incidence of femoral neck fracture – again more marked in women than in men, and much more marked in whites and Asians than in black peoples. However, measurements of bone mass at that age show that there is considerable overlap between those who fracture and those who don't; the assumption is that *qualitative changes* contribute increasingly to bone fragility in old age.

RISK FACTORS Risk factors are similar to those of postmenopausal osteoporosis, with some additions. Prolonged menopausal bone loss may be important; in advanced years there is also a high incidence of chronic illness, mild urinary insufficiency, dietary deficiency, lack of exposure to sunlight, muscular atrophy, loss of balance and an increased tendency to fall. Many old people suffer from vitamin D deficiency and they have mild osteomalacia – which further weakens frail bones.

CLINICAL FEATURES Symptoms and signs are essentially an exaggeration of those seen in postmenopausal osteoporosis. There may be fractures of the ribs or the pubic rami. The classic 'event' is a fracture of the femoral neck, usually after minimal trauma. X-rays may reveal obvious loss of trabecular markings in the femoral neck and the spine, or old vertebral compression fractures. Serum and urinary biochemistry is usually normal, unless there is associated osteomalacia.

TREATMENT Initially, treatment is directed at management of the fracture. This will often require internal fixation; the sooner these patients are mobilized and rehabilitated the better. Patients with muscle weakness and/or poor balance may benefit from gait training and, if necessary, the use of walking aids and rail fittings in the home.

Thereafter the question of general treatment must be considered. Obvious factors such as concurrent illness, dietary deficiencies, lack of exposure to sunlight and lack of exercise will need attention. If there is any doubt about the adequacy of vitamin D and calcium intake, dietary supplements should be prescribed. Beyond this, treatment is hampered by two factors: very few drugs have any positive effect on bone formation; and at that age bone turnover is so slow that metabolic manipulation takes a long time to produce any noticeable increase in bone mass. Nevertheless, if bone mass is markedly reduced, it may still be worthwhile administering bisphosphonates or HRT; although bone mass will not be restored, at least further loss may be slowed.

SECONDARY OSTEOPOROSIS

There are numerous causes of secondary osteoporosis (Table 7.1). The most important are hypercortisonism, gonadal hormone deficiency, hyperthyroidism, multiple myeloma, chronic alcoholism and immobilization. It is impractical to screen all osteoporotic patients for these conditions, but those under 50 years – and older patients with rapidly increasing osteoporosis – should be fully investigated to exclude any potentially reversible disorder.

Hypercortisonism

Glucocorticoid overload occurs in endogenous Cushing's disease or after prolonged treatment with corticosteroids. This often results in severe osteoporosis, especially if the condition for which the drug is administered is itself associated with bone loss – for example, rheumatoid arthritis. The deleterious effect on bone is mainly by suppression of osteoblast function, but there is also reduced calcium absorption, increased calcium excretion and stimulation of PTH secretion (Hahn, 1980). Bone resorption is markedly increased and formation is suppressed.

Treatment presents a problem, because the drug may be essential for the control of some generalized disease. However, forewarned is forearmed: corticosteroid dosage should be kept to a minimum, and it should not be forgotten that intra-articular preparations and cortisone ointments are absorbed and may have systemic effects if given in high dosage or for prolonged periods. Patients on long-term glucocorticoid treatment should, ideally, be monitored for bone density.

Preventive measures include the use of calcium supplements (at least 1500mg per day) and vitamin D. In postmenopausal women and elderly men, HRT is important. Bisphosphonates may also be effective in reducing bone resorption.

In late cases general measures to control bone pain may be required. Fractures are treated as and when they occur.

Gonadal hormone insufficiency

Oestrogen lack is an important factor in postmenopausal osteoporosis. It also accounts for osteoporosis in younger women who have undergone oophorectomy, and in pubertal girls with ovarian agenesis and primary amenorrhoea (Turner's syndrome). Further bone loss can be prevented by long-term HRT. Amenorrhoeic female athletes, and adolescents with anorexia nervosa, may become osteoporotic; fortunately these conditions are usually self-limiting.

A decline in testicular function probably contributes to the continuing bone loss and rising fracture rate in

Table 7.1 Some causes of osteoporosis

Nutritional	*Malignant disease*
Scurvy	Carcinomatosis
Malnutrition	Mutiple myeloma
Malabsorption	Leukaemia

Endocrine disorders	*Non-malignant disease*
Hyperparathyroidism	Rheumatoid arthritis
Gonadal insufficiency	Ankylosing spondylitis
Cushing's disease	Tuberculosis
Thyrotoxicosis	Chronic renal disease

Drug-induced	*Idiopathic*
Corticosteroids	Juvenile osteoporosis
Alcohol	Postclimacteric osteoporosis
Heparin	

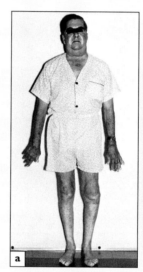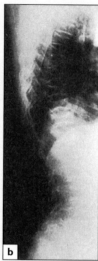

7.13 Hypercortisonism (a) Cushing's syndrome, due in this instance to prolonged corticosteroid treatment for rheumatoid disease. (b) On x-ray the bones look 'washed-out' and there may be spontaneous compression fractures.

men over 70 years of age. A more obvious relationship is found in young men with overt hypogonadism; this may require long-term treatment with testosterone.

Hyperthyroidism

Thyroxine speeds up the rate of bone turnover, but resorption exceeds formation. Osteoporosis is quite common in hyperthyroidism, but fractures usually occur only in older women who suffer the cumulative effects of the menopause and thyroid overload. However, in the worst cases there may be severe and widespread osteoporosis with spontaneous fractures, a marked rise in serum alkaline phosphatase, hypercalcaemia and hypercalciuria. Treatment is needed for both the osteoporosis and the thyrotoxicosis.

Multiple myeloma and carcinomatosis

Generalized osteoporosis, anaemia and a high erythrocyte sedimentation (ESR) are characteristic features of myelomatosis and metastatic bone disease. Bone loss is due to overproduction of local osteoclast-activating factors (see page 191).

Alcohol abuse

This is a common (and often neglected) cause of osteoporosis at all ages, with the added factor of an increased tendency to falls and other injuries. Bone changes are due to a combination of decreased calcium absorption, liver failure and a toxic effect on osteoblast function. Alcohol also has a mild glucocorticoid effect.

Immobilization

The worst effects of stress reduction are seen in states of weightlessness; bone resorption, unbalanced by formation, leads to hypercalcaemia, hypercalciuria and severe osteoporosis. Lesser degrees of osteoporosis are seen in bedridden patients, and regional osteoporosis is common after immobilization of a limb. The effects can be mitigated by encouraging mobility, exercise and weightbearing.

Other conditions

There are many other causes of secondary osteoporosis, including hyperparathyroidism (which is considered below), rheumatoid arthritis, ankylosing spondylitis and even subclinical forms of osteogenesis imperfecta (page 153). The associated clinical features usually point to the diagnosis.

RICKETS AND OSTEOMALACIA

Rickets and osteomalacia are different expressions of the same disease: inadequate mineralization of bone. Bone tissue throughout the skeleton is incompletely calcified, and therefore 'softened' (*osteomalacia*). In children there are also effects on physeal growth and ossification, resulting in deformities of the endochondral skeleton (*rickets*).

The inadequacy may be due to calcium deficiency, hypophosphataemia or defects anywhere along the metabolic pathway for vitamin D: nutritional lack, underexposure to sunlight, intestinal malabsorption, decreased 25-hydroxylation (liver disease, anticonvulsants) and reduced 1α-hydroxylation (renal disease, nephrectomy, 1α-hydroxylase deficiency). The rate of bone formation is slowed down and unmineralized osteoid accumulates along the surfaces of the new bone.

Pathology

The characteristic pathological changes in *rickets* arise from the inability to calcify the intercellular matrix in the deeper layers of the physis. The proliferative zone is as active as ever, but the cells, instead of arranging themselves in orderly columns, pile up irregularly; the entire physical plate increases in thickness, the zone of calcification is poorly mineralized and bone formation is sparse in the zone of ossification. The new trabeculae are thin and weak, and with joint loading the juxta-epiphyseal metaphysis becomes broad and cup-shaped.

Away from the physis the changes are essentially those of *osteomalacia*. Sparse islands of bone are lined by wide osteoid seams, producing ghost trabeculae that are not very strong. The cortices also are thinner than normal and may show signs of new or older stress fractures. If the condition has been present for a long time there may be stress deformities of the bones: indentation of the pelvis, bending of the femoral neck (coxa vara) and bowing of the femora and tibiae.

Clinical features

CHILDREN The infant with *rickets* may present with tetany or convulsions. There is failure to thrive, listlessness and muscular flaccidity. Early bone changes are deformity of the skull (craniotabes) and thickening of the knees, ankles and wrists from physeal overgrowth. Enlargement of the costochondral junctions ('rickety rosary') and lateral indentation of the chest (Harrison's sulcus) may also appear. Distal tibial bowing has been attributed to sitting or lying cross-legged.

Children who are already walking usually present with bow legs or knock knees, swollen joints and disturbed gait. They also lag in growth. In severe rickets there may be coxa vara, spinal curvature and long-bone fractures.

ADULTS *Osteomalacia* has a much more insidious course and patients may complain of bone pain, backache and muscle weakness for many years before the diagnosis is made. Vertebral collapse causes loss of height, and existing deformities such as mild kyphosis or knock knees – themselves perhaps due to adolescent rickets – may increase in later life. Unexplained pain in the hip or one of the long bones may presage a stress fracture.

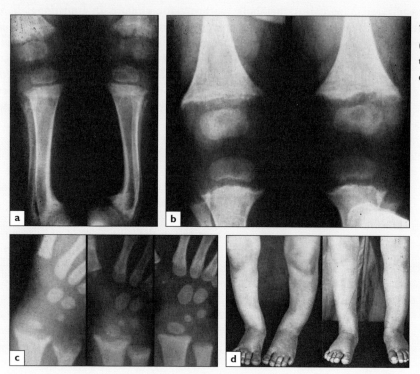

7.14 Rickets (**a**, **b**) Florid disease; (**c**) series showing the response to treatment; (**d**) before and after osteotomy for the neglected case.

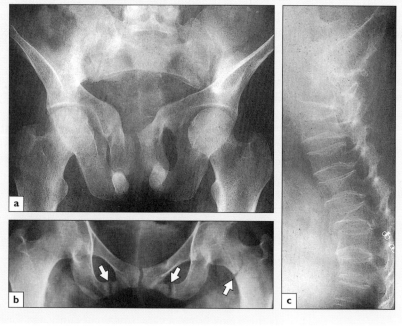

7.15 Osteomalacia Three characteristic features of osteomalacia: (**a**) indentation of the acetabula producing the trefoil or champagne-glass pelvis; (**b**) Looser's zones in the pubic rami and left femoral neck; (**c**) biconcave (codfish) vertebrae.

X–rays

In active *rickets* there is thickening and widening of the growth plate, cupping of the metaphysis and, sometimes, bowing of the diaphysis. The metaphysis may remain abnormally wide even after healing has occurred.

The classic lesion of *osteomalacia* is the Looser zone, a thin transverse band of rarefaction in an otherwise normal-looking bone. These zones, seen especially in the shafts of long bones and the axillary edge of the scapula, are due to incomplete stress fractures which heal with callus lacking in calcium. More often, however, there is simply a slow fading of skeletal structure, resulting in biconcave vertebrae (from disc pressure), lateral indentation of the acetabula ('trefoil' pelvis) and spontaneous fractures of the ribs, pubic rami, femoral neck or the metaphyses above and below the knee.

120

Table 7.2 Osteomalacia and osteoporosis

Osteomalacia	Osteoporosis
	Common in ageing women
	Prone to pathological fracture
	Decreased bone density
Unwell	Well
Generalized chronic ache	Pain only after fracture
Muscles weak	Muscles normal
Looser's zones	No Looser's zones
Alkaline phosphatase increased	Normal
Serum phosphorus decreased	Normal
Ca × P <2.4mmol/l	Ca × P >2.4mmol/l

Secondary hyperparathyroidism occurs if the serum calcium is persistently low. In children the resulting subperiosteal erosions are at the sites of maximal remodelling (medial borders of the proximal humerus, femoral neck, distal femur and proximal tibia, lateral borders of the distal radius and ulna). In adults the middle phalanges of the fingers are more often affected, and in severe cases brown tumours ('cysts') are seen in the long bones.

Biochemistry

Changes common to almost all types of rickets and osteomalacia are diminished levels of serum calcium and phosphate, increased alkaline phosphatase and diminished urinary excretion of calcium. In vitamin D deficiency the 25-HCC levels also are low. The 'calcium phosphate product' (derived by multiplying calcium and phosphorus levels expressed in mmol/l), normally about 3, is diminished in rickets and osteomalacia, and values of less than 2.4 are virtually diagnostic.

Bone biopsy

With clear-cut clinical and x-ray features the diagnosis is obvious. In less typical cases a bone biopsy will provide the answer. Osteoid seams are both wider and more extensive, and tetracycline labelling shows that mineralization is defective.

CLINICAL VARIETIES OF RICKETS AND OSTEOMALACIA

Vitamin D deficiency

Vitamin D deficiency may be due to dietary lack, underexposure to sunlight, malabsorption or a combination of these. Dietary lack of vitamin D (less than 100IU per day) is common in strict vegetarians and in old people who often eat very little; if there is also reduced exposure to sunlight, osteomalacia may result. Even mild osteomalacia can be harmful if it is superimposed on postmenopausal or senile osteoporosis. Treatment with vitamin D (400–1000IU per day) and calcium supplements is usually effective; however, elderly people often require larger doses of vitamin D (up to 2000IU per day).

Intestinal malabsorption – especially fat malabsorption - can cause vitamin D deficiency (fat and vitamin D absorption normally go hand in hand). If vitamin D supplements are administered they have to be given in very large doses (50,000IU per day). Gastrectomy is sometimes followed by osteomalacia; why this should be is unknown, as intestinal absorption is not affected.

Deficiency of vitamin D metabolites

Some patients with typical osteomalacia have no obvious vitamin lack and fail to respond to physiological doses of vitamin D. In some cases there is defective conversion to (or too-rapid breakdown of) the liver metabolite 25-HCC. This is seen in severe liver disease or after long-term administration of anticonvulsants or rifampicin; if these drugs are prescribed it is wise to give vitamin D at the same time. Established osteomalacia requires treatment with vitamin D in large doses.

Patients with early renal failure sometimes develop osteomalacia; this is thought to be due to reduced 1α-hydroxylase activity resulting in deficiency of 1,25-DHCC. It can be treated with 1,25-DHCC (or else with very large doses of vitamin D). Patients with advanced renal disease treated by haemodialysis develop a more complex syndrome – renal osteodystrophy. This is considered below.

Hypophosphataemic rickets and osteomalacia

Chronic hypophosphataemia occurs in a number of disorders in which there is impaired renal tubular reabsorption of phosphate. Calcium levels are normal but bone mineralization is defective.

Familial hypophosphataemic rickets (vitamin D-resistant rickets) This is probably the commonest form of rickets seen today. It is an X-linked genetic disorder with dominant inheritance, starting in infancy or soon after and causing severe bony deformity. The condition is characterized by excessive urinary excretion of phosphate and deficient mineralization of bone. This has, in the past, been attributed to renal tubular disease but it is now thought that there may also be a circulating hormonal factor which acts on the kidney to restrict tubular reabsorption of phosphate. The errant gene, which is normally responsible for phosphate regulation, has been identified (Hyp Consortium, 1995). The present hypothesis is that gene mutation results in a failure to control or inactivate the normally synthesized phosphatonin

Table 7.3 Characteristics of different types of rickets

	Vitamin D deficiency	Renal tubular	Renal glomerular
Family history	−	+	−
Myopathy	+	−	+
Growth defect	±	++	++
Serum:			
Ca	↓	N	↓
P	↓	↓	↑
Alk. phos.	↑	↑	↑
Urine:			
Ca	↓	↓	↓
P	↓	↑	↓
Osteitis fibrosa	±	+	++
Other	Dietary deficiency or malabsorption	Amino-aciduria	Renal failure Anaemia

hormone, which then exerts an unrestrained action on the kidney tubules resulting in excessive phosphate loss.

The children lag in growth, boys more so than girls, and secondary deformities (genu valgum or genu varum) are common. There is no myopathy. X-rays show marked epiphyseal changes but, because the serum calcium is normal, there is no secondary hyperparathyroidism.

Treatment requires the use of phosphate (to replace that which is lost in the urine) and vitamin D (to prevent secondary hyperparathyroidism due to phosphate administration). Large doses of vitamin D are required, or better still 1,25-DHCC (calcitriol). Treatment is continued until growth ceases.

Bony deformities may require bracing or osteotomy. If the child needs to be immobilized, vitamin D must be stopped temporarily to prevent hypercalcaemia from the combined effects of treatment and disuse bone resorption.

Adult-onset hypophosphataemia Although rare, this must be remembered as a cause of unexplained bone loss in adults. Patients also complain of joint pains. It responds dramatically to treatment with phosphate, vitamin D and calcium.

More severe *renal tubular defects* can produce a variety of biochemical abnormalities, including chronic phosphate depletion and osteomalacia. If there is acidosis, this must be corrected; in addition, patients may need phosphate replacement, together with calcium and vitamin D.

Oncogenic osteomalacia Hypophosphataemic vitamin D-resistant rickets or osteomalacia may be induced by certain tumours, particularly vascular tumours such as haemangiopericytomas, and also fibrohistiocytic lesions such as giant cell tumours and pigmented villonodular synovitis. The patient is usually an adult and osteomalacia may appear before the tumour is discovered. Clinical and biochemical features are similar to those of other types of hypophosphataemic disorder and (as in the latter) the condition is believed to be mediated by phosphatonin (Sundaram and McCarthy, 2000).

HYPERPARATHYROIDISM

Excessive secretion of PTH may be primary (usually due to an adenoma or hyperplasia), secondary (due to persistent hypocalcaemia) or tertiary (when secondary hyperplasia leads to autonomous overactivity).

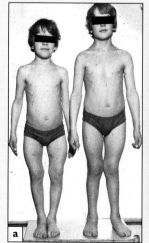 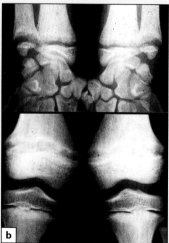 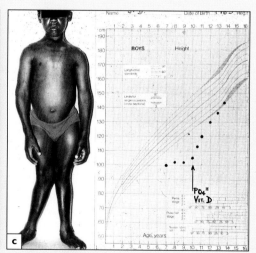

7.16 Renal tubular rickets – familial hypophosphataemia (a) These brothers presented with knee deformities; their x-rays (b) show defective juxta-epiphyseal calcification. (c) Another example of hypophosphataemic rickets; his growth chart shows that he was well below the normal range in height, but improved dramatically on treatment with vitamin D and inorganic phosphate.

Pathology

Overproduction of PTH enhances calcium conservation by stimulating tubular absorption, intestinal absorption and bone resorption. The resulting hypercalcaemia so increases glomerular filtration of calcium that there is hypercalciuria despite the augmented tubular reabsorption. Urinary phosphate also is increased, due to suppressed tubular reabsorption. The main effects of these changes are seen in the kidney: calcinosis, stone formation, recurrent infection and impaired function. There may also be calcification of soft tissues.

There is a general loss of bone substance. In more severe cases, osteoclastic hyperactivity produces subperiosteal erosions, endosteal cavitation and replacement of the marrow spaces by vascular granulations and fibrous tissue (osteitis fibrosa cystica). Haemorrhage and giant-cell reaction within the fibrous stroma may give rise to brownish, tumour-like masses, whose liquefaction leads to fluid-filled cysts.

PRIMARY HYPERPARATHYROIDISM

Primary hyperparathyroidism is quite common; the usual cause is a solitary adenoma in one of the small glands.

Patients are middle-aged (40–65 years) and women are affected twice as often as men. Many remain asymptomatic and are diagnosed only because routine biochemistry tests unexpectedly reveal a raised serum calcium level.

Clinical features are mainly due to hypercalcaemia: anorexia, nausea, abdominal pain, depression, fatigue and muscle weakness. They may develop polyuria, kidney stones or nephrocalcinosis due to chronic hypercalciuria. Some complain of joint symptoms, due to chondrocalcinosis. Only a minority (probably less than 10%) present with bone disease – and this is usually generalized osteoporosis rather than the classic features of osteitis fibrosa, bone cysts and pathological fractures.

X-rays show signs of osteoporosis (sometimes including vertebral collapse), and areas of cortical erosion. Hyperparathyroid 'brown tumours' should be considered in the differential diagnosis of atypical cyst-like lesions of long bones. However, the classic – and almost pathognomonic – feature, which should always be sought, is subperiosteal cortical resorption of the middle phalanges. Non-specific features of hypercalcaemia are renal calculi, nephrocalcinosis and chondrocalcinosis.

Biochemical tests show hypercalcaemia, hypophosphataemia and a raised serum PTH concentration. Serum alkaline phosphatase is raised with osteitis fibrosa.

Diagnosis involves the exclusion of other causes of hypercalcaemia (multiple myeloma, metastatic disease, sarcoidosis) in which PTH levels are usually depressed. Hyperparathyroidism also comes into the differential diagnosis of all types of osteoporosis and osteomalacia.

Treatment is usually conservative and includes adequate hydration and decreased calcium intake. The indications for parathyroidectomy are marked and unremitting hypercalcaemia, recurrent renal calculi, progressive nephrocalcinosis and severe osteoporosis.

Postoperatively there is a danger of severe hypocalcaemia due to brisk formation of new bone (the 'hungry bone syndrome'). This must be treated promptly, with one of the fast-acting vitamin D metabolites.

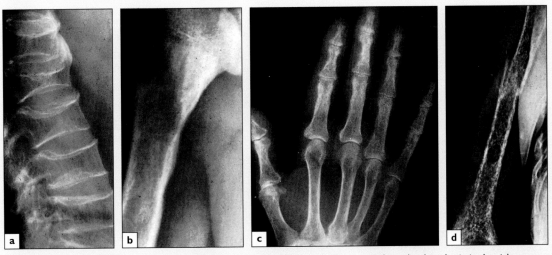

7.17 Hyperparathyroidism (**a**) This hyperparathyroid patient with spinal osteoporosis later developed pain in the right arm; an x-ray (**b**) showed cortical erosion of the humerus; he also showed (**c**) typical erosions of the phalanges. (**d**) Another case, showing 'brown tumours' of the humerus and a pathological fracture.

SECONDARY HYPERPARATHYROIDISM

Parathyroid oversecretion is a predictable response to chronic hypocalcaemia. Secondary hyperparathyroidism is seen, therefore, in various types of rickets and osteomalacia, and accounts for some of the radiological features in these disorders. Treatment is directed at the primary condition.

RENAL OSTEODYSTROPHY

Patients with chronic renal failure are liable to develop diffuse bone changes which are a variable combination of rickets or osteomalacia, secondary hyperparathyroidism, osteoporosis and osteosclerosis. Uraemia and phosphate retention are accompanied by a fall in serum calcium which is due partly to the hyperphosphataemia and partly to 1,25-DHCC deficiency. It is now recognized that the bone changes are aggravated by aluminium retention or contamination of dialysing fluids.

Renal abnormalities precede the bone changes by several years. Children are clinically more severely affected than adults: they are stunted, pasty-faced and have marked rachitic deformities. Myopathy is common.

X-rays show widened and irregular epiphyseal plates. In older children with long-standing disease there may be displacement of the epiphyses (epiphyseolysis). Osteosclerosis is seen mainly in the axial skeleton and is more common in young patients: it may produce a 'rugger jersey' (striped) appearance in lateral x-rays of the spine, due to alternating bands of increased and decreased bone density. Signs of secondary hyperparathyroidism may be widespread and severe.

Biochemical features are low serum calcium, high serum phosphate and elevated alkaline phosphatase levels. Urinary excretion of calcium and phosphate is diminished. Plasma PTH levels may be raised. The renal failure, if irreversible, may require haemodialysis or renal transplantation.

Treatment is difficult. The osteodystrophy should be dealt with, in the first instance, by giving large doses of vitamin D (up to 500,000IU daily); in resistant cases, small doses of 1,25-DHCC may be effective. Epiphyseolysis may need internal fixation and residual deformities can be corrected once the disease is under control.

SCURVY

Vitamin C (ascorbic acid) deficiency causes failure of collagen synthesis and osteoid formation. The result is osteoporosis, which in infants is most marked in the juxta-epiphyseal bone. Spontaneous bleeding is common.

The infant is irritable and anaemic. The gums may be spongy and bleeding. Subperiosteal haemorrhage causes excruciating pain and tenderness near the large joints. Fractures or epiphyseal separations may occur.

X-rays show generalized bone rarefaction, most marked in the long bone metaphyses. The normal calcification in growing cartilage produces dense transverse bands at the juxta-epiphyseal zones and around the ossific centres of the epiphyses (the 'ring

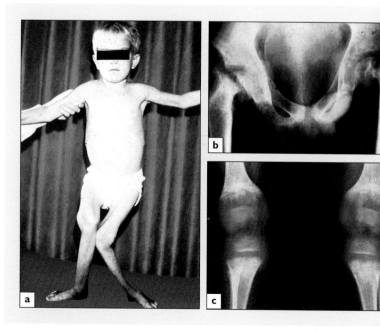

7.18 Renal glomerular osteodystrophy This young boy with chronic renal failure has severe abnormality of epiphyseal growth: the upper femoral epiphyses are grossly displaced.

124

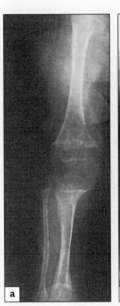
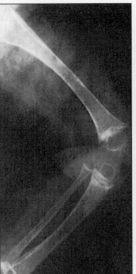
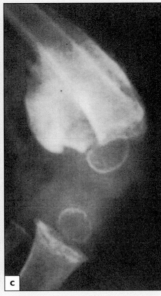

7.19 Scurvy (**a, b**) The epiphyseal ring sign and small subperiosteal haemorrhages; (**c**) the femoral epiphysis has displaced and the subperiosteal haemorrhage has calcified.

sign'). The metaphyses may be deformed or fractured. Subperiosteal haematomas show as soft-tissue swellings or periosseous calcification.

HYPERVITAMINOSIS

Hypervitaminosis A occurs in children following excessive dosage; in adults it seldom occurs except in explorers who eat Polar bear livers. There may be bone pain, and headache and vomiting due to raised intracranial pressure. X-ray shows increased density in the metaphyseal region and subperiosteal calcification.

Hypervitaminosis D occurs if too much vitamin D is given. It exerts a PTH-like effect and so, as in the underlying rickets, calcium is withdrawn from bones; but metastatic calcification occurs. In treatment the dose of vitamin D must be properly regulated and the infant given a low-calcium diet but plentiful fluids.

FLUOROSIS

Fluorine in very low concentration – 1 part per million (ppm) or less – has been used to reduce the incidence of dental caries. At slightly higher levels (2–4ppm) it may produce mottling of the teeth, a condition which is fairly common in those parts of the world where fluorine appears in the soil and drinking water. In some areas – notably parts of India and Africa where fluo-

rine concentrations in the drinking water may be above 10ppm – chronic fluorine intoxication (fluorosis) is endemic and widespread skeletal abnormalities are occasionally encountered in the affected population. Mild bone changes are also sometimes seen in patients treated with sodium fluoride for osteoporosis.

Fluorine directly stimulates osteoblastic activity; fluoroapatite crystals are laid down in bone and these are unusually resistant to osteoclastic resorption. Other effects are thought to be due to calcium retention, impaired mineralization and secondary hyperparathyroidism. The characteristic pathological features in severe cases are subperiosteal new-bone accretion and osteosclerosis, most marked in the vertebrae, ribs, pelvis and the forearm and leg bones, together with hyperostosis at the bony attachments of ligaments, tendons and fascia in these areas. Despite the apparent thickening and 'density' of the skeleton, tensile strength is reduced and the bones fracture more easily under bending and twisting loads.

Patients complain of backache, bone pain and joint stiffness. Examination may show thickening of the tubular bones. Sometimes the first clinical manifestation is a stress fracture. In the worst cases there may be deformities of the spine and lower limbs; hyperostosis can lead to vertebral canal encroachment and resultant neurological defects.

The typical x-ray features are osteosclerosis, osteophytosis and ossification of ligamentous and fascial attachments. Changes are most marked in the spine and pelvis, where the bones become densely opaque.

In a full-blown case the diagnosis should be obvious, but the rarity of the condition leads to it being overlooked. X-ray features at individual sites can be mistaken for those of Paget's disease, idiopathic skeletal hyperostosis, renal osteodystrophy or osteopetrosis.

There is no specific treatment for this condition. After exposure ceases it still takes years for bone fluoride to be excreted. If there is evidence of osteomalacia and secondary hyperparathyroidism, this can be treated with calcium and vitamin D.

PAGET'S DISEASE (OSTEITIS DEFORMANS)

Paget's disease is characterized by enlargement and thickening of the bone, but the internal architecture is abnormal and the bone is unusually brittle. The condition has a curious ethnic and geographic distribution, being relatively common in North America, Britain, Germany and Australia (more than 3% of people aged over 40 years) but rare in Asia, Africa and the Middle East. There is a tendency to familial aggregation. The cause is unknown, although the discovery of inclusion bodies in the osteoclasts has suggested a viral infection (Rebel *et al.*, 1980).

Pathology

The disease may appear in one or several sites; in the tubular bones it starts at one end and progresses slowly towards the diaphysis, leaving a trail of altered architecture behind. The characteristic cellular change is a marked increase in osteoclastic and osteoblastic activity. Bone turnover is accelerated, plasma alkaline phosphatase is raised (a sign of osteoblastic activity) and there is increased excretion of hydroxyproline in the urine (due to osteoclastic activity).

In the osteolytic (or 'vascular') stage there is avid resorption of existing bone by large osteoclasts, the excavations being filled with vascular fibrous tissue. In adjacent areas osteoblastic activity produces new woven and lamellar bone, which in turn is attacked by osteoclasts. This alternating activity extends on both endosteal and periosteal surfaces, so the bone increases in thickness but is structually weak and easily deformed. Gradually, osteoclastic activity abates and the eroded areas fill with new lamellar bone, leaving an irregular pattern of cement lines that mark the limits of the old resorption cavities; these 'tidemarks' produce a marbled or mosaic appearance on microscopy. In the late, osteoblastic, stage the thickened bone becomes increasingly sclerotic and brittle.

Clinical features

Paget's disease affects men and women equally. Only occasionally does it present in patients under 50 years, but from that age onwards it becomes increasingly common. The disease may for many years remain localized to part or the whole of one bone – the pelvis and tibia being the commonest sites, and the femur, skull, spine and clavicle the next commonest.

Most people with Paget's disease are asymptomatic, the disorder being diagnosed when an x-ray is taken for some unrelated condition or after the incidental discovery of a raised serum alkaline phosphatase level. When patients do present, it is usually because of pain or deformity, or some complication of the disease.

The pain is a dull constant ache, worse in bed when the patient warms up, but rarely severe unless a fracture occurs or sarcoma supervenes.

Deformities are seen mainly in the lower limbs. Long bones bend across the trajectories of mechanical stress; thus the tibia bows anteriorly and the femur anterolaterally. The limb looks bent and feels thick, and the skin is unduly warm – hence the term 'osteitis deformans'. If the skull is affected, it enlarges; the patient may complain that old hats no longer fit. The skull base may become

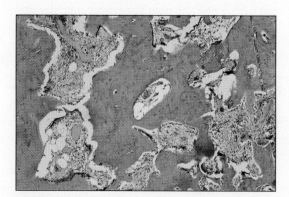

7.20 Paget's disease - histology Section from pagetic bone, showing the mosaic pattern due to overactive bone resorption and bone formation. The trabeculae are thick and patterned by cement lines. Some surfaces are excavated by osteoclastic activity whilst others are lined by rows of osteoblasts. The marrow spaces contain fibrovascular tissue.

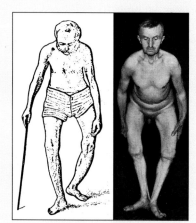

7.21 Paget's disease Paget's original case compared with a modern photograph.

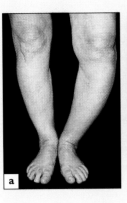
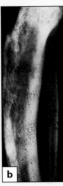
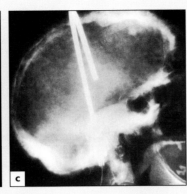

7.22 Paget's disease (**a, b**) The typical thick, bent tibia. (**c**) The skull is enlarged, the vault thickened and the base flattened (x-ray or not, he clung to his hearing aid).

flattened (platybasia), giving the appearance of a short neck. In generalized Paget's disease there may also be considerable kyphosis, so the patient becomes shorter and ape-like, with bent legs and arms hanging in front of him.

Cranial nerve compression may lead to impaired vision, facial palsy, trigeminal neuralgia or deafness. Another cause of deafness is otosclerosis. Vertebral thickening may cause spinal cord or nerve root compression.

Steal syndromes, in which blood is diverted from internal organs to the surrounding skeletal circulation, may cause cerebral impairment and spinal cord ischaemia. If there is also spinal stenosis the patient develops typical symptoms of 'spinal claudication' and lower limb weakness.

X-rays

The appearances are so characteristic that the diagnosis is seldom in doubt. During the resorptive phase there may be localized areas of osteolysis; most typical is the flame-shaped lesion extending along the shaft of the bone, or a circumscribed patch of osteoporosis in the skull (osteoporosis circumscripta). Later the bone becomes thick and sclerotic, with coarse trabeculation. The femur or tibia sometimes develops fine cracks on the convex surface – stress fractures that heal with increasing deformity of the bone. Occasionally the diagnosis is made only when the patient presents with a pathological fracture. Silent lesions are revealed by increased activity in the radionuclide scan.

Biochemistry

Serum calcium and phosphate levels are usually normal. The most useful test is measurement of the serum alkaline phosphatase level, which correlates with the activity and extent of disease.

Twenty-four hour urinary excretion of pyridinoline cross-links is a good indicator of disease activity and bone resorption. However, the test is expensive and is therefore not used routinely.

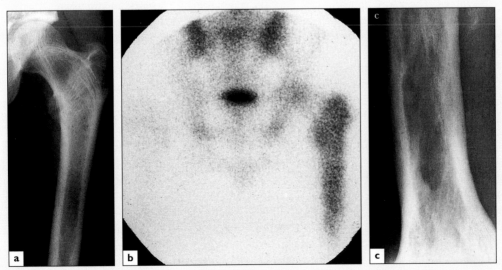

7.23 Paget's disease (**a, b**) In this early case the x-ray is almost normal, but the radionuclide scan of the same femur shows increased activity. (**c**) Flame-shaped area of osteopenia.

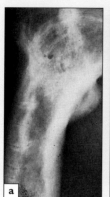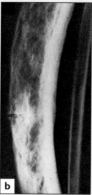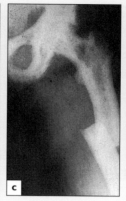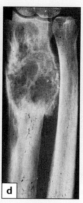

7.24 Paget' disease – complications (a) Fine cracks (microfractures) on the convex aspect, often associated with pain. (b) Incomplete fracture. (c) Complete fracture. This patient also has 'Paget's arthritis' of the hip. (d) Osteosarcoma.

Patients who are immobilized may develop hypercalcaemia.

Complications

FRACTURES Fractures are common, especially in the weightbearing long bones. In the femoral neck they are often vertical; elsewhere the fracture line is usually partly transverse and partly oblique, like the line of section of a felled tree. In the femur there is a high rate of non-union; for femoral neck fractures prosthetic replacement and for shaft fractures early internal fixation are recommended. Small stress fractures may be very painful; they resemble Looser's zones on x-ray, except that they occur on convex surfaces.

OSTEOARTHRITIS Osteoarthritis of the hip or knee is not merely a consequence of abnormal loading due to bone deformity; in the hip it seldom occurs unless the innominate bone is involved. The x-ray appearances suggest an atrophic arthritis with sparse remodelling, and at operation joint vascularity is increased.

NERVE COMPRESSION AND SPINAL STENOSIS Occasionally this is the first abnormality to be detected, and may call for definitive surgical treatment.

BONE SARCOMA Osteosarcoma arising in an elderly patient is almost always due to malignant transformation in Paget's disease. The frequency of malignant change is probably around 1%. It should always be suspected if a previously diseased bone becomes more painful, swollen and tender. Occasionally it presents as the first evidence of Paget's disease. The prognosis is extremely grave.

HIGH-OUTPUT CARDIAC FAILURE Though rare, this is an important general complication. It is due to prolonged, increased bone blood flow.

HYPERCALCAEMIA Hypercalcaemia may occur if the patient is immobilized for long.

In spite of all these complications, patients with Paget's disease usually come to terms with the condition and live to a ripe old age.

Treatment

Most patients with Paget's disease never have any symptoms and require no treatment. Sometimes pain is due to an associated arthritis rather than bone disease, and this may respond to non-steroidal anti-inflammatory therapy.

Patients should be examined, and the alkaline phosphatase level measured, at least once a year. Any change in symptoms, or a rise in alkaline phosphatase, calls for further investigation and, if necessary, more active treatment.

The indications for specific treatment are: (1) persistent bone pain; (2) repeated fractures; (3) neurological complications; (4) high-output cardiac failure; (5) hypercalcaemia due to immobilization; and (6) for some months before and after major bone surgery where there is a risk of excessive haemorrhage.

Drugs that suppress bone turnover, notably calcitonin and bisphosphonates, are most effective when the disease is active and bone turnover is high.

Calcitonin is the most widely used. It reduces bone resorption by decreasing both the activity and the number of osteoclasts; serum alkaline phosphatase and urinary pyridinoline cross-link levels are lowered. Salmon calcitonin is more effective than the porcine variety; subcutaneous injections of 50–100 MRC units are given daily until pain is relieved and the alkaline phosphatase levels are reduced and stabilized. Maintenance injections once or twice weekly may have to be continued indefinitely, but some authorities advocate stopping the drug and resuming treatment if symptoms recur. Drug resistance due to antibody formation may occur, but this will be avoided when human calcitonin is more generally available.

Bisphosphonates bind to hydroxyapatite crystals, inhibiting their rate of growth and dissolution. It is claimed that the reduction in bone turnover following their use is associated with the formation of lamellar rather than woven bone and that, even after treatment is stopped, there may be prolonged remission of disease (Bickerstaff *et al.*, 1990). Etidronate can be given orally (always on an empty stomach) but dosage should be kept low (e.g. 5mg/kg per day for up to 6 months) lest impaired bone mineralization results in osteomalacia.

The newer bishosphonates, such as pamidronate and alendronate, are more effective and produce remissions even with short courses of 1 or 2 weeks. They do not impair bone mineralization and can be repeated if necessary.

SURGERY The main indication for operation is a pathological fracture, which (in a long bone) usually requires internal fixation. When the fracture is treated the opportunity should be taken to straighten the bone. Other indications for surgery are painful osteoarthritis (total joint replacement), nerve entrapment (decompression) and severe spinal stenosis (decompression). *Beware – blood loss is likely to be excessive in these cases.*

An osteosarcoma, if detected early, may be resectable, but generally the prognosis is grave.

ENDOCRINE DISORDERS

The endocrine system plays an important part in skeletal growth and maturation, as well as the maintenance of bone turnover. The anterior lobe of the pituitary gland directly affects growth; it also controls the activities of the thyroid, the gonads and the adrenal cortex, each of which has its own influence on bone; and the pituitary itself is subject to feedback stimuli from the other glands. The various mechanisms are, in fact, part of an interactive system in which balance is more important than individual activity. For example: pituitary growth hormone stimulates cell proliferation and growth at the physes. Gonadal hormone promotes growth plate maturation and fusion. While pituitary activity is in the ascendant, the bones elongate; after sexual maturation, the rise in gonadal hormone activity simultaneously 'feeds back' on the pituitary and also directly closes down further physeal growth.

When the system goes out of balance abnormalities occur. They are often complex, with several levels of dysfunction, due to (a) the local effects of the lesion which upsets the endocrine gland (e.g. pressure on cranial nerves from a pituitary adenoma); (b) oversecretion or undersecretion by the gland affected; and (c) over or under-activity of other glands that are dependent on the primary dysfunctional gland.

For the sake of clarity, the descriptions which follow have been somewhat simplified.

PITUITARY DYSFUNCTION

The *posterior lobe* of the pituitary gland has no influence on the musculoskeletal system.

The *anterior lobe* is responsible for the secretion of pituitary growth hormone, as well as the thyrotropic, gonadotropic and adrenocorticotropic hormones. Abnormalities may affect the production of some of these hormones and not others; thus there is no single picture of 'pituitary deficiency' or 'pituitary excess'. Moreover, the clinical effects are determined in part by the stage in skeletal maturation at which the abnormality occurs.

HYPOPITUITARISM

Anterior pituitary hyposecretion may be caused by *intrinsic disorders* such as infarction or haemorrhage in the pituitary, infection and intrapituitary tumours, or by *extrinsic lesions* (such as a craniopharyngioma) which press on the anterior lobe of the pituitary. In some cases there may also be features due to posterior lobe dysfunction (e.g. diabetes insipidus); and space-occupying lesions are likely to have other intracranial pressure effects, such as headache or visual field defects.

Children In childhood and adolescence two distinct clinical disorders are encountered. In the *Lorain syndrome* the predominant effect is on growth. The body proportions are normal but the child fails to grow (proportionate dwarfism). Sexual development may be unaffected. The condition must be distinguished from other causes of short stature: hereditary or constitutional shortness, which is not as marked; childhood illness or malnutrition; rickets; and the various bone dysplasias, which generally result in disproportionate dwarfism.

In *Fröhlich's adiposogenital syndrome* the effects include those of gonadal hormone deficiency. There is delayed skeletal maturation associated with adiposity and immaturity of the secondary sexual characteristics. Weakness of the physes combined with disproportionate adiposity may result in epiphyseal displacement (epiphysiolysis or 'slipped epiphysis') at the hip or knee.

Adults Panhypopituitarism causes a variety of symptoms and signs, including those of cortisol and sex hormone deficiency. The only important skeletal effect is premature osteoporosis.

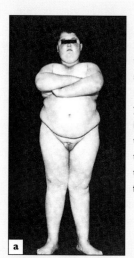

7.25 Endocrine disorders
(a) A boy of 12 with the unmistakable build of Frolich's adiposogenital syndrome.
(b) This young giant, only 16 years old, suffered from a pituitary adenoma; comparison with the photographer is quite startling. His peculiar stance is due to an undetected slipped upper femoral epiphysis on the left.

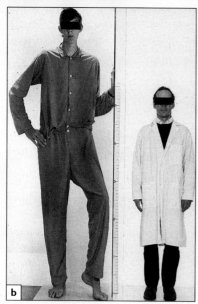

INVESTIGATIONS These should include direct assays and tests for hormone function.

X-RAYS X-rays of the skull may show expansion of the pituitary fossa and erosion of the adjacent bone. *CT and MRI* may reveal the tumour.

TREATMENT Treatment will depend on the cause and the degree of dwarfism. If a tumour is identified, it can be removed or ablated. A word of warning: the sudden reactivation of pituitary function after removal of a tumour may result in slipping of the proximal femoral epiphysis. Awareness of this risk will make for early diagnosis and, if necessary, surgical treatment of the epiphysiolysis.

Growth hormone deficiency has been successfully treated by the administration of biosynthetic growth hormone (somatotropin). The response should be checked by serial plots on the growth chart.

HYPERPITUITARISM

Oversecretion of pituitary growth hormone is usually due to an acidophil adenoma. However, there are rare cases of growth hormone secretion by pancreatic (and other) tumours. The effects vary according to the age of onset.

Gigantism Growth hormone oversecretion in childhood and adolescence causes excessive growth of the entire skeleton. The condition may be suspected quite early, and it is important to track the child's development by regular clinical and x-ray examination. In addition to being excessively tall, patients may develop deformity of the hip due to epiphyseal displacement (epiphysiolysis). There may be mental retardation and sexual immaturity.

Treatment is directed at early removal of the pituitary tumour.

Acromegaly Oversecretion of pituitary growth hormone in adulthood causes enlargement of the bones and soft tissues, but without the very marked elongation which is seen in gigantism. The bones are thickened, rather than lengthened, due to appositional growth; there is also hypertrophy of articular cartilage, which leads to enlargement of the joints. Bones such as the mandible, the clavicles, ribs, sternum and scapulae, which develop secondary growth centres in late adolescence or early adulthood, may go on growing longer than usual. Thickening of the skull, prominence of the orbital margins, overgrowth of the jaw and enlargement of the nose, lips and tongue produce the characteristic facies of acromegaly. The chest is broad and barrel-shaped and the hands and feet are large. Thickening of the bone ends may cause secondary osteoarthritis. About 10% of acromegalics develop diabetes, and cardiovascular disease is more common than usual.

TREATMENT The indications for operation are the presence of a tumour in childhood and cranial nerve pressure symptoms at any age. Trans-sphenoidal surgery has a high rate of success, provided the diagnosis is made reasonably early and the tumour is not too large.

Mild cases of acromegaly can be treated by administering growth hormone suppressants (a somatostatin analogue or bromocriptine, a dopamine agonist).

ADRENOCORTICAL DYSFUNCTION

The adrenal cortex secretes both mineralocorticoids (aldosterone) and glucocorticoids (cortisol). The latter has profound effects on bone and mineral metabolism, causing suppression of osteoblast activity, reduced calcium absorption, increased calcium excretion and enhanced PTH activity. Bone resorption is increased and formation is suppressed.

HYPERCORTISONISM (CUSHING'S SYNDROME)

Glucocorticoid excess may be caused by increased pituitary secretion of adrenocorticotropic hormone (ACTH) (the original Cushing's disease), by independent oversecretion by the adrenal cortex (usually due to a steroid-secreting tumour) or by excessive treatment with glucocorticoids (probably the commonest cause). Whatever the cause, the clinical picture is much the same and is generally referred to as Cushing's syndrome.

Patients have a characteristic appearance: the face is rounded and looks somewhat puffy ('moon face') and the trunk is distinctly obese, often with abdominal striae. However, the legs are quite thin and there may be proximal wasting and weakness.

X-rays show generalized osteoporosis; fractures of the vertebrae and femoral neck are common. A CT scan may show an adrenal tumour.

Biochemical tests are usually normal, but there may be a slight increase in urinary calcium.

MANAGEMENT
Problems for the orthopaedic surgeon are manifold: fractures and wounds heal slowly, bones provide little purchase for internal fixation, wound breakdown and infection are more common than usual and the patients are generally less fit.

Prevention means using systemic corticosteroids only when essential and in low dosage. If treatment is prolonged, calcium supplements (at least 1500mg per day) and vitamin D should be given. In post-menopausal women and elderly men, HRT is important. Bisphosphonates may also be effective in slowing the rate of bone loss and preventing further fractures.

Treatment includes the management of fractures and general measures to control bone pain. If a tumour is found, this will need surgical removal.

THYROID DYSFUNCTION

HYPOTHYROIDISM

Hypothyroidism takes various forms, depending on the age of onset.
Congenital hypothyroidism (cretinism) may be caused by developmental abnormalities of the thyroid, but it also occurs in endemic form in areas of iodine deficiency. Unless the condition is treated immediately (and diagnosis at birth is not easy!) the child becomes severely dwarfed and mentally retarded. X-rays may show irregular epiphyseal ossification. Treatment with thyroid hormone is essential.

Juvenile hypothyroidism is usually less severe than the congenital type. Growth and sexual development are retarded and the child may be mentally subnormal. X-rays show the typical epiphyseal 'fragmentation' appearance. Treatment with thyroid hormone may reverse these changes.

Adult hypothyroidism (myxoedema) may result from some primary disorder of thyroid function (including Hashimoto's disease) or from iatrogenic suppression following treatment for hyperthyroidism. The onset is slow and there may be a long period of non-specific symptoms such as weight increase, a general lack of energy and depression. Later complications include deafness, thinning of the hair, muscle weakness, nerve entrapment syndromes and joint pain, sometimes associated with calcium pyrophosphate dihydrate crystal deposition.

Treatment with thyroxine is effective and will have to be continued for life.

HYPERTHYROIDISM

Hyperthyroidism is an important cause of osteoporosis. This is dealt with on page 118.

PREGNANCY

Pregnancy can hardly be described as an endocrine disorder. However, pregnant women often develop musculoskeletal symptoms, some of which have been ascribed to hormonal changes; others are due to the increased weight and unusual posture.

Backache is common during the latter months. The lordotic posture may be to blame and postural exercises are a help. But there is also increased laxity of the pelvic joints due to secretion of relaxin, and this may play a part. Back pain may persist after childbirth and x-rays sometimes show increased sclerosis near the sacroiliac joint – *osteitis condensans ilii*. This is, in all probability, due to increased stress or minor trauma to the bone associated with sacroiliac laxity.

Carpal tunnel syndrome is common; it is probably due to fluid retention and soft-tissue swelling. Operation should be avoided; symptoms can be controlled with a wrist splint and the condition does not recur after the end of pregnancy.

Rheumatic disorders respond in unusual ways. Patients with rheumatoid arthritis often improve dramatically, while those with systemic lupus erythematosus sometime develop a severe exacerbation of the disease.

REFERENCES AND FURTHER READING

Bickerstaff DR, Douglas DL, Burke PH *et al.* (1990) Improvement in the deformity of the face in Paget's disease treated with diphosphonates. *Journal of Bone and Joint Surgery* **72B**, 132-136

Black DM, Cummings SR, Karpf DB *et al.* (1996) Randomised trial of effect of alendronate on risk of fracture in women with existing vertebral fractures. *Lancet* **348**, 1535-1541

Brighton CT, McCluskey WP (1986) Cellular response and mechanisms of action of electrically induced osteogenesis. In: *Bone and Mineral Research/4* (ed WA Peck). Elsevier, Amsterdam

Chapuy MC, Arlot ME, Delmas PD *et al.* (1994) Effect of calcium and cholecalciferol treatment for three years on hip fractures in elderly women. *British Medical Journal* **308**, 1081-1082

Cummings SR, Black DM, Nevitt MC *et al.* (1993) Bone density at various sites for prediction of hip fractures. *Lancet* **341**, 72-75

El Hajj Fuleihan G, Testa MA, Angell JE *et al.* (1995) Reproducibility of DXA absorptiometry: a model for bone loss estimates. *Journal of Bone Mineral Research* **10**, 1004-1014

Geneant HK, Engelke K, Fuerst T *et al.* (1996) Noninvasive assessment of bone mineral and structure: State of the art. *Journal of Bone and Mineral Research* **11**, 707-730

Hahn TJ (1980) Drug-induced disorders of vitamin D and mineral metabolism. *Clinics in Endocrinology and Metabolism* **9**, 107-129

Horowitz MC (1993) Cytokines and estrogen in bone: anti-osteoporotic effects. *Science*, **260**, 626-627

HYP Consortium (1995) A gene (PEX) with homologies to endopeptidases is mutated in patients with X-linked hypophosphatemic rickets. *Nature Genet* **11**, 130-136

Liberman UA, Downs RW Jr, Dequeker J *et al.* (1995) Effect of oral alendronate on bone mineral density and the incidence of fractures in postmenopausal osteoporosis. *New England Journal of Medicine* **333**, 1437-1443

Lindsay R, Hart DM, Clark DM (1984) The minimum effective dose of estrogen for prevention of postmenopausal bone loss. *Obstetrics and Gynecology* **63**, 759-763

Mirsky EC, Einhorn TA (1998) Bone densitometry in orthopaedic practice. *Journal of Bone and Joint Surgery* **80A**, 1687-1698

Nesbitt T, Drezner MK (1996) Hepatocyte production of phosphatonin in HYP mice. *Journal of Bone and Mineral Research* (Supplement 1), S136

Pak CYC, Sakhall K, Adams-Huet B *et al.* (1995) Treatment of postmenopausal osteoporosis with slow-release sodium fluoride. *Annals of Internal Medicine* **123**, 401-408

Parfitt AM (1988) Bone remodelling: relationship to the amount and structure of bone, and the pathogenesis and prevention of fractures. In: *Osteoporosis* (eds BL Riggs, LJ Nelton III). Raven Press, New York, 45-93

Peck WA, Woods WL (1988) The cells of bone. In: *Osteoporosis* (eds BL Riggs, LJ Melton III). Raven Press, New York, 1-44

Rebel A, Basle M, Poulard A *et al.* (1980) Towards a viral aetiology for Paget's disease of bone. *Metabolic Bone Disorders and Related Research* **3**, 235-238

Rosen HN, Dresner-Pollak R, Moses AC *et al.* (1994) Specificity of urinary excretion of cross-linked N-telopeptides of type I collagen as a marker of bone turnover. *Calcified Tissue International* **54**, 26-29

Skerry TM, Bitensky L, Chayen J, Lanyon LE (1989) Early strain-related changes in enzyme activity in osteocytes following bone loading in vivo. *Journal of Bone and Mineral Research* **4**, 783-788

Sundaram M, McCarthy M (2000) Oncogeneic osteomalacia. *Skeletal Radiology* **29**, 117-124

8 Genetic disorders, skeletal dysplasias and malformations

There can be few diseases in which genetic factors do not play a role – if only in creating a background favourable to the operation of some more proximate pathogen. Sometimes, however, a genetic defect is the major – or the only – determinant of an abnormality that is either present at birth (i.e. congenital) or inevitably evolves in later years. Such conditions can be broadly classified into three categories: *chromosome disorders, single gene disorders* and *polygenic or multifactorial disorders*. Various anomalies may also result from *injury to the formed embryo*. Many of these conditions affect the musculoskeletal system, producing cartilage and bone dysplasia (abnormal bone growth and/or modelling), *malformations* (e.g. absence or duplication of certain parts) or *structural defects of connective tissue*. In some a specific *metabolic abnormality* has been identified.

Genetic influences also contribute to the development of many *acquired disorders*. Osteoporosis, for example, is the result of a multiplicity of endocrine, dietary and environmental factors, yet twin studies have shown a significantly closer concordance in bone mass between identical twins than between non-identical twins.

Before considering the vast range of developmental disorders, it may be helpful to review certain general aspects of genetic abnormalities.

Genetic order

The life-imparting material in the nucleus of every cell is *deoxyribonucleic acid* (DNA). Each of the 46 chromosomes in the human cell consists of a single molecule of DNA; unravelled it would be several centimetres long, a double-stranded chain along which thousands of segments are defined and demarcated as genes.

The *genes* are the basic units of inherited biological information, each one coding for the synthesis of a specific protein. Working as a set (*or genome*) they tell the cells how to develop, differentiate and function in specialized ways.

Chromosomes can be identified and numbered by microscopic examination of suitably prepared blood cells or tissue samples. Of the 46 chromosomes in human cells, 44 (the *autosomes*) are disposed in 22 homologous pairs: one of each pair, carrying the same type of genetic information, is derived from each parent. The remaining two are the *sex chromosomes*: females have two X chromosomes (one from each parent); males have one X chromosome (from the mother) and one Y chromosome (from the father).

Gene studies are more complicated and involve the mapping of molecular sequences by specialized techniques after fragmenting the chains of DNA by means of restriction enzymes. Each gene occurs at a specific point, or locus, on the chromosome. The chromosomes being paired, there are two forms, or *alleles*, of each gene (one maternal, one paternal) at each locus; if the two alleles coding for a particular trait are identical, the person is said to be homozygous for that trait; if they are not identical, the individual is *heterozygous*.

The full genetic make-up of an individual is called the *genotype*. The finished person – a product of inherited traits and environmental forces – is the *phenotype*.

An important part of the unique human genotype is the *major histocompatibility complex* (MHC), also known as the HLA *system* (after human leucocyte antigen). This is a cluster of genes on chromosome 6 that is responsible for immunological specificity. The proteins for which they code are attached to cell surfaces and act as 'chaperones' for foreign antigens, which have to be accompanied by HLA before they are recognized and engaged by the body's T-cells.

HLA proteins can be identified by serological tests and are registered according to their corresponding genetic loci on the short arm of chromosome 6. HLA typing is particularly important in tissue transplantation: acceptance or rejection of the transplant hinges on the degree of matching between the HLA genes of donor and recipient.

Genetic disorder

Any serious disturbance of either the quantity or the arrangement of genetic material may result in disease. Three broad categories of abnormality are recognized: chromosome disorders, single gene disorders and polygenic or multifactorial disorders.

CHROMOSOME DISORDERS Additions, deletions and changes in chromosomal structure usually have serious effects; affected fetuses are either still-born or become infants with severe physical and mental abnormalities. In live-born children a few chromosome disorders have significant orthopaedic abnormalities: *Down's syndrome*, in which there is one extra chromosome 21 (trisomy 21), *Turner's syndrome*, in which one of the X chromosomes is lacking (monosomy X), and *Klinefelter's syndrome*, in which there is one Y but several X chromosomes.

SINGLE GENE DISORDERS Gene mutation may occur by insertion, deletion, substitution or fusion of amino acids

133

or nucleotides in the DNA chain. This can have profound consequences for cartilage growth, collagen structure, matrix patterning and marrow cell metabolism. The abnormality is then passed on to future generations according to simple mendelian rules (see below). There are literally thousands of single gene disorders, accounting for over 5% of child deaths, yet it is rare to see any one of them in an orthopaedic practice.

POLYGENIC AND MULTIFACTORIAL DISORDERS Many normal traits (body build, for example) derive from the interaction of multiple genetic and environmental influences. Likewise, certain diseases have a polygenic background, and some occur only when a genetic predisposition combines with an appropriate environmental 'trigger'. *Gout*, for example, is more common than usual in families with hyperuricaemia: the uric acid level is a polygenic trait, reflecting the interplay of multiple genes; it is also influenced by diet and may be more than usually elevated after a period of overindulgence. Finally, a slight bump on the toe acts as the proximate trigger for an acute attack of pain and swelling.

NON-GENETIC DISORDERS Many developmental abnormalities occur sporadically and have no genetic background. Most of these are of unknown aetiology, but some have been linked to specific teratogenic agents which damage the embryo or the placenta during the first few months of gestation. Suspected or known teratogens include viral infections (e.g. rubella), certain drugs (e.g. thalidomide) and ionizing radiation. The clinical features are usually asymmetrical and localized, ranging from mild morphological defects to severe malformations such as spina bifida or phocomelia ('congenital amputations').

Patterns of inheritance

The single gene disorders have characteristic patterns of inheritance, which may be autosomal or X-linked, and dominant or recessive.

AUTOSOMAL DOMINANT DISORDERS are inherited even if only one of a pair of alleles on a non-sex chromosome is abnormal; the condition is said to be *heterozygous*. A typical example is hereditary multiple exostoses. Either parent may be affected and half the children of both sexes develop exostoses. The pedigree shows a 'vertical' pattern of inheritance, with several affected siblings in successive generations (Fig.8.1a).

Sometimes both parents appear to be normal: the patient may be the first member of the family to suffer the effects of a mutant gene; or (as often happens) the disease shows variable expressivity, some members of the family (in the above example) developing many large exostoses and severe bone deformities, while others have only a few small and well-disguised nodules.

AUTOSOMAL RECESSIVE DISORDERS appear only when both alleles of a pair are abnormal – i.e. the condition is always *homozygous*. Each parent contributes a faulty gene, though if both are heterozygous they themselves will be clinically normal. Theoretically one in four of the children will be homozygous and will therefore develop the disease; two out of four will be *heterozygous carriers* of the faulty gene. The typical pedigree shows a 'horizontal' pattern of inheritance: several siblings in one generation are affected but neither their parents nor their children have the disease (Fig.8.1b).

X-LINKED DISORDERS are caused by a faulty gene in the X chromosome. Characteristically, therefore, they never pass directly from father to son because the father's X chromosome inevitably goes to the daughter, and the Y chromosome to the son. *X-linked dominant disorders* (e.g. hypophosphataemic rickets) pass from an affected mother to half of her daughters and half of her sons, or from an affected father to all of his daughters but none of his sons. Not surprisingly, they are twice as common in girls as in boys. *X-linked recessive disorders* – of which one of the most notorious is haemophilia – have a highly distinctive pattern of inheritance (Fig.8.1c): an affected male will pass the gene only to his daughters, who will become unaffected heterozygous carriers; they, in turn, will transmit it to half of their daughters (who will likewise be carriers) and half of their sons (who will be bleeders).

In-breeding

All types of genetic disease are more likely to occur in the children of consanguineous marriages or in closed communities where many people are related to each other. The rare recessive disorders, in particular, are seen in these circumstances, in which there is an increased risk of a homozygous pairing between two heterozygous carriers.

Genetic heterogenicity

The same phenotype (i.e. a patient with a set of clinical features) can result from widely different gene mutations. For example, there are four different types of osteogenesis imperfecta (OI; brittle bone disease), some showing autosomal dominant and some autosomal recessive inheritance. For such phenotypes, the recessive form is usually the more severe. Subtleties of this kind must be borne in mind when counselling parents.

Genetic markers

Many common disorders show an unusually close association with certain blood groups, tissue types

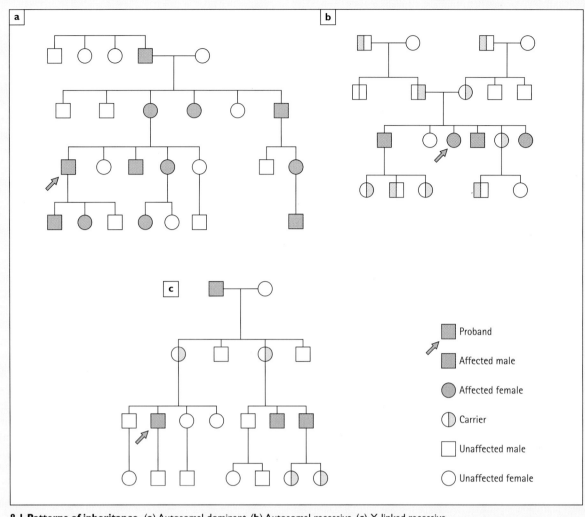

8.1 Patterns of inheritance (**a**) Autosomal dominant. (**b**) Autosomal recessive. (**c**) X-linked recessive.

or other serum proteins that occur with higher than expected frequency in the patients and their relatives. These are referred to as genetic markers; they arise from gene sequences that do not cause the disease but are either 'linked' to other (abnormal) loci or else express some factor that predisposes the individual to a harmful environmental agent. A good example is ankylosing spondylitis: over 90% of patients, and 60% of their first-degree relatives, are positive for HLA-B27. In this case (as in other autoimmune diseases) the HLA marker gene may provide the necessary conditions for invasion by a foreign viral fragment.

Gene mapping

With advancing recombinant DNA technology, the genetic disorders are gradually being mapped to specific loci. In some cases the mutant gene has been cloned, holding out the possibility of replacing flawed genes with correctly functioning versions. This and other aspects of genetics and musculoskeletal disease are reviewed in a paper by Jaffurs and Evans (1998).

PRENATAL DIAGNOSIS

Many genetic disorders can be diagnosed before birth, thus improving the chances of treatment or, at worst, giving the parents the choice of selective abortion. Ultrasound imaging is harmless and is now done almost routinely. On the other hand, tests that involve amniocentesis or chorionic villus sampling carry a risk of injury to the fetus and are therefore used only when there is reason to suspect some abnormality. Indications are: (1) maternal age over 35 years (increased risk of Down's syndrome) or an unduly high paternal age (increased risk of achondroplasia); (2) a previous history of chromosomal abnormalities (e.g. Down's syndrome) or genetic abnormalities amenable to biochemical diagnosis (neural tube defects, or inborn errors of metabolism); or (3) to confirm non-invasive tests suggesting an abnormality.

Maternal screening

Fetal neural tube defects are associated with increased levels of alpha-fetoprotein (AFP) in the amniotic fluid and, to a lesser extent, the maternal blood. Women with positive blood tests may be given the option of further investigation by amniocentesis. It has also been noted that abnormally low levels of AFP are associated with Down's syndrome.

Amniocentesis

Under local anaesthesia, a small amount (about 20ml) of fluid is withdrawn from the amniotic sac with a needle and syringe. (It is best to determine the position of the fetus beforehand by ultrasonography.) The procedure is usually carried out between the 14th and 18th weeks of pregnancy. The fluid can be examined directly for AFP, and desquamated fetal cells can be collected and cultured for chromosomal studies and biochemical tests for enzyme disorders.

Chorionic villus sampling

Under ultrasound screening, a fine catheter is passed through the cervix and a small sample of chorion is sucked out. This is usually done between the 8th and 10th weeks of pregnancy. Mesenchymal fibroblasts can be cultured and used for *chromosomal studies, biochemical tests* and DNA *analysis.* Rapid advances in DNA technology have made it possible to diagnose sickle-cell anaemia and haemophilia (among other disorders) during early pregnancy.

Fetal imaging

By the 18th week of pregnancy, *high resolution ultrasonography* may show anatomical abnormalities such as open neural tube defects and short limbs. In late pregnancy, *x-ray* examination will reveal any marked change in bone density (osteopetrosis) and multiple fractures (OI).

DIAGNOSIS IN CHILDHOOD

Clinical features

Tell-tale features suggesting skeletal dysplasia are:
- retarded growth and shortness of stature

- disproportionate length of trunk and limbs
- localized malformations (dysmorphism)
- soft-tissue contracture
- childhood deformity

All the skeletal dysplasias affect growth, although this may not be obvious at birth. Children should be measured at regular intervals and a record kept of height, length of lower segment (top of pubic symphysis to heel), upper segment (pubis to cranium), span, head circumference and chest circumference. Failure to reach the expected height for the local population group should be noted, and marked shortness of stature is highly suspicious.

Bodily proportion is as important as overall height. The normal upper segment:lower segment ratio changes gradually from about 1.5:1 at the end of the first year to about 1:1 at puberty. *Shortness of stature with normal proportions* is not necessarily abnormal, but it is also seen in endocrine disorders which affect the different parts of the skeleton more or less equally (e.g. hypopituitarism). By contrast, *small stature with disproportionate shortness of the limbs* is characteristic of skeletal dysplasia, the long bones being more markedly affected than the axial skeleton.

The different segments of the limbs also may be disproportionately affected. The subtleties of dysplastic growth are reflected in terms such as *rhizomelia* – unusually short proximal segments (humeri and femora), *mesomelia* – short middle segments (forearms and legs) and *acromelia* – stubby hands and feet.

Dysmorphism (a misshapen part of the body) is most obvious in the face and hands. There is a remarkable consistency about these changes, which makes for a disturbing similarity of appearance in members of a particular group.

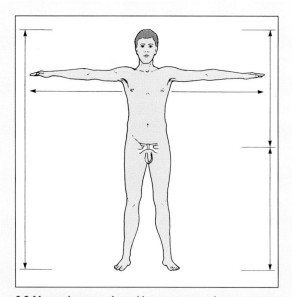

8.2 Normal proportions Upper segment = lower segment. Total height = span.

Local deformities – such as kyphosis, valgus or varus knees, bowed forearms and ulnar deviated wrists – result from disturbed bone growth.

X-rays

The presence of any of the above features calls for a limited radiographic survey: anteroposterior views of the pelvis, knees and hands, and lateral views of the skull and thoracolumbar spine. Fractures, bent bones, exostoses, epiphyseal dysplasia and spinal deformities may be obvious, especially in the older child. Sometimes a complete survey is needed and it is important to note which portion of the long bones (epiphysis, metaphysis or diaphysis) is affected. With severe and varied changes in the metaphyses, periosteal new bone formation or epiphyseal separation always consider the possibility of non-accidental fractures – the battered baby syndrome.

Special investigations

In most cases the diagnosis can be made without laboratory tests; however, *routine blood and urine analysis* may be helpful in excluding metabolic and endocrine disorders such as rickets and pituitary or thyroid dysfunction. Special tests are also available to identify specific excretory metabolites in the storage disorders, and specific enzyme activity can be measured in serum, blood cells or cultured fibroblasts.

Bone biopsy is occasionally helpful in disorders of bone density.

Direct testing for gene mutations is already available for a number of conditions and is rapidly being extended to others. It is a useful adjunct to clinical diagnosis. Still somewhat controversial is its application to pre-clinical diagnosis of late onset disorders and neonatal screening for potentially dangerous conditions such as sickle-cell disease.

ADULT PRESENTATION

In the worst of the genetic disorders the fetus is still-born or survives for only a short time. Those who reach adulthood, though recognizably abnormal, may lead active lives, marry and have children of their own. Nevertheless, they often seek medical advice for several reasons:
- short stature – especially disproportionate shortness of the lower limbs
- local bone deformities or exostoses
- spinal stenosis
- repeated fractures

- secondary osteoarthritis (e.g. due to epiphyseal dysplasia)
- joint laxity or instability

The family history

A careful family history should be obtained. However, the fact that a parent or relative is said to be 'normal' does not exclude the possibility that they are either very mildly affected or have a biochemical defect without any physical abnormality. Many developmental disorders have characteristic patterns of inheritance which may be helpful in diagnosis.

The family history should include information about similar disorders in close relatives, previous deaths in the family (and the cause of death), abortions and intermarriage.

Racial background is important: some diseases are particularly common in certain communities, for example, sickle-cell disease in black African peoples and Gaucher's disease in Ashkenazi Jews.

Previous medical history

Always ask about exposure to teratogenic agents during the early months of pregnancy: x-rays, cytotoxic drugs or virus infections.

MANAGEMENT

Management of the individual patient depends on the diagnosis, the pattern of inheritance, the type and severity of deformity or disability, mental capacity and social aspirations. However, it is worth noting some general principles.

Communication

Once the diagnosis has been made, the next step is to explain as much as possible about the disorder to the patient (if old enough) and the parents. The rare developmental disorders are best treated in a centre that offers a 'special interest' team consisting of a paediatrician, medical geneticist, orthopaedic surgeon, psychologist, social worker, occupational therapist, orthotist and prosthetist.

Counselling

Patients and families may need expert counselling about (1) the likely outcome of the disorders; (2) what will be required of the family; and (3) the risk of siblings or children being affected. Where there are severe deformities or mental retardation, the entire family may need psychological help.

Intrauterine surgery

The concept of operating on the unborn fetus is already a reality and is likely to be extended in the future. At present, however, it is still too early to say whether the advantages (e.g. prenatal skin closure for dysraphism) will outweigh the risks.

Correction of deformities

Anomalies such as coxa vara, genu valgum, club foot, radial club hand or scoliosis (and many others outside the field of orthopaedics) are amenable to corrective surgery. In recent years, with advances in methods of limb lengthening, many short-limbed patients have benefited from this operation; however, the risks should be carefully explained and the expected benefits should not be exaggerated.

Spinal surgery

Several developmental disorders are associated with potentially dangerous spinal anomalies: for example, spinal stenosis and cord compression in achondroplasia; atlantoaxial instability, due to odontoid aplasia, in any disorder causing vertebral dysplasia; or severe kyphoscoliosis, which occurs in a number of conditions. Cord decompression or occipitocervical fusion are perfectly feasible, but surgical correction of congenital kyphoscoliosis carries considerable risks and should be undertaken only in specialized units.

Joint reconstruction

Some of the generalized skeletal dysplasias cause joint incongruity and secondary osteoarthritis – especially of the hip or knee. This may need corrective surgery at a later stage.

Gene therapy

Rapid advances in gene research have brought much closer the prospect of eliminating or counteracting the harmful abnormality. The modification of defective genes in germ-line cells, though possible in some cases, is prohibited for ethical reasons in countries which have the resources for such treatment. However, gene transfer via somatic cells has been in progress for several years and this opens the door to implanting molecular 'factories' which would turn out therapeutically active proteins, a process which may soon come to be seen as nothing more nor less than 'a sophisticated type of drug-delivery system' (Evans and Robbins, 1995).

Theoretically genes could be transferred to any of the musculoskeletal tissues, and success has already been achieved in obtaining gene expression in synovial tissue by both *in vivo* and *ex vivo* techniques using either viral vectors or genetically modified cells which are introduced into the joint. Evans and Robbins (1995) have pointed out that bone disorders could be treated by aiming the therapeutic genes at precursor cells in the bone marrow. Single gene disorders in which the mutant gene has been identified would be amenable to treatment, provided the negative mutation is not expressed as dominant. Acquired diseases, also, could theoretically be treated by delivering therapeutic proteins directly to affected tissues (e.g. synovium or cartilage).

CLASSIFICATION OF DEVELOPMENTAL DISORDERS

There is no completely satisfactory classification of developmental disorders. The same genetic abnormality may be expressed in different ways, while a variety of gene defects may cause almost identical clinical syndromes. The grouping used in Table 8.1 is no more than a convenient way of dividing the various clinical syndromes.

THE CHONDRO–OSTEODYSTROPHIES

The chondro-osteodystrophies, or skeletal dysplasias, are a large group of disorders characterized by abnormal cartilage and bone growth. Since the various conditions are caused by different gene defects, it would be scientifically correct to classify them according to their basic molecular pathology. However, the orthopaedic surgeon faced with a patient will seek first to categorize the disorder according to recognizable clinical and x-ray appearances; it is with this in mind that the conditions are presented here in clinical rather than etiological groups, as follows:
- those with predominantly physeal and metaphyseal changes
- those with predominantly epiphyseal and/or vertebral body changes
- those with mainly diaphyseal changes; and
- those with a mixture of abnormalities

DYSPLASIAS WITH PREDOMINANTLY PHYSEAL AND METAPHYSEAL CHANGES

In these disorders there is abnormal physeal growth, defective metaphyseal modelling and shortness of the tubular bones. The axial skeleton is affected too, but the limbs are disproportionately short compared to the spine.

Table 8.1 A practical grouping of generalized developmental disorders

1 Disorders of cartilage and bone growth	**2 Connective tissue disorders**
1.1 Dysplasias with predominantly physeal and metaphyseal changes	***2.1 Generalized joint laxity***
	2.2 Ehlers–Danlos syndrome
1.1.1 Hereditary multiple exostosis	
1.1.2 Achondroplasis	***2.3 Larsen's syndrome***
1.1.3 Hypochondroplasia	
1.1.4 Metaphyseal chondrodysplasia	***2.4 Osteogenesis imperfecta (brittle bones)***
1.1.5 Dyschondroplasia (enchodromatosis, Ollier's disease)	
	2.4.1 Mild
1.2 Dysplasias with predominantly epiphyseal changes	2.4.2 Lethal
	2.4.3 Severe
1.2.1 Multiple epiphyseal dysplasia	2.4.4 Moderate
1.2.2 Spondyloepiphyseal dysplasia	
1.2.3 Dysplasia epiphysealis hemimelica (Trevor's disease)	***2.5 Fibrodysplasia ossificans progressiva***
1.2.4 Chondrodysplasia punctata (stippled epiphysis)	
	3 Storage disorders and other metabolic defects
1.3 Dysplasias with predominantly metaphyseal and diaphyseal changes	***3.1 Mucopolysaccharidoses***
1.3.1 Metaphyseal dysplasia (Pyle's disease)	3.1.1 Hurler's syndrome (MPS I)
1.3.2 Craniometaphyseal dysplasia	3.1.2 Hunter's syndrome (MPS II)
1.3.3 Diaphyseal dysplasia (Engelmann's disease, Camurati's disease)	3.1.3 Morquio–Brailsford syndrome (MPS IV)
1.3.4 Craniodiaphyseal dysplasia	***3.2 Gaucher's disease***
1.3.5 Osteopetrosis (marble bones, Albers–Shönberg disease)	
1.3.6 Pyknodysostosis	***3.3 Homocystinuria***
1.3.7 Candle bones, spotted bones and striped bones	
	3.4 Alkaptonuria
1.4 Combined and mixed dysplasias	
	3.5 Congenital hyperuricaemia
1.4.1 Spondylometaphyseal dysplasia	
1.4.2 Pseudoachondroplasia	**4 Chromosome disorders**
1.4.3 Diastrophic dysplasia	
1.4.4 Cleidocranial dysplasia	***4.1 Down's syndrome***
1.4.5 Nail–patella syndrome	
1.4.6 Craniofacial dysplasia	***4.2 Thoracospinal anomalies***
	4.3 Elevation of the scapula (Sprengel's deformity)
	4.4 Limb anomalies

HEREDITARY MULTIPLE EXOSTOSIS (DIAPHYSEAL ACLASIS)

The most common, and least disfiguring, of the skeletal dysplasias is multiple exostosis.

Clinical features

The condition is usually discovered in childhood; hard lumps appear at the ends of the long bones and along the apophyseal borders of the scapula and pelvis. As the child grows, these lumps enlarge and some may become hugely visible, especially around the knee. The more severely affected bones are abnormally short; this is seldom very marked, but on measurement the lower body segment is shorter than the upper and span is less than height (Solomon, 1963). In the forearm and leg, the thinner of the two bones (the ulna or fibula) is usually the more defective, resulting in typical deformities: ulnar deviation of the wrist, bowing of the radius, subluxation of the radial head, valgus knees and valgus ankles. Bony lumps may cause pressure on nerves or vessels. Occasionally

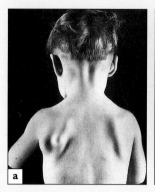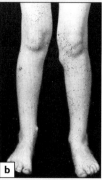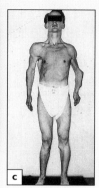

8.3 Hereditary multiple exostoses Clinical presentation at (**a**) 3 years, (**b**) 6 years and (**c**) 28 years. In (**c**) note the numerous small exostoses, the one large tumour near the right shoulder, bowing of the left radius, shortening of the left forearm and valgus deformity of the right knee.

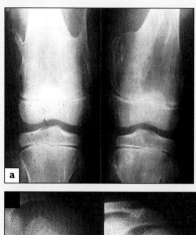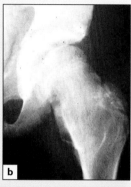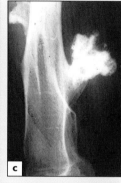

8.4 Hereditary multiple exostoses – x-rays
(**a**) Typical x-ray appearances of the knees.
(**b**) Sessile exostoses of the femoral neck. (**c**) A large pedunculated exostosis of the distal femur.

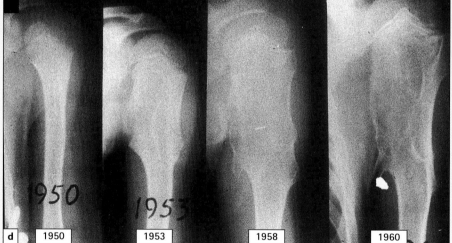

(**d**) Evolution of the wide metaphysis during growth.

1950	1953	1958	1960

one of the cartilage-capped exostoses continues to grow into adult life and transforms to a chrondrosarcoma; this is said to occur in 1–2% of patients.

X-RAY

Typically the long-bone metaphyses are broad and poorly modelled, with sessile or pedunculated exostoses arising from the cortices – almost as if longitudinal growth has been squandered in profligate lateral expansion. A mottled appearance around a bony excrescence indicates calcification in the cartilage cap. The distal end of the ulna is sometimes tapered or carrot-shaped and the bone may be markedly reduced in length; in these cases the radius is usually bowed, or the discrepancy in length may lead to subluxation of the radiohumeral joint.

The cuboidal carpal and tarsal bones show little or no change on x-ray. This is simply because the ossified parts of these bones (which is all that is visible on x-ray) are completely surrounded by cartilage during early development, and any cartilage irregularities are subsumed in the overall expansion of the bone.

Pathology

The underlying fault in multiple exostosis is unrestrained transverse growth of the cartilaginous physis (growth plate). The condition affects only the endochondral bones. Cartilaginous excrescences appear at the peripheri of the physes and proceed, in the usual way, to endochondral ossification. If the abnormal physeal proliferation ceases at that point, but the bone continues to grow in length, the exostosis is left behind where it arose (now part of the metaphysis), but its cartilage cap is still capable of autonomous growth. If the physeal abnormality persists, further growth proceeds in the new abnormal mould, without remodelling of the broadened and misshapen metaphysis. The process finally comes to a stop when endochondral proliferation ceases at the end of the normal period of growth for that bone; any further growth of the exostotic cartilage cap after that suggests neoplastic change.

Genetics

The condition is transmitted as autosomal dominant; half the children are affected, boys and girls equally. However, expression is variable and some people are so mildly affected as to be unaware of the disorder.

Hereditary multiple exostosis is a genetically heterogeneous disorder, with involvement of at least three separate genes (on chromosomes 8, 11 and 19), mutations of which cause very similar phenotypes.

Management

Exostoses may need removal because of pressure on a nerve or vessel, because of their unsightly appearance or because they tend to be bumped during everyday activities. Deformities of the legs or forearms may be severe enough to warrant treatment by osteotomy; this is best postponed till late adolescence.

Exostoses should stop growing when the parent bone does; any subsequent enlargement suggests malignant change and calls for advanced imaging and wide local resection (see page 171).

ACHONDROPLASIA

This is the commonest form of abnormally short stature. Adult height is usually around 122cm (48 inches). Severe, disproportionate shortening of the limb bones may be diagnosed by x-ray before birth.

Clinical features

The abnormality is obvious in childhood: growth is severely stunted; the limbs (particularly the proximal segments) are disproportionately short and the skull is quite large with prominent forehead and saddle-shaped nose. The fingers appear stubby and somewhat splayed (trident hands). Joint laxity is common. Many infants have a thoracolumbar kyphos, but this almost always disappears in a year or two. Mental development is normal.

By early childhood the trunk is obviously disproportionately long in comparison with the limbs. The

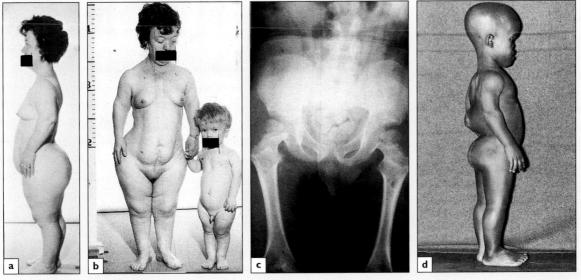

8.5 Achondroplasia (a) A typical achondroplastic patient with disproportionate shortening of the limbs. (b) Her son has obviously inherited the condition. (c) X-ray showing the short femora and flared pelvis. (d) Some children develop a persistent kyphosis.

posture when standing is typical: the back is excessively lordotic, the buttocks prominent, the hips flexed, the legs bowed and the elbows bent.

During adulthood, shortening of the vertebral pedicles may lead to lumbar spinal stenosis, and disc prolapse (which is quite common) has exceptionally severe effects. Cervical spine stenosis may cause typical features of cord compression (see page 365).

X-RAY

The tubular bones are short, the metaphyses wide and the physeal lines somewhat irregular; however, the epiphyses are usually normal. Although the proximal limb bones are disproportionately affected (rhizomelia), changes are also seen in the wrists and hands, where the metaphyses are broad and cup-shaped. The pelvic cavity is small (too small for normal delivery) and the iliac wings are flared, producing an almost horizontal acetabular roof. The skull vault is large but the base rather short and the foramen magnum smaller than usual. The vertebrae also are abnormal and the spinal canal reduced in size. These features are best defined on computed tomography (CT) or magnetic resonance imaging (MRI).

Diagnosis

Achondroplasia should not be confused with other types of short-limbed dwarfism. In some (e.g. Morquio's disease) the shortening affects distal segments more than proximal and there may be widespread associated abnormalities. Others (e.g. pseudoachondroplasia and the epiphyseal dysplasias) are distinguished by the fact that the head and face are quite normal whereas the epiphyses show characteristic changes on x-ray examination.

Pathology

This is essentially an abnormality of endochondral longitudinal growth. The physes show diminished, and less regular, cell proliferation, which accounts for the diminished length of the tubular bones. Membrane bone formation is unaffected, hence the normal growth of the skull vault and the periosteal contribution to bone width.

Genetics

Achondroplasia occurs in about 1 in 25,000 births. There is autosomal dominant inheritance; however, because few achondroplastic people have children, over 80% of cases are sporadic. The fault has been shown to be point mutation in the gene coding for fibroblast growth factor receptor 3, which apparently plays a role in endochondral cartilage growth (Shiang *et al.*, 1994).

Management

During childhood, operative treatment may be needed for lower limb deformities (usually genu varum). Occasionally the thoracolumbar kyphosis fails to correct itself; if there is significant deformity (angulation of more than 40 degrees) by the age of 5 years, there is a risk of cord compression and operative correction may be needed.

During adulthood, spinal stenosis may require decompression. Intervertebral disc prolapse superimposed on a narrow spinal canal should be treated as an emergency.

Advances in methods of external fixation have made leg lengthening a feasible option. This is best achieved by chondrodiatasis of the physis or callotasis of the shaft (see page 264). However, there are drawbacks: complications, including non-union, infection and nerve palsy, may be disastrous; and the cosmetic effect of long legs and short arms may be less pleasing than anticipated. It is essential that the details of the operation, its aims and limitations and the potential complications be fully discussed with the patient (and, where appropriate, with the parents).

Anaesthesia carries a greater than usual risk and requires expert supervision.

HYPOCHONDROPLASIA

This has been described as a very mild form of achondroplasia. However, apart from shortness of stature (with the emphasis on proximal limb segments) and noticeable lumbar lordosis, there is little to suggest any abnormality; the head and face are not affected and many of those with hypochondroplasia pass for normal stocky individuals. X-rays may show slight pelvic flattening

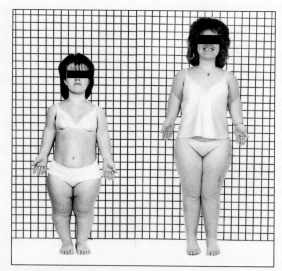

8.6 Achondroplasia The smile reflects the patient's satisfaction with the increased height achieved by lengthening the lower limbs. (Courtesy of Mr M. Saleh.)

and thickening of the long bones. The condition is transmitted as autosomal dominant. Those affected sometimes ask for limb lengthening; after careful discussion, this may be done with a considerable chance of success.

DYSCHONDROSTEOSIS

In this disorder there is also disproportionate shortening of the limbs, but it is mainly the middle segments (forearms and legs) which are affected. It is the commonest of the mesomelic dysplasias and is transmitted as an autosomal dominant defect. Stature is reduced but not as markedly as in achondroplasia. The most characteristic x-ray changes are shortening of the forearms and leg bones, bowing of the radius and Madelung's deformity of the wrist, which may require operative treatment (see page 318).

METAPHYSEAL CHONDRODYSPLASIA (OR DYSOSTOSIS)

This term describes a type of short-limbed dwarfism in which the bony abnormality is virtually confined to the metaphyses. The epiphyses are unaffected but the metaphyseal segments adjacent to the growth plates are broadened and mildly scalloped, somewhat resembling rickets. There may be bilateral coxa vara and bowed legs; patients tend to walk with a waddling gait. Apart from a lordotic posture, the spine is normal. The main deformities are around the hips and knees.

There are several forms of metaphyseal chondrodysplasia. The best known (Schmid type) has the classic features described above, with autosomal

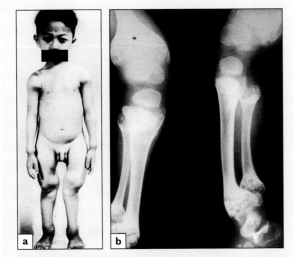

8.7 Metaphyseal chondrodysplasia This boy with the rare Jansen type shows the typical shortening of the lower limbs and metaphyseal enlargement of the long bones. The x-rays show that the changes are confined to the metaphyses.

dominant inheritance. Another group (McKusick type) is associated with sparse hair growth and is sometimes complicated by Hirschsprung's disease; inheritance shows an autosomal recessive pattern. It is thought that these cases may represent an entirely distinct entity. The rarest (and most severe) of all (Jansen type) is usually sporadic and may be associated with deafness.

Operative correction (osteotomy) may be needed for coxa vara or tibia vara.

DYSCHONDROPLASIA (ENCHONDROMATOSIS; OLLIER'S DISEASE)

This is a rare, but easily recognized, disorder in which there is defective transformation of physeal cartilage columns into bone.

Clinical features

Typically the disorder is unilateral; indeed only one limb or even one bone may be involved. An affected limb is short, and if the growth plate is asymmetrically involved the bone grows bent; bowing of the distal end of the femur or tibia is not uncommon and the patient may present with valgus or varus deformity at the knee and ankle. Shortening of the ulna may lead to bowing of the radius and, sometimes, dislocation of the radial head. The fingers or toes frequently contain *multiple enchondromata*, which are characteristic of the disease and may be so numerous that the hand is crippled. A rare variety of dyschondroplasia is associated with *multiple haemangiomata (Maffucci's syndrome)*; this is described below.

The condition is not inherited; indeed, it is probably an embryonal rather than a genetic disorder.

X-RAYS
The characteristic change in the long bones is radiolucent streaking extending from the physis into the metaphysis – the appearance of persistent, incompletely ossified cartilage columns trapped in bone. If only half the physis is affected, growth is asymmetrically retarded and the bone becomes curved. With maturation the radiolucent columns eventually ossify but the deformities remain. In the hands and feet the cartilage islands characteristically produce *multiple enchondromata*. Beware of any change in the appearance of the lesions after the end of normal growth; this may be a sign of *malignant change*, which occurs in 5–10% of cases.

Treatment

Bone deformity may need correction, but this should be deferred until growth is complete; otherwise it is likely to recur.

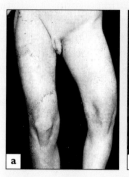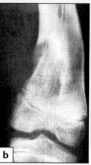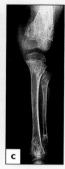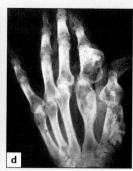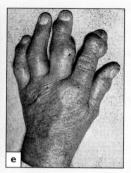

8.8 Dyschondroplasia (**a, b**) The bent femur in this boy is due to slow growth of half the lower femoral physis. (**c**) Incomplete ossification of the cartilage columns accounts for the curious metaphyseal appearance. (**d, e**) Two patients with multiple chondromas.

MAFFUCCI'S SYNDROME

This rare disorder is characterized by the development of multiple enchondromas and soft-tissue haemangiomas of the skin and viscera. Lesions appear during childhood; boys and girls are affected with equal frequency.

There is a strong tendency for malignant change to occur in both soft-tissue and bone lesions; the incidence of sarcomatous transformation in one of the enchondromas is probably greater than 50%, but fortunately these tumours are not highly malignant.

Patients with Maffucci's syndrome should be monitored regularly throughout life for any change in either the bone or the visceral lesions.

DYSPLASIAS WITH PREDOMINANTLY EPIPHYSEAL CHANGES

This group of disorders is characterized by abnormal development and ossification of the epiphyses, resulting in distortion of the bone ends. Limb length may be affected, though usually not as severely as in achondroplasia.

MULTIPLE EPIPHYSEAL DYSPLASIA

Multiple epiphyseal dysplasia (MED) varies in severity from a trouble-free disorder with mild anatomical abnormalities to a severe crippling condition. There is widespread involvement of the epiphyses but the vertebrae are not at all, or only mildly, affected.

Clinical features

Children are below average height and the parents may have noticed that the lower limbs are disproportionately short compared to the trunk. They sometimes walk with a waddling gait and they may complain of hip or knee pain. Some develop progressive deformities of the knees and/or ankles. The hands and feet may be short and broad. The face, skull and spine are normal.

In some cases only one or two pairs of joints are involved, while in others the condition is widespread; these are probably expressions of several different disorders. In adult life, residual epiphyseal defects may lead to joint incongruity and secondary OA. If the changes are mild, the underlying abnormality may be missed and the patient is regarded as 'just another case of OA'.

X-RAY

Changes are apparent from early childhood. Epiphyseal ossification is delayed, and when it appears it is irregular or abnormal in outline. In the growing child the epiphyses are misshapen, and in the hips this may be mistaken for bilateral Perthes' disease. The vertebral ring epiphyses may be affected, but only mildly. At maturity the femoral heads, femoral condyles and humeral heads are flattened; secondary OA may ensue and, if many joints are involved, the patient can be severely crippled.

Genetics

This appears to be a heterogeneous disorder but most cases have an autosomal dominant pattern of inheritance.

The abnormality identified in some cases is in the gene which codes for cartilage oligometric matrix protein (COMP). In ways which are not fully understood, this results in defective chondrocyte function.

Diagnosis

MED is often confused with other childhood disorders which are associated with either lower-limb shortness or Perthes-like changes in the epiphyses.

Achondroplasia and hypochondroplasia should not be difficult to exclude. The former is marked by a more severe degree of dwarfism and characteristic facial changes; the latter by the absence of epiphyseal changes. *Dyschondrosteosis*, likewise, is associated with normal epiphyses.

Pseudoachondroplasia shows widespread epiphyseal abnormalities. However, the skeletal deformities are more severe than those of MED and they also involve the spine.

Perthes' disease is confined to the hips and shows a typical cycle of changes from epiphyseal irregularity to fragmentation, flattening and healing.

Cretinism, if untreated, causes progressive and widespread epiphyseal dysplasia. However, these children have other clinical and biochemical abnormalities and they are mentally retarded.

Management

Children may complain of slight pain and limp, but little can (or need) be done about this. At maturity, deformities around the hips, knees or ankles sometimes require corrective osteotomy.

In later life, secondary OA may require reconstructive surgery.

SPONDYLOEPIPHYSEAL DYSPLASIA

The term 'spondyloepiphyseal dysplasia' (SED) encompasses a heterogeneous group of disorders in which

MED is associated with well-marked vertebral changes – delayed ossification, flattening of the vertebral bodies (platyspondyly), irregular ossification of the ring epiphyses and indentations of the end-plates (Schmorl's nodes). The mildest of these disorders is indistinguishable from MED; the more severe forms have characteristic appearances.

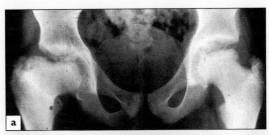
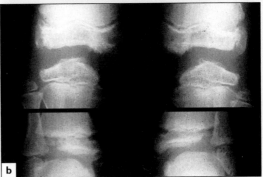

8.9 Multiple epiphyseal dysplasia (a) The grossly abnormal epiphyses led to a mistaken diagnosis of late Perthes' disease. (b) This girl had many epiphyses involved; her sister was similarly affected. Note the characteristic flattening of the femoral condyles.

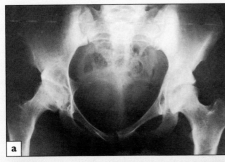
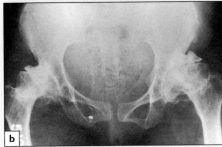
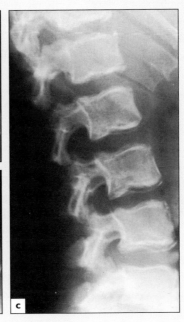

8.10 Multiple epiphyseal dysplasia (a) The typical irregular shape of the upper femoral epiphyses. This may lead to (b) severe osteoarthritis at a relatively young age. (c) The appearance of the vertebral ring epiphyses.

Clinical features

SED CONGENITA

This autosomal dominant disorder can be diagnosed in infancy: the limbs are short, but the trunk is even shorter and the neck hardly there. Older children develop a dorsal kyphosis and a typical barrel-shaped chest; they stand with the hips flexed and the lumbar spine in marked lordosis. By adolescence they often have scoliosis.

X-rays show widespread epiphyseal dysplasia and the characteristic vertebral changes. Odontoid hypoplasia is common and may lead to atlanto-axial subluxation and cord compression.

Diagnosis is not always easy; there are obvious similarities to Morquio's disease but, in the latter, shortening is in the distal limb segments and urinalysis shows increased excretion of keratan sulphate.

8.11 Spondyloepiphyseal dysplasia

(a, b) Adolescent boys with marked lumbar lordosis, vertebral deformities, flexed hips and epiphyseal dysplasia affecting all the limbs.

(c) Widespread deformities and barrel chest in adulthood. X-rays show severe secondary osteoarthritis of the hips.

Management may involve corrective osteotomies for severe coxa vara or knee deformities. Odontoid hypoplasia increases the risks of anaesthesia; if there is evidence of subluxation atlantoaxial fusion may be advisable.

SED TARDA

An X-linked recessive disorder, SED tarda is much less severe and may become apparent only after the age of 5 years when the child fails to grow normally and develops a kyphoscoliosis. Adult men show disproportionate shortening of the trunk and a tendency to barrel chest. They may develop backache or secondary OA of the hips.

X-rays show the characteristic platyspondyly and abnormal ossification of the ring epiphyses, together with more widespread dysplasia.

Treatment may be needed for backache or (in older adults) for secondary OA of the hips.

DYSPLASIA EPIPHYSEALIS HEMIMELICA (TREVOR'S DISEASE)

This is a curious 'hemidysplasia' affecting only one limb and only one-half (the medial or lateral half) of each epiphysis. It is a sporadic disorder which usually appears at the ankle or knee. The child (most often a boy) presents with a bony swelling on one side of the joint; several sites may be affected – all on the same side in the same limb, but rarely in the upper limb.

X-rays show an asymmetrical enlargement of the bony epiphysis and distortion of the adjacent joint. At the ankle, this may give the appearance of an abnormally large medial malleolus.

Treatment is called for if the deformity interferes with joint function. The excess bone is removed, taking care not to damage the articular cartilage or ligaments.

CHONDRODYPLASIA PUNCTATA (STIPPLED EPIPHYSES)

Chrondrodysplasia punctata (or Conradi's disease) is a generalized, multisystem disorder producing facial abnormalities, vertebral anomalies, asymmetrical epiphyseal changes and bone shortening. In severe cases there may also be cardiac anomalies, congenital cataracts and mental retardation; some of these children die during infancy.

The characteristic *x-ray* feature is a punctate stippling of the cartilaginous epiphyses and apophyses. This disappears by the age of 4 years but is often followed by epiphyseal irregularities and dysplasia. It is unlikely that these changes will be confused with those of MED, Down's syndrome or cretinism.

Orthopaedic management is directed at the deformities that develop in older children: joint contractures, limb length inequality or scoliosis.

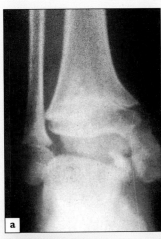

8.12 Epiphyseal dysplasia (a) Trevor's disease. (b) Conradi's disease – the spots disappeared later.

DYSPLASIAS WITH PREDOMINANTLY DIAPHYSEAL CHANGES

Most of the 'metaphyseal' and 'diaphyseal dysplasias' appear to be the result of defective bone modelling. Unlike the physeal and epiphyseal disorders, dwarfing is not a feature. There may be associated thickening of the skull bones, with the risk of foraminal occlusion and cranial nerve entrapment.

Fibrous dysplasia is dealt with on page 174.

METAPHYSEAL DYSPLASIA (PYLE'S DISEASE)

The only significant clinical feature in this disorder is genu valgum – or rather valgus angulation of the bones on either side of the knee. X-rays show a typical 'bottle shape' of the distal femur or proximal tibia – the so-called Erlenmeyer flask deformity – suggesting a failure of bone modelling. Inheritance pattern is autosomal recessive. Treatment is seldom needed.

CRANIOMETAPHYSEAL DYSPLASIA

This condition, of autosomal dominant inheritance, is similar to Pyle's disease, but here the tubular defect is associated with progressive thickening of the skull and mandible resulting in a curiously prominent forehead, a large jaw and a squashed-looking nose. Foraminal occlusion may cause cranial nerve compression – sometimes severe enough to require operative treatment.

OSTEOPETROSIS (MARBLE BONES, ALBERS-SCHÖNBERG DISEASE)

Osteopetrosis is one of several conditions which are characterized by thickening and increased radiographic density of the bones. Differences in the pattern of inheritance, the age of presentation and the distribution of the clinical and x-ray changes show that they are genetically distinct conditions.

OSTEOPETROSIS TARDA

The common form of osteopetrosis is a fairly benign, autosomal dominant disorder that seldom causes symptoms and may only be discovered in adolescence or adulthood after a pathological fracture or when an x-ray is taken for other reasons – hence the designation *tarda*. Appearance and function are unimpaired, unless there are complications: pathological fracture or cranial nerve compression due to bone encroachment on foramina. Sufferers are also prone to bone infection, particularly of the mandible after tooth extraction.

X rays show increased density of all the bones: cortices are widened, leaving narrow medullary canals;

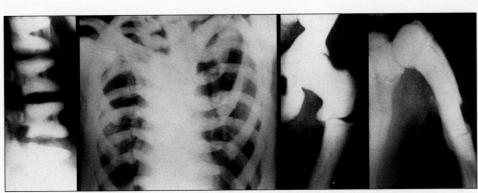

8.13 Marble bones Despite the remarkable density, the bones break easily; but, as in this humerus, union occurs, although rather slowly.

sclerotic vertebral end-plates produce a striped appearance ('rugger-jersey spine'); the skull is thickened and the base densely sclerotic.

Treatment is required only if complications occur.

OSTEOPETROSIS CONGENITA

This rare, autosomal recessive form of osteopetrosis is present at birth and causes severe disability. Bone encroachment on marrow results in pancytopenia, haemolysis, anaemia and hepatosplenomegaly. Foraminal occlusion may cause optic or facial nerve palsy. Repeated haemorrhage or infection usually leads to death in early childhood.

Treatment, in recent years, has focused on methods of enhancing bone resorption. This has been achieved by transplanting marrow from normal donors, suggesting that the condition is due to lack of marrow cells that control osteoclastic activity.

DIAPHYSEAL DYSPLASIA (ENGELMANN'S OR CAMURATI'S DISEASE)

This is another rare childhood disorder in which x-rays show fusiform widening and sclerosis of the shafts of the long bones, and sometimes thickening of the skull. The condition is notable because of its association with muscle pain and weakness. Children complain of 'tired legs' and have a typical wide-based or waddling gait. There may be muscle wasting and failure to thrive.

Muscle pain may need symptomatic treatment. Milder cases usually clear up spontaneously by the age of 25 years.

CRANIODIAPHYSEAL DYSPLASIA

This rare autosomal recessive disorder is characterized by cylindrical expansion of the long bones and gross thickening of the skull and facial bones. Prominent facial contours may appear in early childhood and are the most striking feature of the condition – giving rise to the name *'leontiasis'*. Foraminal occlusion may cause deafness or visual impairment.

PYKNODYSOSTOSIS

Interest in this rare disorder owes something to the suggestion that the French impressionist, Toulouse-Lautrec, was a victim (Maroteaux and Lamy, 1965). Clinical features are shortness of stature, frontal bossing, underdevelopment of the mandible and abnormal dentition. The presence of blue sclerae and proneness to fracture may cause confusion with OI. The condition is inherited as an autosomal recessive trait.

On x-ray the bones are dense; the skull is enlarged, with wide suture lines and open fontanelles, but the facial bones and mandible are hypoplastic, thus accounting for the typical 'triangular' facies.

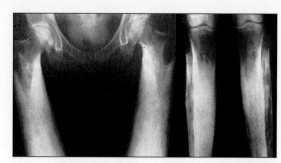

8.14 Engelmann's disease This patient had considerable discomfort from her long bones – all of which were wide and looked dense on x-ray.

Despite appearances, it causes little trouble (apart from the odd pathological fracture) and needs no treatment.

CANDLE BONES, SPOTTED BONES AND STRIPED BONES

CANDLE BONES (MELORHEOSTOSIS, LERI'S DISEASE) This rare, non-familial, condition is sometimes discovered (almost accidentally) in patients who complain of pain and stiffness in one limb. *X-rays* show irregular patches of sclerosis, usually distributed in linear fashion through the limb; the appearance is reminiscent of the wax that congeals on the side of a burning candle. Some patients also develop scleroderma and joint contractures.

SPOTTED BONES (OSTEOPOIKILOSIS) Routine x-rays sometimes show (quite incidentally) numerous white spots distributed throughout the skeleton. Closer examination occasionaly reveals whitish spots in the skin (disseminated lenticular dermatofibrosis). The condition is inherited as an autosomal dominant trait.

STRIPED BONES (OSTEOPATHIA STRIATA) X-rays show lines of increased density parallel to the shafts of long bones, but radiating like a fan in the pelvis. The condition is symptomless. Some cases show autosomal dominant inheritance.

COMBINED AND MIXED DYSPLASIAS

A number of disorders show a mixture of epiphyseal, physeal, metaphyseal and vertebral defects – i.e. dwarfism combined with epiphyseal maldevelopment, abnormal modelling of the metaphyses and platyspondyly.

SPONDYLOMETAPHYSEAL DYSPLASIA
This is the commonest of the 'mixed' dysplasias. There may be severe vertebral flattening and kyphoscoliosis.

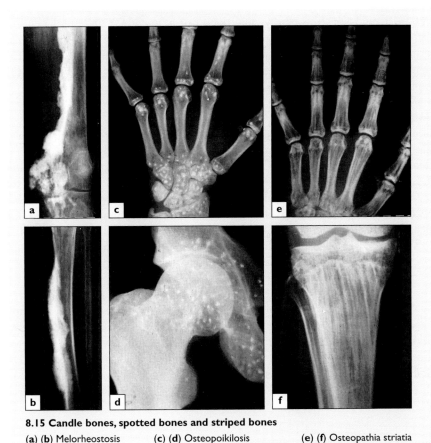

8.15 Candle bones, spotted bones and striped bones
(a) (b) Melorheostosis   (c) (d) Osteopoikilosis   (e) (f) Osteopathia striatia

Epiphyseal changes are usually mild but the metaphyses are broad and ill-formed. Patients may need treatment for spinal deformity or malalignment of the hip or knee.

PSEUDOACHONDROPLASIA

This rare disorder resembles achondroplasia in that it is characterized by short-limbed dwarfism associated with ligamentous laxity, exaggerated lumbar lordosis and bow-leg deformities. In contrast to achondroplasia, clinical features are not evident at birth but become apparent only a year or two later, and the head and face look normal. Transmission is autosomal dominant.

The characteristic x-ray features are underdevelopment and flattening of the epiphyses, widening of the metaphyses, shortening of the tubular bones and oval-shaped vertebral bodies. By the end of growth, the hips may be dysplastic and the vertebral bodies often show defects of the bony end-plates. Spinal stenosis is not a feature.

Deformities sometimes require surgical correction. In adults, secondary OA may call for reconstructive surgery.

DIASTROPHIC DYSPLASIA

This autosomal recessive disorder affects all types of cartilage. Infants are severely dwarfed and distorted, with deformities of the hands ('hitch-hiker's thumb'), club feet, joint contractures, dislocations, 'cauliflower' ears and cleft palate. Softening of the laryngeal cartilage may produce respiratory distress. In older children the main problems are scoliosis and joint contractures.

X-rays show epiphyseal hypoplasia and maldevelopment, metaphyseal thickening, flattening of the pelvis and kyphoscoliosis. Odontoid hypoplasia is usual.

Management involves early correction of joint contractures and treatment of club foot and hand deformities. Scoliosis may require correction and spinal fusion.

CLEIDOCRANIAL DYSPLASIA

This disorder, of autosomal dominant inheritance, is characterized by hypoplasia of the clavicles and flat bones. In a typical case the patient is somewhat short, with a large head, frontal prominence, a flat-looking face and drooping shoulders. The teeth appear late and develop poorly. Because the clavicles are hypoplastic or absent, the chest seems narrow and the patient can bring his shoulders together anteriorly. The pelvis is narrow but the symphysis pubis may be unduly wide and there may be some disproportion of the forearm or finger bones.

X-rays show a brachycephalic skull and persistence of wormian bones. Characteristically there is underdevelopment of the clavicles, scapulae and pelvis. Much of the clavicle may be missing, leaving a nubbin of bone at the medial or lateral end. Scoliosis and coxa vara are common.

Treatment is unnecessary unless the patient develops severe coxa vara or scoliosis; dental anomalies may need attention.

NAIL–PATELLA SYNDROME

This curious condition is relatively common and is inherited as an autosomal dominant trait. The nails are hypoplastic and the patellae unusually small or absent. The radial head is subluxed laterally and the elbows may lack full extension. Congenital nephropathy may be associated. The characteristic *x-ray* features are hypoplastic or absent patellae and the presence of bony protuberances ('horns') on the lateral aspect of the iliac blades.

CRANIOFACIAL DYSPLASIA

Many disorders – some inherited, some not – are distinguished primarily by the abnormal appearance of the face and skull. Other bones may be affected as well, but it is the odd facial appearance that is most striking. Premature fusion of the cranial sutures may lead to exophthalmos and mental retardation. Orthopaedic problems arise from the associated anomalies of the hands and feet.

The best-known of these conditions is *Apert's syndrome* (acrocephalosyndactyly). The head is somewhat egg-shaped: flat at the back, narrow anteroposteriorly, with a broad, towering forehead, depressed face, bulging eyes and prominent jaw. The hands and feet are misshapen, with syndactyly or

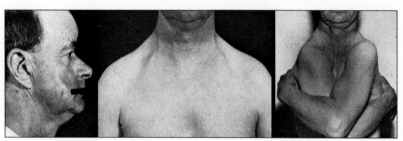

8.16 Cleidocranial dysplasia The 'squashed face' and sloping shoulders which can be brought together anteriorly are pathognomonic.

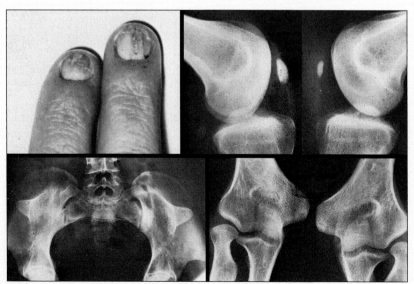

8.17 The nail–patella syndrome The dystrophic nails, minute patellae, pelvic 'horns' and subluxed radii combine to give an unmistakable picture.

synostosis of the medial rays. The condition sometimes shows autosomal dominant inheritance, but most cases are sporadic.

Cerebral compression can be prevented by early craniotomy and the facial appearance may be improved by maxillofacial reconstruction. Syndactyly usually needs operative treatment.

CONNECTIVE TISSUE DISORDERS

Collagen is the commonest form of body protein, making up 90% of the non-mineral bony matrix and 70% of the structural tissue in ligaments and tendons. Some 20 types of collagen, produced by 30 or more genes, have been identified; those distributed most abundantly in the musculoskeletal system are *type I* (in bone, ligament, tendon and skin), *type II* (in cartilage) *and type* III (in blood vessels, muscle and skin).

Heritable defects of collagen synthesis give rise to a number of disorders involving either the soft connective tissues or bone, or both. In many cases the specific collagen defect has now been identified.

GENERALIZED (FAMILIAL) JOINT LAXITY

About 5% of normal people have joint hypermobility, as manifested by the following tests: (1) passive hyperextension of the metacarpophalangeal joints to beyond 90°; (2) passive stretching of the thumb to touch the front of the forearm; (3) hyperextension of the elbows and knees; and (4) the ability to bend forward and place the hands flat on the floor with the knees held perfectly straight. The trait runs in families and is inherited as a mendelian dominant. The condition is not in itself disabling but it may predispose to congenital dislocation of the hip in the newborn or recurrent dislocation of the patella or shoulder in later life. Transient joint pains are common and there is an increased risk of ankle sprains.

MARFAN'S SYNDROME

This is a generalized disorder affecting the skeleton, joint ligaments, eyes and cardiovascular structures. It is thought to be due to a cross-linkage defect in collagen and elastin. The genetic abnormality has been mapped to the fibrillin gene on chromosome 15. It is transmitted as autosomal dominant but sporadic cases also occur. Males and females are affected equally.

Clinical features

Patients are tall, with disproportionately long legs and arms, and often with flattening or hollowing of the chest (pectus excavatum). Typically, the upper body segment is shorter than the lower (a ratio of less than 0.8 is suggestive) and arm span exceeds height by 5cm or more. The digits are unusually long, giving rise to the term 'arachnodactyly' (spider fingers). Spinal abnormalities include spondylolisthesis and scoliosis. There is an increased incidence of slipped upper femoral epiphysis. Generalized joint laxity is usual and patients may develop flat feet or dislocation of the patella or shoulder.

Associated abnormalities include a high arched palate, hernias, lens dislocation, retinal detachment, aortic aneurysm and mitral or aortic incompetence. Cardiovascular complications are particularly serious and account for most of the deaths in severe cases.

X-RAY
Bone structure appears normal (apart from excessive length), but x-ray may reveal complications such as scoliosis, spondylolisthesis or slipped epiphysis.

Diagnosis

'Marfanoid' features are quite common and it is now thought that there are several variants of the underlying condition. Mild cases are easily missed or mistaken for uncomplicated joint laxity; it is important to look for ophthalmic and cardiovascular defects.

Homocystinuria, an inborn error of methionine metabolism, has in the past been confused with Marfan's syndrome (see page 159).

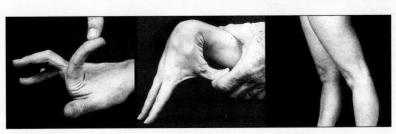

8.18 Generalized joint laxity The hypermobility in this girl was symptomless.

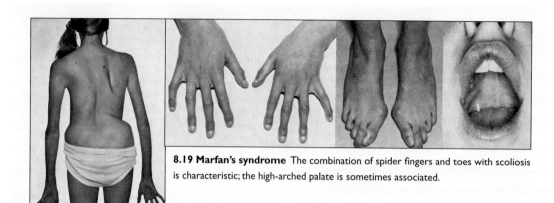

8.19 Marfan's syndrome The combination of spider fingers and toes with scoliosis is characteristic; the high-arched palate is sometimes associated.

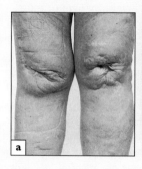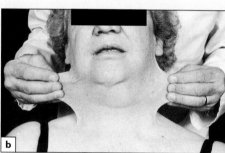

8.20 Ehlers–Danlos syndrome (a) This woman presented with these unpleasant but characteristic scars. (b) She also shows the usual remarkable skin hyperextensibility.

Management

Patients occasionally need treatment for progressive scoliosis or flat feet. The heart should be carefully checked before operation.

EHLERS–DANLOS SYNDROME

Ehlers–Danlos syndrome (EDS) is a heterogeneous condition characterized by unusual skin laxity, joint hypermobility and vascular fragility, expressions of underlying abnormalities of elastin and collagen formation. The syndrome comprises at least 10 distinct disorders in which the individual clinical features appear with varying emphasis (Ainsworth and Aulicino, 1993).

Clinical features

Babies may show marked hypotonia and joint laxity. Hypermobility persists and older patients are often capable of bizarre feats of contortion. The skin is soft and hyperextensible; it is easily damaged and vascular fragility may give rise to 'spontaneous' bruising. Joint laxity, recurrent dislocations and scoliosis are common. Of the many types of EDS so far described, over 90% show autosomal dominant inheritance.

Management

Complications (e.g. recurrent dislocation or scoliosis) may need treatment. However, if joint laxity is marked, soft-tissue reconstruction usually fails to cure the tendency to dislocation. Beware! Blood vessel fragility may cause severe bleeding at operation, and wound healing is often poor.

Joint instability may lead to OA in later life.

LARSEN'S SYNDROME

This is a heterogeneous condition, the more severe (recessive) forms presenting in infancy with marked joint laxity and dislocation of the hips, instability of the knees, subluxation of the radial head, equinovarus deformities of the feet and 'dish-face' appearance. Spinal deformities are common in older children. Mild forms of the same condition show autosomal dominant inheritance.

Operative treatment may be needed for joint instability and dislocation.

OSTEOGENESIS IMPERFECTA (BRITTLE BONES)

Osteogenesis imperfecta (OI) is one of the commonest of the genetic disorders of bone, with an estimated incidence of 1 in 20,000. Abnormal synthesis and structural defects of type I collagen result in abnormalities of the bones, teeth, ligaments, sclerae and skin. The defining clinical features are (1) osteopenia, (2) liability to fracture, (3) laxity of ligaments, (4) blue coloration of the sclerae and (5) dentinogenesis imperfecta ('crumbling teeth'). However, there are considerable variations in the severity of expression of these features and in the pattern of inheritance and it is now recognized that the condition embraces a heterogeneous group of collagen abnormalities resulting from many different genetic mutational defects (Kocher and Shapiro, 1998).

Pathology

The genetic abnormality in OI expresses itself as an alteration in the structural integrity, or a reduction in the total amount of type I collagen, one of the major components of fibrillar connective tissue in skin, ligaments and bone. Even small alterations in the composition of type I collagen can lead to weakening of these tissues and imperfect ossification in all types of bone. Bone formation is initiated in the normal way but it progresses abnormally, the fully formed tissue consisting of a mixture of woven and lamellar bone, and in the worst cases almost entirely of immature woven bone. There is thinning of the dermis, laxity of ligaments, increased corneal translucency and (in some cases) loss of dentin leading to tooth decay.

Clinical features

The clinical features vary considerably, according to the severity of the condition. The most striking abnormality is the propensity to fracture, generally after minor trauma and often without much pain or swelling. In the classic case fractures are discovered during infancy and they recur frequently throughout childhood. Callus formation is florid, so much so that the lump has occasionally been mistaken for an osteosarcoma; however, the new bone also is abnormal and it remains 'pliable' for a long time, thus predisposing to malunion. By the age of 6 years there may be severe deformities of the long bones, and vertebral compression fractures often lead to kyphoscoliosis.

The skin is thin and somewhat loose and the joints are hypermobile. Blue or grey sclerae, when they occur, are due to uveal pigment showing through the hypertranslucent cornea. The teeth may be discoloured and carious.

In milder cases fractures develop a year or two after birth – perhaps when the child starts to walk; they are also less frequent and deformity is not a marked feature.

In the most severe types of OI fractures are present before birth and the infant is either stillborn or lives only a few weeks, death being due to respiratory failure, basilar indentation or intracranial haemorrhage following injury.

X-RAY

There is generalized osteopenia, thinning of the long bones, fractures in various stages of healing, vertebral compression and spinal deformity. The type of abnormality varies with the severity of the disease. The skull may be enlarged and shows the presence of wormian bones – areas of vicarious ossification in the calvarium.

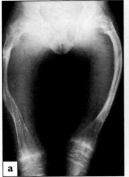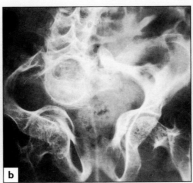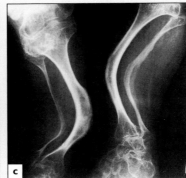

8.21 Osteogenesis imperfecta (**a**) Moderately severe (type IV) disease. (**b**, **c**) Severe deformities in type III disease.

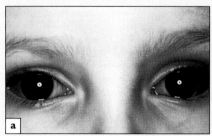 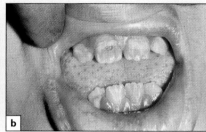

8.22 Osteogenesis imperfecta
(a) The typical deep blue sclerae in type I disease. (b) Faulty dentine in a patient with type IV disease.

After puberty, fractures occur less frequently, but in those who survive the incidence rises again after the climacteric. It is thought that very mild ('subclinical') forms of OI may account for some cases of recurrent fractures in adults.

Diagnosis

In most cases the clinical and radiological features are so distinctive that the diagnosis is not in doubt. However, mistakes have been made and rare disorders causing multiple fractures may have to be excluded by laboratory tests. In hypophosphatasia, for example, the serum alkaline phosphatase level is very low.

In older children with atypical features it is essential to look for evidence of physical abuse.

Classification

The clinical variants of OI can be divided into subgroups showing well-defined differences in the pattern of inheritance, age of presentation and severity of changes in the bones and extra-skeletal tissues. This is helpful in assessing the prognosis and planning treatment for any particular patient.

The most widely use classification is that of Sillence (1981), which defines four clinical types of OI. The principal features are summarized in the Box:

OI type I (mild)
- The commonest variety; over 50% of all cases.
- Fractures usually appear at 1–2 years of age.
- Healing is reasonably good and deformities are not marked.
- Sclerae deep blue.
- Teeth usually normal but some have dentino genesis imperfecta .
- Impaired hearing in adults.
- Quality of life good; normal life expectancy.
- Autosomal dominant inheritance.

OI type II (lethal)
- 5–10% of cases.

- Intra-uterine and neonatal fractures.
- Large skull and wormian bones.
- Sclerae grey.
- Rib fractures and respiratory difficulty.
- Stillborn or survive for only a few weeks.
- Most due to new dominant mutations; some autosomal recessive.

OI type III (severe deforming)
- The 'classic', but not the most common, form of OI.
- Fractures often present at birth.
- Large skull and wormian bones; pinched-looking face.
- Marked deformities and kyphoscoliosis by 6 years.
- Sclerae grey, becoming white.
- Dentinogenesis imperfecta.
- Marked joint laxity.
- Respiratory problems.
- Poor quality of life; few survive to adulthood.
- Sporadic, or autosomal recessive inheritance.

OI type IV (moderately severe)
- Uncommon; less than 5% of cases.
- Frequent fractures during early childhood.
- Deformities common.
- Sclerae pale blue or normal.
- Dentinogenesis imperfecta.
- Survive to adulthood with fairly good function.
- Autosomal dominant inheritance.

Management

There is no medical treatment which will counteract the effects of this abnormality, and genetic manipulation is no more than a promise for the future.

Conservative treatment is directed at preventing fractures – if necessary by using lightweight orthoses during physical activity – and treating fractures when they occur. However, splintage should not be overdone as this may contribute further to the prevailing osteopenia. General measures to prevent recurrent trauma, maintain movement and encourage social adaptation are very important.

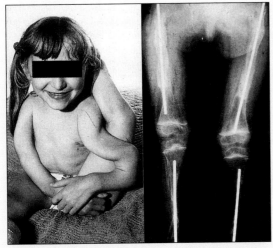

8.23 Osteogenesis imperfecta This patient had severe deformities of both legs; these were corrected by multiple osteotomies and 'rodding'.

Most of the long-term orthopaedic problems are encountered in types III and IV. Fractures are treated conservatively, but immobilization must be kept to a minimum. Long-bone deformities are common, due either to malunion of complete fractures or breaking of recurrent incomplete fractures; these may require operative correction, usually by 4 or 5 years of age. Multiple osteotomies are performed and the bone fragments are then realigned on a straight intramedullary rod; the same effect can be achieved by closed osteoclasis. The problem of the bone outgrowing the rod has been addressed by using telescoping nails; however, these carry a fairly high complication rate.

Spinal deformity is also common and is particularly difficult to treat. Bracing is ineffectual and progressive curves require operative instrumentation and spinal fusion.

After adolescence, fractures are much less common and patients may pursue a reasonably comfortable and useful life.

FIBRODYSPLASIA OSSIFICANS PROGRESSIVA

This rare condition, formerly known as myositis ossificans progressiva, is characterized by widespread ossification of the connective tissue of muscle, mainly in the trunk. It starts in early childhood with episodes of fever and soft-tissue inflammation around the shoulders and trunk. As this subsides the tissues harden and plaques of ossification extend throughout the affected areas. In the worst cases movements are restricted and the patient is severely disabled. Associated anomalies are shortening of the big toe and thumb. The condition is probably transmitted as an autosomal dominant but, since affected individuals seldom have children, most cases result from new mutations. Treatment with diphosphonates may prevent progression.

NEUROFIBROMATOSIS

Neurofibromatosis is one of the commonest single gene disorders affecting the skeleton. Two types are recognized: *Type 1 (NF-1) – also known as von Recklinghausen's disease* – has an incidence of about 1 in 3500 live births. The abnormality is located in the gene which codes for neurofibromin, on chromososme 17. It is transmitted as autosomal dominant, with almost 100% penetrance, but more than 50% of cases are due to new mutation. The most characteristic lesions are neurofibromata (Schwann cell tumours) and patches of skin pigmentation (*café-au-lait* spots), but other features are remarkably protean and musculoskeletal abnormalities are seen in almost half of those affected.

Type 2 (NF-2) is much less common, with an incidence of 1 in 50,000 births. It is associated with the gene which codes for schwannomin, located on chromosome

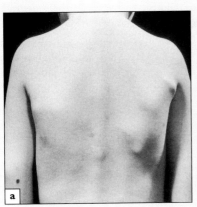

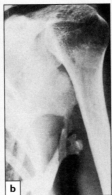

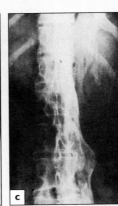

8.24 Fibrodysplasia ossificans progressiva (**a**) The lumps in this boy's back were hard and his back movements were limited. (**b, c**) This adult shows the extensive soft-tissue ossification.

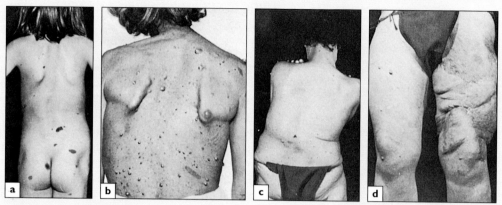

8.25 Neurofibromatosis (a) Café-au-lait spots; (b) multiple neurofibromata and slight scoliosis; (c, d) a patient with scoliosis and soft-tissue overgrowth ('elephantiasis').

22. Like NF-1, it is transmitted as autosomal dominant. Unlike NF-1, intracranial lesions (e.g. acoustic neuromas and meningiomas) are usual while musculoskeletal manifestations are rare.

Clinical features of NF-1

Almost all patients have the typical widespread patches of skin pigmentation and multiple cutaneous neurofibromata which usually appear before puberty. Less common is a single large plexiform neurofibroma, or an area of soft-tissue overgrowth in one of the limbs.

The orthopaedic surgeon is most likely to encounter the condition in a child or adolescent who presents with *scoliosis* (the most suggestive deformity is a very short, sharp curve) or with *localized vertebral abnormalities* such as scalloping of the posterior aspects of the vertebral bodies, erosion of the pedicles, intervertebral foraminal enlargement and pencilling of the ribs at affected levels. *Dystrophic spinal deformities*, including deformities of the cervical spine, are also seen.

Congenital tibial dysplasia and pseudarthrosis are rare conditions, but almost 50% of patients with these lesions have some evidence of neurofibromatosis (see page 164).

Malignant change occurs in 2–5% of affected individuals and is the most common complication in older patients.

Treatment

The orthopaedic conditions associated with neurofibromatosis are dealt with on page 164 of this chapter and in the section on scoliosis in Chapter 18.

METABOLIC DEFECTS

Many single gene disorders are expressed as undersecretion of an enzyme that controls a specific stage in the metabolic chain; the undegraded substrate accumulates and may be stored, with harmful effects, in various tissues or be excreted in the urine. Conditions involving the musculoskeletal system are the mucopolysaccharidoses (MPS), Gaucher's disease, homocystinuria, alkaptonuria and congenital hyperuricaemia. All these inborn errors of metabolism are inherited as recessive traits.

MUCOPOLYSACCHARIDOSES

The polysaccharide glycosaminoglycans (GAGs) form the side-chains of macromolecular proteoglycans, a major component of the matrix in bone, cartilage, intervertebral discs, synovium and other connective tissues. Defunct proteoglycans are degraded by lysosomal enzymes. Deficiency of any of these enzymes causes a hold-up on the degradative pathway. Partially degraded GAGs accumulate in the lysosomes in the liver, spleen, bones and other tissues, and spill over in the blood and urine where they can be detected by suitable biochemical tests. Confirmation of the enzyme lack can be obtained by tests on cultured fibroblasts or leucocytes.

Clinical features

Depending on the specific enzyme deficiency and the type of GAG storage, a number of different clinical syndromes have been defined. All except Hunter's syndrome (an X-linked recessive disorder) are transmit-

Table 8.2 Enzyme defect and GAG excretion in the commoner mucopolysaccharidoses

Syndrome	Enzyme defect	GAG excretion
Hurler (MPS I)	Iduronidase	Dermatan sulphate Heparan sulphate
Hunter (MPS II)	Iduronate sulphatase	Dermatan sulphate Heparan sulphate
Morquio (MPS IV)	N-Acetylgalactosamine-4-sulphate	Keratan sulphate

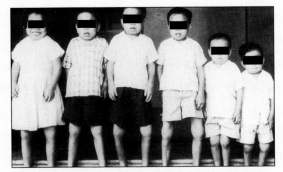

8.26 Mucopolysaccharidoses The appearance of a group of children with Hurler's syndrome. (Courtesy of Prof. K. Bose of Singapore.)

ted as autosomal recessive. As a group they have certain recognizable features: excessively short stature with vertebral deformity, coarse facies, hepatosplenomegaly and (in some cases) mental retardation. X-rays show bone dysplasia affecting the vertebral bodies, epiphyses and metaphyses; typically the bones have a spatulate appearance.

There is a superficial similarity to SED and spondylometaphyseal dysplasia. However, careful observation reveals several points of difference, and the diagnosis can be confirmed by testing for abnormal GAG excretion or demonstrating the enzyme deficiency in blood cells or cultured fibroblasts.

At least 10 different disorders are recognized; here only the three least rare conditions will be described.

HURLER'S SYNDROME (MPS I)

Infants look normal at birth but over the next 2–3 years they gradually develop a typical appearance: they are undersized, with increasing kyphosis, hepatosplenomegaly, coarse facies, protruding tongue, defective hearing and mental retardation. Speech is very poor. Joints are stiff and walking is delayed. There may be corneal opacities, respiratory difficulty and cardiac anomalies. X-rays usually show unmistakable features such as hypoplastic epiphyses and vertebral bodies, poorly modelled metaphyses, short but wide metacarpals, underdeveloped mandible, spatulate ribs and clavicles, flared iliac blades, shallow acetabuli and coxa valga. Cardiac or respiratory complications usually cause death in later childhood.

HUNTER'S SYNDROME (MPS II)

This is also a recessive disorder, but X-linked – so all patients are male. Clinical features are similar to those of Hurler's syndrome, but less severe. Suspicious features usually appear at about 3 years, cardiorespiratory complications gradually become more severe and death usually occurs in the middle or late teens.

MORQUIO–BRAILSFORD SYNDROME (MPS IV)

Development seems normal for the first year or two, although walking may be delayed. Thereafter the child beings to look dwarfed, with a moderate kyphosis, short neck and protuberant sternum. There is marked joint laxity and progressive genu valgum. Suitable tests will reveal a conductive hearing loss. However, the face is unaffected and intelligence is normal. X-rays of the spine show the typical ovoid, hypoplastic vertebral bodies, which end up abnormally flat (platyspondyly) and peculiarly pointed anteriorly.

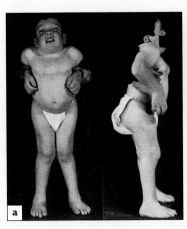
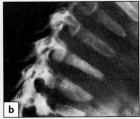
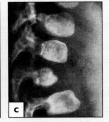
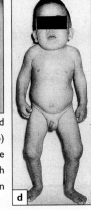

8.27 Mucopolysaccharidoses (a) Morquio–Brailsford syndrome – note the manubriosternal angle. (b) Platyspondyly in a similar patient, contrasted with (c) the sabot appearance in Hurler's syndrome. (d) A boy with Hunter's syndrome; his appearance is similar to that in Hurler's syndrome.

Odontoid hypoplasia is usual. A marked manubriosternal angle (almost 90°) is pathognomonic. By the age of 5 years the femoral head epiphyses are underdeveloped and flat, and the acetabula abnormally shallow. The long bones are of normal width but the metacarpals may be short and broad, and pointed at their proximal ends.

Management

There is, as yet, no specific treatment for the mucopolysaccharide disorders. However, enzyme replacement and gene manipulation are possible in the future.

Hurler's syndrome has a very poor prognosis but the complications (e.g. respiratory infection) may need treatment.

Morquio's syndrome presents several orthopaedic problems. Genu valgum may need correction by femoral osteotomy, though this should be delayed till growth has ceased. Coxa valga and subluxation of the hips, if symmetrical, may cause little disability; unilateral subluxation may need femoral or acetabular osteotomy. Atlanto-axial instability may threaten the cord and require occipitocervical fusion. All the 'spondylodysplasias' carry a risk of atlantoaxial subluxation during anaesthesia and intubation, and special precautions are needed during operation.

GAUCHER'S DISEASE

The genetic disorder first described by Gaucher over 100 years ago is now known to be caused by lack of a specific enzyme which is responsible for the breakdown and excretion of cell membrane products from defunct cells. This is a classic example of a lipid storage disease for which the pathogenesis has been painstakingly worked out, leading to the development of effective treatment.

Each time one of the cells in the body dies, a glucocerebroside is released from the cell membrane; before it can be excreted, the glycoside bond holding the glucose molecule has to be split by a specific enzyme – glucosylceramide β-glucosidase. If this enzyme is lacking, the glucocerebroside cannot be excreted and instead is stored in the lysosomal bodies of macrophages of the reticuloendothelial system, notably in the marrow, spleen and liver. Accumulation of these abnormal macrophages leads to enlargement of the spleen and liver, and secondary changes in the marrow and bone.

Most patients suffer from a chronic form of the disorder, with changes predominantly in the marrow, bone and spleen, and varying degrees of pancytopenia (Type I). A rare form of the disease affecting the central nervous system (Type II) appears in infancy and usually causes death within a year. Type III is a subacute disorder characterized by the appearance of hepatosplenomegaly in childhood and skeletal and neurological abnormalities during adolescence.

Like other storage disorders, Gaucher's disease is transmitted as an autosomal recessive trait. Males and females are affected equally, with a relatively high incidence in Jewish people of Ashkenazi descent. The phenotype is associated with a large number of different gene defects, five of which appear in the majority of cases.

Clinical features

In the commonest form of the disease (Type I), patients present in childhood or adult life with anaemia, thrombocytopenia, hepatosplenomegaly or bone pain; about two thirds of affected people develop skeletal abnormalities. Older patients may develop back pain, due to vertebral osteopenia and compression fractures. Femoral neck fractures also are not uncommon; however, diaphyseal fractures are rare. The haematocrit and platelet count are usually diminished. A suggestive finding (when positive) is elevation of the serum acid phosphatase level. The diagnosis can be confirmed by demonstrating low glucocerebrosidase activity in the blood or by identifying the abnormal gene mutations in DNA tests.

A common complication is osteonecrosis, usually of the femoral head but sometimes in the femoral condyles, the proximal end of the humerus or the bones around the ankle. The patient (usually a child or adolescent) may present with an acute 'bone crisis': unrelenting pain, local tenderness and restriction of movement accompanied by pyrexia, leucocytosis and an elevated erythrocyte sedimentation rate (ESR). The clinical features resemble those of osteomyelitis or septic arthritis; indeed, Gaucher's disease predisposes to bone infection and this may be a source of confusion.

IMAGING

X-rays show a variable pattern of radiolucency or patchy density, more marked in cancellous bone. The distal end of the femur may be expanded, producing the Erlenmeyer flask appearance. A skeletal survey may reveal osteonecrosis of the femoral head, femoral condyles, talus or humeral head.

A radioisotope bone scan may help to distinguish a crisis episode from infection: the former is usually 'cold', the latter 'hot'.

MRI is the most reliable way of defining marrow involvement.

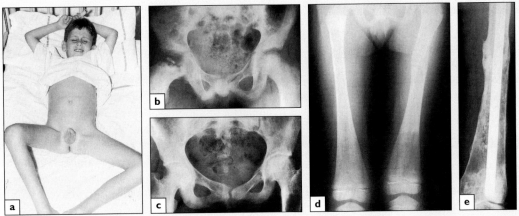

8.28 Gaucher's disease (a) A distressed young boy during an acute Gaucher crisis. The right hip is intensely painful and abduction is restricted. The x-ray (b) shows avascular necrosis of the right femoral head. (c) X-ray of an older patient with a sclerotic left femoral head, the result of previous ischaemic necrosis. (d) Bilateral failure of femoral tubularization – the Erlenmeyer flask appearance. (e) Pathological fracture is uncommon but it does occur. There are also sclerotic 'islands' in the distal femur, typical of old medullary infarcts.

Treatment

Bone pain may need symptomatic treatment. For the acute crisis, analgesic medication and bed rest followed by non-weightbearing walking with crutches is recommended. Specific therapy is now available (albeit costly) in the form of the replacement enzyme, alglucerase. This has been shown to reverse the blood changes and reduce the size of the liver and spleen. The bone complications also are diminished (Pastores *et al.*, 1993, 1996).

Osteonecrosis of the femoral head usually results in progressive deformity of the hip. However, most patients manage quite well with symptomatic treatment and surgery should be deferred for as long as possible (Katz *et al*, 1996).

HOMOCYSTINURIA

This rare disorder is due to deficiency of the enzyme cystathionine β-synthetase and accumulation of homocysteine and methionine. Patients are tall and thin and may develop features reminiscent of Marfan's disease (page 151). However, unlike Marfan's disease, homocystinuria is of autosomal recessive inheritance and is associated with marked osteoporosis and mental retardation. Joint laxity is unusual but there may be muscle weakness. Thromboembolic disease is common and may be fatal. Homocysteine levels are raised in the blood and urine. The enzyme deficiency may be detected in fibroblast cultures. Though rare, the condition should be diagnosed because it can be treated: about half the patients are 'cured' by pyridoxine (vitamin B$_6$) administered from early childhood. Others may be helped by a low methionine, cysteine-supplemented diet.

ALKAPTONURIA

Deficiency of the enzyme homogentisic acid oxidase leads to accumulation of homogentisic acid, which is deposited in connective tissue and excreted in the urine. On standing the urine turns dark (hence the name, alkaptonuria); cartilage and other connective tissues are stained grey – a condition referred to as ochronosis. Clinical problems arise from degenerative changes in articular cartilage with the development of OA, and from calcification of the intervertebral discs.

CONGENITAL HYPERURICAEMIA

The Lesch–Nyhan syndrome is a rare, X-linked recessive disorder causing absence of the enzyme hypoxanthine-guanine phosphoribosyltransferase (HGPRT). This enzyme controls a 'salvage pathway' in the complex purine metabolic chain; absence of HGPRT results in excessive uric acid formation and gout. The young boys are mentally retarded and prone to self-mutilation (gnawing the ends of their fingers). Milder cases present simply as early-onset severe gout. Diagnosis can be confirmed by measuring HGPRT in red cell preparations.

Chromosome disorders are common but usually result in fetal abortion. Of the non-lethal conditions, several produce bone or joint abnormalities.

DOWN'S SYNDROME (TRISOMY 21)

This condition results from having an extra copy of chromosome 21. It is much more common than any of the skeletal dysplasias, with an overall incidence of 1 per 800 live births – and 1 in 250 if the mother is over 37 years of age. Affected infants can be recognized at birth: the head is foreshortened and the eyes slant upwards, with prominent epicanthic folds; the nose is flattened, the lips are parted and the tongue protrudes. There may be abnormal palmar creases, clinodactyly and spreading of the first and second toes. The babies are unusually floppy (hypotonic) and skeletal development is delayed. Children are short and, because of their characteristic facial appearance, they tend to resemble each other. They show varying degrees of mental retardation. Joint laxity may lead to sprains or subluxation (e.g. of the patella).

Adults have a significant incidence of atlanto-axial instability, though fortunately this seldom causes neurological complications. Associated anomalies, particularly cardiac defects, are common, and there is diminished resistance to infection. Life expectancy is about 35 years.

There is no specific treatment but surgery can offer considerable cosmetic improvement, and attentive care will allow many of these individuals to pursue a pleasant and productive life. Atlanto-axial fusion is occasionally needed for patients with neurological symptoms.

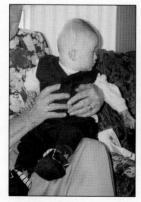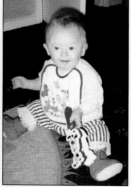

8.29 Down's syndrome Head shape and facial features in an eleven-month old child with Down's syndrome.

TURNER'S SYNDROME

Congenital female hypogonadism is a rare abnormality caused by a defect in one of the X chromosomes. Those affected are phenotypically female, with a normal vagina and uterus, but the ovaries are markedly hypoplastic or absent. Patients are short, with webbing of the neck, barrel chest and increased carrying angle of the elbows. Cardiovascular and renal abnormalities are common. They have primary amenorrhoea, and hypogonadism leads to early-onset osteoporosis. Treatment consists of oestrogen replacement from puberty onwards.

KLINEFELTER'S SYNDROME

Klinefelter's syndrome, a form of male hypogonadism, occurs in about 1 per 1000 males. Those affected have more than one X chromosome (as well as the usual Y chromosome). They are recognizably male, but they have eunuchoid proportions, with gynaecomastia and underdeveloped testicles. The condition should be borne in mind as a cause of osteoporosis in men. Treatment with androgens may improve bone mass.

LOCALIZED MALFORMATIONS

Localized congenital malformations of the vertebrae or limbs are common. The majority cause no disability and may be discovered incidentally during investigation of some other disorder. Some have a genetic background and similar malformations are seen in association with generalized skeletal dysplasia. Most are sporadic and probably non-genetic – i.e. caused by injury to the developing embryo, especially during the first 3 months of pregnancy. In some cases there is a known teratogenic agent; for example, maternal infection or drug administration. Usually, however, the exact cause is unknown.

VERTEBRAL ANOMALIES

These are of three main kinds: (1) agenesis, with total absence of vertebrae; (2) dysgenesis, with hemivertebrae, or with vertebrae fused together (sometimes called errors of segmentation); and (3) dysraphism, with deficiencies of the neural arch. These are considered in the sections on spinal deformity and spina bifida.

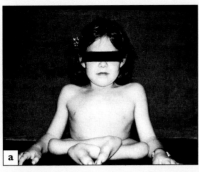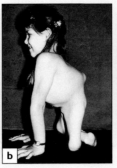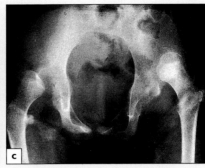

8.30 Sacral agenesis This girl shows (**a**) the characteristic sitting posture and (**b**) the spinal hump. (**c**) The sacrum is absent and the hips are dislocated.

Corresponding sacral anomalies are also encountered and associated visceral anomalies (lower intestinal and urogenital defects) are common in sacral dysgenesis and dysraphism.

KLIPPEL–FEIL SYNDROME (CONGENITAL SHORT NECK)

In this segmentation defect there is fusion of two or more cervical vertebrae. The patient has an unusually short neck, and neck movements are restricted or absent. Prominence of the trapezius muscles gives the appearance of webbing at the base of the neck. The posterior hairline is much lower than normal. Associated anomalies are common and include hemivertebrae, posterior arch defects, cervical meningomyelocele, thoracic defects, scapular elevation and visceral abnormalities.

X-rays may show fusion of the lower cervical vertebrae and various combinations of the associated disorders, together with scoliosis or kyphosis.

Treatment is usually not necessary, but scoliosis may require correction and fusion; occasionally, operative relief is needed for threatened cord compression.

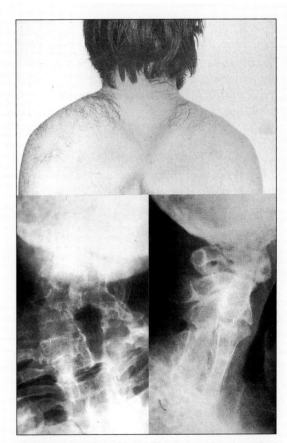

8.31 Klippel–Feil syndrome The short neck and vertebral anomalies in a typical patient.

ELEVATION OF THE SCAPULA (UNDESCENDED SCAPULA; SPRENGEL'S DEFORMITY)

Mild degrees of congenital elevation of the scapula are common. In the full-blown Sprengel deformity the child has obvious asymmetry of the shoulders, with elevation and underdevelopment of the affected side. The scapula is abnormally small and too high. Sometimes the clavicle is affected as well. Shoulder movements may be restricted and on abduction or elevation the scapula moves very little or not at all. Occasionally both sides are involved.

Sprengel's deformity may be associated with other defects of the cervical spine, and high thoracic kyphosis or scoliosis is quite common.

This condition, which usually occurs sporadically, represents a failure of scapular descent from the cervical spine. The high scapula may still be attached to the spine by a tough fibrous band or a cartilaginous bar (the omovertebral bar). Associated vertebral or rib anomalies are quite common.

Treatment is required only if shoulder movements are severely limited or if the deformity is particularly unsightly. Operation is best performed before the age of 6 years. The vertebroscapular muscles are released from the spine, the supraspinous part of the scapula is excised together with the omovertebral bar and the scapula is repositioned by tightening the lower muscles. Great care is needed as there is a risk of injury to the accessory nerve or the brachial plexus.

THORACOSPINAL ANOMALIES

Segmentation defects in the thoracic region usually involve the ribs as well; for example, hemivertebrae may be associated with fusion of adjacent ribs or other types of dysplasia. Some of these disorders are of autosomal dominant inheritance. Clinically, patients present in childhood with scoliosis or kyphoscoliosis, sometimes leading to paraplegia. X-rays may show various combinations of thoracic vertebral fusion or dysgenesis and rib anomalies, together with scoliosis and marked distortion of the thorax. Operative treatment may be needed for threatened cord compression.

LIMB ANOMALIES

Localized malformations of the limbs include extra bones, absent bones, hypoplastic bones and fusions. Complete absence of a limb is called *amelia*, almost complete absence (a mere stub remaining) *phocomelia* and partial absence *ectromelia*; defects may be transverse or axial. In the hands and feet brachydactyly, syndactyly, polydactyly and symphalangism are among the many possibilities.

The embryonal limb buds appear at about the 26th day of gestation; by the 30th day the upper limb has started differentiating into its three segments (upper arm, forearm and hand) and in the lower limb the same process occurs shortly afterwards. By the end of the 6th week the embryo has acquired a recognizable human form. The upper limb is fully formed by 12 weeks and the lower limb by 14 weeks. During this period the muscles and nerves also develop and by the 20th week joint movement is possible.

Most of the malformations involving limb reductions are due to embryonal insults between the 4th and 6th weeks of gestation. Some are genetically determined and these usually have an autosomal dominant pattern of inheritance.

Classification

Various classifications of limb deficiencies have been proposed; none is completely satisfactory. Some veer towards the purely descriptive; others go into almost obsessive detail based on topographical and morphological features. Their usefulness lies in the elaboration of an agreed terminology which will aid communication and permit sensible auditing of the results of various forms of treatment.

Some of the important disorders are referred to below and further details appear in the section on Regional Orthopaedics.

Clinical features

RADIAL DEFICIENCY

Absence or hypoplasia of the radius may occur alone or in association with visceral anomalies or (more rarely) certain blood dyscrasias. Sometimes the thumb is missing too, and the elbow is often abnormal. In about half the cases the condition is bilateral.

The forearm is short and bowed; the hand is underdeveloped and markedly deviated towards the radial side (radial club hand). In some cases the thumb is absent.

The clinical deformity may look bizarre but children often acquire excellent function. If this seems unlikely, operative reconstruction may be advisable (see page 317).

ULNAR DEFICIENCY

Hypoplasia of the distal end of the ulna is usually seen as part of a generalized dysplasia, but occasionally it occurs alone. The radius is bowed (as if growth is tethered on the ulnar side) and the radial head may dislocate; the wrist is deviated medially. Only if function is severely disturbed should wrist stabilization be advised.

Congenital absence of the ulna is extremely rare. The forearm deformity is not as marked as in radial deficiency but overall function is severely restricted. Operative reconstruction may provide some improvement.

TRANSVERSE DEFICIENCY OF THE ARM

Transverse deficiency of the distal part of the arm will leave a simple stump below a normal elbow. This can be managed by fitting a prosthesis with a mechanical facility for grasp.

FEMORAL DEFICIENCY (CONGENITAL SHORT FEMUR)

In its most benign form, femoral dysplasia consists merely of *shortening of the bone with a normal hip and knee*. This can be dealt with by limb lengthening procedures or, if shortening is very marked, by adding a distal orthosis.

Dysplasia of the distal third – sometimes with synostosis of the knee – is uncommon. Since the hip permits normal weightbearing, this condition also can be managed by limb lengthening operations.

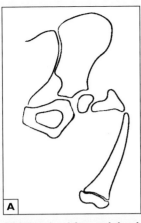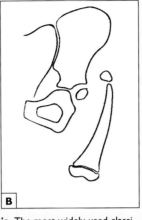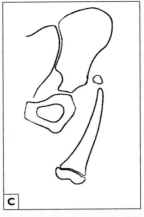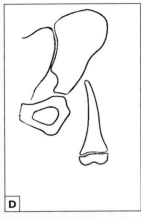

8.32 Proximal femoral dysplasia The most widely used classification of proximal femoral focal deficiency is that of Aitken. *Type A:* the child is born with a 'gap' between the proximal part of the femur and the diaphysis but this usually ossifies by the end of growth. *Type B:* the femoral head is present (though hypoplastic) but there is a 'gap' which fails to ossify. *Type C:* the femoral head and neck are absent and the acetabulum is under-developed. *Type D:* the acetabulum and proximal femur are absent. Congenital coxa vara is not included in this classification although it may also be a variant of the same disorder (see page 420).

In most cases it is the proximal third which is under-developed or absent. This results in a two-fold problem: shortening of the limb and defective weightbearing at the hip.

Various grades of proximal femoral dysplasia are encountered. There may be *coxa vara* with moderate shortening of the shaft; this can be dealt with by corrective osteotomy and limb lengthening (see page 421). Severe degrees of coxa vara, sometimes associated with pseudarthrosis of the neck, may result in marked shortening of the femur. In the worst cases most of the femoral shaft is missing, the knee is situated at thigh level and the foot hangs where the knee is normally expected to be. If the deformity is bilateral and symmetrical, walking is possible and some individuals acquire remarkable agility; however, they may still seek treatment to overcome the severe cosmetic problem. Unilateral deformities are not only unsightly but also very disabling. Effective limb lengthening is out of the question; and fitting a prosthesis to a short limb with flexion deformities of the 'hip' and knee and a foot jutting forwards where the knee-hinge of the prosthesis will lie is a daunting prospect. In the past there was some enthusiasm for the Van Nes operation: fusion of the knee and 180° rotational osteotomy of the leg bones to get the foot facing back-to-front and the ankle substituting for the knee, followed by fitting an 'above-knee' prosthesis. However, the trick is easier, and looks better, in drawings than in real life and the procedure is seldom done nowadays. One alternative is to fuse the knee in a functional position, amputate the foot and fit a suitable prosthesis. The earlier this is done the better.

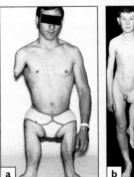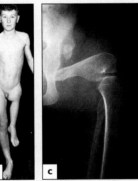

8.33 Proximal femoral dysplasia (a) This man was born with transverse deficiency of the right arm and bilateral proximal femoral focal deficiency. Though unhappy with his appearance, because the lower limb defects were symmetrical he was able to get about remarkably well. **(b)** By contrast, this young man with a similar but unilateral dysplasia, was severely disabled. **(c)** X-ray showing the proximal femoral deficiency.

TIBIAL DEFICIENCY

Congenital absence of the tibia is extremely rare; when it does occur it is usually associated with other anomalies of the limbs. The ankle is non-existent and the foot is in varus. It is quite possible to construct a functioning one-bone leg by transposing the fibula and fusing it to the centre of the femoral articular surface; once fusion is achieved, a Syme's amputation can be performed. This should be done as soon as the fibula has developed sufficiently to permit fusion at the knee. If the procedure fails, or if the associated abnormalities turn out to be more severe than expected, proximal amputation can be undertaken at a later stage.

FIBULAR DEFICIENCY

Mild fibular dysplasia causes little shortening or deformity. However, complete absence of the fibula leads to considerable shortening of the leg, bowing of the tibia and valgus deformity of the unsupported ankle. There may also be absence of the fourth and fifth rays of the foot and underdevelopment of the entire limb. Sometimes, if only the distal fibula is absent, there is a fibrous band in its place. Excision of this remnant may permit correction of the valgus deformity. If overall limb length is markedly affected and the foot deformity intractable, distal amputation of the leg may be needed.

CONGENITAL PSEUDARTHROSIS OF THE TIBIA

This rare condition is usually diagnosed in early infancy. The child may be born with a fractured tibia, or the bone may be attenuated and then fracture some months later. In either case, the fracture fails to unite, or heals very poorly only to fracture again shortly afterwards. By the age of 2 years the leg is noticeably short and bowed anteriorly. By then it has become obvious that this is an intractable condition which will not yield to ordinary forms of fracture treatment. *X-ray* shows a gap, or marked thinning of the tibial shaft. Sometimes the fibula also is affected.

Biopsy of the abnormal segment may show histological features of neurofibromatosis, and other stigmata of this condition are present in about half of those affected.

Treatment is likely to be prolonged and fraught with difficulty. Simple immobilization will certainly fail, and internal fixation with bone grafting succeeds only very occasionally. Better results have been achieved by correcting the deformity, bone grafting the fracture and immobilizing the tibial fragments in a circular external fixator (the Ilizarov technique). Success has also been claimed for excision of the abnormal segment and replacement by a vascularized fibular graft (Weiland *et al*, 1990).

CONGENITAL TIBIAL BOWING

Congenital tibial bowing comprises a spectrum of disorders with significant differences in both etiology and prognosis for the different types (Crawford and Schorry, 1999).

Posteromedial tibial bowing is a relatively benign condition which usually resolves spontaneously as the child grows. However, the leg may end up shorter than normal, requiring epiphysiodesis on the opposite side to counteract the limb length inequality.

Anteromedial bowing is almost always associated with fibular deficiency and congenital defects of the foot, or some type of femoral dysplasia. Treatment depends on the presence or absence (and severity) of the associated disorders and varies from reconstructive procedures of the ankle to – in the very worst cases – amputation.

Anterolateral tibial bowing with failure of normal tubularization may be the forerunner of localized osteolysis and eventual fracture with persistent non-union and pseudarthrosis of the tibia. Corrective osteotomy should be avoided because of the high risk of non-union. While the bone is intact, treatment consists of bracing until the bone matures. If a fracture occurs, treatment is the same as for congenital pseudarthrosis.

PSEUDARTHROSIS OF THE CLAVICLE

A child sometimes presents with a painless lump over the clavicle and x-rays confirm the presence of an ununited fracture, or pseudarthrosis. The condition is not really comparable to pseudarthrosis of the tibia and is thought to be due to pressure by the subclavian artery on the developing bone. In every reported unilateral case the right side has been affected – except in the presence of dextrocardia.

Treatment, if required, is by excision and grafting.

SYNOSTOSIS

The various types of interosseous fusion (radioulnar, tibiofibular, carpal or tarsal) are discussed in the relevant chapters. They rarely cause significant disability, excepting tarsal synostosis (which may be associated with spastic flat foot) or radioulnar fusion which limits forearm supination (a considerable disability if both forearms are affected). In spastic flat foot, division or removal of the bony bridge may improve symptoms. Radioulnar fusion resists any form of operative mobilization, because of

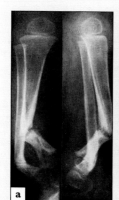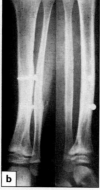

8.34 Congenital pseudoarthrosis of the tibia (**a**) The tibia may at first be bowed or thinned; it usually fractures before the age of 3 years and then fails to unite. (**b**) Treatment is always difficult; happily in this case bone grafting was successful.

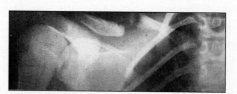

8.35 Pseudoarthrosis of the clavicle It is always the right side which is affected.

the associated soft-tissue involvement. However, the bones can be osteotomized and rotated to leave the hand in a more functional position.

DIGITAL ANOMALIES

There are numerous digital anomalies – missing digits, extra digits, fused digits, short digits or split deformities of the hand or foot – which may occur in isolation, in combination with each other or as part of a generalized dysplasia. Short digits seldom require any form of treatment. Extra digits, if simply hanging by a neck of skin, can be amputated at any time. The more complex anomalies, which involve not only bone but also the associated muscle and neurovascular structures, may be treated by operative reconstruction when the child is 3–4 years old – but only after painstaking assessment and by someone experienced in this branch of surgery.

REFERENCES AND FURTHER READING

Ainsworth SR, Aulicino PL (1993) A survey of patients with Ehlers–Danlos syndrome. *Clinical Orthopaedics* **286**, 250-256

Crawford AH, Schorry EK (1999) Neurofibromatosis in children: the role of the orthopaedist. *Journal of the American Academy of Orthopaedic Surgeons* **7**, 217-230

Evans CH, Robbins PD (1995) Possible orthopaedic applications of gene therapy. *Journal of Bone and Joint Surgery* **77**A, 1103-1114

Jaffurs D, Evans CH (1998) The human genome project: Implications for the treatment of musculoskeletal disease. *Journal of the American Academy of Orthopaedic Surgeons* **6**, 1-14

Katz K, Horev G, Grunebaum M *et al.* (1996) The natural history of osteonecrosis of the femoral head in children and adolescents who have Gaucher's disease. *Journal of Bone and Joint Surgery* **78**A, 14-19

Kocher MS, Shapiro F (1998) Osteogenesis imperfecta. *Journal of the American Academy of Orhopaedic Surgeons* **6**, 225-236

Maroteaux P, Lamy M (1965) The malady of Toulouse–Lautrec. *Journal of the American Medical Association* **191**, 715-717

Pastores GM, Sibille AR, Grabowski GA (1993) Enzyme therapy in Gaucher's disease type 1: dosage efficacy and adverse effect in 33 patients treated for 6 to 24 months. *Blood* **82**, 408-416

Pastores GM, Hermann G, Norton KI *et al.* (1996) Regression of skeletal changes in Type I Gaucher disease with enzyme replacement therapy. *Skeletal Radiology* **25**, 485-488

Shiang R, Thompson LM, Zhu Y-Z *et al.* (1994) Mutations in the transmembrane domain of FGFR3 cause the most common genetic form of dwarfism, achondroplasia. *Cell* **78**, 335-342

Sillence D (1981) Osteogenesis imperfecta: an expanding panorama of variants. *Clinical Orthopaedics and Related Research* **159**, 11-25

Solomon L (1963) Hereditary multiple exostosis. *Journal of Bone and Joint Surgery* **45**B, 292-304

Weiland AJ, Weiss APC, Moore JR, Tolo VT (1990) Vascularized fibular grafts in the treatment of congenital pseudarthrosis of the tibia. *Journal of Bone and Joint Surgery* **72**A, 654-662

9 Tumours

Tumours, tumour-like lesions and cysts are considered together, partly because their clinical presentation and management are similar and partly because the definitive classification of bone tumours is still evolving and some disorders may yet move from one category to another. Benign lesions are quite common, primary malignant ones rare; yet so often do they mimic each other, and so critical are the decisions on treatment, that a working knowledge of all the important conditions is necessary.

Table 9.1 A classification of the less rare primary bone tumours

Cell type	Benign	Malignant
Bone	Osteoid osteoma	Osteosarcoma
Cartilage	Chondroma	Chondrosarcoma
	Osteochondroma	
Fibrous tissue	Fibroma	Fibrosarcoma
Marrow	Haemangioma	Angiosarcoma
Uncertain	Giant cell tumour	Malignant giant cell tumour

CLASSIFICATION

Most classifications of bone tumours are based on the recognition of the dominant tissue in the various lesions (Table 9.1). This is helpful in assembling and comparing data, but there are some drawbacks: (1) the most pervasive tissue is not necessarily the tissue of origin; (2) there is no pathological or clinical connection between the conditions in any particular category; (3) there is often no relationship between benign and malignant lesions with similar tissue elements (e.g. osteoma and osteosarcoma); and (4) some tumours named as single entities (e.g. osteosarcoma) comprise several lesions with different behaviour patterns. Furthermore, the commonest malignant tumours in bone are not, strictly speaking, 'bone' tumours – i.e. not of mesenchymal origen (e.g. metastatic tumours and myeloma).

CLINICAL PRESENTATION

History

The history is often prolonged, and this unfortunately results in a delay in obtaining treatment.

Age may be a useful clue. Many benign lesions present during childhood and adolescence – but so do some primary malignant tumours, notably Ewing's tumour and osteosarcoma. Chondrosarcoma and fibrosarcoma typically occur in older people (4th to 6th decades); and myeloma, the commonest of all primary malignant bone tumours, is seldom seen before the 6th decade. *In patients over 70 years of age, metastasis is more common than all primary tumours together.*

Patients may be completely *asymptomatic* until the abnormality is discovered on x-ray. This is more likely with benign lesions; and, since some of these (e.g. non-ossifying fibroma) are common in children but rare after the age of 30 years, they must be capable of spontaneous resolution. Malignant tumours, too, may remain silent if they are slow-growing and situated where there is room for inconspicuous expansion (e.g. the cavity of the pelvis).

Pain is a common complaint and gives little indication of the nature of the lesion; however, progressive and unremitting pain is a sinister symptom. It may be caused by rapid expansion with stretching of surrounding tissues, central haemorrhage or degeneration in the tumour, or an incipient pathological fracture. However, even a tiny lesion may be very painful if it is encapsulated in dense bone (e.g. an osteoid osteoma).

Swelling, or the appearance of a *lump,* may be alarming. Often, though, patients seek advice only when a mass becomes painful or continues to grow.

A *history of trauma* is offered so frequently that it cannot be dismissed as having no significance. Yet, whether the injury initiates a pathological change or merely draws attention to what is already there remains unanswered.

Neurological symptoms (paraesthesiae or numbness) may be caused by pressure upon or stretching of a peripheral nerve. Progressive dysfunction is more ominous and suggests invasion by an aggressive tumour.

Pathological fracture may be the first (and only) clinical signal. Suspicion is aroused if the injury was slight; in elderly people, whose bones usually fracture at the corticocancellous junctions, any break in the mid-shaft should be regarded as pathological until proved otherwise.

Examination

If there is a *lump*, where does it arise? Is it discrete or ill-defined? Is it soft or hard, or pulsatile? And is it tender? *Swelling* is sometimes diffuse, and the overlying skin warm and inflamed; it can be difficult to distinguish a tumour from infection or a haematoma.

If the tumour is near a joint there may be an *effusion* and/or *limitation of movement*. Spinal lesions, whether benign or malignant, often cause *muscle spasm* and *back stiffness*, or a *painful scoliosis*.

The examination will focus on the symptomatic part, but it should include also the area of lymphatic drainage and, often, the pelvis, abdomen, chest and spine.

IMAGING

X-rays

Plain x-rays are still the most useful of all imaging techniques. There may be an obvious abnormality in the bone – cortical thickening, a discrete lump, a 'cyst' or ill-defined destruction. Where is the lesion: in the bone end, the metaphysis or the diaphysis? Is it solitary or are there multiple lesions? Are the margins well-defined or ill-defined? Are there signs of cortical destruction?

Remember that 'cystic' lesions are not necessarily hollow cavities: any radiolucent material (e.g. a fibroma or a chondroma) may look like a cyst. If the boundary of the 'cyst' is sharply defined it is probably benign; if it is hazy and diffuse it suggests an invasive tumour. Stippled calcification inside a cystic area is characteristic of cartilage tumours.

Questions to ask when looking at an x-ray (Watt, 1985)
Is the lesion solitary or multiple?
What type of bone is involved?
Where is the lesion in the bone?
Are the margins of the lesion well- or ill-defined?
Is there cortical destruction?
Is there a bony reaction?
Is the centre calcified?

Look carefully at the bone surfaces: periosteal new-bone formation and extension of the tumour into the soft tissues are suggestive of malignant change.

Look also at the soft tissues: are the muscle planes distorted by swelling? Is there calcification?

For all its informative detail, the x-ray alone can seldom be relied on for a definitive diagnosis. With some notable exceptions, in which the appearances are pathognomonic (e.g osteochondroma, non-ossifying fibroma, osteoid osteoma), further investigations will be

needed. *If other forms of imaging are planned [bone scans, computed tomography (CT) or magnetic resonance imaging (MRI)], they should be done before undertaking a biopsy* which itself may distort the appearances.

Other imaging

Radionuclide scanning with ^{99m}Tc-HDP shows non-specific reactive changes in bone; this can be helpful in revealing the site of a small tumour (e.g. an osteoid osteoma) that does not show up clearly on x-ray. Skeletal scintigraphy is also useful for detecting skip lesions or 'silent' secondary deposits.

CT extends the range of x-ray diagnosis; it is an excellent method for showing cortical erosion or fracture; it shows more accurately both intra-osseous and extra-osseous extension of the tumour and the relationship to surrounding structures. It may also reveal suspected lesions in inaccessible sites, like the spine or pelvis; and it is a reliable method of detecting pulmonary metastases.

MRI provides further information. Its greatest value is in the assessment of tumour spread – (a) within the bone, (b) into a nearby joint and (c) into the soft tissues (Pettersson *et al.*, 1987). Blood vessels and the relationship of the tumour to the perivascular space are well defined. MRI is far and away the best method for evaluating soft-tissue tumours.

LABORATORY INVESTIGATIONS

Blood tests are often necessary to exclude other conditions, e.g infection or metabolic bone disorders, or a 'brown tumour' in hyperparathyroidism. *Anaemia*, increased *erythrocyte sedimentation rate (ESR)* and elevated *serum alkaline phosphatase* levels are non-specific findings, but if other causes are excluded they may help in differentiating between benign and malignant bone lesions. *Serum protein electrophoresis* may reveal an abnormal globulin fraction and the urine may contain *Bence-Jones protein* in patients with myeloma. A raised *serum acid phosphatase* suggests prostatic carcinoma.

BIOPSY

With few exceptions, biopsy is essential for the accurate diagnosis and planning of treatment. If sufficient expertise is available, the biopsy can be done with a *large-bore needle*. However, this does not always yield sufficient material, and when it does the tissue may not be representative or suitable for accurate diagnosis; its greatest value is in sampling inaccessible tumours or tumours in a site where open biopsy might jeopardize subsequent limited surgery.

Open biopsy is more reliable. The site is selected so that it can be included in any subsequent ablative operation. As little as possible of the tumour is exposed and a block of tissue is removed – ideally in the boundary zone, so as to include normal tissue, pseudocapsule and abnormal tissue. A *frozen section* should be examined – not so much to make a definitive diagnosis but to ensure that representative tissue has been obtained. If necessary, several samples can be taken. If bone is removed the raw area is covered with bone wax or methylmethacrylate cement. If a tourniquet is used, it should be released and full haemostasis achieved before closing the wound. Drains should be avoided, so as to minimize the risk of tumour contamination.

Tumour biopsy should never be regarded as a 'minor' procedure. Complications include haemorrhage, wound breakdown, infection and pathological fracture. The person doing the biopsy should have a clear idea of what may be done next and where operative incisions or skin flaps will be placed. Errors and complications are far less likely if the biopsy is performed in a specializing centre (Mankin *et al.*, 1982).

For tumours that are almost certainly benign, an *excisional biopsy* is permissible (the entire lesion is removed); with cysts that need operations, representative tissue can be obtained by careful curettage. In either case, histological confirmation of the diagnosis is essential.

When dealing with tumours that could be malignant, there is a strong temptation to perform the biopsy as soon as possible; as this may alter the CT and MRI appearances, it is important to delay the biopsy until all the imaging studies have been completed.

DIFFERENTIAL DIAGNOSIS

A number of conditions may mimic a tumour, either clinically or radiologically, and the histopathology may be difficult to interpret. It is important not to be misled by the common dissemblers.

Soft-tissue haematoma A large, clotted subperiosteal or soft-tissue haematoma may present as a painful lump in the arm or lower limb. Sometimes the x-ray shows an irregular surface on the underlying bone. Important clues are the history and the rapid onset of symptoms.

Myositis ossificans Though rare, this may be a source of confusion. Following an injury the patient develops a tender swelling in the vicinity of a joint; the x-ray shows fluffy density in the soft tissue adjacent to bone. Unlike a malignant tumour, however, the condition soon becomes less painful and the new bone better defined and well demarcated.

Stress fracture Some of the worst mistakes have been made in misdiagnosing a stress fracture. The patient is often a young adult with localized pain near a large joint; x-rays show a dubious area of cortical 'destruction' and overlying periosteal new bone; if a biopsy is performed the healing callus may show histological features resembling those of osteosarcoma. If the pitfall is recognized, and there is adequate consultation between surgeon, radiologist and pathologist, a serious error can be prevented.

Tendon avulsion injuries Children and adolescents – especially those engaged in vigorous sports – are prone to avulsion injuries at sites of tendon insertion, particularly around the hip and knee (Donnelly *et al.*, 1999). The best known example is the tibial apophyseal stress

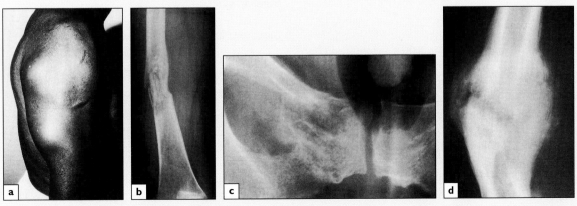

9.1 Tumours – differential diagnosis (1) (**a**) This huge swelling was simply a clotted haematoma. (**b**) Fracture through an area of osteomyelitis. (**c**) Stress fracture in an old woman. (**d**) Florid callus.

lesion of Osgood–Schlatter's disease (see page 478), but lesions at less familiar sites (the iliac crest, the ischial tuberosity, the lesser trochanter of the femur, the hamstring insertions, the attachments of adductor magnus and longus and the distal humeral apophyses) may escape immediate recognition.

Bone infection Osteomyelitis typically causes pain and swelling near one of the larger joints; as with primary bone tumours, the patients are usually children or young adults. X-rays may show an area of destruction in the metaphysis, with periosteal new bone. Systemic features, especially if the patient has been treated with antibiotics, may be mild. If the area is explored, tissue should be submitted for both bacteriological and histological examination.

Gout Occasionally a large gouty tophus causes a painful swelling at one of the bone ends, and x-ray shows a large, poorly defined excavation. If this is kept in mind the diagnosis will be easily confirmed – if necessary by obtaining a biopsy from the lump.

Other bone lesions Non-neoplastic bone lesions such as fibrous cortical defects, medullary infarcts and 'bone islands' are occasionally mistaken for tumours.

STAGING THE LESION

In treating tumours we strive to reconcile two conflicting principles: the lesion must be removed as widely as is necessary; but damage must be kept to a minimum. Choosing the boundary between these objectives depends on knowing (a) how the tumour usually behaves (i.e. how aggressive it is) and (b) how far it has spread. The answers to these two questions are embodied in the staging system developed by Enneking (1986) and subsequently adapted by the American Joint Committee on Cancer (1997).

Aggressiveness

Tumours are graded not only on their cytological characteristics but also on their clinical behaviour; i.e. the likelihood of recurrence and spread after surgical removal. *Benign lesions*, by definition, occupy the lowest grade: the meekest of them either remain quiescent or disappear spontaneously (e.g. non-osteogenic fibroma); the worst of them are difficult to distinguish from a low-grade sarcoma and sometimes undergo malignant change (e.g. aggressive osteoblastoma). They are usually amenable to local (marginal) excision with little risk of recurrence.

Sarcomas are divided into 'low-grade' and 'high-grade'; the former are only moderately aggressive (the estimated risk of metastasis is less than 25%) and take

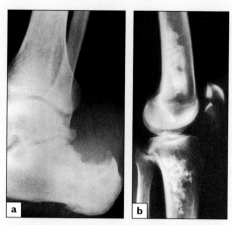

9.2 Tumours – differential diagnosis (2)
(**a**) Tophaceous gout. (**b**) Bone infarcts.

a long time to metastasize (e.g. secondary chondrosarcoma or parosteal osteosarcoma), while the latter are usually very aggressive and metastasize early (e.g. osteosarcoma or fibrosarcoma).

Spread

Assuming that there are no metastases, the local extent of the tumour is the most important factor in deciding how much tissue has to be removed. Lesions that are confined to an enclosed tissue space (e.g. a bone, a joint cavity or a muscle group within its fascial envelope) are called '*intracompartmental*'. Those that extend into interfascial or extrafascial planes with no natural barrier to proximal or distal spread (e.g. perivascular sheaths, pelvis, axilla) are designated '*extracompartmental*'. The extents of the tumour and adjacent 'contaminated' tissue are best shown by CT and MRI; skip lesions can be detected by scintigraphy.

Surgical stage

Sarcomas are broadly divided as follows:

- *Stage I* – all low-grade sarcomas
- *Stage II* – histologically high-grade lesions
- *Stage III* – sarcomas which have metastasized

Following Enneking's original classiffication, each category can be further subdivided into *Type A* (intracompartmental) and *Type B* (extracompartmental). Thus, a localized chondrosarcoma arising in a cartilage-capped exostosis would be designated IA, suitable for wide excision without exposing the tumour. An osteosarcoma confined to bone would be IIA – operable by wide excision or amputation with a low risk of local recurrence;

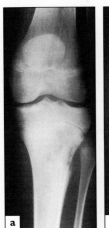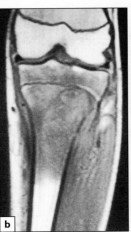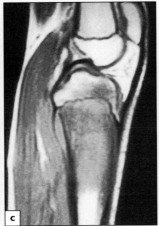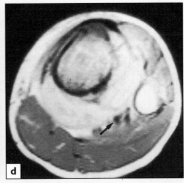

9.3 Staging (**a**) Plain x-ray shows a destructive lesion of the proximal tibia, almost certainly an osteosarcoma; but is it locally resectable? (**b, c**) Coronal and sagittal MR images show the tumour extending medially and laterally, and posteriorly into the soft tissue.

(**d**) Transectional MRI shows that the abnormal tissue extends posteriorly right up to the vascular compartment (arrow). This tumour would be assessed as Stage IIB.

if it has spread into the soft tissues it would be IIB – less suitable for wide excision and preferably treated by radical resection or disarticulation through the proximal joint. If there are pulmonary metastases it would be classified as stage III.

The point of the staging exercise was to select the operation best suited to that particular patient, and carrying a low risk of recurrence. Locally recurrent sarcomas tend to be more aggressive, more often extracompartmental and more likely to metastasize than the original tumour. With the advent of markedly improved imaging and chemotherapy, the above guidelines have been relaxed somewhat and the margins can be placed much closer without significantly increasing the risk of recurrence (Peabody *et al.*, 1998).

PRINCIPLES OF MANAGEMENT

For all but the simplest and most obvious of benign tumours, management calls for consultation and co-operation between the orthopaedic surgeon, radiologist, pathologist and (certainly in the case of malignant tumours) the oncologist, prosthetic designer and rehabilitation therapist as well. Clinical and x-ray examination having suggested the most likely diagnosis, and further management proceeds as follows.

BENIGN, ASYMPTOMATIC LESIONS If the diagnois is beyond doubt (e.g a non-ossifying fibroma or a small osteochondroma) one can afford to temporize; treatment may never be needed. However, if the appearances are not pathognomonic, a biopsy is advisable and this may take the form of excision or curettage of the lesion.

BENIGN, SYMPTOMATIC OR ENLARGING TUMOURS Painful lesions, or tumours that continue to enlarge after the end of normal bone growth, require biopsy and confirmation of the diagnosis. Unless they are unusually aggressive, they can generally be removed by local (marginal) excision or (in the case of benign cysts) by curettage.

SUSPECTED MALIGNANT TUMOURS If the lesion is thought to be a primary malignant tumour, the patient is admitted for more detailed examination, blood tests, chest x-ray, further imaging (including pulmonary CT) and biopsy. This should allow a firm diagnosis and staging. The various treatment options can then be discussed with the patient (or the parents, in the case of a young child). There are choices between amputation, limb-sparing operations and different types of adjuvant therapy, and the patient must be fully informed about the pros and cons of each (Mankin and Gebhardt, 1985).

METHODS OF TREATMENT

TUMOUR EXCISION

The more aggressive the lesion the more widely it needs to be excised, in order to ensure that the tumour as well as any dubious marginal tissue is completely removed.

Intracapsular (intralesional) excision and curettage are manifestly incomplete forms of tumour ablation and therefore applicable only to benign lesions with a very low risk of recurrence, or to incurable tumours which need debulking to relieve local symptoms.

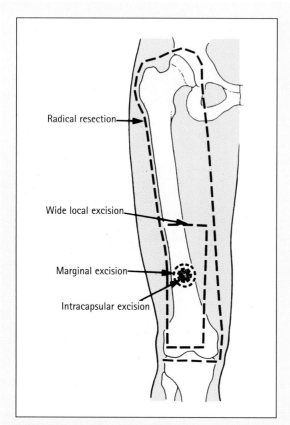

9.4 Tumour excision The more aggressive a tumour is, and the wider it has spread, the more widely it needs to be excised. Local excision is suitable only for low-grade tumours that are confined to a single compartment. Radical resection may be needed for high-grade tumours and this often means amputation at a level above the compartment involved.

Marginal excision goes beyond the tumour, but only just. If the dissection of a malignant lesion is carried through the reactive zone, there is a significant risk of recurrence (up to 50%). For benign lesions, however, this is a suitable method; the resulting cavity can be filled with graft bone.

Wide excision implies that the dissection is carried out well clear of the tumour, through normal tissue. This is appropriate for low-grade intracompartmental lesions (stage IA), with a risk of local recurrence below 10%. However, wide excision is also used *in conjunction with chemotherapy* for stage IIA lesions.

Radical resection means that the entire compartment in which the tumour lies is removed *en bloc* without exposing the lesion. It may be possible to do this while still sparing the limb, but the surrounding muscles will have to be sacrificed; in other cases a true radical resection can be achieved only by amputating at a level above the compartment involved. This method is required for high-grade tumours which have spread beyond the confines of the original compartment (IIB).

Limb-sparing surgery

With more accurate staging procedures and advances in chemotherapy (to control tumour spread), amputation is no longer the automatic choice for stage II sarcomas. The preferred treatment for intracompartmental lesions is now wide excision together with pre- and post-operative chemotherapy.

The resulting defect is dealt with in one of several ways. Short diaphyseal segments can be replaced by *vascularized or non-vascularized bone grafts*. Longer gaps may require *custom-made implants*. Osteo-articular segments can be replaced by large allografts, custom-made prostheses *or allograft–prosthetic composites*. In growing children, *extendible implants* have been used in order to avoid the need for repeated operations; however, they usually need to be replaced at the end of growth. Other procedures, such as *grafting and arthrodesis or distraction osteosynthesis,* are suitable for some situations.

Sarcomas around the hip and shoulder present special problems. Complete excision is difficult and reconstruction involves complex grafting and replacement procedures.

Whatever the method employed, two conditions need to be fulfilled: there must be no skip lesions and the limb must be viable and functional. It goes without saying, also, that expert facilities for prosthetic and graft replacement must be available.

OUTCOME Tumour replacement by massive prosthesis carries a high risk of complications such as wound breakdown and infection. However, in most cases the prostheses function well and the incidence of local recurrence of the tumour is similar to that following amputation (Roberts *et al.*, 1991; Horowitz *et al.*, 1993).

Amputation

Considering the difficulties of limb-sparing surgery – particularly for high-grade tumours or if there is doubt about whether the lesion is intracompartmental – amputation and early rehabilitation may be preferred. However, nowadays this approach is uncommon in specialized units.

MULTI-AGENT CHEMOTHERAPY

This is now the preferred neoadjuvant and adjuvant treatment for malignant bone and soft-tissue tumours. For some years following its introduction in the 1970s there was doubt as to whether it really improved the chances of long-term survival. Evidence is now available to show that, for sensitive tumours, modern chemotherapy regimes effectively reduce the size of the primary lesion, prevent metastatic seeding and improve the chances of survival. Drugs currently in use are methotrexate, doxorubicin (adriamycin), cyclophos-

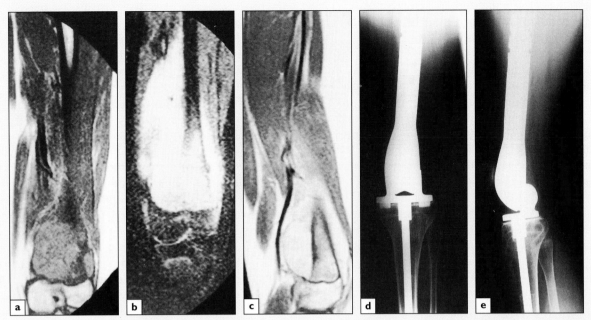

9.5 Staging and treatment (**a**) MRI T$_1$ sequence showing the tumour (an osteosarcoma) in the distal femur but not penetrating the joint. (**b**) STIR sequence (fat suppression) gives a more realistic picture of spread into the soft tissues. (**c**) Proton density sequence showing posterior extension of the tumour up to (but not into) the vascular compartment. (**d, e**) Wide excision and replacement with large 'extending' prosthesis. (Courtesy of Mr John Dixon.)

phamide, vincristine and cisplatin. Treatment is started 8-12 weeks preoperatively and the effect is assessed by examining the resected tumour. If there is little or no necrosis, a different drug is selected for postoperative treatment; otherwise maintenance chemotherapy is continued for another 6–12 months.

RADIOTHERAPY

High-energy irradiation has long been used to destroy radiosensitive tumours or as adjuvant therapy before operation. Nowadays the indications are more restricted.

For highly sensitive tumours (such as Ewing's sarcoma) it offers an alternative to amputation; it is then combined with adjuvant chemotherapy. The same combination can be used for tumours in inaccessible sites, lesions that are inoperable because of size or local spread, metastatic deposits and marrow-cell tumours such as myeloma and malignant lymphoma. It is usually given in divided doses over 4 weeks up to a total of 6000cGy.

BENIGN BONE LESIONS

NON-OSSIFYING FIBROMA (FIBROUS CORTICAL DEFECT)

This, the commonest benign lesion of bone, is a developmental defect in which a nest of fibrous tissue appears within the bone and persists for some years before ossifying. It is asymptomatic and is almost always encountered in children as an incidental finding on x-ray. The commonest sites are the metaphyses of long bones; occasionally there are multiple lesions.

The *x-ray* appearance is unmistakable. There is a more or less oval radiolucent area surrounded by a thin margin of dense bone; views in different planes may

9.6 Non-ossifying fibroma (**a**) The x-ray always shows a cortical defect, although in some projection planes this looks deceptively like a medullary lesion (**b**). The bone may fracture through the weakened area (**c**).

show that a lesion that appears to be 'central' is actually adjacent to or within the cortex, hence the alternative name 'fibrous cortical defect'.

PATHOLOGY Although it looks cystic on x-ray, it is a solid lesion consisting of unremarkable fibrous tissue with a few scattered giant cells.

As the bone grows the defect becomes less obvious and it eventually heals spontaneously. However, it sometimes enlarges to several centimetres in diameter and there may be a pathological fracture. There is no risk of malignant change.

TREATMENT Treatment is usually unnecessary. If the defect is very large or has led to repeated fractures, it can be treated by curettage and bone grafting.

FIBROUS DYSPLASIA

Fibrous dysplasia is a developmental disorder in which areas of trabecular bone are replaced by cellular fibrous tissue containing flecks of osteoid and woven bone. It may affect one bone (monostotic), one limb (monomelic) or many bones (polyostotic). If the lesions are large, the bone is considerably weakened and pathological fractures or progressive deformity may occur.

Small, single lesions are asymptomatic. Large, monostotic lesions may cause pain or may be discovered only when the patient develops a pathological fracture. Patients with polyostotic disease present in childhood or adolescence with pain, limp, bony enlargment, deformity or pathological fracture. Untreated, the characteristic deformities persist through adult life.

Occasionally the bone disorder is associated with *cafe-au-lait* patches on the skin and (in girls) precocious sexual development (*Albright's syndrome*).

X-rays show radiolucent 'cystic' areas in the metaphysis or shaft; because they contain fibrous tissue with diffuse spots of immature bone, the lucent patches typically have a slightly hazy or 'ground-glass' appearance. The weight-bearing bones may be bent, and one of the classic features is the 'shepherd's crook' deformity of the proximal femur. *Radioscintigraphy* shows marked activity in the lesion.

PATHOLOGY At operation the lesional tissue has a coarse, gritty feel (due to the specks of immature bone). The histological picture is of loose, cellular fibrous tissue with widespread patches of woven bone and scattered giant cells.

Both clinically and histologically the monostotic condition may resemble either a bone-forming tumour or hyperparathyroidism. However, detailed x-ray and laboratory studies will exclude these disorders.

Malignant transformation to fibrosarcoma occurs in 5–10% of patients with polyostotic lesions, but only rarely in monostotic lesions.

TREATMENT Treatment depends on the extent of the defect and the presence or absence of deformities. Small lesions need no treatment. Those that are large and painful or are threatening to fracture (or have

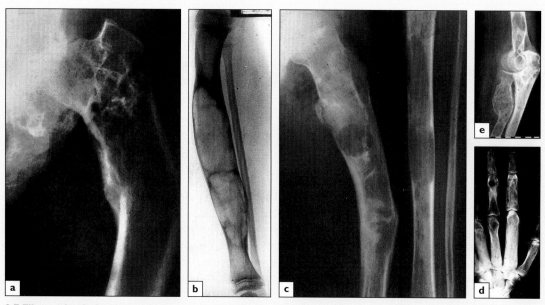

9.7 Fibrous dysplasia Monostotic fibrous dysplasia of (**a**) the upper femur (with the so-called 'shepherd's crook' appearance) and (**b**) of the tibia. (**c, d, e**) From three patients with polyostotic fibrous dysplasia.

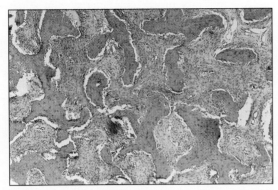

9.8 Fibrous dysplasia – histology Microscopic islands of woven bone lie scattered in a bed of cellular fibrous tissue. Occasional giant cells are seen. (×120)

PATHOLOGY The excised lesion appears as a dark-brown or reddish 'nucleus' surrounded by dense bone; the central area consists of unorganized sheets of osteoid and bone cells.

There is no risk of malignant transformation.

TREATMENT The only effective treatment is complete removal of the nidus. The lesion is carefully localized by x-ray and/or CT and then excised in a small block of bone; the specimen should be x-rayed immediately to confirm that it does contain the little tumour. If the excision is likely to weaken the host bone (especially in the vulnerable medial cortex of the femoral neck), prophylactic internal fixation may be needed.

Less destructive methods, such as laser coagulation or coring out the lesion under CT control, are also being used.

fractured) can be curetted and grafted, but there is a strong tendency for the abnormality to recur. A mixture of cortical and cancellous bone grafts may provide added strength even if the lesion is not eradicated. For very large lesions, the grafts can be supplemented by methylmethacrylate cement. Deformities may need correction by suitably designed osteotomies.

With large cysts, the bone often bleeds profusely at operation: forewarned is forearmed.

OSTEOID OSTEOMA

This tiny bone tumour causes symptoms out of all proportion to its size. Patients are usually under 30 years of age and males predominate. Any bone except the skull may be affected, but over half the cases occur in the femur or tibia. The patient complains of persistent pain, sometimes well localized but sometimes referred over a wide area. Typically the pain is relieved by salicylates. If the diagnosis is delayed, other features appear: a limp or muscle wasting and weakness; spinal lesions may cause intense pain, muscle spasm and scoliosis.

The important *x-ray* feature is a small radiolucent area, the so-called 'nidus'. Lesions in the diaphysis are surrounded by dense sclerosis and cortical thickening; this may be so marked that the nidus can be seen only in tomograms. Lesions in the metaphysis show less cortical thickening. Further away the bone may be osteoporotic. ^{99m}Tc-HDP scintigraphy reveals intense, localized activity.

It is sometimes difficult to distinguish an osteoid osteoma from a small Brodie's abscess without biopsy. Ewing's sarcoma and chronic periostitis must also be excluded.

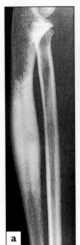

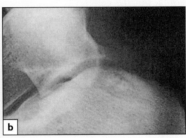

9.9 Osteoid osteoma The x-ray appearance depends on the site of the lesion. **(a)** With cortical tumours there is marked reactive bone thickening leaving a small lucent nidus, which may itself have a central speck of ossification. **(b)** Lesions in cancellous bone produce far less periosteal reaction and are easily mistaken for a Brodie's abscess.

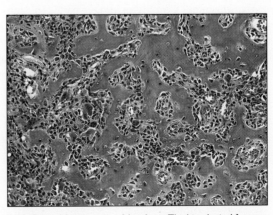

9.10 Osteoid osteoma – histology The histological features are characteristic: the nidus consists of sheets of pink-staining osteoid in a fibrovascular stroma. Giant cells and osteoblasts are prominent. (×300)

OSTEOBLASTOMA (GIANT OSTEOID OSTEOMA)

This tumour is similar to an osteoid osteoma but it is larger, more cellular and sometimes more ominous in appearance. It is usually seen in young adults, more often in men than in women. It tends to occur in the spine and the flat bones; patients present with pain and local muscle spasm.

X-ray shows a well-demarcated osteolytic lesion which may contain small flecks of ossification. There is surrounding sclerosis but this is not always easy to see, especially with lesions in the flat bones or the vertebral pedicle. A *radioisotope scan* will reveal the 'hot' area. Larger lesions may appear cystic, and sometimes a typical aneurysmal bone cyst appears to have arisen in an osteoblastoma.

PATHOLOGY When the tumour is exposed it has a somewhat fleshy appearance. Histologically it resembles an osteoid osteoma, but the cellularity is more striking. Occasionally the picture may suggest a low-grade osteosarcoma.

TREATMENT Treatment consists of excision and bone grafting. With lesions in the vertebral pedicle or the floor of the acetabulum, this is not always easy and removal may be incomplete; local recurrence is common and malignant transformation has been reported (McLeod *et al.*, 1976).

COMPACT OSTEOMA (IVORY EXOSTOSIS)

This rare benign 'tumour' appears as a localized thickening on the outer or inner surface of compact bone. An adolescent or young adult presents with a painless, ivory-hard lump, usually on the outer surface of the skull, occasionally on the subcutaneous surface of the tibia. If it occurs on the inner table of the skull, it may cause focal epilepsy; sometimes it protrudes into the paranasal sinuses. On x-ray a sessile plaque of exceedingly dense bone with a well-circumscribed edge is seen. This might suggest a parosteal osteosarcoma, but the long history, the absence of pain and the smooth outline will dispel this suspicion.

TREATMENT Unless the tumour impinges on important structures, it need not be removed. However, the patient may want to be rid of it; excision is easier if a margin of normal bone is taken with it.

CHONDROMA (ENCHONDROMA)

Islands of cartilage may persist in the metaphyses of bones formed by endochondral ossification; sometimes they grow and take on the characteristics of a benign tumour. Chondromas are usually asymptomatic and are discovered incidentally on x-ray or after a pathological fracture. They are seen at any age (but mostly in young people) and in any bone preformed in cartilage (most commonly the tubular bones of the hands and feet). Lesions may be solitary or multiple and part of a generalized dysplasia (see page 143).

X-ray shows a well-defined, centrally placed radiolucent area at the junction of metaphysis and diaphysis; sometimes the bone is slightly expanded. In mature lesions there are flecks or wisps of calcification within the lucent area; when present, this is a pathognomonic feature.

PATHOLOGY When it is exposed the lesion is seen to consist of pearly-white cartilaginous tissue, often with a central area of degeneration and calcification. Histologically the appearances are those of simple hyaline cartilage.

TREATMENT Treatment is not always necessary, but if the tumour appears to be enlarging, or if it presents as a pathological fracture, it should be removed as thoroughly as possible by curettage; the defect is filled with bone graft. There is a fairly high recurrence rate and the tissue may be seeded in adjacent bone or soft tissues. Chondromas in expendable sites are better removed en bloc.

There is a small but significant risk of *malignant change* (probably less than 2% and hardly ever in a child). Signs of malignant transformation in patients over 30 years are (1) the onset of pain; (2) enlargement of the lesion; and (3) cortical erosion. Unfortunately, biopsy is of little help in this regard as the cartilage

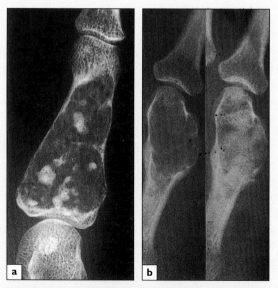

9.11 Chondroma (a) The hand is a common site. **(b)** Another chondroma before and after curettage and bone grafting.

usually looks benign during the early stages of malignant transformation. If the other features are present, and especially in older patients, the lesion should be treated as a stage IA malignancy; the biopsy then serves chiefly to confirm the fact that it is a cartilage tumour.

PERIOSTEAL CHONDROMA

These are rare developmental lesions arising in the deep layer of the periosteum. A cartilaginous lump bulges from the bone into the soft tissues and causes some alarm when it is discovered by the patient.

Since the cartilage remains uncalcified, the lesion itself does not show on x-ray, but the surface of the bone may be irregular or scalloped. MRI may reveal the full extent of the tumour. Histologically the lesion is composed of highly cellular cartilage.

TREATMENT   As it has a propensity to recur, it is best removed by marginal excision (taking a rim of normal bone). Recurrent lesions may look more aggressive but the lesion probably does not undergo malignant change.

CHONDROBLASTOMA

This benign tumour of immature cartilage cells is one of the few lesions to appear primarily in the epiphysis, usually of the proximal humerus, femur or tibia. Patients are affected around the end of the growth period or in early adult life; there is a predilection for males. The presenting symptom is a constant ache in the joint; the tender spot is actually in the adjacent bone.

X-ray shows a rounded, well-demarcated radiolucent area in the epiphysis; this site is so unusual that the diagnosis springs readily to mind. However, sometimes the lesion extends across the physeal line. Occasionally the articular surface is breached. Like

osteoblastoma, the lesion sometimes expands and acquires the features of an aneurysmal bone cyst.

PATHOLOGY   The histological appearances are fairly typical – there are large collections of chondroblasts set off by the surrounding matrix of immature fibrous tissue. Within the stroma are scattered giant cells. In expansile lesions, the edge may resemble that of an aneurysmal bone cyst. These tumours do not undergo malignant change but they may be locally aggressive and extend into the joint.

TREATMENT   In children the risk of damage to the physis makes one hesitate to remove the lesion. After the end of the growth period the lesion can be removed – by marginal excision wherever possible or (less satisfactorily) by curettage – and replaced with autogenous bone grafts. There is a high risk of recurrence after incomplete removal, and if this happens repeatedly there may be serious damage to the nearby joint. Occasionally one is forced to excise the recurrent lesion with an adequate margin of bone and accept the inevitable need for joint reconstruction.

CHONDROMYXOID FIBROMA

Like other benign cartilaginous lesions, this is seen mainly in adolescents and young adults. It may occur in any bone but is more common in those of the lower limb.

Patients seldom complain and the lesion is usually discovered by accident or after a pathological fracture.

X-rays are very characteristic: there is a rounded or ovoid radiolucent area placed eccentrically in the metaphysis; in children it may extend up to or even slightly across the physis. The endosteal margin may be scalloped, but is almost always bounded by a dense zone of reactive bone extending tongue-like towards the diaphysis. The cortex may be asymmetrically expanded. Sometimes there is calcification in the 'vacant' area.

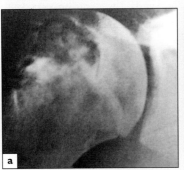

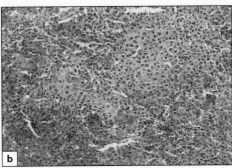

9.12 Chondroblastoma (a) X-ray shows a cyst-like lesion occupying the epiphysis, and sometimes extending across the physis into the adjacent bone. **(b)** The characteristic features in this photomicrograph are the more faintly staining islands of chondroid tissue composed of round cells ('chondroblasts') and scattered multinucleated giant cells. (×300)

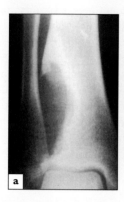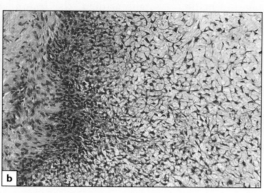

PATHOLOGY Although the lesion looks 'cystic' on x-ray, it contains mucinous material and bits of cartilage. Histologically three types of tissue can usually be identified: patches of myxomatous tissue with delicate, stellate cells; islands of hyaline cartilage; and areas of fibrous tissue with cells of varying degrees of maturity.

Malignant change has been recorded but this must be extremely rare.

TREATMENT Where feasible, the lesion should be excised but often one can do no more than a thorough curettage – followed by autogenous bone grafting. There is considerable risk of recurrence; if repeated operations are needed, care should be taken to prevent damage to the physis (in children) or the nearby joint surface.

OSTEOCHONDROMA (CARTILAGE-CAPPED EXOSTOSIS)

This, one of the commonest 'tumours' of bone, is a developmental lesion which starts as a small overgrowth of cartilage at the edge of the physeal plate and develops by endochondral ossification into a bony protuberance still covered by the cap of cartilage. Any bone that develops in cartilage may be involved; the commonest sites are the fast-growing ends of long bones and the crest of the ilium. In long bones, growth leaves the bump stranded further down the metaphysis. Here it may go on growing but at the end of the normal growth period for that bone it stops enlarging. *Any further enlargement after the end of the growth period is suggestive of malignant transformation.*

The patient is usually a teenager or young adult when the lump is first discovered. Occasionally there is pain due to an overlying bursa or impingement on soft tissues, or, rarely, paraesthesia due to stretching of an adjacent nerve.

The *x-ray* appearance is pathognomonic. There is a well-defined exostosis emerging from the metaphysis, its base co-extensive with the parent bone. It looks smaller than it feels because the cartilage cap is not seen on x-ray; however, large lesions undergo cartilage degeneration and calcification and then the x-ray shows the bony exostosis surrounded by clouds of calcified material.

Multiple lesions may develop as part of a heritable disorder – *hereditary multiple exostosis* – in which there is abnormal bone growth resulting in characteristic deformities (see page 139).

PATHOLOGY At operation the cartilage cap is seen surmounting a narrow base or pedicle of bone. The cap consists of simple hyaline cartilage; in a growing exostosis the deeper cartilage cells are arranged in columns, giving rise to the formation of endochondral new bone. Large lesions may have a 'cauliflower' appearance, with degeneration and calcification in the centre of the cartilage cap. The incidence of malignant transformation is difficult to assess because troublesome lesions are so often removed before they show histological features of malignancy. Figures usually quoted are 1% for solitary lesions and 6% for multiple.

TREATMENT If the tumour causes symptoms it should be excised; if, in an adult, it has recently become bigger or painful then operation is urgent, for these features suggest malignancy. This is seen most often with pelvic exostoses – not because they are inherently different but because considerable enlargement may, for long periods, pass unnoticed. If there are suspicious features, further imaging and staging should be carried out before doing a biopsy. If the histology is that of 'benign' cartilage but the tumour is known for certain to be enlarging after the end of the growth period, it should be treated as a chondrosarcoma.

SIMPLE BONE CYST

This lesion (also known as a *solitary cyst* or *unicameral bone cyst*) appears during childhood, typically in the

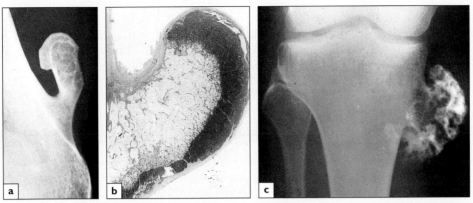

9.14 Osteochondroma (**a**) The lesion is a cartilage-capped exostosis but the cartilage does not show on x-ray unless it is calcified. The bony part may be pedunculated, sessile or cauliflower-like. (**b**) A section through the exostosis shows that it is always covered by hyaline cartilage from which the bony excrescence grows. (**c**) A large exostosis with calcification in the cartilage cap.

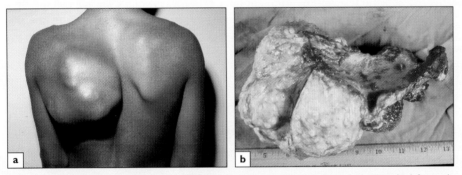

9.15 Osteochondroma – treatment (**a**) This 20-year-old man had known about the lump on his left scapula for many years. He stopped growing at the age of 18 but the tumour continued to enlarge. (**b**) Despite the benign histology in the biopsy, the tumour together with most of the scapula was removed; sections taken from the depths of the lesion showed atypical cells suggestive of malignant change.

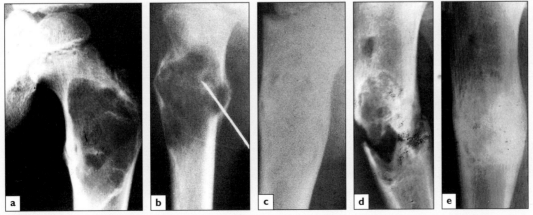

9.16 Simple bone cysts (**a**) A typical solitary (or unicameral) cyst – on the shaft side of the physis and expanding the cortex. (**b**) Injection with methylprednisolone, and (**c**) healing. (**d**) Fracture through a cyst, leading to (**e**) healing.

metaphysis of one of the long bones and most commonly in the proximal humerus or femur. It is not a tumour, tends to heal spontaneously and is seldom seen in adults. The condition is usually discovered after a pathological fracture or as an incidental finding on x-ray.

X-rays show a well-demarcated radiolucent area in the metaphysis, often extending up to the physeal plate; the cortex may be thinned and the bone expanded.

Diagnosis is usually not difficult but other cyst-like lesions may need to be excluded. Non-osteogenic fibroma, fibrous dysplasia and the benign cartilage tumours are solid and merely look cystic on x-ray. In doubtful cases a needle can be inserted into the lesion under x-ray control: with a simple cyst, straw-coloured fluid will be withdrawn. Very seldom will there be any need for biopsy. However, if curettage is thought to be necessary, material from the cyst should be submitted for examination.

PATHOLOGY The lining membrane consists of flimsy fibrous tissue, often containing giant cells. In an actively growing cyst, there is osteoclastic resorption of the adjacent bone.

TREATMENT Treatment depends on whether the cyst is symptomatic, actively growing or involved in a fracture. Asymptomatic lesions in older children can be left alone but the patient should be cautioned to avoid injury which might cause a fracture. 'Active' cysts (those in young children, usually abutting against the physeal plate and obviously enlarging in sequential x-rays) should be treated, in the first instance, by aspiration of fluid and injection of 80-160mg of methylprednisolone. This often stops further enlargement and leads to healing of the cyst. If the cyst goes on enlarging, or if there is a pathological fracture, the cavity should be thoroughly cleaned by curettage and then packed with bone chips. There is a considerable risk of recurrence and more than one operation may be needed. Care should be taken not to damage the nearby physeal plate.

ANEURYSMAL BONE CYST

Aneurysmal bone cyst may be encountered at any age and in almost any bone, though more often in young adults and in the long-bone metaphyses. Usually it arises spontaneously but it may appear after degeneration or haemorrhage in some other lesion .

With expanding lesions, patients may complain of pain. Occasionally, a large cyst may cause a visible or palpable swelling of the bone.

X-rays show a well-defined radiolucent cyst, often trabeculated and eccentrically placed. In a growing tubular bone it is always situated in the metaphysis and therefore may resemble a simple cyst or one of the other cyst-like lesions. Occasional sites include verte-

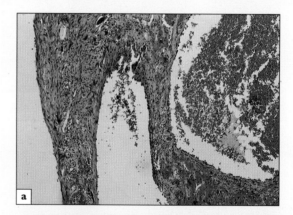

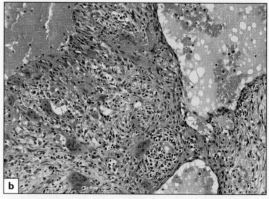

9.18 Aneurysmal bone cyst – histology (a) The cyst contained blood and was lined by loose fibrous tissue containing numerous giant cells. (×120) (b) A high-power view of the same. (×300)

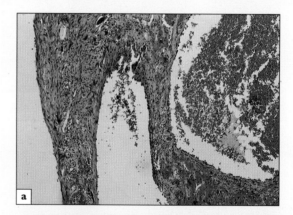

9.17 Aneurysmal bone cyst (a) The outer wall of this cyst is so thin that it barely shows on the x-ray. (b) The soap-bubble appearance in this lesion is produced by ridges on the walls of the cyst. (c) After curettage and packing with bone chips the lesion healed.

180

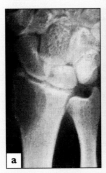
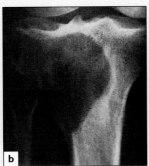
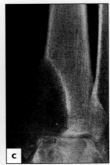
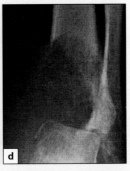

9.19 Giant-cell tumours (**a, b, c**) In each of these the tumour abuts against the joint margin, and is asymmetrically placed – these are characteristic features; in (**d**) malignant change has supervened and the inner margin of the tumour is no longer well defined.

brae and the flat bones. In an adult an aneurysmal bone cyst may be mistaken for a giant-cell tumour but, unlike the latter, it usually does not extend right up to the articular margin. Occasionally it causes marked ballooning of the bone end.

PATHOLOGY When the cyst is opened it is found to contain clotted blood, and during curettage there may be considerable bleeding from the fleshy lining membrane. Histologically the lining consists of fibrous tissue with vascular spaces, deposits of haemosiderin and multinucleated giant cells. Occasionally the appearances so closely resemble those of giant-cell tumour that only the most experienced pathologists can confidently make the diagnosis. Malignant transformation does not occur.

TREATMENT The cyst should be carefully opened, thoroughly curetted and then packed with bone grafts. Sometimes the graft is resorbed and the cyst recurs, necessitating a second or third operation. In these cases, packing with methylmethacrylate cement may be more effective. However, if the cyst is in a 'safe' area (i.e. where there is no risk of fracture) there is no hurry to re-operate; the lesion occasionally heals spontaneously (Malghem *et al.*, 1989).

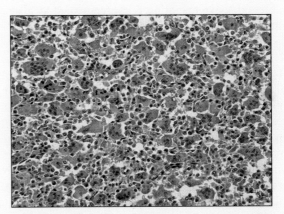

9.20 Giant-cell tumour – histology A low-power view of the biopsy shows the abundant multinucleated giant cells lying in a stroma composed of round and polyhedral tumour cells. There are numerous mitotic figures.

GIANT-CELL TUMOUR

Giant-cell tumour is a lesion of uncertain origin that appears in mature bone, most commonly in the distal femur, proximal tibia, proximal humerus and distal radius, but other bones may be affected. It is hardly ever seen before closure of the physis in that region and characteristically it extends up to the subarticular bone plate. Rarely, there are multiple lesions.

The patient is usually a young adult who complains of pain at the end of a long bone; sometimes there is slight swelling. A history of trauma is not uncommon and pathological fracture occurs in 10–15% of cases. On examination there may be a palpable mass with warmth of the overlying tissues.

X-rays show a radiolucent area situated eccentrically at the end of a long bone and bounded by the subchondral bone plate. The endosteal margin may be quite obvious, but in aggressive lesions it is ill-defined. The centre sometimes has a soap-bubble appearance due to ridging of the surrounding bone. The cortex is thin and sometimes ballooned; aggressive lesions extend into the soft tissue. The appearance of a 'cystic' lesion in mature bone, extending right up to the subchondral plate, is so characteristic that the diagnosis is seldom in doubt.

Considering the tumour's potential for aggressive behaviour, *detailed staging procedures* are essential. CT scans and MRI will reveal the extent of the tumour, both within the bone and beyond. It is important to establish whether the articular surface has been

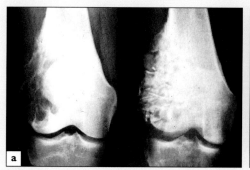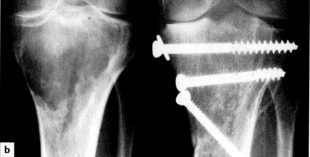

9.21 Giant-cell tumour – treatment (a) Excision and bone grafts. (b) Block resection and replacement with a large allograft.

broached; arthroscopy may be helpful. Biopsy is essential. This can be done either as a frozen section before proceeding with operative treatment or (especially if a more extensive operation is contemplated) as a separate procedure.

PATHOLOGY The tumour has a reddish, fleshy appearance; it comes away in pieces quite easily when curetted, but is difficult to remove completely from the surrounding bone. Aggressive lesions have a poorly defined edge and extend well into the surrounding bone. Histologically the striking feature is an abundance of multinucleated giant cells scattered on a background of stromal cells with little or no visible intercellular tissue. Aggressive lesions tend to show more cellular atypia and mitotic figures, but histological grading is unreliable as a predictor of tumour behaviour.

TREATMENT Well-confined, slow-growing lesions with benign histology can safely be treated by thorough curettage and 'stripping' of the cavity with burrs and gouges, followed by swabbing with hydrogen peroxide or by the application of liquid nitrogen; the cavity is then packed with bone chips. More aggressive tumours, and recurrent lesions, should be treated by excision followed, if necessary, by bone grafting or prosthetic replacement. Tumours in awkward sites (e.g.

the spine) may be difficult to eradicate; supplementary radiotherapy is sometimes recommended, but it carries a significant risk of causing malignant transformation.

GIANT CELL SARCOMA

Giant-cell sarcoma is an unequivocally malignant lesion with x-ray features like those of a highly aggressive benign giant-cell tumour. There is a high risk of metastasis and treatment requires wide, or even radical, resection.

EOSINOPHILIC GRANULOMA AND HISTIOCYTOSIS

Histiocytosis-X defines an unusual group of disorders in which cells of the reticuloendothelial system (histiocytes and eosinophils) form granulomatous collections which may cause osteolytic lesions resembling bone tumours.

Eosinophilic granuloma is the commonest of these conditions, and the only one presenting as a pure bone lesion. Marrow-containing bone is resorbed and one or

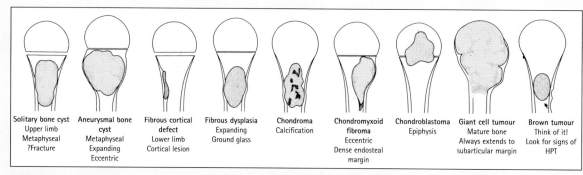

9.22 **Cysts and cyst-like lesions of bone** Thumb-nail sketches of lesions which appear as 'cysts' on x-ray examination.

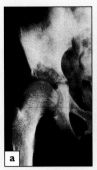
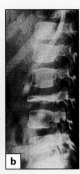
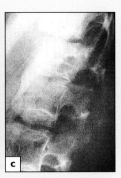
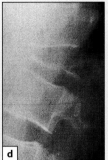
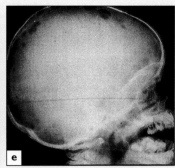

9.23 Lipid storage disorders (a) An eosinophilic granuloma which went on to spontaneous healing. (b) Calve's disease with a flattened vertebral body but discs of normal height. (c, d) The development of Calve's disease from an eosinophilic granuloma. (e) Hand–Schüller–Christian disease.

more lytic lesions may appear in the flat bones or the metaphyses of long bones. The patient is usually a child; there is seldom any complaint of pain and the condition is discovered incidentally or after a pathological fracture.

X-ray shows a well-demarcated oval area of radiolucency within the bone; sometimes this is associated with marked reactive sclerosis. There may be multiple lesions and in the skull they have a characteristic punched-out appearance. Vertebral collapse may result in a flat wedge (*vertebra plana*) which is pathognomonic.

The condition usually heals spontaneously and is therefore rarely seen in adults. Occasionally, however, a solitary lesion may herald the onset of one of the generalized disorders (see below). Operation is usually done to obtain a biopsy; if the lesion is easily accessible it may be completely excised or curetted; if not, radiotherapy is effective.

Hand-Schüller-Christian disease is a disseminated form of the same condition. The patient is a child, usually with widespread lesions involving the skull, vertebral bodies, liver and spleen. There may be anaemia and a tendency to recurrent infection.

Individual lesions can be treated by curettage or radiotherapy; however, complete remission is very unlikely.

Letterer–Siwe disease is an extremely rare (and severe) form of histiocytosis. It is seen in infants and usually progresses rapidly to a fatal outcome.

HAEMANGIOMA

Osseous haemangiomas consist of vascular channels (capillary, venous or cavernous) and are usually seen in middle-aged patients, the spine being the commonest site. They are usually symptomless and discovered accidentally when the back is x-rayed for some other

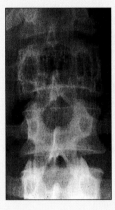

9.24 Haemangioma This haemangioma was symptomless and discovered accidentally. Note the coarse vertical trabeculation and slight loss of definition.

reason. However, if the patient does have backache, the haemangioma is likely to be blamed.

The *x-ray* shows coarse vertical trabeculation (the so-called 'corduroy appearance') in the vertebral body. Other sites include the skull and pelvis where the appearance occasionally suggests malignancy, but there is no associated cortical or medullary destruction. Rarely the presenting feature may be a pathological fracture.

If operation is needed there is a risk of profuse bleeding, and embolization may be a useful preliminary.

OSTEOLYSIS ('DISAPPEARING BONES')

In massive osteolysis (Gorham's disease) there is progressive disappearance of bone, associated with haemangiomatosis or multiple lymphangiectases. Usually the progression involves contiguous bones, but occasionally multiple sites are affected. Patients may present with mild pain or with a pathological fracture. No effective treatment is known, but spontaneous arrest has been described. Occasionally, however, the process spreads to vital structures and the outcome is fatal (Cannon, 1986).

PRIMARY MALIGNANT BONE TUMOURS

CHONDROSARCOMA

Chondrosarcoma can occur either as a primary tumour or as a secondary change in a pre-existing cartilaginous lesion. Both types have their highest incidence in the fourth and fifth decades, and men are affected more often than women. The tumours are slow growing and are usually present for many months before being discovered. Patients may complain of a dull ache or a gradually enlarging lump. Medullary lesions may present as a pathological fracture.

Primary chondrosarcoma can occur in any bone that develops in cartilage but is usually seen in the metaphysis of one of the tubular bones. X-rays show a radiolucent area with central flecks of calcification. Rarely, the tumour appears as a globular mass on the surface of the bone; this distinguishes the so-called 'peripheral chondrosarcoma' from the more common 'central chondrosarcoma'.

Secondary chondrosarcoma usually arises in the cartilage cap of an exostosis (osteochondroma) that has been present since childhood. Exostoses of the pelvis and scapula seem to be more susceptible than others to malignant change, but perhaps this is simply because the site allows a tumour to grow without being detected and removed at an early stage. X-rays show the bony exostosis, often surmounted by clouds of patchy calcification in the otherwise unseen lobulated cartilage cap. A tumour that is very large and calcification that is very fluffy and poorly outlined are suspicious features, but the clearest sign of malignant change is a demonstrable progressive enlargement of an osteochondroma after the end of normal bone growth.

A benign medullary chondroma (enchondroma) may also undergo malignant transformation, but it is difficult to be sure that the lesion was not a slowly evolving sarcoma from the outset.

Staging

If a chondrosarcoma is suspected, full staging procedures should be employed. CT scans and MRI must be carried out before performing a biopsy.

PATHOLOGY A biopsy is essential to confirm the diagnosis. However, low-grade chondrosarcoma may show histological features no different from those of an aggressive benign cartilaginous lesion. High-grade tumours are more cellular, and there may be obvious

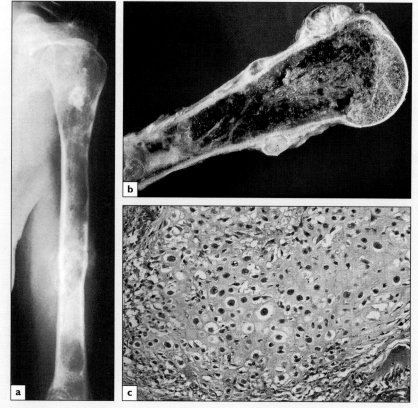

9.25 Chondrosarcoma (**a**) This patient presented with a suspected pathological fracture of the humerus. X-rays showed rarefaction of the bone with central flecks of calcification. At the fracture site the lesion extends into the soft tissues. (**b**) Radical resection was carried out. Pale, glistening cartilage tissue was found in the medullary cavity and, in several places, spreading beyond the cortex. Much of the bone is occupied by haemorrhagic tissue. (**c**) The histological sections show lobules of highly atypical cartilage cells, including binucleate cells.

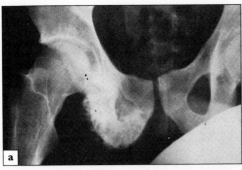 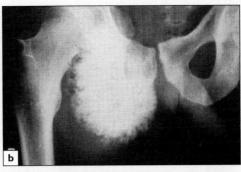

9.26 Chondrosarcoma At the age of 20 years this young man complained of pain in the right groin; x-ray showed an osteochondroma of the right inferior pubic ramus (**a**). A biopsy showed 'benign cartilage' but a year later the tumour had doubled its size (**b**), a clear sign that it was a chondrosarcoma.

abnormal features of the cells, such as plumpness, hyperchromasia and mitoses. The term 'dedifferentiated' chondrosarcoma is used when the usual appearances are associated with areas that look more malignant.

Treatment

Chondrosarcomas are usually slow-growing and metastasize late. They present the ideal case for wide excision and prosthetic replacement, provided it is certain that the lesion can be completely removed without exposing the tumour and without causing an unacceptable loss of function. In that case amputation may be preferable.

The tumour does not respond to either radiotherapy or chemotherapy.

OSTEOSARCOMA

In its classic (intramedullary) form, osteosarcoma is a highly malignant tumour arising within the bone and spreading rapidly outwards to the periosteum and surrounding soft tissues. It is said to occur predominantly in children and adolescents, but epidemiological studies suggest that between 1972 and 1981 the age of presentation rose significantly (Stark *et al.*, 1990). It may affect any bone but most commonly involves the long-bone metaphyses, especially around the knee and at the proximal end of the humerus.

Clinical features

Pain is usually the first symptom; it is constant, worse at night and gradually increases in severity. Sometimes the patient presents with a lump. Pathological fracture is rare. On examination there may be little to find except local tenderness. In later cases there is a palpable mass and the overlying tissues may appear swollen and inflamed. The ESR is usually raised and there may be an increase in serum alkaline phosphatase.

X-RAYS The x-ray appearances are variable: hazy osteolytic areas may alternate with unusually dense osteoblastic areas. The endosteal margin is poorly defined. Often the cortex is breached and the tumour extends into the adjacent tissues; when this happens, streaks of new bone appear, radiating outwards from the cortex – the so-called 'sunburst' effect. Where the tumour emerges from the cortex, reactive new bone forms at the angles of periosteal elevation (Codman's triangle). While both the sunburst appearance and Codman's triangle are typical of osteosarcoma, they may occasionally be seen in other rapidly growing tumours.

Diagnosis and staging

In most cases the diagnosis can be made with confidence on the x-ray appearances. However, atypical lesions can cause confusion. Conditions to be excluded are post-traumatic swellings, infection, stress fracture and the more aggressive 'cystic' lesions.

Other imaging studies are essential for staging purposes. Radioisotope scans may show up skip lesions, but a negative scan does not exclude them. CT and MRI reliably show the extent of the tumour. Chest x-rays are done routinely, but pulmonary CT is a much more sensitive detector of lung metastases. About 10% of patients have pulmonary metastases by the time they are first seen.

A biopsy should always be carried out before commencing treatment; it must be carefully planned to allow for complete removal of the track when the tumour is excised.

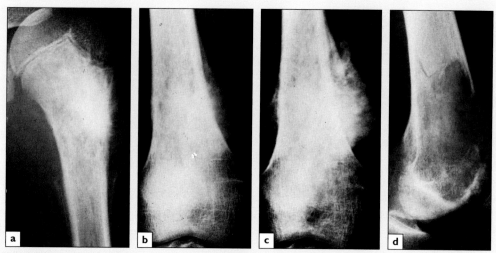

9.27 Osteosarcoma (a) The metaphyseal site, increased density, cortical erosion and periosteal reaction are characteristic. (b) Sunray spicules and Codman's triangle; (c) the same patient after radiotherapy. (d) A predominantly osteolytic tumour.

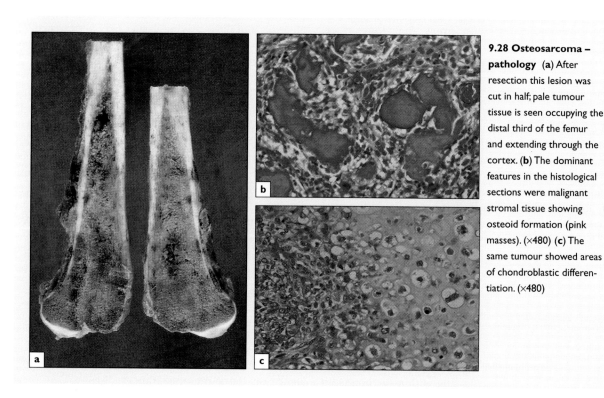

9.28 Osteosarcoma – pathology (a) After resection this lesion was cut in half; pale tumour tissue is seen occupying the distal third of the femur and extending through the cortex. (b) The dominant features in the histological sections were malignant stromal tissue showing osteoid formation (pink masses). (×480) (c) The same tumour showed areas of chondroblastic differentiation. (×480)

Pathology

The tumour is usually situated in the metaphysis of a long bone, where it destroys and replaces normal bone. Areas of bone loss and cavitation alternate with dense patches of abnormal new bone. The tumour extends within the medulla and across the physeal plate. There may be obvious spread into the soft tissues with ossification at the periosteal margins and streaks of new bone extending into the extra-osseous mass.

The histological appearances show considerable variation: some areas may have the characteristic spindle cells with a pink-staining osteoid matrix; others may contain cartilage cells or fibroblastic tissue with little or no osteoid. Several samples may have to be examined; pathologists are reluctant to commit themselves to the diagnosis unless they see evidence of osteoid formation.

Treatment

The appalling prognosis that formerly attended this tumour has markedly improved, partly as a result of better diagnostic and staging procedures, and possibly

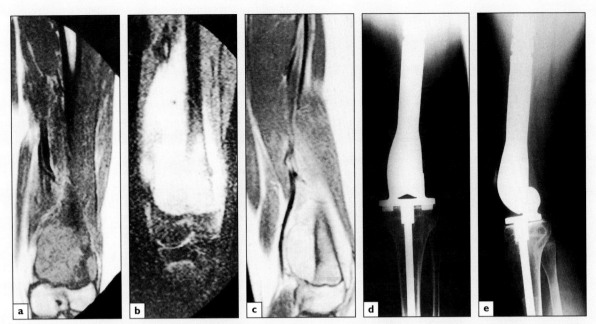

9.29 Staging and treatment (a) MRIT$_1$ sequence showing the tumour (an osteosarcoma) in the distal femur but not penetrating the joint. (b) STIR sequence (fat suppression) gives a more realistic picture of spread into the soft tissues. (c) Proton density sequence showing posterior extension of the tumour up to (but not into) the vascular compartment. (d, e) Wide excision and replacement with large 'extending' prosthesis. (Courtesy of Mr John Dixon.)

because the average age of the patients has increased, but mainly because of advances in chemotherapy to control metastatic spread. However, it is still important to eradicate the primary lesion completely; the mortality rate after local recurrence is far worse than following effective ablation at the first encounter.

The principles of treatment are outlined on page 171. After clinical assessment and advanced imaging, the patient is admitted to a special centre for biopsy. The lesion will probably be graded IIA or IIB. Multi-agent chemotherapy is given for 8–12 weeks and then, provided the tumour is resectable and there are no skip lesions, a wide resection is carried out. Depending on the site of the tumour, preparations would have been made to replace that segment of bone with either a large bone-graft or a custom-made implant; in some cases an amputation may be more appropriate.

The pathological specimen is examined to assess the response to pre-operative chemotherapy. If tumour necrosis is marked, chemotherapy is continued for another 6–12 months; if the response is poor, a different chemotherapeutic agent is substituted.

Pulmonary metastases, especially if they are small and peripherally situated, may be completely resected with a wedge of lung tissue.

OUTCOME Long-term survival after wide resection and chemotherapy is now 50–60% (Rosen *et al.*, 1982). Tumour-replacement implants usually function well. There is a fairly high complication rate (mainly wound

breakdown and infection) but in patients who survive, the incidence of local tumour recurrence is about the same as after amputation.

VARIANTS OF OSTEOSARCOMA

PAROSTEAL OSTEOSARCOMA

This is a low-grade sarcoma situated on the surface of one of the tubular bones, usually at the distal femoral or proximal tibial metaphysis. The patient is a young adult who presents with a slowly enlarging mass near the bone end.

X-ray shows a dense bony mass on the surface of the bone or encircling it; the cortex is not eroded and usually a thin gap remains between cortex and tumour. The picture is easily mistaken for that of a benign bone lesion and the diagnosis is often missed until the tumour recurs after local excision. *CT* and *MRI* will show the boundary between tumour and surrounding soft tissues. Although the lesion is outside the bone, it does not spread into the adjacent muscle compartment until fairly late. Staging, therefore, often defines it as a low-grade intracompartmental tumour (Stage IA).

PATHOLOGY At biopsy the tumour appears as a hard mass. On microscopic examination the lesion consists of well-formed bone but without any regular trabecular arrangement. The spaces between trabeculae are

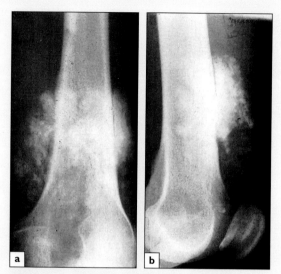

9.30 Parosteal osteosarcoma (a, b) X-rays show an ill-defined extra-osseous tumour – note the linear gap between cortex and tumour.

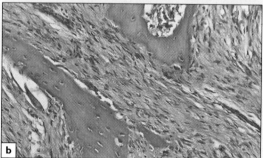

9.31 Parosteal osteosarcoma – histology (a) Histologically there were bony trabeculae and spindle-shaped, well-differentiated fibrous tissue cells with occasional mitotic figures. (×120) **(b)** High-power view of the same. (×300)

filled with cellular fibroblastic tissue; a few atypical cells and mitotic figures can usually be found. Occasionally the tumour has a much more aggressive appearance (*dedifferentiated parosteal osteosarcoma*).

TREATMENT For a low-grade parosteal osteosarcoma, wide excision without adjuvant therapy is sufficient to ensure a recurrence rate below 10%. Dedifferentiated parosteal osteosarcoma should be treated in the same way as intramedullary sarcoma.

PERIOSTEAL OSTEOSARCOMA

This rare tumour is quite distinct from parosteal osteosarcoma. It is more like an intramedullary osteosarcoma, but situated on the surface of the bone. It occurs in young adults and causes local pain and swelling.

X-ray shows a superficial defect of the cortex, but *CT and MRI* may reveal a larger soft-tissue mass. The appearances sometimes suggest a periosteal chondroma and the diagnosis may not be certain until a biopsy is performed.

PATHOLOGY Histologically this is a true osteosarcoma, but characteristically the sections show a prominent cartilaginous element.

TREATMENT Treatment is the same as that of classic osteosarcoma.

PAGET'S SARCOMA

Although malignant transformation is a rare complication of Paget's disease, most osteosarcomas appearing after the age of 50 years fall into this category. Warning signs are the appearance of pain or swelling in a patient with long-standing Paget's disease. In late cases, pathological fracture may occur.

X-ray shows the usual features of Paget's disease, but with areas of bone destruction and soft tissue invasion.

This is a high-grade tumour – if anything even more malignant than classic osteosarcoma. Staging usually shows that extracompartmental spread has occurred; most patients have pulmonary metastases by the time the tumour is diagnosed.

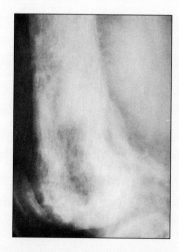

9.32 Paget's sarcoma The lesion, superimposed on Paget's disease, looks malignant – and it was.

TREATMENT Even with radical resection or amputation and chemotherapy the 5-year survival rate is low. If the lesion is definitely extracompartmental, palliative treatment by radiotherapy may be preferable; chemotherapy is usually difficult because of the patient's age and uncertainty about renal and cardiac function.

TREATMENT Low-grade, well-confined tumours (Stage IA) can be treated by wide excision with prosthetic replacement. High-grade lesions (IIA or IIB) require radical resection or amputation; if this cannot be achieved, local excision must be combined with radiation therapy. The value of adjuvant chemotherapy is still uncertain.

FIBROSARCOMA OF BONE

Fibrosarcoma is rare in bone, and is more likely to arise in previously abnormal tissue (a bone infarct, fibrous dysplasia or after irradiation). The patient – usually an adult – complains of pain or swelling; there may be a pathological fracture.

X-ray shows an undistinctive area of bone destruction. *CT or MRI* will reveal the soft-tissue extension.

PATHOLOGY Histologically the lesion consists of masses of fibroblastic tissue with scattered atypical and mitotic cells. Appearances vary from well-differentiated to highly undifferentiated, and the tumours are sometimes graded accordingly.

MALIGNANT FIBROUS HISTIOCYTOMA

Like fibrosarcoma, this tumour tends to occur in previously abnormal bone (old infarcts or Paget's disease). Patients are usually middle-aged adults and x-rays may reveal a destructive lesion adjacent to an old area of medullary infarction. Staging studies almost invariably show that the tumour has spread beyond the bone.

Histologically it is a fibrous tumour, but the arrangement of the tissue is in interweaving bundles, and the presence of histiocytes and of giant cells distinguishes it from the more uniform fibrosarcoma.

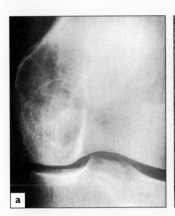 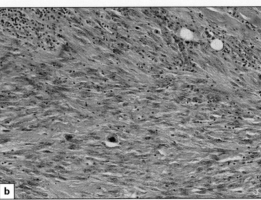

9.33 Fibrosarcoma (a) The area of bone destruction in the femoral condyle has no special distinguishing features. (b) The biopsy showed highly atypical fibroblastic tissue.

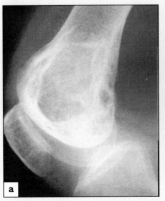 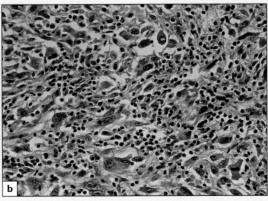

9.34 Malignant fibrous histiocytoma (a) X-ray showing a large 'cystic' lesion in the distal femur. The lesion may occur in an area of old 'bone infarct', which may account for the flecks of increased density in this x-ray. (b) Histology shows abnormal fibrohistiocytic cells, many of which are unusually large and some of which are binucleate or multinucleate. (×480)

TREATMENT Treatment consists of wide or radical resection (or amputation) and adjuvant chemotherapy. For inaccessible lesions, local radiotherapy may be needed.

EWING'S SARCOMA

Ewing's sarcoma is believed to arise from endothelial cells in the bone marrow. It occurs most commonly between the ages of 10 and 20 years, usually in a tubular bone and especially in the tibia, fibula or clavicle.

The patient presents with pain – often throbbing in character – and swelling. Generalized illness and pyrexia, together with a warm, tender swelling and a raised ESR, may suggest a diagnosis of osteomyelitis.

X-rays usually show an area of bone destruction which, unlike that in osteosarcoma, is predominantly in the mid-diaphysis. New bone formation may extend along the shaft and sometimes it appears as fusiform layers of bone around the lesion – the so-called 'onion-peel' effect. Often the tumour extends into the surrounding soft tissues, with radiating streaks of ossification and reactive periosteal bone at the proximal and distal margins. These features (the 'sunray' appearance and Codman's triangles) are usually associated with osteosarcoma, but they are just as common in Ewing's sarcoma.

CT and MRI reveal the large extra-osseous component. *Radioisotope scans* may show multiple areas of activity in the skeleton.

PATHOLOGY Macroscopically the tumour is lobulated and often fairly large. It may look grey (like brain) or red (like redcurrant jelly) if haemorrhage has occurred into it.

Microscopically, sheets of small dark polyhedral cells with no regular arrangement and no ground substance are seen.

DIAGNOSIS The condition which should be excluded as rapidly as possible is bone infection. On biopsy the essential step is to recognize this as a malignant round-cell tumour, distinct from osteosarcoma. Other round-cell tumours that may resemble Ewing's are reticulum-cell sarcoma (see below) and metastatic neuroblastoma.

TREATMENT The prognosis is always poor and surgery alone does little to improve it. Radiotherapy has a dramatic effect on the tumour but overall survival is not much enhanced. Chemotherapy is much more effective, offering a 5-year survival rate of about 50% (Souhami and Craft, 1988). The best results are achieved by a combination of all three methods: a course of preoperative chemotherapy; then wide excision (or amputation) if the tumour is in a favourable site, or radiotherapy followed by local excision if it is less accessible; and then a further course of chemotherapy for 1 year.

RETICULUM-CELL SARCOMA (NON-HODGKIN'S LYMPHOMA)

Like Ewing's sarcoma, this is a round-cell tumour of the reticuloendothelial system. It is usually seen in sites with abundant red marrow: the flat bones, the spine and the long-bone metaphyses. The patient, usually an adult of 30–40 years, presents with pain or a pathological fracture.

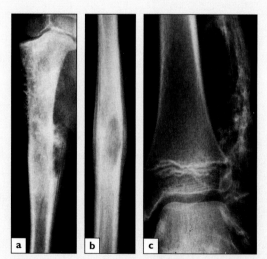

9.35 Ewing's tumour Examples of Ewing's tumour in (**a**) the humerus, (**b**) the mid-shaft of the fibula and (**c**) the lower end of the fibula.

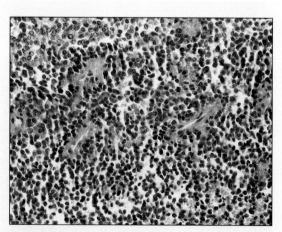

9.36 Ewing's sarcoma – histology There is a monotonous pattern of small round cells clustered around blood vessels. (×480)

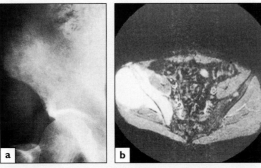

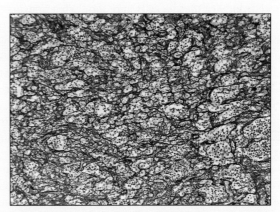

9.37 Reticulum-cell sarcoma (**a**) X-ray showing a rather nondescript mottled appearance of the ilium. (**b**) MRI reveals the extent of the soft-tissue lesion.

9.38 Reticulum-cell sarcoma – histology There is dense infiltration of abnormal lymphocytes (a typical 'round-cell tumour'), which is distinguished from Ewing's by the characteristic distribution of reticulin around collections of cells and between individual cells. (×200; special reticulin stain)

X-ray shows a mottled area of bone destruction in areas that normally contain red marrow; the *radioisotope scan* may reveal multiple lesions.

PATHOLOGY Histologically this is a marrow-cell tumour with collections of abnormal lymphocytes. Special reticulin stains are needed to show the fine fibrillar network that helps to distinguish the picture from that of Ewing's sarcoma.

TREATMENT The preferred treatment is by chemotherapy and radical resection; radiotherapy is reserved for less accessible lesions.

MULTIPLE MYELOMA

Multiple myeloma is a malignant B-cell lymphoproliferative disorder of the marrow, with plasma cells predominating. The effects on bone are due to marrow cell proliferation and increased osteoclastic activity, resulting in *osteoporosis* and the appearance of discrete *lytic lesions* throughout the skeleton. A particularly

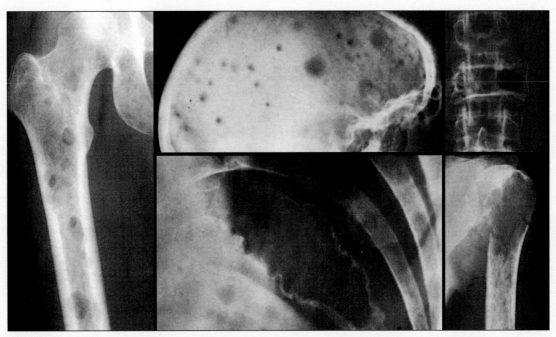

9.39 Myeloma The characteristic x-ray features are bone rarefaction, expanding lesions (typically in the ribs and pelvis) and punched-out areas in the skull and the long bones.

large colony of plasma cells may form what appears to be a solitary tumour *(plasmacytoma)* in one of the bones, but sooner or later most of these cases turn out to be unusual examples of the same widespread disease.

Associated features of the marrow cell disorder are *plasma protein abnormalities, increased blood viscosity* and *anaemia*. Bone resorption leads to *hypercalcaemia* in about one-third of cases. Late secondary features are due to *renal dysfunction* and *spinal cord or root compression* caused by vertebral collapse.

The patient, typically aged 45–65 years, presents with weakness, backache, bone pain or a pathological fracture. Hypercalcaemia may cause symptoms such as thirst, polyuria and abdominal pain. Clinical signs (apart from a pathological fracture) are often unremarkable. Localized tenderness and restricted hip movements could be due to a plasmacytoma in the proximal femur. In late cases there may be signs of cord or nerve root compression, chronic nephritis and recurrent infection.

X-RAYS X-rays often show nothing more than generalized osteoporosis; but remember that *myeloma is one of the commonest causes of osteoporosis and vertebral compression fracture in men over the age of 45 years.* The 'classic' lesions are multiple punched-out defects with 'soft' margins (lack of new bone) in the skull, pelvis and proximal femur, a crushed vertebra, or a solitary lytic tumour in a large-bone metaphysis.

INVESTIGATIONS Mild anaemia is common, and an almost constant feature is a high ESR. Blood chemistry may show a raised creatinine level and hypercalcaemia. Over half the patients have Bence–Jones protein in their urine, and serum protein electrophoresis shows a characteristic abnormal band. A sternal marrow puncture may show plasmacytosis, with typical 'myeloma' cells.

DIAGNOSIS If the only x-ray change is osteoporosis, the differential diagnosis must include all the *other causes of bone loss.* If there are lytic lesions, the features can be similar to those of *metastatic bone* disease.

Paraproteinaemia is a feature of other (benign) *gammopathies*; it is wise to seek the help of a haematologist before reaching a clinical diagnosis.

PATHOLOGY At operation the affected bone is soft and crumbly. The typical microscopic picture is of sheets of plasmacytes with a large eccentric nucleus containing a spoke-like arrangement of chromatin.

TREATMENT The immediate need is for pain control and, if necessary, treatment of pathological fractures. General supportive measures include correction of fluid balance and (in some cases) hypercalcaemia.

Limb fractures are best managed by internal fixation and packing of cavities with methylmethacrylate cement (which also helps to staunch the profuse bleed-

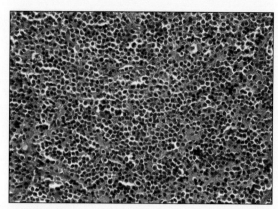

9.40 Myeloma – histology There are dense sheets of plasma cells with eccentric nuclei. (×480)

ing that sometimes occurs). Perioperative antibiotic prophylaxis is important as there is a higher than usual risk of infection and wound breakdown.

Spinal fractures carry the risk of cord compression and need immediate stabilization – either by effective bracing or by internal fixation. Unrelieved cord pressure may need decompression.

Solitary plasmacytomas can be treatment by radiotherapy.

Specific therapy is with alkylating cytotoxic agents (e.g. melphalan). Corticosteroids are also used – especially if bone pain is marked – but this probably does not alter the course of the disease. Treatment should be carried out in a specialized unit where dosages and response parameters can be properly monitored.

The *prognosis* in established cases is poor, with a median survival of 2–3 years.

CHORDOMA

This rare malignant tumour arises from primitive notochordal remnants. It affects young adults and usually presents as a slow-growing mass in the sacrum; however, it may occur elsewhere along the spine.

The patient complains of long-standing backache. The tumour expands anteriorly and, if it involves the sacrum, may eventually (after months or even years) cause rectal or urethral obstruction; rectal examination may disclose the presacral mass. In late cases there may also be neurological signs.

X-ray shows a radiolucent lesion in the sacrum. *CT and MRI* reveal the extent of intrapelvic enlargement.

TREATMENT This is a low-grade tumour, though often with extracompartmental spread. After wide excision there is little risk of recurrence. However, attempts to

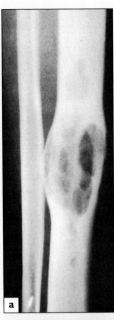

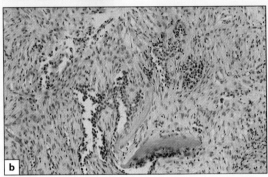

9.41 Adamantinoma (a) The bubble-like appearance in the mid-shaft of the tibia is typical. (b) Histology typically shows epithelial-like cells, sometimes with an acinar arrangement. (×300)

PATHOLOGY The histological picture varies considerably but the most typical features are islands of epithelial-like cells on a densely-populated stroma of spindle cells; the 'epithelial' nests may have an acinar arrangement.

TREATMENT If the diagnosis is made reasonably early, wide local excision with a substantial margin of normal bone is adequate. Preoperative CT and MRI are essential to determine how deep the tumour penetrates; if it is confined to the anterior cortex, the posterior cortex can be preserved and this makes reconstruction much easier. If the lesion extends to the endosteal surface, a full segment of bone must be excised; the gap is filled with a vascularized graft.

If there has been more than one recurrence, or if the tumour extends into the surrounding soft tissues, radical resection or amputation is advisable.

METASTATIC BONE DISEASE

The skeleton is one of the commonest sites of secondary cancer; *in patients over 50 years bone metastases are seen more frequently than all primary malignant bone tumours together.* The commonest source is carcinoma of the breast; next in frequency are carcinomas of the prostate, kidney, lung, thyroid, bladder and gastrointestinal tract. In about 10% of cases no primary tumour is found.

The commonest sites for bone metastases are the vertebrae, pelvis, the proximal half of the femur and the humerus. Spread is usually via the blood stream; occasionally, visceral tumours spread directly to adjacent bones (e.g. the pelvis or ribs).

Metastases are usually osteolytic, and pathological fractures are common. Bone resorption is due either to the direct action of tumour cells or to tumour-derived factors that stimulate osteoclastic activity. Osteoblastic lesions are uncommon; they usually occur in prostatic carcinoma.

prevent damage to the pelvic viscera usually result in inadequate surgery. If there are doubts in this regard, operation should be combined with local radiotherapy.

ADAMANTINOMA

This rare tumour has a predilection for the anterior cortex of the tibia but is occasionally found in other long bones. The patient is usually a young adult who complains of aching and mild swelling in the front of the leg. On examination there is thickening and tenderness along the subcutaneous border of the tibia.

X-ray shows a typical bubble-like defect in the anterior tibial cortex; sometimes there is thickening of the surrounding bone.

Adamantinoma is a low-grade tumour which metastasizes late – and usually only after repeated and inadequate attempts at removal. Early on it is confined to bone; later, *CT* may show that the tumour has extended inwards to the medullary canal or outwards beyond the periosteum.

Clinical features

The patient is usually aged 50-70 years; with any destructive bone lesion in this age group, the differential diagnosis must include metastasis.

Pain is the commonest – and often the only – clinical feature. The sudden appearance of backache or thigh pain in an elderly person (especially someone known to have been treated for carcinoma in the past) is always suspicious. If x-rays do not show anything, a radionuclide scan might.

Some deposits remain clinically silent and are discovered incidentally on x-ray, or after a pathological fracture. Sudden collapse of a vertebral body or a fracture of the mid-shaft of a long bone in an elderly

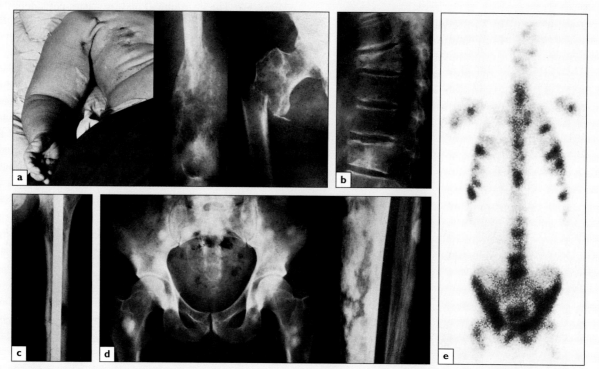

9.42 Metastatic deposits (a) This woman presents an all-too-familiar picture – breast cancer and mastectomy, followed by metastasis and pathological fracture. (b) Spinal secondary deposits. (c) Osteolytic deposits are liable to fracture and invite prophylactic fixation. (d) Osteoblastic deposits in the pelvis and tibia, from prostatic carcinoma. (e) Radioscintigraphy revealed some silent deposits in this patient.

person are ominous signs; if there is no history and no clinical clue pointing to a primary carcinoma, a biopsy of the fracture area is essential.

In children under 6 years of age, metastatic lesions are most commonly from adrenal neuroblastoma. The child presents with bone pain and fever; examination reveals the abdominal mass.

Symptoms of hypercalcaemia may occur (and are often missed) in patients with skeletal metastases. These include anorexia, nausea, thirst, polyuria, abdominal pain, general weakness and depression.

Imaging

X-ray Most skeletal deposits are osteolytic and appear as rarified areas in the medulla or produce a moth-eaten appearance in the cortex; sometimes there is marked bone destruction, with or without a pathological fracture. Osteoblastic deposits suggest a prostatic carcinoma; the pelvis may show a mottled increase in density which has to be distinguished from Paget's disease or lymphoma.

Radioscintigraphy Bone scans with ^{99m}Tc-HDP are the most sensitive method of detecting 'silent' metastatic deposits in bone; areas of increased activity are selected for x-ray examination.

Special investigations

The ESR may be increased and the haemoglobin concentration is usually low. The serum alkaline phosphatase concentration is often increased, and in prostatic carcinoma the acid phosphatase also is elevated.

Patients with breast cancer can be screened by measuring blood levels of tumour-associated antigen markers.

Treatment

By the time a patient has developed secondary deposits the prognosis for survival is almost hopeless. Occasionally, radical treatment (by combined surgery and radiotherapy) of a solitary secondary deposit and of its parent primary may be rewarding and even apparently curative. This applies particularly to hypernephroma and thyroid tumours; but in the great majority of cases, and certainly in those with multiple secondaries, treatment is entirely symptomatic. For that reason, elaborate witch-hunts to discover the source of an occult primary tumour are avoided, though it may be worthwhile investigating for tumours that are amenable to hormonal manipulation.

Despite the ultimately hopeless prognosis, patients deserve to be made comfortable, to enjoy (as far as possible) their remaining months or years, and to die in a peaceful and dignified way. The active treatment of skeletal metastases contributes to this in no small measure. In addition, patients need sympathetic counselling and practical assistance with their material affairs.

CONTROL OF PAIN AND METASTATIC ACTIVITY Most patients require analgesics, but the more powerful narcotics should be reserved for the terminally ill.

Unless specifically contraindicated, *radiotherapy* is used both to control pain and to reduce metastatic growth. This is often combined with other forms of treatment (e.g. internal fixation).

Secondary deposits from breast or prostate can often be controlled by *hormone therapy:* stilboestrol for prostatic secondaries and androgenic drugs or oestrogens for breast carcinoma. Disseminated secondaries from breast carcinoma are sometimes treated by oophorectomy combined with adrenalectomy or by hypophyseal ablation.

Hypercalcaemia may have serious consequences, including renal acidosis, nephrocalcinosis, unconsciousness and coma. It should be treated by ensuring adequate hydration, reducing the calcium intake and, if necessary, administering bisphosphonates.

TREATMENT OF FRACTURES Surgical timidity may condemn the patient to a painful lingering death, so shaft fractures should almost always be treated by internal fixation and (if necessary) packing with methylmethacrylate cement. If there are multiple fractures, more than one bone may be fixed at the same sitting, though one must bear in mind that the risk of fat embolism increases with multiple intramedullary nailing. Pain is immediately relieved, nursing is made easier and the patient can get up and about or attend for other types of treatment without unnecessary discomfort. Shaft fractures usually unite satisfactorily.

In most cases intramedullary nailing is the most effective method; fractures near joints (e.g. the distal femur or proximal tibia) may need fixation with plates or blade-plates.

Fractures of the femoral neck rarely, if ever, unite. They are best treated by prosthetic replacement: a hemiarthroplasty if the pelvis is intact, or total joint replacement if the acetabulum is involved. If the pelvic wall is destroyed, it can be reconstructed by large bone grafts or a custom-made prosthesis; however, if such extensive surgery is contraindicated, one may have to settle for a simple excisional arthroplasty.

Postoperative irradiation is essential to prevent further extension of the metastatic lesion.

PROPHYLACTIC FIXATION Large deposits that threaten to result in fracture should be treated by internal fixation while the bone is still intact. The principles are the same as for the management of fractures. A preoperative radionuclide scan will show whether other lesions are present in that bone, thus calling for more extensive fixation and postoperative radiotherapy.

SPINAL STABILIZATION Vertebral fractures usually require some form of support. If the spine is stable, a well-fitting brace may be sufficient. However, spinal instability may cause severe pain, making it almost impossible for the patient to sit or stand – with or without a brace. For these patients, operative stabilization is indicated – usually a posterior spinal fusion – followed by radiotherapy.

Preoperative assessment should include CT or MRI, and sometimes myelography, to establish whether the cord is threatened; if it is, spinal decompression should be carried out at the same time.

If there are overt symptoms and signs of cord compression, treatment is urgent. If the patient is expected to live for some time, surgical decompression and fusion are indicated. With improved methods of fixation, the results of posterior decompression and stabilization are probably as good as those of (the more difficult) anterior spinal surgery (Bauer, 1997). If the patient is in a terminal stage, it may be more humane to give radiotherapy, alone or together with corticosteroids and narcotics, to control oedema and pain.

SOFT-TISSUE TUMOURS

Benign soft-tissue tumours are common, malignant ones rare. The distinction between these two groups is not always easy, and some lesions, treated confidently as 'benign', recur in more aggressive form after inadequate removal. Features suggestive of malignancy are: pain in a previously painless lump; a rapid increase in size; poor demarcation; and attachment to the surrounding structures. Sonograms of malignant lesions are said to show a discrete echo pattern, whereas with benign lesions the pattern may be ill-defined (Lange *et al.*, 1987). When doubt exists, a biopsy is essential. Wherever possible this should take the form of an excisional biopsy, including a wide margin of normal tissue around the tumour. As with bone tumours, special imaging and staging should be carried out before the field is disturbed by operation (Sim *et al.*, 1994). Chest x-rays and blood investigations may be necessary as well.

The account that follows is intended as a summary of those soft-tissue tumours likely to be encountered in orthopaedics.

FATTY TUMOURS

LIPOMA

A lipoma, one of the commonest of all tumours, may occur almost anywhere; sometimes there are multiple lesions. The tumour usually arises in the subcutaneous layer. It consists of lobules of fat with a surrounding

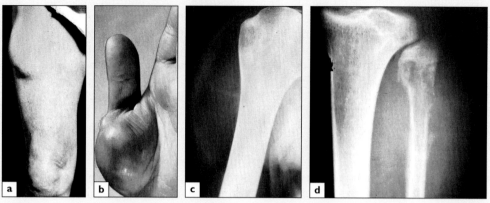

9.43 Fatty tumours (a) Subcutaneous lipoma – like so many lipomas, this one felt almost fluctuant; (b) intramuscular lipoma; (c) subperiosteal lipoma; (d) liposarcoma – the cortex of the fibula has been eroded.

capsule which may become tethered to neighbouring structures. The patient, usually aged over 50 years, complains of a painless swelling. The lump is soft and almost fluctuant; the well-defined edge and lobulated surface distinguish it from a chronic abscess. Fat is notably radiotranslucent, a feature that betrays the occasional subperiosteal lipoma.

If the lump is troublesome it may be removed by marginal excision. Prior biopsy is usually unnecessary; however, one should never be complacent about a 'lipoma' and if there are any atypical features, preoperative staging and biopsy are essential in order to avoid the risk of performing a marginal excision and then discovering that the lesion was malignant.

LIPOSARCOMA

Liposarcoma is rare but should be suspected if a fatty tumour (especially in the buttock or thigh) goes on growing and becomes painful. The lump may feel quite firm and is usually not translucent. CT or MRI is essential to determine the extent of the tumour.

Treatment depends on the degree of malignancy. Low-grade lesions can be removed by wide excision; high-grade tumours need radical resection. For liposarcomas in inaccessible sites, radiation therapy is often effective.

FIBROUS TUMOURS

FIBROMA

The common fibroma is a solitary, benign tumour of fibrous tissue. It is usually discovered as a small asymptomatic nodule or lump. Treatment is not essential; if it is removed, a marginal excision is adequate.

FIBROMATOSIS

This term is applied to lesions that are more aggressive than simple fibromas and have a strong tendency to recur after excision. They appear, usually in young adults, as thick cords or plaques in the subcutaneous tissues of the limbs or trunk. If left, they grow into featureless masses with ill-defined margins, sometimes extending proximally up the limb or along the trunk. After local excision they tend to recur, and new lesions appear more and more proximally. Pressure on nerves may cause paraesthesiae. CT and MRI are useful to show the extent of this invasive tumour.

Although not malignant in the true sense of the term, the lesion can be highly aggressive. Local excision is often performed too timidly, and the recurrences are more and more invasive and difficult to eradicate without damage to nerves or blood vessels. Wide excision is essential, especially if the lesion threatens to involve the pelvis or axilla; once this has occurred, complete removal may be impossible. Occasionally, amputation is the only solution.

Microscopically these lesions vary from those with clearly benign cells to some whose appearance suggests malignancy (multinucleated cells with many mitoses). The differentiation from fribrosarcoma is difficult and demands considerable histological expertise; but it is important because fibromatosis does not metastasize and can be eradicated if surgery is sufficiently thorough.

FIBROSARCOMA

Fibrosarcoma may occur in any area of connective tissue but is more common in the extremities. It presents as an ill-defined, painless mass and may grow to a considerable size. The diagnosis is usually made only after biopsy and histological examination. Local extension can be shown on MRI. There may be metastases in the lungs.

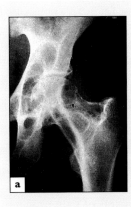
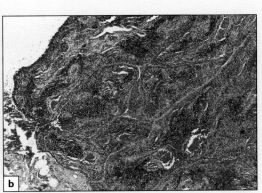

9.44 Pigmented villonodular synovitis
(**a**) A farmer presented with pain in the hip. The x-rays showing cystic excavations on both sides of the joint at first suggested tuberculosis. However, there were no signs of infection. At operation the synovium was thick and golden in colour. (**b**) The biopsy showed dense proliferation of the synovium with scattered multinucleated giant cells. (×120)

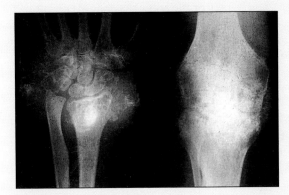

9.45 Malignant synoviomas X-rays showing the so-called snowstorm appearance.

High-grade lesions showing atypical spindle cells are usually easy to diagnose. Low-grade lesions may be difficult to distinguish from fibromatosis.

For *low-grade lesions*, wide excision is usually sufficient. For *high-grade lesions*, wide excision should be supplemented by preoperative and postoperative radiation therapy.

SYNOVIAL TUMOURS

PIGMENTED VILLONODULAR SYNOVITIS AND GIANT-CELL TUMOUR OF TENDON SHEATH

These are two forms of the same condition – a benign disorder that occurs wherever synovial membrane is found: in joints, tendon sheaths or bursae.

Pigmented villonodular synovitis (PVNS) presents as a long-standing boggy swelling of the joint – usually the hip, knee or ankle – in an adolescent or young adult. X-ray may show excavations in the juxta-articular bone on either side of the joint. When the joint is opened, the synovium is swollen and hyperplastic, often covered with villi and golden-brown in colour – the effect of haemosiderin deposition. The juxta-articular excavations contain clumps of friable synovial material.

Tendon sheath lesions are seen mainly in the hands and feet, where they cause nodular thickening of the affected sheath. X-ray may show pressure erosion of an adjacent bone surface – for example, on one of the phalanges. At operation the boggy synovial tissue is often yellow; this type of lesion is sometimes called *xanthoma of tendon sheath*.

PATHOLOGY Histologically, joint and tendon sheath lesions are identical. There is proliferation and hypertrophy of the synovium, which contains fibroblastic tissue with foamy histiocytes and multinucleated giant cells. These features have engendered yet another name for the same condition: *giant-cell tumour of tendon sheath*.

TREATMENT The only effective treatment is synovectomy. Although the tumour does not undergo malignant change, the recurrence rate is high unless excision is complete. This may be unattainable and subtotal synovectomy is then sometimes combined with local radiotherapy. If, despite such aggressive treatment, there are repeated recurrences, it may be necessary to sacrifice the joint and carry out arthroplasty or arthrodesis.

SYNOVIAL SARCOMA (MALIGNANT SYNOVIOMA)

This rare malignant tumour of synovium causes rapid enlargement of the joint, usually around the knee, hip or shoulder. Occasionally it presents as a small swelling in the hand or foot and the histological diagnosis comes as a complete surprise. X-ray shows a soft-tissue mass, sometimes with extensive calcification. MRI will help to outline the tumour.

Biopsy reveals a fleshy lesion composed of proliferative synovial cells and fibroblastic tissue; characteristically the cellular areas are punctured by vacant slits that give the tissue an acinar appearance. Cellular abnormality and mitoses reflect the degree of malignancy.

Small, well-defined lesions can be treated by wide excision. High-grade lesions, which usually have ill-defined margins, require radical resection – and this may mean radical amputation – combined with radiotherapy and chemotherapy.

BLOOD VESSEL TUMOURS

HAEMANGIOMA

This benign lesion, probably a hamartoma, is usually seen during childhood but may be present at birth. It occurs in two forms. The *capillary haemangioma* is more common; it usually appears as a reddish patch on the skin, and the congenital naevus or 'birthmark' is a familiar example. A *cavernous haemangioma* consists of a sponge-like collection of blood spaces; superficial lesions appear as blue or purple skin patches, sometimes overlying a soft subcutaneous mass; deep lesions may extend into the fascia or muscles, and occasionally an entire limb is involved. X-rays may show calcified phleboliths in the cavernous lesions.

There is no risk of malignant change and treatment is needed only if there is significant discomfort or disability. Local excision carries a high risk of recurrence, but more radical procedures seem unnecessarily destructive.

GLOMUS TUMOUR

This rare tumour usually occurs around fine peripheral neurovascular structures, and especially in the nail beds of fingers or toes. A young adult presents with recurrent episodes of intense pain in the fingertip. A small bluish nodule may be seen under the nail; the area is sensitive to cold and exquisitely tender. X-rays sometimes show erosion of the underlying phalanx. Treatment is excision; the tumour, never larger than a pea, is easily shelled out of its fibrous capsule.

NERVE TUMOURS

NEUROMA

A neuroma is not a tumour but an overgrowth of fibrous tissue and randomly sprouting nerve fibrils following injury to a nerve. It is often tender and local percussion may induce paraesthesiae distal to the lesion (Tinel's sign).

Treatment can be frustrating. Many techniques have been described, suggesting that none is uniformly satisfactory; they include resection followed by nerve grafting, resection with implantation of the stump into muscle, bone or vein, and 'capping' with tissue glue within the epineural sleeve.

NEURILEMMOMA

Neurilemmoma is a benign tumour of the nerve sheath. It is seen in the peripheral nerves and in the spinal nerve roots. The patient complains of pain or paraesthesiae; sometimes there is a small palpable swelling along the course of the nerve.

Growth on a spinal nerve root is a rare cause of 'sciatica', and x-rays of the spine may show erosion of the intervertebral foramen at that level. MRI or high-resolution ultrasound will demonstrate the eccentric swelling on a peripheral nerve.

With careful dissection the tumour can be removed from its capsule without damage to the nerve.

NEUROFIBROMA

This is a benign tumour of fibrous and neural elements; its origin in a peripheral nerve may be obvious, but it is also seen as a nodule in the skin or subcutaneous tissues where it presumably originates in fine nerve fibrils. Occasionally it arises directly in bone; more often it causes pressure erosion of an adjacent surface.

Lesions may be solitary or multiple. Curiously, they are sometimes associated with skeletal abnormalities (scoliosis, pseudarthrosis of the tibia) or overgrowth of a digit or an entire limb, in which there is no obvious neural pathology.

The patient may present with a lump overlying one of the peripheral nerves, or with neurological symptoms such as paraesthesiae or muscle weakness. If a nerve root is involved, symptoms can mimic those of a disc prolapse; x-rays may show erosion of a vertebral pedicle or enlargement of the intervertebral foramen.

Multiple neurofibromatosis (von Recklinghausen's disease) is transmitted by autosomal dominant inheritance (see page 155). Patients (usually children) develop numerous skin nodules and café-au-lait patches; there may be associated skeletal abnormalities. Malignant transformation is said to occur in 5–10% of cases.

The pathological appearances are characteristic: on cross-section the tumour consists of pale fibrous tissue with nerve elements running into and through the substance of the tumour. Microscopically, the fibrillar and cellular elements are arranged in a wavy pattern.

Treatment is needed only if pain or paraesthesiae become troublesome, or if a tumour becomes very large. The tumour cannot be separated from intact

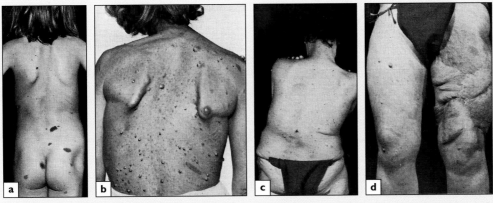

9.46 Neurofibromatosis (**a**) Café-au-lait spots, (**b**) multiple fibromata and slight scoliosis; (**c, d**) a patient with scoliosis and elephantiasis.

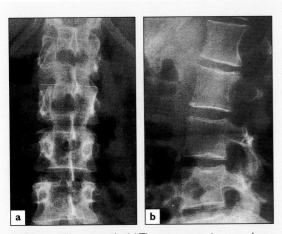

9.47 Neurofibromatosis (**a**) The anteroposterior x-ray shows erosion of the pedicles of L1 and L2. Compare the appearance with the well-marked pedicles (like staring eyes) at L3 and L4. (**b**) The lateral view shows scalloping of the backs of L1 and L1.

nerve fibres; if it involves an unimportant nerve, it can be excised en bloc; if nerve damage is not acceptable, intracapsular shelling out is preferable, notwithstanding the risk of recurrence.

NEUROSARCOMA (MALIGNANT SCHWANNOMA)

Malignant tumours may arise from the cells of the nerve sheath or from a pre-existing neurofibroma. Symptoms are due to local pressure. There may be a visible or palpable swelling and percussion causes distal paraesthesiae.

Histologically this is a cellular fibrous lesion.

If the tumour arises in the neurovascular bundle, spread is inevitable and local excision is not feasible without severe damage to important structures. For this reason, treatment usually involves amputation.

MUSCLE TUMOURS

Tumours of muscle are rare; only those that occur in the striped muscle of the extremities are considered here.

RHABDOMYOMA

Rhabdomyoma is a rare cause of a lump in the muscle. It is occasionally confused with the 'lump' that appears after muscle rupture: both are in the line of a muscle, can be moved across but not along it, and harden with muscle contraction. However, with muscle rupture symptoms appear quite suddenly, there is a depression proximal or distal to the lump and the swelling does not grow any bigger. If a tumour is suspected, early exploration and biopsy are advisable because malignant change may occur. If the diagnosis is confirmed, the tumour should be excised.

RHABDOMYOSARCOMA

Malignant tumours are occasionally seen in the muscles around the shoulder or hip. The patient – usually a young adult – presents with ache and an enlarging, ill-defined lump that moves with the affected muscle. CT and MRI show that the mass is in the muscle, but the edge may be poorly demarcated because the tumour tends to spread along the fascial planes. At biopsy the tissue looks and feels different from normal muscle and microscopic examination shows clusters of highly abnormal muscle cells.

This is a high-grade lesion which requires radical resection of the affected muscle – i.e. from its origin to its insertion. If this cannot be assured or if the tumour has spread beyond the fascial sheath, amputation is advisable. Recurrent lesions are also treated by amputation. If complete removal is impossible, adjunctive radiotherapy may lessen the risk of recurrence.

REFERENCES AND FURTHER READING

American Joint Committee on Cancer (1997) Bone. In: *AJCC Cancer Staging Manual*, 5th edn, ed ID Fleming *et al.* Lippincott-Raven, Philadelphia

Bauer HCF (1997) Posterior decompression and stabilization for spinal metastases: Analysis of sixty-seven consecutive patients. *Journal of Bone and Joint Surgery* 79A, 514–522

Cannon, S.R. (1986) Massive osteolysis. Journal of Bone and Joint Surgery 68B, 24–28

Donnelly LF, Bisset GF, Helms CA *et al.* (1999) Chronic avulsive injuries of childhood. *Skeletal Radiology* 28, 138-144

Enneking WF (1986) A system of staging musculoskeletal neoplasms. *Clinical Orthopaedics and Related Research* 204, 9-24

Horowitz SM, Glasser DB, Lane JM, Healy JH (1993) Prosthetic and extremity survivorship after limb salvage for sarcoma. *Clinical Orthopaedics* 295, 280-286

Lange TA, Austin CW, Siebert JJ *et al.* (1987) Ultrasound imaging as a screening study for malignant soft tissue tumours. *Journal of Bone and Joint Surgery* 69A, 100-105

Malghem J, Maldague B, Esselinckx W *et al.* (1989) Spontaneous healing of aneurysmal bone cysts. *Journal of Bone and Joint Surgery* 71B, 645-650

Mankin HJ, Gebhardt MC (1985) Advances in the management of bone tumours. *Clinical Orthopaedics and Related Research* 200, 73-84

Mankin HJ, Lange TA, Spanier SS (1982) The hazards of biopsy in patients with malignant primary bone and soft-tissue tumors. *Journal of Bone and Joint Surgery* 64A, 1121-1127

McLeod RA, Dahlin DC, Beabout JW (1976) The spectrum of osteoblastoma. *American Journal of Roentgenology* 126, 321-335

Peabody TD, Gibbs CP, Simon MA (1998) Evaluation and staging of musculoskeletal neoplasms. *Journal of Bone and Joint Surgery* 80A, 1204-1218

Pettersson H, Gillespy T, Hamlin DJ *et al.* (1987) Primary musculoskeletal tumors: examination with MR imaging compared with conventional modalities. *Radiology* 164, 237-241

Roberts P, Chan D, Grimer RJ *et al.* (1991) Prosthetic replacement of the distal femur for primary bone tumours. *Journal of Bone and Joint Surgery* 73B, 762-769

Rosen G (1987) Neoadjuvant chemotherapy for osteogenic sarcoma. In: *Limb Salvage in Musculoskeletal Oncology*, ed WF Enneking. Churchill Livingstone, New York

Rosen G, Caparrow B, Huvos AG *et al.* (1982) Pre-operative chemotherapy for osteogenic sarcoma: selection of post-operative chemotherapy based on the response of the primary tumor to pre-operative chemotherapy. *Cancer* 49, 1221-1230

Souhami RL, Craft AW (1988) Annotation: Progress in management of malignant bone tumours. *Journal of Bone and Joint Surgery* 70B, 345-347

Stark A, Kreicbergs A, Nilsonne U, Sillvensward L (1990) The age of osteosarcoma patients is increasing. *Journal of Bone and Joint Surgery* 72, 89-93

Sim FH, Frassica FJ, Frassica DA (1994) Soft-tissue tumours: Diagnosis, evaluation and management. *Journal of the American Academy of Orthopaedic Surgeons* 2, 202-211

Watt I (1985) Radiology in the diagnosis and management of bone tumours. *Journal of Bone and Joint Surgery* 67B, 520-529

NERVES AND MUSCLES

The neuron

The neuron is the specialized cell of the nervous system, capable of electrical excitation and conduction of impulses (action potentials) along one of its thread-like extensions – the axon. Motor axons carry efferent impulses to the periphery; sensory axons carry afferent impulses to the spinal cord or brain.

Peripheral nerves carry motor, sensory and autonomic fibres. Motor axons run from cells in the anterior horn of the spinal cord to striated muscle throughout the body. Sensory neurons have their cells in the dorsal root (or cranial nerve) ganglia; they carry impulses from receptors in the skin and deep structures. Autonomic sympathetic axons arise from cells in the thoracolumbar cord; preganglionic fibres leave with the ventral roots to enter the sympathetic chain and synapse with postganglionic fibres that supply blood vessels and sweat glands in the periphery. Parasympathetic fibres pass from the cord and synapse in ganglia close to their target organs.

Peripheral nerve structure is described in Chapter 11. Here it should merely be noted that nerves carry a mixture of myelinated and unmyelinated axons; the former include all motor axons and the larger sensory axons serving touch, pain and proprioception, while the latter (much the more numerous) are small-diameter sensory fibres serving crude touch, pain and warmth and sympathetic vasomotor and sudomotor fibres. Damage to the myelin sheath – by either disease or injury – will cause slowing of conduction and, eventually, loss of sensory and motor functions.

Axons carry the impulse along the nerve pathway by a series of relays, or synapses, where the message is passed on by chemical neurotransmitters – chiefly acetylcholine. For a motor neuron the cell body is in the anterior horn of the spinal cord and the terminal synapse is at the neuromuscular junction. Sensory neurons have their cell bodies in the dorsal root ganglia and their synapses in the spinal cord.

Each motor neuron innervates hundreds of muscle fibres. Normal resting muscle tone is maintained by a reflex arc consisting of fast-conducting sensory fibres from the muscle spindles (stretch receptors) and alpha motor neurons. Sudden stretching of the muscle (e.g. by tapping the tendon sharply) induces an involuntary muscle contraction – the stretch reflex. This reflex is normally monitored or controlled by impulses passing from the brain down the spinal cord. Interruption of the central nervous pathways (the upper motor neurons) results in undamped reflex contraction and spastic paralysis. Damage to the anterior horn cells or peripheral motor nerves causes flaccid paralysis.

Muscle

Skeletal muscle is striated muscle. Each muscle belly consists of thousands of muscle fibres, each of which is made up of many tiny (1μm diameter) myofibrils. The motor neuron and the group of muscle fibres supplied by it make up a motor unit.

Muscle fibres are of different types, which can be distinguished by histochemical staining. Type I fibres contract slowly and are not easily fatigued; their prime function is postural control. Type II fibres are fast contracting and are rapidly fatigued; they are ideally suited to intense

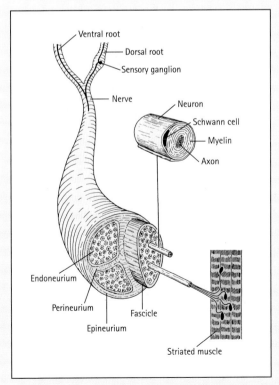

10.1 Nerve structure Diagram of the structural elements of a peripheral nerve.

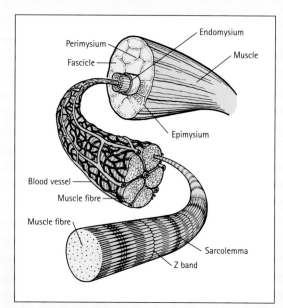

10.2 Muscle structure Diagrams showing the structural elements of striated muscle.

activities of short duration. The muscles of the body comprise a mixture of fibre types, the proportions varying from person to person. The average individual has 50% type I and 50% type II fibres, and long-distance runners have more type I fibres.

Muscle contraction is a complex activity. Individual myofibrils respond to electrical stimuli in much the same way as do motor neurons. However, muscle fibres (which consist of bundles of myofibrils), and the muscle as a whole, are activated by overlap and summation of contractile responses. When the fibres contract, internal tension in the muscle increases. In *isometric contraction* there is increased tension without actual shortening of the muscle or movement of the joint controlled by that muscle. In *isotonic contraction* the muscle shortens and moves the joint, but tension within the muscle fibres remains constant.

Muscle tone is the state of tension in a resting muscle when it is passively stretched; characteristically tone is increased in upper motor neuron (UMN) lesions (spastic paralysis) and decreased in lower motor neurone (LMN) lesions (flaccid paralysis).

Muscle contracture (as distinct from contraction) is the adaptive change which occurs when a normally innervated muscle is held immobile in a shortened position for some length of time. If a joint is allowed to be held flexed for a long time, it may be impossible to straighten it passively without injuring the muscle. Active exercise will eventually overcome the muscle contracture, unless the muscle has been permanently damaged.

Muscle wasting follows either disuse or denervation; in the former, the fibres are intact but thinner; in the latter, they degenerate and are replaced by fibrous tissue or fat.

CLINICAL ASSESSMENT

History

Age is important. Cerebral palsy and spina bifida present during infancy. Poliomyelitis usually occurs in childhood but may be seen at any age. Spinal cord lesions and peripheral neuropathies are more common in adults. However, the orthopaedic surgeon deals mainly with the residual effects of neurological disease, and these may require diagnosis and treatment throughout life.

Muscle weakness may be due to UMN lesions (spastic paresis), LMN (flaccid paresis) or muscle disorders. The type of weakness, its distribution and rate of onset are important clues to diagnosis.

Numbness and paraesthesiae may be the main complaints. It is important to establish their exact distribution as this will often localize the lesion accurately. The rate of onset and the relationship to posture may, likewise, suggest the cause.

Deformity is a common complaint in long-standing disorders. It arises from muscle imbalance (see below) and therefore usually goes hand in hand with other symptoms. However, minor degrees of weakness in one muscle group may go unnoticed and the deformity appears so insidiously that its cause may escape detection (e.g. claw toes or scoliosis).

Other features such as headache, dizziness, loss of balance, change in visual acuity or hearing, disorder of speech and loss of bladder or bowel control may be significant.

Examination

Examination should include a complete neurological assessment. Particular attention should be paid to the patient's mental state, natural posture, gait, sense of balance, involuntary movements, muscle wasting, muscle tone and power, reflexes, skin changes, the various modes of sensibility and autonomic functions such as sphincter control, peripheral blood flow and sweating.

The back should be examined for skin changes, local deformities (e.g. a kyphos) and mobility.

Table 10.1 Nerve root supply and actions of main muscle groups

Sternomastoids	Spinal accessory C2, 3, 4
Trapezius	Spinal accessory C3, 4
Diaphragm	C3, 4, 5
Deltoid	C5, 6
Supra- and infraspinatus	C5, 6
Serratus anterior	C5, 6, 7
Pectoralis major	C5, 6, 7, 8
Elbow flexion	C5, 6
extension	C7
Supination	C5, 6
Pronation	C6
Wrist extension	C6, (7)
flexion	C7, (8)
Finger extension	C7
flexion	C7, 8, T1
ab- and adduction	C8, T1
Hip flexion	L1, 2, 3
extension	L5, S1
adduction	L2, 3, 4
abduction	L4, 5, S1
Knee extension	L(2), 3, 4
flexion	L5, S1
Ankle dorsiflexion	L4, 5
plantarflexion	S1, 2
inversion	L4, 5
eversion	L5, S1
Toe extension	L5
flexion	S1
abduction	S1, 2

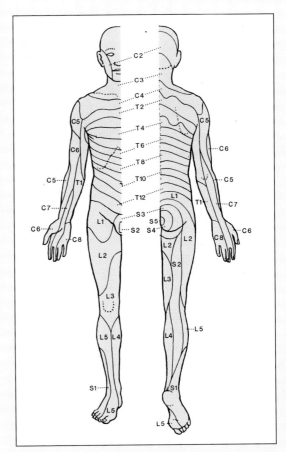

10.3 Examination Dermatomes supplied by the spinal nerve roots.

GRADING MUSCLE POWER

In assessment it is important to examine not only *individual muscles* but also *functional groups*. Grading muscle power is most valuable in the flaccid paralysis associated with spina bifida and poliomyelitis; in cerebral palsy, grading is useful but difficult because spasticity of the muscle obscures the inherent weakness.

Muscle charting pinpoints the site and severity of paralysis; repetition enables progress to be recorded. The following grades are standard:

0 total paralysis
1 barely detectable contracture
2 not enough power to act against gravity
3 strong enough to act against gravity
4 still stronger but less than normal
5 full power

DEFORMITY

In long-standing disorders, deformity may become a major problem. It arises when one group of muscles is too weak to balance the pull of antagonists (*unbalanced paralysis*). At first it can be corrected passively but with

time the active muscles and joint structures contract and the deformity becomes fixed.

When all muscle groups are equally weak (*balanced paralysis*) the joint simply assumes the position imposed on it by gravity. The joint is unstable and, on examination, the limb feels floppy or flail.

Paralysis arising in childhood seriously affects bone growth. The bone is both thinner and shorter than normal and, in the absence of the mechanical stresses normally imposed by muscle pull, modelling is defective. The bone ends may appear dysplastic and there may be loss of joint congruity. A good example is the common valgus deformity of the femoral neck, with acetabular dysplasia and hip subluxation, resulting from childhood weakness of the hip abductors.

GAIT AND POSTURE

Watching the patient walk is most valuable. With experience, certain typical patterns will be recognized.

A spastic gait is stiff and jerky, often with the feet in equinus, the knees somewhat flexed and the hips adducted ('scissoring').

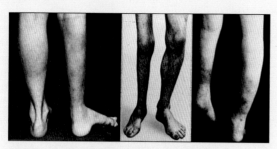

10.4 Some effects of neurological lesions These patients, all of whom had polio, illustrate some of the effects of paralysis – deformity, wasting and shortening; the trophic changes in the patient on the right suggest that, in her, the anterolateral horn cells also may have been damaged.

The term *dystonia* refers to abnormal posturing of any part of the body, often aggravated when the patient concentrates on movement (see box).

Causes of dystonia
Generalized
1 Cerebral disorders, most commonly cerebral palsy, stroke and Huntington's disease
2 Drug-induced
Focal dystonia
1 Stroke (hemiplegia of monoplegia)
2 Spasmodic torticollis
3 Writer's cramp

A *high-stepping gait*, where the legs are lifted unnecessarily high off the ground, signifies either a problem with proprioception and balance or bilateral foot drop.

A *drop-foot gait* is due to peripheral neuropathy or injury of the nerves supplying the dorsiflexors of the ankle. During the swing phase the foot falls into equinus ('drops') and if it were not lifted higher than usual the toes would drag along the ground.

A *waddling gait*, in which the trunk is thrown from side to side with each step, may be due to dislocation of the hips or to weakness of the abductor muscles.

Ataxia produces a more obvious and irregular loss of balance, which is compensated for by a broad-based gait, or sometimes uncontrollable staggering.

Imaging studies

Plain x-rays of the skull and/or spine are routine for all disorders of the central nervous system. If the diagnosis is not obvious, further studies by myelography, computed tomography (CT) or magnetic resonance imaging (MRI) may be necessary.

Imaging of the spine is essentially aimed at demonstrating compression of the spinal cord or nerve roots.

Fractures and dislocations usually show on the plain x-rays but a CT scan will reveal the exact relationship of bone fragments to nerve structures.

Prolapsed intervertebral disc is usually diagnosed on clinical examination, but myelography, CT and MRI will help to establish the extent of the lesion and its exact site.

Narrowing of the spinal canal is best demonstrated by CT. The commonest cause is osteophytic overgrowth following disc degeneration and osteoarthritis of the facet joints. This is even worse when the spinal canal is congenitally narrow or trefoil-shaped (spinal stenosis).

Destructive lesions of the bones may be due to infection or tumour (usually metastatic lesions). These may show on plain x-rays but CT, MRI and myelography are helpful.

Electrodiagnosis

Neurophysiological studies, though hardly part of the routine examination, can be extremely helpful in elucidating less obvious syndromes. Electromyography (EMG) records the motor response to nerve stimuli. It is of greatest use in deciding whether muscle weakness is due to nerve or muscle disorder. Nerve conduction studies help in establishing the site of compression in peripheral nerve entrapment.

Other special investigations

Depending on the type of disorder, diagnostic investigations may include blood tests [cell counts, erythrocyte sedimentation rate (ESR), serology, blood sugar, muscle enzymes], cerebrospinal fluid (CSF) examination and specialized tests for vision, hearing, speech and mental capacity.

MUSCLE BIOPSY A biopsy may yield valuable information in diagnosing muscle disorders. However, for the findings to be reliable, certain precautions are necessary. The sample should be taken from an affected muscle, but one that is still working; the muscle itself must not be injected with local anaesthetic; the specimen, about 2cm long and 1cm wide, should be handled gently and kept at the natural fibre length by laying it on a wooden spatula and securing the two ends with stitches before placing it in fixative.

Specimens for light microscopy are fixed in 10% formalin; those for electron microscopy in glutaraldehyde; and those for histochemical staining are frozen at $-160°C$.

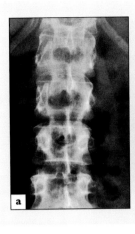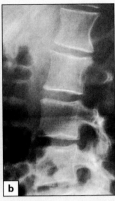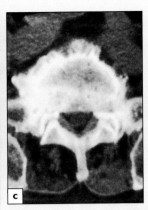

10.5 Imaging (**a**) In the lower two vertebrae the pedicles are seen end on and look like eyes; the upper two vertebrae are 'blind' because the pedicles have been destroyed by tumour. (**b**) The scalloping at the back of the upper two vertebrae is typical of a neurofibroma. (**c**) This CT shows degeneration of the facet joints with encroachment on the intervertebral foramina and spinal canal.

CEREBRAL PALSY

The term 'cerebral palsy' includes a group of disorders that result from non-progressive brain damage during early development. The incidence is about 2 per 1000 live births. Known causal factors are maternal toxaemia, prematurity, perinatal anoxia, kernicterus and postnatal brain infections or injury; birth injury, though often blamed, is a distinctly unusual cause. The main consequence is the development of neuromuscular incoordination, dystonia, weakness and spasticity; in addition there may be convulsions, perceptual problems, speech disorder and mental retardation or behavioural problems.

Classification

Cerebral palsy is usually classified according to the type of motor dysfunction, with further subdivisions referring to the topographical distribution of the clinical signs.

TYPE OF MOTOR DYSFUNCTION
- *Spastic palsy* is the commonest variety, accounting for over 60% of all cases. It is characterized by increased muscle tone and hyperactive reflexes; the resistance to passive movement may obscure a basic weakness of the affected muscles.

- *Athetosis* manifests as continuous, involuntary, writhing movements. The patient's body seems to be out of control, yet he or she is usually capable of surprisingly good function. Tongue and speech muscles may be involved and this can give a mistaken impression of mental retardation.

- *Ataxia* appears in the form of muscular incoordination during voluntary movements. Balance is poor and the patient walks with a characteristic wide-based gait.

- *Rigid palsy* differs from spastic palsy in that the muscles are in a constant state of contraction and do not 'give' on passive movement.

- *Mixed palsy* appears as a combination of spasticity and athetosis.

TOPOGRAPHIC DISTRIBUTION
- *Hemiplegia* is the commonest. This usually appears as a spastic palsy of the upper and lower limbs on one side of the body. Most of these children can walk and they respond reasonably well to treatment.

- *Diplegia* affects mainly the lower limbs; almost invariably there are also milder features in the upper limbs.

- *Total body involvement* describes a general disorder affecting all four limbs, the trunk, neck and face with varying degrees of severity. Patients usually have a low intelligence quota (IQ), they are unable to walk and the response to treatment is poor.

- *Other terms*, such as monoplegia, triplegia and tetraplegia, are also used but they are too specific and careful examination will almost always show that other areas are involved as well.

Early diagnosis

The full-blown clinical picture may take months or even years to develop. Diagnosis in infancy calls for painstaking examination. A history of prenatal toxaemia, haemorrhage, premature birth, difficult labour, fetal distress or kernicterus should arouse suspicion. Early symptoms include difficulty in sucking and swallowing, with dribbling at the mouth. The mother may notice that the baby feels stiff or wriggles awkwardly.

Gradually it becomes apparent that the milestones are delayed (the normal child holds up its head at 3 months, sits up at 6 months and begins walking at about 1 year).

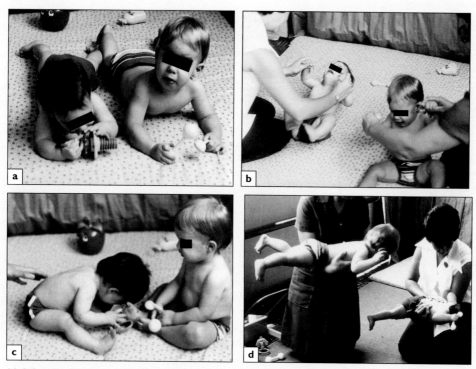

10.6 Cerebral palsy – early diagnosis By 6 months these twin brothers had developed quite differently, the one being smaller and showing (**a**) lack of head and arm control, (**b**) lack of body control when helped to the sitting position, (**c**) inability to sit unaided, and (**d**) lack of the normal extension response when turned face downwards.

Neonatal reflexes (e.g. the grasp reflex, withdrawal reflexes and sucking reflexes) may be delayed.

Bleck (1987) has described seven tests for children over 1 year; these give an idea of severity and of the prognosis for walking. The primitive neck-righting reflex, asymmetrical and symmetrical tonic neck reflexes, the Moro reflex and the extensor thrust response should all have disappeared at 1 year. The 'parachute reflex' and the stepping reflex should be present. If several of these are abnormal, the prognosis for walking is poor.

Clinical features in children over 1 year

Since cerebral palsy is essentially a disorder of posture and movement, the child should be carefully observed sitting, standing, walking and lying. Dystonia (abnormal posture of some part of the body, aggravated by attempts at movement) may be obvious but it is essential to carry out a detailed examination of the limbs and trunk. It is important also to assess speech, hearing, visual acuity, intelligence, psychological attitude and social adjustment. Optimal management is provided by a multidisciplinary team consisting of a paediatrician, orthopaedic surgeon, neurologist, psychologist, speech therapist, physiotherapist, occupational therapist, remedial teacher and social worker.

SITTING POSTURE The child may find it difficult to sit unsupported; hypotonic children will slump forward. The lower limbs may be thrust into extension. Note also whether there is scoliosis or a skew pelvis.

STANDING POSTURE Scoliosis and pelvic obliquity are common; it is important to establish whether these deformities are fixed or correctable when the spine is flexed. In the typical spastic posture the child stands with the hips flexed, adducted and internally rotated, the knees bent and the feet in equinus. If the hamstrings are tight there may be flattening of the normal lumbar lordosis and the child may have difficulty standing unsupported. Indeed, any attempt to correct one spastic deformity may aggravate another and it is important to establish whether the deformity is primary or compensatory.

Equilibrium reactions are tested by gently pushing the child forwards, backwards or sideways; normal children take a step to maintain balance, spastic children may simply topple over.

GAIT If the child can walk unsupported, the elements of gait are analysed; it is important to observe limb movement in the swing phase as well as limb posture in the stance phase. In hemiplegics asymmetric flexed-knee toe-walking is characteristic. Ataxia or athetoid movement also may now be obvious.

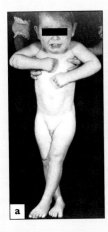
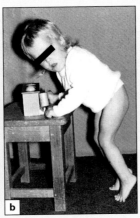
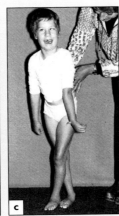

10.7 Cerebral palsy (**a**) Scissors stance; (**b**) flexion deformity of hips and knees with equinus of the feet; (**c**) characteristic facial expression and limb deformities.

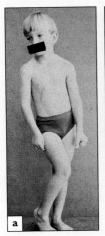
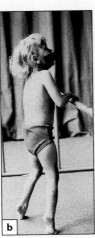
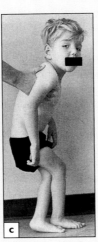
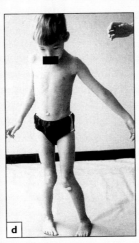

10.8 Spastic palsy Common types of spastic palsy: (**a**) hemiplegic, (**b**) diplegic, (**c**) tetraplegic and (**d**) ataxic.

In spastic diplegia a common gait abnormality is a tendency to walk with the hips flexed and adducted (scissors gait); the trunk leans forward, the knees are bent and the feet are held in equinus. The lack of free rotation at the hip makes it necessary to swivel the trunk from side to side as each leg swings through. The narrow walking base (due to hip adduction) and the tendency to fall forward (due to hip and knee flexion and equinus) are often dealt with by using crutches. Correction of these deformities is therefore an important objective.

A good account of gait patterns in cerebral palsy is given by Sutherland and Davids (1995).

Computerized gait analysis, including video sequences, force plate studies and EMG, provides more detailed information than simple observation, and energy expenditure can be measured at the same time. Where these facilities are available they may be helpful in the detailed planning of treatment.

NEUROMUSCULAR EXAMINATION Examination of the limbs shows the typical features of upper motor neuron or spastic paresis. Passive movements are resisted, the reflexes are exaggerated and there is a positive Babinski

response. However, spasticity may obscure the fact that muscle power is actually weak.

DEFORMITIES Deformity at one level may be markedly influenced by the positions of the joints above or below. Equinus is often correctable if the knee is flexed; and knee flexion deformity (due to tight hamstrings) is made worse by flexing and abducting the hips. Flexion deformity of the hip may be unmasked by Thomas' test.

In the upper limb, fingers may be tightly flexed with the wrist in extension, but uncurl quite easily when the wrist is flexed. The child uses these fixed-length reactions to manipulate the hands and fingers in a variety of ways (so-called trick movements).

In total body palsy spinal deformity is common. This is usually a scoliosis, which may be associated with marked pelvic obliquity. Kyphosis is also quite common and may be severe enough to require surgical correction.

SENSATION Skin sensibility is usually present, if not completely normal. However, stereognosis may be repaired – an important factor which contributes to upper limb disability.

Overall assessment

A full assessment of the complex abnormalities and alterations in function in the child with cerebral palsy requires experience and patience. The reader is referred to the monograph by Bleck (1987). Repeated examination will be necessary as the child develops. Late abnormalities are due mainly to fixed muscle 'contractures' and secondary bony deformities.

Secondary defects

MUSCLE 'CONTRACTURE' Long-standing spasticity leads to apparent fixed contraction or shortening of the muscle. Whether this is true shortening or a failure of muscle to grow along with skeletal growth remains unanswered. Unopposed, it will eventually lead to fixed deformities and alterations in joint congruity.

BONY DEFORMITY Persistent adduction of the hip leads to valgus of the femoral neck, acetabular dysplasia and subluxation of the hip. At the knee, flexion deformity is associated with upward displacement of the patella and patellofemoral pain. External tibial torsion may result in planovalgus deformity of the foot. Fixed deformities of the toes and foot may become painful.

STRUCTURAL SCOLIOSIS This is most likely to occur in children with whole body involvement and adds greatly to the problems of rehabilitation.

Management

Any serious approach to treatment demands multidisciplinary skills; the team of therapists should meet as often as necessary to work out realistic objectives, discuss progress and plan further management. The objective is not merely to improve physical performance but to increase overall functional ability as well.

SETTING GOALS Based on the extent and severity of the neuromuscular disorder, realistic goals should be defined as early as possible. Even if the child is unlikely ever to walk, active treatment may enable him or her to sit and get about in a wheelchair – an infinitely better prospect than spending a lifetime lying flat. Children with cerebral diplegia and adequate trunk control can be treated as potential walkers, and the objectives then are to overcome or prevent progressive deformity and to provide stability and balance.

PHYSIOTHERAPY Although it is usually impossible to assess prognosis in children under a year old, physical treatment is begun early (1) to provide a setting for repeated observation and assessment, (2) to establish contact between patient and therapist, and (3) to provide a source of counselling and support for the parents.

Special methods abound, but there is a paucity of objective comparative studies of outcome; any controlled trial is, for ethical reasons, impossible. What is agreed is that treatment should be concerned with broad functional patterns of movement and postural reactions. The most widely practised methods have been reviewed by Bleck (1987). Whatever line is followed, the physiotherapist must be skilled in neurophysiological assessment, in modern methods of movement therapy and in the conduct of interpersonal relationships. Physiotherapy continues throughout childhood and early adolescence. Walking patterns are normally established by the age of 7 years and children with spastic diplegia show a levelling off of motor development after that. However, physiotherapy goes hand in hand with other methods of treatment at all stages of development. Every decision on surgery is a combined decision by both surgeon and therapist.

SPLINTAGE Splints are widely used to prevent fixed deformity, to facilitate improved patterns of movement and to hold position after corrective surgery. In the short term (1–2 years) they are certainly useful, but whether they have a long-term effect on the development of muscle contractures is controversial. If they are used, they require careful supervision and adjustment. They should be removed intermittently for physiotherapy. Splintage may be abandoned altogether (a) because it cannot control the deformity or (b) because a permanent correction is achievable by operation.

OPERATIONS The indications for surgery are (1) a spastic deformity which cannot be controlled by conservative measures; (2) fixed deformity that interferes with function; (3) secondary complications such as bony deformities, dislocation of the hip and joint instability.

Patients with *hemiplegia* respond well to both conservative and operative treatment, and all of them should eventually be able to walk unaided. Those with *diplegia* are more difficult to manage but most of them will eventually be able to walk. Patients *with total body involvement* have a poor prognosis for walking, yet even in this group surgery may be needed to improve spinal stability to enable the patient to sit and to facilitate perineal hygiene by providing adequate hip abduction. Low intelligence is no bar to surgery.

Timing is crucial. That is why it is important for patients to be seen and reassessed repeatedly. As long as the dynamic spastic deformity is controlled by lesser measures, there is no urgency about operations; indeed, one approach is to deliberately put off all operations until the condition plateaus off after the age of 6 or 7 years and then do all the necessary corrective surgery at one or two sittings. However, if it becomes increasingly difficult to regain or maintain position, it may be better to operate before function deteriorates and certainly before fixed deformity supervenes. The physiotherapist's advice is often the most valuable.

Operative strategies are limited. (1) Tight muscles can be released or their tendons lengthened but remember that this will also diminish muscle power and may therefore affect overall function. (2) Weak muscles can be augmented by tendon transfers, but beware the combined effect of enhancing power on one side of a joint and taking away the spastic antagonist – the patient may end up with severe overcorrection! (3) Fixed deformities can be corrected by osteotomy, by reshaping the bone ends and performing an arthrodesis, or by arthroplasty; but always consider what effect this will have on the position of other joints and on overall function.

A general rule should be to tackle soft-tissue problems first and bony problems later.

REGIONAL SURVEY

Lower limb

In most patients (those with spastic diplegia) treatment is concentrated on the lower limbs. In the very young child, treatment consists of physiotherapy and splintage to prevent fixed contractures. Surgery is indicated either to correct structural defects (e.g. a fixed contracture or hip subluxation) or to improve gait. By 3–4 years of age the walking pattern can be observed and the functional needs assessed. Operative treatment should be completed, if possible, between 4 and 8 years of age.

Although each individual deformity should be given its due attention, it is important not to lose sight of the interrelationship between the various postural defects, especially lumbar lordosis, hip flexion, knee flexion and ankle equinus.

Hip adduction deformity The child walks with the thighs together and sometimes even with the knees crossing ('scissors gait'). This may be combined with spastic internal rotation. Adductor release is indicated if passive abduction is less than 20° on each side (Hoffer, 1986). If medial hamstring lengthening is planned (see below) it should be done first because this alone may restore some hip abduction.

For most patients open tenotomy of adductor longus and division of gracilis will suffice. Only if this fails to restore passive abduction (a rare occurrence) should the other adductors be released. Anterior branch obturator neurectomy is hardly ever indicated.

Hip flexion deformity This is often associated with fixed knee flexion (the child walks with a 'sitting' posture) or else hyperextension of the lumbar spine. Operative correction is indicated if the hip deformity is more than 20°. This consists of psoas tendon lengthening; an associated fixed flexion deformity of the knee may require medial hamstring lengthening as well.

Hip internal rotation deformity Internal rotation is usually combined with flexion and adduction. If so, adductor release and psoas lengthening are combined with division of the anterior half of the gluteus medius. If, after a few years, rotation is still excessive, a derotation osteotomy of the femur (subtrochanteric or supracondylar) may be considered; however, be warned that this may have to be followed by compensatory rotation osteotomy of the tibia.

Hip subluxation A persistent flexion–adduction deformity leads to femoral neck anteversion. If the abductors are weak and the child is not fully weightbearing, there is a risk of subluxation and acetabular dysplasia; in non-walkers there may be complete dislocation. *Correction of flexion and adduction deformities (see above) before the age of 6 years is the surest way of preventing subluxation.* Older children may need varus-derotation osteotomy of the femur, perhaps combined with acetabular reconstruction. Long-standing dislocation in a non-walker may be irreducible; if discomfort makes operation imperative, the proximal end of the femur can be excised.

Knee flexion deformity This is one of the commonest deformities and is usually due to hamstring spasticity or contracture; however, it is aggravated by any associated hip flexion deformity or weakness of ankle plantarflexion. All three factors must be considered in planning treatment. Spastic flexion deformity may be revealed only when the hip is flexed to 90° so that the hamstrings are tightened. Flexion deformity with the patient lying flat (hip extended) must be due to capsular contracture.

Hamstring lengthening is indicated if there is spastic flexion of more than 20° during the stance phase of walking – but only after carefully assessing the hip and foot. There are three important preconditions: (1) the hip extensors must be working, otherwise the weakened hamstrings will cause anterior tilting of the pelvis and excessive lumbar lordosis; (2) if there is any marked hip flexion deformity this must be corrected at the same time; (3) knee extension is aided by plantarflexion of

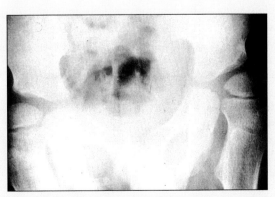

10.9 Spastic hips X-ray of a boy with spastic adducted hips showing acetabular dysplasia and coxa valga, worse on the left side.

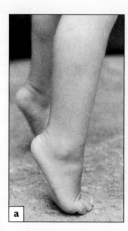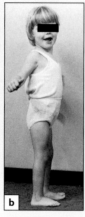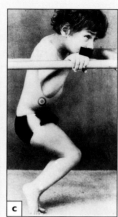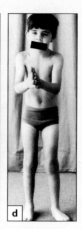

10.10 Spastic knee and foot (**a**) This young girl had true spastic equinus deformities. (**b**) Tendo Achillis lengthening resulted in complete correction and a balanced posture. (**c**) This boy is also standing on his toes but he has a much more complex problem. He has spastic flexion of the knees due to tight hamstrings; close observation shows that the hindfeet are not really in equinus, and lengthening of the tendo Achillis would be disastrous. (**d**) Here he is after a simple hamstring release.

the foot in walking, so it is important not to weaken the triceps surae by overzealous lengthening of the Achilles tendon (see below).

Sometimes hamstring contracture is associated with rectus femoris spasticity (co-spasticity) which prevents knee flexion during the swing phase; this may be corrected by combined hamstring lengthening and rectus femoris release at its distal end.

Spastic knee extension This can usually be corrected by simple tenotomy of the proximal end of rectus femoris.

External tibial torsion This is easily corrected by supra-malleolar osteotomy.

Equinus of the foot Spastic equinus in the young child can be treated by physiotherapy and intermittent splintage. Active plantar flexion is needed to assist knee extension in the stance phase of walking (see above), so Achilles tendon lengthening should be considered only if there is severe spastic deformity or fixed contracture, and should never be overdone.

Pes varus Varus deformity of the foot is associated with tightness of tibialis posterior and tibialis anterior. This can be corrected by tibialis posterior lengthening and tibialis anterior tendon transfer to the outer side of the foot. But only half the tendon is transferred, so as to avoid the risk of overcorrection into valgus. Older children with fixed deformity may need bone operations – calcaneal osteotomy or triple arthrodesis.

Pes valgus (pronated foot) Fixed flat-foot may require subtalar arthrodesis.

Upper limb

Upper limb deformities are seen most typically in the child with spastic hemiplegia and consist of flexion of the elbow, pronation of the forearm, flexion of the

wrist, clenched fingers and adduction of the thumb. In the mildest cases, spastic postures emerge only during exacting activities. Proprioception is often disturbed and this may preclude any marked improvement of function, whatever the kind of treatment. Operative treatment is usually delayed till after the age of 8 years; it is aimed at improving the resting position of the limb and restoring grasp.

Elbow flexion deformity Provided the elbow can extend to a right angle, no treatment is needed.

Forearm pronation deformity This is fairly common and may give rise to subluxation or dislocation of the radial head. Simple release of pronator teres may improve the position, or the tendon can be rerouted round the back of the forearm in the hope that it may act as a supinator. If the wrist is flexed, pronator release may be combined with flexor carpi ulnaris lengthening.

Wrist flexion deformity This can be improved by lengthening or releasing flexor carpi ulnaris; if extension is weak, the release flexor tendon is transferred into one of the wrist extensors.

Flexion deformity of the fingers Spasticity of the long flexor muscles may give rise to clawing. The flexor tendons can be lengthened individually, but if the deformity is severe a forearm muscle slide may be more appropriate. If the fingers can be unclenched only by simultaneously flexing the wrist, it is obviously important not to extend the wrist by tendon transfer or fusion.

Thumb-in-palm deformity This is due to spasticity of the thumb adductors or flexors (or both), but later there is also contracture of flexor pollicis longus. In mild cases, function can be improved by splinting the thumb away from the palm, or by operative release of the adductor pollicis and first dorsal interosseous muscles. Resistant deformity is best treated by Matev's procedure: first the flexor pollicis longus is lengthened; then, through a palmar incision, all the thenar muscles are released; finally abduction and extension are reinforced by tendon transfers.

Spine and pelvis

Scoliosis is common in children with cerebral palsy and is evidently due to involvement of the trunk muscles. The curve is usually thoracolumbar; sometimes (especially in patients unable to walk) it incorporates the pelvis, which is tilted obliquely so that one hip is in abduction and one in adduction and threatening to dislocate. Deformity is usually progressive and treatment is more difficult than with idiopathic scoliosis. If the child can walk and there is little or no pelvic obliquity, treatment is the same as that of idiopathic scoliosis. If the child is unable to walk, or if there is marked pelvic obliquity, combined anterior and posterior fusion with internal instrumentation is recommended. Even in those with severe whole body involvement, if the child is alert and intelligent, corrective surgery may make it easier to sit upright, use a wheelchair and attend to hygiene and dressing. For those who need a wheelchair permanently, the Matrix seating system is useful (Trail and Galasko, 1990).

STROKE – ADULT SPASTIC PARESIS

Cerebral damage following a stroke may cause persistent spastic paresis in the adult; disturbance of proprioception and stereognosis may coexist.

In the early recuperative stage, physiotherapy and splintage are important in preventing fixed contractures; all affected joints should be put through a full range of movement every day, and deformities should be corrected and splinted until controlled muscle power returns. Proprioception and co-ordination can be improved by occupational therapy. Once maximal motor recovery has been achieved – usually by 9 months – residual deformity or joint instability may need surgical correction or permanent splinting.

In the lower limbs the principal deformities requiring correction are equinus or equinovarus of the foot, flexion of the knee and adduction of the hip. In the upper limb (where the chances of regaining controlled movement are less) the common residual deformities are adduction and internal rotation of the shoulder (often accompanied by shoulder pain), and flexion of the elbow, wrist and metacarpophalangeal joints. Treatment is similar to that of spastic deformity in the child, and is summarized in Table 10.1.

FRIEDREICH'S ATAXIA

Friedreich's ataxia, though itself rare, is the commonest of the hereditary ataxias. It is an autosomal recessive disorder in which there is degeneration of the spinocerebellar tracts, the corticospinal tracts, the posterior columns of the cord and part of the cerebellum. It usually presents at the age of 5–6 years, with an awkward unsteady gait, a tendency to fall and clumsiness. Typical deformities are pes cavovarus with claw toes, and scoliosis, sometimes very mild. Neurological examination reveals ataxia and loss of vibration sense and two-point discrimination. There is marked slowing of sensory conduction. In severe cases there is progressive disability and cardiac involvement; patients eventually take to a wheelchair and may die before they are 30 years, usually from cardiac failure. In milder cases operative correction of the foot and spine deformities is well worth while.

LESIONS OF THE SPINAL CORD

The three major pathways in the spinal cord are the corticospinal tracts (in the anterior columns) carrying motor neurons, the spinothalamic tracts carrying sensory neurons for pain, touch and temperature, and

Table 10.2 Treatment of the principal deformities of the limbs

	Deformity	Splintage	Surgery
Foot	Equinus	Spring-loaded dorsiflexion	Lengthen tendo Achillis
	Equinovarus	Bracing in eversion and dorsiflexion	Lengthen tendo Achillis and transfer lateral half of tibialis anterior to cuboid
Knee	Flexion	Long caliper	Hamstring release
Hip	Adduction	–	Obturator neurectomy
			Adductor muscle release
Shoulder	Adduction	–	Subscapularis release
Elbow	Flexion	–	Release elbow flexors
Wrist	Flexion	Wrist splint	Lengthen or release wrist flexors

the posterior column tracts serving deep sensibility (joint position and vibration).

Clinical features

With lesions of the spinal cord, patients complain of muscle weakness, numbness or loss of balance; bladder and bowel control may be impaired and men may complaint of impotence. Examination reveals a spastic UMN paresis, with exaggerated reflexes and a Babinski response; there may be a fairly precise boundary of sensory change, suggesting the level of cord involvement. However, it should be remembered that extradural compressive lesions often involve the nerve roots as well, so there may be a combination of UMN and LMN signs. Several typical patterns are recognized.

Cervical cord compression causes LMN weakness and paraesthesiae or numbness in the arms, with UMN signs in the lower limbs. Bladder symptoms are usually frequency and incontinence but acute lesions may cause retention.

Thoracic cord lesions cause UMN paresis in the lower limbs and variable types of sensory impairment, depending on whether there is involvement of the spinothalamic tracts or posterior columns.

Lumbar lesions may involve the conus medullaris (L1) or the cauda equina (below L1) or both. Thus there may be a combination of UMN paresis and LMN signs. The typical cauda equina syndrome consists of lower limb weakness, depressed reflexes, impaired sensation and urinary retention with overflow.

The Brown–Séquard syndrome occurs with asymmetrical (hemisectional) lesions: below the lesion there is ipsilateral UMN weakness and posterior column dysfunction, with contralateral loss of skin sensibility; at the level of the lesion there is ipsilateral loss of sensibility.

Acute cord lesions at any level may present with flaccid paralysis which only later changes to the more typical UMN picture.

Diagnosis and management

The more common causes of spinal cord dysfunction are listed in Table 10.3. Traumatic and compressive lesions are the ones most likely to be seen by orthopaedic surgeons. Plain x-rays will show structural abnormalities of the spine; cord compression can be visualized by myelography, alone or combined with CT. Intrinsic lesions of the cord require further investigation by blood tests, CSF examination and MRI.

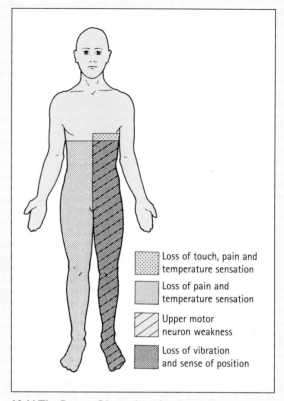

Loss of touch, pain and temperature sensation

Loss of pain and temperature sensation

Upper motor neuron weakness

Loss of vibration and sense of position

10.11 The Brown–Séquard syndrome

Acute compressive lesions require urgent diagnosis and treatment if permanent damage is to be prevented. Bladder dysfunction is ominous: whereas motor and sensory signs may improve after decompression, loss of bladder control, if present for more than 24 hours, is usually irreversible.

Spinal injury is dealt with in Chapter 25. It is important to remember that (1) any spinal injury may be associated with cord damage, and great care is needed in transporting and examining the patient; (2) in the early period of 'spinal shock' the usual picture is one of flaccid paralysis; and (3) plain x-rays seldom show the full extent of bone displacement, which is much better displayed on CT. Unstable injuries usually need operative treatment; stable injuries can be treated conservatively. Corticosteroids are sometimes used to treat acute cord injuries and there is some evidence that this can reduce the degree of permanent damage. However, the matter is highly controversial and patients should be informed that high-dosage corticosteroids may have serious side effects, including widespread avascular necrosis.

Epidural abscess is a surgical emergency. The patient rapidly develops acute pain and muscle spasm, with fever, leucocytosis and elevation of the ESR. X-rays may show disc space narrowing and bone erosion. Treatment is by immediate decompression and antibiotics.

Table 10.3 Causes of spinal cord dysfunction

Acute injury
Vertebral fractures
Fracture–dislocation

Infection
Epidural abscess
Poliomyelitis

Intervertebral disc prolapse
Sequestrated disc
Disc prolapse in spinal stenosis

Vertebral canal stenosis
Congenital stenosis
Acquired stenosis

Spinal cord tumours
Neurofibroma
Meningioma

Intrinsic cord lesions
Tabes dorsalis
Syringomyelia
Other degenerative disorders

Miscellaneous
Spina bifida
Vascular lesions
Multiple lesions
Multiple sclerosis
Haemorrhagic disorders

Acute disc prolapse usually causes unilateral symptoms and signs. However, complete lumbar disc prolapse may present as a cauda equina syndrome with urinary retention and overflow; spinal canal obstruction is demonstrated by myelography or CT; operative discectomy is urgent.

Chronic discogenic disease is often associated with narrowing of the intervertebral foramina and compression of nerve roots (radiculopathy), and occasionally with bony hypertrophy and pressure on the spinal cord (myelopathy). Diagnosis is usually obvious on x-ray and transectional imaging.

Spinal stenosis produces a typical clinical syndrome – due partly to direct pressure on the cord or nerve roots and partly to vascular obstruction and ischaemic neuropathy during hyperextension of the lumbar spine. The patient complains of 'tiredness', weakness and sometimes aching or paraesthesia in the lower limbs after standing or walking for a few minutes, symptoms that are completely relieved by bending forward, sitting or crouching so as to flex the lumbar spine. Congenital

narrowing of the spinal canal is rare, except in developmental disorders such as achondroplasia. But a moderately narrow canal may be further constricted by osteophytes, thus compromising the cord and nerve roots. Treatment calls for laminectomy and bony decompression of the nerve structures.

Vertebral disease, such as tuberculosis or metastatic disease, may cause cord compression and paraparesis. The diagnosis is usually obvious on x-ray, but a needle biopsy may be necessary for confirmation. Management is usually by anterior decompression and, if necessary, internal stabilization. However, in metastatic disease, if the prognosis is poor it may be wise to use radiotherapy and corticosteroids, plus narcotics for pain.

Spinal cord tumours are a comparatively rare cause of progressive paraparesis. X-rays may show bony erosion, widening of the spinal canal or flattening of the vertebral pedicles. Widening of the intervertebral foramina is typical of neurofibromatosis. Treatment usually involves operative removal of the tumour.

Intrinsic lesions of the cord produce slowly progressive neurological signs. Two conditions in particular – tabes dorsalis and syringomyelia – may present with orthopaedic problems because of neuropathic joint destruction.

Tabes dorsalis is a late manifestation of syphilis causing degeneration ('tabes' means wasting) of the posterior columns of the spinal cord. A pathognomonic feature is 'lightning pains' in the lower limbs. Much later other neurological features appear: sensory ataxia, which causes a stamping gait; loss of position sense and sometimes of pain sensibility; trophic lesions in the lower limbs; progressive joint instability; and almost painless destruction of joints (Charcot joints). There is no treatment for the cord disorder.

Syringomyelia In syringomyelia a long cavity (the syrinx) filled with CSF develops within the spinal cord, most commonly in the cervical region. Usually the cause is unknown but the condition is sometimes associated with prolapse of the cerebellar tonsils and hydrocephalus or, in later life, with spinal cord injury or tumour. Symptoms and signs are most evident in the upper limbs. The expanding cyst presses on the anterior horn cells, producing weakness and wasting of the hand muscles. And destruction of the decussating spinothalamic fibres in the centre of the cord produces a characteristic dissociated sensory loss in the upper limbs – impaired response to pain and temperature but preservation of touch. There may be trophic lesions in the fingers and neuropathic arthropathy ('Charcot joints') in the upper limbs. CT may reveal an expanded cord and the syrinx can be defined on MRI. Deterioration may be slowed down by decompression of the foramen magnum.

SPINA BIFIDA

Spina bifida is a congenital disorder in which the two halves of the posterior vertebral arch (or several arches) have failed to fuse. This embryonic defect, which probably occurs within the first 6 weeks of gestation, is often associated with maldevelopment of the neural tube and the overlying skin; the combination of faults is called *dysraphism.* It usually occurs in the lumbar or lumbosacral region. If neural elements are involved there may be paralysis and loss of sensation and sphincter control.

Pathology

SPINA BIFIDA OCCULTA In the mildest forms of dysraphism there is a midline defect between the laminae and nothing more; hence the term 'occulta'. However, in some cases – and especially if several vertebrae are affected – there are telltale defects in the overlying skin; for example, a dimple, a pit or a tuft of hair. Occasionally there are associated intraspinal anomalies, such as tethering of the conus medullaris below L1, splitting of the spinal cord (*diastematomyelia*) and cysts or lipomas of the cauda equina.

SPINA BIFIDA CYSTICA In severe forms of dysraphism the vertebral laminae are missing and the contents of the vertebral canal prolapse through the defect. The abnormality takes one of several forms. The least disabling is a *meningocele,* which accounts for about 5% of cases of spina bifida cystica. The spinal cord and nerve roots remain in their normal position; the dura mater is open posteriorly and a CSF-filled meningeal sac protrudes under the skin. There is usually no neurological abnormality.

The most common abnormality is a *myelomeningocele,* in which part of the spinal cord and nerve roots prolapse together with the meningeal sac. In some cases the neural tube is fully formed and covered by membrane and skin – a *'closed' myelomeningocele.* In others the cord is in its primitive state, the unfolded neural plate forming part of the roof of the sac – an *'open' myelomeningocele* or *rachischisis.* Myelomeningocele is always associated with neurological deficit below the level of the lesion. If neural tissue is exposed to the air, it may become infected, leading to more severe abnormality and even death.

HYDROCEPHALUS Distal tethering of the cord may cause herniation of the cerebellum and brainstem through the foramen magnum, resulting in obstruction to CSF circulation and hydrocephalus. The ventricles dilate and the skull enlarges by separation of the cranial sutures. Persistently raised intracranial pressure may cause cerebral atrophy and mental retardation.

Incidence and screening

Isolated laminar defects are seen in over 5% of lumbar spine x-rays. By comparison, cystic spina bifida is rare at 2–3 per 1000 live births, but if one child is affected the risk for the next child is ten times greater.

Neural tube defects are associated with high levels of alpha-fetoprotein in the amniotic fluid and serum. This offers an effective method of antenatal screening during the 15th to 18th weeks of pregnancy.

Folic acid, 400μg daily before conception and continuing through the first 12 weeks of pregnancy, has been shown to reduce the risk of neural tube defects in the foetus.

Clinical features

SPINA BIFIDA OCCULTA
Isolated laminar defects are often seen in normal people, and usually they can be ignored. However, a posterior midline dimple, a tuft of hair or a pigmented naevus signifies something more serious. Patients may present at any age with neurological symptoms – usually a partial cauda equina syndrome with enuresis, urinary frequency or incontinence; neurological examination may reveal weakness and some loss of sensibility in the lower limbs. X-rays will show the laminar defect and any associated vertebral anomalies. A midline ridge of bone suggests bifurcation of the cord (diastematomyelia). Intraspinal anomalies are best shown by myelography, CT and MRI.

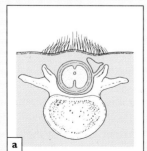 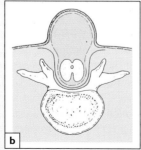 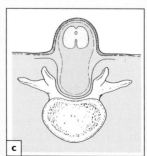 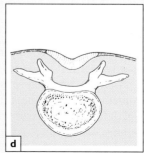

10.12 Dysraphism (a) Spina bifida occulta. (b) Meningocele. (c) Myelomeningocele. (d) Open myelomeningocele.

SPINA BIFIDA CYSTICA

The saccular lesion over the lumbosacral spine is obvious at birth. It may be covered only with membrane, or with membrane and skin. In open myelomeningoceles the neural elements form the roof of the cyst, which merges into plum-coloured skin at its base. Meningoceles are covered by normal looking skin.

Hydrocephalus may be present at birth; with a communicating hydrocephalus the intracranial pressure may not be elevated until leakage from the spinal lesion is arrested by surgical closure.

The baby's posture may suggest the type of paralysis and sometimes indicates its neurological level. Deformities are common, especially hip dislocation, genu recurvatum, talipes and claw toes. Such deformities may be due to muscle imbalance, to abnormal positioning of the limbs in utero or after birth, or to associated anomalies that are independent of the paralysis.

Muscle charting (page 203) should be performed within 24 hours of birth in order to establish both the type and the level of neurological defect. Sharrard has shown convincingly that this is perfectly practicable; he suggests that the untreated child may, within a few days, become increasingly paralysed as enlargement of the meningeal sac exerts traction on adherent nerve roots. In about one-third of infants with myelomeningocele there is complete lower motor neuron paralysis and loss of sensation and sphincter control below the affected level. In one-third there is a complete lesion at some level but a distal segment of cord is preserved, giving a mixed neurological picture with intact segmental reflexes and spastic muscle groups. In one-third the cord lesion is incomplete and some movement and sensation are preserved.

X-rays and CT will show the extent of the bony lesion as well as other vertebral anomalies. MRI may be helpful to define the neurological defects.

Older children with neurological lesions are liable to suffer fractures after minor injuries. These may not always be obvious; suspicion should be raised by the appearance of swelling, warmth and redness in the limb.

Initial treatment

Selection of patients for operative closure of the spinal lesion is ethically controversial. Some centres avoid urgent operation if the neurological level is high (above L1), if spinal deformities are severe or if there is marked hydrocephalus. In the majority of cases, however, the defect should be closed within 48 hours of birth in order to prevent drying and ulceration, or infection, of the lesion. All neural tissue should be carefully preserved and covered with dura. The skin is then widely undercut to facilitate complete closure.

A few weeks later, when the back has healed, the degree of hydrocephalus is assessed and, if necessary, it is treated by drainage of CSF. A one-way valve is inserted (under the skin, behind the ear) to connect the ventricles (via the jugular vein) with the right atrium. Ventriculoatrial drainage can be maintained (if necessary, by changing the valve as the baby grows) for 5 or 6 years, by which time the tendency to hydrocephalus usually ceases.

Orthopaedic management

Optimal treatment of spina bifida calls for a team approach with input from paediatrics, orthopaedic surgery, neurosurgery, urology, physiotherapy, occupational therapy and orthotics. The orthopaedic surgeon is usually not called upon for several weeks, and then

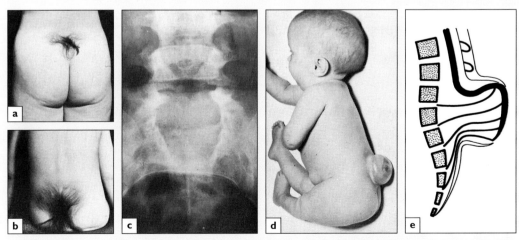

10.13 Dysraphism (**a, b**) Examples of the hairy patches which suggest a bony defect such as that in (**c**). (**d**) Spina bifida cystica. (**e**) Why traction lesions of the nerve roots develop with growth.

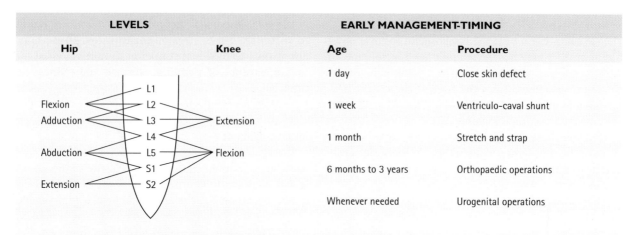

LEVELS		EARLY MANAGEMENT-TIMING	
Hip	**Knee**	**Age**	**Procedure**
		1 day	Close skin defect
Flexion	L1 L2	1 week	Ventriculo-caval shunt
Adduction	L3 — Extension		
	L4	1 month	Stretch and strap
Abduction	L5 — Flexion		
	S1	6 months to 3 years	Orthopaedic operations
Extension	S2		
		Whenever needed	Urogenital operations

10.14 Spina bifida The diagram shows the root levels concerned with hip and knee movements. The table is a simple guide to the timing of operations.

only if the child is thriving, the back healed and a shunt (if needed) working. At this stage muscle charting is repeated and a programme of stretching and strapping begun: stretching to keep deformity at a minimum; elastic strapping (or simple splints) to hold correction.

The goals of treatment are reviewed, bearing in mind the following observations:

- Except in the mildest cases, the late functional outcome cannot be predicted with any confidence until the child's neuromuscular condition is assessed at the age of 3 or 4 years.
- Most patients with myelomeningocele will never be functionally independent (Beaty and Canale, 1990).
- More important than walking is the development of upper limb function and intellectual skills and the ability to cope with the basic activities of daily living. These objectives can be achieved from a wheelchair just as well as from unsteady legs. For many patients the ability to sit comfortably is more important than the ability to stand.

- Joint deformities should be corrected – initially by gentle physiotherapy (beware of causing iatrogenic fractures!) and later by splintage with lightweight orthoses. Surgical correction may be needed if these measures fail.
- Prolonged immobilization carries the risk of pathological fracture and should therefore be avoided.
- Children with lesions below L4 will have quadriceps control and active knee extension; they should therefore be encouraged to walk. Children with high lumbar lesions may start off walking with the aid of lower limb braces but they will eventually opt for a wheelchair.
- *Urinary problems* develop in 90% of cases; they range from poor control to bladder paralysis, urinary retention and hydronephrosis. Simple measures such as manual expression may be needed from an early age. In males, urinary retention with overflow can be managed by fitting a penile appliance; in females, bladder neck resection or urinary diversion may be necessary.

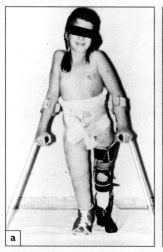
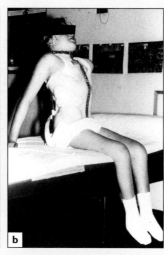
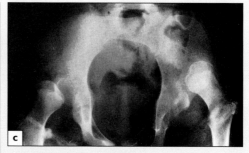

10.15 Spina bifida (a) Paralysis may require permanent splintage in a caliper, and crutch-walking for life. (b) Scoliosis is common and is treated in a brace until the child is old enough for fusion. (c) Muscle imbalance may lead to bilateral hip dislocation.

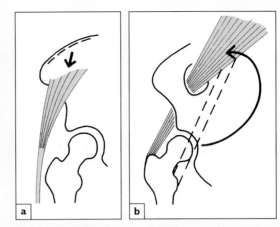

10.16 Spina bifida Two procedures for hip deformity:
(a) Soutter's muscle slide; **(b)** Sharrard's iliopsoas transfer.

REGIONAL SURVEY

Spine

Spinal deformity (scoliosis and/or kyphosis) is common in children with myelomeningocele, due to a combination of muscle weakness and imbalance, associated congenital vertebral anomalies (in about 20% of cases) and the so-called tethered cord syndrome (Banta and Lubicky, 1990).

Distal tethering of the cord or other neural elements is almost inevitable after repair of a myelomeningocele; this may be harmless, but it can cause pain and progression of neurological dysfunction during phases of rapid growth, and in some cases it gives rise to scoliosis. Diagnosis may be aided by CT and myelography. Indications for operative release of the tethered cord are increasing pain and neurological dysfunction or progressive spinal deformity.

Kyphosis may result in stretching and breakdown, or chronic ulceration, of the overlying skin and compression of the abdominal and thoracic viscera. Treatment is difficult and may require localized vertebral resection and arthrodesis.

Spinal deformities which are not associated with the above complications can be treated, in the first instance, by bracing; this is unlikely to correct the deformity but it may prevent or slow down progression so that surgery can be put off until the child is 10 or 12 years old. Those with high lesions who are confined to a wheelchair may require moulded chair inserts.

The main indication for operative correction and spinal stabilization is progression of the deformity. This is likely to occur in over 80% of children with scoliosis. If a tethered cord syndrome is present, this should be dealt with first. Stabilization of the spine requires either advanced posterior instrumentation or combined anterior and posterior instrumentation and fusion. If there is marked pelvic obliquity, the fusion should include the pelvis.

Hip

The aim is to secure hips straight enough to enable the child to stand in calipers, and flexible enough for him or her to sit. If the neurological level of the lesion is above L1, all muscle groups are equally paralysed (balanced); the hips are flail and no treatment other than splintage is needed; in the long term, the child will probably use a wheelchair. With a lesion from S1 downwards there may be pure flexion deformity; this can be corrected by elongation of the psoas tendon combined with detachment of the flexors from the ilium (Soutter).

Usually the lesion is between these levels and the commonest hip problem is dislocation: 50% of spina bifida children have subluxed or dislocated hips by the age of 2 years. Some may be coincidental congenital dislocations but most result from unbalanced paralysis; if the flexors and adductors can overpower the extensors and abductors, dislocation is almost inevitable. In infancy, reduction (closed or open) is usually possible, perhaps aided by adductor tenotomy; but, because postoperative splintage must be minimized, it is important to improve muscle balance. This is achieved by transferring the psoas tendon from the lesser to the greater trochanter through an opening in the ilium (Sharrard's operation); flexor power is reduced and extensor–abductor power may be increased. The Sharrard operation is often combined with open reduction of the hip and capsulorrhaphy; if the acetabulum is dysplastic, proximal femoral and/or pelvic osteotomy also may be necessary to secure a stable hip.

Knee

Unlike the hip, the knee usually presents no problem, because the aim is simple – a straight knee suitable for straight calipers. Occasionally, recurvatum develops and cautious elongation of the quadriceps may be called for. In older children fixed flexion may follow prolonged sitting. If stretching and splintage fail, one or more of the hamstrings may be lengthened, divided or reinserted into the femur or patella. Not uncommonly the knees are straight and will not bend, making sitting difficult; extensive soft-tissue release may be needed if subcutaneous tenotomy proves inadequate.

Foot

The aim is a plantigrade foot with plantar skin strong enough not to break down easily. The floppy foot of balanced paralysis needs no surgery; accurately fitting

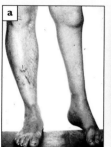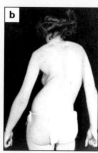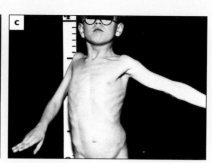

10.17 Poliomyelitis (a) Shortening and wasting of the left leg, with equinus of the ankle. (b) This long curve is typical of a paralytic scoliosis. (c) This boy is trying to abduct both arms, but the right deltoid and supraspinatus are paralysed.

footwear with strong external bracing is adequate. The same is true of any deformity that can be corrected passively, though in every case the patient and parents must be taught an elaborate ritual of skin care; pressure sores must, at all costs, be prevented.

Fixed deformities are common and varied. Tendon operations are often helpful and are best performed at or before the age of 6 months; preoperative electrical testing may help in deciding if the short tendon is paralysed but contracted (in which case simple division is satisfactory) or is active but unopposed (in which case transfer is better). The common equinovarus deformity is usually more severe (and more resistant to treatment) than the 'ordinary' clubfoot; it often requires extensive posteromedial release, preferably at the age of 6–12 months. Residual deformity may have to be tackled by bony procedures at a later stage.

Vertical talus is not uncommon, with a rigid boat-shaped foot and possibly skin ulceration. Operative reduction is important and preferable to talectomy; it is performed at the age of 3 years or over. Still older children may need bone operations to restore a plantigrade foot. Should claw toes prove troublesome, flexor-to-extensor transfer is suitable for the outer four toes, and tenodesis of the long flexor (anchoring it to the proximal phalanx) for the hallux.

ANTERIOR POLIOMYELITIS

Poliomyelitis is a viral infection of the anterior horn cells of the spinal cord and brainstem, which may lead to LMN paralysis of the affected muscle groups. In countries where vaccination is encouraged, it has become a rare disease, though the victims of earlier epidemics continue to pose challenging problems.

Pathology

The virus gains entry through the gut and usually produces no more than a mild influenza-like illness.

Sometimes, however, it attacks the anterior horn cells, causing varying degrees of paralysis in isolated muscles or muscle groups. Some motor neuron cells, merely damaged by inflammation or oedema, survive, and the muscles they supply can regain their lost power. Residual paralysis 6 months after the infection will be permanent.

Clinical features

Poliomyelitis typically passes through several clinical phases, from an acute illness resembling meningitis, to paralysis, then slow recovery or convalescence and finally the stage of residual paralysis. The disease strikes at any age but most commonly in children.

The acute illness begins with fever and headache; in about one-third of cases the patient gives a history of a minor illness with sore throat, mild headache and slight pyrexia 5–7 days before. As the symptoms increase in severity, neck stiffness appears and meningitis may be suspected. The patient lies curled up with the joints flexed; the muscles are painful and tender, and passive stretching provokes painful spasms.

Paralysis soon follows and reaches its maximum in 2–3 days. The limbs are weak and there may be difficulty with breathing and swallowing. If the patient does not succumb from respiratory paralysis, pain and pyrexia subside after 7–10 days and the patient enters the convalescent stage. However, he or she should be considered to be infective for at least 4 weeks from onset.

The stage of recovery and convalescence is prolonged. The return of muscle power is most noticeable during the first 6 months, but there may be continuing improvement for up to 2 years.

Residual paralysis is by no means inevitable. Some cases did not progress beyond the early stage of meningeal irritation. In others, however, recovery is incomplete and the patient is left with some degree of asymmetric flaccid (LMN) paralysis or muscle weakness. With time, unbalanced muscle weakness may lead to joint deformities and growth defects. Sensation is intact but the limb is often cold and blue.

NB Although it is generally held that the pattern of muscle weakness is firmly established by 2 years, experience has shown that power may continue to deteriorate very slowly over many years. Around the menopause there may also be a noticeable loss of energy and easier fatiguability in the affected muscles.

Early treatment

During the acute phase the patient is isolated and kept at complete rest, with symptomatic treatment for pain and muscle spasm. Active movement is avoided but gentle passive stretching helps to prevent contractures. Respiratory paralysis calls for artificial respiration. Once the acute illness settles, physiotherapy is stepped up, active movements are encouraged and every effort is made to regain maximum power. Between exercise periods, splintage may be necessary to prevent fixed deformities.

Muscle charting (see page 203) is carried out at monthly intervals until no further recovery is detected.

Late treatment

During the stage of residual paralysis there are five types of problem that may require treatment.

ISOLATED MUSCLE WEAKNESS WITHOUT DEFORMITY Quadriceps paralysis may make walking impossible; it is best managed with a splint (or caliper) which holds the knee straight. Elsewhere, isolated weakness (e.g. of thumb opposition) may be treated by tendon transfer.

DEFORMITY Unbalanced paralysis may lead to deformity. At first this is passively correctable and can be counteracted by a splint (e.g. a caliper with corrective strap to control valgus or varus of the foot). However, an appropriate tendon transfer may solve the problem permanently.

Fixed deformity cannot be corrected by either splintage or tendon transfer alone; it is also necessary to restore alignment operatively, and to stabilize the joint (if necessary, by arthrodesis). This is especially applicable to fixed deformities of the ankle and foot, but the same principle applies in treating paralytic scoliosis.

Occasionally, fixed deformity is an advantage. Thus, an equinus foot may help to compensate mechanically for quadriceps weakness; stepping on an equinus foot automatically forces the knee into full extension. If this has occured, the equinus should not be corrected.

FLAIL JOINT Balanced paralysis, because it causes no deformity, may need no treatment. However, if the joint is unstable or flail it must be stabilized, either by permanent splintage or by arthrodesis.

SHORTENING Lack of muscle activity undermines normal bone growth. Leg length inequality of up to 3cm can be compensated for by building up the shoe. Anything more is unsightly, and operative lengthening of the limb (or shortening of the opposite limb) may be preferable (see page 264).

VASCULAR DYSFUNCTION Sensation is intact but the paralysed limb is often cold and blue. Large chilblains sometimes develop and sympathectomy may be needed.

REGIONAL SURVEY

Shoulder

Provided the scapular muscles are strong, *abduction* at the shoulder can be restored by arthrodesing the glenohumeral joint (50° abducted and 25° flexed). Contracted adductors may need division.

Elbow and forearm

At the elbow, *flexion* can be restored in one of two ways. If there is normal power in the anterior forearm muscles (wrist and finger flexors) the common flexor origin can be moved more proximally on the distal humerus to provide better leverage across the elbow. Alternatively, if the pectoralis major is strong, the lower half of the muscle can be detached at its origin on the rib-cage, swung down and joined to the biceps tendon.

Pronation of the forearm can be strengthened by transposing an active flexor carpi ulnaris tendon across the front of the forearm to the radial border. Loss of *supination* may be countered by transposing flexor carpi ulnaris across the back of the forearm to the distal radius.

Wrist and hand

Wrist deformity or instability can be markedly improved by arthrodesis. Any active muscles can then be used to restore finger movement.

In the thumb, weakness of opposition can be overcome by a superficialis transfer. The tendon (usually of the ring finger) is wound round that of flexor carpi ulnaris (which acts as a pulley), threaded across the palm and fixed to the distal end of the first metacarpal.

Trunk

Unbalanced paralysis causes scoliosis, frequently a long thoracolumbar curve which may involve the lumbosacral junction, causing pelvic obliquity. Operative treatment is often needed, the most effective being a combination of anterior and posterior instrumentation and fusion (see page 379).

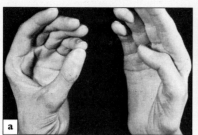
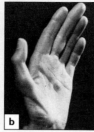
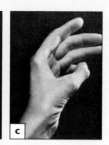

10.18 Poliomyelitis – tendon transfer (a) In both hands the opponens pollicis was paralysed; in the left hand a superficialis transfer has restored opposition. **(b, c)** The transferred tendon in action.

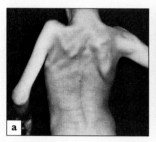
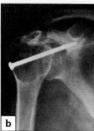
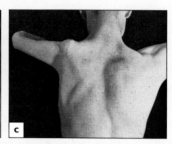

10.19 Poliomyelitis – arthrodesis (a) This patient had paralysis of the left deltoid; after arthrodesis **(b)** he could lift his arm **(c)** by using his scapular muscles.

Hip

Hip deformities are usually complex and difficult to manage; the problem is often aggravated by the gradual development of subluxation or dislocation due either to muscle imbalance (abductors weaker than adductors) or pelvic obliquity associated with scoliosis. Furthermore, since paralysis usually occurs before the age of 5 years, growth of the proximal femur is abnormal and this may result in secondary deformities such as persistent anteversion of the femoral neck, coxa valga and underdevelopment of the acetabular socket – all of which will increase the tendency to instability and dislocation.

The keys to successful treatment are (1) to reduce any scoliotic pelvic obliquity by correcting or improving the scoliosis; (2) to overcome or improve the muscle imbalance by suitable tendon transfer (e.g. iliopsoas to the lateral aspect of the greater trochanter); (3) to correct the proximal femoral deformities by intertrochanteric or subtrochanteric osteotomy; and (4) to deepen the acetabular socket, if necessary, by an acetabuloplasty which will prevent posterior displacement of the femoral head.

Fixed flexion can be treated by Soutter's muscle slide operation or by transferring psoas to the greater trochanter. For fixed abduction with pelvic obliquity the fascia lata and iliotibial band may need division; occasionally, for severe deformity, proximal femoral osteotomy may be required as well. With this type of obliquity the 'higher' hip tends to be unstable and the 'lower' hip to have fixed abduction; if the abducted hip

is corrected first the pelvis may level and the other hip become normal.

Knee

Instability due to relative weakness of the knee extensors is a major problem. Unaided walking may still be possible provided the hip has good extensor power and the foot good plantar-flexion power (or fixed equinus); with this combination the knee is stabilized by being thrust into hyperextension as body weight comes onto the leg. The patient often learns to help matters by putting a finger on the front of the thigh and pushing the knee into extension with each step. In the absence of such passive stabilization a full-length caliper may be needed. In some cases stability can be achieved by carrying out a supracondylar extension osteotomy.

Fixed flexion with flexors stronger than extensors is more common and must be corrected. Flexor-to-extensor transfer (e.g. hamstring muscles to the patella or the quadriceps tendon) is feasible if the flexor muscles are normal; however, quadriceps power is unlikely to be improved by more than one grade. If the flexors are not strong enough, the deformity can be corrected by supracondylar extension osteotomy.

Marked hyperextension (genu recurvatum) sometimes occurs, either as a primary deformity or secondary to fixed equinus. It can be improved by supracondylar flexion osteotomy, provided quadriceps power is sufficient to stablize the knee; an alternative is to excise the patella and slot it into the upper tibia where it acts as a bone block (Hong-Xue Men *et al.*, 1991).

Foot

Instability can be controlled by a below-knee caliper, and *foot-drop* by a toe-raising spring. Often there is imbalance causing varus, valgus or calcaneocavus *deformity*; fusion in the corrected position should be combined with tendon rerouting to restore balance, otherwise there is risk of the deformity recurring.

For varus or valgus the simplest procedure is to slot bone grafts into vertical grooves on each side of the sinus tarsi (Grice); alternatively, a triple arthrodesis (Dunn) of subtalar and mid-tarsal joints is performed, relying on bone carpentry to correct deformity. With associated foot drop, Lambrinudi's modification is valuable; triple arthrodesis is performed but the fully plantar-flexed talus is slotted into the navicular with the forefoot in only slight equinus: foot drop is corrected because the talus cannot plantar-flex further, and slight equinus helps to stabilize the knee. With calcaneocavus deformity, Elmslie's operation is useful: triple arthrodesis is performed in the calcaneus position, but corrected at a second stage by posterior wedge excision combined with tenodesis using half of the tendo Achillis.

Claw toes, if the deformity is mobile, are corrected by transferring the toe flexors to the extensors; if the deformity is fixed, the interphalangeal joints should be arthrodesed in the straight position and the long extensor tendons reinserted into the metatarsal necks.

MOTOR NEURON DISORDERS

Rare degenerative disorders of the large motor neurons may cause progressive and sometimes fatal paralysis.

MOTOR NEURON DISEASE (AMYOTROPHIC LATERAL SCLEROSIS)

This is a degenerative disease of unknown aetiology. It affects both cortical (upper) motor neurons and the anterior horn cells of the cord, causing widespread UMN and LMN symptoms and signs. Patients usually present in middle age with dysarthria and difficulty in swallowing or, if the limbs are affected, with muscle weakness (e.g. clumsy hands or unexplained foot drop) and wasting in the presence of exaggerated reflexes. Sensation and bladder control are normal. Some of the features are also seen in spinal cord compression, which may have to be excluded by myelography. The disease is progressive and incurable. Patients usually end up in a wheelchair and have increasing difficulty with speech and eating. Most of them die within 5 years from a combination of respiratory weakness and aspiration pneumonia.

SPINAL MUSCULAR ATROPHY

In this rare group of heritable disorders there is widespread degeneration of the anterior horn cells in the cord, leading to progressive LMN weakness. The commonest form (*Werdnig–Hoffmann disease*) is inherited as an autosomal recessive and is diagnosed at birth or soon afterwards. The baby is floppy and weak, feeding is difficult and breathing is shallow. Death occurs, usually within a year.

A less severe form (*Kugelberg–Welander disease*), of either dominant or recessive inheritance, is usually seen in adolescents or young adults who present with limb weakness, proximal muscle wasting and 'paralytic' scoliosis. However, it sometimes appears in early childhood as a cause of delayed walking. Patients may live to 30–40 years of age but are usually confined to a wheelchair. Spinal braces are used to improve sitting ability; if this cannot prevent the spine from collapsing, operative instrumentation and fusion is advisable.

ARTHROGRYPOSIS MULTIPLEX CONGENITA

Arthrogryposis is included in the neuromuscular disorders for want of certainty about its pathogenesis. It is a non-specific term applied to congenital disorders in which there is non-progressive restriction of movement due to soft-tissue contractures. Neuropathic and myopathic varieties are described. In addition to the contractures there is stiffness of several joints, shapeless, cylindrical limbs and absence of skin creases.

Typically the shoulders are not rotated, elbows are either flexed or extended and the wrists are stiff in flexion. The knees are usually hyperextended and the ankles either flexed or extended.

Rigid equinovarus is common and difficult to treat; operative correction is often necessary and even then there is a high risk of recurrence. Displacement or dislocation of the hip, likewise, often defies conservative treatment and open reduction is often needed. In the rarer myopathic form of the disease, children may develop spinal deformities.

The deformities are associated with unbalanced muscle weakness which follows a neurosegmental distribution, and necropsy specimens show sparseness of anterior horn cells in the cervical and lumbar cord. Deformities and contractures develop in utero and remain largely unchanged throughout life.

Treatment begins soon after birth and initially consists of manipulation and splintage of deformed joints. Later, if progress is slow, tendon release, tendon transfers and osteotomies may become necessary. The

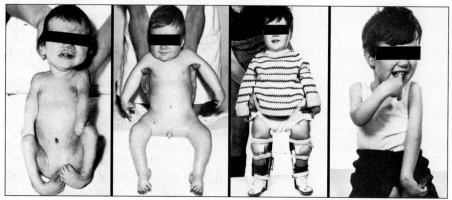

10.20 Arthrogryposis multiplex congenita Severe deformities are present at birth but surgery is possible and, as this bright lad shows, worth while. The lower limbs are tackled first (aiming at straight legs with plantigrade feet), then the upper limbs (where the minimum aim is to enable a hand to reach the mouth).

contractures are notoriously resistant to all forms of treatment and recurrences or deformity are the rule rather than the exception.

PERIPHERAL NEUROPATHY

Disorders of the peripheral nerves may affect motor, sensory or autonomic functions, may be localized to a short segment or may involve the full length of the nerve fibres including their cell bodies in the anterior horn (motor neurons), posterior root ganglia (sensory neurons) and autonomic ganglia. In some cases spinal cord tracts are involved as well.

Pathology

There are essentially three types of nerve pathology: (1) acute interruption of axonal continuity; (2) axonal degeneration; and (3) demyelination. In all three, conduction is disturbed or completely blocked, with consequent loss of motor and/or sensory function.

Axonal degeneration occurs most typically after nerve division and is described in Chapter 11. Recovery, when it occurs, is slow (a new axon grows by 1–2 mm per day) and is often incomplete. Demyelination is less damaging and may be localized to a short segment of nerve; recovery usually takes less than 6 weeks. Most of the chronic neuropathies show a mixture of degeneration and demyelination.

Classification

The clinical disorders are divided into:

1. *Mononeuropathy* – Involvement of a single nerve (e.g. nerve entrapment).

2. *Multiple mononeuropathy* – Involvement of several isolated nerves (e.g. leprosy).
3. *Polyneuropathy* – Widespread symmetrical dysfunction (e.g. diabetic neuropathy, alcoholic myopathy, vitamin deficiency or – perhaps the most common – idiopathic neuropathy (Table 10.3).

Disorders may be predominantly sensory (e.g. diabetic polyneuropathy), predominantly motor (e.g. peroneal muscular atrophy) or mixed. Chronic motor loss with no sensory component is usually due to anterior horn cell disease rather than polyneuropathy.

Clinical features

Patients usually complain of sensory symptoms: 'pins and needles', numbness, a limb 'going to sleep', 'burning', shooting pains or restless legs. They may also notice weakness or clumsiness, or loss of balance in walking. Occasionally (in the predominantly motor neuropathies) the main complaint is of progressive deformity; for example, claw hand or cavus foot. The onset may be rapid (over a few days) or very gradual (over weeks or months). Sometimes there is a history of injury, infection, a known disease such as diabetes or malignancy, alcohol abuse or nutritional deficiency.

Examination may reveal motor weakness in a particular muscle group. In the polyneuropathies the limbs are involved symmetrically, usually legs before arms and distal before proximal parts. Reflexes are usually depressed, though in small-fibre neuropathies (e.g. diabetes) this occurs very late. In mononeuropathy, sensory loss follows the 'map' of the affected nerve. In polyneuropathy, there is a symmetrical 'glove' or 'stocking' distribution. Trophic skin changes may be present. Deep sensation is also affected and some patients develop ataxia. If pain sensibility and proprioception are depressed there may be joint instability or breakdown of the articular surfaces ('Charcot' joints).

Table 10.4 Causes of polyneuropathy

Hereditary
Hereditary motor and sensory neuropathy
Friedreich's ataxia
Hereditary sensory neuropathy

Infections
Viral infections
Herpes zoster
Neuralgic amyotrophy
Leprosy

Inflammatory
Acute inflammatory polyneuropathy
Gullain–Barré syndrome
Systemic lupus erythematosus
Sarcoidosis

Nutritional and metabolic
Vitamin deficiencies
Diabetes
Myxoedema
Amyloidosis

Neoplastic
Primary carcinoma
Myeloma

Toxic
Alcohol
Lead

Drugs
Various

Clinical examination alone may establish the diagnosis. Further help is provided by electromyography (which may suggest the type of abnormality) and nerve conduction studies (which may show exactly where the lesion is).

The *mononeuropathies* – mainly nerve injuries and entrapment syndromes – are dealt with in Chapter 11. The more common polyneuropathies are listed in Table 10.4 and some are described below. In over 50% of cases no specific cause is found.

HEREDITARY NEUROPATHIES

These rare disorders present in childhood and adolescence, usually with muscle weakness and deformity.

Hereditary motor and sensory neuropathy (HMSN)

This is the preferred name for a group of conditions which *includes peroneal muscular atrophy* and *Charcot–Marie–Tooth disease*, the commonest of the inherited neuropathies, which are usually passed on as autosomal dominant disorders. HMSN type I is seen in young children who have difficulty walking and develop claw toes and pes cavus or cavovarus. There may be severe wasting of the legs and (later) the upper limbs. Spinal deformity is common. This is a demyelinating disorder and nerve conduction velocity is markedly slowed. The diagnosis can be confirmed by finding demyelination on sural nerve biopsy. Type II HMSN occurs in adolescents and young adults and is much less disabling than type I; it affects only the lower limbs, causing mild pes cavus and wasting of the peronei. Nerve conduction velocity is only slightly reduced, indicating primary axonal degeneration.

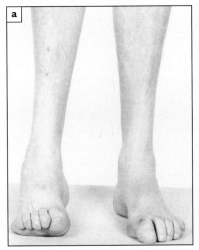
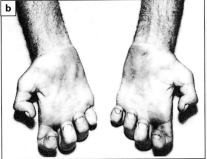
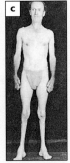

10.21 Hereditary neuropathies (a) This patient with peroneal muscular atrophy presented with cavus feet and claw toes; his lower legs were abnormally thin (due to muscle wasting). Further examination showed that he had similar wasting and clawing of his hands (b). The patient in (c) was even more severely affected, with marked changes in all the extremities.

If foot deformities are progressive or disabling, operative correction may bring marked improvement. Claw toes (due to intrinsic muscle weakness) can be corrected by transferring the toe flexors to the extensors, with or without fusion of the interphalangeal joints. Clawing of the big toe is best corrected by the Robert Jones procedure – transfer of the extensor hallucis longus to the metatarsal neck and fusion of the interphalangeal joint. The cavus deformity often needs no treatment, but if it causes pain it can be improved by calcaneal or dorsal mid-tarsal osteotomy.

Friedreich's ataxia

This autosomal recessive disorder is characterized by spinocerebellar dysfunction, but there may also be degeneration of the posterior root ganglia and peripheral nerves. Patients present at around the age of 6 years with gait ataxia, lower limb weakness and deformities similar to those of severe Charcot–Marie–Tooth disease. The muscle weakness, which may also involve the upper limbs and the trunk, is progressive; by the age of 20 years the patient has usually taken to a wheelchair and is likely to die of cardiomyopathy before the age of 40. Despite the poor prognosis, surgical correction of deformities is worthwhile.

Hereditary sensory neuropathy

Congenital insensitivity to pain and temperature is inherited as either a dominant or a recessive trait. Patients develop Charcot joints and ulceration of the feet.

Diabetic neuropathy

Diabetes is one of the commonest causes of peripheral neuropathy. Hyperglycaemia interferes with Schwann cell function, leading to demyelination and axonal degeneration. Microvascular occlusion may also play a part. Patients complain of numbness and paraesthesiae in the foot and hands. The onset is insidious and the condition often goes undiagnosed until complications arise – neuropathic ulcers of the feet, regional osteoporosis and fractures of the foot bones, or Charcot joints in the ankles and feet. There may be muscular weakness and loss of reflexes. A late feature is loss of balance.

Treatment consists of skin care, management of fractures and splintage or arthrodesis of grossly unstable or deformed joints. The underlying disorder should, of course, be controlled. The orthopaedic surgeon is most likely to encounter problems in the foot. Management of the diabetic foot is discussed on page 507.

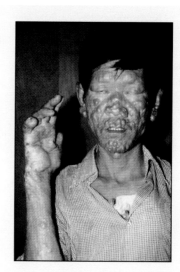

10.22 Leprosy
A patient severly affected by leprosy. Note the claw hand, due to advanced ulnar neuropathy.

Leprosy

Although uncommon in Europe and North America, this is still a frequent cause of peripheral neuropathy in Africa and Asia.

Mycobacterium leprae, an acid-fast organism, causes a diffuse inflammatory disorder of the skin, mucous membranes and peripheral nerves. Depending on the host response, several forms of disease may evolve. The most severe neurological lesions are seen in tuberculoid leprosy. Anaesthetic skin patches develop over the extensor surfaces of the limbs; loss of motor function leads to weakness and deformities of the hands and feet. Thickened nerves may be felt as cords under the skin or where they cross the bones (e.g. the ulnar nerve behind the medial epicondyle of the elbow). Trophic ulcers are common and may predispose to osteomyelitis. *Lepromatous leprosy* is associated with a symmetrical polyneuropathy, which occurs late in the disease.

Treatment by combined chemotherapy (mainly rifampicin and dapsone) is continued for 6 months to 2 years, depending on the response. Muscle weakness – particularly the intrinsic muscle paralysis due to ulnar nerve involvement – may require multiple tendon transfers.

Herpes zoster (shingles)

This common disorder is caused by varicella (chickenpox) virus infection of the dorsal root ganglia. Elderly or immunosuppressed patients are particularly susceptible. Following an injury or intercurrent illness, the patient develops severe unilateral pain in the distribution of several adjacent nerve roots. Involvement of the lumbar roots may closely mimic sciatica. Days or weeks later an irritating vesicular rash appears; characteristically it trails out along the dermatomes corresponding to affected nerves. The condition usually subsides spontaneously but

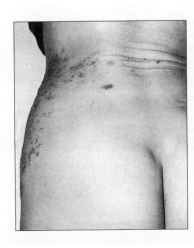

10.23 Herpes zoster This patient was treated for several weeks for 'sciatica' – then the typical rash of shingles appeared.

10.24 Neuralgic amyotrophy A young nurse complained of acute neck and shoulder pain on the left. She had weakness of levator scapulae (**a**) and slight winging of the left scapula (**b**). The neurological defect usually returns to normal but occasionally wasting and weakness are permanent.

neuralgia may persist for months or years. Treatment is symptomatic, though in severe cases systemic antiviral therapy may be justified.

Neuralgic amyotrophy (acute brachial neuritis)

This unusual cause of severe cervicobrachial pain and weakness is believed to be a viral infection of the cervical nerve roots; there is often a history of an antecedent viral infection and sometimes a small epidemic occurs among inmates of an institution.

The history alone often suggests the diagnosis. Pain in the shoulder and arm is intense and sudden in onset. It may extend into the neck and down as far as the hand; usually it lasts a few days but may continue for weeks. Other symptoms are paraesthesia in the arm or hand, and weakness of the muscles of the shoulder, forearm and hand.

Wasting of the deltoid or the small muscles of the hand may be obvious after a few days, and winging of the scapula (due to serratus anterior weakness) is common. Shoulder movement is limited by pain but this limitation is invariably transient. Sensory loss in one or more of the cervical dermatomes is not uncommon.

The feature that distinguishes neuralgic amyotrophy from an acute cervical disc herniation is the involvement of multiple nerve root levels.

There is no specific treatment; pain is controlled with analgesics. The prognosis is usually good but full neurological recovery may take months or years.

PAIN

Many – perhaps most – musculoskeletal disorders are accompanied by pain. Whatever the nature of the underlying condition, pain usually requires treatment in its own right; sometimes it becomes the main focus

of attention even after the initiating factors have disappeared or subsided.

PAIN PERCEPTION

Pain is confounding. The same receptors that appreciate discomfort also respond to tickling with feelings of pleasure. The electrical discharge in 'mild' pain is no different from that in 'severe' pain. That the degree of discomfort is related to the magnitude of the physical stimulus cannot be doubted, but ultimately both the severity of the pain and its character are experienced subjectively and cannot be measured.

Pain receptors (nociceptors) in the form of free nerve endings are found in almost all tissues. They are stimulated by mechanical distortion, by chemical, thermal or electrical irritation, or by ischaemia. Musculoskeletal pain associated with trauma or inflammation is due to both tissue distortion and chemical irritation (local release of kinins, prostaglandins and serotonin). Visceral nociceptors respond to stretching and anoxia. In nerve injuries the regenerating axons may be hypersensitive to all stimuli.

Pain transmission occurs via both myelinated axons (the large-diameter A-0d fibres), which carry well-defined and well-localized sensation, and the far more numerous unmyelinated axons (small-diameter C fibres) which are responsible for crude, poorly defined pain. From the dorsal horn synapses in the cord, fibres run via the spinothalamic tracts to the thalamus and cortex (where pain is appreciated and localized) as well as the reticular system, which may be responsible for reflex autonomic and motor responses to pain.

Pain modulation Pain impulses may be suppressed or inhibited by (1) simultaneous sensory impulses travelling via adjacent axons or (2) impulses descending from the brain. Thus, it is posited that pain impulses are 'sorted out' – some of them blocked, some allowed through – in the dorsal horn of the cord (the 'gate-control' theory of Melzak and Wall, 1965). This could explain why counter-stimulation sometimes reduces pain perception. In addition, certain morphine-like compounds (endorphins and enkephalins), normally elaborated in the brain and spinal cord, can inhibit pain sensibility. These neurotransmitters are activated by a variety of agents, including severe pain itself, other neurological stimuli, psychological messages and placebos.

Pain threshold is the level of stimulus needed to induce pain. There is no fixed 'threshold' for any individual; pain perception is the result of all the factors mentioned above, operating against a complex and changing psychological background. The threshold is lowered by fear, anxiety, depression, lack of self-esteem and mental or physical fatigue; and it is elevated by relaxation, diversion, reduction of anxiety and general psychological support. The management of pain involves not only the elimination of noxious stimuli, or the administration of painkillers, but also the care of the whole person.

ACUTE PAIN

Severe acute pain, as seen typically after injury, is accompanied by an autonomic 'fight or flight' reaction: increased pulse rate, peripheral vasoconstriction, sweating, rapid breathing, muscle tension and anxiety. Similar features are seen in pain associated with acute neurological syndromes or in malignant disease. Lesser degrees of pain may have negligible side effects.

Treatment is directed at (1) removing or counteracting the painful disorder; (2) splinting the painful area; (3) making the patient feel comfortable and secure; (4) administering analgesics, anti-inflammatory drugs or – if necessary – narcotic preparations; and (5) alleviating anxiety.

CHRONIC PAIN

Chronic pain usually occurs in degenerative and arthritic disorders or in malignant disease and is accompanied by vegetative features such as fatigue and depression. Treatment again involves alleviation of the underlying disorder if possible and general analgesic therapy, but there is an increased need for rehabilitative and psychologically supportive measures.

COMPLEX REGIONAL PAIN SYNDROME (ALGODYSTROPHY)

A number of clinical syndromes appear under this heading, including *reflex sympathetic dystrophy, algodystrophy, Sudeck's atrophy, shoulder–hand syndrome* and –

particularly after a nerve injury – *causalgia*. What they have in common is pain, vasomotor instability, trophic skin changes, functional impairment and osteoporosis. Precipitating causes are trauma (often trivial), operation or arthroscopy, a peripheral nerve lesion, myocardial infarction or stroke. The cause is unknown but peripheral sympathetic overactivity is an important component.

The incidence of post-traumatic reflex sympathetic dystrophy (RSD) is unknown, largely because there are no agreed criteria for diagnosing mild cases. However, the condition is more common than is generally recognized and it has been suggested that as many as 30% of patients with fractures of the extremities develop features of RSD. Fortunately, in the majority of cases these features are very mild and they recover spontaneously.

Clinical features

Following some precipitating event, the patient complains of persistent pain, and sometimes cold intolerance, in the affected area – usually the hand or foot, sometimes the knee, hip or shoulder. In the mild or early case there may be no more than slight swelling, with tenderness and stiffness of the nearby joints. More suspicious are local redness and warmth, sometimes changing to cyanosis with a blotchy, cold and sweaty skin. X-rays are usually normal but triple-phase radionuclide scanning at this stage shows increased activity.

Later, or in more severe cases, trophic changes become apparent: a smooth shiny skin with scanty hair and atrophic brittle nails. Swelling and tenderness persist and there may be marked loss of movement. X-rays now show patchy osteoporosis, which may be quite diffuse.

In the most advanced stage, there may be severe joint stiffness and fixed deformities. The acute symptoms may subside after a year or 18 months, but some degree of pain often persists indefinitely.

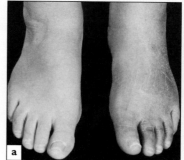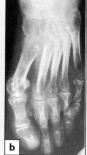

10.25 Complex regional pain syndrome (a) A 53-year old woman fractured her left tibia. The fracture healed but she developed pain, swelling and stiffness of the left foot. The skin became smooth and atrophic; x-ray showed regional osteoporosis of the foot. (b) This is the typical picture of complex regional pain syndrome (algodystrophy; Sudeck's atrophy).

Causalgia is a severe form of regional pain, usually seen after nerve injury. Pain is intense, often 'burning' or 'penetrating' and exacerbated by touching, jarring or sometimes even by a loud noise. Symptoms may start distally and progress steadily up the limb to involve an entire quadrant of the body.

Treatment

Treatment should be started as early as possible; if the condition is allowed to persist for more than a few weeks it may become irreversible.

Mild cases often respond to a simple regimen of reassurance, anti-inflammatory drugs and physiotherapy. Other conservative measures include the administration of corticosteroids, calcium channel blockers and tricyclic antidepressants.

If there is no improvement after a few weeks, and as a first measure in severe cases, sympathetic blockade often helps. This can be done by one or more local anaesthetic injections to the stellate or the appropriate lumbar sympathetic ganglia, or by regional block with guanethidine given intravenously to the affected limb.

A small percentage of patients go on complaining of pain and impaired function almost indefinitely. Psychological treatment may help them to deal with the emotional distress and to develop better coping strategies.

'CHRONIC PAIN SYNDROME'

In a minority of patients with chronic pain there is an apparent mismatch between the bitterness of complaint and the degree of physical abnormality. The most common example is the patient with discogenic disease and prolonged, unresponsive, disabling low back pain. Labels such as 'functional overlay', 'compensitis', 'supratentorial reaction' and 'illness behaviour' are introduced and both patient and doctor are overtaken by a sense of hopelessness. Sometimes there are well-marked features of depression, or complaints of widespread somatic illness (pain in various parts of the body, muscular weakness, paraesthesiae, palpitations and impotence).

Treatment is always difficult and should, ideally, be managed by a team that includes a specialist in pain control, a psychotherapist, a rehabilitation specialist and a social worker. Pain may be alleviated by a variety of measures: (1) analgesics and anti-inflammatory drugs; (2) local injections to painful areas; (3) local counterirritants; (4) acupuncture; (5) transcutaneous nerve stimulation; (6) sympathetic block; and, occasionally, (7) surgical interruption of pain pathways. These methods, as well as psychosocial assessment and therapy, are best applied in a dedicated pain clinic.

MUSCULAR DYSTROPHIES

The muscular dystrophies are rare hereditary disorders causing progressive muscle weakness and wasting.

DUCHENNE MUSCULAR DYSTROPHY

This is a progressive disease of X-linked inheritance. It is therefore seen only in boys (or in girls with sex chromosome disorders). The defective gene at locus p21 on the X chromosome fails to produce normal levels of dystrophin, which is necessary for calcium transport. The condition is usually unsuspected until the child starts to walk; he has difficulty standing and climbing stairs; he cannot run properly and he falls frequently. The muscles look bulky, but much of this is due to fat and the pseudohypertrophy belies the weakness, which is progressive and generalized. Compensatory postural deformities produce a typical stance and gait, with the feet in equinus, the pelvis tilted forward, the back arched in lordosis and the neck extended. A characteristic feature is the method of rising from the floor by climbing up his legs (Gowers' sign); this is due to weakness of the gluteus maximus and thigh muscles. By 10 years of age the child is unable to walk and by 20 he may be dying of cardiac or respiratory failure.

Diagnostic tests are a raised level of serum creatinine phosphokinase, characteristic EMG signs and histochemical abnormalities on muscle biopsy.

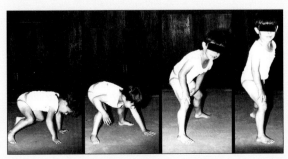

10.26 Muscle dystrophy This boy, with a Duchenne type of dystrophy, has to climb up his legs in order to achieve the upright position.

While the child can still walk, physiotherapy and splintage or even tendon operations may help to prevent and correct joint deformities and so prolong the period of mobility. Muscle weakness makes it difficult to use crutches. When he is wheelchair-bound, spinal deformity must be prevented and physiotherapy is directed at retaining muscle power for as long as possible. If scoliosis is marked (more than 30°), instrumentation and spinal fusion may be necessary.

BECKER'S DYSTROPHY

This condition is similar to, but milder than, Duchenne's dystrophy; affected boys retain the ability to walk in their teens and patients may survive into the 4th or 5th decade. Dystrophin is decreased and/or abnormal in character.

LIMB GIRDLE DYSTROPHY

This disorder, of autosomal recessive inheritance, is even rarer than the Duchenne type and much less disabling. Symptoms usually start in late adolescence. Pelvic girdle weakness causes a waddling gait and difficulty in rising from a low chair; pectoral girdle weakness makes it difficult to raise the arms above the head. The disease is slowly progressive and by the 5th decade disability is usually marked. Treatment consists of physiotherapy and splintage to prevent contractures, and operative correction when necessary. Because the deltoid muscles are spared, shoulder movements can be improved by fixing the scapula to the ribs posteriorly, so improving deltoid leverage.

FACIOSCAPULOHUMERAL DYSTROPHY

This condition, of autosomal dominant inheritance, presents in adolescence or early adult life with facial muscle weakness and winging of the scapulae. There may also be slight pelvic girdle weakness and foot drop. Deterioration is slow and the life span normal. Treatment is the same as for limb girdle dystrophy.

MYOTONIC DISORDERS

Myotonia is persistent muscle contraction after cessation of voluntary effort. It is a prominent feature in certain autosomal dominant genetic disorders.

DYSTROPHIA MYOTONICA

Patients present in adult life with distal muscle weakness and myotonia. Later there is more widespread involvement and the face and tongue may be affected as well. Patients usually have low intelligence. Complications are dysphagia, respiratory difficulty and cardiomyopathy. Foot deformities may need manipulation and splintage.

MYOTONIA CONGENITA

Myotonia is present at birth and may cause feeding problems. Children have 'stiff joints' and muscle cramps, which are usually worse after rest. Limb muscles are quite bulky and in mild cases function is not severely disturbed.

REFERENCES AND FURTHER READING

Banta JV, Lubicky JP (1990) Orthopaedic aspects of myelomeningocele: Spinal deformities. *Journal of Bone and Joint Surgery* **72A**, 628-629

Beaty JH, Canale JT (1990) Orthopaedic aspects of myelomeningocele: Current concepts review. *Journal of Bone and Joint Surgery* **72A**, 626-630

Bleck EE (1987) *Orthopaedic Management in Cerebral Palsy.* Blackwell Scientific, Oxford; Lippincott, Philadelphia

Hoffer MM (1986) Management of the hip in cerebral palsy. *Journal of Bone and Joint Surgery* **68A**, 629-631

Hong-Xue Men, Chan-Hua Bian, Chan-Dou Yang *et al.* (1991) Surgical treatment of the flail knee after poliomyelitis. *Journal of Bone and Joint Surgery* **73B**, 195-199

Lau JHK, Parker JC, Hsu LCS *et al.* (1986) Paralytic hip instability in poliomyelitis. *Journal of Bone and Joint Surgery* **68B**, 528-533

Louis DS, Hensinger RM, Fraser BA *et al.* (1989) Surgical management of the severely multiply handicapped individual. *Journal of Pediatric Orthopedics* **9**, 15-18

Mazur JM, Shurtleff D, Merelaus M *et al.* (1989) Orthopaedic management of high level spina bifida. *Journal of Bone and Joint Surgery* **71A**, 56-61

Melzac R, Wall P (1965) Pain mechanisms: a new theory. *Science* **150**, 971-979

Rang M, Wright J (1989) What have 30 years of medical progress done for cerebral palsy? *Clinical Orthopaedics and Related Research* **247**, 55-60

Roper BA, Tibrewal SB (1989) Soft tissue surgery in Charcot–Marie–Tooth disease. *Journal of Bone and Joint Surgery* **71B**, 17-20

Scrutton D (1989) The early management of hips in cerebral palsy. *Developmental Medicine and Child Neurology* **31**, 108-116

Sharrard WJW (1992) *Paediatric Orthopaedics and Fractures.* Blackwell Scientific, Oxford

Sutherland DH, Ohlson R, Cooper L, Woo SK (1980) The development of mature gait. *Journal of Bone and Joint Surgery* **62A**, 336-353

Sutherland DH, Davids JR (1995) Common gait abnormalities of the knee in cerebral palsy. *Clinical Orthopaedics and Related Research* **288**, 139-147

Trail IA, Galasko CSB (1990) The matrix seating system. *Journal of Bone and Joint Surgery* **73B**, 666-669

NERVE STRUCTURE AND FUNCTION

Peripheral nerves are bundles of *axons* conducting efferent (motor) impulses from cells in the anterior horn of the spinal cord to the muscles, and afferent (sensory) impulses from peripheral receptors via cells in the posterior root ganglia to the cord. They also convey sudomotor and vasomotor fibres from ganglion cells in the sympathetic chain. Some nerves are predominantly motor, some predominantly sensory; the larger trunks are mixed, with motor and sensory axons running in separate bundles.

Each axon is, in reality, an extension or elongated process of a nerve cell, or *neuron*. The cell bodies of the motor neurons supplying the peripheral muscles are clustered in the anterior horn of the spinal cord; a single motor neuron with its axon may, therefore, be more than a metre long. The cell bodies of the sensory neurons serving the trunk and limbs are situated in the dorsal root ganglia and each neuron has one process (axon) extending from the periphery to the cell body and another from the cell body up the spinal cord.

The peripheral ends of all the neurons are branched. A single motor neuron may supply anything from 10 to several thousand muscle fibres, the ratio depending on the degree of dexterity demanded of the particular muscle (the smaller the ratio, the finer the movement). Similarly, the peripheral branches of each sensory neuron may serve anything from a single muscle spindle to a comparatively large patch of skin; here again, the fewer the end receptors served the greater the degree of discrimination.

The signal, or action potential, carried by motor neurons is transmitted to the muscle fibres by the release of a chemical transmitter, acetylcholine, at the terminal bouton of the nerve. Sensory signals are similarly conveyed to the dorsal root ganglia and from there up the ipsilateral column of the spinal cord, through the brain-stem and thalamus, to the opposite (sensory) cortex. Proprioceptive impulses from the muscle spindles and joints bypass this route and are carried to the anterior horn cells as part of a local reflex arc. The economy of this system ensures that 'survival' mechanisms like balance and sense of position in space are activated with great speed.

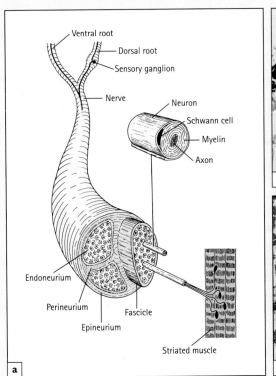

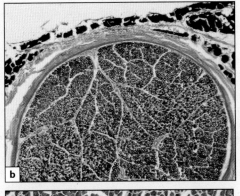

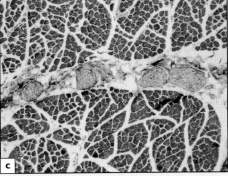

11.1 Nerve structure (a) Diagram of the structural elements of a peripheral nerve. (b) Histological section through a large nerve. (c) High-power view of the same, showing blood vessels in the perineurium.

In the peripheral nerves, all motor axons and the large sensory axons serving touch, pain and proprioception are coated with *myelin*, a multilayered lipoprotein membrane derived from the accompanying *Schwann cells*. Every few millimetres the myelin sheath is interrupted, leaving short segments of bare axon called the *nodes of Ranvier*. Nerve impulses leap from node to node at the speed of electricity, much faster than would be the case if these axons were not insulated by the myelin sheaths. Consequently, depletion of the myelin sheath causes slowing – and eventually complete blocking – of axonal conduction.

Most axons – in particular the small-diameter fibres carrying crude sensation and the efferent sympathetic fibres – are unmyelinated but wrapped in Schwann cell cytoplasm. Damage to these axons causes unpleasant or bizarre sensations and various sudomotor and vasomotor effects.

Outside the Schwann cell membrane the axon is covered by a connective tissue stocking, the *endoneurium*. The axons that make up a nerve are separated into bundles – or fascicles – by fairly dense membranous tissue, the *perineurium*. In a transected nerve, these fascicles are seen pouting from the cut surface, their perineurial sheaths well defined and strong enough to be grasped by fine instruments. The groups of fascicles that make up a nerve trunk are enclosed in an even thicker connective tissue coat, the *epineurium*. The epineurium varies in thickness and is particularly strong where the nerve is subjected to movement and traction, for example near a joint.

The nerve is richly supplied by *blood vessels* that run longitudinally in the epineurium before penetrating the various layers to become the *endoneurial capillaries*. These fine vessels may be damaged by stretching or rough handling of the nerve; however, they can withstand extensive mobilization of the nerve, making it feasible to repair or replace damaged segments by operative transposition or nerve transfer. The tiny blood vessels have their own *sympathetic nerve supply* coming from the parent nerve, and stimulation of these fibres (causing intraneural vasoconstriction) may be important in conditions such as reflex sympathetic dystrophy and other unusual pain syndromes.

PATHOLOGY

Nerves can be injured by ischaemia, compression, traction, laceration or burning. Damage varies in severity from transient and quickly recoverable loss of function to complete interruption and degeneration. There may be a mixture of types of damage in the various fascicles of a single nerve trunk.

Transient ischaemia

Acute nerve compression causes numbness and tingling within 15 minutes, loss of pain sensibility after 30 minutes and muscle weakness after 45 minutes. Relief of compression is followed by intense paraesthesiae lasting up to 5 minutes (the familiar 'pins and needles' after a limb 'goes to sleep'); feeling is restored within 30 seconds and full muscle power after about 10 minutes. These changes are due to transient anoxia and they leave no trace of nerve damage.

Neurapraxia

Seddon (1942) coined the term 'neurapraxia' to describe a reversible physiological nerve conduction block in which there is loss of some types of sensation and muscle power followed by spontaneous recovery after a few days or weeks. It is due to mechanical pressure causing segmental demyelination and is seen typically in 'crutch palsy', pressure paralysis in states of drunkenness (*'Saturday night palsy'*) and the milder types of tourniquet palsy.

Axonotmesis

This is a more severe form of nerve injury, seen typically after closed fractures and dislocations. The term means, literally, axonal interruption. There is loss of conduction but the nerve is in continuity and the neural tubes are intact. Distal to the lesion, and for a few millimetres retrograde, axons disintegrate and are resorbed by phagocytes. This *wallerian degeneration* (named after the physiologist, Augustus Waller, who described the process in 1851) takes only a few days and is accompanied by marked proliferation of Schwann cells and fibroblasts lining the endoneurial tubes. The denervated target organs (motor end-plates and sensory receptors) gradually atrophy, and if they are not reinnervated within 2 years they will never recover.

Axonal *regeneration* starts within hours of nerve damage, probably encouraged by neurotropic factors produced by Schwann cells distal to the injury. From the proximal stumps grow numerous fine unmyelinated tendrils, many of which find their way into the cell-clogged endoneurial tubes. These axonal processes grow at a speed of about 1mm per day, the larger fibres slowly acquiring a new myelin coat. Eventually they join to end-organs, which enlarge and start functioning again.

Neurotmesis

In Seddon's original classification, neurotmesis meant division of the nerve trunk, such as may occur in an

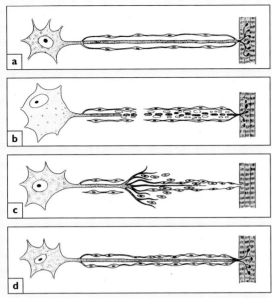

11.2 Nerve injury and repair (**a**) Normal axon and target organ (striated muscle). (**b**) Following nerve injury the distal part of the axon disintegrates and the myelin sheath breaks up. The nerve cell nucleus becomes eccentric and Nissl bodies are sparse. (**c**) New axonal tendrils grow into the mass of proliferating Schwann cells. One of the tendrils will find its way into the old endoneurial tube and (**d**) the axon will slowly regenerate.

here the endoneurial tubes are destroyed over a variable segment and scarring thwarts any hope of regenerating axons entering the distal segment and regaining their target organs. Instead, regenerating fibres mingle with proliferating Schwann cells and fibroblasts in a jumbled knot, or 'neuroma', at the site of injury. Even after surgical repair, many new axons fail to reach the distal segment, and those that do may not find suitable Schwann tubes, or may not reach the correct end-organs in time or may remain incompletely myelinated. Function may be adequate but is never normal.

The 'double crush' phenomenon

There is convincing evidence that proximal compression of a peripheral nerve renders it more susceptible to the effects of a second, more peripheral injury (Osterman, 1991). This may explain why peripheral entrapment syndromes are often associated with cervical or lumbar spondylosis. A similar type of 'sensitization' is seen in patients with peripheral neuropathy due to diabetes or alcoholism.

open wound. It is now recognized that severe degrees of damage may be inflicted without actually dividing the nerve. If the injury is more severe, whether the nerve is in continuity or not, recovery will not occur. As in axonotmesis, there is rapid wallerian degeneration, but

CLASSIFICATION OF NERVE INJURIES

Seddon's description of the three different types of nerve injury (neurapraxia, axonotmesis and neurotmesis) served as a useful classification for many years. Increasingly, however, it has been recognized that many

Table 11.1 The five grades of nerve injury

GRADE		CONTINUITY OF STRUCTURES				CLINICAL FEATURES			
Sunder-land	Seddon	Epineurium	Perineurium	Endoneurium	Axon	Outcome	Treatment	Tinel's	Electro-physiology
1	Neurapraxia	+	+	+	Block	Good	Expectant	Absent	Conduction block at injury site, normal conduction distally
2	Axonotmesis	+	+	+	–	Good/fair	Expectant	Advancing	Conduction block at site of injury and distally Denervation on EMG
3	Axonotmesis	+	+	–	–	Fair/poor	Expectant/repair/graft	Advancing	As 2
4	Axonotmesis	+	–	–	–	Poor	Repair/graft	Advancing	As 2
5	Neurotmesis	–	–	–	–	Poor	Repair/graft	Static	As 2

cases fall into an area somewhere between axonotmesis and neurotmesis. Therefore, following Sunderland, a more practical classification is offered here.

First degree injury This embraces transient ischaemia and neurapraxia, the effects of which are reversible.

Second degree injury This corresponds to Seddon's axonotmesis. Axonal degeneration takes place but, because the endoneurium is preserved, regeneration can lead to complete, or near complete, recovery without the need for intervention.

Third degree injury This is worse than axonotmesis. The endoneurium is disrupted but the perineurial sheaths are intact and internal damage is limited. The chances of the axons reaching their targets are good, but fibrosis and crossed connections will limit recovery.

Fourth degree injury Only the epineurium is intact. The nerve trunk is still in continuity but internal damage is severe. Recovery is unlikely; the injured segment should be excised and the nerve repaired or grafted.

Fifth degree injury The nerve is divided and will have to be repaired.

CLINICAL FEATURES

Acute nerve injuries are easily missed, especially if associated with fractures or dislocations, the symptoms of which may overshadow those of the nerve lesion. *Always test for nerve injuries following any significant trauma.* And if a nerve injury is present, it is crucial also to look for an accompanying vascular injury.

Ask the patient if there is numbness, paraesthesia or muscle weakness in the related area. Then examine the injured limb systematically for signs of abnormal posture (e.g. a wrist drop in radial nerve palsy), weakness in specific muscle groups and changes in sensibility.

Areas of altered sensation should be accurately mapped. Each spinal nerve root serves a specific dermatome and peripheral nerves have more or less discrete sensory territories, which are illustrated in the relevant sections of this chapter. Despite the fact that there is considerable overlap in sensory boundaries, the area of altered sensibility is usually sufficiently characteristic to provide an anatomical diagnosis. Sudomotor changes may be found in the same topographic areas; the skin feels dry due to lack of sweating. If this is not obvious, the 'plastic pen test' may help. The smooth barrel of the pen is brushed across the palmar skin: normally there is a sense of slight stickiness, due to the thin layer of surface sweat but in denervated skin the pen slips along smoothly with no sense of stickiness in the affected area.

The neurological examination must be repeated at intervals so as not to miss signs which appear hours after the original injury, or following manipulation or operation.

In chronic nerve injuries, there are other characteristic signs. The anaesthetic skin may be smooth and shiny, with evidence of diminished sensibility such as cigarette burns of the thumb in median nerve palsy or foot ulcers with sciatic nerve palsy. Muscle groups will be wasted and postural deformities may become fixed. Beware of trick movements which give the appearance of motor activity where none exists.

Assessment of nerve recovery

The presence or absence of distal nerve function can be revealed by simple clinical tests of power and light touch; remember that motor recovery is slower than sensory recovery. More specific assessment is required to answer two questions: How severe was the lesion? And how well is the nerve functioning now?

THE DEGREE OF INJURY *The history* is most helpful. A low energy injury is likely to have caused a neurapraxia; the

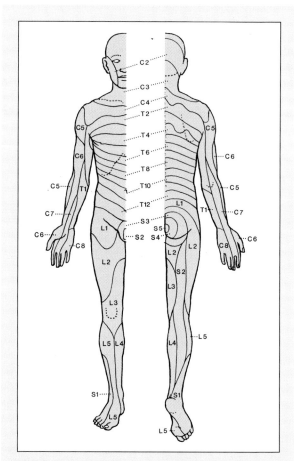

11.3 Examination Dermatomes supplied by spinal nerve roots. The sensory distribution of peripheral nerves is illustrated in the relevant sections.

patient should be observed and recovery anticipated. A high energy injury is more likely to have caused axonal and endoneurial disruption (Sunderland third and fourth degree) and so recovery is less predictable. An open injury, or a very high-energy closed injury, will probably have divided the nerve and early exploration is called for.

Tinel's sign – peripheral tingling or dysaesthesia provoked by percussing the nerve – is important. In a neurapraxia, Tinel's sign is negative. In axonotmesis, it is positive at the site of injury because of sensitivity of the regenerating axon sprouts. After a delay of a few days or weeks, the Tinel sign will then advance at a rate of about 1mm each day as the regenerating axons progress along the Schwann-cell tube. *Motor activity* also should progress down the limb. Failure of Tinel's sign to advance suggests a fourth or fifth degree injury and the need for early exploration. If the Tinel sign proceeds very slowly, or if muscle groups do not sequentially recover as expected, then a good recovery is unlikely and here again exploration must be considered.

Electromyogram (EMG) studies can be helpful (Campion, 1996). If a muscle loses its nerve supply, the EMG will show denervation potentials at the third week. This excludes neurapraxia but of course it does not distinguish between axonotmesis and neurotmesis; this remains a clinical distinction, but if one waits too long to decide then the target muscle may have failed irrecoverably and the answer hardly matters.

THE LEVEL OF NERVE FUNCTION *Two-point discrimination* is a measure of innervation density. After nerve regeneration or repair, a proportion of proximal sensory axons will fail to reach their appropriate sensory end-organ; they will either have regenerated down the wrong Schwann-cell tube or will be entangled in a neuroma at the site of injury. Therefore, two-point discrimination (measured with a bent paper clip and compared with the opposite normal side) gives an indication of how completely the nerve has recovered. *Static two-point discrimination* measures slowly adapting sensors (Merkel cells) and moving two-point discrimination measures rapidly adapting sensors (Meissner corpuscles and Pacinian corpuscles). *Moving two-point discrimination* is more sensitive and returns earlier. Normal static two point discrimination is about 6mm and moving is about 3mm at the finger tips.

Threshold-tests measure the threshold at which a sensory receptor is activated. They are more useful in nerve-compression syndromes, where individual receptors fail to send impulses centrally; two-point discrimination is preserved because the innervation density is not affected. Fine nylon monofilaments of varying widths are placed perpendicularly on the skin and the size of the lightest perceptible filament is recorded.

The Moberg pick-up test measures tactile gnosis. The patient is blindfolded and instructed to pick up and identify nine objects as rapidly as possible.

Motor power is graded on the Medical Research Council scale as:

0 no contraction
1 a flicker of activity
2 muscle contraction but unable to overcome gravity
3 contraction able to overcome gravity
4 contraction against resistance
5 normal power

PRINCIPLES OF TREATMENT

Nerve exploration

Closed low energy injuries usually recover spontaneously and it is worth waiting until the most proximally supplied muscle should have regained function. Exploration is indicated: (1) if the nerve was seen to be divided and needs to be repaired; (2) if the type of injury (e.g. a knife wound or a high energy injury) suggests that the nerve has been divided or severely damaged; (3) if recovery is inappropriately delayed and the diagnosis is in doubt.

Vascular injuries, unstable fractures, contaminated soft tissues and tendon divisions should be dealt with before the nerve lesion. The incision will be long, as the nerve must be widely exposed above and below the lesion before the lesion itself is cleared. The nerve must be handled gently with suitable instruments. Bipolar diathermy is used. Magnification helps; an operating microscope is ideal but a loupe or watchmaker's headpiece is better than nothing. A nerve stimulator is essential if scarring makes recognition uncertain. If microsurgical equipment and expertise are not available, then the nerve lesion should be identified and the wound closed pending transferral to an appropriate facility.

Primary repair

A divided nerve is best repaired as soon as this can be done safely. Primary suture at the time of wound toilet has considerable advantages: the nerve ends have not retracted much; their relative rotation is usually undisturbed; and there is no fibrosis.

A clean cut nerve is sutured without further preparation; a ragged cut may need paring of the stumps with a sharp blade, but this must be kept to a minimum. The stumps are anatomically orientated and fine (10/0) sutures are inserted in the epineurium. There should be no tension on the suture line. Opinions are divided on the value of fascicular repair with perineurial sutures.

Sufficient relaxation of the tissues to permit tension-free repair can usually be obtained by positioning the nearby joints or by mobilizing and re-routing the nerve. If this does not solve the problem then a primary nerve graft must be considered. A traction lesion – especially of the brachial plexus – may leave a gap too wide to close. These injuries are best dealt with in specialized

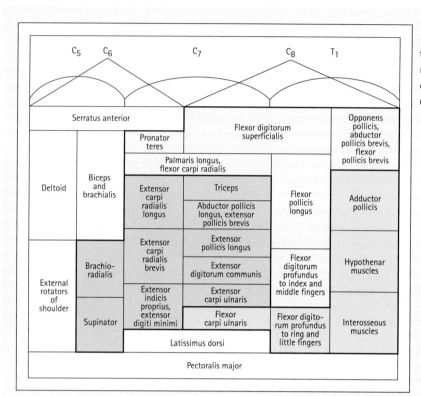

11.4 Examination Type of form used for recording muscle power in new and recovering nerve lesions (after Merle d'Aubigné). Power is recorded in individual blocks on the MRC Scale 1–5.

centres, where primary grafting or nerve transfer can be carried out.

If a tourniquet is used it should be a pneumatic one; it must be released and bleeding stopped before the wound is closed.

The limb is splinted in a position to ensure minimal tension on the nerve; if flexion needs to be excessive, a graft is required. The splint is retained for 2–3 weeks and thereafter physiotherapy is encouraged.

Delayed repair

Late repair – i.e. weeks or months after the injury – may be indicated because (1) a closed injury was left alone but shows no sign of recovery at the expected time, (2) the diagnosis was missed and the patient presents late or (3) primary repair has failed. The options must be carefully weighed: if the patient has adapted to the functional loss, if it is a high lesion and reinnervation is unlikely within the critical 2-year period, or if there is a pure motor loss which can be treated by tendon transfers, it may be best to leave well alone. Excessive scarring and intractable joint stiffness may, likewise, make nerve repair questionable; yet in the hand it is still worthwhile simply to regain protective sensation.

The lesion is exposed, working from normal tissue above and below towards the scarred area. When the nerve is in continuity it is difficult to know whether resection is necessary or not. If the nerve is only slightly thickened and feels soft, or if there is conduc-

tion across the lesion, resection is not advised; if the 'neuroma' is hard and there is no conduction on nerve stimulation, it should be resected, paring back the stumps until healthy fascicles are exposed.

How to deal with the gap? The nerve must be sutured without tension. The stumps may be brought together by gently mobilizing the proximal and distal segments, by flexing nearby joints to relax the soft tissues, or (in the case of the ulnar nerve) by transposing the nerve trunk to the flexor aspect of the elbow. In this way, gaps

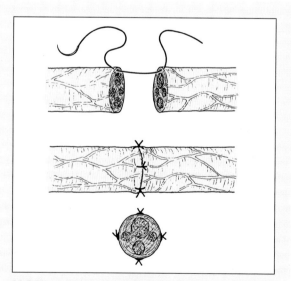

11.5 Nerve repair The stumps are correctly orientated and attached by fine sutures through the epineurium.

of 2cm in the median nerve, 4–5cm in the ulnar nerve and 6–8cm in the sciatic nerve can usually be closed, the limb being splinted in the 'relaxing' position for 4–6 weeks after the operation. Elsewhere, gaps of more than 1–2cm usually require grafting.

Nerve grafting

Free autogenous nerve grafts can be used to bridge gaps too large for direct suture. The sural nerve is most commonly used; up to 40cm can be obtained from each leg. Because the nerve diameter is small, several strips may be used (cable graft). The graft should be long enough to lie without any tension, and it should be routed through a well-vascularized bed. The graft is attached at each end either by fine sutures or with fibrin glue.

It is crucial that the motor and sensory fascicles are appropriately connected by the graft. There are various techniques which can help. Careful inspection of the fascicular alignment, structure and vascular markings is often helpful. Enzyme-staining techniques can be used.

Vascularized grafts are used in special situations. If the ulnar and median nerves are both damaged (e.g. in Volkmann's ischaemia) a pedicle graft from the ulnar nerve may be used to bridge the gap in the median. It is also possible to use free vascularized grafts for certain brachial plexus lesions.

Nerve transfer

In root avulsions of the upper brachial plexus, too proximal for direct repair, nerve transfer can be used. The spinal accessory nerve can be transferred to the suprascapular nerve, and intercostal nerves can be transferred to the musculocutaneous nerve. If biceps has failed because too much time has passed since the injury, an entire muscle (gracilis or latissimus dorsi) can be transferred as a free flap, attached between elbow and shoulder and then innervated by joining intercostal nerves or the spinal accessory nerve to the stump of the original nerve supplying that muscle.

Care of paralysed parts

While recovery is awaited the skin must be protected from friction damage and burns. The joints should be moved through their full range twice daily to prevent stiffness and minimize the work required of muscles when they recover. 'Dynamic' splints may be helpful.

Tendon transfers

Motor recovery may not occur if the axons, regenerating at about 1mm per day, do not reach the muscle within

18–24 months of injury. This is most likely when there is a proximal injury in a nerve supplying distal muscles. In such circumstances, tendon transfers should be considered. The principles can be summarized as follows:

1. Assess the problem
- Which muscles are missing?
- Which muscles are available?

2. The donor muscle should
- Be expendable
- Have adequate power
- Be an agonist or synergist

3. The recipient site should
- Be stable
- Have mobile joints and supple tissues

4. The transferred tendon should
- Be routed subcutaneously
- Have a straight line of pull
- Be capable of firm fixation

Recommended transfers are discussed under the individual nerve lesions.

PROGNOSIS

Type of lesion Neurapraxia always recovers fully; axonotmesis may or may not; neurotmesis will not unless the nerve is repaired.

Level of lesion The higher the lesion, the worse the prognosis.

Type of nerve Purely motor or purely sensory nerves recover better than mixed nerves, because there is less likelihood of axonal confusion.

Size of gap Above the critical resection length, end-to-end suture is not successful and a graft is needed.

Age Children do better than adults.

Delay in suture This is a most important adverse factor. The best results are obtained with early nerve repair. After a few months, recovery following suture becomes progressively less likely.

Associated lesions Damage to vessels, tendons and other structures makes it more difficult to obtain recovery of a useful limb even if the nerve itself recovers.

Surgical techniques Skill, experience and suitable facilities are needed to treat nerve injuries. If these are lacking, it is wiser to perform the essential wound toilet and then transfer the patient to a specialized centre.

REGIONAL SURVEY OF NERVE INJURIES

BRACHIAL PLEXUS INJURIES

Pathological anatomy

The brachial plexus is formed by the confluence of nerve roots from C5 to T1; the network and its branches are shown diagrammatically below. The plexus, as it passes from the cervical spine between the muscles of the neck and beneath the clavicle en route to the arm, is vulnerable to injury – either a stab wound or severe traction caused by a fall on the side of the neck or the shoulder.

Traction injuries are generally classed as supraclavicular (65%), infraclavicular (25%) and combined (10%). *Supraclavicular lesions* typically occur in motorcycle accidents: as the cyclist collides with the ground or another vehicle his or her neck and shoulder are wrenched apart. In the most severe injuries the arm is practically avulsed from the trunk, with rupture of the subclavian artery. *Infraclavicular lesions* are usually associated with fractures or dislocations of the shoulder; in about one-quarter of cases the axillary artery also is torn. Fractures of the clavicle rarely damage the plexus and then only if caused by a direct blow.

The injury may affect any level, or several levels within the plexus, often involving a mixture of nerve root(s), trunk(s) and nerve(s). An important distinction is made between preganglionic and postganglionic lesions. Avulsion of a nerve root from the spinal cord is a *preganglionic lesion*, i.e. disruption proximal to the dorsal root ganglion; this cannot recover and it is surgically irreparable. Rupture of a nerve root distal to the ganglion, or of a trunk or peripheral nerve, is a *postganglionic lesion*, which is surgically reparable and potentially capable of recovery. *Lesions in continuity*, from first to fourth degree, generally have a better prognosis than complete ruptures. *Mild lesions (neurapraxia)* are fairly common and may be caused by comparatively trivial trauma such as sudden compression by a tight harness or motor vehicle seatbelt; these recover spontaneously but mild residual symptoms may prove a nuisance for many months.

Clinical features

Brachial plexus injuries are often overshadowed by other, life-threatening trauma which needs immediate attention. Associated injuries, such as rupture of the subclavian or axillary artery, should be sought and attended to, otherwise a poor outcome is inevitable.

Neurological dysfunction soon becomes obvious. Detailed clinical examination is directed at answering specific questions: What is the level of the lesion? Is it preganglionic or postganglionic? If postganglionic, what type of lesion is it?

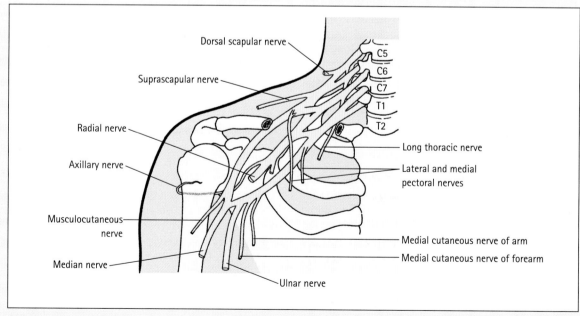

11.6 Brachial plexus Diagram of the brachial plexus and its relationship to the clavicle (some of the less important nerve branches and the posterior attachment of the second rib have been omitted).

THE LEVEL OF THE LESION

In upper plexus injuries (C5 and 6) the shoulder abductors and external rotators and the forearm supinators are paralysed. Sensory loss involves the outer aspect of the arm and forearm.

Pure lower plexus injuries are rare. Wrist and finger flexors are weak and the intrinsic hand muscles are paralysed. Sensation is lost in the ulnar forearm and hand.

If the entire plexus is damaged, the whole limb is paralysed and numb. Sometimes the scapular muscles and one side of the diaphragm too are involved. By examining systematically for each component of the brachial plexus (roots, trunks, divisions, cords and branches) the exact site of the lesion may be identified. For instance, preservation of the dorsal scapular nerve (rhomboids), long thoracic nerve (serratus anterior) and suprascapular nerve (supraspinatus), but loss of musculocutaneous nerve function (biceps), radial nerve (triceps) and axillary nerve (deltoid) suggest a lateral and posterior cord injury.

PRE- OR POST-GANGLIONIC?

It is crucial to establish how far from the cord the lesion is. Preganglionic lesions (root avulsions) are irreparable; postganglionic lesions may either recover (axonotmesis) or may be amenable to repair. Features suggesting root avulsion are: (1) crushing or burning pain in an anaesthetic hand, (2) paralysis of scapular muscles or diaphragm, (3) Horner's syndrome ptosis, miosis (small pupil), enopthalmos and anhidrosis, (4) severe vascular injury, (5) associated fractures of the cervical spine and (6) spinal cord dysfunction (e.g. hyper-reflexia in the lower limbs).

The *histamine test* is helpful. Intradermal injection of histamine usually causes a triple response in the surrounding skin (central capillary dilatation, a wheal and a surrounding flare). If the flare reaction persists in an anaesthetic area of skin, the lesion must be proximal to the posterior root ganglion – i.e. it is probably a root avulsion. With a postganglionic lesion the test will be negative because nerve continuity between the skin and the dorsal root ganglion is interrupted.

Computed tomography (CT) myelography or magnetic resonance imaging (MRI) may show pseudomeningocoeles produced by root avulsion. Note that during the first few days a 'positive' result is unreliable because the dura can be torn without there being root avulsion.

Nerve conduction studies need careful interpretation. If there is sensory conduction from an anaesthetic dermatome, this suggests a preganglionic lesion (i.e. the nerve distal to the ganglion is not interrupted). This test becomes reliable only after a few weeks, when Wallerian degeneration in a postganglionic lesion will block nerve conduction.

THE TYPE OF LESION

Once a postganglionic lesion has been diagnosed, it becomes important to decide how severely the nerve has been damaged. The history is informative: the mechanism of injury and the impact velocity may suggest either a mild (first or second degree) or a severe (fourth or fifth degree) injury. With the former a period of observation is justified; a first or second degree lesion may show signs of recovery by 6 or 8 weeks. If a neurotmesis seems likely then early operative exploration is called for. Since there may be different degrees of injury within the plexus, some muscles may recover while others fail to do so.

Management

The patient is likely to be admitted to a general unit where fractures and other injuries will be given priority. Emergency surgery is required for brachial plexus lesions associated with penetrating wounds, vascular injury or severe (high energy) soft-tissue damage whether open or closed; clean cut nerves should be repaired or grafted. This is best performed by a team specializing in this field of work.

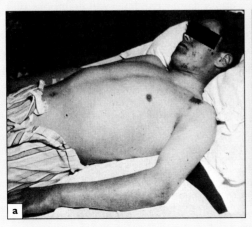 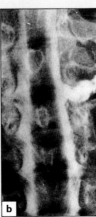

11.7 Brachial plexus (a) Telltale abrasions on the face and shoulder show how this motorcyclist pulled his entire plexus apart. (b) The myelogram shows leakage of the contrast medium, indicating root avulsion.

All other closed injuries are left until detailed examination and special investigations have been completed. Patients with root avulsion or severe, mutilating injuries of the limb will be unsuitable for nerve surgery, at least until the prognosis for limb function becomes clear.

Progress of the neurological features is carefully monitored. As long as recovery proceeds at the expected rate, watchful conservation is the byword. If recovery falters, or if special investigations show that it is more than a second degree lesion, then the patient should be referred to a special centre for surgical exploration of the brachial plexus and nerve repair, grafting or nerve transfer procedures. The sooner this decision is made, the better: during the early days operative exposure is easier and the response to repair more reliable. Repairs performed after 6 months are unlikely to succeed.

THE PATTERN OF INJURY

Surgical exploration reveals three typical patterns of injury:

- *C5,6(7) avulsion or rupture with C(7)8, T1 intact:* this group has the most favourable outcome as hand function is preserved and muscles innervated from the upper roots often recover after plexus repair or nerve transfer.
- *C5,6(7) rupture with avulsion of C7,8,T1:* these may recover shoulder and elbow movement after repair and grafting of the upper levels, but hand function is irretrievably lost.
- *C5–T1 avulsion:* these cases have a poor outcome. There are few donor axons available to neurotize the upper levels (shoulder and elbow function) and no recovery will take place in the hand.

The implication is that all efforts for nerve repair or nerve transfer are directed towards lesions involving C5 and 6. The objectives are to regain shoulder abduction, elbow flexion, wrist extension, finger flexion, and sensibility over the lateral (radial) side of the hand.

These and other aspects of brachial plexus injuries are discussed in the review paper by Birch (1996).

NERVE GRAFTING AND NERVE TRANSFER

Nerve grafting is often necessary and the results for restoration of shoulder and elbow function are quite good; however, the outcome for lesions affecting the forearm and hand are disappointing (Ochiai *et al.*, 1996).

Nerve transfer is a more recent development. If C5 and C6 are avulsed, then the spinal accessory nerve can be transferred to the suprascapular nerve; or two or three intercostal nerves can be tansferred to the musculocutaneous nerve.

If one nerve root is available (e.g. C5) then this should be grafted on to the lateral cord which will supply elbow flexion, finger flexion and sensation over the radial side of the hand. If two roots are available (e.g. C5, C6) these can be grafted on to the lateral and posterior cords. These procedures bypass the suprascapular nerve which is joined to the spinal accessory nerve.

Two or three years must pass before the final results of plexus reconstruction are apparent.

LATER RECONSTRUCTION

The best results of plexus reconstruction are obtained after very early operation. If the patient is not seen until very late after injury, or if plexus reconstruction has failed, then there are a number of options.

Tendon transfer to achieve elbow flexion: Various muscles can be transferred as elbow flexors: pectoralis major (Clarke's transfer), the common flexor origin (Steindler transfer), latissimus dorsi or triceps. The nerve supply to these muscles must remain intact, so they are suitable only for certain patterns of injury.

Free muscle transfer: Gracilis, rectus femoris or the contralateral latissimus dorsi can be transferred as a free flap and innervated with two or three intercostal nerves. Elbow flexion and wrist extension can be regained.

Shoulder arthrodesis: Arthrodesis is usually reserved for an unstable or painful shoulder, perhaps after failure of re-innervation of the supraspinatus. The position must be tailored to the needs of the particular patient.

OBSTETRICAL BRACHIAL PLEXUS PALSY

Obstetrical palsy is caused by excessive traction on the brachial plexus during childbirth. Two patterns are seen: (1) *upper root injury (Erb's palsy)*, typically in overweight babies with shoulder dystocia at delivery; or (2) *complete plexus injury (Klumpke's palsy)*, usually after breech delivery of smaller babies.

Clinical features

The diagnosis is usually obvious at birth: after a difficult delivery the baby has a floppy or flail arm. Further examination a day or two later will define the type of brachial plexus injury.

Erb's palsy is caused by injury of C5, C6 and (sometimes) C7. The abductors and external rotators of the shoulder and the supinators are paralysed. The arm is held to the side, internally rotated and pronated. There may also be loss of finger extension. Sensation cannot be tested reliably in a baby.

Klumpke's palsy is much less common, but more severe. This is a complete plexus lesion. The arm is flail and pale; all finger muscles are paralysed and there may also be vasomotor impairment and a unilateral Horner's syndrome.

X-rays should be taken to exclude fractures of the shoulder or clavicle.

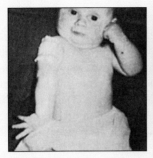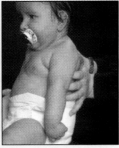

11.8 Obstetric palsy Two babies with Erb's palsy.

Management

Over the next few weeks one of several things may happen.

Paralysis may recover completely Many (perhaps most) of the upper root lesions recover spontaneously. A fairly reliable indicator is return of biceps activity by the third month. However, absence of biceps activity does not completely rule out later recovery.

Paralysis may improve A total lesion may partially resolve, leaving the infant with either an upper or a complete root syndrome which is unlikely to change.

Paralysis may remain unaltered This is more likely with complete lesions, especially in the presence of a Horner's syndrome.

While waiting for recovery, physiotherapy is applied to keep the joints mobile.

OPERATIVE TREATMENT

If there is no biceps recovery by 3 months, operative intervention should be considered. Unless the roots are avulsed, it may be possible to excise the scar and bridge the gap with free sural nerve grafts; if the roots are avulsed, nerve transfer may give a worthwhile result. This is highly demanding surgery which should be undertaken only in specialized centres.

The shoulder is prone to fixed internal rotation and adduction deformity. If diligent physiotherapy does not prevent this, then a subscapularis release will be needed, sometimes supplemented by a tendon transfer. In older children, the deformity can be treated by rotation ostotomy of the humerus.

LONG THORACIC NERVE

The long thoracic nerve of Bell (C5, C6, C7) may be damaged in shoulder or neck injuries (usually an axonotmesis) or during operations such as first rib resec-

tion, transaxillary sympathectomy or radical mastectomy. However, serratus anterior palsy is also seen after comparatively benign events, such as carrying loads on the shoulder, and even viral illnesses or toxoid injections.

Clinical features

Paralysis of serratus anterior is the commonest cause of winging of the scapula. The patient may complain of aching and weakness on lifting the arm. Examination shows little abnormality until the arm is elevated in flexion or abduction. The classic test for winging is to have the patient pushing forwards against the wall or thrusting the shoulder forwards against resistance.

Treatment

Except after direct injury or division, the nerve usually recovers spontaneously, though this may take a year or longer. Persistent winging of the scapula occasionally requires operative stabilization by transferring pectoralis minor or major to the lower part of the scapula.

SPINAL ACCESSORY NERVE

The spinal accessory nerve (C2–6) supplies the sternomastoid muscle and then runs obliquely across the posterior triangle of the neck to innervate the upper half of the trapezius. Contrary to general belief, the nerve appears also to have sensory functions, including pain sensibility (Bremner-Smith *et al.*, 1999). Because of its superficial course, it is easily injured in stab wounds and operations in the posterior triangle of the neck (e.g. lymph node biopsy). It is occasionally injured in whiplash injuries (Bodack *et al.*, 1998).

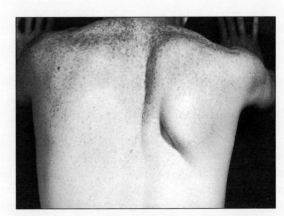

11.9 Long thoracic nerve palsy Winging of the scapula is demonstrated by having the patient push forwards against the wall.

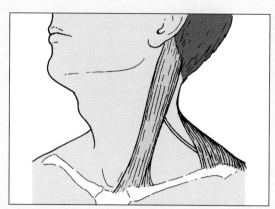

11.10 Accessory nerve The accessory nerve is embedded in the fascia which covers the posterior triangle and is easily damaged during lymph node biopsy or excision (and in stab wounds).

Clinical features

Following an open wound or operation, the patient complains of pain and 'stiffness' of the shoulder. Examination reveals asymmetry or drooping of the shoulder, reduced ability to hitch or hunch the shoulder and weakness on abduction of the arm; typically there is mild winging of the scapula on attempting active abduction against resistance; unlike the deformity in serratus anterior palsy, this disappears on flexion or forward thrusting of the shoulder. Often the true nature of the problem is not appreciated and diagnosis is delayed for weeks or months. In late cases there may be wasting of the trapezius.

Treatment

Stab injuries and surgical injuries should be explored immediately and the nerve repaired. If the exact cause of injury is uncertain, it is prudent to wait for about 8 weeks for signs of recovery. If this does not occur, the nerve should be explored (a) to confirm the diagnosis and (b) to repair the lesion by direct suture or grafting. While waiting for recovery the arm is held in a sling to prevent dragging on the neck muscles. The results of early nerve repair are generally good but some patients continue to complain of shoulder fatigue during lifting and overhead activities.

SUPRASCAPULAR NERVE

The suprascapular nerve, which arises from the upper trunk of the brachial plexus (C5,6), runs through the suprascapular notch (beneath the superior transverse scapulae ligament) to supply the supra- and infraspinatus muscles. It may be injured in fractures of the clavicle or scapula, by a direct blow or sudden traction, or simply by carrying heavy loads over the shoulder.

Clinical features

There may be a history of injury, but more often patients present with unexplained pain in the suprascapular region or at the back of the shoulder, and weakness of shoulder abduction – symptoms readily mistaken for a rotator cuff syndrome or a cervical radiculopathy. There is usually wasting of the supraspinatus and diminished power of abduction and external rotation. EMG may help to establish the diagnosis.

Treatment

This is usually a neurapraxia or an axonotmesis which clears up spontaneously after 3 months. In the absence of trauma one might suspect a nerve entrapment syndrome, and decompression by division of the suprascapular ligament often brings improvement. The operative approach is through a posterior incision above and parallel to the spine of the scapula.

AXILLARY NERVE

The axillary nerve (C5,6) arises from the posterior cord of the brachial plexus, runs along subscapularis and across the axilla just inferior to the shoulder joint. It emerges behind the humerus, deep to the deltoid; after supplying the teres minor, it divides into a medial branch which supplies the posterior part of the deltoid and a patch of skin over the muscle and an anterior branch that curls round the surgical neck of the humerus to innervate the anterior two-thirds of the deltoid. The landmark for this important branch is 5cm below the tip of the acromion.

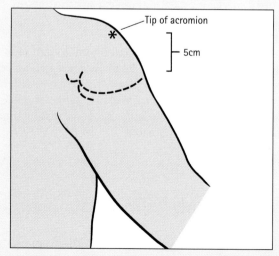

11.11 Axillary nerve Surface marking of the axillary nerve.

The nerve is sometimes ruptured in a brachial plexus injury. More often it is injured during shoulder dislocation or fractures of the humeral neck. Iatrogenic injuries occur in transaxillary operations on the shoulder and with lateral deltoid-splitting incisions.

Clinical features

The patient complains of shoulder 'weakness', and the deltoid is wasted. Although abduction can be initiated (by supraspinatus), it cannot be maintained. Retropulsion (extension of the shoulder with the arm abducted to 90°) is impossible. Careful testing will reveal a small area of numbness over the deltoid.

Treatment

Nerve injury associated with fractures or dislocations recovers spontaneously in about 80% of cases. If the deltoid shows no sign of recovery by 6 or 8 weeks, EMG should be performed; if the tests suggest denervation then the nerve should be explored through a combined deltopectoral and posterior (quadrilateral space) approach. Excision of the nerve ends and grafting are usually necessary; a good result can be expected if the nerve is explored within 3 months of injury. However, if the operation fails, provided that trapezius and serratus anterior are functioning, shoulder arthrodesis can provide both stability and some degree of 'abduction'.

RADIAL NERVE

The radial nerve may be injured at the elbow, in the upper arm or in the axilla.

Clinical features

Low lesions are usually due to fractures or dislocations at the elbow, or to a local wound. Iatrogenic lesions of the posterior interosseous nerve where it winds though the supinator muscle are sometimes seen after operations on the proximal end of the radius. The patient complains of clumsiness and, on testing, cannot extend the metacarpophalangeal joints of the hand. In the thumb there is also weakness of abduction and interphalangeal extension. Wrist extension is preserved because the branch to the extensor carpi radialis longus arises proximal to the elbow.

High lesions occur with fractures of the humerus or after prolonged tourniquet pressure. There is an obvious wrist drop, due to weakness of the radial extensors of the

wrist, as well as inability to extend the metacarpophalangeal joints. Sensory loss is limited to a small patch on the dorsum around the anatomical snuffbox.

Very high lesions may be caused by trauma or operations around the shoulder. More often, though, they are due to chronic compression in the axilla; this is seen in drink and drug addicts who fall into a stupor with the arm dangling over the back of a chair ('Saturday-night palsy') or in thin elderly patients using crutches ('crutch palsy'). In addition to weakness of the wrist and hand, the triceps is paralysed and the triceps reflex is absent.

Treatment

Open injuries should be explored and the nerve repaired or grafted as soon as possible.

Closed injuries are usually first or second degree lesions, and function eventually returns. In patients with fractures of the humerus it is important to examine for a radial nerve injury on admission, before treatment and again after manipulation or internal fixation.

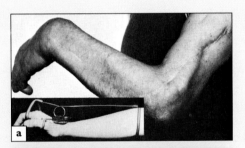
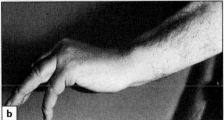
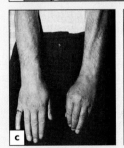
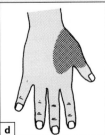

11.12 Radial nerve lesions (a) High lesion, producing a drop wrist. The inset shows a type of drop wrist splint. (b) Low lesion: the wrist extensors are spared but the patient cannot extend his metacarpophalangeal joints. (c) Muscle wasting due to a long-standing posterior interosseous nerve lesion. (d) Area of sensory loss.

If the palsy is present on admission, one can afford to wait for 6 weeks to see if it starts to recover. If it does not, then EMG should be performed; if this shows denervation potentials then a neurapraxia is excluded and the nerve should be explored.

If it is certain that there was no nerve injury on admission, and the signs appear only after manipulation or internal fixation, then the chances of an iatrogenic injury are high and the nerve should be explored and – if necessary – repaired or grafted without delay.

While recovery is awaited, the small joints of the hand must be put through a full range of passive movements. The wrist is splinted in extension. 'Lively' hand splints are avoided as they tend to hold the metacarpophalangeal joints in extension and this will lead to fixed contractures.

If recovery does not occur, the disability can be largely overcome by tendon transfers: pronator teres to the short radial extensor of the wrist, flexor carpi radialis to the long finger extensors and palmaris longus to the long thumb abductor.

ULNAR NERVE

Injuries of the ulnar nerve are usually either near the wrist or near the elbow, although open wounds may damage it at any level.

Clinical features

Low lesions are often caused by cuts on shattered glass. There is numbness of the ulnar one and a half fingers. The hand assumes a typical posture in repose – the claw hand deformity – with hyperextension of the metacarpophalangeal joints of the ring and little fingers, due to weakness of the intrinsic muscles. Hypothenar and interosseous wasting may be obvious by comparison with the normal hand. Finger abduction is weak and this, together with the loss of thumb adduction, makes pinch difficult. The patient is asked to grip a sheet of paper forcefully between thumbs and index fingers while the examiner tries to pull it away; powerful flexion of the thumb interphalangeal joint signals weakness of adductor pollicis and overcompensation by the flexor pollicis longus (Froment's sign).

Entrapment of the ulnar nerve in the pisohamate tunnel (Guyon's canal) is often seen in long-distance cyclists who lean with the pisiform pressing on the handlebars. Unexplained lesions of the distal (motor) branch of the nerve may be due to compression by a deep carpal ganglion or ulnar artery aneurysm.

High lesions occur with elbow fractures or dislocations. The hand is not markedly deformed because the ulnar half of flexor digitorum profundus is paralysed and the fingers are therefore less 'clawed' (the *'high*

ulnar paradox'). Otherwise, motor and sensory loss are the same as in low lesions.

'Ulnar neuritis' may be caused by compression or entrapment of the nerve in the medial epicondylar (cubital) tunnel, especially where there is severe valgus deformity of the elbow or prolonged pressure on the elbows in anaesthetized or bed-ridden patients (see page 249). It is important to be aware of this condition in patients who start complaining of ulnar nerve symptoms some weeks after an upper limb injury; one can easily be misled into thinking that the nerve lesion is due to the original injury!

Treatment

Exploration and suture of a divided nerve are well worthwhile, and anterior transposition at the elbow permits closure of gaps up to 5cm. While recovery is awaited, the skin should be protected from burns. Passive physiotherapy keeps the hand supple and useful.

If there is no recovery after nerve division, hand function is significantly impaired. Grip strength is diminished because the primary metacarphophalangeal flexors are lost, and pinch is poor because of the weakened thumb adduction and index finger abduction. Fine, coordinated finger movements are also affected.

Metacarpophalangeal flexion can be improved by extensor carpi radialis longus to intrinsic tendon transfers (Brand), or by looping a slip of flexor digitorum superficialis around the flexor sheath. Index abduction is improved by transferring extensor pollicis brevis or extensor indicis to the interosseous insertion on the radial side of the finger.

MEDIAN NERVE

The median nerve is most commonly injured near the wrist or high up in the forearm.

Clinical features

Low lesions may be caused by cuts in front of the wrist or by carpal dislocations. The patient is unable to abduct the thumb, and sensation is lost over the radial three and a half digits. In long-standing cases the thenar eminence is wasted and trophic changes may be seen.

High lesions are generally due to forearm fractures or elbow dislocation, but stabs and gunshot wounds may damage the nerve at any level. The signs are the same as those of low lesions but, in addition, the long flexors to the thumb, index and middle fingers, the radial wrist

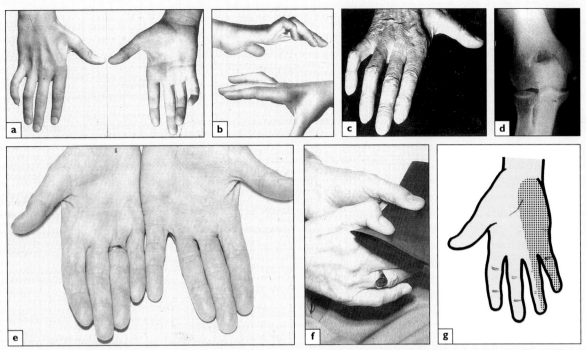

11.13 Ulnar nerve lesions (**a, b**) Low ulnar palsy: intrinsic muscle wasting; in the ring and little fingers the knuckle joints are hyperextended (paralysed lumbricals) and the interphalangeal joints are flexed (paralysed interossei). (**c**) High ulnar palsy: profundus action is lost, so the terminal interphalangeal joints are not flexed (ulnar paradox). He had cut his elbow on some glass. (**d**) The x-ray shows the glass fragment. (**e**) When the patient tries to push his little fingers apart, weakness of one abductor digiti minimi is displayed. (**f**) Froment's sign – because adductor pollicis is weak, the flexor pollicis longus is being used. (**g**) Sensory loss.

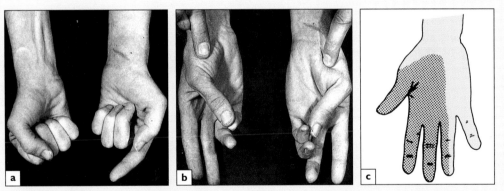

11.14 Cut median nerve (**a**) The pointing index when trying to clench the fist. (**b**) Abductor pollicis brevis wasting. (**c**) Sensory loss.

flexors and the forearm pronator muscles are all paralysed. Typically the hand is held with the ulnar fingers flexed and the index straight (the 'pointing sign'). Also, because the thumb and index flexors are deficient, there is a characteristic pinch defect: instead of pinching with the thumb and index finger-tips flexed, the patient pinches with the distal joints in full extension.

Isolated anterior interosseous nerve lesions are extremely rare. The signs are similar to those of a high median nerve injury, but without any sensory loss.

Treatment

If the nerve is divided, suture or nerve grafting should always be attempted. Postoperatively the wrist is splinted in flexion to avoid tension; when movements are commenced, wrist extension should be prevented.

Late lesions are sometimes seen. If there has been no recovery, the disability is severe because of sensory loss and deficient opposition. If sensation recovers but not opposition, abductor digiti minimi or extensor indicis can be re-routed to the distal end of the opponens pollicis. Extensor carpi radialis longus is available as a transfer for flexor digitorum profundus and brachioradialis for flexor pollicis longus.

LUMBROSACRAL PLEXUS

Any part of the plexus may be injured by sacroiliac dislocation or fractures of the sacrum. These lesions are usually incomplete and often missed; the patient may complain of no more than patchy muscle weakness and some difficulty with micturition. Sensation is diminished in the perineum or in one or more of the lower limb dermatomes. *Plexus injuries should always be looked for in patients with fractures of the pelvis.*

Recovery is usually quite good and no purpose is served by operative exploration.

FEMORAL NERVE

The femoral nerve may be injured by a gunshot wound, by pressure or traction during an operation or by bleeding into the thigh.

Clinical features

Quadriceps action is lacking and the patient is unable to extend the knee actively. There is numbness of the anterior thigh and medial aspect of the leg. The knee reflex is depressed.

Treatment

This is a fairly disabling lesion and, where possible, counter-measures should be undertaken. A thigh haematoma may need to be evacuated. A clean cut of the nerve may be treated successfully by suturing or grafting. The alternative would be a caliper to stabilize the knee, or tendon transfers of hamstrings to quadriceps.

SCIATIC NERVE

Division of the main sciatic nerve is rare except in gunshot wounds. Traction lesions may occur with traumatic hip dislocations and with pelvic fractures. Intraneural haemorrhage in patients receiving anticoagulants is a rare cause of intense pain and partial loss of function.

Iatrogenic lesions are sometimes discovered after total hip replacement – due either to direct trauma, compression by bone levers or possibly thermal injury from extruded acrylic cement; in most cases, though, no specific cause can be found and injury is assumed to be due to traction (see below).

Clinical features

In a complete lesion the hamstrings and all muscles below the knee are paralysed; the ankle jerk is absent. Sensation is lost below the knee, except on the medial side of the leg which is supplied by the saphenous branch of the femoral nerve. The patient walks with a drop foot and a high-stepping gait to avoid dragging the insensitive foot on the ground.

Sometimes only the deep part of the nerve is affected, producing what is essentially a common peroneal (lateral popliteal) nerve lesion (see below). This is the usual presentation in patients suffering foot-drop after hip replacement; however, careful examination will often reveal minor abnormalities also in the tibial (medial popliteal) division. Electrodiagnostic studies will help to establish the level of the injury.

If sensory loss extends into the thigh and the gluteal muscles are weak, suspect an associated lumbosacral plexus injury.

In late cases the limb is wasted, with fixed deformities of the foot and trophic ulcers on the sole.

Treatment

If the nerve is known to be divided, suture or nerve grafting should be attempted even though it may take more than a year for leg muscles to be reinnervated. While recovery is awaited, a below-knee drop foot splint is fitted. Great care is taken to avoid damaging the insensitive skin and to prevent trophic ulcers.

The chances of recovery are generally poor and, at best, will be long delayed and incomplete. Partial lesions, in which there is protective sensation of the sole, can sometimes be managed by transferring tibialis posterior to the front in order to counteract the drop foot. The deformities should be corrected if they threaten to cause pressure sores. If there is no recovery whatever, amputation may be preferable to a flail, deformed, insensitive limb.

SCIATIC PALSY AFTER TOTAL HIP REPLACEMENT

The incidence of overt sciatic nerve dysfunction is reported as 0.5–3% following primary hip replacement and about twice as high after revision. However, subclinical electromyographic changes are quite common and intra-operative electrical conduction tests have detected

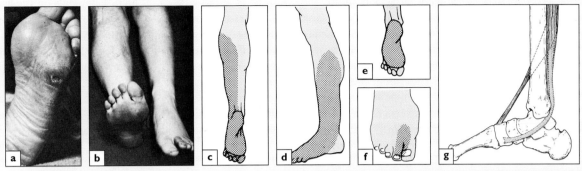

11.15 Two problems in sciatic nerve lesions are (**a**) trophic ulcers because of sensory loss and (**b**) foot drop. Sensory loss following division of (**c**) complete sciatic nerve, (**d**) lateral popliteal nerve, (**e**) posterior tibial nerve and (**f**) anterior tibial nerve. (**g**) Drop foot can be treated by rerouting tibialis posterior so that it acts as a dorsiflexor.

abnormalities in 18% of patients (mostly women) undergoing routine hip replacement (Black *et al.*, 1991). The vast majority of these resolve fairly quickly and do not manifest as postoperative nerve lesions. The less fortunate patients present soon after operation with weakness of ankle dorsiflexion, or a foot-drop, and abnormal sensibility in the distribution of the common peroneal nerve – a combination which is readily mistaken for a peroneal nerve lesion (wishful thinking in almost every case!). The reason for this is that the 'peroneal' portion of the sciatic nerve lies closest to the acetabulum and is most easily damaged. Careful examination will often show minor abnormalities also in the tibial nerve. If there is any doubt about the level of the lesion, EMG and nerve conduction tests will help.

X-rays may show a bone fragment or extruded cement (with the possibility of thermal damage) in the soft tissues; MRI may be needed to establish its proximity to the sciatic nerve. However, in most cases no cause is identified and one is left guessing whether the nerve was inadvertently injured by a scalpel point, haemostat, electrocautery, suture knot or traction levers. Delayed onset palsy may be due to a haematoma.

In about half the cases the lesion proves to be a first or second degree injury; some of these recover within weeks, others take months and may not recover completely. Unless a definite cause is known or strongly suspected, it is usually worth waiting for 6 weeks to see if the condition improves. During this time the patient is fitted with a drop-foot splint and physiotherapy is begun.

There is no agreement about the indications for immediate operation. Those who argue against it say they are unlikely to find any specific pathology and anyway if they do discover evidence of nerve damage, the chances of functional recovery after nerve repair are probably no better than those of waiting for spontaneous improvement. Our own indications for early operation are: (1) total sciatic palsy; (2) a partial lesion associated with severe burning pain; and (3) strong evidence of a local, and possibly reversible, cause such as a bone fragment, acrylic cement or haematoma near the nerve. If the exploratory operation reveals a local cause, it should be corrected. If the nerve is divided or shows full thickness damage, repair or grafting may be worthwhile. At best, recovery will take several years and will be incomplete. Partial lesions are better left alone and the resulting disability managed by splintage and/or tendon transfers.

PERONEAL NERVES

Injuries may affect either the common peroneal (lateral popliteal) nerve or one of its branches, the deep or superficial peroneal nerves.

Clinical features

The common peroneal nerve is often damaged at the level of the fibular neck by severe traction when the knee is forced into varus (e.g. in lateral ligament injuries and fractures around the knee, or during operative correction of gross valgus deformities), or by pressure from a splint or a plaster cast, from lying with the leg externally rotated, by skin traction, by an intraneural ganglion or by wounds. The patient has a drop foot and can neither dorsiflex nor evert the foot. He or she walks with a high-stepping gait to avoid catching the toes. Sensation is lost over the front and outer half of the leg and the dorsum of the foot. In late cases, pain may be a major feature.

The deep peroneal nerve runs between the muscles of the anterior compartment of the leg and emerges at the lower border of the extensor retinaculum of the ankle. It may be threatened in an anterior compartment syndrome, causing pain and weakness of dorsiflexion and sensory loss in a small area of skin between the first and second toes. Sometimes the distal portion is cut during operations on the ankle, resulting in paraesthesia and numbness on the dorsum around the first web space.

The *superficial peroneal nerve* descends along the fibula, innervating the peroneal muscles and emerging through the deep fascia 5–10cm above the ankle to supply to the skin over the dorsum of the foot and the medial four toes. The muscular portion may be involved in a lateral compartment syndrome. The patient complains of pain in the lateral part of the leg and numbness or paraesthesia of the foot; there may be weakness of eversion and sensory loss on the dorsum of the foot. The cutaneous branches alone may be trapped where the nerve emerges from the deep fascia, or stretched by a severe inversion injury of the ankle, causing pain and sensory symptoms without muscle weakness.

Treatment

Direct injuries of the common peroneal nerve and its branches should be explored and repaired or grafted wherever possible. While recovery is awaited a splint may be worn to control ankle weakness. Pain may be relieved and drop foot is improved in almost 50% of patients, especially those who are operated on early (Wilkinson and Birch, 1995). If there is no recovery, the disability can be minimized by tibialis posterior tendon transfer or by foot stabilization; the alternative is a permanent splint.

An acute compartment syndrome calls for immediate decompression by splitting the fascia (see page 564).

Chronic compartment syndromes, in which symptoms are triggered by exercise, may likewise need decompression. However, even after fasciectomy, patients may still have symptoms following very strenuous activity.

TIBIAL NERVES

The tibial (medial popliteal) nerve is rarely injured except in open wounds. The distal part (posterior tibial nerve) is sometimes involved in injuries around the ankle.

Clinical features

The tibial nerve supplies the flexors of the ankle and toes. With division of the nerve, the patient is unable to plantar-flex the ankle or flex the toes; sensation is absent over the sole and part of the calf. Because both the long flexors and the intrinsic muscles are involved, there is not much clawing. With time the calf and foot become atrophic and pressure ulcers may appear on the sole.

The posterior tibial nerve runs behind the medial malleolus under the flexor retinaculum, gives off a small calcaneal branch and then divides into *medial and lateral plantar nerves* which supply the intrinsic muscles and the skin of the sole. Fractures and dislocations around the ankle may injure any of these branches and the resultant picture depends on the level of the lesion. Thus, posterior tibial nerve lesions cause wide sensory loss and clawing of the toes due to paralysis of the intrinsics with active long flexors; but injury to one of the smaller branches causes only limited sensory loss and less noticeable motor weakness. A compartment syndrome of the foot (e.g. following metatarsal fractures) is easily missed if one fails to test specifically for plantar nerve function.

Treatment

A complete nerve division should be sutured as soon as possible. A peculiarity of the tibial nerve is that injury or repair (especially delayed repair) may be followed by causalgia.

While recovery is awaited, a suitable orthosis is worn (to prevent excessive dorsiflexion) and the sole is protected against pressure ulceration. In suitable cases, weakness of plantar flexion can be treated by hindfoot fusion or transfer of the tibialis anterior to the back of the foot.

NERVE COMPRESSION (ENTRAPMENT) SYNDROMES

Pathophysiology

Wherever peripheral nerves traverse fibro-osseous tunnels they are at risk of entrapment and compression, especially if the soft tissues increase in bulk (as they may in pregnancy, myxoedema or rheumatoid arthritis) or if there is a local obstruction (e.g. a ganglion or osteophytic spur).

Nerve compression impairs epineural blood flow and axonal conduction, giving rise to symptoms such as numbness, paraethesia and muscle weakness; the relief of ischaemia explains the sudden improvement in symptoms after decompressive surgery. Prolonged or severe compression leads to segmental demyelination, target muscle atrophy and nerve fibrosis; symptoms are then less likely to resolve after decompression.

Peripheral neuropathy associated with generalized disorders such as diabetes or alcoholism may render a nerve more sensitive to the effects of compression. There is evidence, too, that proximal compression (e.g. discogenic root compression) impairs the synthesis and transport of neural substances, so predisposing the nerve to the effects of distal entrapment – the so-called *double-crush syndrome* (Osterman, 1991).

Common sites for nerve entrapment are the *carpal tunnel* (median nerve) and the *cubital tunnel* (ulnar nerve); less common sites are the *tarsal tunnel* (posterior tibial nerve), the *inguinal ligament* (lateral cutaneous nerve of the thigh), the *suprascapular notch* (suprascapular nerve), *the neck of the fibula* (common peroneal nerve) and the *fascial tunnel of the superficial peroneal nerve.* A special case is the *thoracic outlet*, where the subclavian vessels and roots of the brachial plexus cross the first rib between the scalenus anterior and medius muscles. In these cases there may be vascular as well as neurological signs.

Clinical features

The patient complains of unpleasant tingling or pain or numbness. Symptoms are usually intermittent and sometimes related to specific postures which compromise the nerve. Thus, in the *carpal tunnel syndrome* they occur at night when the wrist is held still in flexion, and relief is obtained by moving the hand 'to get the circulation going'. In *ulnar neuropathy*, symptoms recur whenever the elbow is held in acute flexion for long periods. In the *thoracic outlet syndrome*, paraesthesia in the distribution of C8 and T1 may be provoked by holding the arms in abduction, extension and external rotation.

Areas of altered sensation and motor weakness are mapped out. In long-standing cases there may be obvious muscle wasting. The likely site of compression should be carefully examined for any local cause. MRI and ultrosonography are useful for excluding compression by a soft-tissue mass (e.g. a ganglion).

EMG and nerve conduction tests help to confirm the diagnosis, establish the level of compression and estimate the degree of nerve damage. Conduction is slowed across the compressed segment and EMG may show abnormal action potentials in muscles that are not obviously weak or wasted, or fibrillation in cases with severe nerve damage.

Treatment

In early cases splintage may help (e.g. holding the wrist or elbow in extension) and corticosteroid injection into the entrapment area can reduce local tissue swelling. If symptoms persist, operative decompression will usually be successful. However, in long-standing cases with muscle atrophy there may be endoneurial fibrosis and axonal degeneration; tunnel decompression may then fail to give complete relief.

MEDIAN NERVE COMPRESSION

Three separate syndromes are recognized: (1) carpal tunnel syndrome (far and away the most common); (2) proximal median nerve compression (the 'pronator syndrome'); and (3) anterior interosseous nerve compression.

CARPAL TUNNEL SYNDROME

This is the best known of all the entrapment syndromes. In the normal carpal tunnel there is barely room for all the tendons and the median nerve; consequently, any swelling is likely to result in compression and ischaemia of the nerve. Usually the cause eludes detection; the syndrome is, however, common at the menopause, in rheumatoid arthritis, in pregnancy and in myxoedema.

CLINICAL FEATURES The history is most helpful in making the diagnosis. Pain and paraesthesia occur in the distribution of the median nerve in the hand. Night after night the patient is woken with burning pain, tingling and numbness. Hanging the arm over the side of the bed, or shaking the arm, may relieve the symptoms. In advanced cases there may be clumsiness and weakness, particularly with tasks requiring fine manipulation such as fastening buttons.

The condition is eight times more common in women than in men. The usual age group is 40–50 years; in younger patients it is not uncommon to find related factors such as pregnancy, rheumatoid disease, chronic renal failure or gout.

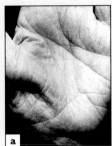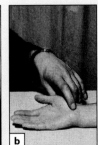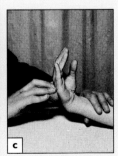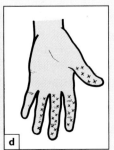

11.16 Carpal tunnel syndrome (**a**) Wasting of the thenar eminence is not usually as obvious as this. (**b**) Pressure of the tunnel or (**c**) forced flexion of the wrist may induce the patient's symptoms. (**d**) Area of diminished sensibility.

Sensory symptoms can often be reproduced by percussing over the median nerve (Tinel's sign) or by holding the wrist fully flexed for a minute or two (Phalen's test). In late cases there is wasting of the thenar muscles, weakness of thumb abduction and sensory dulling in the median nerve territory.

Electrodiagnostic tests, which show slowing of nerve conduction across the wrist, are reserved for those with atypical symtoms.

Radicular symptoms of cervical spondylosis may confuse the diagnosis and may coincide with carpal tunnel syndrome.

TREATMENT Light splints that prevent wrist flexion can help those with night pain or with pregnancy-related symptoms. Corticosteroid injection into the carpal canal, likewise, provides temporary relief.

Open surgical division of the transverse carpal ligament usually provides a quick and simple cure. The incision should be kept to the ulnar side of the thenar crease so as to avoid accidental injury to the palmar cutaneous (sensory) and thenar motor branches of the median nerve. Internal neurolysis is not recommended. Endoscopic carpal tunnel release offers an alternative with slightly quicker post-operative rehabilitation; however, the complication rate is higher (Agee *et al.*, 1995).

PROXIMAL MEDIAN NERVE COMPRESSION

The median nerve can be compressed beneath one of several structures around the elbow including the ligament of Struthers (a connection between the medial epicondyle and the humerus), the bicipital aponeurosis or the arch-like origins of either pronator teres or flexor digitorum superficialis. This variability is not well conveyed by the more common term *'pronator syndrome'*. Symptoms are similar to those of carpal tunnel syndrome, although night pain is unusual and forearm pain is more common. Phalen's test will obviously be negative; instead, symptoms can be provoked by resisted elbow flexion with the forearm supinated (tightening the bicipital aponeurosis), by resisted forearm pronation with the elbow extended (pronator tension) or by resisted flexion of the middle finger proximal interphalangeal joint (tightening the superficialis arch). Pain may be felt in the forearm and there may be altered sensation in the territory of the palmar cutaneous branch of the median nerve (which originates proximal to the carpal tunnel). Tinel's sign may be positive over the nerve proximally but not at the carpal tunnel. Nerve conduction studies will help to localize the level of the compression. X-ray may show a bony spur at the attachment of Struthers' ligament.

Surgical decompression involves division of the bicipital aponeurosis and any other restraining structure; great care is needed in the dissection.

ANTERIOR INTEROSSEOUS NERVE SYNDROME

The anterior interosseous nerve can be selectively compressed at the same sites as the proximal median nerve. There is motor weakness without sensory symptoms. The patient is unable to make the 'OK sign' – pinching with the thumb and index finger joints flexed, like a ring – because of weakness of the flexor pollicis longus and flexor digitorum profundus. Isolated loss of flexor pollicis longus can occur. Pressure over the belly of this muscle in the forearm will flex the thumb-tip, thus excluding tendon rupture.

Many patients will settle spontaneously within 3 months or so. If not, then electrodiagnostic studies should be performed to localize the site of compression prior to surgical exploration and release.

ULNAR NERVE COMPRESSION

This occurs most commonly at the elbow and less commonly at the wrist.

CUBITAL TUNNEL SYNDROME

The ulnar nerve is easily felt behind the medial epicondyle of the humerus (the 'funny bone'). It can be trapped or compressed within the cubital tunnel (by bone abnormalities, ganglia or hypertrophied synovium), proximal to the cubital tunnel (by the fascial arcade of Struthers) or distal to the cubital tunnel as it passes through the two heads of flexor carpi ulnaris to enter the forearm. Sometimes it is 'stretched' by a cubitus valgus deformity or simply by holding the elbow flexed for long periods.

CLINICAL FEATURES The patient complains of numbness and tingling in the little and the ulnar half of the ring finger; symptoms may be intermittent and related to specific elbow postures (e.g. they may appear only while the patient is lying down with the elbows flexed, or while holding the newspaper – again with the elbows flexed). Initially there is little to see but in late cases there may be weakness of grip, slight clawing, intrinsic muscle wasting and diminished sensibility in the ulnar nerve territory. Froment's sign and weakness of abductor digiti minimi can often be demonstrated.

Bone or soft tissue abnormalities may be obvious. Tinel's percussion test, tenderness over the nerve behind the medial epicondyle, reproduction of the symptoms with flexion of the elbow, and weakness of flexor carpi ulnaris and the flexor digitorum profundus to the little finger all suggest compression at the elbow rather than at the wrist.

The diagnosis may be confirmed by nerve conduction tests; however, since the symptoms are often postural or activity-related, a negative test does not exclude the diagnosis.

TREATMENT Conservative measures such as modification of posture and splintage of the elbow in mid-extension at night should be tried.

If symptoms persist, and particularly if there is intrinsic wasting, operative decompression is indicated. Options include simple release of the roof of the cubital tunnel, anterior transposition of the nerve into a subcutaneous or submuscular plane, or medial epicondylectomy (Geutjens *et al.*, 1996). It is essential that the nerve is released entirely from the arcade of Struthers right down to the aponeurosis beneath the flexor carpi ulnaris.

COMPRESSION IN GUYON'S CANAL

The ulnar nerve can be compressed as it passes through Guyon's canal at the ulnar border of the wrist. The symptoms can be pure motor, pure sensory or mixed, depending on the precise location of entrapment. A ganglion from the triquetrohamate joint is the most common cause; a fractured hook of hamate and ulnar artery aneurysm (seen with overuse of a hammer) are much rarer causes. Preservation of sensation in the dorsal branch of the ulnar nerve (which leaves the nerve proximal to Guyon's canal) suggests entrapment at the wrist rather than elbow; similarly power to flexor carpi ulnaris and flexor digitorum profundus to the little finger will be maintained.

After electrophysiological localization of the lesion to the wrist, further investigations should be considered: MRI may demonstrate a ganglion, CT a carpal fracture and Doppler studies an ulnar artery aneurysm. Depending on the results of these investigations, surgery can be planned.

RADIAL (POSTERIOR INTEROSSEOUS) NERVE COMPRESSION

The radial nerve itself is rarely the source of 'entrapment' symptoms. Just above the elbow, it divides into a superficial branch (sensory to the skin over the anatomical snuffbox) and the posterior interosseous nerve which dives between the two heads of the supinator muscle before supplying motor branches to extensor carpi ulnaris and the metacarpophalangeal extensors (branches to extensor carpi radialis longus and brevis arise above the elbow). Posterior interosseous nerve compression may occur at the proximal edge or within the substance of the supinator muscle. Two clinical patterns are encounterd: the posterior interosseous syndrome and the radial tunnel syndrome.

POSTERIOR INTEROSSEOUS SYNDROME

CLINICAL FEATURES This is a pure motor disorder and there are no sensory symptoms. Gradually emerging weakness of metacarpophalangeal extension affects first one or two and then all the digits. Wrist extension is preserved (the nerves to extensor carpi radialis longus and brachioradialis arise proximal to the supinator) but the wrist veers into abduction because of the weak extensor carpi ulnaris. This feature helps to distinguish posterior interosseous nerve entrapment from conditions such as neuralgic amyotrophy, in which the more proximally supplied muscles are often affected.

Compression usually occurs at the arcade of Frohse (a thickening of the proximal edge of supinator) but it may also be caused by swellings (a lipoma, a ganglion or synovial proliferation) in or around the radial tunnel. MRI may help to pinpoint the diagnosis.

TREATMENT Surgical exploration is warranted if the condition does not resolve spontaneously within 3 months. Recovery after surgery is slow; if there is no improvement by the end of a year, and if muscle weakness is disabling, tendon transfer is needed.

RADIAL TUNNEL SYNDROME

This syndrome is controversial; it has been aptly labelled 'resistant tennis elbow'. Although a motor nerve is involved the patient presents with pain, often work-related or at night, just distal to the lateral aspect of the elbow. Wrist movements may precipitate the pain. Electrodiagnostic tests are not helpful. If the symptoms do not resolve with prolonged non-operative measures (modification of activities and splintage), then surgery is considered. The nerve is freed beneath the extensor carpi radialis brevis and supinator muscle. However, the patient should be warned that surgery often fails to relieve the symptoms.

SUPRASCAPULAR NERVE COMPRESSION

Chronic or repetitive compression of the suprascapular nerve and its branches is much more common than is generally recognized. The peculiar anatomy of the nerve makes it unusually vulnerable to both traction and compression. However, the symptoms of this condition closely mimic those of rotator cuff lesions and cervical radiculopathy; unless the diagnosis is kept in mind in all such cases, it is likely to be missed.

The suprascapular nerve arises from the upper trunk of the brachial plexus (see Fig. 11.6), passes across the posterior triangle of the neck and then courses through the suprascapular notch beneath the superior transverse scapular ligament to supply the supraspinatus and infraspinatus muscles; it also sends sensory branches to the posterior part of the gleno-humeral joint, the acromioclavicular joint, the subacromial bursa, the ligaments around the shoulder and (in a small proportion of people) the skin on the outer, upper aspect of the arm (Ajmani, 1994). Compression or entrapment occurs at two sites: (a) the suprascapular notch and (b) a fibro-osseous tunnel where the infraspinatus branch curves around the edge of the scapular spine. Causes are continuous pressure or intermittent impact on the supraclavicular muscles (e.g. by carrying loads on the shoulder) or repetitive traction due to forceful shoulder movements (e.g. in games which involve pitching and throwing). In some cases nerve compression may be produced by a soft-tissue mass such as a large 'ganglion' at the back of the shoulder joint (Cummins *et al.*, 2000).

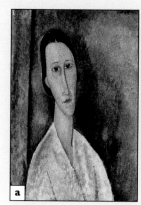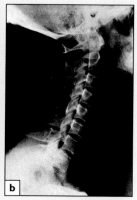

11.17 Thoracic outlet syndrome (a) Amadeo Modigliani's painting of Madame Zborowska (Coutesy of the Tate Gallery, London). (b) X-ray of a long-necked woman: all the vertebrae down to T1 are above the clavicle.

CLINICAL FEATURES There may be a history of injury to the pectoral girdle; more often, though, patients present with unexplained pain in the suprascapular region or at the back of the shoulder, and weakness of shoulder and upper arm movements – symptoms readily mistaken for cervical radiculopathy or a rotator cuff disorder. There is usually wasting of the supraspinatus muscle and diminished power of abduction and external rotation. Tensing the nerve by forceful adduction (pulling the arm across the front of the chest) causes increased pain.

EMG and measurement of nerve conduction velocity may help to establish the diagnosis. Ultrasonography and MRI are useful in excluding a soft-tissue mass.

TREATMENT The first step is to stop any type of activity which might stress the suprascapular nerve; after a few weeks, this can be combined with graded muscle strengthening exercises. If the condition is likely to settle, it will do so within 3–6 months.

If there is no improvement, or if imaging studies have revealed a soft-tissue mass, operative decompression is justified. The nerve is approached through a posterior incision above and parallel to the spine of the scapula. Provided the diagnosis was correct, there is a good chance that symptoms will be improved; muscle wasting, however, will probably remain.

THORACIC OUTLET SYNDROME

Neurological and vascular symptoms and signs in the upper limbs may be produced by compression of the lower trunk of the brachial plexus (C8 and T1) and subclavian vessels between the clavicle and the first rib (Oates and Daley, 1996; Novak and MackKinnon, 1996).

The subclavian artery and lower brachial trunk pass through a triangle based on the first rib and bordered by scalenus anterior and medius. These neurovascular structures are made taut when the shoulders are braced back and the arms held tightly to the sides; an extra rib (or its fibrous equivalent extending from a large costal process), or an anomalous scalene muscle, exaggerates this effect by forcing the vessel and nerve upwards.

These anomalies are all congenital; yet symptoms are rare before the age of 30 years. This is probably because, with increasing age, the shoulders sag, thus putting more traction on the neurovascular bundle; indeed drooping shoulders alone may cause the syndrome and symptoms are characteristically posture-related.

Stretching or compression of the lower nerve trunk produces sensory changes along the ulnar side of the forearm and hand, and weakness of the intrinsic hand muscles. The subclavian artery is rarely compressed but the lumen may contract due to irritation of its sympathetic supply, or else its wall may be damaged leading to the formation of small emboli. Even more unusual are signs of venous compression – oedema, cyanosis or thrombosis.

Clinical features

The patient, typically a woman in her thirties, complains of pain and paraesthesia extending from the shoulder, down the ulnar aspect of the arm and into the medial two fingers. Symptoms tend to be worse at night and are aggravated by bracing the shoulders (wearing a back-pack) or working with the arms above shoulder height. Examination may show mild clawing of the ulnar two fingers with wasting and weakness of the intrinsic muscles. If a female, the patient is often long-necked with sloping shoulders (like a Modigliani painting).

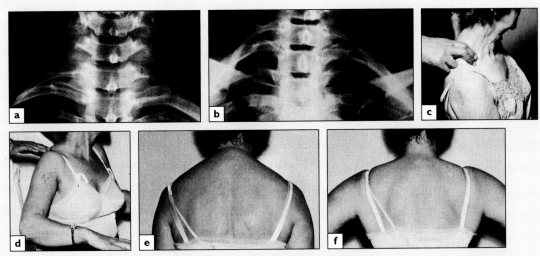

11.18 Cervical ribs (**a**) Unilateral; (**b**) bilateral. (**c**) Feeling for a pulsating lump near the subclavian artery. (**d**) Teaching the patient shrugging exercises. (**e, f**) Before and after improvement of shoulder posture.

Vascular signs are uncommon, but there may be cyanosis, coldness of the fingers and increased sweating. *Unilateral Raynaud's phenomenon should make one think 'thoracic outlet'.*

Symptoms and signs may be reproduced by various provocative manoeuvres. In *Adson's test* the patient's neck is extended and turned towards the affected side while he or she breathes in deeply; this compresses the interscalene space and may cause paraesthesia and obliteration of the radial pulse. In *Wright's test* the arms are abducted and externally rotated; again the symptoms recur and the pulse disappears on the abnormal side. Continue the examination by asking the patient to hold his or her arms high above the head and then open and close the fingers rapidly; this may cause cramping pain on the affected side *(Roos's test)*.

Investigations

X-rays of the neck occasionally demonstrate a cervical rib or an abnormally long C7 cervical process. X-rays should also be obtained of the lungs (is there an apical tumour?) and the shoulders (to exclude any painful local lesion).

Angiography and venography are reserved for the few patients with vascular symptoms.

Electodiagnostic tests are helpful mainly to exclude peripheral nerve lesions such as ulnar or median nerve compression which may confuse the diagnosis.

Diagnosis

The diagnosis of thoracic outlet syndrome is not easy. Some of the symptoms occur as transient phenomena in *normal individuals*, and 'cervical ribs' are sometimes discovered as incidental findings in patients who are x-rayed for other reasons. Postural obliteration of the radial pulse, likewise, may be quite normal; the provocative tests should be interpreted as positive only if they affect the pulse *and* reproduce the sensory symptoms.

The early symptoms and signs are almost identical to those *of ulnar nerve compression.* In fact, ulnar neuropathy may accompany thoracic outlet compression as a manifestation of the double-crush syndrome.

Cervical spondylosis is sometimes discovered on x-ray. However, this disorder seldom involves the T1 nerve root.

Pancoast's syndrome, due to apical carcinoma of the bronchus with infiltration of the structures at the root of the neck, includes pain, numbness and weakness of the hand. A hard mass may be palpable in the neck and x-ray of the chest shows a characteristic opacity.

Rotator cuff lesions sometimes cause pain radiating down the arm. However, there are no neurological symptoms and shoulder movement is likely to be abnormal.

Treatment

Most patients can be managed by *conservative treatment*: exercises to strengthen the shoulder girdle muscles, postural training and instruction in work practices and ways of preventing shoulder droop and muscle fatigue. Analgesics may be needed for pain.

Operative treatment is indicated if pain is severe, if muscle wasting is obvious or if there are vascular disturbances. The thoracic outlet is decompressed by removing the first rib (or the cervical rib). This is accomplished by either a supraclavicular approach or a transaxillary approach; in the latter, care must be taken to prevent injury to the brachial plexus and subclavian vessels, or perforation of the pleura.

LOWER LIMB COMPRESSION SYNDROMES

COMPRESSION OF LATERAL CUTANEOUS NERVE OF THE THIGH

The lateral cutaneous nerve can be compressed as it runs through the inguinal ligament just medial to the anterior superior iliac spine.

The patient complains of numbness, tingling or burning discomfort over the anterolateral aspect of the thigh (*meralgia paraesthetica*).

If the symptoms are troublesome the nerve can be released.

TARSAL TUNNEL SYNDROME

Pain and sensory disturbance over the plantar surface of the foot may be due to compression of the posterior tibial nerve behind and below the medial malleolus. The pain may be precipitated by prolonged weight-bearing. It is often worse at night and the patient may seek relief by walking around or stamping his or her foot. Paraesthesia and numbness should follow the characteristic sensory distribution, but these symptoms are not as well defined as in other entrapment syndromes. Tinel's percussion test may be positive behind the medial malleolus. The diagnosis is difficult to establish but nerve conduction studies may show slowing of motor or sensory conduction.

Treatment Tarsal tunnel entrapment may be relieved by fitting a medial arch support that holds the foot in slight varus. If this fails, surgical decompression is indicated. The nerve is exposed behind the medial malleolus and followed into the sole; sometimes it is trapped by the belly of abductor hallucis arising more proximally than usual. Unfortunately symptoms are not consistently relieved by this procedure.

DIGITAL NERVE COMPRESSION IN THE FOOT

Compression neuropathy of the digital nerve (Morton's metatarsalgia) is dealt with in Chapter 21.

OTHER PERIPHERAL NERVE DISORDERS

COMPARTMENT SYNDROMES

Capillary perfusion of a nerve may be markedly reduced by swelling within an osteofascial compartment. Direct trauma, prolonged compression or arterial injury may result in muscle swelling and a critical rise in compartment pressure; if unrelieved, this causes further impedance of blood flow, more prolonged ischaemia and so on into a vicious circle of events ending in necrosis of nerve and muscle. This may occur after proximal arterial injury, soft-tissue bleeding from fractures or operations, circular compression by tight dressings or plasters, and even direct pressure in a comatose person lying on a hard surface. Lesser, self-relieving effects are sometimes produced by muscle swelling due to strenuous exercise. Common sites are the forearm and leg; less common are the foot, upper arm and thigh.

ACUTE COMPARTMENT SYNDROME   Acute compartment syndrome and its late effects (Volkmann's contracture) are described in Chapter 23.

CHRONIC COMPARTMENT SYNDROME   Long-distance runners sometimes develop pain along the anterolateral aspect of the calf, brought on by muscular exertion. Swelling of the the anterior calf muscles contained within the inexpansile deep fascia causes ischaemia of the deep peroneal nerve as it traverses the compartment. The condition is diagnosed from the history and can be confirmed by measuring the compartment pressure before and after exercise. Release of the fascia is curative.

IATROGENIC INJURIES

Positioning the patient for diagnostic or operative procedures needs careful attention so as to avoid compression or traction on nerves at vulnerable sites. The brachial plexus, radial nerve, ulnar nerve and common peroneal nerve are particularly at risk. Recovery may take anything from a few minutes to several months; permanent loss of function is unusual.

During operation an important nerve may be injured by accidental scalpel or diathermy wounds, excessive traction, compression by instruments, snaring by sutures or heating and compression by extruded acrylic cement. Nerves most frequently involved are the spinal accessory or the trunks of the brachial plexus (during operations in the posterior triangle of the neck), the axillary and musculocutaneous nerves (during operations for recurrent dislocation of the shoulder), the posterior interosseous branch of the radial nerve (during approaches to the proximal end of the radius), the median nerve at the wrist (in tendon surgery), the palmar cutaneous branch of the median nerve (in carpal tunnel release), the cutaneous branch of the radial nerve (when operating for de Quervain's disease), the digital nerves (in operations for Dupuytren's contracture), the sciatic nerve (in hip arthroplasty), the common peroneal nerve (in operations around the knee) and the sural nerve (in operations on the calcaneum).

Tourniquet pressure is an important cause of nerve injury in orthopaedic operations. Damage is due to direct pressure rather than prolonged ischaemia; injury is therefore more likely with very high cuff pressure (it need never be more than 75mmHg above systolic pressure), a non-pneumatic tourniquet or a very narrow cuff. However, ischaemic damage may occur at 'acceptable' pressures if the tourniquet is left on for more than 3 hours.

Manipulative pressure or traction – e.g. during reduction of a fracture or dislocation – may injure a nerve coursing close to the bone or across the joint. Shoulder abduction and varus angulation of the knee under anaesthesia are particularly dangerous. Even moderate pressure or traction can be harmful in patients with peripheral neuropathy; this is always a risk in alcoholics and diabetics.

Injections are occasionally misdirected and delivered into a nerve – usually the radial or sciatic during intramuscular injection, the median nerve during non-operative treatment of carpal tunnel syndrome or the brachial plexus during axillary blockade.

Irradiation may cause irreparable nerve damage, a mishap not always avoidable when treating cancer. The effects may not appear until a year or two after exposure.

Diagnosis

Following operations in 'high-risk' areas of the body, local nerve function should always be tested as soon as the patient is awake. Even then it may be difficult to distinguish true weakness or sensory change from the 'normal' postoperative discomfort and unwillingness to move.

Initially it may be impossible to tell whether the lesion is a neurapraxia, axonotmesis or neurotmesis. With closed procedures it is more likely to be a lesser injury, with open ones a greater. If there is no recovery after a few weeks, EMG may be helpful. The demonstration of denervation potentials suggests either axonotmesis or neurotmesis. Surgical exploration at this early stage gives the best chance of a favourable outcome.

Prevention and treatment

Awareness is all. Knowing the situations in which there is a real risk of nerve injury is the best way to prevent the calamity. The operative exposure should be safe and well rehearsed; important nerves should be given a wide berth or otherwise kept under vision and out of harm's way; retraction should be gentle and intermittent; hidden branches (such as the posterior interosseous nerve in the supinator muscle) should be retracted with their muscular covering. It goes without saying that self-retaining retractors should never be used to retract nerves.

If a nerve is seen to be divided, it should be repaired immediately. If the injury is discovered only after the operation, it is wiser to wait for signs that might clarify the diagnosis; however, if nerve division seems likely, if there is a marked loss of function and no flicker of recovery by 6 weeks, the nerve should be explored. Even then, fibrosis may make diagnosis difficult; nerve stimulation will show whether there is conduction across the injured segment. Partial lesions, injuries that cause only minor disability and those that can be salvaged by effective tendon transfers are probably best left alone. More serious lesions may need excision and repair or grafting.

REFERENCES AND FURTHER READING

Ajmani ML (1994) The cutaneous branch of the human suprascapular nerve. *Journal of Anatomy* **185**, 439-442

Agee JM, Peimer CA, Pyrek JD, Walsh WE (1995) Endoscopic carpal tunnel release: a prospective study of complications and surgical experience. *Journal of Hand Surgery* **20A**, 165-71

Birch R (1996) Brachial plexus injuries. *Journal of Bone and Joint Surgery* **78B**, 986-992

Birch R, Bonney G, Wynn Parry CB (1998) *Surgical Disorders of the Peripheral Nerves*. Churchill Livingstone, Edinburgh

Black DL, Reckling FW, Porter SS (1991) Somatosensory evoked potential monitored during total hip arthroplasty. *Clinical Orthopaedics and Related Research* **262**, 170–177

Bodack MP, Tunkel RS, Marini SG, Nagler W (1998) Spinal accessory nerve palsy as a cause of pain after whiplash injury: case report. *Journal of Pain Symptom Management* **15**, 321-328

Bremner-Smith AT, Unwin AJ, Williams WW (1999) Sensory pathways in the spinal accessory nerve. *Journal of Bone and Joint Surgery* **81B**, 226-228

Campion D (1996) Electrodiagnostic testing in hand surgery. *Journal of Hand Surgery* **21A**, 947-956

Cummins CA, Messer TM, Nuber GW (2000) Suprascapular nerve entrapment. *Journal of Bone and Joint Surgery* **82A**, 415-424

Gelberman RH (1991) *Operative Nerve Repair and Reconstruction*. Lippincott, New York

Gelberman RH, Eaton R, Urbaniak JR (1993) Peripheral nerve compression. *Journal of Bone and Joint Surgery* 75A, 1854-1878

Geutjens GG, Longstaff RJ, Smith NJ *et al.* (1996) Medial epicondylectomy or ulnar nerve transposition for ulnar neuropathy at the elbow. *Journal of Bone and Joint Surgery* 78B, 777-779

Green DP, Hotchkis RN, Pedersen WC (1998) *Green's Operative Hand Surgery, 4th edition.* Churchill Livingstone, Edinburgh, Philadelphia

MRC Memorandum *Aids to the Examination of the Peripheral Nervous System, MRC Memorandum no. 45.* London, HM Stationery Office

Novak CB, Mackinnon SE (1996) Thoracic outlet syndrome. *Orthopaedic Clinics of North America* 27, 747-762

Oates SD, Daley RA (1996) Thoracic outlet syndrome. *Hand Clinics* 12, 705-718

Ochiai N, Nagano A, Sugioka H, Hara T (1996) Nerve grafting in brachial plexus injuries. *Journal of Bone and Joint Surgery* 78B, 754-758

Osterman AL (1991) Double crush phenomenon; the double crush syndrome. *Orthopaedic Clinics of North America* 19, 147-155

Seddon HJ (1942) A classification of nerve injuries. *British Medical Journal* 2, 237-239

Seddon H (1972) *Surgical Disorders of the Peripheral Nerves.* Churchill Livingstone, Edinburgh

Seror P (1996) Anterior interosseous nerve lesions: Clinical and electrophysiological features. *Journal of Bone and Joint Surgery* 78B, 238-41

Simon SR (1994) *Orthopaedic Basic Science.* American Academy of Orthopaedic Surgeons

Wilkinson MCP, Birch R (1995) Repair of the common peroneal nerve. *Journal of Bone and Joint Surgery* 77B, 501-3

12 Orthopaedic operations

To operate on bone requires the tools of a carpenter, but orthopaedic surgery is not carpentry; biological imperatives ensure that it never can be. *The art and skill of orthopaedic surgery is directed not to constructing a particular arrangement of parts but to restoring function to the whole.*

In this chapter certain principles applying to orthopaedic operations will be discussed. For detailed descriptions of the various operative procedures the reader is referred to well-known reference texts such as *Campbell's Operative Orthopaedics* and *Chapman's Operative Orthopaedics*, or monographs dealing with specific regional subjects.

PREPARATION

PLANNING

Operations upon bone must be carefully planned in advance, when accurate measurements can be made and bones can be compared for symmetry with those of the opposite limb. X-rays, magnetic resonance imaging (MRI) and computed tomography (CT), (if necessary with three-dimensional reformation) are helpful; transparent templates may be needed to help select the most appropriate implant. Complex corrective osteotomies should be simulated on paper cut-outs before the operation is undertaken; best of all is a rehearsal of the operation using artificial bones.

EQUIPMENT

The minimum requirements for orthopaedic operations are drills (for boring holes), osteotomes (for cutting cancellous bone), saws (for cutting cortical bone), chisels (for shaping bone), gouges (for removing bone) and plates, screws and screwdrivers (for fixing bone).

Many operations, such as joint replacement, spinal fusion and the various types of internal fixation, require special implants and instruments to ensure that these implants are correctly aligned and fixed. It is well-nigh criminal to attempt these operations without gaining familiarity with the equipment and practising the operation on dry specimens. 'Preparatory surgery' is still sadly neglected; it should be normal practice conducted in every hospital offering an orthopaedic service.

INTRAOPERATIVE RADIOGRAPHY

Intraoperative radiography is often helpful and sometimes essential for certain procedures. Fracture reduction, osteotomy alignments and the positioning of implants and fixation devices can be checked before allowing the patient off the operating table. Angiography may be needed to diagnose a vascular injury or demonstrate the success of a vascular repair.

X-ray cassettes must be wrapped in sterile drapes. They must be positioned accurately and time is lost while the plates are developed. However, they show excellent resolution of bone architecture and provide a permanent record of the procedure. Image intensification and fluoroscopy are more efficient and, although fine features may not be seen in such detail, the resolution is usually adequate. Some machines are fitted with a printer, so that a permanent copy is available.

MAGNIFICATION

Magnification is an integral part of peripheral nerve and hand surgery. The improved view minimizes the trauma of surgery and allows more accurate apposition of tissues during reconstruction.

Operating loupes range in power from 2 times to 6 times magnification. As the magnification increases, the field of view decreases and the interruption by unwanted head movements becomes more apparent. Most surgeons, therefore, choose between 2.5 and 3.5 times magnification.

The operating microscope allows much greater magnification with a stable field of view. It is particularly important when very accurate apposition of tissue is required, for example when aligning nerve fascicles during nerve repair or nerve grafting, or when anastomosing small vessels.

THE 'BLOODLESS FIELD'

Many operations on limbs (and particularly the hand) can be done more rapidly and accurately if bleeding is prevented by the application of a tourniquet.

The tourniquet cuff Only a pneumatic cuff should be used and it should be at least as wide as the diameter of the limb. A tied rubber bandage is a potentially dangerous substitute and should not be used; the pressure beneath the bandage cannot be controlled and there is a real risk of damage to the underlying nerves and muscle. A layer of wool bandage beneath the pneumatic tourniquet will distribute the pressure and prevent wrinkling of the underlying skin. During skin preparation, it is essential that the sterilizing fluid does not leak beneath the cuff as this can cause a chemical burn.

Exsanguination Elevation of the limb for 5 minutes will suffice to 'drain' the tissues if a truly bloodless field is not essential, or when surgery is being undertaken for tumour or infection and forceful exsanguination might squeeze pathological tissue into the proximal part of the limb. If a true bloodless field is required then exsanguination can be achieved by pressure on the palm or foot, followed by sequential squeezing of the limb in a proximal direction by the surgeon and his or her assistant. An Esmarch bandage wrapped from distal to proximal, or a rubber tubular exsanguinator, are also effective.

Tourniquet pressure A tourniquet pressure of 150mmHg above systolic is recommended for the lower limb, and 80–100mmHg above systolic for the upper limb. This may need to be increased in obese or muscular patients. Higher pressures are unnecessary and will increase the risk of damage to underlying muscles and nerves.

Tourniquet time An absolute maximum tourniquet time of 3 hours is allowed, although it is safer to keep this under 2 hours; transient nerve-related symptoms may occur with 3 hour tourniquet times but full recovery is usual by the fifth day. Time can be saved by ensuring that the limb is shaved, prepared, draped and marked before inflating the cuff. The time of application of the tourniquet should be recorded and the surgeon should be informed of the elapsed time at regular intervals, particularly as the two-hour period is approached. Recent work suggests that reperfusion of tissue after ischaemia causes damage, part of which is mediated by free radicals; this has questioned the practice of deflating tourniquets and allowing a period of reperfusion before reinflating – the ischaemic injury may be compounded by two or more episodes of reperfusion (Bushell *et al.*, 1995; Klenerman *et al.*, 1995). If further tourniquet time is required, and if this is anticipated due to the complexity of surgery to be undertaken, then it is wise to warn the patient of the possibility of transient nerve-related symptoms and to obtain their consent to use the absolute maximum period of 3 hours.

Finger tourniquet This is suitable for relatively minor hand operations. The finger is exsanguinated by wrapping the digit from distal to proximal with an opened gauze swab or with a rubber drain prior to applying the tourniquet at the base of the finger. A sterile rubber glove-finger makes a good cuff; the tip is cut and the margin is then rolled back proximally. This has the combined effect of exsanguinating the finger and acting as a tourniquet. A stretched rubber catheter is sometimes used but this may damage the underlying structures.

SKIN PREPARATION AND DRAPING

Hair removal Shaving the limb is more likely to be harmful than helpful. If the skin is shaved some time before the operation then the resulting superficial skin damage can cause proliferation of local bacteria. If shaving is thought to be necessary, it is better done in the operating theatre.

Skin cleaning The limb may benefit from washing with soap or a grease remover, particularly in open trauma cases. Various cleansing agents are available, usually based on alcohol, iodine or chlorhexidine. The use of colouring in the preparation fluid will help to ensure that the limb is fully covered. However, the use of red colouring should be avoided if a tourniquet is used, since it may make it difficult to determine whether blood-flow has returned after releasing the tourniquet.

Drapes Plastic adhesive coverings, perhaps impregnated with iodine, exclude some of the resident bacteria surrounding the skin incision and also secure the drapes. A variety of water resistant or absorbent drapes are available. Since a bloodstained drape will act as a conduit for bacteria, there should be a waterproof layer between the operating site and the operating table or patient.

GOWNS, GLOVES AND MASKS

Occlusive materials should be used for gowns; older types of cloth gowns become permeable to microorganisms when wet. Face masks are regarded (especially by the lay public) as the surgeon's trademark. They protect the operation wound from direct droplet contamination by personnel in the immediate vicinity. Sterile gloves should be worn for all operations, and double gloves are recommended for long or difficult procedures, with frequent changes of the outer pair.

GENERAL MEASURES TO REDUCE THE RISK OF INFECTION

Despite the use of ultraclean air systems in the operating theatre, shortening of operating times, limiting the number of people in the theatre and the various other precautions referred to above, the ideal of complete asepsis has still not been achieved. For long and complex operations, joint replacement procedures and all operations in which the risk of tissue contamination or infection is considered to be high, it is wise to use prophylactic antibiotics immediately before, during and after the operation. Complacency should be dispelled by a recent study which showed that 'sterile' drapes, instruments and the operation field itself are contaminated in most joint replacement operations performed under modern hospital conditions (Davis *et al.*, 1999).

SURGEON PROTECTION

There is increasing concern about the risk of transmitting viral infections from the patient to the surgeon. Hepatitis B vaccination is effective and is recommended, and in many centres is mandatory, for all operating theatre personnel. Vaccination is not available for hepatitis C nor for the HIV virus. Therefore, mechanical protection should be considered at all times. When a patient with an open injury is being examined, the surgeon should wear protective clothing; as a minimum, this should include rubber examination gloves and eye protection.

A waterproof gown should be used to prevent transmission of infective organisms between the surgeon and the patient. Eye protection should be worn at all times to avoid contamination of the conjunctivae with bone or blood.

The use of double gloves will decrease the risk of needle stick injury and of contamination of the finger tips from glove puncture, and this is now more or less routine for fracture and arthroplasty surgery. However, the loss of dexterity may make it inappropriate for undertaking fine procedures.

THROMBOPROPHYLAXIS

Thromboembolism is the commonest complication of lower limb surgery. It comprises three associated disorders: *deep vein thrombosis (DVT), pulmonary embolism (PE)* and the later complication of *chronic venous insufficiency*. The most important risk factors are increasing age, obesity and a history of previous thrombosis.

Pathophysiology

According to Virchow, thrombosis results from an interaction between vessel wall damage, alterations in blood components and venous stasis. Following major orthopaedic operations, there is activation of the coagulation cascade and restricted fibrinolysis lasting for several days. During hip replacement, femoral vein blood flow is temporarily interrupted when the acetabulum and femoral medulla are exposed. There is also more prolonged stasis as the patient recovers from surgery and begins to mobilize. DVT occurs most frequently in the veins of the calf, and less often in the proximal veins of the thigh and pelvis. It is from the larger thrombi that fragments sometimes break off and get carried to the lungs where they may give rise to symptomatic PE and, in a small percentage of cases, fatal pulmonary embolism (FPE).

Incidence of symptomatic events

Prophylaxis is aimed at reducing the likelihood *of clinically manifested thromboembolism.* Recommendations for thromboprophylaxis have usually been based on randomized clinical trials and meta-analyses using objective radiological tests, particularly venography. However, it must be appreciated that the correlation between 'venographic DVT' and symptomatic events has not been validated. A further problem in considering incidence is that different operations carry different risks, and for some of these procedures there are, as yet, no reliable statistics.

Hip replacement Figures usually quoted for the incidence of FPE following hip replacement without thromboprophylaxis are 2%–3%. These were derived from series in the early 1970s and do not reflect the risk associated with modern practice, which is probably around 0.4%. The incidence of clinically detectable DVT and PE together is perhaps around 4%. Symptomatic chronic venous insufficiency occurs mainly after symptomatic DVT, but it may also arise from the larger asymptomatic thromboses (Warwick *et al.*, 1995).

Knee replacement The incidence of FPE after total knee replacement without prophylaxis is around 0.2%, and of symptomatic DVT and PE together about 10%.

Hip fracture About 20% of patients die within 3 months of hip fracture and PE causes perhaps 5% of these deaths; i.e. the incidence of FPE is about 1%. The incidence of non-fatal symptomatic thromboembolism is not known.

Major limb trauma The incidence of FPE in polytraumatized patients is about 1%. There is some evidence that tibial fractures are associated with an increased risk of chronic venous insufficiency. The overall incidence of symptomatic thromboembolism after lower limb trauma, whether treated with a plaster cast or by surgical fixation, is unknown.

Other limb surgery The incidence of thromboembolism after other types of limb surgery is unknown. However, it is very rare following upper limb operations.

Clinical features and diagnosis

DVT is, in the main, an occult disease, considerably more common than the symptoms and signs suggest. There may be pain in the calf or thigh; however, following trauma or operation even those patients who do not complain should be examined regularly for swelling and soft-tissue tenderness. Some patients also develop a sudden slight increase in temperature and pulse rate. Homans' sign – increased pain on passive dorsiflexion of the foot – is unreliable. The final diagnosis of DVT should not be made on clinical grounds alone – false positives and false negatives are common – but should always be confirmed by venography or ultrasound scanning.

Patients with symptomatic DVT, and also asymptomatic patients who develop pain in the chest or shortness of breath during the postoperative period, should be examined for signs of pulmonary embolism. The diagnosis can be confirmed by ventilation–perfusion (V/Q) scanning.

Chronic venous insufficiency occurs some years after the DVT. The patient presents with leg discomfort, swelling, skin changes and/or frank ulceration. The diagnosis is usually obvious. This is a debilitating condition which places huge demands on health resources.

Prevention

The overall risk of DVT and PE can be reduced by prophylactic treatment. However, there is considerable controversy over which procedures, and which type of patient, should be covered; the estimated risk of symptomatic thromboembolism after any particular operation must be balanced against the likely effectiveness, safety and cost of prophylactic measures.

PHYSICAL METHODS
Simple physical routines include elevation of the foot of the bed, the use of elastic stockings or graduated compression stockings, postoperative exercises and early mobilization.

Intermittent plantar venous compression takes advantage of the fact that blood from the sole of the foot is normally expressed during weightbearing by intermittent pressure on the venous plexus around the lateral plantar arteries; this, in turn, increases venous blood-flow in the leg. A mechanical foot-pump can reproduce this physiological mechanism in patients who are confined to bed. Clinical trials have shown that this provides effective thromboprophylaxis without the risk of soft-tissue side effects (Warwick et al., 1998).

Intermittent pneumatic compression of the leg has been shown to reduce the risk of 'radiological DVT' after hip and knee replacement. It is, however, impractical for patients undergoing operations at or below the knee.

The use of spinal epidural anaesthesia reduces the incidence of DVT by improving venous blood-flow and possibly also by a local fibrinolytic effect.

CHEMICAL METHODS
Unfractionated heparin In the past, the usual prophylactic regimen was to give subcutaneous low-dose heparin, 5000 units preoperatively and then three times a day postoperatively until the patient became mobile. Unfortunately, this carries a risk of increased bleeding after operation and it is contraindicated in elderly people. Moreover, there are doubts about its efficacy in preventing proximal DVT.

Low molecular weight heparin This class of drug has haematological and pharmacokinetic advantages over unfractionated heparin. Dose adjustment and monitoring are not required. Randomized studies have shown that it effectively reduces the prevalence of venographic DVT in hip and knee replacement surgery.

Warfarin Warfarin has been widely used, particularly in North America. It reduces the prevalence of DVT after hip and knee replacement and FPE is extremely rare. Drawbacks are the difficulty in establishing appropriate dosage levels and the need for constant monitoring; there is also a risk of interaction with other drugs and alcohol.

Aspirin This reduces the frequency of FPE and thromboembolism after sugery.

BLEEDING WITH CHEMICAL PROPHYLAXIS.
Surgeons are intuitively concerned about increased bleeding, particularly with knee replacement where the soft tissue envelope is unforgiving. At *prophylactic* dosages the risk is very low; however, *therapeutic* anticoagulation (following either failure or absence of prophylaxis) carries a very high risk of bleeding complications, emphasizing the need for effective and safe prophylaxis. Mechanical methods, of course, are free of such concerns.

TIMING
Although risk factors for thromboembolism are most pronounced during surgery, it is not clear whether prophylaxis should be started before the operation or whether it can be safely deferred until after surgery.

DURATION OF PROPHYLAXIS
The ideal duration of thromboprophylaxis is not known. Traditional recommendations suggest that it should be continued until the patient is fully mobile. The risk of radiographic thrombosis persists for at least 5 weeks following surgery and the death rate after hip replacement does not return to 'normal' until 3 months. Theoretically, therefore, thromboprophylaxis

should be prolonged for some time after discharge from hospital. This is easy with methods using elastic stockings, or aspirin, and even warfarin, although it is prudent to point out that there is no support from randomized trials for doing so. The prolonged use of low molecular weight heparin reduces the incidence of radiographic DVT after hip replacement but the clinical relevance, risk benefit and cost effectiveness of such a strategy is not so clear.

Treatment of thromboembolism

Particularly after major lower limb surgery, patients may present with symptoms that suggest DVT or PE. Whenever possible, the clinical diagnosis should be confirmed by imaging (venography or ultrasound for DVT, V/Q scanning or pulmonary angiography for PE) before treatment is started. This is important because the clinical diagnosis of these complications is notoriously unreliable and full therapeutic anticoagulation carries a high complication rate soon after major surgery.

Once the diagnosis of DVT has been confirmed, treatment is started with a loading dose of 5000 units of heparin intravenously. This is followed by a daily weight-adjusted dose of low molecular weight heparin subcutaneously. Warfarin is started with a loading dose of 10mg daily for 3 days. Thereafter the dose is adjusted until the International Normalized Ratio (INR) is stable at 2.0–3.0, and the heparin is then discontinued.

If low molecular weight heparin is not available, then unfractionated heparin can be given by continuous intravenous infusion, or twice daily subcutaneously, adjusted to maintain the activated partial thromboplastin (APTT) at 1.5–2 times normal.

Acute, severe PE demands cardiorespiratory resuscitation, vasopressors for shock, oxygen and a large intravenous dose (15 000 units) of heparin. Streptokinase is used both to dissolve clots and to prevent more forming. Antibiotics may be given to prevent lung infection. Anticoagulant treatment is continued for at least 6 months.

OPERATIONS ON BONES

OSTEOTOMY

Osteotomy may be used to correct deformity, to change the shape of the bone or to relieve pain in arthritis by redirecting the load trajectories. Preoperative planning is essential, with precise measurements of the patient and the x-rays (see above under 'Planning'). The following must be determined.

The exact site of bone division For corrective osteotomy this should be as near as possible to the site of deformity. For joint realignment, local geometry dictates the level.

The amount of correction required The intended angular, translational or rotational shift must be measured in degrees.

The method of correction To change an angular deformity a wedge of bone may have to be removed ('closing wedge') or inserted ('opening wedge'). The size of the wedge should be calculated accurately and reproduced precisely by using suitable templates. An alternative is to apply an adjustable external fixation device which will permit progressive correction over time. The aim of correction is not only to restore the alignment of the bone but also to adjust the position of the mechanical axis of the limb.

The method of fixation Sometimes plaster splintage alone will suffice. Usually internal or external fixation is preferred. Weightbearing is allowed if fixation is stable; otherwise it is deferred until healing is sufficiently advanced.

Complications

General As with all bone operations, *thromboembolism* and *infection* are calculated risks.

Undercorrection and overcorrection Under and overcorrection of the deformity can be avoided by undertaking careful preoperative planning. In difficult cases, intra-operative x-ray or fluoroscopy is essential. If the fault is recognized while the patient is still under the anaesthetic, it should be corrected straight away. If it is discovered on a postoperative x-ray check, it may still be advisable to re-do the procedure rather than hope that 'nature' will come to the rescue.

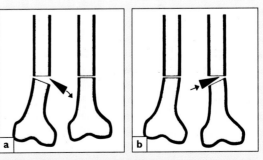

12.1 Osteotomy A bent bone can be straightened **(a)** by removing a wedge of bone (an opening wedge osteotomy), or **(b)** by inserting one (a closing wedge osteotomy).

Nerve tension Correction of severe deformities may put excessive tension on a nearby nerve. The commonest example is peroneal nerve palsy after corrective osteotomy for a marked valgus deformity of the knee. In general, acute long-bone corrections greater than 20° should be avoided and if there is a known risk of nerve injury it should be limited to 10°. If greater correction is needed it can be done gradually in an appropriate external fixator (see the Ilizarov method).

Compartment syndrome Osteotomy of the tibia or forearm bones may be followed by oozing of blood from the cut bone surfaces into the surrounding muscle compartments. The limb should be checked repeatedly for signs of ischaemia and prompt action taken if danger signals appear (see page 564).

Non-union Non-union may occur if fixation is inadequate or if the soft tissues are damaged by excessive stripping during surgical exposure. Gentle handling of tissues and respect for the blood supply to bone, together with sound fixation techniques, will minimize the risk.

BONE FIXATION

Bone fragments can be firmly joined by simple *screwing* (especially if a small piece has to be fixed back in position), by transfixing the fragments with *pins* or stiff *wires*, by securing the pieces with *malleable wire*, by *stapling* the pieces together (only in cancellous bone), by *attaching a bridging plate* to the bone with a row of screws on each side of the break, by passing a *long nail* down the medullary canal, by using an *external fixator* (transfixing pins on either side of the break, connected by a rigid frame outside the body), or by a *combination* of these methods. All will eventually loosen or break unless natural union occurs.

BONE GRAFTS

Bone grafts are both *osteoinductive* and *osteoconductive*, i.e. they are able to stimulate osteogenesis and they also provide linkage across defects and a scaffold upon which new bone can form. Osteogenesis is brought about partly by the activity of cells surviving on the surface of the graft, but mainly by the stimulation of osteoprogenitor cells in the host bed – an effect that is due to the presence of bone morphogenetic protein in the graft matrix (Urist, 1970). Cancellous grafts are more rapidly incorporated into host bone than cortical grafts, but sometimes the greater strength of cortical bone is needed to provide structural integrity.

AUTOGRAFTS (AUTOGENOUS GRAFTS) In these, bone is moved from one place to another in the same individual. They are the most commonly used grafts and are satisfactory provided that sufficient bone of the sort required is available and that, at the recipient site, there is a clean vascular bed. Vascularized grafts are theoretically ideal. Bone is transferred complete with its blood supply, which is anastomosed to vessels at the recipient site. The technique is difficult and time consuming, requiring microsurgical skill. Available donor sites include the iliac crest (complete with one of the circumflex arteries), the fibula (with the peroneal artery) and the radial shaft.

Cancellous autografts can be obtained from the thicker portions of the ilium, the greater trochanter, the proximal metaphysis of the tibia, the lower radius, the olecranon or from an excised femoral head. Cortical grafts can be harvested from any convenient long bone or from the iliac

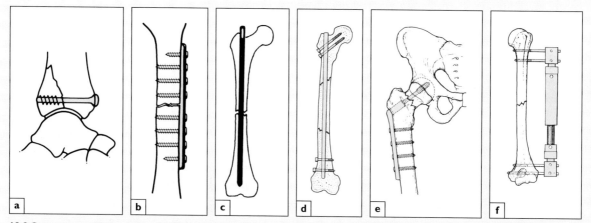

12.2 Some ways of fixing bone (**a**) With a single screw – this is a lag screw (threaded only distally) and therefore achieving interfragmentary compression. (**b**) Plate and screws. (**c**) Intramedullary nail. (**d**) Locked intramedullary nail. (**e**) Dynamic hip screw. (**f**) External fixator.

crest; they usually need to be fixed with screws, sometimes reinforced by a plate, and can be placed on the host bone, or inlaid or slid along the long axis of the bone.

Vascularized grafts remain completely viable and become incorporated by a process analogous to fracture healing. All other autografts undergo necrosis, though a few surface cells remain viable. The graft stimulates an inflammatory response with the formation of a fibrovascular stroma; through this, blood vessels and osteoprogenitor cells can pass from the recipient bone to the graft. Apart from providing a stimulus for bone growth (osteoinduction), the graft also provides a passive scaffold for the new growth (osteoconduction). Cancellous grafts become incorporated more quickly and more completely than cortical grafts.

ALLOGRAFTS (HOMOGRAFTS) With these, bone is transferred from one individual (alive or dead) to another of the same species. They can be stored in a bone bank and, as supplies can be plentiful, are particularly useful when large defects have to be filled.

Fresh allografts, though dead, are not immunologically acceptable. They induce an inflammatory response in the host and this may lead to rejection. However, the antigenicity can be reduced by freezing or freeze-drying, or by ionizing radiation.

The process of incorporation (when it occurs) is similar to that with autografts but slower and less complete. Demineralization is another way of reducing antigenicity and it may also enhance the osteoinductive properties of the graft. The best way of ensuring the incorporation of foreign grafts of all kinds is to impregnate the graft with marrow obtained from the host (Nade and Burwell, 1977).

Allografts are plentiful and can be stored for long periods. However, sterility must be ensured. This can be done by exposure to ethylene oxide or by ionizing radiation, but their physical properties and potential for osteoinduction are considerably altered by doses that are high enough to ensure sterility (Friedlaender, 1987; Aspenberg *et al.*, 1990). Freezing the grafts and storing them at –70°C is much less harmful but the graft must then be harvested under sterile conditions and the donor must be cleared for malignancy, venereal disease, hepatitis and human immunodeficiency virus (HIV); this requires prolonged (several months) testing of the donor before the graft is used.

OTHER VARIETIES *Xenografts* are obtained from another mammalian species, such as pigs or cows. After treatment for antigenicity they should, theoretically, behave like allografts, but in practice they are much less effective unless host marrow is added to the graft. 'Artificial bone' made of *hydroxyapatite (HA) composites* can be used in the same way to fill a cavity or bridge a small gap.

Bioactive bone cements (injectable calcium phosphate preparations) offer a simple alternative, e.g. for replacing metaphyseal bone loss in Colles' fractures.

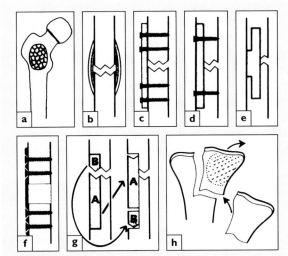

12.3 Bone grafts (a) Chip grafts to fill a cavity; (b) onlay strips of cancellous bone (Phemister technique); (c) onlay cortical graft; (d) inlay cortical graft; (e) latch graft; (f) cancellous block graft plus plating (Nicoll technique); (g) sliding graft – the portion marked A is slid up to bridge the fracture; (h) large cadaveric osteocartilaginous graft obtained fresh and sterile from an organ donor.

Applications

Vascularized grafts tend to be used only in exceptional circumstances such as congenital pseudarthrosis of the tibia or non-union of a fractured femoral neck. They are also useful in treating large bone defects, although techniques based on the Ilizarov method are becoming more popular for this purpose (see below).

Cortical or corticocancellous grafts are needed where bone has been lost as a result of trauma or has been removed because it contained a tumour. When reinforced by metallic implants, large gaps can be filled.

Cancellous grafts have a wide variety of uses, including: (1) filling cavities; (2) filling the space after the crushing of a metaphysis; (3) augmenting the compression side of a long-bone fracture which is being fixed internally; (4) as part of the treatment for atrophic non-union of a fracture; (5) to fill spaces left when revising a loose prosthesis; (6) to augment a deficient acetabulum during hip surgery; and (7) as part of a fusion operation, particularly of the spine.

DISTRACTION HISTOGENESIS AND LIMB RECONSTRUCTION – THE ILIZAROV METHOD

Present day limb reconstruction is founded on the principle of tension-stress, which is the generation of new tissue in response to gradual increases in tension. Discovered in the 1950s by Gavril Ilizarov in Russia, the application of this principle to orthopaedic conditions represents a significant departure from old; it has opened opportunities for treatment in conditions which hitherto were poorly treated or even untreatable. The term 'Ilizarov method' embraces the various applications of this principle and its emphasis on minimally invasive surgery (many of the techniques are performed percutaneously), coupled to an early return of function. In many ways, it has redefined deformity correction in the late 20th century.

DISTRACTION HISTOGENESIS

CALLOTASIS

Callus distraction, or callotasis, is perhaps the single most important application of the tension-stress principle. It is used for limb lengthening or the filling of large defects in bone, either through bone transport or other strategies. The basis of the technique is to produce a careful fracture of bone, followed by a short wait before the young callus is gradually distracted via a circular or unilateral external fixator.

The initial fracture can be accomplished by several methods. In a corticotomy, the bony cortex is partially divided with a sharp osteotome through a small skin incision and the break completed by osteoclasis, leaving the medullary blood supply and endosteum largely intact. Alternatively, the periosteum can be incised and elevated and the bone then drilled several times before using an osteotome to complete the division; the periosteum is then repaired. Both techniques are exacting – simply dividing the bone with a power saw results in nothing being formed in the gap. Transfixing wires or screws are introduced proximal and distal to the corticotomy site and the external frame is set in place.

After an initial wait of 5–10 days, distraction is begun and it proceeds at 1mm a day, with small (usually 0.25mm) increments spaced out evenly. The first callus is usually seen on x-ray after 3 weeks; in optimum conditions, it forms up as an even column of young callus in the gap between the bone fragments (this is called the *regenerate*). If the distraction rate is too fast, or the osteotomy performed poorly, the regenerate may be thin with an hourglass appearance; conversely if distraction is too slow, it may appear bulbous or worse still may consolidate prematurely, thereby preventing any further lengthening. Regular x-rays allow the surgeon to check on the quality of regenerate.

When the desired length is reached, a second waiting period follows which allows the regenerate callus to consolidate and harden. Weight-bearing is permitted throughout this period and the consolidation process is helped by dynamizing the external fixator, thereby allowing greater transfer of load across the column of new bone. When cortices of even thickness are seen in the regenerate on x-ray, the fixator is ready to be removed. Throughout treatment, physiotherapy is important to preserve joint movement and avoid contractures.

CHONDRODIATASIS

Bone lengthening can also be achieved by distracting the growth plate (chondrodiatasis) (De Bastiani *et al.*, 1986). No osteotomy is needed but the distraction rate is slower, usually 0.25mm twice daily. Although a wide even column of regenerate is usually seen, the fate of the physis is sealed – the growth plate frequently closes after the process; it is a technique best reserved for children close to the end of growth.

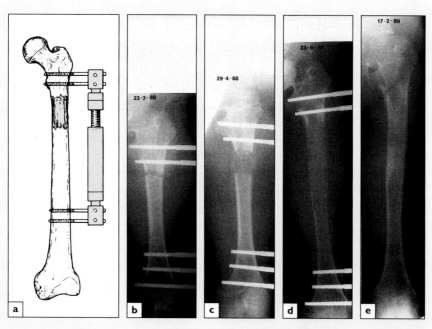

12.4 Callotasis At any age, bone lengthening can be achieved by callotasis (callus 'stretching') after osteotomy. (**a**) Shows one technique. (**b**) 10cm was gained in this achondroplastic patient. (Courtesy of Professor M. Saleh.)

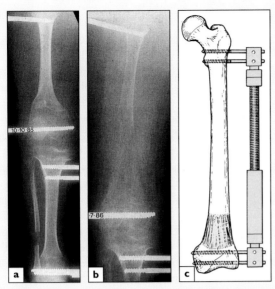

12.5 Chondrodiatasis The shorter leg can, in a child, be lengthened by chondrodiatasis; the interval between the two films (**a, b**) is 9 months. (Courtesy of Professor M. Saleh.) The drawing (**c**) shows where the growth plate has been 'stretched'.

BONE TRANSPORT

The principle of callotasis is used not only for limb lengthening but also as a means of filling defects in bone. In bone *transport*, the defect (or gap) is filled gradually by creating a 'floating' segment of bone through a corticotomy either proximal or distal to the defect, and slowly moving this segment across the defect. An external fixator provides the stability during this process. As the segment is transported from the corticotomy site to the new docking site, new bone is created which fills the defect.

A variant of the bone transport technique is bifocal compression-distraction. With this method the defect is closed by instantly bringing the bone ends together; a corticotomy is then performed at a different level and length is restored by callotasis. In this case the limb is shortened temporarily, whereas in bone transport overall limb length remains unchanged.

CORRECTING BONE DEFORMITIES AND JOINT CONTRACTURES

Angular deformities can usually be corrected by carefully planned closing or opening wedge osteotomies (see above). However, the degree of correction is limited by the effect on soft-tissue tension, in particular nerves. With the Ilizarov method, it is now possible to undertake large corrections with much lower risk to the soft tissues. The correction is performed gradually with the aid of an external fixator; length, rotation and translation deformities can be dealt with simultaneously.

The principle of tension stress can also be applied to correcting soft-tissue contractures. For example, an intractable club-foot deformity is dealt with by applying gradual tension loads to the contracted soft tissue structures and slowly altering the position of the ankle, subtalar and midtarsal joints until a normal position is achieved. The assembly of the external fixator to accomplish this technique is complex, but the results are often gratifying.

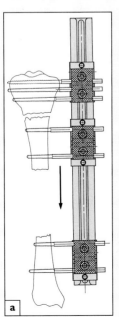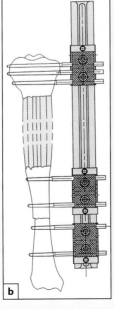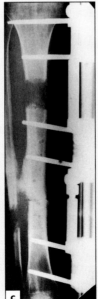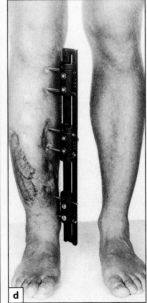

12.6 Bone transport (**a**) Bone loss or excision may leave a gap in the shaft. Proximal osteotomy and callotasis allows a segment of the diaphysis to be moved distally (**b**), thus restoring continuity. The proximal gap gradually fills first with callus and then with new bone. (**c, d**) The situation at the end of transport and 'docking' is shown in this patient.

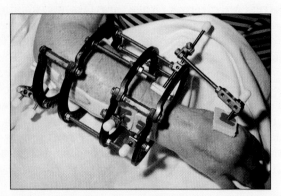

12.7 Correcting bone and soft-tissue deformity Here the Ilizarov principles are applied in the correction of post-traumatic deformities of the forearm and wrist. (Courtesy of Mr RM Atkins.)

LEG LENGTH EQUALIZATION

Inequality of leg length may result from many causes, including congenital anomalies, malunited fractures, epiphyseal and physeal injuries, infections and paralysis. Inequality greater than 2.5cm needs treatment; this may be no more than a shoe-raise, or it may involve surgery to either the shorter or the longer leg.

Consequences of leg length inequality

Unequal leg lengths leads to inefficient walking. The longer leg has to be lifted higher to clear the ground during swing-through, and the pelvis and shoulders dip noticeably during the stance phase on the shorter side; both of these adjustments increase energy consumption. Pelvic tilt and compensatory scoliosis tend to cause backache, and there is a higher reported incidence of osteoarthritis of the hip on the longer side – possibly because of the 'uncovering' of the femoral head due to pelvic obliquity.

Techniques for correcting leg length

There are four choices:

- shortening the longer leg
- slowing growth in the longer leg
- lengthening the shorter leg
- speeding up growth in the shorter leg

The timing of surgery for limb length inequality in children is important. The rate of change in length difference is charted and the discrepancy at the end of growth can then be predicted by reference to suitable charts or tables. This allows the surgeon to plan a timely intervention which will result in limb length equality at skeletal maturity.

Operations of the longer leg

In children, epiphyseal arrest is an effective method of slowing the rate of growth of the longer leg; it can be temporary, using removable staples fixed across the growth plate, or permanent, by drilling across the physis and curetting out the growth plate. Another method is to excise a rectangular block of bone across the physis, rotate the block through 90° and then reinsert it into the original bed. When the physis fuses (epiphyseodesis), longitudinal growth at that site ceases and the overall gain in length of the limb is retarded. In due course the difference in lengths should be reduced.

The timing and technique of epiphyseodesis is important; if inaccurately timed, a difference in leg lengths will remain, and if improperly done, deformity may occur. In deciding when to operate, Menelaus' formula, though approximate, is useful; he assumed that each year the lower femoral and upper tibial epiphyses contribute 1.0cm and 0.6cm, respectively, in length; and that these epiphyses fuse at 16 years of age in boys and 14 years in girls. However, this simple formula may trap unwary surgeons and result in the procedure being done too early in an attempt to equalize large predicted differences – this carries the risk of creating disproportionate lower limb segments or unequal knee levels. Chart-based methods are probably safer, provided they are used to equalize no more than 5cm of predicted discrepancy at the end of growth. (Eastwood *et al.*, 1995)

In adults it is obviously necessary to excise a segment of bone, preferably from the femur, since tibial shortening is more complicated and is cosmetically unattractive; up to 7.5cm of femoral shortening can be achieved without permanent loss of function. The safest technique is to excise a segment from between the lesser trochanter and the femoral isthmus (a step cut may be preferred), to approximate the cut ends and to fix them together with a locking intramedullary nail or plate. Open excision of bone segments from the long leg has several disadvantages, among which scarring and poor muscle tone are important. The scarring results from a longitudinal incision being suddenly subjected to a concertina effect, which causes the wound to gape widely. Shorter segments can be removed by 'closed' intramedullary techniques which rely on an intramedullary saw and bone splitter and thereby avoid the problem with scars. In general, shortening of the long leg is reserved for situations where the patient is too old for an epypiphyseodesis or where lengthening the short leg is deemed too risky, e.g. in the presence of unstable joints or infection.

Shortening should, of course, be applied only if the patient's residual height will still be acceptable. It should also be remembered that, since the longer leg is usually the normal one, if a serious complication such as non-union ensues, the patient may 'not have a leg to stand on'!

Lengthening the shorter leg

Lengthening, the commonest method of equalizing leg length, is most easily accomplished by wearing a raised shoe, but this is often inadequate or unacceptable – a shoe-raise of more than 5cm risks injury to the ankle!

Stimulation of the growth plate can be achieved by the technique of periosteal division (Wilde and Baker, 1987). A circumferential 5mm strip is excised from around the distal femoral or proximal tibial physis. The physis responds with an accelerated growth rate which may last for up to 2 years. However, like epiphyseodesis, poor technique may produce deformity; the method is probably best reserved for young children (under 6 years) as the effects on older children are less predictable.

Limb lengthening by the Ilizarov method is an appropriate solution for predicted length discrepancies of greater than 5cm. Chondrodiatasis and callotasis have become much safer since it has been appreciated how slow the distraction must be if neural or vascular damage is to be avoided (see above). Major length corrections can be tackled by staging the treatment process over several years, or by attempting to lengthen at two levels within the same bone (bifocal *lengthening*). The latter method, although attractive, has a higher rate of complications largely from the soft tissues being distracted too quickly.

OPERATIONS TO INCREASE STATURE

Bilateral leg lengthening is a feasible procedure for achondroplastics and other individuals of short stature, but detailed consultation is an essential preliminary. The prospective patient must understand that treatment is painful, prolonged, and may be associated with a substantial number of complications such as pintrack sepsis, angulatory deformity or fracture. Morever, gain in height is not the same as 'normality'. Nevertheless, successful treatment is so rewarding ('People no longer look at me in the street'; 'I can now get things off a shelf without having to climb up') that it should not be with-held if the patient is otherwise normal and is psychologically prepared. Referral to a specialized centre is wise.

The techniques of lengthening described above are used and two bones at a time can be dealt with. Simultaneous lengthening of the ipsilateral femur and tibia has been advocated as a means of ensuring that the patient will complete the treatment programme, but it is kinder to lengthen both tibiae at one procedure and both femora at another. Gains in height averaging 30cm have been achieved by combining the bone lengthening with soft-tissue releases (Vilarrubias *et al.*, 1990).

OPERATIONS ON JOINTS

ARTHROTOMY

Arthrotomy (opening a joint) may be indicated: (1) to inspect the interior or perform a synovial biopsy; (2) to drain a haematoma or an abscess; (3) to remove a loose body or damaged structure (e.g. a torn meniscus); and (4) to excise inflamed synovium. The intra-articular tissues should be handled with great care, and if postoperative bleeding is expected (e.g. after synovectomy) a drain should be inserted – postoperative haemarthrosis predisposes to infection. Following the operation the joint should be rested for a few days, but thereafter movement must be encouraged.

REALIGNMENT

Osteotomies around a joint may be carried out for several reasons. In children, realignment of an abnormal joint may encourage normal development, e.g. in

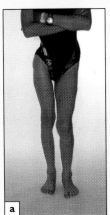
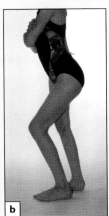
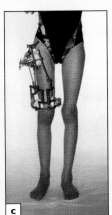
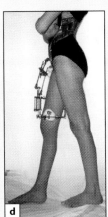

12.8 Leg lengthening (a, b) Following a childhood infection of the right hip and destruction of the proximal femoral epiphysis, this patient ended up with marked shortening of the right femur and an awkward gait. **(c, d)** Here she is seen, markedly improved, after femoral lengthening by the Ilizarov method. The frame was in place for 18 months.

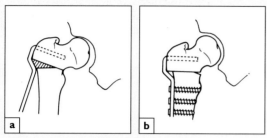

12.9 Joint realignment (a) The joint space is not congruent; (b) an osteotomy has realigned it – now it is nearly equal throughout.

dysplastic hips. In early osteoarthritis of the hip or knee, realignment osteotomy can be used to redistribute stress to less damaged areas of the joint and thereby relieve pain for some years.

ARTHRODESIS

The most reliable operation for a painful or unstable joint is arthrodesis; where stiffness does not seriously affect function, this is often the treatment of choice. Examples are the spine, the tarsus, the ankle, the wrist and the interphalangeal joints. Arthrodesis is useful also for a knee that is already fairly stiff (provided the other knee has good movement) and for a flail shoulder. More controversial is arthrodesis of the hip. Though it is a reasonable alternative to arthroplasty or osteotomy for joint disease in young patients, there is an understandable resistance to sacrificing all movement in such an important joint. It is difficult to convey to the patient that a fused hip can still 'move' by virtue of pelvic tilting and rotation; the best approach is to introduce the patient to someone who has had a successful arthrodesis.

The principles of arthrodesis are straightforward and involve four stages: (1) exposure – both joint surfaces need to be well visualized, and often this means an extensile incision, but some smaller joints are now accessible by arthroscopic means; (2) preparation – both articular surfaces are denuded of cartilage and sometimes the subchondral bone is 'feathered' to increase the contact area; (3) coaptation – the prepared surfaces are apposed in the optimum position, ensuring good contact; and (4) fixation – the surfaces are held rigidly by some form of internal or external fixation. Success will depend on every stage being completed well – sometimes bone grafts are added in the larger joints to promote osseous bridging.

The main complication is non-union with the formation of a pseudarthrosis. Rigid fixation lessens this risk; where feasible (e.g. the knee and ankle), the bony parts are squeezed together by compression-fixation devices.

ARTHROPLASTY

Arthroplasty, the surgical refashioning of a joint, aims to relieve pain and to retain or restore movement. The following are the main varieties.

EXCISION ARTHROPLASTY Sufficient bone is excised to create a gap at which movement can occur (e.g. Girdlestone's hip arthroplasty). In some situations (e.g. after excising the trapezium) a shaped 'spacer' can be inserted; this may be tissue from another part (e.g. tendon) or artificial material like Silastic.

PARTIAL REPLACEMENT One articular component only is replaced (e.g. Moore's prosthesis for a fractured femoral neck); or one compartment of a joint is replaced (e.g. the medial or the lateral half of the tibiofemoral joint). The prosthesis is kept in position either by acrylic cement or by a cementless fit between implant and bone.

TOTAL REPLACEMENT Both articular bone ends are replaced by prosthetic implants; for biomechanical reasons, the convex component is usually metal and the concave

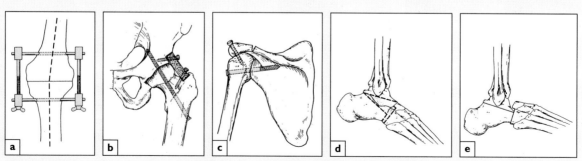

12.10 Arthrodesis (a) Compression arthrodesis; (b) screw plus bone graft; (c) similar technique using the acromion. (d, e) Subtalar mid-tarsal fusion.

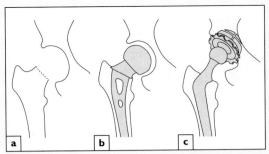

12.11 Arthroplasty The main varieties as applied to the hip joint: (**a**) excision arthroplasty (Girdlestone); (**b**) partial replacement – an Austin Moore prosthesis has been inserted after removing the femoral head; (**c**) total replacement – both articular surfaces are replaced.

high-density polyethylene. They are fixed to the host bone, either with acrylic cement or by a cementless press-fit technique. The rationale, indications and complications of total joint replacement are discussed in detail on page 443.

MICROSURGERY AND LIMB REPLANTATION

Microsurgical techniques are used in repairing nerves and vessels, transplanting bone with a vascular pedicle, substituting a less essential digit (e.g. a toe) for a more essential one (e.g. a thumb) and – occasionally – for reattaching a severed limb or digit. Essential prerequisites are an operating microscope, special instruments, microsutures, a chair with arm supports and – not least – a surgeon well practised in microsurgical techniques.

For replantation, the severed part should be kept cool during transport. The more muscle in the amputated part, the shorter the period it will last; a finger tip may survive for 24 hours, a forearm only a few hours. Two teams dissect, identify and mark each artery, nerve and vein of the stump and the limb. Following careful debridement the bones are shortened to reduce tension and fixed together by wires, nails or plates. Next the vessels are sutured – veins first and (if possible) two veins for each artery. A vessel of 1mm diameter needs seven or eight sutures around the circumference! Nerves and tendons next need suturing; only healthy ends of approximately equal diameter should be joined; tension, kinking and torsion must be prevented. Decompression of skin and fascia, as well as thrombectomy, may be needed in the postoperative period.

Replantation surgery is time consuming, expensive and often unsuccessful. It should be carried out only in centres specially equipped, and by teams specially trained, for this work.

AMPUTATIONS

Indications

Colloquially speaking, the indications are three Ds: Dead, Dangerous and Damn nuisance.

DEAD (OR DYING) *Peripheral vascular disease* accounts for almost 90% of all amputations. Other causes of bone death are *severe trauma, burns and frostbite.*

DANGEROUS 'Dangerous' disorders are *malignant tumours*, potentially *lethal sepsis* and *crush injury*. In crush injury, releasing the compression may result in renal failure (the crush syndrome).

DAMN NUISANCE Retaining the limb may be worse than having no limb at all. This may be because of *pain*, gross *malformation*, recurrent *sepsis* or severe *loss of function*. The combination of deformity and loss of sensation is particularly trying, and in the lower limb is likely to result in pressure ulceration.

Varieties

A provisional amputation may be necessary because primary healing is unlikely. The limb is amputated as distal as the causal conditions will allow. Skin flaps sufficient to cover the deep tissues are cut and sutured loosely over a pack. Re-amputation is performed when the stump condition is favourable.

Definitive end-bearing amputation is performed when weight is to be taken through the end of a stump. Therefore the scar must not be terminal, and the bone end must be solid, not hollow, which means it must be cut through or near a joint. Examples are through-knee and Syme's amputations.

Definitive non-end-bearing amputations are the commonest variety. All upper limb and most lower limb amputations come into this category. Because weight is not to be taken at the end of the stump, the scar can be terminal.

AMPUTATIONS AT THE SITES OF ELECTION

Most lower limb amputations are for ischaemic disease and are performed through the site of election below the most distal palpable pulse. Sometimes, especially in transtibial (below-knee) amputations, the level can be modified by measurement of the transcutaneous oxygen pressure (Christensen and Clarke, 1986). The 'sites of election' are determined by the demands of prosthetic design and local function. Too short a stump may tend

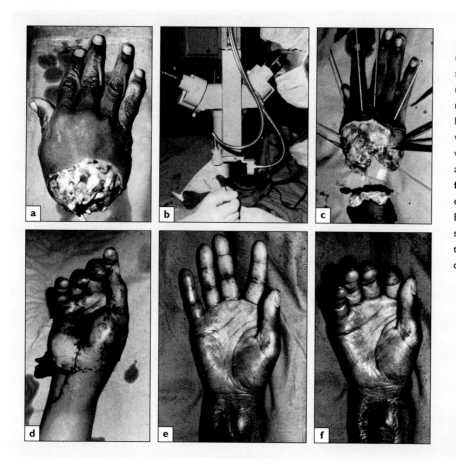

12.12 Microsurgery and limb replantation (**a**) The problem – a severed hand. (**b**) The solution – replantation with microsurgical techniques. (**c**) The bones of the severed hand have been fixed with Kirschner wires as a preliminary to suturing vessels and nerves. (**d**) The appearance at the end of the operation. (**e, f**) The limb 1 year later; the fingers extend fully and bend about half-way. But the hand survived, has moderate sensation and the patient was able to return to work (as a guillotine operator in a paper works!).

to slip out of the prosthesis. Too long a stump may have inadequate circulation and can become painful, or ulcerate; moreover, it complicates the incorporation of a joint in the prosthesis. For all that, the skill of the modern prosthetist has made it possible to amputate at almost any site.

Principles of technique

A tourniquet is used unless there is arterial insufficiency. Skin flaps are cut so that their combined length equals one and a half times the width of the limb at the site of amputation. As a rule anterior and posterior flaps of equal length are used for the upper limb and for transfemoral (above-knee) amputations; below the knee a long posterior flap is usual.

Muscles are divided distal to the proposed site of bone section; subsequently, opposing groups are sutured over the bone end to each other and to the periosteum (myoplasty), thus providing better muscle control as well as better circulation. Nerves are divided proximal to the bone cut. Great care is taken to ensure that a raw nerve end will not bear weight.

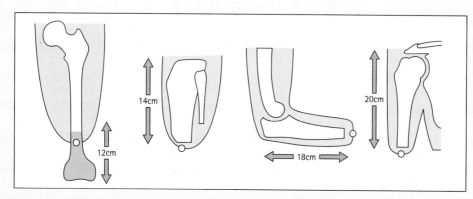

12.13 Amputations The traditional sites of election; the scar is made terminal because these are not end-bearing stumps.

The bone is sawn across at the proposed level. In transtibial amputations the front of the tibia is usually bevelled and filed to create a smoothly rounded contour; the fibula is cut 3cm shorter.

The main vessels are tied, the tourniquet is removed and every bleeding point meticulously ligated. The skin is sutured carefully without tension. Suction drainage is advised and the stump firmly bandaged.

Aftercare

If a haematoma forms, it is evacuated as soon as possible. Repeated elastic bandaging is applied to help shrink the stump and produce a conical limb-end. The muscles must be exercised, the joints kept mobile and the patient taught to use his or her prosthesis.

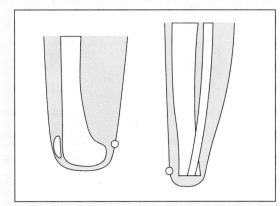

12.14 Amputations Through-knee and Syme's amputations are end-bearing; consequently the scars are not terminal.

AMPUTATIONS OTHER THAN AT THE SITES OF ELECTION

INTERSCAPULO-THORACIC (FOREQUARTER) AMPUTATION This mutilating operation should be done only for traumatic avulsion of the upper limb (a rare event), when it offers the hope of eradicating a malignant tumour or as palliation for otherwise intractable pain.

DISARTICULATION AT THE SHOULDER This is rarely indicated, and if the head of the humerus can be left, the appearance is much better. If 2.5cm of humerus can be left below the anterior axillary fold, it is possible to hold the stump in a prosthesis.

TRANSRADIAL AMPUTATION The shortest forearm stump that will stay in a prosthesis is 2.5cm, measured from the front of the flexed elbow. However, an even shorter stump may be useful as a hook to hang things from.

AMPUTATIONS IN THE HAND These are discussed on page 641.

HEMIPELVECTOMY (HINDQUARTER AMPUTATION) This operation is performed only for malignant disease.

DISARTICULATION THROUGH THE HIP This is rarely indicated and prosthetic fitting is difficult. If the femoral head, neck and trochanters can be left, it is possible to fit a tilting-table prosthesis in which the upper femur sits flexed; if, however, a good prosthetic service is available, a disarticulation and moulding of the torso is preferable.

TRANSFEMORAL AMPUTATIONS A longer stump offers the patient better control of the prosthesis, but at least 12cm must be left below the stump for the knee mechanism. With less than 18cm from the top of the greater trochanter it is difficult to keep the stump in the socket.

AROUND THE KNEE The *Stokes–Gritti operation* (in which the trimmed patella is apposed to the trimmed femoral condyle) is rarely performed because the bone may not unite securely, the end-bearing stump is rarely satisfactory and there is no room for a sophisticated knee mechanism.

Amputation through the knee is commonly used, especially for vascular insufficiency. A long anterior or equal medial and lateral flaps are used. The patella is left *in situ* and the patellar ligament sutured to the cruciate ligaments. Through-knee amputations are also of value in children, because the lower femoral growth disc is preserved.

A very short below-knee amputation (less than 3cm) is worse than a through-knee amputation and should be avoided.

TRANSTIBIAL (BELOW-KNEE) AMPUTATIONS Healthy below-knee stumps can be fitted with excellent prostheses allowing good function and nearly normal gait. Even a 5–6cm stump may be fittable in a thin patient; more makes fitting easier, but there is no advantage in prolonging the stump beyond the conventional 14cm. With a long posterior flap and suction drainage, healing can often be achieved even when the blood supply is impaired.

ABOVE THE ANKLE *Syme's amputation* is sometimes very satisfactory, provided the circulation of the limb is good. It gives excellent function in children and is well accepted by men, but women find it cosmetically undesirable. The indications are few, and the operation is difficult to do well. Because the stump is designed to be end-bearing, the scar is brought away from the end by cutting a long posterior flap. The flap must contain not only the skin of the heel but also all the fibrofatty tissue, to provide a good pad for weightbearing, and therefore in cutting the flap the bone must be picked clean. The bones are divided just above the malleoli to provide

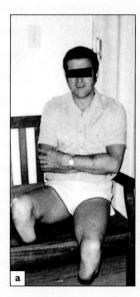
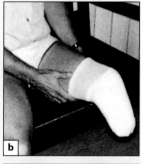
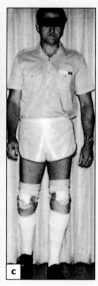
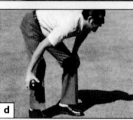

12.15 Amputations – fitting the prosthesis
(**a**) This man had severe congenital deformities which necessitated bilateral below-knee amputations. (**b**) A cast was made of each stump, and from this the stump socket was fashioned and fitted into a prosthesis. (**c**) The prosthesis (held on in this case by straps above the knee) is patellar-tendon-bearing. (**d**) After rehabilitation he has excellent balance and has resumed a near-normal life.

a broad area of cancellous bone, to which the flap should stick firmly, otherwise the soft tissues tend to wobble about. *Pirogoff's amputation* is similar in principle to Syme's but is rarely performed. The back of the os calcis is fixed onto the cut end of the tibia and fibula.

PARTIAL FOOT AMPUTATION The problem here is that the tendo Achillis tends to pull the foot into equinus; this can be prevented by splintage, tenotomy or tendon transfers. The foot may be amputated at any convenient level; for example, through the mid-tarsal joints (Chopart), through the tarsometatarsal joints (Lisfranc), through the metatarsal bones or through the metatarsophalangeal joints. It is best to disregard the classic descriptions and to leave as long a foot as possible provided it is plantigrade and that an adequate flap of plantar skin can be obtained. The only prosthesis needed is a specially moulded slipper worn inside a normal shoe.

IN THE FOOT Where feasible, it is better to amputate through the base of the proximal phalanx rather than through the metatarsophalangeal joint. With diabetic gangrene, septic arthritis of the joint is not uncommon; the entire ray (toe plus metatarsal bone) should be amputated.

PROSTHESES

All prostheses must fit comfortably; they should also function well and look presentable. The patient accepts and uses a prosthesis much better if it is fitted soon after operation; delay is unjustifiable now that modular components are available and only the socket need be made individually.

In the upper limb, the distal portion of the prosthesis is detachable and can be replaced by a 'dress hand' or by a variety of useful terminal devices. Electrically powered limbs are available for both children and adults.

In the lower limb, weight can be transmitted through the ischial tuberosity, the patellar tendon, the upper tibia or the soft tissues. Combinations are permissible; recent developments in silicon and gel materials provide improved comfort in total-contact self-suspending sockets.

COMPLICATIONS OF AMPUTATION STUMPS

Early complications

In addition to the complications of any operation (especially secondary haemorrhage from infection), there are two special hazards: breakdown of skin flaps and gas gangrene.

Breakdown of skin flaps This may be due to ischaemia, to suturing under excessive tension or (in below-knee amputations) to an unduly long tibia pressing against the flap.

Gas gangrene Clostridia and spores from the perineum may infect a high above-knee amputation (or re-amputation), especially if performed through ischaemic tissue.

Late complications

Skin Eczema is common, and tender purulent lumps may develop in the groin. A rest from the prosthesis is indicated.

Ulceration is usually due to poor circulation, and re-amputation at a higher level is then necessary. If, however, the circulation is satisfactory and the skin around an ulcer is healthy, it may be sufficient to excise 2.5cm of bone and resuture.

Muscle If too much muscle is left at the end of the stump, the resulting unstable 'cushion' induces a feeling of insecurity which may prevent proper use of a prosthesis; if so, the excess soft tissue must be excised.

Artery Poor circulation gives a cold, blue stump which is liable to ulcerate. This problem chiefly arises with below-knee amputations and often re-amputation is necessary.

Nerve A cut nerve always forms a bulb ('neuroma') and occasionally this is painful and tender. Excising 3cm of the nerve above the bulb sometimes succeeds. Alternatively, the epineural sleeve of the nerve stump is freed from nerve fascicles for 5mm and then sealed with a synthetic tissue adhesive or buried within muscle or bone away from pressure points.

'Phantom limb' is the term used to describe the feeling that the amputated limb is still present. The patient should be warned of the possibility; eventually the feeling recedes or disappears.

A painful phantom limb is very difficult to treat. Intermittent percussion to the end of the stump has been recommended for phantom limb and for painful nerve bulb; it sounds brutal but success is claimed.

Joint The joint above an amputation may be stiff or deformed. A common deformity is fixed flexion and fixed abduction at the hip in above-knee stumps (because the adductors and hamstring muscles have been divided). It should be prevented by exercises. If it becomes established, subtrochanteric osteotomy may be necessary. Fixed flexion at the knee makes it difficult to walk properly and should also be prevented.

Bone A spur often forms at the end of the bone, but is usually painless. If there has been infection, however, the spur may be large and painful and it may be necessary to excise the end of the bone with the spur.

If the bone is transmitting little weight, it becomes osteoporotic and liable to fracture. Such fractures are best treated by internal fixation.

IMPLANT MATERIALS

METAL

Metal used in implants (screws, plates, prostheses) should be tough, strong, non-corrodible, biologically inert and easily sterilizable. Those commonly used are stainless steel, cobalt–chromium alloys and titanium alloys.

No one material is ideal for all purposes. Stainless steel, because of its relative plasticity, can be cold worked; not only is it easier to manufacture such implants, but also cold working is a way of hardening and strengthening the material. Moreover, its tensile plasticity (ductility) makes it possible to bend stainless steel plates to required shapes during an operation without seriously disturbing their strength.

Cobalt-based alloys (Vitallium, Vinertia) must be cast or wrought. The implants are therefore difficult to manufacture, but they are stronger, more rigid and less liable to corrosion than steel.

Titanium alloys can be worked and shaped like steel, and are corrosion-resistant; however, in metal-on-metal prostheses they are liable to adhesive wear and sludge formation.

IMPLANT FAILURE
Metal implants may not be strong enough to resist local bending forces, and fatigue fractures of plates and screws are common. In some cases, tough, even strong implants fail because they are wrongly placed or inadequately fixed and cannot withstand repetitive bending movement; if used to treat a fracture, protection may be needed until the bone has joined.

CORROSION
Corrosion is rarely a problem, except with plates and screws, where it may be initiated by abrasive damage to polished oxide surfaces, or minute surface cracks due to fatigue failure. Crevice corrosion weakens the metal ('stress corrosion cracking') and may cause a local inflammatory reaction and osteoclastic bone resorption; the result is breakage or loosening of the implant.

All metallic implants corrode to some extent; the corrosion products are biologically active and they permeate every tissue of the body (Black, 1988). Whether this might prove harmful only time will tell, but clearly there is justification for removing fracture implants when they are no longer needed.

DISSIMILAR METALS
Dissimilar metals immersed in solution in contact with one another may set up galvanic corrosion with accelerated destruction of the more reactive (or 'base') metal. In the early days of implant surgery when highly corrodible metals were used, the same thing happened in the body. However, the passive alloys now used for implants do not exhibit this phenomenon and the traditional fear of using dissimilar metals in bone implants is probably exaggerated.

FRICTION AND WEAR
The *coefficient of friction* is constant for any two surfaces regardless of their size. However, shape has a marked influence on this property: in a ball-and-socket

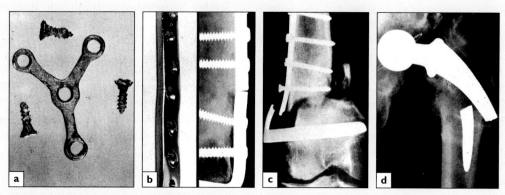

12.16 Implant failure (a) An old metal implant, showing corrosion of the plate and screws; (b) the tiny defect in this plate, due to stress corrosion cracking, is just visible in the x-ray; (c) complete implant failure; (d) the implant is not necessarily to blame – this man was being taken home after a small celebration; he alighted from the car, unhappily without waiting for it to stop.

joint the frictional moment is related to the degree of congruity and the size of the ball (the larger the ball, the greater the frictional resistance). The type of material also is important: metal-on-metal may cause adhesive wear ('seizing'), whereas metal-on-plastic has a low coefficient of friction and has therefore predominated in joint replacement surgery. Ceramic bearing surfaces provide both low friction and low wear. With improved manufacturing techniques metal-on-metal prostheses may again come into their own.

Wear particles sometimes cause local inflammation and scarring, and occasionally a toxic or allergic reaction; most importantly, however, they may cause implant loosening following their uptake by macrophages and subsequent activation of osteoclastic bone resorption. Wear particles have also been demonstrated in lymph nodes and other organs far distant from the implant; the significance of this finding is uncertain but there is increasing evidence that this can produce chromosomal damage.

INFECTION
Metal does not cause infection, but implants may encourage the persistence of infection (1) by offering an acceptable substrate for bacterial growth and (2) by impeding drainage.

MALIGNANCY
A few cases of malignancy at the site of metal implants have been reported, but the number is so small in comparison with the number of implants that the risk can probably be discounted.

HIGH-DENSITY POLYETHYLENE

High-density polyethylene (HDPE) is an inert thermoplastic polymer modified to provide increased strength and wear resistance. In contact with polished metal it has a low coefficient of friction and it therefore seemed ideal for joint replacement. This has proved to be true in hip reconstruction with a simple ball-and-socket articulation. However, it has one major disadvantage – a tendency to viscoelastic deformity (stretching) and creep; this occurs particularly at the knee, probably because of its complex and demanding load characteristics. HDPE is also easily abraded, and hard chips of bone or acrylic cement trapped on its surface cause it to disintegrate. Even in the absence of severe surface abrasion, wear products may find their way into the bone–cement interface and stimulate bone resorption and prosthesis loosening.

SILICON COMPOUNDS

There is a wide variety of silicon polymers, of which silicone rubber (Silastic) is particularly useful. It is firm, tough, flexible and inert, and is used to make hinges for replacing finger and toe joints, and for spacers to replace resected bone (e.g. the head of the radius or the trapezium). Silastic wears well but may fracture if the implant surface is nicked or torn by a sharp instrument or piece of bone. The presence of silicon in the body may induce a giant cell synovitis; sometimes bone erosion and 'cyst' formation are seen at some distance from the implant.

CERAMICS

Ceramic materials are being used, either alone or bonded to metal, for joint replacement prostheses. They are more brittle than other materials but they are also hard and strong, and their low coefficient of friction makes them particularly suitable for younger patients in whom wear problems are more significant. Porous ceramic implants may allow bone ingrowth as a means of fixation.

CARBON

This eminently biocompatible material is looking for a purpose. As graphite it has wear and lubricant properties that might fit it for joint replacement. As carbon fibre it is sometimes used to replace ligaments; it induces the formation of longitudinally aligned fibrous tissue which substitutes for the natural ligament. However, the carbon fibres tend to break up and if particles find their way into the synovial cavity they induce a synovitis. Carbon composites are also used to manufacture plates and joint prostheses; these have a lower modulus of elasticity than metal and may therefore be more compatible with the bone to which they are attached.

ACRYLIC CEMENT

In joint replacements the prostheses are often fixed to the bone with acrylic cement (polymethylmethacrylate), which acts as a grouting material (Charnley, 1970). It is applied to the bone as a partially polymerized dough, in which the prosthesis is embedded. With sufficient pressure the pasty material is forced into the bony interstices and, when fully polymerized, the hard compound prevents all movement between prosthesis and bone. It can withstand large compressive loads but is easily broken by tensile stress.

When the partially polymerized cement is forced into the bone there is often a drop in blood pressure; this is attributed to the uptake of residual monomer, which can cause peripheral vasodilatation, but there may also be fat embolization from the bone marrow. This is seldom a problem in fit patients with osteoarthritis, but in elderly people who are also osteoporotic, monomer and marrow fat may enter the circulation very rapidly when the cement is compressed and the fall in blood pressure can be alarming (and occasionally fatal).

With good cementing technique osseointegration can and does take place on the acrylic surface. However, if the initial cement application is not perfect, a fibrous layer forms at the cement–bone interface, its thickness depending on the degree of cement penetration into the bone crevices. In this flimsy membrane fine granulation tissue and foreign body giant cells can be seen. This relatively quiescent tissue remains unchanged under a wide range of biological and mechanical conditions, but if there is excessive movement at the cement–bone interface, or if polyethylene or metallic wear products track down into the cement–bone interface, an aggressive reaction produces bone resorption and disintegration of the interlocking surface; occasionally this is severe enough to justify the term 'aggressive granulomatosis' or 'aggressive osteolysis' (Eskola *et al.*, 1990). Bone resorption and cement loosening may also be associated with low-grade infection which can manifest for the first time many years after the operation; whether the infection in these cases precedes the loosening or vice versa is still not known for certain.

HYDROXYAPATITE

The mineral phase of bone exists largely in the form of crystalline HA. It is not surprising, therefore, that this material has been used to reproduce the osteoinductive and osteoconductive properties of bone grafts. Porous HA obtained from coral exoskeleton is rapidly incorporated in living bone (Holmes *et al.*, 1986) and synthetic implants consisting of HA, tricalcium phosphate and fibrillar collagen, when mixed with host marrow, have been used successfully as graft substitutes in humans (Kocialkowski *et al.*, 1990). HA can also be plasma sprayed onto titanium alloy implants; the HA coating is a highly acceptable substrate for bone cells and promotes rapid osseointegration (Stephenson *et al.*, 1991). This principle has been applied in the use of uncemented hip replacement prostheses; however, a final verdict on its value must await long-term follow-up studies.

REFERENCES AND FURTHER READING

Aspenberg P, Johnsson E, Thirngren KG (1990) Dose-dependent reduction of bone inductive properties by ethylene oxide. *Journal of Bone and Joint Surgery* **72B**, 1036-1037

Black J (1988) Editorial. Does corrosion matter? *Journal of Bone and Joint Surgery* **70B**, 517-519

Bushell AJ, Klenerman L, Davies HM *et al* (1995) Damage to skeletal muscle induced by prolonged ischemia and reperfusion. *Transplantation Proceedings* **27**, 2834-2835

Charnley J (1970) *Acrylic Cement in Orthopaedic Surgery*. Churchill Livingstone, Edinburgh and London

Christensen KS, Clarke M (1986) Transcutaneous oxygen measurement in peripheral occlusive disease. *Journal of Bone and Joint Surgery* **68B**, 423-426

Davis N, Curry A, Gambhir AK *et al* (1999) Intraoperative bacterial contamination in operations for joint replacement. *Journal of Bone and Joint Surgery* **81B**, 886-889

de Bastiani G, Aldegheri R, Brivio LR *et al* (1986) Chondrodiatasis – controlled symmetrical distraction of the epiphyseal plate. *Journal of Bone and Joint Surgery* **68B**, 550-556

Eastwood DM, Cole WG (1995) A graphic method for timing the correction of leg-length discrepancy. *Journal of Bone and Joint Surgery* **77B**, 743-747

Eskola A, Santavirta S, Konttinen YT *et al* (1990) Cementless revision of aggressive granulomatous lesions in hip replacement. *Journal of Bone and Joint Surgery* **72B**, 212-216

Friedlaender GE (1987) Bone grafts. *Journal of Bone and Joint Surgery* **69A**, 786-790

Holmes RE, Bucholz RW, Mooney V (1986) Porous hydroxyapatite as a bone graft substitute in metaphyseal defects. *Journal of Bone and Joint Surgery* **68A**, 904-911

Ilizarov GA (1992) *Transosseous Osteosynthesis*. Springer, Berlin, Heidelberg and New York

Klenerman L, Lowe NM, Miller I *et al* (1995). Dantrolene sodium protects against experimental ischemia and reperfusion damage to skeletal muscle. *Acta Orthopaedica Scandinavica* **66**, 352-358

Kocialkowski A, Wallace WA, Price HG (1990) Clinical experience with a new artificial bone graft. *Injury* **21**, 142–144

Leyvras PF, Bachmann F, Hoek J *et al* (1991) Prevention of deep vein thrombosis after hip replacement: randomised comparison between unfractionated heparin and low molecular weight heparin. *British Medical Journal* **303**, 543-548

Nade S, Burwell RG (1977) Decalcified bone as a substrate for osteogenesis. *Journal of Bone and Joint Surgery* **59B**, 189-196

O'Brien MD (2000) Editor. Aids to the Examination of the Peripheral Nervous System (4th Edition). WB Saunders, London

Saleh M, Sharrard WJW (1989) Leg lengthening in achondroplasia. In *External Fixation and Functional Bracing* (eds Coombs R, Green S, Sarmiento A). Orthotext, London

Stephenson PK, Freeman MAR, Revell PA *et al* (1991) The effect of hydroxyapatite coating on ingrowth of bone into cavities in an implant. *Journal of Arthroplasty* **6**, 51-58

Urist MR (1970) Bone formation in implants of partially and wholly demineralized bone matrix. *Clinical Orthopaedics and Related Research* **71**, 271-278

Vilarrubias JM, Ginebreda I, Jimeno E (1990) Lengthening of the lower limbs and correction of lumbar hyperlordosis in achondroplasia. *Clinical Orthopaedics and Related Research* **250**, 143-149

Warwick DJ, Williams MH, Bannister GC (1995) Death and thromboembolic disease after total hip replacement without routine chemical prophylaxis *Journal of Bone and Joint Surgery* **77B**, 6-10

Warwick DJ, Harrison J, Glew *et al.* (1998) Comparison of the use of a foot pump and low molecular weight heparin for the prevention of deep vein thrombosis after total hip replacement. *Journal of Bone and Joint Surgery* **80A**, 1158–1116

Wilde GP, Baker GCW (1987) Circumferential periosteal release in the treatment of children with leg length inequality. *Journal of Bone and Joint Surgery* **69B**, 817-821

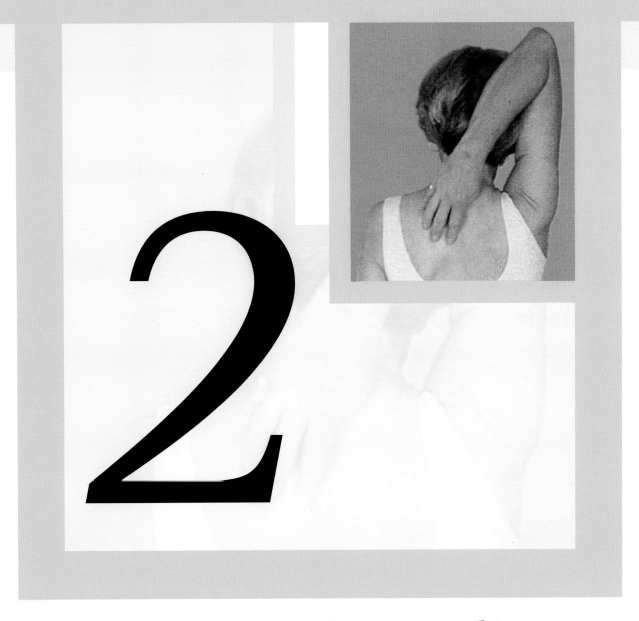

2

Regional Orthopaedics

In This Section

13 **The shoulder and pectoral girdle**   277

14 **The elbow**   303

15 **The wrist**   315

16 **The hand**   333

17 **The neck**   357

18 **The back**   371

19 **The hip**   405

20 **The knee**   449

21 **The ankle and foot**   485

The shoulder and pectoral girdle

CLINICAL ASSESSMENT

SYMPTOMS

Pain is the commonest symptom. But 'pain in the shoulder' is not necessarily 'shoulder pain'! If the patient points to the top of the shoulder, think of the acromioclavicular joint, or referred pain from the neck. Pain from the shoulder joint and the rotator cuff is felt, typically, over the front and outer aspect of the joint, often as far down as the middle of the arm. The relationship to posture may be significant: pain which appears when the arm is in the 'window-cleaning' position is characteristic of rotator cuff impingement; pain which comes on suddenly when the arm is held high overhead suggests instability.

Beware the trap of *referred pain*. Mediastinal disorders, including cardiac ischaemia, can present with aching in either shoulder.

Stiffness may be progressive and severe – so much so as to merit the term 'frozen shoulder'.

Swelling may be in the joint, the muscle or the bone; the patient won't know the difference.

Deformity may consist of muscle wasting, prominence of the acromioclavicular joint, winging of the scapula or an abnormal position of the arm.

Instability symptoms may be gross and alarming ("my shoulder jumps out of its socket when I raise my arm"); more often they are quite subtle: a click or jerk when the arm is held overhead, or the 'dead arm' sensation that overtakes the tennis player as he prepares to serve.

Weakness may appear as a true loss of power, suggesting a neurological disorder, or as a sudden and surprising inability to abduct the shoulder – perhaps due to a tendon rupture.

Loss of function is usually expressed as difficulty with dressing and grooming, or inability to lift objects or work with the arm above shoulder height.

SIGNS

The patient should always be examined from in front and from behind. Both upper limbs, the neck and the chest must be visible.

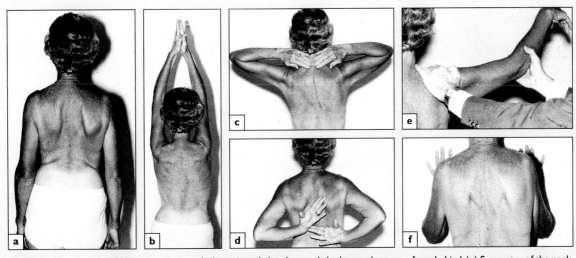

13.1 Examination Small alterations in scapulothoracic and glenohumeral rhythm are best seen from behind. (**a**) Symmetry of the neck, shoulders and scapulae is assessed. (**b**) Full abduction (or 'circumduction'), a combination of scapular and glenohumeral movements. (**c**) Abduction and external rotation. (**d**) Adduction and internal rotation (slightly limited on the right). (**e**) True glenohumeral movement is gauged by pressing down firmly on the scapula to stop scapulothoracic movement. (**f**) When the patient presses against a wall the scapula should remain flat; if serratus anterior is weak it stands out prominently ('winging').

Look

Skin Scars or sinuses are noted; don't forget the axilla!

Shape The two sides should be compared. Asymmetry of the shoulders, winging of the scapula, wasting of the deltoid, supraspinatus and infraspinatus muscles and acromioclavicular dislocation are best seen from behind; swelling of the acromioclavicular or sternoclavicular joint or wasting of the pectoral muscles is more obvious from the front. A joint effusion causes swelling anteriorly and occasionally 'points' in the axilla. Wasting of the deltoid suggests a nerve lesion whereas wasting of the supraspinatus may be due to either a full-thickness tear or a suprascapular nerve lesion. The typical 'Popeye' bulge of a ruptured biceps is more easily seen if the elbow is flexed.

Position If the arm is held internally rotated, think of posterior dislocation of the shoulder.

Feel

Skin As the joint is well covered, inflammation rarely influences skin temperature.

Bony points and soft tissues The deeper structures are carefully palpated, following a mental picture of the anatomy. Start with the sternoclavicular joint, then follow the clavicle laterally to the acromioclavicular joint, and so onto the anterior edge of the acromion and around the acromion. The anterior and posterior margins of the glenoid should be palpated. With the shoulder held in extension, the supraspinatus tendon can be pinpointed just under the anterior edge of the acromion; below this, the bony prominence bounding the bicipital groove is easily felt, especially if the arm is gently rotated so that the hard ridge slips medially and laterally under the palpating fingers. Crepitus over the supraspinatus tendon during movement suggests tendinitis or a tear.

Move

Active movements Movements are observed first from in front and then from behind, with the patient either standing or sitting. Sideways elevation of the arms normally occurs in the plane of the scapula – i.e. about 20° anterior to the coronal plane – with the arm rising through an arc of 180°. However, by convention, abduction is performed in the coronal plane and flexion/extension in the sagittal plane.

Abduction starts at 0°; the early phase of movement takes place almost entirely at the glenohumeral joint, but as the arm rises the scapula begins to rotate on the thorax and in the last 60° of movement is almost entirely scapulothoracic (hence sideways movement beyond 90° is sometimes called 'elevation' rather than 'abduction'). The rhythmic transition from glenohumeral to scapulothoracic movement is disturbed by disorders in the joint or by dysfunction of the stabilizing tendons around the joint. Thus, abduction may be (1) difficult to initiate, (2) diminished in range or (3) altered in rhythm, the scapula moving too early and creating a shrugging effect. If movement is painful, the arc of pain must be noted; pain in the mid-range of abduction suggests a minor rotator cuff tear or supraspinatus tendinitis; pain at the end of abduction is often due to acromioclavicular arthritis.

Flexion and extension are examined by asking the patient to raise the arms forwards and then backwards. The normal range is 180° of flexion and 40° of extension.

Rotation is tested in two ways. The arms are held close to the body with the elbows flexed to 90°; the hands are then separated as widely as possible (external rotation) and brought together again across the body (internal rotation). This is a rather unnatural movement and one learns more by simply asking the patients to clasp their fingers behind their neck (external rotation in abduction) and then to reach up their back with their fingers (internal rotation in adduction); the two sides are compared.

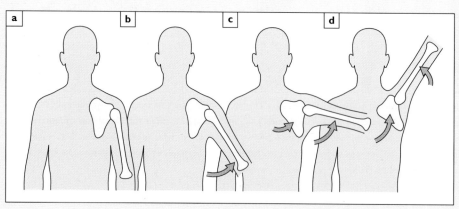

13.2 Scapulohumeral rhythm (**a–c**) During the early phase of abduction, most of the movement takes place at the glenohumeral joint. As the arm rises, the scapula begins to rotate on the thorax (**c**). In the last phase of abduction, movement is almost entirely scapulothoracic (**d**).

Passive movements To test the range of glenohumeral movement (as distinct from combined glenohumeral and scapular movement) the scapula must first be anchored; this is done by the examiner pressing firmly down on the top of the shoulder with one hand while the other hand moves the patient's arm. Grasping the angle of the scapula as a method of anchorage is less satisfactory.

Power The deltoid is examined for bulk and tautness while the patient abducts against resistance. To test serratus anterior (long thoracic nerve, C5,6,7) the patient is asked to push forcefully against a wall with both hands; if the muscle is weak, the scapula is not stabilized on the thorax and stands out prominently (winged scapula). Pectoralis major is tested by having the patient thrust both hands firmly into the waist. Rotator power is tested by asking the patient to stand with his or her arms tucked into his or her side and the elbows flexed, then to externally rotate against resistance. Weakness is associated with a cuff tear, pain or instability.

Other joints Clinical assessment is completed by examining the cervical spine (as a common source of referred pain) and testing for generalized joint laxity (a frequent accompaniment of shoulder instability).

EXAMINATION AFTER LOCAL ANAESTHETIC INJECTION

It is sometimes possible to localize the source of shoulder pain by injecting local anaesthetic into the target site (for example the supraspinatus tendon or the acromioclavicular joint) and thus to see whether there is a temporary reduction in pain on movement. Injection into the subacromial space may help to distinguish loss of movement due to pain from that due to a rotator cuff tear.

IMAGING

X-ray At least two x-ray views should be obtained: an anteroposterior in the plane of the shoulder and an axillary projection with the arm in abduction to show the relationship of the humeral head to the glenoid. Look for evidence of subluxation, or dislocation, joint space narrowing, bone erosion and calcification in the soft tissues. The acromioclavicular joint is best shown by an anteroposterior projection with the tube tilted upwards 20° (the cephalic tilt view). The subacromial space is viewed by tilting the tube downwards 30° (the caudal tilt view).

Arthrography This is useful for detecting rotator cuff tears and some larger Bankart lesions found with anterior instability.

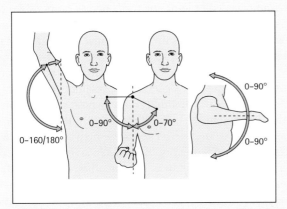

13.3 Normal range of movement (a) Abduction is from 0° to 160° (or even 180°), but only 90° of this takes place at the glenohumeral joint (in the plane of the scapula, 20° anterior to the coronal plane); the remainder is scapular movement. (b) External rotation is usually about 80°, but internal is rather less because the trunk gets in the way. (c) With the arm abducted to a right angle, internal rotation can be assessed without the trunk getting in the way.

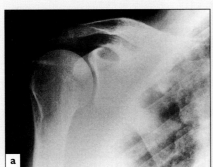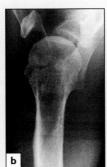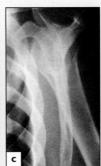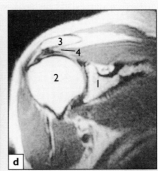

13.4 Imaging (a) Anteroposterior x-ray. (b) Axillary view showing the humeral head opposite the shallow glenoid fossa, and the coracoid process anteriorly. The acromion process shadow overlaps that of the humeral head. (c) Lateral view; the head of the humerus should lie where the coracoid process, the spine of the scapula and the blade of the scapula meet. (d) MRI. Note 1 the glenoid, 2 the head of the humerus, 3 the acromion process and 4 the supraspinatus (with degeneration of the tendon).

CT scan Particularly when enhanced with intra-articular contrast, CT scans can identify cuff tears and labral detachments.

Ultrasound In experienced hands, ultrasound provides a reliable and simple means of identifying rotator cuff tears.

MRI The information provided by MRI depends on the quality of the equipment and the imaging sequences which are chosen. For patients with suspected rotator cuff pathology, MRI gives information on the site and size of a tear, as well as the anatomy of the coracoacromial arch and acromioclavicular joint (Recht and Resnick, 1993). For patients with symptoms and signs suggesting instability, it can demonstrate associated anomalies of the capsule, labrum, glenoid and humeral head. MRI is also useful in detecting osteonecrosis of the head of the humerus and in the diagnosis and staging of tumours.

ARTHROSCOPY

Arthroscopy is useful for to diagnose (and sometimes treat) intra-articular lesions, detachment of the labrum or capsule and impingement or tears of the rotator cuff.

DISORDERS OF THE ROTATOR CUFF

The commonest cause of pain around the shoulder is a disorder of the rotator cuff. This is sometimes referred to rather loosely as 'rotator cuff syndrome'; however, there are at least five conditions with distinct clinical features and natural history:

- the impingement syndrome or supraspinatus tendinitis;
- ruptures of the rotator cuff;
- acute calcific tendinitis;
- biceps tendinitis and/or rupture;
- adhesive capsulitis or 'frozen shoulder'.

IMPINGEMENT SYNDROME (SUPRASPINATUS TENDINITIS)

Pathology

The rotator cuff impingement syndrome is a painful disorder which is thought to arise from repetitive compression or rubbing of the tendons (mainly supraspinatus) under the coracoacromial arch. Normally, when the arm is abducted, the conjoint tendon slides under the coracoacromial arch. As abduction approaches 90°, there is a natural tendency to externally rotate the arm, thus allowing the rotator cuff to occupy the widest part of the subacromial space. If the arm is held persistently in abduction and then moved to and fro in internal and external rotation (as in cleaning a window, painting a wall or polishing a flat surface) the rotator cuff may be compressed and irritated as it comes in contact with the anterior edge of the acromion process and the taut coracoacromial ligament. This attitude (abduction, slight flexion and internal rotation) has been called the 'impingement position'. Perhaps significantly, the site of impingement is also the 'critical area' of diminished vascularity in the supraspinatus tendon about 1cm proximal to its insertion into the greater tuberosity.

Other factors which may predispose to repetitive impingement are osteoarthritic thickening of the acromioclavicular joint, the formation of bony ridges or 'osteophytes' on the anterior edge of the acromion and swelling of the cuff or the subacromial bursa in inflammatory disorders such as gout or rheumatoid arthritis.

The mildest injury is a type of friction, which may give rise to localized oedema and swelling ('tendinitis'). This is usually self-limiting, but with prolonged or repetitive impingement – and especially in older people – minute tears can develop and these may be followed by scarring, fibrocartilaginous metaplasia or calcification in the tendon. Healing is accompanied by a vascular reaction and local congestion (in itself painful) which may contribute to further impingement in the constricted space under the coracoacromial arch whenever the arm is elevated.

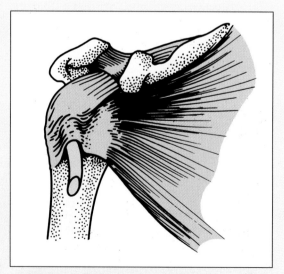

13.5 Anatomy The tough coracoacromial ligament stretches from the coracoid to the underside of the anterior third of the acromion process; the humeral head moves beneath this arch during abduction and the rotator cuff may be irritated or damaged as it glides in this confined space.

Sometimes – perhaps where healing is slow or following a sudden strain – the microscopic disruption extends, becoming a partial or full-thickness tear of the cuff; shoulder function is then more seriously compromised and active abduction may be impossible. The tendon of the long head of biceps, lying adjacent to the supraspinatus, also may be involved and is often torn.

Wear, tear and repair The pathological processes described above may be summed up as 'wear', 'tear' and 'repair'. In the young patient 'repair' is vigorous; consequently, healing is relatively rapid but (because the vascular repair process itself causes pain) it is accompanied by considerable distress. The older patient has more 'wear' but less vigorous 'repair'; healing will be slower but pain less severe. Thus acute tendinitis (which affects younger patients) is intensely painful but rapidly better; chronic tendinitis (a middle group) is only moderately painful but takes many months to recover and may be complicated by partial tears; and a complete tear (which usually occurs in the elderly) becomes painless soon after injury, but never mends. Degenerative changes are extremely common and small tears of the cuff are found at autopsy in about half of those aged over 60 years.

Secondary arthropathy Large tears of the cuff eventually lead to serious disturbance of shoulder mechanics.

The humeral head migrates upwards, abutting against the acromion process, and passive abduction is severely restricted. Abnormal movement predisposes to osteoarthritis (OA) of the glenohumeral joint. Occasionally this progresses to a rapidly destructive arthropathy – the so-called Milwaukee shoulder [named after the city where it was first described by McCarty *et al.* (1981)].

Clinical features

The clinical features depend on the stage of the disorder, the age of the patient and the vigour of the healing response. Three patterns of symptoms are encountered:

- Subacute tendinitis – the 'painful arc syndrome', due to vascular congestion, microscopic haemorrhage and oedema.
- Chronic tendinitis – recurrent shoulder pain due to tendinitis and fibrosis.
- Cuff disruption – recurrent pain, weakness and loss of movement due to tears in the rotator cuff.

SUBACUTE TENDINITIS (PAINFUL ARC SYNDROME)
The patient, usually under 40 years of age, develops anterior shoulder pain after vigorous or unaccustomed activity – e.g. competitive swimming or a weekend of

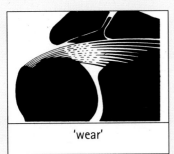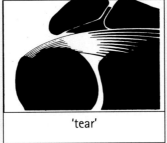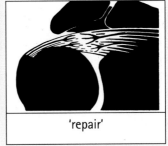

'wear' 'tear' 'repair'

13.6 The progression of rotator cuff lesions

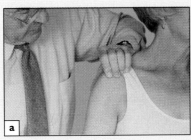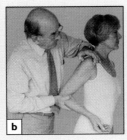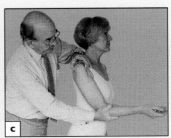

13.7 Supraspinatus tenderness (a) The tender spot is at the anterior edge of the acromion process. When the shoulder is extended (b) tenderness is more marked; with the shoulder slightly flexed (c) the painful tendon disappears under the acromion process and tenderness disappears.

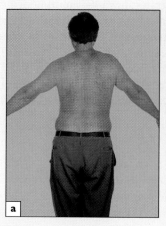 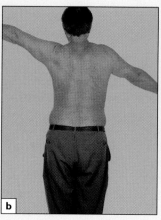 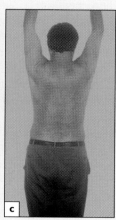

13.8 The painful arc (a, b) In abduction, scapulohumeral rhythm is disturbed on the right and the patient starts to experience pain at about 60°. **(c)** As the arm passes beyond 120° the pain eases and the patient is able to abduct and elevate up to the full 180°.

house decorating. The shoulder looks normal but is acutely tender along the anterior edge of the acromion. Point tenderness is most easily elicited by palpating this spot with the shoulder held in extension, thus placing the supraspinatus tendon in an exposed position anterior to the acromion process; with the arm held in flexion the tenderness disappears.

There are three clinical tests for supraspinatus tendinitis:

- *The painful arc:* On active abduction scapulohumeral rhythm is disturbed and pain is aggravated as the arm traverses an arc between 60° and 120°. Repeating the movement with the arm in full external rotation may be much easier and relatively painless.
- *The impingement sign:* The scapula is stabilized with one hand while the other raises the affected arm in flexion, abduction and internal rotation, thus bringing the greater tuberosity directly under the coracoacromial arch. The test is positive when pain is elicited by this manoeuvre. However, the test is not specific and it may be positive in patients with acromioclavicular osteoarthritis or glenohumeral instability.
- *The impingement test:* If the previous manoeuvre is positive, it may be repeated after injecting 10ml of 1% lignocaine into the subacromial space; if the pain is abolished (or significantly reduced), this will help to confirm the diagnosis.

The condition is often reversible, settling down gradually once the initiating activity is avoided.

CHRONIC TENDINITIS

The patient, usually aged between 40 and 50 years, gives a history of recurrent attacks of subacute tendinitis, the pain settling down with rest or anti-inflammatory treatment, only to recur when more demanding activities are resumed. Characteristically pain is worse at night; the patient cannot lie on the affected side and often finds it more comfortable to sit up out of bed.

Pain and slight stiffness of the shoulder may restrict even simple activities such as hair grooming or dressing. The physical signs described above should be elicited. In addition there may be signs of bicipital tendinitis: tenderness along the bicipital groove and crepitus on moving the biceps tendon.

A disturbing feature is coarse crepitation or palpable snapping over the rotator cuff when the shoulder is passively rotated; this may signify a partial tear or marked fibrosis of the cuff. Small, unsuspected tears are quite often found during arthroscopy or operation.

CUFF DISRUPTION

The most advanced stage of the disorder is progressive fibrosis and disruption of the cuff, resulting in either a partial or full thickness tear. The patient is usually aged over 45 years and gives a history of refractory shoulder pain with increasing stiffness and weakness.

Partial tears may occur within the substance or on the deep surface of the cuff and are not easily detected, even on direct inspection of the cuff. They are deceptive also in that continuity of the remaining cuff fibres permits active abduction with a painful arc, making it difficult to tell whether chronic tendinitis is complicated by a partial tear.

A full-thickness tear may follow a long period of chronic tendinitis, but occasionally it occurs spontaneously after a sprain or jerking injury of the shoulder. There is sudden pain and the patient is unable to abduct the arm. Passive abduction also may, in the early stages, be limited or prevented by pain. If the diagnosis is in doubt, pain can be eliminated by injecting a local anaesthetic into the subacromial space. If active abduction is now possible the tear must be only partial. If active abduction remains impossible, then a complete tear is likely.

If some weeks have elapsed since the injury the two types are more easily differentiated. With a complete tear, pain has by then subsided and the clinical picture is unmistakable: active abduction is impossible and

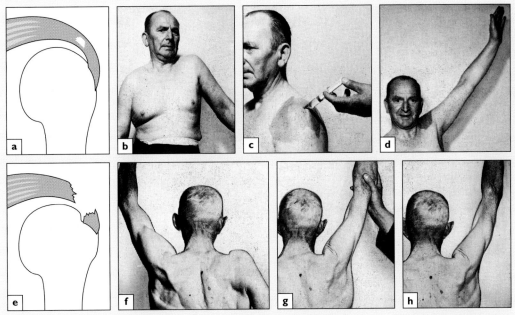

13.9 Torn supraspinatus (**a–d**) Partial tear of left supraspinatus: the patient can abduct actively once pain has been abolished with local anaesthetic. (**e–h**) Complete tear of right supraspinatus: active abduction is impossible even when pain subsides (**f**), or has been abolished by injection; but once the arm is passively abducted (**g**), the patient can hold it up with his deltoid muscle (**h**).

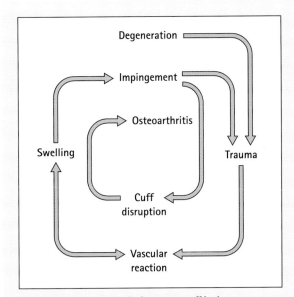

13.10 The vicious spiral of rotator cuff lesions

attempting it produces a characteristic shrug; but passive abduction is full and once the arm has been lifted above a right angle the patient can keep it up by using his or her deltoid (the 'abduction paradox'); when he or she lowers it sideways it suddenly drops (the 'drop arm sign').

With time there may be some recovery of active abduction, though power in both abduction and exter-

nal rotation is weaker than normal. There is usually wasting of the supraspinatus and infraspinatus, and on testing the biceps there may be an old tear of the long head tendon (see below). There is often tenderness of the acromioclavicular joint.

In long-standing cases of partial or complete rupture, secondary OA of the shoulder may supervene and movements are then severely restricted.

Imaging

X-rays are usually normal in the early stages of the cuff syndrome, but with chronic tendinitis there may be erosion, sclerosis or cyst formation at the site of cuff insertion on the greater tuberosity. In chronic cases the caudal tilt view may show roughening or overgrowth of the anterior edge of the acromion, thinning of the acromion process and upward displacement of the humeral head. OA of the acromioclavicular joint is common in older patients and in late cases the glenohumeral joint also may show features of OA. Sometimes there is calcification of the supraspinatus, but this is usually coincidental and not the cause of pain (see below).

Arthrography may reveal a full thickness cuff tear, the opaque medium extending from the joint into the subacromial space. However, it does not detect a bursal-side partial thickness tear or an intra-tendinous tear.

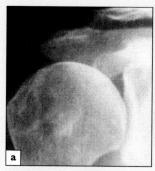 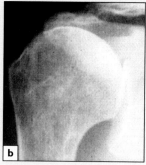 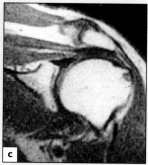

13.11 Chronic tendinitis – imaging (a, b) When the patient attempts to abduct, the head of the humerus rides upwards to abut against the acromion process. Note the marked erosion of the acromioclavicular joint. (c) MRI shows thickening of the supraspinatus and an erosion at its insertion. The acromioclavicular joint is swollen and clearly abnormal.

Ultrasonography can demonstrate large cuff tears, but it is heavily operator dependent.

MRI effectively demonstrates the structures around the shoulder. In patients with rotator cuff pathology, it provides valuable information on the site and size of a cuff tear; it also shows the precise anatomy of the coracoacromial arch and acromioclavicular joint. However, it should be remembered that a third of asymptomatic individuals have abnormalities of the rotator cuff on MRI (Sher *et al.*, 1995).

Treatment

CONSERVATIVE TREATMENT

The uncomplicated impingement syndrome (or tendinitis) is often self-limiting and symptoms settle down once the aggravating activity is eliminated. Patients should be taught ways of avoiding the 'impingement position'. Physiotherapy, including ultrasound and active exercises in the 'position of freedom', may tide the patient over the painful healing phase. A short course of non-steroidal anti-inflammatory tablets sometimes brings relief. If all these methods fail, and before disability becomes marked, the patient should be given one or two injections of depot corticosteroid into the subacromial space. In most cases this will relieve the pain, and it is then important to persevere with protective modifications of shoulder activity for at least 6 months. Healing is slow, and a hasty return to full activity will often precipitate further attacks of tendinitis.

SURGICAL TREATMENT

The indications for surgical treatment are essentially clinical; the presence of a cuff tear does not necessarily call for an operation. Provided the patient has a useful range of movement, adequate strength and well-controlled pain, non-operative measures are adequate. If symptoms do not subside after 3 months of conservative treatment,

or if they recur persistently after each period of treatment, an operation is advisable. Certainly this is preferable to prolonged and repeated treatment with anti-inflammatory drugs and local corticosteroids. The indication is more pressing if there are signs of a partial rotator cuff tear and in particular if there is good clinical evidence of a full thickness tear in a younger patient. The object is to decompress the rotator cuff by excising the coracoacromial ligament, undercutting the anterior part of the acromion process and, if necessary, reducing any bony excrescences at the acromioclavicular joint (Neer, 1972; Rockwood and Lyons, 1993). This can be achieved by open surgery or arthroscopically; the latter is technically demanding but it can produce results equivalent to those of open surgery (Sachs *et al.*, 1994; Nutton *et al.*, 1997).

Open acromioplasty Through an anterior incision the deltoid muscle is split and the part arising from the anterior edge of the acromion is dissected free, exposing the coracoacromial ligament, the acromion and the acromioclavicular joint. The coracoacromial ligament is excised and the anteroinferior portion of the acromion is removed by an undercutting osteotomy. The cuff is then inspected: if there is a defect, it is repaired. Excrescences on the undersurface of the acromioclavicular joint are pared down. If the joint is hypertrophic, the outer 1cm of clavicle is removed; this last step exposes even more of the cuff and permits reconstruction of larger defects. An important step is careful reattachment of the deltoid to the acromion, if necessary by suturing though drill holes in the acromion; failure to obtain secure attachment may lead to postoperative pain and weakness. After the operation, shoulder movements are commenced as soon as pain subsides.

Arthroscopic acromioplasty This should achieve the same basic objectives as open acromioplasty (Nutton *et al.*, 1997). The underside of the acromion (and, if necessary, the acromioclavicular joint) must be trimmed and the coracoacromial ligament divided or removed. If a partial cuff tear is encountered, then it may be possible to repair it; otherwise the edges can be debrided or an open repair undertaken (Gartsman, 1997).

Open repair of the rotator cuff The indications for open repair of the rotator cuff are chronic pain, weakness of the shoulder and significant loss of function. The younger and more active the patient, the greater is the justification for surgery. The operation always includes an acromioplasty as described above. The cuff is mobilized, if necessary by releasing the coracohumeral ligament and the glenoid attachment of the capsule; this dissection should not stray more than 2cm medial to the glenoid rim lest the suprascapular nerve is damaged.

It may be possible to approximate the ends of the cuff defect. Larger tears can be dealt with by suturing the cuff tendon directly to a roughened area on the greater tuberosity using drill holes or soft-tissue anchors.

Postoperatively, movements are restricted for 6–8 weeks and then graded exercises are introduced.

The results of open cuff repair are reasonably good, with satisfactory pain relief in about 80% of patients. This alone usually improves function, even if strength and range of movement are still restricted (Ianotti, 1994).

Massive full-thickness tears that cannot be reconstructed are treated by subacromial decompression and debridement of degenerate cuff tissue; the relief of pain may allow reasonable abduction of the shoulder by the remaining muscles (Rockwood *et al.*, 1995). Other methods to reconstruct irreparable tears in the younger patient include supraspinatus advancement, latissimus dorsi transfer, rotator cuff transposition, fascia lata autograft and synthetic tendon graft.

Acute rupture of the rotator cuff in patients over 70 years usually becomes painless; although movement is restricted, operation is contraindicated.

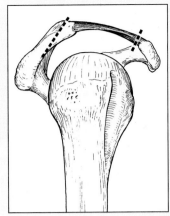

13.12 Impingement syndrome – surgical treatment The coracoacromial ligament and underside of the anterior third of the acromion are removed to enlarge the space for the rotator cuff. This can be performed by open surgery or arthroscopically.

CALCIFICATION OF THE ROTATOR CUFF

ACUTE CALCIFIC TENDINITIS

Acute shoulder pain may follow deposition of calcium hydroxyapatite crystals, usually in the 'critical zone' of the supraspinatus tendon slightly medial to its insertion, occasionally elsewhere in the rotator cuff. The condition is not unique to the shoulder, and similar lesions are seen in tendons and ligaments around the ankle, knee, hip and elbow.

The cause is unknown but it is thought that local ischaemia leads to fibrocartilaginous metaplasia and deposition of crystals by the chondrocytes. Calcification alone is probably not painful; symptoms, when they occur, are due to the florid vascular reaction which produces swelling and tension in the tendon. Resorption

of the calcific material is rapid and it may soften or disappear entirely within a few weeks.

Clinical features

The condition affects 30–50 year olds. Aching, sometimes following overuse, develops and increases in severity within hours, rising to an agonizing climax. After a few days, pain subsides and the shoulder gradually returns to normal. In some patients the process is less dramatic and recovery slower. During the acute stage the arm is held immobile; the joint is usually too tender to permit palpation or movement.

X-ray

Calcification is seen just above the greater tuberosity An initially well-demarcated deposit becomes more 'woolly' and then gradually disappears.

Treatment

If symptoms are not very severe the arm is rested in a sling and the patient is given a short course of non-steroidal anti-inflammatory medication. If pain is more intense a single injection of corticosteroid (methylprednisolone 40mg) and local anaesthetic (lignocaine 1%) is given into the hypervascular area. If this is not rapidly effective, or if symptoms soon recur, relief can be obtained by surgery; through a deltoid-splitting approach the calcific material is scooped out. The coracoacromial ligament is divided at the same time.

CHRONIC CALCIFICATION

Asymptomatic calcification of the rotator cuff is common and often appears as an incidental finding in

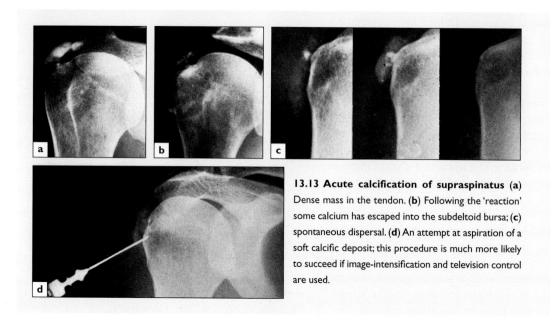

13.13 Acute calcification of supraspinatus (a)
Dense mass in the tendon. (**b**) Following the 'reaction'
some calcium has escaped into the subdeltoid bursa; (**c**)
spontaneous dispersal. (**d**) An attempt at aspiration of a
soft calcific deposit; this procedure is much more likely
to succeed if image-intensification and television control
are used.

shoulder x-rays. When it is seen in association with the impingement syndrome, it is tempting to attribute the symptoms to the only obvious abnormality – supraspinatus calcification. However, the connection is spurious and treatment should be directed at the impingement lesion rather than the calcification.

LESIONS OF THE BICEPS TENDON

TENDINITIS

Bicipital tendinitis usually occurs together with rotator cuff impingement; rarely, it presents as an isolated problem in young people after unaccustomed shoulder strain. Tenderness is sharply localized to the bicipital groove. Two manoeuvres that often cause pain are (1) resisted flexion with the elbow straight and the forearm supinated (Speed's test); and (2) resisted supination of the forearm with the elbow bent (Yergason's test).

Rest, local heat and deep transverse frictions usually bring relief. If recovery is delayed, a corticosteroid injection will help. For refractory cases, anterior acromioplasty is indicated.

RUPTURE

Rupture of the tendon of the long head of biceps usually accompanies rotator cuff disruption, but sometimes the biceps lesion is paramount. The patient is always aged over 50 years. While lifting he or she feels something snap in the shoulder and the upper arm becomes painful and bruised. Ask the patient to flex

the elbow: the detached belly of the biceps forms a prominent lump in the lower part of the arm.

Isolated tears in elderly patients need no treatment. However, if the rupture is part of a rotator cuff lesion – and especially if the patient is young and active – this is an indication for anterior acromioplasty; at the same time the distal tendon stump can be sutured to the bicipital groove. Postoperatively the arm is lightly splinted with the elbow flexed for 4 weeks.

(Avulsion of the distal attachment of the biceps is discussed in Chapter 14.)

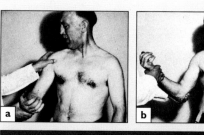

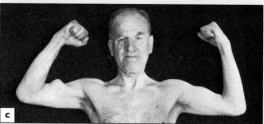

13.14 Biceps tendon *Tendinitis*: localized tenderness (**a**), and pain on flexion against resistance (**b**). (**c**) *Ruptured long head of right biceps*: compared with the normal side, the belly of biceps is lower and rounder.

SLAP LESIONS

Compressive loading of the shoulder in the flexed abducted position (e.g. in a fall on the outstretched hand) can damage the Superior Labrum Anteriorly and Posteriorly (SLAP). Patients complain of a painful 'click' on lifting the arm above shoulder height and loss of power when using the arm in that position. On examination these symptoms can be reproduced by abducting the patient's arm and turning it firmly into external rotation. The diagnosis is best confirmed by arthroscopic examination and at the same time the lesion is treated by debridement or repair. Postoperatively range of motion and muscle strengthening exercises are encouraged.

ADHESIVE CAPSULITIS (FROZEN SHOULDER)

The term 'frozen shoulder' should be reserved for a well-defined disorder characterized by progressive pain and stiffness of the shoulder which usually resolves spontaneously after about 18 months. The cause remains unknown. The histological features are reminiscent of Dupuytren's disease, with active fibroblastic proliferation in the rotator interval, anterior capsule and coracohumeral ligament (Bunker and Anthony, 1995). The condition is particularly associated with diabetes, Dupuytren's disease, hyperlipidaemia, hyperthyroidism, cardiac disease and hemiplegia. It occasionally appears after recovery from neurosurgery.

Clinical features

The patient, aged 40–60 years, may give a history of trauma, often trivial, followed by aching in the arm and shoulder. Pain gradually increases in severity and often prevents sleeping on the affected side. After several months it begins to subside, but as it does so stiffness becomes an increasing problem, continuing for another 6–12 months after pain has disappeared. Gradually movement is regained, but it may not return to normal and some pain may persist.

Apart from slight wasting, the shoulder looks quite normal; tenderness is seldom marked. The cardinal feature is a stubborn lack of active and passive movement in all directions.

X-rays are normal unless they show reduced bone density from disuse. Their main value is to exclude other causes of a painful, stiff shoulder.

Diagnosis

Not every stiff or painful shoulder is a frozen shoulder, and indeed there is some controversy over the criteria for diagnosing "frozen shoulder" (Zuckerman *et al.*, 1994). Stiffness occurs in a variety of conditions – arthritic, rheumatic, post-traumatic and postoperative. The diagnosis of frozen shoulder is clinical, resting on two characteristic features: (1) painful restriction of movement in the presence of normal x-rays, and (2) a natural progression through three successive phases.

When the patient is first seen, a number of conditions should be excluded: infection, post-traumatic stiffness, diffuse stiffness and reflex sympathetic dystrophy.

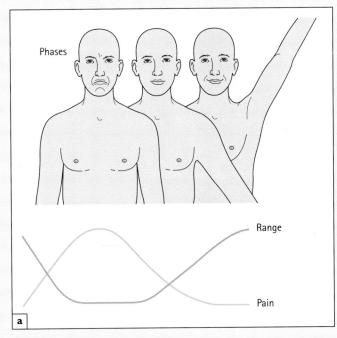
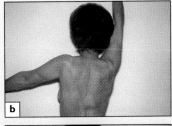
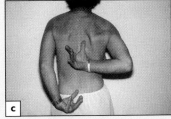

13.15 Frozen shoulder (a) Natural history of frozen shoulder. The face tells the story. (b, c) This patient has hardly any abduction but manages to lift her arm by moving the scapula. She cannot reach her back with her left hand.

INFECTION In patients with diabetes, it is particularly important to exclude infection. During the first day or two, signs of inflammation may be absent.

POST-TRAUMATIC STIFFNESS After any severe shoulder injury, stiffness may persist for some months. It is maximal at the start and gradually lessens, unlike the pattern of a frozen shoulder.

DIFFUSE STIFFNESS If the arm is nursed over-cautiously (e.g. following a forearm fracture) the shoulder may stiffen. Again, the characteristic pattern of a frozen shoulder is absent.

REFLEX SYMPATHETIC DYSTROPHY Shoulder pain and stiffness may follow myocardial infarction or a stroke. The features are similar to those of a frozen shoulder and it has been suggested that the latter is a form of reflex sympathetic dystrophy. In severe cases the whole upper limb is involved, with trophic and vasomotor changes in the hand (the 'shoulder–hand syndrome').

The painful shoulder

Referred pain syndromes	Rotator cuff disorders
Cervical spondylosis	Tendinitis
Mediastinal pathology	Rupture
Cardiac ischaemia	Frozen shoulder
Joint disorders	**Instability**
Glenohumeral arthritis	Dislocation
Acromioclavicular arthritis	Subluxation
Bone lesions	**Nerve injury**
Infection	Suprascapular nerve entrapment
Tumours	

Treatment

CONSERVATIVE TREATMENT

Conservative treatment aims to relieve pain and prevent further stiffening while recovery is awaited. It is important not only to administer analgesics and anti-inflammatory drugs but also to reassure the patient that recovery is certain.

Exercises are encouraged, the most valuable being 'pendulum' exercises in which the patient leans forward at the hips and moves his arm as if stirring a giant pudding (this is really a form of assisted active movement, the assistance being supplied by gravity). However, the patient is warned that moderation and regularity will achieve more than sporadic masochism. The role of physiotherapy is unproven and the benefits of steroid injection are debatable.

Once the acute pain has subsided, manipulation under general anaesthesia may improve the range of movement.

The shoulder is moved gently but firmly into external rotation, then abduction and flexion. Special care is needed in elderly, osteoporotic patients as there is a risk of fracturing the neck of the humerus. At the end, the joint is injected with methylprednisolone and lignocaine.

An alternative method of treatment is to distend the joint by injecting a large volume (50–200ml) of sterile saline under pressure. Arthroscopy has shown that both manipulation and distension achieve their effect by rupturing the capsule.

Postoperative pain can be controlled, if necessary, by an interscalene block. Active exercises are resumed as soon as comfort permits.

The results of conservative treatment are subjectively good, most patients eventually regaining painless and satisfactory function; however, examination is likely to show some residual restriction of movement (especially external rotation) in over 50% of cases (Schaffer *et al.*, 1992).

SURGICAL TREATMENT

Surgery does not have a well-defined role. The main indication is prolonged and disabling restriction of movement which fails to respond to conservative treat-

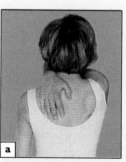
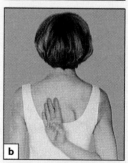
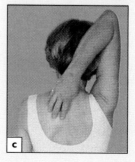

13.16 Shoulder pain – the scratch test 'Shoulder' pain may be due to disorders proximal to the joint (e.g. cervical spondylosis or cardiac ischaemia), disorders distal to the joint (e.g. arthritis of the elbow or carpal tunnel syndrome) or disorders of the shoulder itself (e.g. the rotator cuff syndromes, glenohumeral arthritis, acromioclavicular arthritis or bone disease). If the patient can scratch the opposite scapula in these three ways, the shoulder joint and its tendons are unlikely to be at fault.

ment. The rotator interval and coracohumeral ligament are released and the coracoacromial ligament is excised. This can be achieved arthroscopically, although for difficult cases open operation is safer (Warner, 1997).

INSTABILITY OF THE SHOULDER

The shoulder achieves its uniquely wide range of movement at the cost of stability. The humeral head is held in the shallow glenoid socket by the glenoid labrum, the glenohumeral ligaments, the coracohumeral ligament, the overhanging canopy of the coracoacromial arch and the surrounding muscles. Failure of any of these mechanisms may result in chronic instability of the joint. This can take the form of either recurrent *dislocation* or recurrent *subluxation*. In 95% of cases the displacement is anterior; in the remainder it is either *posterior* or *multidirectional.*

ANTERIOR INSTABILITY

Pathology

This is far and away the commonest type of instability, accounting for over 95% of cases. Traumatic anterior instability usually follows an acute injury in which the arm is forced into abduction, external rotation and extension. In *recurrent dislocation* the labrum and capsule are often detached from the anterior rim of the glenoid (the classic Bankart lesion). In addition there may be an indentation on the posterolateral aspect of the humeral head (the Hill–Sachs lesion), a compression fracture due to the humeral head being forced against the anterior glenoid rim each time it dislocates. In some cases *recurrent subluxation* may alternate with recurrent dislocation. In other cases the shoulder never dislocates completely and in these the labral tear and bone defect may be absent, although the inferior glenohumeral ligament will be stretched.

Clinical features

The patient is usually a young man who gives a history of his shoulder 'coming out', perhaps during a sporting event. The first episode of *acute dislocation* is a landmark and he may be able to describe the mechanism precisely: an applied force with the shoulder in abduction, external rotation and extension. The diagnosis may have been verified by x-ray and the injury treated by closed reduction and 'immobilization' in a bandage or sling for several weeks. This may be the first of many

similar episodes: *recurrent dislocation* requiring treatment develops in about one third of patients under the age of 30 years and in about 20% of older patients (Hovelius *et al.,* 1996). A greater proportion have instability without actual dislocation.

Recurrent subluxation is less obvious. The patient may describe a 'catching' sensation, followed by 'numbness' or 'weakness' – the so-called dead arm syndrome – whenever the shoulder is used with the arm in the overhead position (e.g. throwing a ball, serving at tennis or swimming). Pain with the arm in abduction may suggest a rotator cuff syndrome; it is as well to remember that recurrent subluxation may actually cause supraspinatus tendinitis.

On examination, between episodes of dislocation, the shoulder looks normal and movements are full. Clinical diagnosis rests on provoking subluxation. In the *apprehension test,* with the patient seated or lying, the examiner cautiously lifts the arm into abduction, external rotation and then extension; at the crucial moment the patient senses that the humeral head is about to slip out anteriorly and his body tautens in apprehension. The test should be repeated with the examiner applying pressure to the front of the shoulder; with this manoeuvre, the patient feels more secure and the apprehension sign is negative.

The same effect can be demonstrated by the *fulcrum test.* With the patient lying supine, arm abducted to 90°, the examiner places one hand behind the patient's shoulder to act as a fulcrum over which the humeral head is levered forward by extending and laterally rotating the arm; the patient immediately becomes apprehensive.

If instability is marked the *drawer test* may be positive. Again with the patient supine, the scapula is stabilized with one hand while the upper arm is grasped firmly with the other so as to manipulate the head of the humerus forwards and backwards (like a drawer).

Investigations

Most cases can be diagnosed from the history and examination alone. The Hill–Sachs lesion (when it is present) is best shown by an anteroposterior *x-ray* with the shoulder internally rotated, or in the axillary view. Subluxation is seen in the axillary view.

CT or *CT arthrography* is useful for demonstrating bone lesions and labral tears. *Arthroscopy* is sometimes needed to define the labral tear.

Examination under anaesthesia can help to determine the direction of instability.

Treatment

If dislocation recurs at long intervals, the patient may choose to tolerate the inconvenience and simply try to

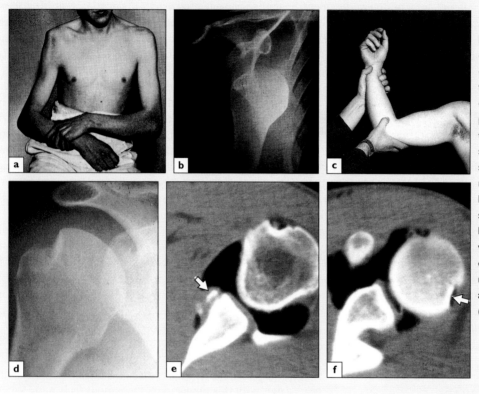

13.17 Anterior instability (a, b) Anterior dislocation of the shoulder. This may be followed by recurrent dislocation and (c) a positive 'apprehension test'. (d) The plain x-ray shows a large depression in the posterosuperior part of the humeral head (the Hill–Sachs sign). (e, f) MRI shows both a Bankart lesion, with a flake of bone detached from the anterior edge of the glenoid, and the Hill–Sachs lesion (arrows).

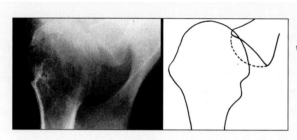

13.18 Recurrent subluxation X-ray showing anterior subluxation; the humeral head is riding on the lip of the glenoid.

avoid vulnerable positions of the shoulder. There is some evidence that dislocation predisposes to OA, although it is probably the initial dislocation rather than recurrence which causes this (Hovelius *et al.*, 1996).

OPERATIVE TREATMENT
The indications for operation are: (1) frequent dislocation, especially if this is painful, and (2) recurrent subluxation or a fear of dislocation sufficient to prevent participation in everyday activities, including sport.
    Operations are of four types:

- those that repair the torn glenoid labrum and capsule – the Bankart procedure (Gill *et al.*, 1997);
- those that shorten the anterior capsule and subscapularis by an overlapping repair (the Putti-Platt operation);
- those that reinforce the antero-inferior capsule by redirecting other muscles across the front of the joint (e.g. the Bristow–Laterjet operation); and

- bone operations: correction of a reduced retroversion angle of the humeral head by osteotomy has been recommended (Kronberg and Brostrum, 1995).

If the labrum and anterior capsule are detached, and there is no marked joint laxity, the Bankart operation combined with anterior capsulorrhaphy is the procedure of choice. The joint is exposed by the deltopectoral approach, the labrum is re-attached to the glenoid rim with suture anchors or drill holes and, if necessary, the capsule is tightened by an overlapping tuck without shortening the subscapularis. The Putti-Platt operation, in which the subscapularis is overlapped and shortened, also gives good results but at the cost of significant loss of external rotation. The Bristow–Laterjet operation, in which the coracoid process with its attached muscles is transposed to the front of the neck of the scapula, gives less loss of external rotation (Singer *et al.*, 1995). Arthroscopic techniques are being developed, but are not as reliable as open procedures and their precise indication needs further definition.

POSTERIOR INSTABILITY

Pathology

This condition is usually due to a violent jerk in an unusual position or following an epileptic fit or a severe electric shock. Dislocation may be associated with fractures of the proximal humerus. The posterior capsule is stripped from the bone or stretched, and there may be an indentation on the anterior aspect of the humeral head. Recurrent instability is almost always a *posterior subluxation* with the humeral head riding back on the posterior lip of the glenoid.

Clinical features

Acute posterior dislocation is rare, and when it does occur it is often missed. There may be a history of fairly violent injury or an electric shock. On examination the arm is held in internal rotation and attempts at external rotation are resisted. The anteroposterior x-ray may show a typical 'light-bulb' appearance of the proximal humerus (the humeral head looks symmetrically bulbous because the shoulder is internally rotated). If the arm can be abducted, an axillary view will show the dislocation quite clearly.

Recurrent posterior instability usually takes the form of subluxation when the arm is used in flexion and internal rotation. On examination, the posterior drawer test (scapular spine and coracoid process in one hand, humeral head pushed backwards with the other) and posterior apprehension test (forward flexion and internal rotation of the shoulder with a posterior force on the elbow) confirm the diagnosis.

Treatment

Recurrent posterior subluxation can usually be treated conservatively, by encouraging muscle strengthening exercises and teaching the patient how to control the position of the shoulder. The results of operative treatment are less predictable than in anterior instability; recurrence of up to 50% can occur.

Surgery should be considered only if (1) the condition is genuinely disabling, (2) there is no gross joint laxity and (3) the patient is emotionally well adjusted. Posterior capsular reconstruction can be augmented by a posterior bone block; postoperatively the shoulder is held abducted and externally rotated in a spica for 6 weeks. If there is excessive glenoid retroversion (shown on CT scan) then glenoid osteotomy should be considered.

MULTIDIRECTIONAL INSTABILITY

Pathology

This condition is associated with capsular and ligamentous laxity, and sometimes with weakness of the shoulder muscles.

Clinical features

Little force is required to displace the joint and it may subluxate even with mildly stressful daily activities. Sometimes anterior or posterior instability changes gradually to inferior and then multidirectional instability (Neer and Foster, 1980). The condition is difficult to diagnose with certainty, but is suggested when both anterior and posterior drawer tests and the apprehension tests are positive, often with joint laxity elsewhere.

Treatment

Muscle strengthening exercises and training in joint control are helpful. Surgical treatment (a capsular shift procedure) is seldom indicated.

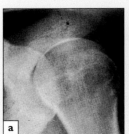 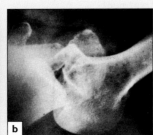 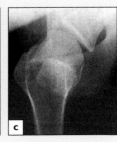

13.19 Posterior instability (a) In the anteroposterior view the humeral head looks globular but may mistakenly be called normal. (b) The lateral view shows the obvious subluxation with impaction of the humeral head; (c) the defect in the anterior part of the head.

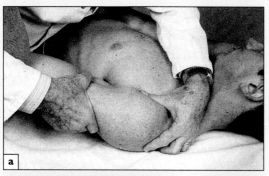

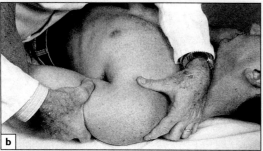

13.20 Multidirectional instability (a) The anterior and (b) the posterior drawer tests are best performed with the patient lying supine. The amount of movement is compared with that on the unaffected side.

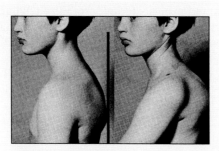

13.21 Habitual subluxation The clue is the unconcerned expression.

ATRAUMATIC DISLOCATION OR SUBLUXATION

Dislocation can occur more or less spontaneously if there are congenital anatomical abnormalities or severe ligamentous laxity. The patient *can voluntarily subluxate* or dislocate the shoulder painlessly, and can just as easily reduce it again; emotionally disturbed people may find the temptation to do so irresistible. Sometimes displacement occurs so frequently as to justify the term *habitual*. Treatment is supportive and surgery should be avoided.

INFERIOR SUBLUXATION

Routine x-ray examination of the shoulder some weeks after an injury may show that the head of the humerus has subluxated inferiorly. This looks worse than it really is! The condition is due to weakness of the shoulder muscles and it eventually corrects itself.

DISORDERS OF THE GLENOHUMERAL JOINT

TUBERCULOSIS

Tuberculosis (see also Chapter 2) of the shoulder is uncommon. It usually starts as an osteitis but is rarely diagnosed until arthritis has supervened. This may proceed to abscess and sinus formation, but in some cases the tendency is to fibrosis and ankylosis. If there is no exudate the term 'caries sicca' is used; however, one suspects that many such cases, formerly diagnosed on the basis of coexisting pulmonary tuberculosis rather than joint biopsy or bacteriological examination, are actually examples of frozen shoulder.

Clinical features

Adults are affected mainly. They complain of a constant ache and stiffness lasting many months or years. The striking feature is wasting of the muscles around the shoulder, especially the deltoid. In neglected cases a sinus may be present over the shoulder or in the axilla. There is diffuse warmth and tenderness and all movements are limited and painful. Axillary lymph nodes may be enlarged.

X-rays show generalized rarefaction, usually with some erosion of the joint surfaces. There may be abscess cavities in the humerus or glenoid, with little or no periosteal reaction.

Treatment

In addition to systemic treatment with antituberculous drugs, the shoulder should be rested until acute symptoms have settled. Thereafter movement is encouraged and, provided the articular cartilage is not destroyed, the prognosis for painless function is good. If there are repeated flares, or if the articular surfaces are extensively destroyed, the joint should be arthrodesed.

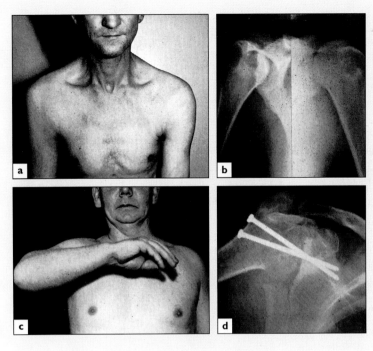

13.22 Tuberculosis (**a**) Marked wasting of right deltoid. (**b**) Bone rarefaction and joint damage in arthritis, compared with the normal. (**c**, **d**) After arthrodesis of the glenohumeral joint scapulothoracic movement remains, permitting useful abduction.

RHEUMATOID ARTHRITIS

Rheumatoid arthritis (see also Chapter 3) is the most common arthropathy to affect the shoulder complex; 90% of patients with rheumatoid arthritis have involvement of the acromioclavicular joint, the shoulder joint and the various synovial pouches around the shoulder.

The acromioclavicular joint develops an erosive arthritis which may go on to capsular disruption and instability. This is sometimes the first site to be diagnosed from routine x-rays of the chest.

The glenohumeral joint, with its lax capsule and folds of synovium, shows marked soft-tissue inflammation. Often there is an accumulation of fluid and fibrinoid particles which may rupture the capsule and extrude into the muscle planes. Cartilage destruction and bone erosion are often severe.

The subacromial bursa and the synovial sheath of the long head of biceps become inflamed and thickened; often this leads to rupture of the rotator cuff and the biceps tendon.

Clinical features

The patient may be known to have generalized rheumatoid arthritis; occasionally, however, acromioclavicular erosion discovered on an x-ray of the chest is the first clue to the diagnosis.

Pain and swelling are the usual presenting symptoms; the patient (usually a woman) has increasing difficulty with simple tasks such as combing her hair or washing her back. Though it may start on one side, the condition usually becomes bilateral.

Synovitis of the joint results in swelling and tenderness anteriorly, superiorly or in the axilla. *Tenosynovitis* produces features similar to those of cuff lesions, including tears of supraspinatus or biceps. Joint and tendon lesions usually occur together and conspire to cause the marked weakness and limitation of movement that are features of the disease.

X-rays

The usual picture is of an erosive arthritis affecting the articular surfaces of both the humeral head and the glenoid fossa.

Treatment

The general treatment of rheumatoid arthritis is discussed in Chapter 3. In the early stages, local treatment in the form of intra-articular injections of methylprednisolone may be needed.

If synovitis persists, operative synovectomy is carried out; at the same time, cuff tears may be repaired. Excision of the lateral end of the clavicle may relieve acromioclavicular pain.

In advanced cases pain and stiffness can be very disabling. Provided the rotator cuff is not completely destroyed and there is still adequate bone stock, joint replacement with an unconstrained prosthesis may be

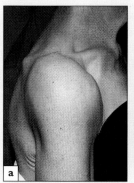
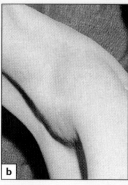
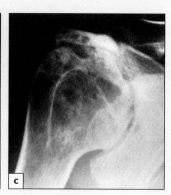

13.23 Rheumatoid arthritis (a) Large synovial effusions cause easily visible swelling; small ones are likely to be missed – especially if they present, like this one (b), in the axilla. (c) X-rays show erosion of the joint and of the periarticular bone.

carried out. This operation provides good pain relief, moderate shoulder function and reasonable durability (Stewart and Kelly, 1997). Even if movement is poor, at least it is relatively painless.

If the rotator cuff is destroyed, or bone erosion very advanced, arthrodesis may be preferable; despite its apparent limitations, it gives improved function because scapulothoracic movement is usually undisturbed.

OSTEOARTHRITIS

OA of the glenohumeral joint is more common than is generally recognized. It is usually secondary to local trauma, recurrent subluxation or long-standing rotator cuff lesions. Often chondrocalcinosis is present as well but it is not known whether this predisposes to OA or appears as a sequel to joint degradation.

Clinical features

The patient is usually aged 50–60 years and may give a history of injury, shoulder dislocation or a previous painful arc syndrome. There is usually little to see but shoulder movements are restricted in all directions.

X-rays show distortion of the joint, bone sclerosis and osteophyte formation; the articular 'space' may be narrowed or may show calcification.

Treatment

Analgesics and anti-inflammatory drugs relieve pain, and exercises may improve mobility. Most patients manage to live with the restrictions imposed by stiffness, provided pain is not severe. However, if both shoulders are involved then the disability can be severe.

In advanced cases, if pain becomes intolerable shoulder arthroplasty is justified. It may not improve

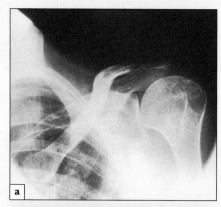
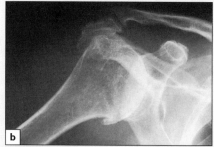
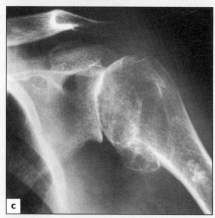

13.24 Osteoarthritis of the shoulder (a) Upward shift of the humeral head due to cuff disruption. (b) Osteoarthritis of both the shoulder and the acromioclavicular joints. (c) Advanced osteoarthritis; this patient had hardly any shoulder movement.

mobility much, but it does relieve pain. The alternative is arthrodesis.

RAPIDLY DESTRUCTIVE ARTHROPATHY (MILWAUKEE SHOULDER)

Occasionally, in the presence of long-standing or massive cuff tears, patients develop a rapidly progressive and destructive form of OA in which there is severe erosion of the glenohumeral joint, the acromion process and the acromioclavicular joint – what Neer *et al.* (1983) called a *cuff tear arthropathy*. The changes are now attributed to hydroxyapatite crystal shedding from the torn rotator cuff and a synovial reaction involving the release of lysosomal enzymes (including collagenases) which lead to cartilage breakdown (McCarty *et al.*, 1981). A similar condition is seen in other joints such as the hip and knee.

Clinical features

The patient is usually aged over 60 years and may have suffered with shoulder pain for many years. Over a period of a few months the shoulder becomes swollen and increasingly unstable. On examination there is marked crepitus in the joint and loss of active movements.

X-rays show severe erosion of the articular surfaces, subluxation of the joint and calcification in the soft tissues.

Treatment

There is no satisfactory treatment for this condition. Resurfacing arthroplasty may relieve pain but will not improve function, because the rotator cuff is disrupted and the joint is unstable.

OSTEONECROSIS

The shoulder is the second most common site of corticosteroid-induced osteonecrosis. The condition may also be seen in association with marrow storage disorders, sickle-cell disease and caisson disease, or following irradiation of the axilla.

The clinical features and diagnosis are discussed in Chapter 6. Articular collapse occurs more slowly than in weightbearing joints and operative treatment can usually be delayed for several years. If this should become necessary, joint replacement is the method of choice.

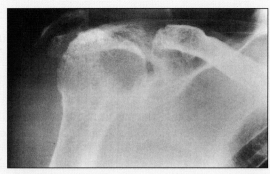

13.25 Milwaukee shoulder X-ray showing a destructive arthropathy with marked swelling and calcification in the soft tissues around the shoulder.

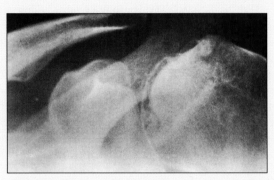

13.26 Osteonecrosis A young woman with systemic lupus erythematosus was treated with large doses of prednisolone. She developed pain in one hip and one shoulder. X-ray of the shoulder shows the classic features of osteonecrosis, including a long subarticular fracture of the humeral head.

DISORDERS OF THE SCAPULA AND CLAVICLE

CONGENITAL ELEVATION OF THE SCAPULA

The scapulae normally complete their descent from the neck by the third month of fetal life; occasionally one or both scapulae remain incompletely descended. Associated abnormalities of the cervical spine are common and sometimes there is a family history of scapular deformity.

Clinical features

Two similar, and possibly related, conditions are encountered.

SPRENGEL'S DEFORMITY Deformity is the only symptom and it may be noticed at birth. The shoulder on the affected side is elevated; the scapula looks and feels abnormally high, smaller than usual and somewhat prominent; occasionally both scapulae are affected. The neck appears shorter than usual and there may be kyphosis or scoliosis of the upper thoracic spine. Shoulder movements are painless but abduction and elevation may be limited by fixation of the scapula. *X-rays* will show the elevated scapula and any associated vertebral anomalies; sometimes there is also a bony bridge between the scapula and the cervical spine (the omovertebral bar).

KLIPPEL–FEIL SYNDROME This is usually a more widespread disorder. There is bilateral failure of scapular descent associated with marked anomalies of the cervical spine and failure of fusion of the occipital bones. Patients look as if they have no neck; there is a low hairline, bilateral neck webbing and gross limitation of neck movement. This condition should not be confused with *bilateral shortness of the sternomastoid muscle* in which the head is poked forward and the chin thrust up; the absence of associated congenital lesions is a further distinguishing feature.

Treatment

Mild cases are best left untreated. Surgical treatment aims to decrease deformity and improve shoulder function. In children under 6 years of age, the scapula can be repositioned by releasing the muscles along the vertebral and superior borders of the scapula, excising the supraspinous portion of the scapula and the omovertebral bar, pulling the scapula down, then reattaching the muscles to hold it firmly in its new position. In older children this carries a risk of brachial nerve compression or traction between the clavicle and first rib; here it is safer merely to excise the supraspinous portion of the scapula in order to improve the appearance but without improving movement. Before undertaking any operation the cervical spine should be carefully imaged in order to identify any abnormalities of the odontoid process or base of skull.

CLEIDOCRANIAL DYSOSTOSIS

This is a heritable disorder (autosomal dominant) characterized by hypoplasia or aplasia of the clavicles and flat bones (pelvis, scapulae and skull). Those affected have a typical appearance, with drooping shoulders, an usually narrow chest and the ability to bring the shoulders together across the front of the chest.

X-rays show hypoplasia or complete absence of the clavicles, and sometimes also of the scapulae. Other skeletal defects, which occur in varying degree, are delayed closure of the fontanelles, brachycephaly, underdevelment of the pelvis, coxa vara and scoliosis.

Treatment is usually unnecessary and, despite the widespread defects, patients enjoy good function.

CONGENITAL PSEUDARTHROSIS OF THE CLAVICLE

The typical clinical picture is that of a child with a painless lump in the mid-shaft of the clavicle. This always occurs on the right side, except in the presence of dextrocardia. X-ray shows the break in the clavicle, which usually heals only after excision of the 'non-union' and bone grafting.

SCAPULAR INSTABILITY

Winging of the scapula causes asymmetry of the shoulders, but the deformity may not be obvious until the patient tries to contract the serratus anterior against resistance.

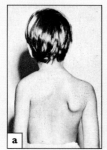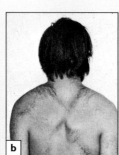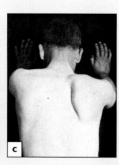

13.27 Scapular disorders (**a**) Sprengel shoulder; (**b**) Klippel–Feil syndrome; (**c**) winged scapula.

Weakness or paralysis of the serratus anterior may arise from:

- neuralgic amyotrophy (see page 225)
- injury to the brachial plexus (a blow to the top of the shoulder, severe traction on the arm or carrying heavy loads on the shoulder)
- direct damage to the long thoracic nerve (e.g. during radical mastectomy)
- fascioscapulohumeral muscular dystrophy.

Disability is usually slight and is best accepted. However, if function is noticeably impaired, it is possible to stabilize the scapula by transferring the sternal portion of pectoralis major and attaching it via a fascia lata graft to the lower pole of the scapula; or the scapula can be fixed to the rib cage to provide the deltoid and the rotator cuff muscles with a stable base from which to control the shoulder.

A less obvious, but sometimes more disabling, form of scapular instability may follow *injury to the spinal accessory nerve* (e.g. following operations in the posterior triangle of the neck). The trapezius muscle is an important stabilizer of the shoulder and loss of this function results in weakness and pain on active abduction against resistance. Early recognition may permit nerve repair or grafting.

GRATING SCAPULA

The patient complains of grating or clicking on moving the arm. It is painless but annoying. Usually no cause is found, though bony, muscular and bursal abnormalities have been blamed. Tangential x-ray views of the scapula should be obtained to exclude an osteochondroma on the undersurface of the scapula; if present, the lesion can be excised. Otherwise no treatment is necessary.

SEPTIC ARTHRITIS OF THE STERNOCLAVICULAR JOINT

This condition is rare except in drug abusers following intravenous injections, and as a secondary complication of sternoclavicular haemarthrosis following trauma. Local signs may be misleadingly mild but persistent pain, swelling and tenderness associated with systemic signs of infection should arouse suspicion. X-rays are usually normal until fairly late when they may show erosion of the sternoclavicular joint and the adjacent bone. Treatment is by antibiotics and local drainage of infected material.

STERNOCLAVICULAR HYPEROSTOSIS

Several individually uncommon disorders are associated with pain and swelling over the clavicle or the sternoclavicular joint. They are often confused, though certain characteristic features permit appropriate differentiation in the majority of cases.

CONDENSING OSTEITIS OF THE CLAVICLE

This is usually seen in women of 20–40 years who present with pain at the medial end of the clavicle, which is aggravated by abducting the arm. The clavicle may be thickened and tender. X-rays reveal sclerosis and radionuclide scanning shows increased activity in the affected bone (Cone *et al.*, 1983). The condition may be no more than a reaction to the mechanical stress of excessive lifting activities, and treatment consists simply of avoiding such activities. Of greater importance is the need to distinguish it from the other hyperostotic disorders.

STERNOCOSTOCLAVICULAR HYPEROSTOSIS

This condition in some ways resembles condensing osteitis, but it is seen in slightly older people (both men and women) and is usually bilateral. Patients develop pain, swelling and tenderness over the sternoclavicular region and x-rays show hyperostosis of the medial ends of the clavicles, the adjacent sternum, the anterior ends of the upper ribs and the soft tissues in between. Vertebrae also may be affected and the erythrocyte sedimentation rate may be increased; little wonder that it has been suggested that this is a type of seronegative spondarthropathy. Biopsy is of little help; the histological changes are non-specific and microorganisms have not been identified. A peculiarity which links this condition with the next is an association with pustular lesions on the palms and soles (palmo-plantar pustulosis) and pustular psoriasis (see also page 34).

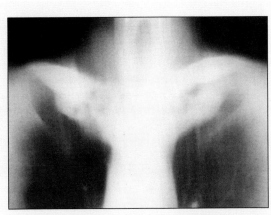

13.28 Sternoclavicular hyperostosis Tomogram showing irregularity and hyperostosis of the sternoclavicular joint.

Multifocal osteomyelitis usually occurs in children and adolescents; the clavicle and lower limb metaphyses are sites of predilection. It may present as a painful, fusiform swelling of the clavicle and x-rays show thickening and sclerosis of the medial third of the bone. Like sternocostoclavicular hyperostosis, it is sometimes associated with palmo-plantar pustulosis. The diagnosis is strongly suggested if pustulosis is present, otherwise it usually emerges gradually as other sites become affected over the course of the next year or two and x-rays show the typical lytic areas in the metaphyses and/or epiphyses close to the physis. The full-blown picture is well described in the paper by Carr *et al.* (1993). There is no effective treatment; the lesions almost invariably heal spontaneously over a period of months or years, the only trace of the condition being the thickened bone ends.

OSTEOARTHRITIS OF THE ACROMIOCLAVICULAR JOINT

OA of the acromioclavicular joint is common in middle-aged and older people. Predisposing factors are trauma (subluxation of the joint) and occupational stress (habitually carrying weights on the shoulder or working with pneumatic hammers and drills), but the condition also occurs in the absence of any suggestive history. The patient may complain of 'shoulder pain', but if you ask him or her to point, your attention is directed to the prominent bump at the outer end of the clavicle; tenderness is sharply localized to this area. Shoulder movements are usually not restricted (unless the shoulder joint itself is involved), but there may be pain at the extremes of abduction and flexion.

X-ray shows the characteristic features of OA; the changes are often bilateral, even though only one side may be hurting. In some cases the condition is discovered while examining the patient for an impingement syndrome; indeed, acromioclavicular OA may *cause* impingement.

Treatment If analgesics or corticosteroid injections are ineffectual, pain may be relieved by excision of the lateral end of the clavicle. This procedure can now be performed arthroscopically. Trimming of the bony roughness, or excision of the outer end of the clavicle, may also be needed during subacromial decompression for rotator cuff impingement.

OPERATIONS

Rotator cuff surgery and shoulder stabilization are described in the relevant sections.

ARTHROSCOPY

Arthroscopy is a useful technique for the *diagnosis* of peri-articular and intra-articular disorders, such as rotator cuff disruption and instability. At the same time a *biopsy* can be taken which may assist in the diagnosis of synovial disorders such as rheumatoid arthritis or pigmented villonoduar synovitis.

Arthroscopic surgery is now well-established, particularly for subacromial decompression, debridement of rotator cuff tears and release of frozen shoulder. Arthroscopic repair of Bankart lesions is more difficult and needs further development.

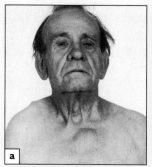 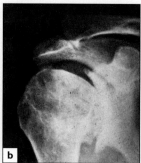 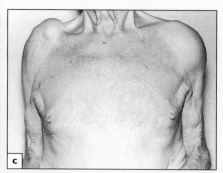

13.29 Osteoarthritis of the acromioclavicular joint (**a, b**) This elderly man has osteoarthritis of both the acromioclavicular and the right shoulder joint. Osteophytic thickening of the acromioclavicular joint has produced a small (but very tender) bump on top of the shoulder. (**b**) Occasionally the joint capsule herniates, producing a large 'cyst' over the acromioclavicular joint.

ARTHROPLASTY OF THE SHOULDER

Since the introduction of unconstrained implants, the results of shoulder replacement have steadily improved. With modern methods, 85–95% of patients are relieved of pain and regain adequate function for 5 years or longer; however, the range of movement is seldom better than 50 or 60% of normal.

Indications The indications for arthroplasty are: (1) chronic arthritis causing pain and loss of movement; (2) severe joint injury; (3) complex fractures of the proximal humerus; (4) destructive lesions of the humeral head; and (5) tumours of the proximal humerus.

Operative problems Glenoid replacement is not always advisable. This is technically difficult and complications often arise. There is minimal cancellous bone for fixation, especially in rheumatoid arthritis. Good results can be achieved in many patients with a humeral implant alone. If glenoid replacement is thought necessary, then a metal-backed polyethylene surface fixed with methylmethacrylate cement is probably the best option.

Complications The commonest, in order of frequency, are loosening of the components, glenohumeral instability, rotator cuff failure, peri-prosthetic fracture, infection and implant failure. Glenoid fixation remains a challenge; lucent lines around the glenoid component are very common, although not always symptomatic (Wirth and Rockwood, 1996).

Outcome This depends largely on the indications for surgery. Arthroplasty for fractures, avascular necrosis or proximal humeral tumours gives good pain relief and shoulder movement, although power is always diminished. Where there is more extensive joint destruction and disruption of the soft tissues (e.g. in rheumatoid arthritis), pain relief is still excellent but the range of movement is only moderately improved. The greater the integrity of the surrounding soft tissues (and especially the rotator cuff), the more stable will the new joint be, and thus the better the outcome of the operation. In severe cuff failure, constrained arthroplasty or arthrodesis should be considered.

ARTHRODESIS

Arthrodesis of the glenohumeral joint is now seldom performed, but it is still a useful operation for severe shoulder dysfunction.

Indications The indications for shoulder arthrodesis are: (1) paralysis of the scapulohumeral muscles; (2) infective disorders of the glenohumeral joint (including tuberculous arthritis); and (3) advanced erosive arthritis with massive disruption of the rotator cuff.

The operation A prerequisite is stable and powerful scapulothoracic movement, because with a fused shoulder 'movement' is achieved entirely by rotation of the scapula on the thorax.

Through a posterior incision the joint is disarticulated, the surfaces are rawed, then fixed together by a heavy nail, screws or a plate. The acromion is osteotomized and hinged into a bed chiselled out of the humerus. The shoulder is held in a plaster spica for 3–6 months. The optimal position is controversial. The position should be tailored for the patient's needs and with consideration of restriction in other joints of the limb.

Outcome Despite the restriction of glenohumeral movement, postoperative function is surprisingly good – and painless.

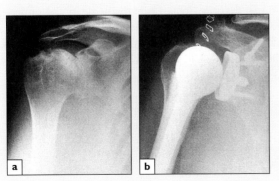

13.30 Arthroplasty X-ray appearances before and after total joint replacement.

NOTES ON APPLIED ANATOMY

JOINTS

The anatomy of the shoulder is uniquely adapted to allow freedom of movement and maximum reach for the hand. Five 'articulations' are involved:

- the glenohumeral joint
- the pseudojoint between the humerus and the coracoacromial arch
- the sternoclavicular joint
- the acromioclavicular joint
- the scapulothoracic articulation.

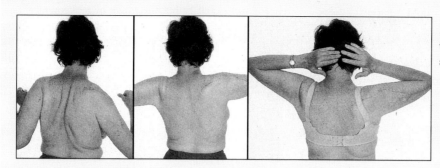

13.31 Arthrodesis The useful function after a successful arthrodesis.

STABILITY

The shallow glenohumeral articulation has little inherent stability because the glenoid surface area is only one-quarter that of the humeral articular surface. The extent to which the socket is deepened by the labrum may seem trivial, but it must be significant because labral tears are associated with dislocation. Stability depends mainly on the integrity of the ligaments and capsule. The muscles provide kinetic stability: during abduction the rotator cuff muscles draw the head of the humerus firmly into its socket while the deltoid elevates the arm.

ROTATOR CUFF

The rotator cuff is a sheet of conjoint tendons closely applied over the top of the shoulder capsule and inserting into the greater tuberosity of the humerus. It is made up of subscapularis in front, supraspinatus above and infraspinatus and teres minor behind. The 'rotator' muscles have an important function in stabilizing the head of the humerus by pulling it firmly into the glenoid whenever the deltoid lifts the arm forwards or sideways. The rotator interval lies between the supraspinatus and infraspinatus tendons.

Arching over the cuff is a fibro-osseous canopy – the coracoacromial arch – formed by the acromion process postero-superiorly, the coracoid process anteriorly and the coracoacromial ligament joining them. Separating the tendons from the arch, and allowing them to glide, is the subacromial bursa. Of the four cuff tendons, the supraspinatus is the most exposed; it runs over the top of the shoulder under the anterior edge of the acromion and the adjacent acromioclavicular joint, with the intra-articular portion of the biceps tendon closely applied to its deep surface.

MOVEMENT

Abduction and flexion of the shoulder look simple; in fact they are very complex movements involving all the joints of the shoulder girdle. Imagine what would happen if the deltoid muscle acted alone in abducting the shoulder. Because of the relatively unstable fulcrum, the deltoid would simply shrug the arm upwards at the side of the body. In reality, the rotator cuff muscles, particularly the supraspinatus, draw the head of the humerus firmly into the socket and slightly downwards, thus allowing the deltoid to act as a true abductor.

The first 30° of abduction occurs almost entirely at the glenohumeral joint with slight movement of the clavicle at the sternoclavicular joint. From 30 to 90° of abduction the scapula gradually comes into play, with about one-third of the movement coming from the scapula rotating on the thorax. From 90 to 180°, the movement is mainly scapulothoracic and for this reason it is termed 'elevation' rather than 'abduction'. As the arm rises above shoulder height, it rolls into external rotation so that the greater tuberosity clears the projecting acromion. The sternoclavicular joint participates in movements close to the trunk (e.g. shrugging or bracing the shoulders); the acromioclavicular joint moves in the last 60° of abduction.

REFERENCES AND FURTHER READING

Bigliani LV, Levine WN (1997) Subacromial impingement syndrome. *Journal of Bone and Joint Surgery* **79**A, 1854-1868

Bunker T, Anthony PP (1995) The pathology of frozen shoulder. *Journal of Bone and Joint Surgery* **77**B, 677–683

Carr AJ, Cole WG, Roberton DM, Chow CW (1993) Chronic multifocal osteomyelitis. *Journal of Bone and Joint Surgery* **75**B, 582-591

Cone RD, Resnick D, Goergen TG *et al* (1983) Condensing osteitis of the clavicle. *American Journal of Roentgenology* **141**, 387-388

Gartsman GM (1995) Arthroscopic treatment of rotator cuff disease. *Journal of Shoulder and Elbow Surgery* **4**, 228-241

Gartsman GM (1997) Combined arthroscopic and open treatment of tears of the rotator cuff. *Journal of Bone and Joint Surgery* **79**A, 776-783

Gill TJ, Micheli LJ, Geghard F, Binder C (1997) Bankart repair for anterior instability of the shoulder. *Journal of Bone and Joint Surgery* **79**A, 850-857

Hertzog R (1997) Magnetic resonance imaging of the shoulder. *Journal of Bone and Joint Surgery* **79**A, 934-953

Hovelius L, Augustini BG, Fredin OH *et al* (1996) Primary anterior dislocation of the shoulder in young patients. *Journal of Bone and Joint Surgery* **78**A, 1677-1684

Ianotti JP (1994) Full thickness rotator cuff tears: factors affecting surgical outcome. *Journal of the American Academy of Orthopaedic Surgeons* **2**, 87-95

Kronberg M, Brostrum L-A (1995) Rotation osteotomy of the proximal humerus to stabilise the shoulder. *Journal of Bone and Joint Surgery* **77**B, 924-927

McCarty DJ, Halverson PB, Carrera GF *et al.* (1981) Milwaukee shoulder: association of microspheroids containing hydroxyapatite crystals, active collagenase and neutral protease with rotator cuff defects. *Arthritis and Rheumatism* **24**, 464-473

Neer CS (1972) Anterior acromioplasty for the chronic impingement syndrome in the shoulder. *Journal of Bone and Joint Surgery* **54**A, 41-50

Neer CS, Foster CR (1980) Inferior capsular shift for involuntary inferior and multidirectional instability of the shoulder. A preliminary report. *Journal of Bone and Joint Surgery* **62**A, 897-908

Neer CS, Craig EV, Fukuda HF (1983) Cuff tear arthropathy. *Journal of Bone and Joint Surgery* **65**A, 1232-1244

Nutton RW, McBirnie JM, Phillips C (1997) Treatment of chronic rotator cuff impingement by arthroscopic subacromial decompression. *Journal of Bone and Joint Surgery* **79**B, 73-76

Recht MP, Resnick D (1993) Magnetic resonance-imaging studies of the shoulder. *Journal of Bone and Joint Surgery* **75**A, 1244-1253

Rockwood CA, Lyons FR (1993) Shoulder impingement syndrome: diagnosis, radiographic evaluation and treatment with a modified Neer acromioplasty. *Journal of Bone and Joint Surgery* **75**A, 409-424

Rockwood CA, Williams GR, Burkhead WZ (1995) Debridement of degenerative, irreparable lesions of the rotator cuff. *Journal of Bone and Joint Surgery* **77**A, 857-866

Sachs RA, Stone ML, Devine S (1994) Open versus arthroscopic acromioplasty – a prospective randomised study. *Arthroscopy* **10**, 248-254

Shaffer B, Tibone JE, Kerlan RK (1992) Frozen shoulder. A long term follow-up. *Journal of Bone and Joint Surgery* **74**A, 738-746

Sher JS, Urbie JW, Posada A *et al* (1995) Abnormal findings on MRI of asymptomatic shoulders. *Journal of Bone and Joint Surgery* **77**A, 10-15

Singer GC, Kirkland PM, Emery RJH (1995) Coracoid transposition for recurrent anterior dislocation of the shoulder. *Journal of Bone and Joint Surgery* **77**B, 73-76

Stewart MPM, Kelly IG (1997) Total shoulder replacement in rheumatoid disease. *Journal of Bone and Joint Surgery* **79**B, 68-72

Warner JJP (1997) Frozen shoulder: diagnosis and management. *Journal of the American Academy of Orthopaedic Surgeons* **5**, 130-140

Wirth MA, Rockwood CA (1996) Complications of total shoulder replacement arthroplasty. *Journal of Bone and Joint Surgery* **78**A, 603-616

Zuckerman JD, Cuomo F, Rokito S (1994) Definition and classification of frozen shoulder – a consensus approach. *Journal of Shoulder and Elbow Surgery* **3**, S72

CLINICAL ASSESSMENT

SYMPTOMS

Pain from the elbow is fairly diffuse and may extend into the forearm. Localized pain over the lateral or medial epicondyle of the humerus is usually due to tendinitis. Remember that the elbow is a common site of referred pain from the cervical spine.

Stiffness, if it is mild, may hardly be noticed. If it is severe, it can be very disabling; the patient may be unable to reach up to the mouth (loss of flexion) or the perineum (loss of extension); limited supination makes it difficult to carry large objects.

Swelling may be due to injury or inflammation; a soft lump on the back of the elbow suggests an olecranon bursitis.

Deformity is uncommon except in rheumatoid arthritis and after trauma. Always ask about previous injuries.

Instability – the feeling that the elbow 'moves out of joint – is due either to previous trauma or to destructive joint disease.

Ulnar nerve symptoms (tingling, numbness and weakness of the hand) may occur in elbow disorders because of the nerve's proximity to the joint.

Loss of function is noticed mainly in grooming, carrying and placing activities.

SIGNS

Both upper limbs should be completely exposed, and is is essential to look at the back of the elbow as well as the front. Often the neck, shoulders and hands also need to be examined.

Look

With both upper limbs completely exposed, the patient holds his or her arms alongside the body with palms forwards. Varus or valgus deformity is then obvious, but it cannot be accurately assessed unless the elbow extends fully. The patient then holds his or her arms out sideways at right angles to the body with palms upwards and elbows straight. In this position, wasting or lumps are easily seen.

Feel

The back of the joint is palpated for warmth, subcutaneous nodules, synovial thickening and fluid (fluctuation on each side of the olecranon); the back and sides are felt for tenderness and to determine whether the bony points are correctly placed.

The joint line can be located laterally by feeling for the head of the radius (pronating and supinating the

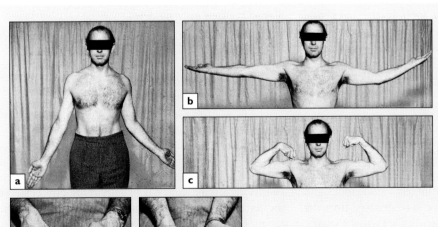

14.1 Examination The signs demonstrated are of osteoarthritis in the left elbow: (**a**) valgus deformity, (**b**) limited extension, (**c**) limited flexion, (**d, e**) limited pronation and supination.

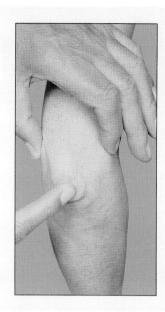

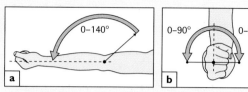

forearm makes this easier), but medially it is difficult to find.

The ulnar nerve is fairly superficial behind the medial condyle and here it can be rolled under the fingers to feel if it is thickened or hypersensitive.

Move

Flexion and extension are compared on the two sides. Then, with the elbows tucked into the sides and flexed to a right angle, the radioulnar joints are tested for pronation and supination.

GENERAL EXAMINATION

Clinical examination should include the neck and shoulder (which are sources of referred pain to the elbow) and the hand (for signs of nerve dysfunction).

X-RAY

The position of each bone is noted, then the joint line and space. Next, the individual bones are inspected for evidence of old injury or bone destruction. Finally, loose bodies are sought.

In children the epiphyses are largely cartilaginous and the articular relations often have to be deduced from the shape and position of the emerging secondary ossific centres. The average ages at which they appear are easily remembered by the mnemonic CRITOE: Capitulum – 2 years; Radial head – 4 years; Internal (medial) epicondyle – 6 years; Trochlea – 8 years; Olecranon – 10 years; External (lateral) epicondyle – 12 years.

CONGENITAL DISORDERS

CONGENITAL DISLOCATION

This may be anterior or posterior and is usually bilateral. The patient may notice the lump, which is easily palpable and can be felt to move when the forearm is rotated. X-rays show that the dislocated radial head is dome-shaped (due to abnormal modelling).

Function is usually surprisingly good and pain is unusual. Surgery is therefore rarely required; however, if the lump limits elbow flexion it can be excised (beware of the posterior interosseous nerve).

CONGENITAL SYNOSTOSIS

Congenital deficiencies of the forearm bones are occasionally associated with fusion of the humerus to the radius or ulna. This disabling condition is, fortunately, very rare. A more useful angle can be achieved by osteotomy.

Proximal radio-ulnar synostosis causes loss of rotation, but elbow flexion is retained and the inconvenience is often only moderate.

ACQUIRED DEFORMITIES

CUBITUS VALGUS

The normal carrying angle of the elbow is 10–15° of valgus; anything more than this is regarded as a valgus deformity, which is usually quite obvious when the patient stands with arms to the sides and palms facing forwards.

The commonest cause is non-union of a fractured lateral condyle; the deformity may be associated with marked prominence of the medial condylar outline.

The importance of cubitus valgus is the liability to delayed ulnar palsy; years after the causal injury the

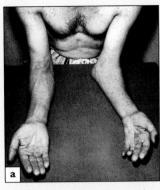
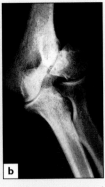

14.4 Cubitus valgus This man's valgus deformity, the sequel to an un-united fracture of the lateral condyle, has resulted in ulnar nerve palsy.

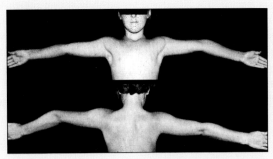

14.5 Cubitus varus This ugly deformity, the sequel to a supracondylar fracture, was later corrected by osteotomy.

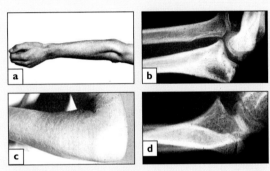

14.6 Dislocated head of radius (**a, b**) Anterior dislocation, from an old Monteggia fracture; (**c, d**) posterior dislocation – the radial head is dome-shaped, suggesting that the dislocation was congenital.

patient notices weakness of the hand, with numbness and tingling of the ulnar fingers. The deformity itself needs no treatment, but for delayed ulnar palsy the nerve should be transposed to the front of the elbow. Great care is needed in performing the operation; damage to the medial collateral ligaments will result in elbow instability.

CUBITUS VARUS ('GUN-STOCK' DEFORMITY)

The deformity is most obvious when the elbow is extended and the arms are elevated. The most common cause is malunion of a supracondylar fracture. The deformity can be corrected by a wedge osteotomy of the lower humerus.

SUBLUXATION OF THE RADIAL HEAD

This is commonly associated with bone dysplasias in which the ulna is disproportionately shortened (e.g. hereditary multiple exostosis). It causes little disability, but if it becomes troublesome the radial head can be excised after all growth has ceased.

UNREDUCED DISLOCATION OF THE HEAD OF RADIUS

An unreduced Monteggia fracture-dislocation will leave the radial head permanently dislocated. Open reduction and stabilization with a Kirschner wire, together with soft-tissue reconstruction, may improve function.

'PULLED ELBOW'

Downward dislocation of the head of the radius from the annular ligament is a fairly common injury in children under the age of 6 years. There may be a history of the child being jerked by the arm and subsequently complain-

ing of pain and inability to use the arm. The limb is held more or less immobile with the elbow fully extended and the forearm pronated; any attempt to supinate the forearm is resisted. The diagnosis is essentially clinical, though x-rays are usually obtained in order to exclude a fracture.

The radial head can be forcibly pulled out of the noose of the annular ligament only when the forearm is pronated; even then the distal attachment of the ligament is sometimes torn.

If the history and clinical picture are suggestive, an attempt should be made to reduce the subluxation or dislocation. While the child's attention is diverted, the elbow is quickly supinated and then slightly flexed; the radial head is relocated with a snap. (This sometimes happens 'spontaneously' while the radiographer is positioning the arm!)

OSTEOCHONDRITIS DISSECANS

The capitulum is one of the common sites of osteochondritis dissecans. This is probably due to repeated stress following prolonged or unaccustomed activity. The pathological changes are described in Chapter 6.

The patient – usually a young boy – complains of aching which is aggravated by activity and relieved by rest. On examination there may be swelling, signs of an effusion, tenderness over the capitulum and slight limitation of movement. If the fragment has separated, there may be intermittent locking.

X-rays may show fragmentation or, at a much later stage, flattening of the capitulum. *Computed tomography (CT)* and *magnetic resonance imaging (MRI)* are more useful for defining the lesion.

Treatment is usually symptomatic. However, if the fragment has separated and is lying free in the joint, it should be removed; this can be done arthroscopically.

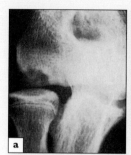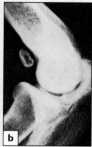

14.7 Osteochondritis dissecans (a) The capitulum is fragmented and slightly flattened. (b) Sometimes the fragment separates and lies in the joint.

LOOSE BODIES

Loose bodies in the elbow may be due to: (1) acute trauma (an osteocartilaginous fracture); (2) osteochondritis dissecans; (3) synovial chondromatosis (a cluster of mainly cartilaginous 'pebbles'); or (4) osteoarthritis (separation of osteophytes).

The patient may complain of sudden locking and unlocking of the joint. Symptoms of osteoarthritis may coexist.

A loose body is rarely palpable. When degenerative changes have occurred, extremes of movement are limited.

X-rays nearly always reveal the loose body or bodies; in the special case of osteochondritis dissecans there is a rarefied cystic area in the capitulum and enlargement of the radial head.

If loose bodies are troublesome, they should be removed.

TUBERCULOSIS

Pathology The elbow is affected in about 10% of patients with skeletal tuberculosis (see also Chapter 2). Although the disease begins as synovitis or osteomyelitis, patients are rarely seen until arthritis supervenes.

Clinical features The onset is insidious with a long history of aching and stiffness. The most striking physical sign is the marked wasting. While the disease is active the joint is held flexed, looks swollen, feels warm and diffusely tender; movement is considerably limited and accompanied by pain and spasm.

X-rays The typical features are peri-articular osteoporosis and joint erosion. There may also be suchondral cystic lesions.

Diagnosis Aspiration, synovial biopsy and microbiological investigation will usually confirm the diagnosis.

Treatment General antituberculous treatment is essential. The elbow is rested until the acute symptoms subside – at first in a splint and positioned at 90° of flexion and mid-rotation, later simply by applying a collar and cuff. As soon as possible, however, movement is encouraged.

Late residual effects – chronic pain, stiffness or deformity – may be troublesome enough to justify arthrodesis or arthroplasty.

RHEUMATOID ARTHRITIS

The elbow is involved in more than 50% of patients with polyarticular rheumatoid arthritis (see also Chapter 3), and in the majority of cases the condition is bilateral.

Clinical features

Ulnar bursitis and rheumatoid nodules are often found on the back of the elbow even if the joint itself is not affected. With true joint involvement, synovitis gives rise to pain and tenderness, especially over the lateral

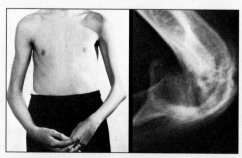

14.8 Tuberculosis of the elbow Muscle wasting is marked and bone destruction extensive.

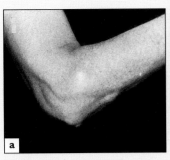
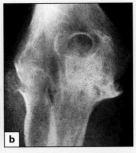
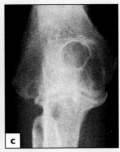

14.9 Rheumatoid arthritis (**a**) This rheumatoid patient has nodules over the olecranon and a bulge over the radiohumeral joint; (**b**) his x-rays show deformity of the radial head and marked erosion of the rest of the elbow. (**c**) Excision of the radial head combined with synovectomy relieved the pain and the joint looks much healthier.

aspect of the radiohumeral joint. Later the entire elbow may be swollen. Movements are restricted but, if bone destruction is marked, the joint becomes unstable.

Synovial swelling occasionally causes ulnar nerve or posterior interosseous nerve compression, with symptoms and signs in the wrist and hand. It is important to distinguish these features from those of local weakness and tendon rupture due to generalized disease.

X-rays reveal bone erosion, with gradual destruction of the radial head and widening of the trochlear notch of the ulna. Sometimes large synovial extensions penetrate the articular surface and appear as cysts in the proximal radius or ulna.

Treatment

In addition to general treatment, the elbow should be splinted during periods of active synovitis. Local injections of corticosteroids or radiocolloids may reduce pain and swelling dramatically.

OPERATIVE TREATMENT If, despite adequate conservative treatment, synovitis persists – and more particularly if this is associated with erosion of the radial head – synovectomy is worthwhile. This is usually performed through a lateral approach, with excision of the radial head. There are two reasons for this: the radiocapitellar surfaces are almost invariably eroded, and radial head excision permits wider access to the hypertrophic synovium. The operation relieves pain and may slow the progress of the disease, but after 5–6 years erosion of the humeroulnar joint often causes increasing instability and recurrence of pain. A drawback of radial head excision is that it may jeopardize the result of joint replacement if this should later become necessary.

Progressive bone destruction and instability may call for reconstructive surgery. There is a dilemma: arthrodesis is very disabling and is unlikely to be accepted by the patient; yet joint replacement is difficult to perform and fraught with complications such as infection, instability and dislocation, ulnar neuropathy and aseptic loosening of the implants. Nevertheless, good 5-year

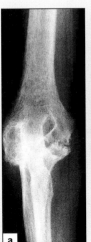
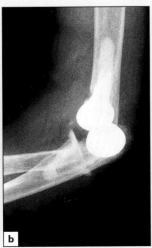
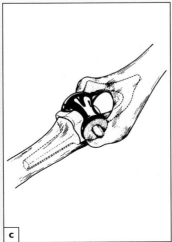

14.10 Total elbow replacement (**a**) Severe rheumatoid arthritis of the elbow. (**b**) X-ray after joint replacement. (**c**) The Souter arthroplasty: a metal humeral prosthesis and polyethylene ulnar implant.

results have been reported in about 90% of patients (Morrey and Adams, 1992; Ewald *et al.*, 1993).

GOUT AND PSEUDOGOUT

The elbow – or more precisely the olecranon bursa – is a favourite site for gout. In an acute attack the area rapidly becomes painful, swollen and inflamed. The swelling and redness may extend well down the forearm and the condition is easily mistaken for cellulitis or joint infection. The serum uric acid level may be raised and the bursal aspirate will contain urate crystals. Treatment is with high dosage anti-inflammatory preparations.

Similar attacks occur in pseudogout, due to the deposition of calcium pyrophosphate dihydrate (CPPD) crystals, which can be identified in the aspirate (see Chapter 4).

Chronic calcium pyrophosphate arthropathy is more serious. This condition should always be suspected when 'osteoarthritic' changes appear spontaneously in an unusal site such as the elbow; x-rays may show additional features such as chondrocalcinosis and peri-articular calcification. The diagnosis can be confirmed by demonstrating the typical positively birefringent crystals in fluid aspirated from the joint. Treatment is as for osteoarthritis (see below).

OSTEOARTHRITIS

Osteoarthritis (see also Chapter 5) of the elbow is uncommon and usually denotes some recognizable underlying pathology – a previous fracture or ligamentous injury, loose bodies in the joint, long-standing occupational stress, inflammatory arthritis or gout. 'Primary' osteoarthritis – especially when it is part of a polyartic-ular disorder – sugggests calcium pyrophosphate deposition disease (see above).

Clinical features The patient usually complains of pain and stiffness, especially following periods of inactivity. Examination shows local tenderness, thickening of the joint, crepitus and restriction of movement. Osteophytic hypertrophy may cause ulnar nerve palsy.

X-rays show narrowing of the joint space with scle-rosis and osteophytes. One or more loose bodies may be seen; chondrocalcinosis and periarticular calcifica-tion are typical of pyrophosphate arthropathy.

Treatment is usually limited to pain control and the use of non-steroidal anti-inflammatory preparations. Loose bodies, if they cause locking, should be removed. If there are signs of ulnar neuritis, the nerve should be transposed.

Debridement of the joint may be helpful (Tsuge and Mizuseki, 1994). In advanced cases joint replacement can

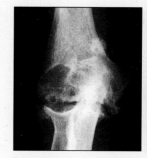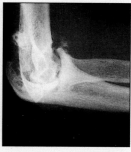

14.11 Pyrophosphate arthropathy Osteoarthritis of the elbow is unusual except after trauma. These x-rays show a destructive arthritis in a patient with generalized pyrophosphate arthropathy.

be considered; however, upper limb activities will have to be permanently restricted in order to reduce the risk of implant loosening.

NEUROPATHIC ARTHRITIS

Neuropathic arthritis (see also Chapter 5) of the elbow is seen in syringomyelia and diabetes mellitus. Sometimes neurological features predominate and the diagnosis may be known; occasionally the patient presents with progressive instability of the elbow. The joint may be markedly swollen and hypermobile, with coarse crepita-tion on passive movement, or it may be completely flail.

The condition must be distinguished from other causes of flail elbow, such as advanced rheumatoid arthritis and unreduced (or un-united) fracture-dislocations.

Treatment consists of splintage to maintain stabil-ity. Arthrodesis usually fails and arthroplasty is tech-nically hazardous.

STIFFNESS OF THE ELBOW

Stiffness of the elbow may be due *congenital abnormali-ties* (various types of synostosis, or arthrogryposis), *infec-tion, inflammatory arthritis, osteoarthritis* or the late effects of *trauma*. Most of these conditions are dealt with in other chapters. Here consideration will be given to post-traumatic stiffness, which is an important cause of disability.

POST-TRAUMATIC STIFFNESS

For reasons that are not entirely clear, the elbow is partic-ularly prone to post-traumatic stiffness. The more obvi-ous causes (as with other joints) are either extrinsic (e.g.

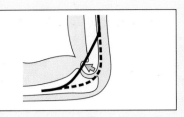

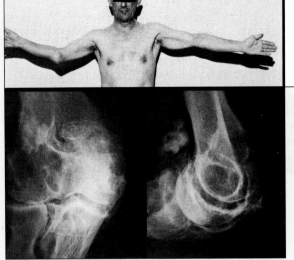

14.12 Osteoarthritis and loose bodies
This patient had osteoarthritis and loose bodies in the elbow; the associated ulnar palsy was treated by transposing the nerve to the front of the elbows (diagram).

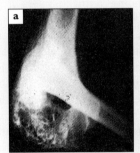 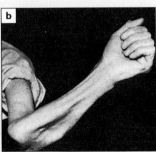 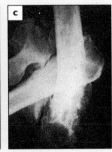 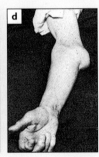

14.13 Flail elbow (a, b) Following gunshot wound; **(c, d)** neuropathic arthritis.

soft-tissue contracture or heterotopic bone formation), intrinsic (e.g. intra-articular adhesions and articular incongruity) or a combination of these. Clinical assessment should include examination of all the joints of the upper limb as well as an evaluation of the functional needs of the particular patient. Most of the activities of daily living can be managed with a restricted range of elbow motion: flexion from 30–130° and pronation and supination of 50° each. Any greater loss is likely to be disabling.

NON-OPERATIVE TREATMENT
The most effective treatment is prevention, by early active movement through a functional range. If movement is restricted and fails to improve with exercise, serial splintage may help; however, it is important to avoid using the splint as a means of forced manipulation.

OPERATIVE TREATMENT
The indication for operative treatment is failure to regain a functional range of movement at 12 months after injury. There are a few caveats: the limb as whole should be useful; there should be no over-riding neurological impairment; and the patient should be cooperative and motivated. If there is heterotopic ossification, it is important to wait until the bone is 'mature' (i.e. showing clear cortical margins and trabecular markings on x-ray).

The objectives are determined by the type of pathology. Heterotopic bone can be excised. Capsular release or capsulectomy may restore a satisfactory range of movement. Intra-articular procedures include fixing of un-united or correction of malunited fractures. The pros and cons of the various operations are discussed in the review paper by Modabber and Jupiter (1995).

Post-traumatic radio-ulnar synostosis sometimes follows internal fixation of fractures of the radius and ulna. It is treated by resection when the synostosis has matured (this takes about 1 year) followed by diligent physiotherapy (Sachar *et al.*, 1994).

RECURRENT ELBOW INSTABILITY

Following a dislocation or severe sprain, the lateral collateral ligament can be stretched or ruptured

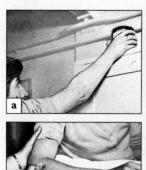
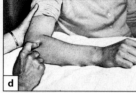
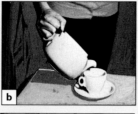
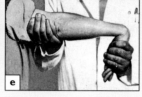
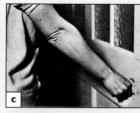
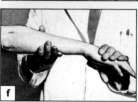
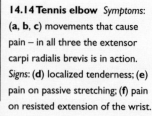

14.14 Tennis elbow *Symptoms:* (**a, b, c**) movements that cause pain – in all three the extensor carpi radialis brevis is in action. *Signs:* (**d**) localized tenderness; (**e**) pain on passive stretching; (**f**) pain on resisted extension of the wrist.

(O'Driscoll *et al.*, 1991). The patient may present with painful clicking and locking. On examination, an apprehension response can be elicited by supinating the forearm whilst applying a valgus force to the elbow during flexion.

The lateral collateral ligament can be directly repaired or reconstructed with a tendon autograft (e.g. palmaris longus).

OVERUSE OR REPETITIVE STRAIN SYNDROMES

The elbow is prone to painful disorders of the tendons or ligaments due to overuse or repetitive strain. These conditions have acquired names derived from the activities in which they were encountered when they were first described.

TENNIS ELBOW (LATERAL EPICONDYLITIS)

Pain and tenderness over the lateral epicondyle of the elbow (or, more accurately, the bony insertion of the common extensor tendon) is a common complaint among tennis players – but even more common in non-players who perform similar activities involving forceful repetitive wrist extension. The condition is probably a chronic tendinitis of the extensor carpi radialis brevis, rather similar to the 'overuse' or 'attrition' lesions of the rotator cuff at the shoulder. Like supraspinatus tendinitis, it may result in small tears, fibrocartilaginous metaplasia, microscopic calcification and a painful vascular reaction in the tendon fibres close to the lateral epicondyle.

Clinical features

The patient is usually an active individual of 30 or 40 years. Pain comes on gradually, often after a period of unaccustomed activity involving forceful gripping and wrist extension. It is usually localized to the lateral epicondyle, but in severe cases it may radiate widely. It is aggravated by movements such as pouring out tea, turning a stiff doorhandle, shaking hands or lifting with the forearm pronated. Among tennis players it is usually blamed on faulty technique.

The elbow looks normal, and flexion and extension are full and painless. Characteristically there is localized tenderness at or just below the lateral epicondyle. Pain can be reproduced by passively stretching the extensor radialis brevis; this is done by extending the elbow, pronating the forearm and then passively flexing the wrist (see Fig. 14.14e). Active extension of the wrist against resistance is also painful.

The x-ray is usually normal, but occasionally shows calcification at the tendon origin.

Diagnosis

In patients with long-standing symptoms which do not respond to treatment, the possibility of a painful radial nerve entrapment ('radial tunnel syndrome' – see page 249) should be considered.

Treatment

Many methods of treatment are available but the benefits of most are unclear (Labelle *et al.*, 1992). The first step is to identify, and then restrict, those activities which cause pain. Injection of the tender area with corticosteroid and local anaesthetic relieves pain but is not curative. The role of physiotherapy and manipulation is unproven (Verhaar *et al.*, 1996).

Operative treatment A few cases are sufficiently persistent or recurrent for operation to be indicated. The origin of the common extensor muscle is detached from the lateral epicondyle. Additional procedures such as division of the orbicular ligament or removal of a 'synovial fringe' are sometimes advocated; they probably make very little difference to the outcome. Surgery is successful in only about 60% of cases.

GOLFER'S ELBOW (MEDIAL EPICONDYLITIS)

This is very similar to tennis elbow except that the flexor origin (not the extensor) is affected. Treatment is the same as for lateral epicondylitis (Kurvers and Verhaar, 1995).

BASEBALL PITCHER'S ELBOW

Repetitive, vigorous throwing activities can cause damage to the bones or soft-tissue attachments around the elbow. Professional baseball players may develop hypertrophy of the lower humerus and incongruity of the joint, or loose-body formation and osteoarthritis. The junior equivalent (*Little Leaguers' elbow*) is a partial avulsion of the medial epicondyle; the only remedy (however grudgingly accepted) is to stay off baseball until the condition clears up completely.

JAVELIN THROWERS' ELBOW

The over-arm action employed by javelin throwers may avulse the tip of the olecranon; with the round-arm action the medial ligament may be avulsed. The pain usually settles down after a period of rest and modification of activities.

AVULSION OF THE DISTAL TENDON OF BICEPS

The typical patient is a man of about 55 years who feels pain and weakness at the front of the elbow after strenuous effort. Feel for the distal biceps tendon while the patient flexes the elbow against resistance (ask him or her to grip the desk or table as if to lift it; normally the biceps tendon stands out as a taut cord across the elbow crease). The tendon may be partially or completely avulsed from its insertion into the bicipital tuberosity of the radius.

The diagnosis is often missed because elbow flexion and supination, although weaker than normal, are preserved by brachialis and supinator action. MRI helps to confirm the diagnosis (Le Huec *et al.*, 1996).

Treatment Operative repair is not always necessary; some patients are content to manage with slightly reduced function. The best results are achieved by early operation before the tendon retracts. A two-incision technique is recommended; tissue anchors can be used to attach the tendon to its insertion point.

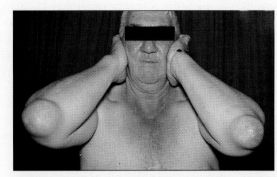

14.15 Olecranon bursitis The enormous red lumps over the points of the elbows are enlarged olecranon bursae; the ruddy complexion completes the typical picture of gout.

BURSITIS

The olecranon bursa sometimes becomes enlarged as a result *of continual pressure or friction* (this used to be called students' elbow); if the enlargement is a nuisance the fluid may be aspirated.

The commonest non-traumatic cause is *gout*; there may be a sizeable lump with calcification on x-ray. In *rheumatoid arthritis*, also, the bursa may become enlarged, and sometimes nodules can be felt in the lump or just distal to it over the proximal ulna. In both conditions other joints are likely to be affected as well.

A chronically enlarged bursa may prove a severe nuisance and need to be excised.

OPERATIONS

ARTHROSCOPY

Arthroscopy of the elbow is technically demanding; its role for diagnosis and treatment continues to evolve. *Indications* include removal of loose bodies, irrigation for infection and trimming of osteophytes. More advanced indications such as synovectomy and capsular release carry a risk of damage to neurovascular structures and should be left to those surgeons very experienced in the technique (Poehling and Ekman, 1994).

ARTHROPLASTY

A complex anatomy and relatively fragile bone structure make it unlikely that elbow arthroplasty will repeat the success stories of hip and knee replacement. Nevertheless, in specific circumstances it may be better than the alternative of a painful and grossly unstable joint.

Indications The most common indication for arthroplasty is rheumatoid arthritis; it is occasionally suitable for the treatment of osteoarthritis or non-union of a distal humerus fracture (Morrey, 1993). One should think carefully before offering elbow replacement to patients who intend to return to heavy work or leisure activities or to those with single-joint disease, i.e. without the protective effect against overuse of other involved joints in the same limb.

Design Earlier constrained (single-axis hinge) implants had a high failure rate due to loosening. Unconstrained designs are associated with instability and dislocation. Semi-constrained implants allow some of the forces to be absorbed by the soft tissues whilst maintaining some intrinsic stability.

Outcome The majority of patients with an elbow replacement can expect relief of pain and a functional range of movement. Five-year survival rates as high as 90% have been achieved in patients with rheumatoid arthritis (perhaps the joint is protected because of poor function in the rest of the limb) whereas the survival rate for those with osteoarthritis or distal humeral non-union is probably no better than 50% (Kraay *et al.*, 1994).

Complications The operation has a relatively high complication rate, particularly ulnar nerve palsy, wound failure and collateral ligament instability.

ARTHRODESIS

Arthrodesis is rarely indicated. It is a technically difficult and very disabling procedure. Even with normal wrist and shoulder function it is not possible to fuse the elbow in a position which would facilitate both feeding (i.e. 100° of flexion) and perineal hygiene (about 45° of flexion). Compression plating is one technique (McAuliffe *et al.*, 1992).

NOTES ON APPLIED ANATOMY

The elbow needs to be able to convey the hand upwards to the head and mouth, downwards to the perineum and legs and also to a wide variety of working positions at bench, desk, wall or table. A varied combination of flexion and extension with pronation and supination is clearly needed. Although the elbow is obviously capable of full extension, flexion to about 130° and 90° of both pronation and supination, the *functional range of movement* is 30–130° of flexion and 50° both pronation and supination.

The forearm is normally in slight valgus in relation to the upper arm, the average carrying angle being about 15°. The complex geometry of the joint allows for the fact that when the elbow is flexed the forearm comes to lie directly upon the upper arm. The carrying angle may be altered by malunion of a fracture or by damage to the physis, resulting in cubitus valgus or cubitus varus.

In some ways the joint acts as a 'sloppy hinge' permitting a few degrees of valgus/varus movement and some rotational laxity. Stability is provided by (1) the relative conformity of the humeral trochlea with the olecranon, (2) the medial collateral ligament (particularly the anterior band) and (3) the lateral collateral ligament (particularly the ulnar part). The radial head is a secondary constraint to valgus instability; it can be excised with impunity as long as the medial collateral ligament and humero-ulnar articulation are intact. The elbow is not really a 'non-weightbearing' joint – forces of up to three times body weight pass across it with normal use.

Pronation and supination take place mainly at the radioulnar joints with a small amount of abduction and adduction between the olecranon and the trochlea. The movement is often supplemented by rotation at the shoulder. The humeroradial joint is held in position by the strong annular (orbicular) ligament which embraces the head and neck of the radius but is not attached to it. The capsule of the elbow is attached to the annular ligament but also is not attached to the radius. The circular and slightly concave upper surface of the radius ensures that in all positions of rotation it retains adequate contact with the capitulum.

NERVES

The ulnar nerve passes behind the medial condyle of the humerus; it may be stretched if there is marked cubitus valgus. Distal to the condyle the nerve is closely applied to the elbow capsule, and there also it may be compromised if the joint is osteoarthritic.

On the lateral side of the elbow the posterior interosseous nerve passes between the two parts of the supinator muscle; it is vulnerable to injury during surgical approaches to the proximal part of the radius.

In front of the elbow lies the brachialis muscle and also the median nerve in company with the great vessels; these relationships make an anterior approach to the elbow somewhat challenging.

REFERENCES AND FURTHER READING

Ewald FC, Simmons ED Jr, Sullivan JA *et al* (1993) Capitello-condylar total elbow replacement in rheumatoid arthritis: long term results. *Journal of Bone and Joint Surgery* **75**A, 498-507

Kraay MJ, Figgie MP, Inglis AE *et al* (1994) Primary semiconstrained total elbow arthroplasty. *Journal of Bone and Joint Surgery* **76**B, 636-640

Kurvers H, Verhaar J (1995) Results of operative treatment of medial epicondylitis. *Journal of Bone and Joint Surgery* **77**A, 1374-1379

Labelle H, Guibert R, Joncas J *et al* (1992) Lack of scientific evidence for the treatment of lateral epicondylitis of the elbow. *Journal of Bone and Joint Surgery* **74**B, 646-651

Le Huec JC, Moinard M, Liquois F *et al* (1996) Distal rupture of the tendon of biceps brachii. *Journal of Bone and Joint Surgery* **78**B, 767-770

McAuliffe JA, Burkhalter WE, Ouellette EA *et al* (1992) Compression plate arthrodesis of the elbow. *Journal of Bone and Joint Surgery* **74**B, 300-304

Modabber MR, Jupiter JB (1995) Reconstruction for post-traumatic conditions of the elbow. *Journal of Bone and Joint Surgery* **77**A, 1431-1446

Morrey BF (1993) *The Elbow and its Disorders*. WB Saunders Company, Philadelphia

Morrey BF, Adams RA (1992) Semiconstrained arthroplasty for the treatment of rheumatoid arthritis of the elbow. *Journal of Bone and Joint Surgery* **74**A, 479-490

O'Driscoll SW, Bell DF, Morrey BF (1991) Posterolateral rotatory instability of the elbow. *Journal of Bone and Joint Surgery* **73**A, 40-446

Poehling GG, Ekman EF (1994) Arthroscopy of the elbow. *Journal of Bone and Joint Surgery* **76**A, 1265-1271

Sachar K, Akelman E, Ehrlich MG (1994) Radioulnar synostosis. *Hand Clinics* **10**, 339-404

Schemitsch EH, Ewald FC, Thornhill TS (1996) Results of total elbow arthroplasty after excision of radial head and synovectomy in patients who had rheumatoid arthritis. *Journal of Bone and Joint Surgery* **78**A, 1541-1547

Stewart NJ, Manzanares MD, Morrey BF (1997) Surgical treatment of aseptic olecranon bursitis. *Journal of Shoulder and Elbow Surgery* **6**, 49-54

Tsuge K, Mizuseki T (1994) Debridement arthroplasty for advanced primary osteoarthritis of the elbow. *Journal of Bone and Joint Surgery* **76**B, 642-646

Verhaar J, Walenkamp G, Kester A *et al* (1993). Lateral extensor release for tennis elbow. *Journal of Bone and Joint Surgery* **75**A, 1034-1043

Verhaar JAN, Walenkamp GHIM, van Mameren H *et al* (1996) Local corticosteroid injection versus Cyriax type physiotherapy for tennis elbow. *Journal of Bone and Joint Surgery* **78**B, 128-132

CLINICAL ASSESSMENT

SYMPTOMS

Pain may be localized to the radial side (especially in tenovaginitis of the thumb tendons), to the ulnar side (possibly from the radioulnar joint) or to the dorsum (the usual site in disorders of the carpus).

Stiffness is often not noticed until it is severe.

Swelling may signify involvement of either the joint or the tendon sheaths.

Deformity is a late symptom except after trauma or radial nerve palsy.

Loss of function refers mainly to the hand – a firm grip is possible only with a strong, stable, painless wrist that also has a reasonable range of movement.

SIGNS

Examination of the wrist is not complete without also examining the elbow, forearm and hand. Both upper limbs should be completely exposed.

Look

The skin is inspected for scars. Both wrists and forearms are compared to see if there is any deformity. If there is swelling, note whether it is diffuse or localized to one of the tendon sheaths. Look also at the hands and fingers to see if there are any related abnormalities.

Feel

Undue warmth is noted. Tender areas must be accurately localized and the bony landmarks compared with those of the normal wrist. The site of tenderness may be diagnostic, for example in de Quervain's disease (tip of radial styloid), scaphoid fracture (anatomical snuffbox), carpometacarpal osteoarthritis (OA) (base of first metacarpal), Kienböck's disease (over the lunate) and localized tenosynovitis of any of the wrist tendons.

Move

To compare passive dorsiflexion of the wrists the patient places his or her palms together in the position of prayer, then elevates his or her elbows. Palmarflexion is examined in a similar way. Radial and ulnar deviation are measured in either the palms-up or the palms-down position. With the elbows at right angles and tucked in to the sides, pronation and supination are assessed.

While testing passive movements, the presence of abnormal 'clicks' should be noted; they may signify one or other form of carpal instability.

Active movements should be tested against resistance; loss of power may be due to pain, tendon rupture or muscle weakness.

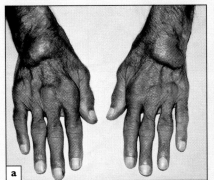
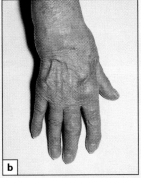

15.1 Examination Look at the wrist *and the hand*. **(a)** This woman has swellings on both wrists, due to tenosynovitis of the extensor tendons. The finger joints also are swollen; she has rheumatoid arthritis. **(b)** In this case it is the wrist joint itself which is swollen due to rheumatoid synovitis.

Grip strength can be gauged by having the patient squeeze the examiner's hand; mechanical instruments allow more accurate assessment of both power grip and pinch.

Provocative tests

Special tests are needed to assess stability of the carpal articulations. The *luno-triquetral joint* is tested by gripping or pinching the lunate with one hand, the trique-tral-pisiform with the other, and then applying a sheer stress: pain or clicking suggests an incompetent luno-triquetral ligament. The *piso-triquetral joint* is tested by pushing the pisiform backwards and ulnarwards against the lunate. Stability of the *scapho-lunate joint* is tested by pressing hard on the palmer aspect of the scaphoid tubercle while moving the wrist alternately in abduction and adduction: pain or clicking on abduction (radial deviation) is abnormal. The *triangular fibrocartilage* is tested by pushing the wrist medially then flexing and extending it. These tests are mentioned again in the section on carpal instability.

IMAGING

X-RAYS Anteroposterior and lateral views are obtained routinely. Note the position and shape of the individual carpal bones and whether there are any abnormal spaces between them. Then look for evidence of joint space narrowing, especially at the radiocarpal joint and the carpometacarpal joint of the thumb. The wrist x-ray should be taken in a standard position of mid-pronation with the elbow at 90°; often both wrists must be x-rayed for comparison. Special views may be necessary to show a scaphoid fracture or carpal instability. Moving the wrist under image intensification is useful to investigate some cases of carpal instability.

ARTHROGRAPHY The wrist contains three separate compartments – the radiocarpal joint, the distal radio-ulnar joint and the midcarpal joint. Defects in the triangular fibrocartilage, scapho-lunate ligaments or luno-triquetral ligaments can be identified by arthrography.

COMPUTED TOMOGRAPHY CT is the ideal method for assessing congruity of the distal radio-ulnar joint.

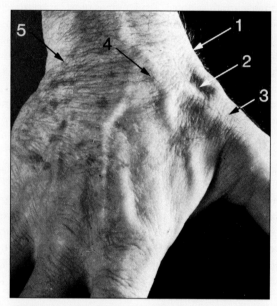

15.2 Tender points at the wrist The exact site of tenderness may be diagnostic for: (1) de Quervain's disease; (2) scaphoid fracture; (3) carpometacarpal osteoarthritis; (4) tenosynovitis of extensor carpi radialis brevis; (5) tenosynovitis of extensor carpi ulnaris.

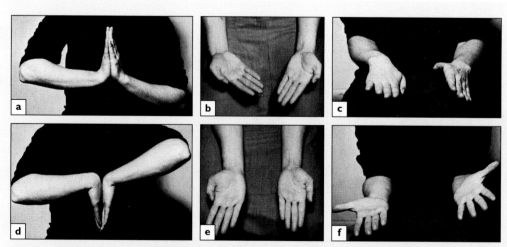

15.3 Examination All movements of the left wrist are limited: (**a**) dorsiflexion, (**b**) palmarflexion, (**c**) ulnar deviation, (**d**) radial deviation, (**e**) pronation, (**f**) supination.

MAGNETIC RESONANCE IMAGING MRI is particularly useful for detecting changes associated with scaphoid fractures, avascular necrosis of the lunate (Kienböck's disease) and intra-osseous ganglia. The thickness of the cuts may be too large to detect injury to thin structures such as the luno-triquetral ligament, scapho-lunate ligament or triangular fibrocartilage.

ARTHROSCOPY

The wrist is suspended by finger traps and inspected through a radiocarpal portal and a midcarpal portal. Ligament tears, articular cartilage damage, synovitis and triangular fibrocartilage lesions can be recognized and in some cases treated.

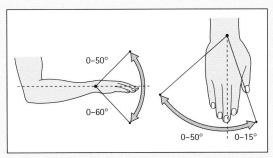

15.4 Normal range of movement From the neutral position dorsiflexion is slightly less than palmarflexion. Most hand functions are performed with the wrist in ulnar deviation; normal radial deviation is only about 15°.

CONGENITAL AND CHILDHOOD DEFORMITIES

CARPAL FUSIONS

Coalition of two or more of the carpal bones is one of the commonest congenital wrist anomalies; it is usually inherited as an autosomal dominant trait and may be bilateral. Often it is associated with other abnormalities. It seldom causes problems and no treatment is necessary.

TRANSVERSE ABSENCE

The commonest site of transverse absence in the upper limb is at the junction of the middle and upper third of the forearm. A static prosthesis is fitted at 6 months. If facilities are available, this is replaced at 18 months by a split hook operated by a cord from the other shoulder, and at about 3 years by a myoelectric prosthesis.

RADIAL LONGITUDINAL DEFICIENCY (RADIAL CLUB HAND)

The infant is born with the wrist in marked radial deviation – hence the *term 'club hand'*. Bilateral deformity is more common than unilateral. There is absence of the whole or part of the radius; often the thumb, scaphoid and trapezium fail to develop normally. It usually occurs as an isolated abnormality but is occasionally associated with other conditions such as thrombocytopaenia and absent radius (TAR), Fanconi anaemia, atrial septal defect (Holt–Oram syndrome) or the VATER syndrome (Vertebral defects, Anal atresia, Tracheo-Esophageal fistula, Renal and Radial dysplasia).

Treatment in the neonate consists of gentle manipulation and splintage. Surgical treatment is intended to improve appearance and improve function. It is undertaken preferably between 6 and 9 months of age. The tight tissues are released, the carpus is 'centralized' on to the ulna and tendons are transferred to prevent recurrence. The correction is held for several weeks with a K-wire; after the wire is removed, prolonged splintage is recommended to avoid recurrence. A deficient thumb can be reconstructed with an opposition transfer and an absent thumb by pollicization of the index

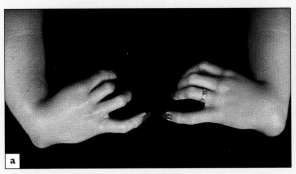

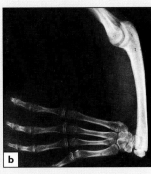

15.5 Radial dysplasia
(a) Bilateral. (b) X-ray showing that the entire radius is absent.

finger. In bilateral cases, elbow stiffness is a contraindication to corrective surgery because radial deviation of the wrist is the only position in which the hand can reach the mouth or perineum.

ULNAR LONGITUDINAL DEFICIENCY

In this rare deformity ulnar deviation is present at birth and is due to partial or complete absence of the ulna; in addition the ulnar rays of the hand may be missing. As the child grows the radial head may dislocate.

Treatment consists of stretching and splintage during the first few months. If deformity is marked, excision of the ulnar anlage and osteotomy of the radius may improve the appearance. If the radial head has dislocated, thus restricting elbow movement, it can be excised; if the forearm is unstable, the distal radius is fused to the proximal ulna (Straub procedure).

DISTAL ULNAR DYSPLASIA

In older children with hereditary multiple exostoses there is often disproportionate shortening of the ulna; its distal end becomes carrot-shaped and the radius is bowed. The same deformity is sometimes seen in dyschondroplasia, and occasionally without any obvious bone disease.

Treatment is seldom necessary. If deformity is marked, ulnar lengthening (with or without osteotomy of the radius) may be advisable.

MADELUNG'S DEFORMITY

In this deformity the lower radius curves forwards, carrying with it the carpus and hand but leaving the lower ulna sticking out as a lump on the back of the wrist. It may be congenital or post-traumatic. The congenital disorder may appear as an isolated entity or as part of a generalized dysplasia; although the abnormality is present at birth, the deformity is rarely seen before the age of 10 years, after which it increases until growth is complete. Function is usually excellent.

Treatment If deformity is severe the lower end of the ulna may be excised (Darrach's procedure); this is sometimes combined with osteotomy of the radius. Excision of the physeal tether and replacement with a free fat graft is an alternative.

ARTHROGRYPOSIS MULTIPLEX CONGENITA

Multiple, non-progressive joint contractures are noted at birth. The cause is unknown; there is an underlying neuropathy or myopathy. The limbs appear atrophic,

with waxy skin lacking normal joint creases. The elbows are extended, the wrists flexed and ulnar deviated, the thumb adducted and clasped, and the fingers flexed.

Treatment is difficult. Serial splintage is started soon after birth; however, correction is often not adequate. Persistent extension deformity of the elbow can be managed by posterior capsulotomy, triceps lengthening and transfer of the pectoralis major into the biceps. Severe wrist deformity may require soft-tissue release, proximal row carpectomy or fusion.

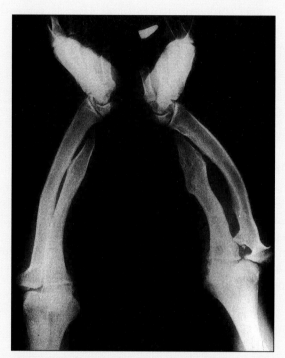

15.6 Distal ulnar deformity The x-ray characteristically shows a tapering, carrot-shaped distal end of ulna. This bilateral case was due to hereditary multiple exostoses; there is bilateral bowing of the radius and on the right side the radial head has subluxated.

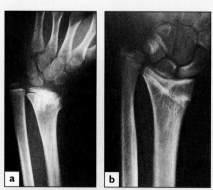

15.7 Madelung's deformity (a) Damage to radial growth disc, which might cause (b) Madelung's deformity.

ACQUIRED DEFORMITIES

PHYSEAL INJURY

Fracture-separation of the distal radial epiphysis may result in partial fusion of the physis, with asymmetrical growth deformity of the wrist. The bony bridge crossing the physis, if it is small, may be excised and replaced by a fat graft. Once growth slows down the deformity can be corrected by a suitable osteotomy, if necessary combined with soft-tissue release; the Ilizarov apparatus can be used for this.

FOREARM FRACTURES

After a Colles' fracture radial deviation and posterior angulation are common. These deformities may be unsightly but cause little disability.

Subluxation of the distal radioulnar joint may result in prominence of the ulnar head and loss of pronation or supination. This can sometimes be treated by reconstructing the distal articulation; otherwise the head of the ulna may need to be excised. In young patients abnormal angulation of the radius may lead to progressive carpal collapse and loss of grip strength. A radial osteotomy is then necessary.

RHEUMATOID DEFORMITIES

The typical rheumatoid deformity is radial deviation of the wrist, with or without radio-ulnar subluxation. With erosion of the radiocarpal joint, forward subluxation of the carpus develops (see below).

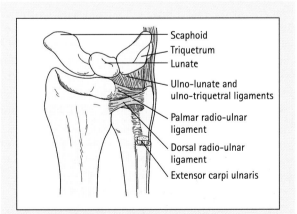

Scaphoid
Triquetrum
Lunate
Ulno-lunate and
ulno-triquetral ligaments
Palmar radio-ulnar
ligament
Dorsal radio-ulnar
ligament
Extensor carpi ulnaris

15.8 The distal radio-ulnar joint The joint incorporates the triangular fibrocartilage complex. The fibrocartilaginous plate is connected at its apex to the base of the ulnar styloid process and laterally to the inferomedial ridge of the radius. Its outer fibres blend with those of the ligaments around the ulnar aspect of the wrist.

DROP WRIST

With radial nerve palsy the wrist drops into flexion and active extension is lost. If the nerve does not recover, tendon transfers may restore function (see page 243).

CHRONIC INSTABILITY OF THE WRIST

Movements of the wrist and hand are closely interdependent, the wrist providing appropriate mobility and stability to position and steady the hand for the remarkable range of actions and tactile sensibility employed in our daily activities. Abnormalities of wrist mechanics are a common source of functional disability.

Articulations of the wrist

The wrist comprises three movable joints: *the distal radio-ulnar joint, the radio-carpal joint* (between the radius and the proximal row of carpal bones) and *the mid-carpal joint* (between the proximal and distal rows of carpal bones).

THE DISTAL RADIO-ULNAR JOINT (DRUJ) The distal radius and ulna are linked to each other by the interosseous membrane, the capsule of the DRUJ *and the triangular fibrocartilage complex (TFCC).* The head of the ulna articulates congruently with the sigmoid notch of the distal radius; movement at the joint occurs by the radius both rotating and sliding in an arc around the head of the ulna during pronation and supination of the forearm. Interposed between the head of the ulna and the carpus is a fibrocartilaginous plate, a fan-shaped structure spreading from an apical attachment at the base of the ulnar styloid process to the rim of the radial sigmoid notch. Its dorsal and volar edges are coextensive with the dorsal and palmar radio-ulnar ligaments; further attachments to the joint capsule, the ulno-triquetral and ulno-lunate ligaments, the ulnar collateral ligament and the sheath of the extensor carpi ulnaris tendon complete the fibrocartilage complex. The peripheral attachments of the TFCC have a good vascular supply and can heal after injury; the central area of the triangular plate is avascular and tears do not heal.

The anatomy of this region and the joint mechanics are well described in the review paper by Chidgey (1995).

THE RADIO-CARPAL AND MID-CARPAL JOINTS Movements in the sagittal plane (flexion and extension) occur at both the radio-carpal and mid-carpal joints. Movements in the frontal plane (adduction or ulnar deviation and abduction or radial deviation) occur mainly at the radio-carpal joint, but they inevitably involve also the scaphoid which has to make way as the trapezium moves towards the radial styloid during abduction.

The bones of the distal carpal row (hamate, capitate, trapezium and trapezoid) are joined by ligaments to each other and to the bases of the metacarpals. Although there is some movement of the fifth carpo-metacarpal joint, there is very little movement in the remaining carpo-metacarpal articulations.

The distal row articulates through the mid-carpal joint with the bones of the proximal row (triquetrum, lunate and scaphoid), which are likewise held together by stout interosseous ligaments. As these bones have no muscles attaching to them, their position is determined by the way they all fit together and by the constraints of the interosseous ligaments. The proximal row is, in a sense, 'interposed' between the forearm bones and the hand bones and is called an *intercalated segment*.

The articular surface of the radius slopes obliquely and faces distally and medially at an angle of 25–30°. With the wrist in the neutral position, tightening of the long muscles will tend to drag the carpus down the slope, and when the wrist is pulled into abduction this tendency is increased. By contrast, when the wrist is adducted about 30°, muscle pull draws the carpus most securely into the radial 'socket'. This is, in fact, the *'position of function'* (or maximum stability) and there is a natural inclination to adopt this position during power grip.

The scaphoid is potentially the most unstable of all the carpal bones. As the wrist flexes and extends, so does the scaphoid bone; the lunate and triquetrum follow passively, guided by the interosseous ligaments. With abduction, the space between the trapezium and radial styloid closes down so the scaphoid moves out of the way by flexing palmarwards and sliding ulnarwards. During adduction, the scaphoid tilts dorsally and slides radially. As the wrist abducts and adducts, the helical surface of the hamate also causes the triquetrum to move.

INSTABILITY OF THE DISTAL RADIO–ULNAR JOINT

Chronic instability of the distal radio-ulnar joint may result from trauma, rheumatoid arthritis (RA) or excision of the distal end of the ulna. The previous history is therefore important. Fracture of the radial shaft may have been associated with dislocation of the distal radio-ulnar joint (Galeazzi fracture-dislocation); after reduction of the radius, one must be certain that the radio-ulnar joint also is reduced.

The patient complains of painful restriction of pronation and supination and undue prominence of the head of the ulna. There may be tenderness directly over the radio-ulnar joint and grip strength is sometimes reduced. The unstable ulna can be 'ballotted' by holding the patient's forearm pronated and pushing sharply upon the prominent head of the ulna (the *piano-key sign*).

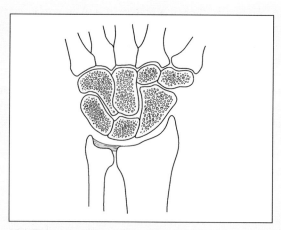

15.9 The carpal joints This schematic section through the wrist shows the *radio-carpal joint* between the radius and the proximal row of carpal bones and the *mid-carpal joint* between the proximal and distal rows of carpal bones. The proximal row is an intercalated segment.

X-ray examination may show evidence of previous injury or arthritis. Special views, with precise positioning of the wrist, have been developed (Chidgey, 1995). However, the most effective way of demonstrating radio-ulnar incongruity or subluxation is by CT.

TREATMENT Chronic instability without joint incongruity and degeneration can be managed by reconstruction of the capsule and ligaments and/or tenodesis of the ulna to the carpus. There is no completely reliable operation for chronic 'degenerative' instability.

LONGITUDINAL INSTABILITY OF THE RADIUS AND ULNA

Fracture of the radial head is sometimes accompanied by disruption of the interosseous membrane and dislocation of the distal radio-ulnar joint. Excision of the radial head can lead to proximal migration of the radius and ulno-carpal impaction (see below); whenever possible the radial head should be preserved or replaced by a titanium or Silastic spacer. Chronic longitudinal instability may cause wrist pain and loss of grip strength.

Treatment of the distal radio-ulnar joint symptoms is generally unsatisfactory. Radio-ulnar fusion is sometimes advocated as a salvage procedure.

DISORDERS OF THE TRIANGULAR FIBROCARTILAGE COMPLEX

Palmer and Werner (1989) described and classified the clinically significant disorders of the TFCC and suggested that they could be divided into traumatic and degenerative conditions.

TRAUMATIC DISRUPTION There may be a history of a fall on the outstretched hand or a twisting injury of the forearm. The patient complains of pain, and sometimes clicking, in the distal radio-ulnar joint, particularly on twisting the wrist. There is tenderness over the ulno-carpal joint and pain on rotation of the forearm. Symptoms can also be reproduced by holding the wrist in adduction and compressing the ulnar head against the carpus. The distal ulna should be tested for instability. The diagnosis is confirmed by contrast arthrography or high-resolution MRI.

Peripheral tears can be reattached by either open or arthroscopic techniques with a reasonable expectation that they will heal (Cooney *et al.*, 1994). Central tears, in the absence of ulno-carpal impaction (see below), are best managed by arthroscopic debridement (Osterman, 1990).

DEGENERATION The TFCC tends to degenerate with age; usually this is asymptomatic. However, progressive degenerative change may be associated with distal migration of the ulna, impaction of the ulnar head against the ulnar side of the lunate and ulno-carpal arthritis (the *ulno-carpal impaction syndrome*). X-ray examination may show distal displacement of the ulnar head ('positive ulnar variance') and in late cases there may be arthritic changes in the ulno-lunate articulation. Similar changes may occur in people born with positive ulnar variance.

Initial treatment is with simple analgesics, splintage and corticosteroid injections. If this is not successful then the long ulna can be shortened.

CHRONIC INSTABILITY OF THE RADIO–CARPAL AND INTERCARPAL JOINTS

Abnormal movement between the carpus and the forearm bones, or between individual carpal bones, results from loss of the bony relationships and/or ligamentous constraints which normally stabilize the wrist. The initiating cause is usually some type of injury – a wrist sprain with ligament damage, subluxation or dislocation at one of the radio-carpal or intercarpal joints or a fracture of one of the wrist bones – but chronic instability may also arise insidiously in erosive joint disorders such as RA.

Patterns of carpal instability

Acute carpal injuries are dealt with in Chapter 25. Here we shall consider the problems associated with chronic carpal instability. The disorder affects mainly the intercalated segment (proximal carpal row) of the wrist. The common patterns are described here.

DORSAL INTERCALATED SEGMENT INSTABILITY (DISI) Following a fracture of the scaphoid or rupture of the scapho-lunate ligament (scapho-lunate dissociation), the lunate no longer passively follows the scaphoid. The scaphoid tends to flex and the lunate assumes its default position of extension (dorsal tilt).

VOLAR INTERCALATED SEGMENT INSTABILITY (VISI) Less commonly, the luno-triquetral ligament is ruptured. The lunate, unrestrained by the triquetrum, but still controlled by the scaphoid, tends to flex whilst the capitate tends to extend.

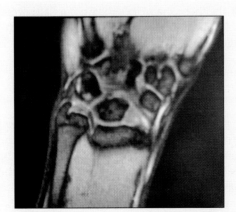

15.10 Ulno-carpal impaction MRI showing positive ulnar variance and impaction of the ulnar head on the side of the lunate. Bone changes are present in the lunate.

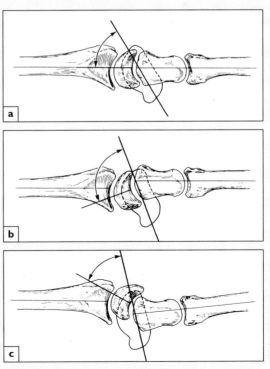

15.11 Carpal instability The relationships of the carpal bones in (**a**) the normal wrist, (**b**) DISI and (**c**) VISI.

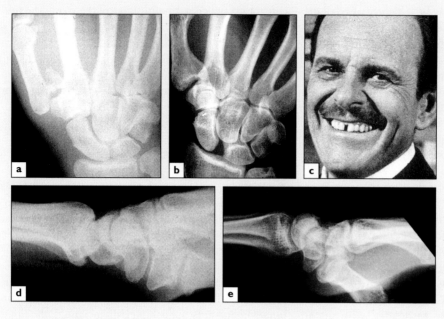

15.12 Carpal instability This patient was first seen after he fell and injured his wrist. **(a)** The x-ray showed a Bennett's fracture of the base of the first metacarpal and no other injury was apparent. A year later he was still complaining of pain in the wrist; x-ray at this stage **(b)** showed rotation of the scaphoid and a gap between the scaphoid and lunate (the Terry Thomas sign) **(c)** The actor, Terry Thomas showing the trademark gap between his front teeth (reproduced by permission; © United Artists Inc.). **(d)** In the lateral view the lunate is tilted dorsally (DISI); compare this with **(e)**, an example of VISI, showing volar tilt of the lunate.

MID-CARPAL INSTABILITY This usually emerges as a chronic problem, associated with generalized ligamentous laxity. The proximal and distal rows become unstable through the mid-carpal joint, probably due to attenuation of the radio-capitate ligament. It is also seen after malunion of a distal radial fracture: if the radial articular surface is left tilted dorsally, then the proximal carpal row tends also to tilt dorsally and the mid-carpal joint may become unstable.

RADIO-CARPAL TRANSLOCATION Chronic synovitis and articular erosion (as in RA) gradually leads to attenuation of the wrist ligaments and subluxation of the entire radiocarpal joint. In advanced RA the carpus usually shifts ulnarwards and simultaneously deviates into abduction.

Clinical features

The patient with scapho-lunate or luno-triquetral incompetence presents with pain and weakness of the wrist, and sometimes also clicking during movement or gripping actions. It is important to enquire about any previous injury, however trivial it may have seemed at the time.

On examination, there may be generalized tenderness over the carpus from synovitis or more localized tenderness, for example at the scapho-lunate junction or over the scaphoid itself. Grip strength is reduced. Provocative tests are useful.

Watson's test for scapho-lunate incompetence Thumb pressure is applied to the volar aspect of the wrist over the distal pole of the scaphoid (this restores the alignment of the volar-tilted scaphoid). While maintaining this position, the wrist is moved alternately into adduction and abduction. A painful 'clunk' occurs as the proximal pole of the scaphoid subluxes dorsally.

Luno-triquetral ballotment With one hand the examiner grasps and stabilizes the lunate between index finger and thumb. With the other thumb he or she presses on the pisiform/triquetrum to produce a shearing motion between lunate and triquetrum. If there is pain and excessive movement, this suggests incompetence of the luno-triquetral ligament.

Pivot shift test The examiner grasps the patient's forearm with one hand and the patient's hand with the other; he or she then compresses the wrist axially while moving it from abduction to adduction. A painful 'clunk' suggests mid-carpal instability.

X-ray

An antero-posterior x-ray may show an old or new scaphoid fracture. There may be widening of the scapho-lunate interval (*the Terry Thomas sign*); if the scaphoid is flexed, it will look foreshortened and the tubercle may appear as a dense 'ring' in the bone.

A true lateral view is examined to assess the relative alignment of the distal radius, the lunate, capitate and scaphoid. In a normal wrist, the articular surfaces of the radius, lunate and capitate are parallel. In the DISI deformity, the capitate axis is shifted dorsally, the lunate tilts backwards and the scaphoid flexes; the scapho-lunate angle is greater than 70°. In a VISI deformity, the lunate is flexed forwards and the scapho-lunate angle is less than 30°; the capitate tilts dorsally.

In an antero-posterior 'clenched fist view' the scaphoid is seen to flex and a scapho-lunate gap becomes more apparent.

Antero-posterior views with the wrist adducted and abducted emphasize scapho-lunate gaps and abnormal scaphoid flexion (the ring sign), particularly when compared with x-rays of the other side.

Further details of radiographic signs and helpful measurements can be found in the review paper by Bednar and Osterman (1993).

Further investigations

Image intensification helps to define the site of instability in difficult cases.

MRI will reveal any associated injuries, such as a scaphoid fracture. The scapho-lunate and luno-triquetral interosseous ligaments are so slim that the resolution of MRI scanning may be inadequate to detect significant injuries.

Arthroscopy of the radio-carpal and mid-carpal joints is the best method for demonstrating carpal instability. Ligament tears, certain patterns of instability, synovitis and damaged articular cartilage can be detected (Dantel *et al.*, 1993).

Treatment

SCAPHO-LUNATE AND LUNO-TRIQUETRAL DISSOCIATION   The best results are obtained if the ligaments heal in an anatomical position. The diagnosis should, therefore, be made as soon as possible after injury; this requires a high index of suspicion. The surgeon should be alerted by a history of wrist pain following a fall on the outstretched hand and a finding of dorsolateral tenderness. The ligaments are repaired, the bones stabilized with Kirschner wires and the wrist held in a cast for at least 2 months.

Patients seen more than 12 months after injury will require a more extensive type of carpal reduction and ligament reconstruction. If the displacement cannot be reduced, or if soft tissue repair fails, then a limited intercarpal fusion may be undertaken. If OA has supervened, a more extended arthrodesis will be needed. All of these procedures carry a high complication rate and relief of symptoms is unpredictable.

SYMPTOMATIC MID-CARPAL INSTABILITY   This is initially managed with forearm strengthening exercises and splinting. If this fails, then either ligament reconstruction or limited intercarpal fusion is worth considering.

DORSAL MALUNIONS OF THE DISTAL RADIUS   A dorsal tilt deformity which is symptomatic may be treated by a corrective osteotomy of the distal radius; normal carpal alignment should be restored.

KIENBÖCK'S DISEASE

Robert Kienböck, in 1910, described what he called 'traumatic softening' of the lunate bone. This is a form of ischaemic necrosis that usually follows chronic stress or injury. It has been suggested that relative shortening of the ulna ('negative ulnar variance') predisposes to stress overload of the lunate between the distal edge of the radius and the carpus, but this has not been proven convincingly.

Pathology

As in other forms of ischaemic necrosis, the pathological changes proceed in four stages: *stage 1*, ischaemia without naked-eye or radiographic abnormality; *stage 2,* trabecular necrosis with reactive new bone formation and increased radiographic density, but little or no distortion of shape; *stage 3,* collapse of the bone; and *stage 4,* disruption of radio-carpal congruence and secondary OA.

Clinical features

The patient, usually a young adult, complains of ache and stiffness; only occasionally is there a history of acute trauma. Tenderness is localized over the lunate and grip strength is diminished. In the later stages wrist movements are limited and painful.

Imaging

X-rays at first show no abnormality, but radioscintigraphy may reveal increased activity. *MRI* is the most reliable way of detecting the early changes. Later, x-rays may show either mottled or diffuse density of the bone. In stage 3 the bone looks squashed and irregular, and in stage 4 there are osteoarthritic changes in the wrist.

Ulnar variance should be assessed by standardized x-ray examination with the shoulder abducted

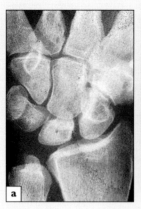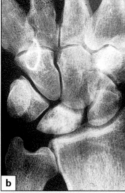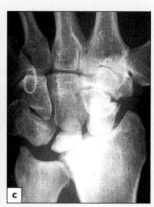

15.13 Kienböck's disease (a) In stage 2 – the bone shows mottled increase of density, but is still normal in shape. **(b)** In stage 3 – density is more marked and the lunate looks slightly squashed. **(c)** In stage 4 – the bone has collapsed and there is radio-carpal osteoarthritis. In all three the ulna looks disproportionately short.

to 90°, the forearm in neutral rotation and the wrist in neutral flexion-extension.

Treatment

NON-OPERATIVE TREATMENT
In early cases, splintage of the wrist for 6–12 weeks relieves pain and possibly reduces mechanical stress. If bone healing catches up with ischaemia, the lunate may remain virtually undistorted; this is more likely in very young patients. However, if pain persists, and even more so if the bone begins to flatten, operative treatment is indicated.

OPERATIVE TREATMENT
While the wrist architecture is only minimally disturbed (i.e. up to early stage 3), it seems rational to aim for a reduction of carpal stress by shortening the radius; the same can be achieved by lengthening the ulna but a bone graft is needed and union is less predictable.

Once the bone has collapsed, the options are limited. Lunate replacement by a silicone prosthesis, once popular, gives poor long-term results and is liable to cause synovitis. Other procedures, such as intercarpal fusion or excision of the proximal row of the carpus, may improve function but in the long term may not prevent the occurrence of OA. If pain and restriction of movement become intolerable, *radio-carpal arthrodesis* is the one reliable way of providing a stable, pain-free wrist.

TUBERCULOSIS

At the wrist, tuberculosis is rarely seen until it has progressed to a true arthritis (see also Chapter 2). Pain and stiffness come on gradually and the hand feels weak. The forearm looks wasted; the wrist is swollen and feels warm. Involvement of the flexor tendon compartment may give rise to a large fluctuant swelling that crosses the wrist into the palm (compound palmar ganglion). In a neglected case there may be a sinus. Movements are restricted and painful.

X-rays show localized osteoporosis and irregularity of the radio-carpal and intercarpal joints, and sometimes bone erosion.

Diagnosis

The condition must be differentiated from RA. Bilateral arthritis of the wrist is nearly always rheumatoid in origin, but when only one wrist is affected the signs resemble those of tuberculosis. X-rays and serological tests may establish the diagnosis, but often a biopsy is necessary.

Treatment

Antituberculous drugs are given and the wrist is splinted. If an abscess forms, it must be drained. If the wrist is destroyed, systemic treatment should be continued until the disease is quiescent and the wrist is then arthrodesed.

RHEUMATOID ARTHRITIS

After the metacarpophalangeal joints, the wrist is the most common site of RA (see also Chapter 3). Wrist and hand should always be considered together when dealing with RA.

Pathology

In the early stages, the cardinal features are synovitis of the radio-carpal and radio-ulnar joints and tenosynovitis of the extensor tendons. If the disease persists, the radio-carpal and intercarpal joints become eroded;

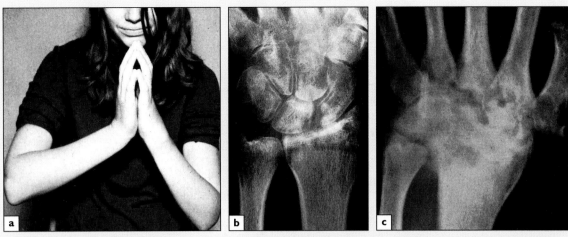

15.14 Tuberculosis (**a**) This girl presented with chronic ache and swelling of her left wrist; the forearm was wasted and extension absent; (**b**) her x-ray shows the washed-out appearance of osteoporosis around the wrist. (**c**) A different patient who had severe tuberculous arthritis; the disease is no longer active (hence the dense appearance), but destruction has been extensive.

this, together with tendon weakness or rupture, often leads to instability. An unstable wrist means a weak hand; deformities of the metacarpophalangeal joints are almost invariably associated with complementary deformities of the wrist.

Clinical features

Early symptoms are pain, swelling and stiffness of the wrists. At first the swelling is usually localized to the common extensor tendon sheath or the extensor carpi ulnaris, but as time progresses the joints become thickened and tender.

Gradually the wrist becomes unstable. Subluxation of the radio-ulnar joint causes the head of the ulna to pop up on the back of the wrist where it can be jogged up and down (the *piano-key sign*). The radio-carpal joint slides into abduction and volar subluxation; this usually precedes, and may contribute to, the classic ulnar drift deformity of the fingers.

Tendon lesions are common in the late stage. The first to rupture is usually the extensor digiti minimi, followed by the extensor communis tendons of the little and ring fingers. The flexor tendons seldom rupture but thickening of the synovium in the carpal tunnel may cause median nerve compression.

X-rays show osteoporosis and erosion of the ulnar styloid and of the radio-carpal and intercarpal joints. In the majority of cases the hands also will be affected, but there is a well-recognized group of patients (mostly elderly men) in whom the wrists carry the brunt of the disease.

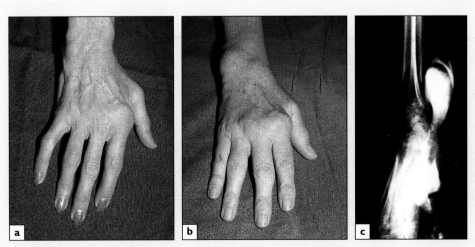

15.15 Rheumatoid arthritis (**a**) The typical deformities in RA: radial deviation at the wrist and ulnar deviation of the fingers. (**b**) In this patient the distal radio-ulnar joint is markedly swollen. (**c**) Contrast radiography showing a large synovial protrusion on the volar aspect of the wrist.

Treatment

Stage 1 In addition to systemic treatment, synovitis of the wrist and/or tendons will be helped by splintage and intrasynovial injections of corticosteroid preparations.

Stage 2 As joint erosion makes its appearance, the focus turns increasingly to the safeguarding of joint stability and the prevention of deformity. Synovectomy and soft-tissue stabilization may forestall further deterioration. Removal of the thickened synovium around the extensor tendons and placement of the extensor retinaculum beneath the tendons improves function and reduces the risk of tendon rupture. If the radio-ulnar joint is involved, synovectomy can be combined with excision of the ulnar head and transposition of the extensor carpi radialis longus to the ulnar side of the wrist (to counteract its tendency to radial drift).

Stage 3 In the late stage tendon rupture, joint destruction, instability and deformity may require reconstructive surgery. Direct repair of tendons is seldom possible; suture to an adjacent tendon, tendon grafting or tendon transfer is much better.

Joint replacement by a silicone 'spacer' has a high failure rate; it is reserved for patients who need to preserve some wrist movement but who have low functional demands, who do not depend on walking aids, have good bone stock and no tendon imbalance. Total wrist replacement with a metal–polyethylene device is generally unreliable. Salvage after a failed arthroplasty is very difficult because bone stock has been lost.

Arthrodesis is considered for pain and instability in the radio-carpal joint. The wrist is stabilized with a Steinman pin passed between the second and third metacarpals, across the carpus and into the distal radius; bone graft from the excised ulnar head is useful.

As a general rule, wrist deformities should be corrected before hand deformities.

OSTEOARTHRITIS OF THE WRIST

RADIO-CARPAL OSTEOARTHRITIS

OA is uncommon except as a sequel to injury. Any fracture into the joint may predispose to OA, but the commonest is a fractured scaphoid, especially with non-union or avascular necrosis. Post-traumatic carpal instability and Kienböck's disease are less frequent causes.

Clinical features

The patient may have forgotten the original injury. Years later he or she complains of pain and stiffness. At first these symptoms occur intermittently after use; later they become more constant, and recurrent 'wrist sprains' are common.

The appearance is usually normal and there is no wasting. Movements are limited and painful.

X-rays show irregular narrowing of the radio-carpal joint, with subchondral sclerosis. A predisposing cause, such as an intra-articular fracture or Kienböck's disease, may be apparent.

Treatment

Rest, in a polythene splint, is often sufficient treatment. Excision of the distal part of the radial styloid process

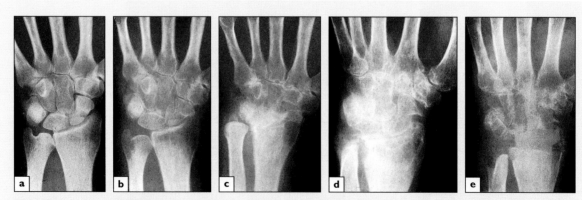

15.16 Rheumatoid arthritis (**a**) At first the x-rays show only soft-tissue swelling; (**b**) 2 years later, this patient shows early bone changes – periarticular osteoporosis and diminution of the joint space; (**c**) 5 years later still, bony erosions and joint destruction are marked. (**d**) Another patient with severe disease, who has been treated by (**e**) excising the diseased surfaces and inserting a Silastic spacer – reasonable stability was restored; this can be done only if the joint has not been too severely distorted.

is helpful when OA has followed a scaphoid fracture and is limited to that part of the joint.

Arthrodesis of the wrist is occasionally necessary. The radio-carpal and intercarpal joints are de-corticated, bone graft is impacted and a compression plate is fixed to the third metacarpal and the distal radius. Contouring the plate to 15° of dorsiflexion may improve grip strength.

DISTAL RADIO–ULNAR ARTHRITIS

Progressive destruction of the distal radio-ulnar joint is a characteristic feature of severe RA. Lesser degenerative changes are seen in secondary OA, possibly following marked and long-standing instability of the joint. If pain and loss of function cannot be controlled by conservative measures, the patient may benefit from resection (or partial resection) of the distal ulna. An alternative approach is to fuse the distal ulna to the radius (the Suavé–Kapandji procedure); forearm rotation is restored by excising a short section of the ulnar shaft proximal to the arthrodesis. The patient should be warned that these procedures usually achieve only a limited improvement in function and may cause instability.

CARPOMETACARPAL OSTEOARTHRITIS

OA of the trapezio-metacarpal joint is common in postmenopausal women. It is often accompanied by Heberden's nodes of the finger joints, in which case it is usually bilateral and part of a generalized OA.

Clinical features

The patient, usually a middle-aged woman, complains of diffuse pain around the base of her thumb. Pinch and grip are weakened. On examination, the joint is swollen and in advanced cases is held in an adducted position,

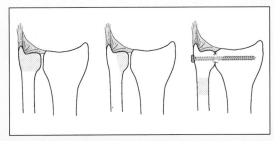

15.17 Distal radio-ulnar joint arthritis Three operations used in the treatment of radio-ulnar arthritis: (**a**) resection of the distal end of the ulna (the Darrach operation); (**b**) partial resection of the distal ulna; (**c**) the Suavé-Kapandji operation – arthrodesis plus ulnar resection.

with prominence of the subluxed metacarpal base. The joint is tender and the 'grind test' (compressing and rotating the metacarpal longitudinally against the trapezium) is painful.

X-rays show narrowing of the trapezio-metacarpal joint. Radioscintigraphy is useful in early cases when the diagnosis is in doubt; increased activity precedes the more obvious x-ray changes.

Treatment

Most patients can be treated by anti-inflammatory preparations, local corticosteroid injections and temporary splintage. If these measures fail to control pain, or if instability becomes marked, operative treatment may be necessary.

Excision of the trapezium (excisional arthroplasty) gives pain relief and return of function, though thumb pinch is always weak. The bone is best removed through the palmar approach rather than the anatomical snuff box. Attempts have been made to prevent postoperative collapse of the joint and proximal migration of the

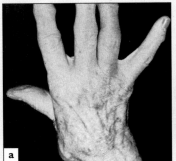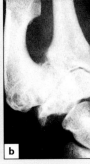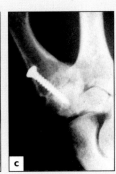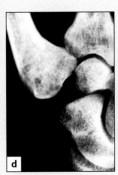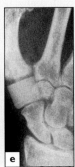

15.18 Osteoarthritis of the traprezio-metacarpal thumb joint (**a**) Typical deformity in an advanced case, with (**b**) narrow joint space and osteophytes. If operation is needed, the possibilities are (**c**) arthrodesis, (**d**) excision of the trapezium, or (**e**) replacement arthroplasty using a Silastic spacer.

metacarpal. A free strip of tendon is coiled up and placed in the empty space; another option is to stabilize the metacarpal by re-routing a slip of flexor carpi radialis or abductor pollicis longus tendon and attaching it to a drill hole in the metacarpal base.

Replacement arthroplasty using a silicone spacer has a high complication rate and the results are unpredictable.

Arthrodesis of the trapezio-metacarpal joint relieves pain, but the restriction of movement is a distinct drawback. The scapho-trapezial joint should be normal.

SCAPHO-LUNATE ADVANCED COLLAPSE (SLAC)

A late complication of unreduced scapho-lunate dissociation is OA which begins between the radial styloid and scaphoid and then progresses to the midcarpal joint. In the earliest stage, excision of the tip of the radial styloid may help if only the distal pole of the scaphoid is involved. In later stages, scaphoid excision and limited intercarpal fusion, or else proximal row excision, may be considered. However, these procedures are not always effective; total radio-carpal fusion is more reliable. The real answer is earlier diagnosis and treatment of scapho-lunate dissociation!

TENOSYNOVITIS AND TENOVAGINITIS

The extensor retinaculum contains six compartments which transmit tendons lined with synovium. Tenosynovitis can be caused by unaccustomed movement, overuse or repetitive minor trauma; sometimes it occurs spontaneously. The resulting synovial inflammation causes secondary thickening of the sheath and stenosis of the compartment, which further compromises the tendon. Early treatment, including rest, anti-inflammatory medication and injection of corticosteroids, may break this vicious circle.

The first dorsal compartment (abductor pollicis longus and extensor pollicis brevis) and the second dorsal compartment (extensor carpi radialis brevis) are most commonly affected.

The flexor tendons are affected far less frequently.

DE QUERVAIN'S DISEASE

Pathology This condition, first described in 1895, is caused by reactive thickening of the sheath around the extensor pollicis brevis and abductor pollicis longus tendons within the first extensor compartment. It may be initiated by overuse but it also occurs spontaneously, particularly in middle-aged women, and sometimes during pregnancy.

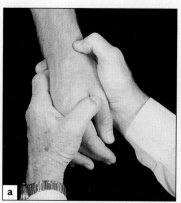
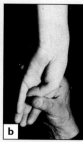

15.19 De Quervain's disease (**a**) There is point tenderness at the tip of the radial styloid process. (**b**) Finkelstein's test – stretching the tendons in the common sheath on the radial side of the wrist causes intense pain.

Clinical features The patient is usually a woman aged 40–50 years, who complains of pain on the radial side of the wrist. There may be a history of unaccustomed activity such as pruning roses or wringing out clothes. Sometimes there is a visible swelling over the distal end of the radius, and the tendon sheath feels thick and hard. Tenderness is most acute at the very tip of the radial styloid.

The pathognomonic sign is elicited by *Finkelstein's test*. The examiner places the patient's thumb across the palm in full flexion and then, holding the patient's hand firmly, turns the wrist sharply into adduction. In a positive test this is acutely painful; repeating the movement with the thumb left free is relatively painless.

The *differential diagnosis* includes arthritis at the base of the thumb, scaphoid non-union and the intersection syndrome (see below).

Treatment The early case can be relieved by a corticosteroid injection into the tendon sheath, sometimes combined with splintage of the wrist. Resistant cases need an operation, which consists of slitting the thickened tendon sheath. Sometimes there is duplication of tendons and even of the sheath, in which case both sheaths need to be divided. Care should be taken to prevent injury to the dorsal sensory branches of the radial nerve, which may cause intractable dysaesthesia.

INTERSECTION SYNDROME

This condition, otherwise known as *crossover syndrome* or *peritendinitis crepitans*, is characterized by pain, swelling and crepitus over the tendons of extensor pollicis brevis and abductor pollicis longus, 4–6cm proximal to the extensor retinaculum. It is found in weight-lifters, canoeists and rowers. It should be distinguished clinically from de Quervain's disease. The condition is generally attributed to friction between these tendons (the so-called 'outcropping tendons') and the underlying longitudinally-aligned extensor tendons, leading to an adventitious bursa or a tenosynovitis. There is always an associated tenosynovitis within the second extensor compartment containing extensors carpi radialis longus and brevis.

Treatment involves rest, splintage, corticosteroid injection and, in resistant cases, surgical release of the second compartment and exploration of the intersection.

OTHER SITES OF EXTENSOR TENOSYNOVITIS

Tenosynovitis of *extensor carpi radialis brevis* (the most powerful extensor of the wrist) or *extensor carpi ulnaris* may cause pain and point tenderness just medial to the anatomical snuffbox or immediately distal to the head of the ulna, respectively (see Figure 15.2). Splintage and corticosteroid injections are usually effective.

The common extensor compartment is occasionally irritated by direct trauma. Patients present with pain and crepitation on the dorsum of the wrist; flexing and extending the fingers produces a fine, palpable crepitus over the common extensor compartment. Treatment is by rest and splintage of the wrist.

FLEXOR TENDINITIS

Except in specific inflammatory disorders such as RA, the flexor tendons are rarely affected.

Flexor carpi radialis tendinitis causes pain on the front of the wrist alongside the scaphoid tubercle; symptoms are reproduced by resisted wrist flexion. Tenderness is sharply localized and should be distinguished from that of de Quervain's disease or OA of the basal joint of the thumb.

Flexor carpi ulnaris can become inflamed near its insertion into the pisiform. Occasionally x-rays show calcific deposits around the sheath.

Treatment of these conditions is the same as for the other types of tenosynovitis.

OCCUPATIONAL PAIN DISORDERS

Terms such as *repetitive stress injury* and *cumulative trauma disorder* have been used for a controversial syndrome comprising ill-defined and unusually disabling pain around the wrist and forearm (and sometimes the entire limb) which is usually ascribed to a particular work practice. In some cases there is undoubted evidence of tenosynovitis, which could

have been caused by unaccustomed or prolonged activity of a particular kind. Epidemiological studies suggest that these conditions are no more common amongst keyboard operators than in the general population. What has fuelled the controversy surrounding the 'occupational' disorders is their apparent severity and intractability compared with other types of overuse syndrome.

SWELLINGS AROUND THE WRIST

GANGLION CYSTS

Pathology The ganglion cyst is the most common swelling in the wrist. It arises from leakage of synovial fluid from a joint or tendon sheath and contains a glairy, viscous fluid. Although it can appear anywhere around the carpus, it usually develops on the dorsal surface of the scapho-lunate ligament. Palmar wrist ganglia usually arise from the scapho-lunate or scapho-trapezio-trapezioid joint.

Clinical features The patient, often a young adult, presents with a painless lump, though occasionally there is slight ache and weakness. The lump is well defined, cystic and not tender; it can sometimes be transilluminated. It does not move with the tendons. The back of the wrist is the commonest site; less frequently a ganglion emerges alongside the radial artery on the volar aspect. Occasionally a small, hidden ganglion is found to be the cause of compression of the deep (muscular) branch of the ulnar nerve.

Treatment Treatment is usually unnecessary. The lump can safely be left alone; it often disappears spontaneously. If it becomes troublesome, and certainly if there is any pressure on a nerve, operative removal is justified. Even then it may recur with embarrassing persistence; it is not easy to ensure that every shred of abnormal tissue is removed.

EXTENSOR TENOSYNOVITIS

Localized swelling of a tendon sheath on the dorsum of the wrist sometimes occurs in rheumatoid disease and can be mistaken for a 'cyst' (see Figure 15.1).

'COMPOUND PALMAR GANGLION'

This lesion is neither a ganglion nor compound. Chronic inflammation distends the common sheath of the flexor tendons both above and below the flexor

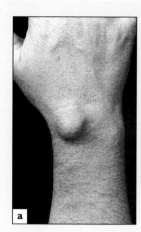
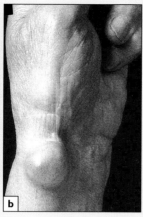
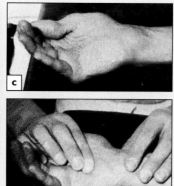

15.20 Wrist swellings
(**a, b**) Common sites of simple ganglion. (**c, d**) 'Compound palmar ganglion' with cross-fluctuation.

retinaculum. RA and tuberculosis are the commonest causes. The synovial membrane becomes thick and villous. The amount of fluid is increased and it may contain fibrin particles moulded by repeated movement to the shape of melon seeds. The tendons may eventually fray and rupture.

Clinical features Pain is unusual but paraesthesia due to median nerve compression may occur. The swelling is hourglass in shape, bulging above and below the flexor retinaculum; it is not warm or tender; fluid can be pushed from one part to the other (cross-fluctuation).

Treatment If the condition is tuberculous, general treatment is begun. The contents of the sac are evacuated, streptomycin is instilled and the wrist rested in a splint. If these measures fail, the entire flexor sheath is dissected out. Complete excision is also the best treatment when the cause is rheumatoid disease.

CARPAL TUNNEL SYNDROME

The carpal tunnel syndrome, due to median nerve compression under the flexor retinaculum of the wrist, is described together with other nerve compression disorders in Chapter 11.

NOTES ON APPLIED ANATOMY

In most positions of the forearm the styloid process of the radius is more distal than that of the ulna, but with the forearm supinated the two processes are at approximately the same level. The relationship may be altered as a result of injury; relative shortness of the ulna also

appears as an anatomical variant in association with Kienböck's disease.

Just distal to the radial styloid is the scaphoid, immediately beneath the anatomical snuffbox, which is one of the key areas for localizing tenderness. Tenderness at the distal end of the snuffbox may incriminate the carpometacarpal joint of the thumb. More proximal tenderness, at the tip of the radial styloid, is characteristic of de Quervain's disease. Dorsal to the snuffbox the oblique course of extensor pollicis longus exposes it to damage by a careless incision.

The carpal bones are arranged in two rows, with the pisiform as the odd man out. The scaphoid, trapezium and thumb combine to function almost as a separate entity, a 'jointed strut', with independent movement; degenerative arthritis of the wrist occurs most commonly in the joints of this strut.

Wrist dorsiflexion takes place at both the radiocarpal joint and at the midcarpal joint. Abduction (radial deviation) of the wrist is much less than adduction. When the wrist is fully dorsiflexed the scaphoid, which straddles the mid-carpal joint, swivels backwards. Even so, it is vulnerable and liable to fracture.

Stability of the carpus depends not only upon bony conformity, joint capsules and overlying tendons but also upon a series of tough ligaments. The volar radiocarpal ligament is the most important of these and, if torn, leads to carpal instability.

On their volar aspect the carpal bones form a concavity roofed over by the carpal ligament; in the tunnel lie the flexor tendons and sheath together with the median nerve. The thenar branch of the nerve (supplying the all-important thenar muscles) is in danger if, during a decompression operation, the carpal ligament is divided too far radially. On the radial side of the wrist, branches of the radial nerve are vulnerable; and on the ulnar side, the close relationship of the ulnar nerve to the pisiform must be borne in mind.

REFERENCES AND FURTHER READING

Bednar JM, Osterman AL (1993) Carpal instability: Evaluation and treatment. *Journal of the American Academy of Orthopaedic Surgeons* 1, 10-17

Chidgey LK (1995) The distal radioulnar joint: Problems and solutions. *Journal of the American Academy of Orthopaedic Surgeons* 3, 95-109

Cooney WP, Linscheid RL, Dobyns JH (1994) Triangular fibrocartilage tears. *Journal of Hand Surgery* 19A, 143-154

Dantel G, Goudot B, Merle M (1993) Arthroscopic diagnosis of scapho-lunate instability in the absence of x-ray abnormalities. *Journal of Hand Surgery* 18B, 403-406

Garcia-Elias M (1997) The treatment of wrist instability. *Journal of Bone and Joint Surgery* 79B, 684-690

Hand Surgery Update (1996) American Society for Surgery of the Hand. AAOS, Illinois

Manske PR (1996) Longitudinal failure of upper-limb formation. *Journal of Bone and Joint Surgery* 78A, 1600-1623

Osterman AL (1990) Arthroscopic debridement of triangular fibrocartilage complex tears. *Arthroscopy* 6, 120-124

Palmer AK, Werner FW (1989) Triangular fibrocartilage complex lesions: A classification. *Journal of Hand Surgery* 14A, 594-606

Richards RR (1996) Chronic disorders of the forearm. *Journal of Bone and Joint Surgery* 78A, 916-930

Stanley JK, Trail IA (1994) Carpal instability. *Journal of Bone and Joint Surgery* 76B, 691-700

Ruby LK (1995) Carpal instability. *Journal of Bone and Joint Surgery* 77A, 476-487

Terrona AL, Feldon PG, Millender LH, Nalebuff EA (1995) Evaluation and treatment of the rheumatoid wrist. *Journal of Bone and Joint Surgery* 77A, 1116-1128

Siegal JM, Ruby LK (1996) A critical look at intercarpal arthrodesis: review of the literature. *Journal of Hand Surgery* 21A, 717-723

Vender MI, Kasdan ML, Truppa KL (1995) Upper extremity disorders: a review of the literature to determine work-relatedness. *Journal of Hand Surgery* 20A, 534-541

The hand

The hand is (in more senses than one) the medium of introduction to the outside world. Its unique repertoire of prehensile movements and tactile acuity sets us apart from all other species. We usually think of the hand as a sophisticated tool, but it is also an organ of communication, used for gesturing and expressing a range of emotions from anxiety and fear to submission and helplessness, scorn and hatred, determination and control, or tenderness and love. We are more aware of our hands than of any other part of the body; when they go wrong we know about it from a very early stage.

CLINICAL ASSESSMENT

SYMPTOMS

Pain is usually felt in the palm or in the finger joints. Remember, though, that a poorly defined ache may be referred from the neck, shoulder or mediastinum.

Deformity may appear suddenly (due to tendon rupture) or slowly (suggesting bone, joint or other pathology).

Swelling may be localized, or may occur in many joints simultaneously. Characteristically, rheumatoid arthritis causes swelling of the proximal joints, and osteoarthritis the distal joints.

Loss of function is particularly troublesome and can take various forms. The patient may have difficulty handling eating utensils, holding a cup or glass, grasping a doorknob (or a crutch), dressing or (most trying of all) attending to personal hygiene.

Sensory symptoms and motor weakness provide well-defined clues to neurological disorders. A precise description of the affected area tells us a great deal about the level of the lesion.

SIGNS

Both upper limbs should be bared for comparison; ask which is the dominant hand. A rapid assessment can be carried out in a few minutes. A full examination needs patience and meticulous attention to detail.

Look

Note how the patient holds the hand and uses it during the interview; the resting posture may be suggestive of nerve or tendon damage (see below). Ask the patient to place both hands on the table in front of you, with the palms first upwards and then downwards. The skin may be scarred, altered in colour, dry or moist, and hairy or smooth. Wasting and deformity, and the presence of any lumps, should be noted. Swelling may be in the subcutaneous tissue, in a tendon sheath or in a joint. The nails may show signs of atrophy or disease (e.g. psoriasis).

Feel

The temperature and texture of the skin are noted and the pulse is felt. If a nodule is felt, the underlying tendon should be moved to discover if it is attached. Swelling or thickening may be in the subcutaneous tissue, a tendon sheath, a joint or one of the bones. Tenderness should be accurately localized to one of these structures.

Move

Active movements With palms facing upwards the fingers are curled into full flexion; a 'lagging finger' is immediately obvious. Individual movements are then examined, first at the metacarpophalangeal joints and then at each interphalangeal joint in turn. The patient is asked to touch the tip of each finger with the tip of the thumb. More detailed examination of active movements is described below.

Passive movements These are examined in a similar manner, noting the range of movement at each joint.

Posture during rest and movement

Normally with the palm upwards, the fingers fall into a gentle 'cascade' with the metacarpophalangeal joints flexed – about 40° in the index finger, ranging to 70° in the little finger. The interphalangeal joints similarly lie in increasing flexion from index to little finger. When the hand is turned palm downwards, the fingers straighten out, again in a gentle cascade with greater extension on the index finger than the little finger. If the cascade is interrupted, then a tendon may be inactive, divided or stuck. If the cascade is normal but active movements are not possible, then a nerve injury should be suspected.

Note the reciprocal relationship between the position of the wrist and the resting position of the fingers. If you allow your wrist to drop into flexion, the fingers

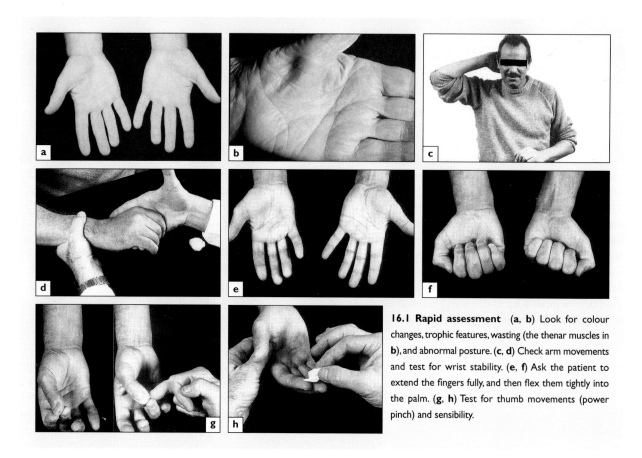

16.1 Rapid assessment (**a**, **b**) Look for colour changes, trophic features, wasting (the thenar muscles in **b**), and abnormal posture. (**c**, **d**) Check arm movements and test for wrist stability. (**e**, **f**) Ask the patient to extend the fingers fully, and then flex them tightly into the palm. (**g**, **h**) Test for thumb movements (power pinch) and sensibility.

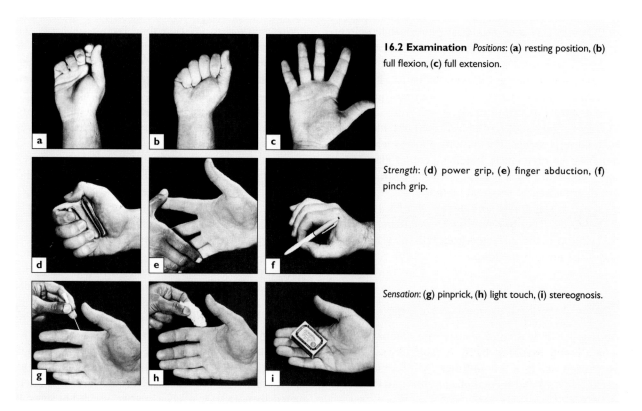

16.2 Examination *Positions*: (**a**) resting position, (**b**) full flexion, (**c**) full extension.

Strength: (**d**) power grip, (**e**) finger abduction, (**f**) pinch grip.

Sensation: (**g**) pinprick, (**h**) light touch, (**i**) stereognosis.

'automatically' tend to straighten and as the wrist is pulled into extension the fingers flex slightly. If the long flexors are shortened, the fingers will curl tightly in flexion as the wrist is extended.

Testing for active movement

Testing *flexor digitorum profundus* is straightforward: the proximal interphalangeal joint is immobilized and the patient is then asked to bend the tip of the finger.

To test *flexor digitorum superficialis,* the flexor profundus must first be inactivated, otherwise one cannot tell which tendon is flexing the proximal interphalangeal joint. This is done by grasping all the fingers, except the one being examined, and holding them firmly in full extension; because the profundus tendons share a common muscle belly, this manoeuvre automatically prevents *all* the profundus tendons from participating in finger flexion. The patient is then asked to flex the isolated finger which is being examined; this movement must be activated by flexor digitorum superficialis. There are two exceptions to this rule. Firstly, the little finger sometimes has no independent flexor digitorum superficialis. Secondly, the index finger often has an entirely separate flexor profundus, which cannot be inactivated by the usual mass action manoeuvre; instead, flexor superficialis is tested by asking the patient to pinch hard with the distal interphalangeal joint in full extension and the proximal interphalangeal joint in full flexion (this position can be maintained only if the superficialis tendon is active and intact).

The *long extensors* are tested by asking the patient to extend the metacarpophalangeal joints. Inability to do this does not necessarily signify either paralysis or tendon rupture: the long extensor tendon may simply have slipped off the knuckle into the interdigital gutter (a common occurrence in rheumatoid arthritis).

Metacarpophalangeal flexion and interphalangeal extension are activated by the *intrinsic muscles (lumbricals and interossei).* Ask the patient to extend the fingers with the metacarpophalangeal joints flexed (the 'duckbill' position). The interossei also motivate finger abduction and adduction.

Thumb movements are somewhat confusing as they also involve the metacarpal. With the hand lying flat, palm upwards, five types of movement are possible: *extension* (sideways movement in the plane of the palm); *abduction* (upwards movement at right angles to the palm); *adduction* (pressing against the palm); *flexion* (sideways movement towards the palm in the plane of the palm) and *opposition* (touching the tips of the fingers). Since the thumb has only a single interphalangeal joint, the *flexor pollicis longus* is tested by immobilizing the thumb metacarpophalangeal joint.

Grip strength

Grip strength is assessed by asking the patient to squeeze the examiner's fingers; it may be diminished because of muscle weakness, tendon damage, finger stiffness or wrist instability. Strength can be measured more accurately by having the patient squeeze a partially inflated sphygmomanometer cuff (normally a pressure of 150mmHg can be achieved easily) or a mechanical dynamometer. Pinch grip also should be measured.

NEUROLOGICAL ASSESSMENT

If symptoms such as numbness, tingling or weakness exist – and in all cases of trauma – a full neurological examination of the upper limb should be carried out,

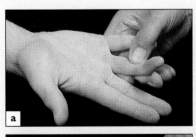
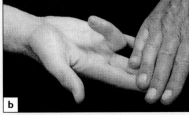
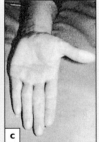
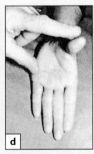
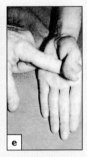

16.3 Finger and thumb movements (a) Testing flexor digitorum profundus; and (b) flexor superficialis. (c, d, e) Thumb movements. With the hand held flat on the table and palm upwards, the patient is asked to (c) stretch the thumb away from the hand (extension), (d) lift it towards the ceiling (abduction) and (e) squeeze down on the examiner's finger (adduction). Opposition is shown in Fig. 16.1g.

testing power, reflexes and sensation. Further refinement is achieved by testing two-point discrimination, sensibility to heat and cold, and stereognosis.

FUNCTIONAL TESTS

Ultimately it is function that counts; patients learn to overcome their defects by ingenious modifications and trick movements. There are several types of grip, which can be tested by giving the patient a variety of tasks to perform: picking up a pin (precision grip), holding a sheet of paper (pinch), holding a key (sideways pinch), holding a pen (chuck grip), holding a bag handle (hook grip), holding a glass (span) and gripping a hammer handle (power grip).

Each finger has its special task: the thumb and index finger are used for pinch. The index finger is also an important sensory organ; slight loss of movement matters little, but if sensation is abnormal the patient probably won't use the finger at all. The middle finger controls the position of objects in the palm. The ring and little fingers are used for power grip; any loss of movement here will affect function markedly.

CONGENITAL VARIATIONS

The hand and foot are much the commonest sites of congenital variations in the musculoskeletal system; the incidence is at least one in 1000 live births. The cause may be an inherited genetic defect, a chromosome disorder or an embryonal insult due to viral infection, nuclear radiation or harmful drug administration during the first 2 months of pregnancy.

Early recognition is important and definitive treatment should be timed to fit in with the developing skills and functional demands of the child. If surgery is contemplated, it should be carried out as soon as it is technically feasible and preferably before the age of 3 years. Often, the procedures have to be staged and this needs careful planning. Psychological support for parents and children is important if problems of social adaptation and self-esteem are to be avoided.

The clinical disorders are conventionally divided into seven groups (see Box).

FAILURE OF FORMATION

The upper limb can fail to develop either *transversely* or *longitudinally*.

Transverse failure

Transverse failure may occur at any level, the commonest being the proximal third of the forearm. Absence of

parts of the fingers (symbrachydactyly) can be managed by non-vascularized bone transfer or microvascular transfer of a toe, or by simply fitting a prosthesis. More proximal defects can, as yet, be dealt with only by prosthetic replacement.

Longitudinal failure

The deficiency can be *radial, ulnar* or *central.*

RADIAL LONGITUDINAL DEFICIENCY (RADIAL CLUB HAND) There is partial or complete absence of the thumb and/or radius; the typical deformity is one of marked radial deviation of the wrist and hand. In some cases the humerus is fused to the ulna. Associated anomalies should be sought, especially in the heart and blood vessels, since these may also need treatment and could compromise the safety of an anaesthetic.

The parents should be taught to manipulate the infant's wrist and elbow regularly from birth. At 6–12 months the wrist is centralized on the end of the ulna: the soft tissues are released, bone is resected and the reduction is held with a K-wire for several weeks. The wrist should not be centralized if the elbow is so stiff that the hand would not then reach the mouth. If the thumb is absent, then the index finger should be pollicised (shortened and rotated to form a new thumb) a few months later.

Classification of congenital variations	
Type	**Example**
Failure of formation	Transverse absence
	Longitudinal absence – radial (radial club hand)
	Longitudinal absence – ulnar (ulnar club hand)
	Longitudinal absence – central (typical cleft hand)
Failure of differentiation	Syndactyly
	Symphalangism
	Camptodactyly
	Clinodactyly
	Flexed thumb
	Arthrogryposis
Duplication	Thumb duplication
Overgrowth	Macrodactyly
Undergrowth	Thumb hypoplasia
Constriction ring syndrome	Simple rings
Generalized skeletal abnormalities	Marfan's, Turner's, Down's etc.

ULNAR LONGITUDINAL DEFICIENCY (ULNAR CLUB HAND) This is much rarer than radial club hand. Digits are absent from the ulnar side of the hand and the remaining digits are often syndactylized. The elbow is frequently unstable or stiff. The condition is associated with skeletal defects such as fibular hemimelia rather than the visceral defects which frequently accompany a radial longitudinal deficiency.

Treatment includes syndactyly release, excision of soft tissue tether ('anlage') and stabilization of the elbow.

CENTRAL LONGITUDINAL DEFICIENCY ('CLEFT HAND') This usually presents as a familial disorder. Typically, the second, third and fourth rays are affected. The condition is bilateral and the feet are often involved. The appearance ranges from a simple cleft, with only the middle ray missing, to absence of all three central rays (unkindly described as a 'lobster claw'). Function is often excellent despite the appearance, and reconstructive surgery should be undertaken only if this offers some definite improvement.

FAILURE OF DIFFERENTIATION

Syndactyly (congenital webbing) is the most common congenital variation in the hand. It may be *simple* (skin only) or *complex* (skin and bone). With *acrosyndactyly*, only the tips are joined. When the fingers are surgically separated, skin grafts are almost always required. If more than two fingers are to be divided, it is wise to stage the procedures in case the blood vessels on each side of a digit are damaged.

Camptodactyly is a flexion deformity of the proximal interphalangeal joint (usually of the little finger). It is hereditary and often bilateral, but deformity is rarely obvious before the age of 10 years. A normal distal interphalangeal joint distinguishes it from a boutonnière deformity. Splintage can help, but surgery is rarely beneficial. In the rare cases which are explored because of a marked, troublesome deformity, an abnormal insertion of either the lumbrical or the superficialis tendon is usually found.

Clinodactyly is the term used for a finger which is bent sideways. Usually the little finger is involved. In mild cases treatment is not needed. In severe deformity, the cause is usually a 'delta' deformity of the middle phalanx, in which the epiphysis curves along one side of the bone; osteotomy may be required.

Kirner's deformity is not congenital but is mentioned here as it could otherwise be mistaken for a camptodactyly or clinodactyly. Presenting in adolescence, the distal phalanx (yet again, the little finger) becomes swollen and curved. Treatment is with splintage and occasionally osteotomy.

Hereditary symphalangism describes congenital stiffness of the proximal interphalangeal joint. The whole finger is small, shiny and stiff. Motion cannot be restored with surgery.

Arthrogryposis is a condition in which there is severe muscle weakness caused by an intrinsic abnormality of the motor nerves and muscle. The joints are stiff and contracted. The overlying skin is smooth, without flexion creases. There may be a single abnormality, such as a pronated forearm, flexed wrist or clasped thumb, or the whole limb may be involved. Treatment includes splintage, tendon transfers and arthrodesis.

Congenital clasped thumb is due to weak or absent extensor tendons (and contractures of the metacarpophalangeal and carpometacarpal joints in severe cases). Simple extensor tendon weakness may respond to splintage in extension for a few months; if this fails, an extensor tendon transfer is needed.

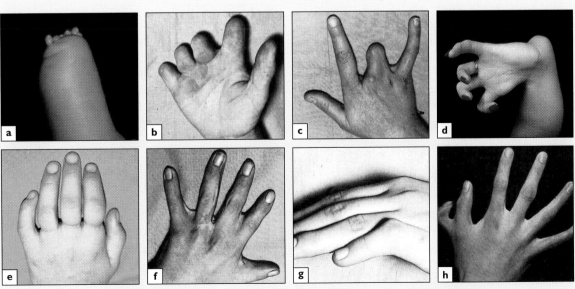

16.4 Congenital variations (**a**) Transverse failure of formation; (**b**) transverse failure in fingers; (**c**) central failure of formation; (**d**) radial longitudinal deficiency ('radial club hand'); (**e**) constriction rings; (**f**) syndactyly; (**g**) camptodactyly; (**h**) extra digits.

The condition must be distinguished from a *'congenital' trigger thumb,* which is due to stenosing tenovaginitis of the flexor pollicis longus. The parents notice that the child's thumb is fixed in flexion; a firm nodule can be felt over the front of the metacarpophalangeal joint. The defect may resolve spontaneously within the first year. If it does not, then surgical release of the pulley at the metacarpophalangeal joint is curative.

DUPLICATION

Polydactyly (extra digits) is nearly as common as syndactyly. An *extra little finger* is usually inherited and other variations may be present. By contrast, an *extra thumb* is usually sporadic. An *extra central digit,* the rarest of the duplications, is often associated with syndactyly and disorganization of the skeleton.

Extra skin tags can be simply excised. Anything more complex needs meticulous surgery because of the altered skin cover and associated variations in the soft tissues and bone.

OVERGROWTH

Macrodactyly has a neurogenic cause. The giant finger is stiff and unsightly, but attempts at operative reduction are fraught with complications. The finger cannot be made normal; several attempts may be needed to reduce the size, each leaving the finger increasingly stiff and scarred.

UNDERGROWTH

The thumb is most commonly affected, the defect ranging from a slightly small digit to complete aplasia. The most severe forms need a pollicization to provide a post to oppose against the fingers; less severe forms may need a web space release, stabilization of

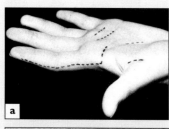
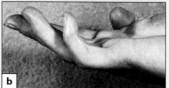

16.5 Acquired deformities – skin (a) Skin incisions should never cross the creases on the flexor surface; those shown are safe; (b) postoperative contracture of a badly placed scar.

the metacarpophalangeal joint, correction of abnormal tendons and a muscle transfer to provide opposition.

CONSTRICTION BANDS

These may occur in any part of the limb. The consequences range from complete amputation to an obvious circumferential constriction with a viable distal part. The latter is treated by multiple Z-plasties.

GENERALIZED SKELETAL ABNORMALITIES

Generalized skeletal disorders often involve the hand, e.g. Marfan's syndrome ('spider hand'), achondroplasia ('trident hand') and Down's syndrome (short little finger, often curved).

ACQUIRED DEFORMITIES

Deformity of the hand may result from disorders of the skin, subcutaneous tissues, muscles, tendons, joints, bones or neuromuscular function. Often there is a history of trauma or infection or concomitant disease; at other times the patient is unaware of any cause.

Problems arise for three reasons: (1) the defect may be very unsightly; (2) function is impaired; and (3) the deformed part becomes a nuisance during daily activities.

Assessment and management of hand deformities demand a detailed knowledge of functional anatomy and, in particular, of the normal mechanisms of balanced movement in the wrist and fingers.

SKIN CONTRACTURE

Cuts and burns of the palmar skin are liable to heal with contracture. *Surgical incisions should never cross skin creases;* they should lie more or less parallel or oblique to them, or in the mid-axial line of the fingers. A useful alternative is a zig-zag incision with the middle part of the Z in the skin crease. Longitudinal wounds can also be closed as Z-plasties.

Established contractures may require excision of the scar, Z-plasty of the remaining skin, skin grafts, a pedicled flap and occasionally a free flap.

SUPERFICIAL PALMAR FASCIA (DUPUYTREN'S) CONTRACTURE

The superficial palmar fascia (palmar aponeurosis) fans out from the wrist towards the fingers, sending extensions across the metacarpophalangeal joints to the fingers. Hypertrophy and contracture of the palmar fascia may lead to puckering of the palmar skin and fixed flexion of the fingers (see page 343).

MUSCLE CONTRACTURE

VOLKMANN'S ISCHAEMIC CONTRACTURE   Contracture of the forearm muscles may follow circulatory insufficiency due to injuries at or below the elbow. Shortening of the long flexors causes the fingers to be held in flexion; they can be straightened only when the wrist is flexed so as to relax the long flexors. Sometimes the picture is complicated by associated damage to the ulnar or median nerve (or both). If disability is marked, some improvement may be obtained by lengthening the shortened tendons, or else by excising the dead muscles and restoring finger movement with tendon transfers.

SHORTENING OF THE INTRINSIC MUSCLES   Shortening of the intrinsic muscles in the hand produces a characteristic deformity: flexion at the metacarpophalangeal joints with extension of the interphalangeal joints and adduction of the thumb (the so-called *'intrinsic-plus' hand*). Slight degrees of deformity may not be obvious, but can be diagnosed by the 'intrinsic-plus' test: with the metacarpophalangeal joints pushed passively into hyperextension (thus putting the intrinsics on stretch), it is difficult or impossible to flex the interphalangeal joints passively. The causes of intrinsic shortening or contracture are: (1) spasticity (e.g. in cerebral palsy); (2) volar subluxation of the metacarpophalangeal joints (e.g. in rheumatoid arthritis); (3) scarring after trauma or infection; and (4) shrinkage due to distal ischaemia. Moderate contracture can be treated by resecting a triangular segment of the intrinsic 'aponeurosis' at the base of the proximal phalanx (Littler's operation).

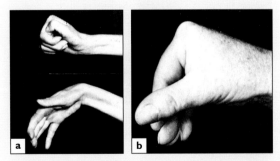

16.6 Deformities – muscle **(a)** Ischaemic contracture of the long flexors in the forearm; with the wrist in extension, the fingers involuntarily curl into flexion; when the wrist flexes, the pull on the finger flexors is released. **(b)** Flexion deformity due to ischaemic contracture of the intrinsic hand muscles (the 'intrinsic-plus' hand).

TENDON LESIONS

MALLET FINGER   This results from injury to the extensor tendon of the terminal phalanx. It may be due to direct trauma but more often follows tendon rupture when the finger tip is forcibly bent during active extension, perhaps while tucking the blankets under a mattress or trying to catch a ball. The terminal joint is held flexed and the patient cannot straighten it, but passive movement is normal. With the extensor mechanism unbalanced, the proximal interphalangeal joint may become hyperextended.

An acute mallet finger should be splinted with the joint in extension for 8 weeks. This treatment may still work if presentation is delayed for a few weeks. Surgery is ill-advised, even with fracture dislocations, as the complication rate is very high and it is unlikely to improve the outcome. Old lesions need treatment only if the deformity is marked, hand function seriously impaired and the joint still mobile. The options include fusion, tendon reconstruction or Fowler's central slip tenotomy.

RUPTURED EXTENSOR POLLICIS LONGUS   The long thumb extensor may rupture after fraying or ischaemia where it crosses the wrist (e.g. after a Colles' fracture, or in rheumatoid arthritis). The distal phalanx drops into flexion; it can be passively extended, and there may still be weak active extension because of thenar muscle insertion into the extensor expansion. Direct repair is unsatisfactory and a tendon transfer, using the extensor indicis, is needed.

DROPPED FINGER   Sudden loss of finger extension at the metacarpophalangeal joint is usually due to tendon rupture at the wrist (e.g. in rheumatoid arthritis). Because direct repair is not usually possible, the distal portion can be attached to an adjacent finger extensor or a tendon transfer performed.

BOUTONNIÈRE DEFORMITY   This lesion (which the French call *'le buttonhole'*) presents as a flexion deformity of the proximal interphalangeal joint. It is due to interruption or stretching of the central slip of the extensor tendon where it inserts into the base of the middle phalanx; the usual causes are direct trauma or rheumatoid disease. The lateral slips separate and the head of the proximal phalanx thrusts through the gap like a button through a buttonhole. Initially deformity is slight and passively correctable; later the soft tissues contract, resulting in fixed flexion of the proximal and hyperextension of the distal interphalangeal joints. Early diagnosis is therefore important; an impending deformity should be suspected in anyone with tenderness or a cut over the dorsum of the proximal interphalangeal joint, especially if they cannot actively extend the interphalangeal joint with the metacarpophalangeal joints and wrist flexed.

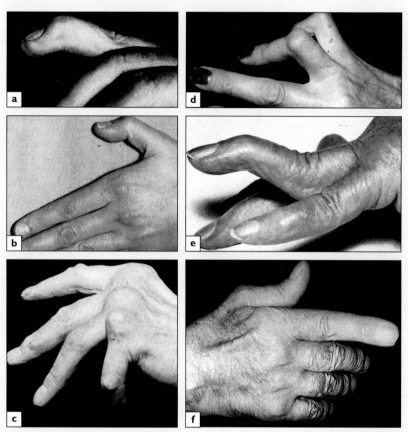

16.7 Deformities – tendons (a) Mallet finger. (b) Mallet thumb. (c) Dropped fingers due to rupture of extensor tendons. (d) Boutonnière. (e) Swan-neck deformity. (f) The so-called 'W-thumb', which results from rupture of the extensor pollicis brevis.

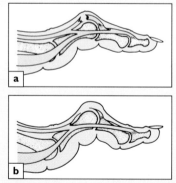

16.8 Deformities – boutonnière (a) When the middle slip of the extensor tendon first ruptures there is no more than an inability to extend the proximal interphalangeal joint. If it is not repaired, (b) the lateral slips slide towards the volar surface, the knuckle 'buttonholes' the extensor hood and the distal joint is drawn into hyperextension.

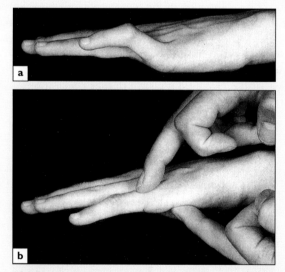

16.9 Pseudo-boutonnière deformity (a) The little finger is typically cocked up at the metacarpal joint and flexed at the proximal interphalangeal joint. (b) If the metacarpophalangeal joint is stabilized, the patient can easily straighten the finger.

In the early post-traumatic case, splinting the proximal interphalangeal joint in full extension for 6 weeks usually leads to healing; the distal interphalangeal joint must be moved passively to prevent the lateral bands from sticking. Open injuries of the central slip should be repaired, with the joint protected by a K-wire for 3 weeks. In later cases in which the joint is still passively correctable, several operations have been invented

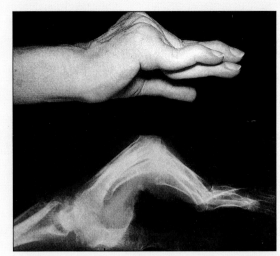

16.10 Swan-neck deformity The typical appearance and x-ray.

(suggesting that none is too reliable). Long-standing fixed deformities are extremely difficult to correct and may be better left alone.

SWAN-NECK DEFORMITY This is the reverse of the boutonnière deformity; the proximal interphalangeal joint is hyperextended and the distal interphalangeal joint flexed. The deformity can be reproduced voluntarily by lax-jointed individuals. The clinical disorder has many causes, with two things in common: imbalance of extensor versus flexor action at the proximal interphalangeal joint and laxity of the palmar plate. Thus it may occur: (1) if the proximal interphalangeal extensors overact (e.g. due to intrinsic muscle spasm or contracture, after disruption of the distal extensor attachment, or following volar subluxation of the metacarpophalangeal joint); (2) if the proximal interphalangeal flexors are inadequate (inhibition or division of the flexor superficialis); or (3) if the palmar plate fails (in rheumatoid arthritis, lax-jointed individuals or trauma). If the deformity is allowed to persist, secondary contractures of the intrinsic muscles, and eventually of the proximal interphalangeal joint itself, make correction increasingly difficult and ultimately impossible.

Treatment depends on the cause and whether or not the deformity has become fixed. If the deformity corrects passively, then a simple ring splint to maintain the proximal interphalangeal joint in a few degrees of flexion may be all that is required; if this works but cannot be tolerated, then tenodesis of the proximal interphalangeal joint with a slip of flexor digitorum superficialis stops the hyperextension. If the intrinsic muscles are tight they are released. If the deformity is fixed, then it may respond to gentle manipulation supplemented by temporary K-wire fixation in a few degrees of flexion; if not then lateral band release from the central slip may be needed. The dorsal skin may not close directly after correction. If the swan neck deformity is secondary to a mallet finger, then the latter should be addressed as described above.

If function is severely impaired and does not respond to one of the above measures, the joint is arthrodesed in a more acceptable position.

JOINT DISORDERS

RHEUMATOID ARTHRITIS Rheumatoid arthritis causes multiple, symmetrical deformities of both hands, typically ulnar deviation of the metacarpophalangeal joints and boutonnière or swan-neck deformities of the proximal finger joints (see page 345).

JUVENILE CHRONIC ARTHRITIS The pattern of involvement is different from that of adult disease. The wrists tend to develop ulnar (rather than radial) deviation, the metacarpophalangeal joints develop flexion contractures (rather than ulnar drift) and the interphalangeal joints also become fixed in flexion (swan-neck deformities are rare). The hands are small because of premature fusion of the physes.

The mainstay of treatment is medical. Long-term splintage of the hand is helpful and synovectomy is sometimes needed. Later, wrist fusion, metacarpophalangeal joint replacement and interphalangeal joint fusion also have a role.

PSORIATIC ARTHRITIS Psoriatic arthritis can devastate the small joints of the hand ('arthritis mutilans') resulting in deformities of the interphalangeal and metacarpophalangeal joints. The nails are often pitted and skin lesions may be evident. Occasionally joint fusion is needed to relieve pain and to provide stability in a functional position.

SYSTEMIC LUPUS ERYTHEMATOSUS Soft tissue slackening leads to extensor tendon dislocation, ulnar deviation at the metacarpophalangeal joints and swan-neck deformity of the fingers. Soft tissue corrections tend to fail with time and eventually fusions may be needed to maintain function.

SCLERODERMA Typically the fingers are smooth-skinned and stiff, with flexion deformities of the interphalangeal joints. Raynaud's phenomenon and painful ulcers may develop. Early on, physiotherapy and splinting help; in the later stages, joint fusion in a functional position and digital sympathectomy to relieve ulcers may be needed.

OSTEOARTHRITIS Osteoarthritis, by contrast, affects mainly the distal interphalangeal joints. It is common in post-menopausal women and may cause deformity. The thumb carpometacarpal joint is another common site, and this may result in adduction of the first metacarpophalangeal joint. Treatment is discussed in Chapter 5.

GOUT Gouty swellings (tophi) and finger deformities are sometimes mistaken for rheumatoid disease. However, the lesions tend to be asymmetrical and the x-ray appearances are distinctive. The diagnosis can be confirmed by identifying urate crystals in the tophaceous material. Curiously, gout and rheumatoid arthritis hardly ever occur in the same patient. In addition to systemic treatment, evacuation of a tophus (or tophi) is sometimes advisable.

TRAUMA Fractures may go on to malunion and joints may become stiff and swollen. This subject is dealt with in Chapter 26).

BONE LESIONS

A variety of bone lesions (acute infection, tuberculosis, malunited fractures, infantile rickets, tumours) may cause metacarpal or phalangeal deformity. X-rays usually show the abnormality. In addition to treating the pathological lesion, deformity may need correction by osteotomy with internal fixation.

NEUROMUSCULAR DISORDERS

SPASTIC PARESIS Cerebral palsy, head injury and stroke may result in typical deformities of the hand. The 'intrinsic-plus' posture is easily recognized. Another common disability is 'thumb-in-palm'; the tendency to adduct and flex the thumb into the palm is increased by activity, especially finger flexion. Releasing the adductor pollicis from the third metacarpal may improve the appearance, but normal thumb pinch is rarely restored.

OTHER NEUROLOGICAL DISORDERS Poliomyelitis, leprosy, syringomyelia and Charcot–Marie–Tooth disease may cause hand deformities. If there is only partial involvement, tendon transfer may be feasible.

PERIPHERAL NERVE LESIONS The postural deformities are so characteristic that the diagnosis should seldom be in doubt (see Chapter 11). The most common are drop wrist and drop fingers (radial nerve palsy), a simian thumb and pointing index finger (median nerve palsy) and partial claw hand (ulnar nerve palsy). The distribution of sensory loss helps to establish the site of the lesion.

THE 'INTRINSIC MINUS' HAND Among the late neurological defects, *intrinsic paralysis* is particularly disabling. The 'intrinsic-minus' hand shows wasting of the small muscles and moderate clawing, with extension of the metacarpophalangeal and partial flexion of the interphalangeal joints. If all the intrinsic muscles are affected (e.g. after poliomyelitis or a combined low median and ulnar nerve injury) the thumb lies flat at the side of the hand and cannot be opposed. In ulnar nerve palsy only the ring and little fingers are clawed, because the index and middle lumbricals are supplied by the median nerve; these muscles continue to flex the metacarpophalangeal joints and extend the interphalangeal joints. Thumb opposition is retained but thumb pinch is unstable

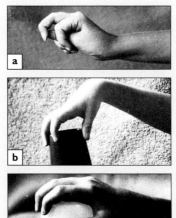

16.11 The hand in cerebral palsy
(a) Typically, when the wrist is extended the fingers flex and the thumb tucks into the palm; the hand unclasps only (b) when the wrist is flexed. After muscle release (c) the hand may be able to open with the wrist in a functional position.

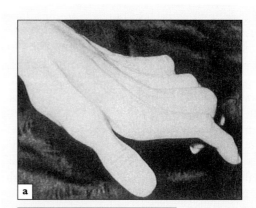

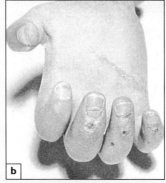

16.12 Two types of claw hand (a) The 'classic' claw-hand deformity of ulnar nerve palsy, due mainly to loss of intrinsic muscle power. (b) Clawing of the fingers, due to Volkmann's contracture of the long flexor muscles.

because index-finger abduction (first dorsal interosseous) is weak, and loss of thumb adduction is compensated for by exaggerated interphalangeal flexion during strong pinch (Froment's sign).

The objectives of treatment are: (1) stabilization of the metacarpophalangeal joints in flexion, which can be achieved dynamically by a tendon transfer (e.g. splitting a flexor superficialis tendon) or statically by looping a slip of flexor digitorum superficialis around the flexor pulley; (2) restoration of index abduction to provide stable pinch (e.g. by extensor tendon transfer to the first dorsal interosseous); (3) restoration of thumb opposition (if it is lost) by a tendon transfer looped around a pisiform pulley and attached to the proximal phalanx of the thumb. *Before any of these operations, stiff finger joints must be made mobile.*

DUPUYTREN'S CONTRACTURE

This is a nodular hypertrophy and contracture of the superficial palmar fascia (palmar aponeurosis). The condition is inherited as an autosomal dominant trait and is most common in people of European (especially Anglo-Saxon) descent. It is more common in males than females; the prevalence increases with age, but onset at an early stage usually means aggressive disease. There is a high incidence in epileptics receiving phenytoin therapy; associations with diabetes, smoking, alcoholic cirrhosis, AIDS and pulmonary tuberculosis have also been described.

Pathology

The essential problem in Dupuytren's disease is proliferation of myofibroblasts; where they come from and why they proliferate remains unclear. After an initial proliferative phase, fibrous tissue within the palmar fascia and fascial bands within the fingers contract, causing flexion deformities of the metacarpophalangeal and proximal interphalangeal joints. Fibrous attachments to the skin lead to puckering. The digital nerve is displaced or enveloped, but not invaded, by fibrous tissue. Occasionally the plantar aponeurosis also is affected.

Clinical features

The patient – usually a middle-aged man – complains of a nodular thickening in the palm. Gradually this extends distally to involve the ring or little finger. Pain may occur but is seldom a marked feature. Often both hands are involved, one more than the other. The palm is puckered, nodular and thick. If the subcutaneous cords extend into the fingers they may produce flexion deformities at the metacarpophalangeal and proximal interphalangeal joints. Sometimes the dorsal knuckle pads are thickened (Garrod's pads).

Similar nodules may be seen on the soles of the feet (Ledderhose's disease). There is a rare, curious association with fibrosis of the corpus cavernosum (Peyronie's disease).

Diagnosis

Dupuytren's contracture must be distinguished from skin contracture (in which the previous laceration is usually obvious), tendon contracture (in which the finger deformity changes with wrist position) and proximal interphalangeal joint contracture (in which there may be a history of clinodactyly or injury).

Treatment

Operation is indicated if the deformity is a nuisance or rapidly progressing. In particular, proximal interphalangeal joint contractures soon become irreversible. The aim is reasonable, not complete, correction. Surgery does not cure the disease, it only partially corrects the deformity and recurrence or extension is common. Correction of the metacarpophalangeal joint is more predictable than improvement of the proximal interphalangeal joint.

Only the thickened part of the fascia is excised (complete fasciectomy is usually unnecessary and fraught with complications). The affected area is approached through a longitudinal or a Z-shaped incision and, after carefully freeing the nerves and blood vessels, the cords are excised. Skin closure may be facilitated by multiple Z-plasties. This has the dual effect of improving the deformity and, if recurrence occurs, preventing a longitudinal wound contracture. The palmar section of the wound can be left open; it will soon heal with dressings. This makes

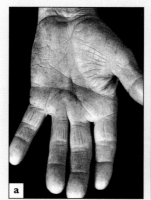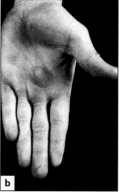

16.13 Dupuytren's contracture (a) In the early case there is usually only a palmar nodule but no deformity. This must be distinguished from (b) an implantation dermoid which produces a more superficial nodule in the skin.

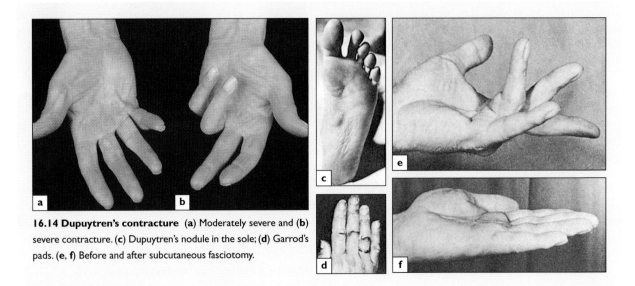

16.14 Dupuytren's contracture (**a**) Moderately severe and (**b**) severe contracture. (**c**) Dupuytren's nodule in the sole; (**d**) Garrod's pads. (**e**, **f**) Before and after subcutaneous fasciotomy.

skin closure easier and allows any haematoma (which may predispose to recurrence) escape. After operative correction a splint is applied, and removed after a few days for active motion exercises. Night splinting for a few months may reduce recurrence.

If there is severe skin involvement, particularly in surgery for recurrent disease, then skin grafting should be considered. Amputation is occasionally advisable for severe, recurrent disease in the little finger.

STENOSING TENOVAGINITIS ('trigger finger')

A flexor tendon may become trapped at the entrance to its sheath; on forced extension it passes the constriction with a snap ('triggering'). The usual cause is thickening of the fibrous tendon sheath (often following local trauma or unaccustomed activity), but a similar hold-up may occur in rheumatoid tenosynovitis. The condition is more common in diabetics and in people with gout.

Clinical features

Although any digit (including the thumb) may be affected, but the ring and middle fingers are most commonly; sometimes several fingers are affected. The patient notices that the finger clicks as he or she bends it; when the hand is unclenched, the affected finger remains bent at the proximal interphalangeal joint, but with further effort it suddenly straightens with a snap. A tender nodule can be felt in front of the metacarpophalangeal joint

INFANTILE TRIGGER THUMB   Babies sometimes develop tenovaginitis of the thumb flexor sheath. The diagnosis is often missed, or the condition is wrongly taken for a 'dislocation'. Very occasionally the child grows up with the thumb permanently bent. This condition must be distinguished from the rare *congenitally clasped thumb* in which both the interphalangeal joint and the metacarpophalangeal joint are flexed because of congenital insufficiency of the extensor mechanism (see page 337).

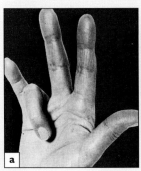

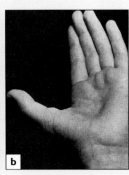

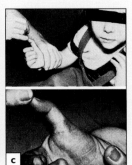

16.15 Stenosing tenovaginitis
(**a**) Trigger finger; (**b**) trigger thumb – the only variety which occurs also in children, in whom (**c**) the thumb may be bent and stuck in that position.

Treatment

Early cases may be cured by an injection of methylprednisolone carefully placed into the tendon sheath. Refractory cases need operation: through an incision over the distal palmar crease, or in the metacarpophalangeal crease of the thumb, the fibrous sheath is incised until the tendon moves freely. The digital neurovascular bundles are at risk during surgery.

In patients with rheumatoid arthritis the fibrous pulley must be carefully preserved; damage to this structure will predispose to ulnar deviation of the fingers. Flexor synovectomy is preferred.

In babies it is worth waiting until the child is a year old, as spontaneous recovery often occurs.

RHEUMATOID ARTHRITIS

The hand, more than any other region, is where rheumatoid arthritis carves its story (see also Chapter 3). In *stage 1* there is synovitis of joints (metacarpophalangeal and proximal interphalangeal) and of tendon sheaths (flexor and extensor). In *stage 2*, joint and tendon erosions prepare the ground for mechanical derangement. And in *stage 3*, joint instability and tendon rupture cause progressive deformity and loss of function.

Clinical features

STAGE 1 (PROLIFERATIVE)
Stiffness and swelling of the fingers are early symptoms; often the wrist also is painful and swollen. Carpal tunnel compression from flexor tenosynovitis sometimes causes the first symptom. Examination may reveal swelling of the metacarpophalangeal joints, the proximal interphalangeal joints (giving the fingers a spindle shape) or the wrists; both hands are affected, more or less symmetrically. Swelling of tendon sheaths is usually seen on the dorsum of the wrist, on its ulnar side (extensor carpi ulnaris) and on the volar aspect of the proximal phalanges. The joints are tender and crepitus may be felt on moving the tendons. Joint mobility and grip strength are diminished.

STAGE 2 (DESTRUCTIVE)
As the disease progresses, early deformities make their appearance: slight radial deviation of the wrist and ulnar deviation of the fingers; correctable swan-necking; an isolated boutonnière; and/or the sudden appearance of a drop finger or mallet thumb (from extensor tendon rupture).

STAGE 3 (REPARATIVE)
In the later stage, long after inflammation may have subsided, established deformities are the rule: the carpus settles into radial tilt and volar subluxation; there is marked ulnar drift of the fingers and volar dislocation of the metacarpophalangeal joints, often associated with multiple swan-neck and boutonnière deformities. When these abnormalities become fixed, functional loss may be so severe that the patient can no longer dress or feed him- or herself.

Z-collapse If one of two adjacent joints changes direction, then the overlying long tendons will pull the other joint into the opposite direction. In rheumatoid arthritis this is typified by radial tilt of the wrist with ulnar drift of the metacarpophalangeal joints, the boutonnière deformity and the swan-neck deformity.

Rheumatoid nodules These are associated with aggressive disease in seropositive patients. They tend to occur at pressure areas (e.g. the pulps of the fingers and the radial side of the index finger).

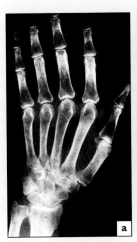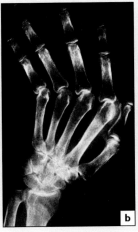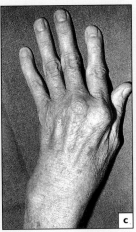

16.16 Rheumatoid arthritis – ulnar drift (a) Early ulnar drift. (b) The same patient 2 years later – the progressive finger deformity is accompanied by (perhaps preceded by) an equal and opposite wrist deformity, in which the entire carpus moves ulnarwards and rotates radialwards. (c) The clinical appearance shows the zig-zag deformity.

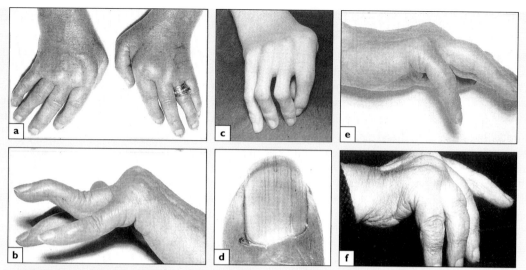

16.17 Rheumatoid arthritis – hands (**a**) Ulnar drift; (**b**) swan-neck deformity; (**c**) boutonnière deformities; (**d**) 'nail-fold lesion' due to arthritis; (**e**) dropped finger; (**f**) three dropped fingers. (NB The extensor tendons rupture where they cross the wrist, not the knuckles.)

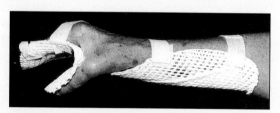

16.18 Rheumatoid arthritis – treatment Lightweight splints are worn to rest the joints, not to correct deformity.

Weakness Rheumatoid hands are weak because of a combination of generalized muscular weakness, pain inhibition, tendon malalignment or rupture, joint stiffness and nerve compression

General features The hand should not be considered in isolation. Its functional interaction with the wrist and elbow is crucial and, in a generalized disorder such as rheumatoid disease, the condition of all the upper limb joints and the cervical spine should be carefully assessed.

X-rays

During *stage 1* the x-rays show only soft-tissue swelling and osteoporosis around the joints. In *stage 2*, joint 'space' narrowing and small periarticular erosions appear; these are commonest at the metacarpophalangeal joints and in the styloid process of the ulna. In *stage 3,* articular destruction may be marked, affecting the metacarpophalangeal proximal interphalangeal and wrist joints almost equally. Joint deformity and dislocation are common.

Treatment

In stage 1 treatment is directed essentially at controlling the systemic disease and the local synovitis. In addition to general measures, static splints may reduce pain and swelling. These splints are not corrective but are designed to rest inflamed joints and tendons; in mild cases they are worn only at night, but in more active cases during the day as well. Persistent synovitis of a few joints or tendon sheaths may benefit from local injections of corticosteroid with local anaesthetic. Only small quantities are injected (e.g. 0.5ml for a metacarpophalangeal joint or flexor tendon sheath and 1ml for the wrist). This should not be repeated more than two or three times. A boggy flexor tenosynovitis may not respond to this limited therapeutic assault; operative synovectomy may be needed. If carpal tunnel symptoms are present, the transverse carpal ligament is divided and, if necessary, a flexor synovectomy performed.

In stage 2 it becomes increasingly important to prevent deformity. Uncontrolled synovitis of joints or tendons requires operative synovectomy followed by physiotherapy. Excision of the distal end of the ulna, synovectomy of the common extensor sheath and the wrist, and reconstruction of the soft tissues on the ulnar side of the wrist may arrest joint destruction and progressive deformity. Early instability and ulnar drift at the metacarpophalangeal joints can be corrected by excising the inflamed synovium, tightening the capsular structures and releasing the ulnar pull of the intrinsic tendons. Mobile boutonnière and swan-neck deformities can be treated with splints; if they progress or are fixed, then surgery may be needed. Isolated tendon ruptures are repaired or bypassed by appropriate tendon transfers. These procedures are followed by dynamic splintage and physiotherapy.

In stage 3 deformity is combined with articular destruction; soft-tissue correction alone will not suffice. For the metacarpophalangeal and interphalangeal joints of the thumb, arthrodesis gives predictable pain relief, stability and functional improvement. The metacarpophalangeal joints of the fingers can be excised and replaced with silastic 'spacers', which improve stability and correct deformity. Replacement of interphalangeal joints gives less predictable results; if deformity is very disabling (e.g. a fixed swan-neck) it may be better to settle for arthrodesis in a more functional position. At the wrist, painless stability can be regained by fusion of the radiocarpal, midcarpal and carpometacarpal joints; a stout pin through the index/middle web and across the wrist is usually sufficient. Wrist replacement with silastic or metal–plastic implants, whilst providing some movement, may well fail; the loss of bone stock that accompanies failure means that salvage can be very difficult.

THE THUMB IN RHEUMATOID ARTHRITIS

Soft tissue failure leads to characteristic deformities: boutonnière at the metacarpophalangeal joint, carpometacarpal instability, swan-neck deformity and ulnar collateral instability.

Depending on the deformity, the patient's demands and the condition of the rest of the hand, treatment may involve various combinations of splintage, fusion, excision arthroplasty and joint replacement.

METACARPOPHALANGEAL DEFORMITIES

Chronic synovitis of the metacarpophalangeal joints results in failure of the palmar plate and the collateral ligaments. The powerful flexor tendons drag the proximal phalanx palmarwards, causing subluxation of the joint. The deformity may be aggravated by primary or secondary intrinsic muscle tightness.

The most obvious deformity of the rheumatoid hand is ulnar deviation of the metacarpophalangeal joints. There are several reasons for this: palmar grip and thumb pressure naturally tend to push the index finger ulnarwards; weakening of the collateral ligaments and the first dorsal interosseous muscle reduces the normal resistance to this force; the wrist is usually involved and, as it collapses into radial deviation, the metacarpophalangeal joints automatically veer in the opposite direction due to the longitudinal pull of the long extensor tendons (the so-called zig-zag mechanism); once ulnar drift begins, it becomes self-perpetuating due to tightening of the ulnar intrinsic muscles and stretching of the radial intrinsics and the adjacent capsular structures.

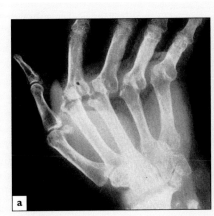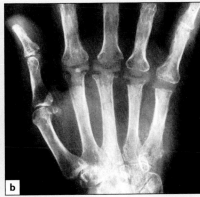

16.19 Rheumatoid arthritis – treatment In advanced rheumatoid arthritis the metacarpophalangeal joints may be completely dislocated, as they were in this patient; joint replacement with flexible silastic spacers corrected her deformity and restored stability.

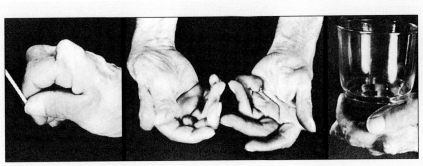

16.20 Rheumatoid arthritis – does it need treatment? Not always. Why interfere if deformities have been present for years and the hand still works? Despite gross deformity this patient can manipulate both tiny objects and large ones.

At an early stage, before joint destruction and soft tissue instability, synovectomy may relieve pain but the joint usually stiffens somewhat. When ulnar drift has started, dynamic splintage may maintain function and retard progression. With marked deformity but little joint damage, a soft tissue reconstruction (reefing of the radial sagittal bands with intrinsic muscle release and transfer) can give a satisfactory and fairly durable correction. Once there is marked damage to the joint surface, replacement with a silastic spacer, along with the soft tissue reconstruction, is recommended. There is no point in correcting the metacarpophalangeal joints unless any wrist deformity is also corrected; the tendency to zig-zag deformity will otherwise lead to recurrence of the ulnar drift.

FINGER DEFORMITIES

Boutonnière Synovitis in the proximal interphalangeal joint causes elongation or rupture of the central slip which passes over the back of the joint before inserting into the base of the middle phalanx. The lateral bands slip away from the central slip and pass in front of the axis of rotation of the proximal joint but remain behind the axis in the distal joint, to form the characteristic deformity. Early, correctable deformity responds to splinting and synovectomy; later, central slip reconstruction (an unpredictable procedure) may be required; simple division of the distal insertion is a simpler, and often effective, alternative. In fixed deformities, or those with joint damage, fusion or replacement is considered.

Swan neck Chronic synovitis may lead to swan-neck deformity by one or more of the following mechanisms: failure of the palmar plate of the proximal interphalangeal joint; rupture of the flexor digitorum superficialis; dislocation or subluxation of the metacarpophalangeal joint and consequent tightening of the intrinsic muscles. Treatment depends on a careful analysis of the cause.

The pathogenesis and management of these finger deformities are well described in the review paper by Boyer and Gelberman (1999).

TENOSYNOVITIS AND TENDON RUPTURE

Extensor tendons Extensor tendon rupture is a common complication of chronic synovitis. Extensor digiti minimi is usually the first to go and presages rupture of the other tendons. Treatment consists of either suturing the distal tendon stump to an adjacent tendon, inserting a bridge graft (e.g. palmaris longus) or performing a tendon transfer (e.g. extensor indicis proprius). Synovectomy and excision of the distal ulna may also be necessary.

Flexor tendons Flexor tenosynovitis is one of the earliest and most troublesome features of rheumatoid disease. The restriction of finger movement is easily mistaken for arthritis; however, careful palpation of the palm and the nearby joints will quickly show where the swelling and tenderness are located. Secondary problems include carpal tunnel syndrome, triggering of one or more fingers and tendon rupture. Synovitis of the flexor digitorum superficialis also contributes to the swan-neck deformity.

If carpal tunnel release is needed, the operation should include a flexor tenosynovectomy. If the flexor tendons are bulky (best felt over the proximal phalanges and the metacarpal heads) and joint movement is limited, then flexor tenosynovectomy should improve movement and, just as important, should prevent tendon rupture. Triggering, likewise, should be treated by tenosynovectomy rather than simple splitting of the sheath. Rupture of flexor digitorum profundus is best treated by distal interphalangeal joint fusion. Rupture of flexor pollicis longus can be treated either by tendon grafting or by fusion of the thumb joint.

A flexor tendon occasionally ruptures from attrition against the underside of the distal radius (Mannerfelt lesion).

OSTEOARTHRITIS

Eighty per cent of people over the age of 65 years have radiological signs of osteoarthritis (OA) in one or more joints of the hand; fortunately, most of them are asymptomatic (see also Chapter 5).

Distal interphalangeal joints OA of the distal interphalangeal joints is very common in postmenopausal women. It often starts with pain in one or two fingers; the distal joints become swollen and tender, the condition usually spreading to all the fingers of both hands. On examination there is bony thickening around the joints (Heberden's nodes) and some restriction of movement. Treatment is usually symptomatic. However, if pain and instability are severe, then fusion is the answer.

Mucous cysts sometimes protrude between the extensor tendon and collateral ligament of an osteoarthritic distal interphalangeal joint. They are unsightly and occasionally ulcerate. If this becomes very troublesome, excision of the cyst and the underlying osteophytes may be necessary.

Proximal interphalangeal joints Not infrequently some of the proximal interphalangeal joints are involved (Bouchard's nodes). These are strongly associated with OA elsewhere in the body (polyarticular OA). The joints are swollen and tend to deviate ulnarwards due to mechanical pressure in daily activities. Treatment is usually non-operative. If the joint is very painful or unstable then fusion may be required, but this will cause some functional restriction.

Metacarpophalangeal joints This is an uncommon site for OA. When it does occur, a specific cause can usually be identified: occupational stress, previous trauma, infection, gout or one of the rarer crystal arthropathies. Treatment is non-operative – splints, injections and analgesics. Fusion has serious functional consequences and silastic replacement is unlikely to withstand long-term usage. New implants are now being developed which may be more robust.

Carpometacarpal joint of the thumb This is discussed on page 327.

ACUTE INFECTIONS OF THE HAND

Infection of the hand is frequently limited to one of several well-defined compartments: under the nail fold (paronychia); the pulp space (felon) and subcutaneous tissues elsewhere; tendon sheaths; the deep fascial spaces; and joints. Usually the cause is a staphylococcus which has been implanted by fairly trivial injury. However, contaminated cuts, with unusual organisms, account for about 10% of cases.

GENERAL PRINCIPLES

Pathology

Here, as elsewhere, the response to infection is an acute inflammatory reaction with oedema, suppuration and increased tissue tension. In closed tissue compartments (e.g. the pulp space or tendon sheath) pressures may rise to levels where the local blood-supply is threatened, with the risk of tissue necrosis. In neglected cases infection can spread from one compartment to another and the end result may be a permanently stiff and useless hand. There is also a danger of lymphatic and haematogenous spread; even apparently trivial infections may give rise to lymphangitis and septicaemia.

Clinical features

Usually there is a history of trauma (a superficial abrasion, laceration or penetrating wound), but this may have been so trivial as to pass unnoticed. A few hours or days later the finger or hand becomes painful and swollen. There may be throbbing and sometimes the patient feels ill and feverish. Ask if he or she can recall any causative incident: a small cut or even a scratch, a prick injury (including plant-thorns) or a local injection. And don't forget to enquire about predisposing conditions such as diabetes mellitus, intravenous drug abuse and immunosuppression.

On examination the finger or hand is red and swollen, and usually exquisitely tender over the site of tension. However, in immune-compromised patients, in the very elderly and in babies, local signs may be mild. With superficial infection the patient can usually be persuaded to flex an affected finger; with deep infections active flexion is not possible. The arm should be examined for lymphangitis and swollen glands, and the patient more generally for signs of septicaemia.

X-ray examination may disclose a foreign body, but is otherwise unhelpful in the early stages of infection. However, a few weeks later there may be features of osteomyelitis or septic arthritis, and later still of bone necrosis.

If pus becomes available, this should be sent for bacteriological examination.

Diagnosis

In making the diagnosis, several conditions must be excluded: an *insect bite or sting* (which can closely mimic a subcutaneous infection), a *thorn prick* (which, itself, can become secondarily infected), acute *tendon rupture* (which may resemble a septic tenosynovitis) and *acute gout* (which is easily mistaken for septic arthritis).

Plant-thorn injuries are extremely common and the distinction between secondary infection and a non-septic reaction to a retained fragment can be difficult. Rose-thorn and black-thorn are the usual suspects in Britain, but any plant-spine (including cactus needles) can be implicated. The local inflammatory response sometimes leads to recurrent arthritis or tenosynovitis, which is arrested only by removing the retained fragment. If the condition is suspected, the fragment may be revealed by ultrasound scanning or MRI (Stevens *et al.*, 2000). Secondary infection with unusual soil or plant organisms may occur.

Principles of treatment

Superficial hand infections are common; if their treatment is delayed or inadequate, infection may rapidly extend, with serious consequences. The essentials of treatment are:

- antibiotics;
- rest, splintage and elevation;
- drainage;
- rehabilitation.

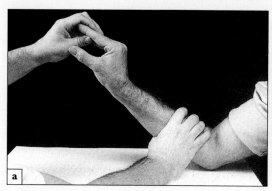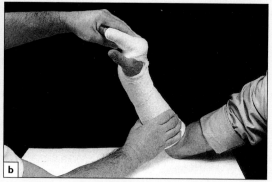

16.21 The position of safe immobilization The knuckle joints are 90° flexed, the finger joints extended and the thumb abducted. This is the position in which the ligaments are at their longest and splintage is least likely to result in stiffness.

ANTIBIOTICS

As soon as the clinical diagnosis is made, and preferably after a specimen has been taken for Gram stain and culture, antibiotic treatment is started – usually with flucloxacillin or a cephalosporin. If bone infection is suspected, fusidic acid may be added. For bites (which should always be assumed to be infected) a broad spectrum penicillin is advisable. Agricultural injuries risk infection by anaerobic organisms and it is therefore prudent to add metranidazole. The interim antibiotic may later be changed when the bacterial sensitivity is known.

REST, SPLINTAGE AND ELEVATION

In a mild case the hand is rested in a sling. In a severe case the patient is admitted to hospital; the arm is held elevated in an overhead sling while the patient is kept under observation. Analgesics are given for pain. *The hand must be splinted in the position of safe immobilization ('POSI'), that is with the wrist slightly extended, the metacarpophalangeal joints in full flexion, the interphalangeal joints extended and the thumb in abduction* (see Fig. 16.21).

DRAINAGE

If treated within the first 24 to 48 hours, many hand infections will respond to antibiotics, rest, elevation and splintage.

If there are signs of an abscess – throbbing pain, marked tenderness and toxaemia – the pus should be drained. A tourniquet and either general or regional block anaesthesia are essential. The hand should be exsanguinated by elevation only; an exsanguinating bandage can spread the sepsis. The incision should be planned to give access to the abscess without causing injury to other structures – *but never at right angles across a skin crease*. When pus is encountered it must be carefully wiped away and a search made for deeper pockets of infection. Necrotic tissue should be excised. The area is thoroughly washed out and, in some cases, a catheter may be left in place for further, postoperative,

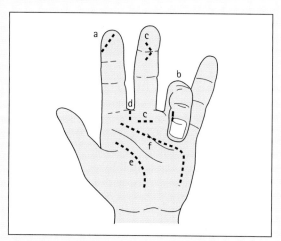

16.22 Infections The incisions for surgical drainage are shown here: (**a**) pulp space (directly over the abscess); (**b**) nailfold (it may also be necessary to excise the edge of the nail); (**c**) tendon sheath; (**d**) web space; (**e**) thenar space; (**f**) mid-palmar space.

irrigation (e.g. in cases of flexor tenosynovitis). The wound is either left open or lightly sutured, and then covered with a non-stick dressing and betadine-soaked gauze. The pus obtained is sent for culture.

At the end of the operation the hand is splinted in the position of safe immobilization. A removable splint will permit betadine soaks, repeated wound dressings and exercises. A suitable sling is used to keep the arm elevated.

The hand should be re-examined within the next 24 hours to ensure that drainage is effective; if it is not, further operative drainage may be needed. Inadequate drainage of acute infection may lead to chronic infection.

POST-OPERATIVE REHABILITATION

As soon as the signs of acute inflammation have settled, movements must be started under the guidance

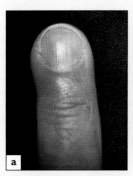
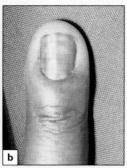
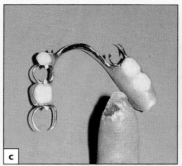
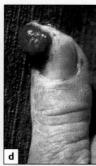

16.23 Acute infections (1) (**a**) Acute nail-fold infection (paronychia); and (**b**) chronic paronychia. (**c**) Pulp-space infection (felon or whitlow) of the thumb due to a prick-injury on the patient's own denture. (**d**) Septic granuloma. (Courtesy of Professor S. Biddulph).

of a hand therapist, otherwise the joints are liable to become stiff. For the first few days the resting splint is re-applied between exercise sessions.

NAIL-FOLD INFECTION (PARONYCHIA)

Infection under the nail fold is the commonest hand infection; it is seen most often in children, or in older people after rough nail-trimming. The edge of the nail-fold becomes red and swollen and increasingly tender. A tiny abscess may form in the nail-fold; if this is left untreated, pus can spread under the nail.

At the first sign of infection, treatment with antibiotics alone may be effective. However, if pus is present it must be released by an incision at the corner of the nail-fold in line with the edge of the nail; a pledget of paraffin gauze is used to keep the nail-fold open. If pus has spread under the nail, part or all of the nail may need to be removed.

Chronic paronychia Chronic nail-fold infection may be due to (1) inadequate drainage of an acute infection, or (2) a fungal infection, which requires specific treatment. The nail bed may have to be laid open ('marsupialized'); care should be taken to avoid damaging the more proximal nail matrix.

PULP INFECTION (FELON)

The distal finger pad is essentially a closed fascial compartment filled with compact fat and subdivided by radiating fibrous septa. A rise in pressure within the pulp space causes intense pain and, if unrelieved, may threaten the terminal branches of the digital artery which supply most of the terminal phalanx.

Pulp-space infection is usually caused by a prick injury. The most common organism is *Staphylococcus aureus*. The patient complains of throbbing pain in the finger-tip, which becomes tensely swollen, red and acutely tender.

If the condition is recognized very early, antibiotic treatment and elevation of the hand may suffice. Once an abscess has formed, the pus must be released through a small incision over the site of maximum tenderness. If treatment is delayed, infection may spread to the bone, the joint or the flexor tendon sheath.

Postoperatively the finger is dressed with a loose packing of gauze; antibiotic treatment is modified if the results of culture and sensitivity so dictate, and is continued until all signs of infection have cleared. The wound will gradually heal by secondary intention.

Herpetic whitlow The herpes simplex virus may enter the finger-tip, possibly by auto-inoculation from the patient's own mouth or genitalia, or by cross infection during dental surgery. Small vesicles form on the finger-tip, then coalesce and ulcerate. The condition is self-limiting and usually subsides after about 10 days, but may recur from time to time. Herpes whitlow should not be confused with a staphylococal felon. Surgery is unhelpful and may be harmful, exposing the finger to secondary infection. Acyclovir may be effective in the early stages.

OTHER SUBCUTANEOUS INFECTIONS

Anywhere in the hand a blister, a superficial cut or an insect 'bite' may become infected, causing redness, swelling and tenderness. A local collection of pus should be drained through a small incision over the site of maximal tenderness (but never crossing a skin crease or the web edge); in the finger, a mid-lateral incision is suitable. It is important to exclude a deeper pocket of pus in a nearby tendon sheath or in one of the deep fascial spaces.

TENDON SHEATH INFECTION (SUPPURATIVE TENOSYNOVITIS)

The tendon sheath is a closed compartment extending from the distal palmar crease to the distal interphalangeal joint. In the thumb and fifth finger, the sheaths

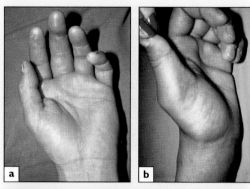

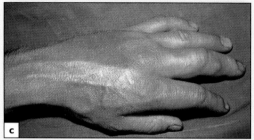

16.24 Acute infections (2) (a) Flexor tenosynovitis of the middle finger following a cortisone injection. (b) Tuberculous synovitis of flexor pollicis longus. (c) Diffuse septic extensor tendinitis. (Courtesy of Professor S. Biddulph.)

are co-extensive with the radial and ulnar bursae, which envelope the flexor tendons in the proximal part of the palm and across the wrist; these bursae also communicate with Parona's space in the lower forearm.

Pyogenic tenosynovitis is uncommon but dangerous. It usually follows a penetrating injury, the commonest organism being *Staphylococcus aureus*; however, streptococcus and Gram negative organisms are also encountered.

The affected digit is painful and swollen; it is usually held in slight flexion, is very tender and the patient will not move it or permit it to be moved. Early diagnosis is based on clinical findings; x-rays are unhelpful but ultra-sound scanning may be useful.

Delayed diagnosis results in a progressive rise in pressure within the sheath and a consequent risk of vascular occlusion and tendon necrosis. In neglected cases infection may spread proximally within the radial or ulnar bursa, or from one to the other (a 'horse-shoe abscess); it can also spread proximally to the flexor compartment at the wrist and into Parona'space in the forearm. Occasionally this results in median nerve compression.

Treatment must be started as soon as the diagnosis is suspected. The hand is elevated and splinted and antibiotics are administered intravenously – ideally a broad-spectrum penicillin or a systemic cephalosporin. If there is no improvement after 24 hours, surgical drainage is essential. Two incisions are needed, one at the proximal end of the sheath and one at the distal end; using a fine catheter, the sheath is then irrigated (always from proximal to distal) with Ringer's lactate solution. Additional, proximal, incisions may be needed if the synovial bursae are infected.

Postoperatively the hand is swathed in absorbent dressings and splinted in the position of safe immobilization. The dressings should not be too bulky, as this will make it difficult to ensure correct positioning of the joints. The flexor sheath catheter is left in place; using a syringe, the sheath is irrigated with 20ml of saline three or four times a day for the next 2 days. The catheter and dressings are then removed and finger movements are started. Splintage is retained until the operation wounds are healed, but is interrupted for daily betadine soaks and supervized physiotherapy.

DEEP FASCIAL SPACE INFECTION

The large thenar and mid-palmar fascial spaces may be infected directly by penetrating injuries or by secondary spread from a web space or an infected tendon sheath.

Clinical signs can be misleading; the hand is painful but, because of the tight deep fascia, there may be little or no swelling in the palm while the dorsum bulges like an inflated glove. There is extensive tenderness and the patient holds the hand as still as possible.

As with other infections, splintage and intravenous antibiotics are commenced as soon as the diagnosis is made. For drainage, an incision is made directly over the abscess (being careful not to cross the flexor creases) and sinus forceps inserted; if the web space is infected it, too, should be incised. A *thenar space* abscess can be approached through the first web space (but do not incise in the line of the skin-fold) or through separate dorsal and palmar incisions around the thenar eminence. Great care must be taken to avoid damage to the tendons, nerves and blood vessels. A thorough knowledge of anatomy is essential. The deep *mid-palmar space* (which lies between the flexor tendons and the metacarpals) can be drained through an incision in the web space between the middle and ring fingers, but wider exposure through a transverse or oblique palmar incision is preferable, taking care not to cross the flexor creases directly. Above all, do not be misled by the swelling on the back of the hand into attempting drainage through the dorsal aspect.

Occasionally, deep infection extends proximally across the wrist, causing symptoms of median nerve compression. Pus can be drained by anteromedial or anterolateral approaches; incisions directly over the flexor tendons and median nerve are avoided.

Operation wounds are either loosely stitched or left open. Bulky dressings and saline irrigation are employed, more or less as described for tendon sheath infections.

SEPTIC ARTHRITIS

Any of the metacarpophalangeal or finger joints may be infected, either directly by a penetrating injury or intra-articular injection, or indirectly from adjacent structures (and occasionally by haematogenous spread from a distant site). *Staphylococcus* and *Streptococcus* are the usual organisms; *Haemophilus influenzae* is a common pathogen in children.

Pain, swelling and redness are localized to a single joint, and all movement is resisted. The presence of lymphangitis and/or systemic features may help to clinch the diagnosis; in their absence, the early symptoms and signs are indistinguishable from those of acute gout. Joint aspiration may give the answer.

Intravenous antibiotics are administered and the hand is splinted. If the inflammation does not subside within 24 hours, or if there are overt signs of pus, open drainage is needed. For the interphalangeal and thumb metacarpophalangeal joints, mid-lateral incisions are recommended (avoiding damage to the collateral ligaments); for the other metacarpophalangeal joints and the wrist, dorsal incisions (avoiding the extensor tendons) are preferred. The wounds are left open, to heal by secondary intention. Copious dressings are applied and the hand is splinted in the 'position of safety' for 48 hours; thereafter, movement is encouraged.

Intravenous antibiotics are continued until all signs of sepsis have disappeared; it is prudent to follow this with another two-week course of oral antibiotics.

BITES

Animal bites are usually inflicted by cats, dogs, farm animals or rodents. Many become infected and, although the common pathogens are staphylococci and streptococci, unusual organisms like *Pasteurella multocida* are often reported.

Human bites are generally thought to be even more prone to infection. A wide variety of organisms (including anaerobes) are encountered, the commonest being *Staphylococcus aureus*, *Streptococcus Group A* and *Eikenella corrodens*.

Bites can involve any part of the hand, fingers or thumb; tell-tale signs of a human bite are lacerations on both volar and dorsal surfaces of the finger. Often, though, the 'bite' consists only of a dorsal wound over one of the metacarpophalangeal knuckles, sustained during a fist-fight. *All such wounds should be assumed to be infected.* Moreover, it should be remembered that a laceration of the clenched fist may have penetrated the extensor apparatus and entered the metacarpophalangeal joint; this will not be apparent if the wound is examined with the fingers in extension because the extensor hood and capsule will have retracted proximally.

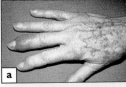
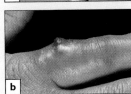
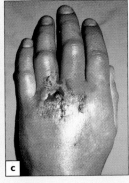

16.25 Acute infections (3) (**a**) Septic arthritis of the terminal interphalangeal joint following a cortisone injection. (**b**) Infected insect 'bite'. (**c**) Septic human bite resulting in acute infection of the fourth metacaropophalangeal joint. (Courtesy of Professor S. Biddulph.)

X-rays should be obtained (to exclude a fracture or foreign body) and swabs taken for bacterial culture and sensitivity.

Fresh wounds should be carefully examined in the operating theatre and, if necessary, extended and debrided. Search for a fragment of tooth or – with a knuckle bite – for a divot of articular cartilage from the joint. The hand is splinted and elevated and antibiotics are given prophylactically until the laboratory results are obtained.

Infected bites will need debridement, wash-outs and intravenous antibiotic treatment. The common infecting organisms are all sensitive to broad-spectrum penicillins (e.g. amoxycillin with clavulanic acid) and cephalosporins. With animal bites one should also consider the possibility of rabies.

Postoperative treatment consists, as usual, of copious wound dressings, splintage in the 'safe' position and encouragement of movement once the infection has resolved. Tendon lacerations can be dealt with when the tissues are completely healed.

MYCOBACTERIAL INFECTIONS

Tuberculous tenosynovitis is uncommon even in countries where tuberculosis is still rife. The diagnosis should be considered in patients with chronic synovitis once the alternatives such as rheumatoid disease have been excluded; it can be confirmed by synovial biopsy. Treatment is by synovectomy and then prolonged chemotherapy.

'Fishmonger's infection' is a chronic infection of the hand caused by *Mycobacterium marinum*. The organism is introduced by prick-injuries from fish spines or hard fins in people working with fish or around fishing

boats. It may appear as no more than a superficial granuloma, but deep infection can give rise to an intractable synovitis of tendon or joint (Hurst *et al.*, 1987). Other causes of chronic synovitis must be excluded; definitive diagnosis usually requires biopsy for histological examination and special culture.

Superficial lesions often heal on their own; if not, they can be excised. Deep lesions usually require surgical synovectomy. Prolonged antibiotic treatment is needed to avoid recurrence; the recommended drug is a broad-spectrum tetracycline, or else chemotherapy with ethambutol and rifampicin (Hausman and Lisser, 1992).

FUNGAL INFECTIONS

Superficial tinea infection of the palm and interdigital clefts (similar to 'athlete's foot') is fairly common and can be controlled by topical preparations. Tinea of the nails can be more difficult to eradicate and may require oral anti-fungal medication and complete removal of the nail.

Subcutaneous infection by *Sporothrix schenkii* (sporotrichosis) is rarely seen in Britain but is not uncommon in North America, where it is usually caused by a thorn-prick. Chronic ulceration at the prick site, unresponsive to antibiotic treatment, may suggest the diagnosis, which can be confirmed by microbiological culture. The recommended treatment is oral potassium iodide.

Deep mycotic infection may involve tendons or joints. The diagnosis should be confirmed by microscopy and microbiological culture. Treatment is by local excision and administration of an intravenous anti-fungal agent. Resistant cases occasionally require limited amputation.

Opportunistic fungal infections are more likely to occur in debilitated and immunosuppressed patients.

VASCULAR DISORDERS OF THE HAND

Emboli

Arising from the heart or from aneurysms in the arteries of the upper limb, emboli can lodge in distal vessels causing splinter haemorrhages, or in larger, more proximal vessels causing ischaemia of the arm. A large embolus leads to the classic signs of pain, pulselessness, paraesthesia, pallor and paralysis. Untreated, gangrene or ischaemic contracture ensues.

Raynaud's disease

Raynaud's syndrome is produced by a vasospastic disorder which affects mainly the hands and fingers. Attacks are usually precipitated by cold; the fingers go pale and icy, then dusky blue (or cyanotic) and finally red. Between attacks the hands look normal. The condition is most commonly seen in young women who have no underlying or predisposing disease.

Raynaud's phenomenon is the term applied when these changes are associated with an underlying disease such as scleroderma or arteriosclerosis. Similar, though milder, changes are also seen in thoracic outlet syndrome. The hands must be kept warm; calcium channel blockade or digital sympathectomy (surgical removal of the sympathetic plexus around the digital arteries) may be needed.

Vibration white finger

Excessive and prolonged use of vibrating tools can damage the nerves and vessels in the fingers, leading to pain, cold intolerance and colour changes. Treatment is generally unsatisfactory.

Ulnar artery thrombosis

Repeated blows to the hand, especially using the hypothenar eminence as a hammer, can damage the intima of the ulnar artery, leading to either thrombosis or an aneurysm. The patient presents with cold intolerance in the little finger. Microvascular reconstruction of the ulnar artery is needed.

NOTES ON APPLIED ANATOMY

Function

The hand serves three basic functions: *sensory perception, precise manipulation* and *power grip.* The first two involve the thumb, index and middle fingers; without normal sensation and the ability to oppose these three digits, manipulative precision will be lost. The ring and little fingers provide power grip, for which they need full flexion; sensation is less important for these.

With the wrist flexed the fingers and thumb fall naturally into extension. With the wrist extended the fingers curl into flexion and the tips of the thumb, index and middle fingers form a functional tripod; this is the *position of function*, because it is best suited to the actions of prehension.

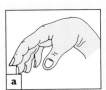
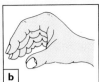
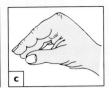

16.26 Three positions of the hand (**a**) The position of relaxation, (**b**) the position of function (ready for action) and (**c**) the position of safe immobilization, with the ligaments taut.

Finger flexion is strongest when the wrist is powerfully extended; normal grasp is possible only with a painless, stable wrist. Spreading the fingers produces abduction to either side of the middle finger; bringing them together, adduction. Abduction and adduction of the thumb occur in a plane at right angles to the palm (i.e. with the hand lying palm upwards, abduction points the thumb to the ceiling). By a combination of movements the thumb can also be opposed to each of the other fingers. Functionally, the thumb is 40% of the hand.

Skin

The palmar skin is relatively tight and inelastic; skin loss can be ill-afforded and wounds sutured under tension are liable to break down. The acute sensibility of the digital palmar skin cannot be achieved by any skin graft. Although the dorsal skin seems lax and mobile with the fingers extended, flexion will show that there is very little spare skin. Loss of skin therefore often requires a graft or flap.

Just deep to the palmar skin is the palmar aponeurosis, the embryological remnant of a superficial layer of finger flexors; attachment to the bases of the proximal phalanges explains part of the deformity of Dupuytren's contracture. Incisions on the palmar surface are also liable to contracture unless they are placed in the line of the skin creases, along the mid-lateral borders of the fingers or obliquely across the creases.

Joints

THE CARPOMETACARPAL JOINTS
The second and third metacarpals have very little independent movement; the fourth and fifth have more, allowing greater closure of the ulnar part of the hand during power grip. The metacarpal of the thumb is the most mobile and the first carpometacarpal joint is a frequent target for degenerative arthritis.

THE METACARPOPHALANGEAL JOINTS
These flex to about 90°. The range of extension increases progressively from the index to the little finger. The collateral ligaments are lax in extension (permitting abduction) and tight in flexion (preventing abduction).

If these joints are immobilized they should always be in flexion, so that the ligaments are at full stretch and therefore less likely to shorten if they should fibrose.

THE INTERPHALANGEAL JOINTS
The interphalangeal joints are simple hinges, each flexing to about 90°. Their collateral ligaments send attachments to the volar plate and these fibres are tight in extension and lax in flexion; *immobilization of the interphalangeal joints, therefore, should always be in extension.*

Muscles and tendons

Two sets of muscles control finger movements: the *long extrinsic muscles* (extensors, deep flexors and superficial flexors), and the *short intrinsic muscles* (interossei, lumbricals and the short thenar and hypothenar muscles). The extrinsics extend the metacarpophalangeal joints (long extensors) and flex the interphalangeal joints (long flexors). The intrinsics flex the metacarpophalangeal and extend the interphalangeal joints; the dorsal interossei also abduct and the palmar interossei adduct the fingers from the axis of the middle finger. Spasm or contracture of the intrinsics causes the *intrinsic-plus* posture – flexion at the metacarpophalangeal joints, extension at the interphalangeal joints and adduction of the thumb. Paralysis of the intrinsics produces the *intrinsic-minus* posture – hyperextension of the metacarpophalangeal and flexion of the interphalangeal joints ('claw hand').

Tough *fibrous sheaths* enclose the flexor tendons as they traverse the fingers; starting at the metacarpophalangeal joints (level with the distal palmar crease) they extend to the distal interphalangeal joints. They serve as runners and pulleys, so preventing the tendons from bowstringing during flexion. Scarring within the fibro-osseous tunnel prevents normal excursion.

The long extensor tendons are prevented from bowstringing at the wrist by the extensor retinaculum; here they are liable to frictional trauma. Over the metacarpophalangeal joints each extensor tendon widens into an expansion which inserts into the proximal phalanx and then splits in three; a central slip inserts into the middle phalanx, the two lateral slips continue distally, join and end in the distal phalanx. Division of the middle slip causes a flexion deformity of the proximal interphalangeal joint (boutonnière); rupture of the distal conjoined slip causes flexion deformity of the distal interphalangeal joint (mallet finger).

Nerves

The median nerve supplies the abductor pollicis brevis, opponens pollicis and lumbricals to the middle and index fingers; it also innervates the palmar skin of the thumb, index and middle fingers and the radial half of the ring finger.

The ulnar nerve supplies the hypothenar muscles, all the interossei, lumbricals to the little and ring fingers, flexor pollicis brevis and adductor pollicis. Sensory branches innervate the palmar and dorsal skin of the little finger and the ulnar half of the ring finger.

The radial nerve supplies skin over the dorsoradial aspect of the hand.

REFERENCES AND FURTHER READING

ASSH Hand Surgery Update (1996) American Academy of Orthopaedic Surgeons, Rosemount

Boyer MI, Gelberman RH (1999) Operative correction of swan-neck and boutonnière deformities in the rheumatoid hand. *Journal of the American Academy of Orthopaedic Surgeons* 7, 92-100

Brand PW, Hollister A (1993) *Clinical Mechanics of the Hand.* Mosby, St Louis

Green DP (1998) *Operative Hand Surgery.* Churchill Livingstone, Edinburgh

Flatt AE (1995) *The Care of the Arthritic Hand.* QMP, St Louis

Hausman MR, Lisser SP (1992) Hand infections. *Orthopaedic Clinics of North America* 23, 171-185

Hurst LC, Amadio PC, Badalamente MA *et al.* (1987) *Mycobacterium marinum* infections of the hand. *Journal of Hand Surgery* 12A, 428-435

Lister G (1993) *The Hand - Diagnosis and Indications.* Churchill Livingstone, Edinburgh

Stevens KJ, Theologis T, McNally EG (2000) Imaging of plant-thorn synovitis. *Skeletal Radiology* 29, 605-608

CLINICAL ASSESSMENT

SYMPTOMS

Pain is felt in the neck itself, but it may also be referred to the shoulders or arms. If it starts suddenly after exertion, and is exaggerated by coughing or straining, think of a disc prolapse. Chronic or recurrent pain in older people is usually due to chronic disc degeneration and spondylosis. Always enquire if any posture or movement makes it worse; or better.

Stiffness may be either intermittent or continuous. Sometimes it is so severe that the patient can scarcely move the head.

Deformity usually appears as a wry neck; occasionally the neck is fixed in flexion.

Numbness, tingling and weakness in the upper limbs may be due to pressure on a nerve root; weakness in the lower limbs may result from cord compression in the neck.

Headache sometimes emanates from the neck, but if this is the only symptom other causes should be suspected.

'*Tension*' is often mentioned as a cause of neck pain and occipital headache. The neck and back are common target zones for psychosomatic illness.

SIGNS

No examination of the neck is complete without examination of the upper trunk and both upper limbs.

Look

Any deformity is noted. Wry neck, due to muscle spasm, may suggest a disc lesion, an inflammatory disorder or cervical spine injury; but it also occurs with intracranial lesions and disorders of the eyes or semi-circular canals. Neck stiffness is usually fairly obvious.

Feel

The front of the neck is most easily palpated with the patient seated and the examiner standing behind him or her. The best way to feel the back of the neck is with the patient lying prone and resting his or her head over a pillow; this way the patient can relax and the bony structures are more easily palpated. Feel for tender areas or lumps and note if the paravertebral muscles are in spasm.

Move

Forward flexion, extension, lateral flexion and rotation are tested, and then shoulder movements. Range of motion normally diminishes with age, but even in the older patient movement should be smooth and pain free.

Tests for arterial compression

If the thoracic outlet is tight, the radial pulse may disappear if, when the patient holds a deep breath, the

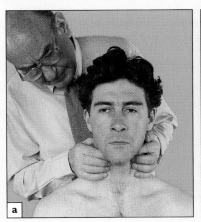
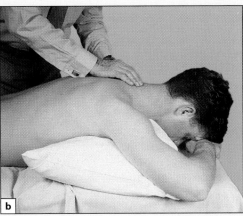

17.1 Examination – feel
(a) The front of the neck is felt with the patient seated and the examiner standing behind him. The back of the neck can be palpated with the patient standing, (b) but the bony structures are better felt with the patient lying prone over a pillow; this way muscle spasm is reduced and the neck is relaxed.

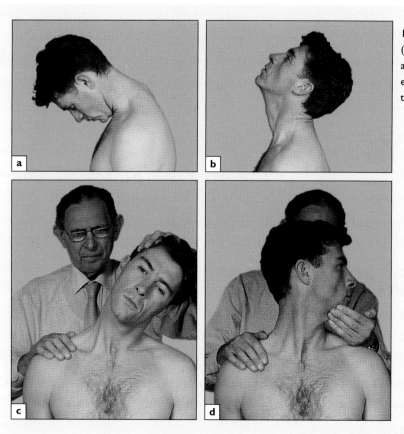

neck is turned towards the affected side and extended (Adson), or if the shoulder is abducted and externally rotated (Wright). These tests are described on page 250.

NEUROLOGICAL EXAMINATION

Neurological examination of the upper limbs is mandatory in all cases; in some the lower limbs also should be examined. Muscle power, reflexes and sensation should be carefully tested; even small degrees of abnormality may be significant.

IMAGING

X-RAYS

The standard radiographic series for the cervical spine comprises anteroposterior, lateral, and open-mouth views.

The anteroposterior view should show the regular, undulating outline of the lateral masses; their symmetry may be disturbed by destructive lesions or fractures. A projection through the mouth is required to show the upper two vertebrae.

When looking at the lateral view, *make sure that all seven vertebrae can be seen;* patients have been paralysed, and some have lost their lives, because a fracture-dislocation at C6/7 or C7/T1 was missed. The normal

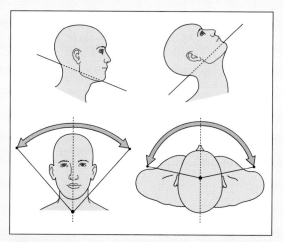

17.3 Normal range of movement In full flexion the chin normally touches the chest; in full extension the imaginary line joining the chin to the posterior occipital protuberance (the occipitomental line) forms an angle of at least 45° with the horizontal, and usually over 60° in young people. Lateral flexion and rotation are equal in both directions.

cervical lordotic curve shows four parallel lines: one along the anterior surfaces of the vertebral bodies, one along their posterior surfaces, one along the posterior borders of the lateral masses and one along the bases of the spinous processes; any malalignment suggests

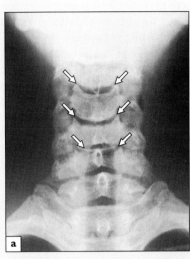
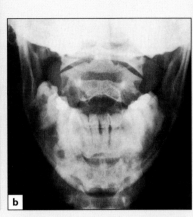
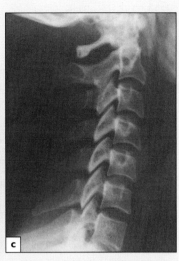

17.4 Imaging – normal x-rays (**a**) Anteroposterior view – note the smooth, symmetrical outlines and the clear, wide uncovertebral joints (arrows). (**b**) Open mouth view – to show the odontoid process and atlantoaxial joints. (**c**) Lateral view – showing all seven cervical vertebrae.

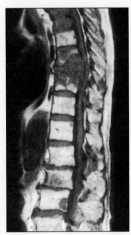

17.5 Magnetic resonance imaging MRI of the lower cervical and upper thoracic spine, showing metastatic deposits (dark grey areas in this T1-weighted image) in several vertebral bodies. The large tumour deposit at T2/3 is encroaching perilously on the spinal canal.

subluxation. The disc spaces are inspected; loss of disc height and the presence of osteophytic spurs at the margins of adjacent vertebral bodies suggest chronic intervertebral disc degeneration. The posterior interspinous spaces are compared; if one is wider than the rest, this may signify chronic instability of that segment, possibly due to a previously undiagnosed subluxation. Flexion and extension views may be needed to demonstrate instability, though after an acute injury this is best avoided!

Children's x-rays present special problems. Because the ligaments are relatively lax and the bones incompletely ossified, flexion views may show unexpectedly large shifts between adjacent vertebrae; this is sometimes mistaken for abnormal subluxation. Thus, during flexion, the lateral x-ray may show an atlanto-dental interval of 4 or 5mm (which in an adult would suggest rupture of the transverse ligament), or anterior 'subluxation' at C2/3. Note also that the retropharyngeal space between the cervical spine and pharynx at the level of C3 increases markedly on forced expiration (e.g. when crying) and this can be misinterpreted as a soft tissue mass. Another error is to mistake the normal synchondrosis between the dens and the arch of C2 (which only fuses at about 6 years) for an odontoid fracture. Finally, remember that normal-looking radiographs in children do not exclude the possibility of a spinal cord injury.

COMPUTED TOMOGRAPHY

In the cervical spine, CT (computed tomography) is particularly helpful for demonstrating the shape and size of the spinal canal and intervertebral foramena, as well as the integrity of the bony structures.

MYELOGRAPHY

Changes in the contour of the contrast-filled thecal sac suggest intra-dural and extra-dural compression. However this is an invasive investigation and fairly non-specific. Its usefulness is enhanced by performing a post-contrast CT scan.

MAGNETIC RESONANCE IMAGING

This is non-invasive, does not expose the patient to radiation and provides excellent resolution of the intervertebral disc and neural structures. It is the most sensitive method of demonstrating tumours and infection. It provides information on the size of the spinal canal and neural foramena. Its sensitivity can be a drawback: 20% of asymptomatic patients show significant abnormalities and the scans must therefore be interpreted alongside the clinical assessment.

DEFORMITIES OF THE NECK IN CHILDREN

A variety of deformities are encountered, some reflecting postural adjustments to underlying disorders and others due to developmental anomalies.

TORTICOLLIS

This is a description rather than a diagnosis. The chin is twisted upwards and towards one side. There are many causes. The condition may be either *congenital* or *acquired*.

Infantile (congenital) torticollis

This condition is common. The sternomastoid muscle on one side is fibrous and fails to elongate as the child grows; consequently, progressive deformity develops. The cause is unknown; the muscle may have suffered ischaemia from a distorted position *in utero* (the association with breech presentation and hip dysplasia is supporting evidence), or it may have been injured at birth.

A history of difficult labour or breech delivery is common. A lump may be noticed in the first few weeks of life; it is well defined and involves one or both heads of the sternomastoid. At this stage there is neither deformity nor obvious limitation of movement and within a few months the lump has disappeared. Deformity does not become apparent until the child is 1–2 years old. The head is tilted to one side, so that the ear approaches the shoulder; the sternomastoid on that side may feel tight and hard. There may also be asymmetrical development of the face (plagiocephaly). These features become increasingly obvious as the child grows.

Other causes of wry neck (bony anomalies, discitis, lymphadenitis) should be excluded. The history and the typical facial appearance are helpful clues. Radiographs must be taken to exclude a bone abnormality or fracture.

Treatment If the diagnosis is made during infancy, daily muscle stretching by the parents may prevent the incipient deformity. Non-operative treatment is successful in most cases. If the condition persists beyond 1 year, operative correction is required to avoid progressive facial deformity. The contracted muscle is divided (usually at its lower end but sometimes at the upper end or at both ends) and the head is manipulated into the neutral position. After operation, correction must be maintained, with a temporary rigid orthosis followed by stretching exercises.

Secondary torticollis

Childhood torticollis may be secondary to congenital bone anomalies, atlantoaxial rotatory displacement, infection (lymphadenitis, retropharyngeal abscess, tonsillitis, discitis, tuberculosis), trauma, juvenile rheumatoid arthritis, posterior fossa tumours, intraspinal tumours, dystonia (benign paroxysmal torticollis) or ocular dysfunction.

ATLANTOAXIAL ROTATORY DISPLACEMENT The aetiology of this condition is unclear, but it is thought to be due to muscle spasm resulting from inflammation of the ligaments, capsule and synovium of the atlantoaxial

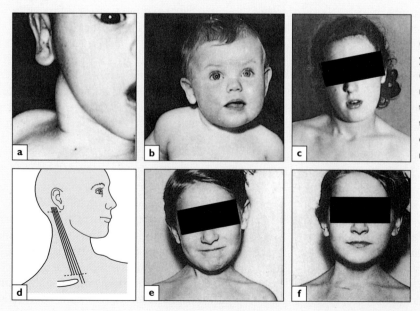

17.6 Torticollis Natural history: **(a)** sternomastoid tumour in a young baby; **(b)** early wry neck; **(c)** deformity with facial hemiatrophy in the adolescent. Surgical treatment: **(d)** two sites at which the sternomastoid may be divided; **(e, f)** before and a few months after operation.

region. There may be a history of trauma or upper respiratory tract infection. The child presents with a painful wry neck. Plain x-rays are difficult to interpret; a CT scan in both neutral and maximum lateral rotation is the most helpful investigation.

Most cases are mild and can be managed expectantly with a soft collar and analgesics. If there is no resolution after a week, halter traction, bed rest and analgesics should be prescribed. In more resistant cases, halo traction may be required. Occasionally there is anterior displacement of C1 on C2; the articulation may not stabilize following traction and a C1/2 fusion is then indicated.

VERTEBRAL ANOMALIES

There are many vertebral anomalies and most are very rare. Three are described here.

KLIPPEL–FEIL SYNDROME (CERVICAL-VERTEBRAL SYNOSTOSIS)

This developmental disorder represents a failure of segmentation of the cervical somites; it is often associated with abnormalities in the genito-urinary, nervous or cardiovascular systems. Some children have a hearing impediment.

Children with synostosis have a characteristic appearance: the neck is short or non-existent and there may be webbing; the hairline is low; and neck movements are limited. About one in three children with Klippel–Feil syndrome also has Sprengel's deformity of the scapula. Scoliosis is present in about 60% and rib anomalies in about 30%. Hand deformities such as syndactyly, thumb hypoplasia and extra digits are often present. X-rays reveal fusion of two or more cervical vertebrae.

Symptoms tend to arise in the second or third decades, not from the fused segments but from the adjacent mobile segments. There may be pain due to joint hypermobility, or neurological symptoms from instability.

Children with symptoms may need cervical fusion. For asymptomatic patients, treatment is unnecessary but parents should be warned of the risks of contact sports; sudden catastrophic neurological compromise can occur after minor trauma.

BASILAR IMPRESSION

In this condition the floor of the skull is indented by the upper cervical spine. The odontoid can impinge upon the brain stem. The cause is either a primary bone abnormality (associated with other bone defects such as odontoid abnormalities, Morquio syndrome and Klippel–Feil syndrome) or secondary to softening of the bones (osteomalacia, rickets, rheumatoid arthritis, neurofibromatosis, etc.). The relationship between the odontoid and the foramen magnum can be ascertained on plain radiographs; further information is acquired with CT or MRI. Patients may present – often in the second or third decade – with symptoms of raised intracranial pressure (because the aqueduct of Sylvius becomes blocked), weakness and paraesthesia of the limbs (because of direct compression or ischaemia of the cord). Treatment involves surgical decompression and stabilization.

ODONTOID ANOMALIES

The odontoid may be absent or hypoplastic, or there may be a separate ossicle (the os odontoideum). The anomaly should be suspected (and looked for even if the child does not complain) in skeletal dysplasias which involve the spine. This is especially important in patients undergoing operation; the atlantoaxial joint may subluxate under anaesthesia. Some patients present with pain or torticollis, or neurological complications such as transient paralysis, myelopathy with upper motor neurone signs or sphincter disturbances. In the majority of cases the anomaly is discovered by chance in a routine cervical spine x-ray following trauma. Open-mouth radiographs show the abnormality; lateral flexion/extension views may show instability of the C1–C2 articulation.

Patients with symptoms should have surgical stabilization; the prophylactic treatment of asymptomatic patients is controversial.

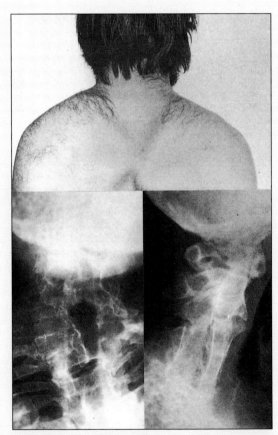

17.7 Klippel–Feil syndrome The short neck and vertebral anomalies in a typical patient.

ACUTE INTERVERTEBRAL DISC PROLAPSE

Acute disc prolapse is not as common in the neck as in the lower back; both segments of the spine are mobile but loading stresses in the cervical region are not as high as in the lumbosacral region. The pathological features are similar; these are described in some detail on page 390.

The acute prolapse may be precipitated by local strain or injury, especially sudden unguarded flexion and rotation, and usually occurs immediately above or below the sixth cervical vertebra. In many cases (perhaps in all) there is a predisposing abnormality of the disc with increased nuclear tension. Prolapsed material may press on the posterior longitudinal ligament or dura mater, causing neck pain and stiffness as well as pain referred to the upper limb. Pressure on the nerve roots causes paraesthesia, and sometimes weakness, in one or both arms – usually in the distribution of C6 or C7.

Clinical features

The original attack can usually be related to a specific strain episode, e.g. acute flexion of the neck during intense physical exertion, or (occasionally) a 'whiplash' injury. Subsequent attacks may be sudden or gradual in onset, and with trivial cause. The patient complains of (a) pain and stiffness of the neck, the pain often radiating to the scapular region and sometimes to the occiput; and (b) pain and paraesthesia in one upper limb (rarely both), often radiating to the outer elbow, back of the wrist and the index and middle fingers. Weakness is rare. Between attacks the patient feels well, although the neck may feel a bit stiff.

The neck may be held tilted forwards and sideways. The muscles are tender and movements are restricted. The arms should be examined for neurological deficit. The C6 root innervates the biceps reflex, the biceps muscle and wrist extensors, and sensation of the lateral forearm, thumb and index finger; C7 innervates the triceps and radial reflexes, the triceps muscle, wrist flexors and finger extensors, and sensation in the middle finger. Rotation and tilting of the neck to the affected side, combined with a Valsalva manoeuvre, may provoke radicular symptoms.

IMAGING

X-rays may reveal straightening out of the normal cervical lordosis (due to muscle spasm) and narrowing of the disc space (although this is unlikely during a first attack). The most useful form of imaging is *MRI*, which will show the disc and its relationship to the nerve root in most cases. Even more accurate, but not used routinely because it involves intrathecal injection of contrast medium, is *CT myelography*.

Differential diagnosis

Acute soft-tissue strain Acute strains of the neck are often associated with pain, stiffness and vague 'tingling' in the upper limbs. It is important to bear in mind that pain radiating into the arm is not necessarily due to nerve root pressure.

Neuralgic amyotrophy This condition can closely resemble an acute disc prolapse and should always be thought of if there is no definite history of a strain episode. Pain is sudden and severe, and situated over the shoulder rather than in the neck itself. Careful examination will show that more than one level is affected – an extremely rare event in disc prolapse.

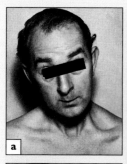
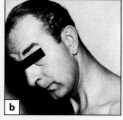
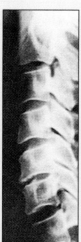
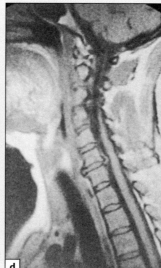

17.8 Acute disc prolapse (**a, b**) Acute wry neck due to a prolapsed disc. (**c**) A reduced disc space at C5/6 is not necessary for the diagnosis; (**d**) MRI showing a prolapsed disc at C5/6.

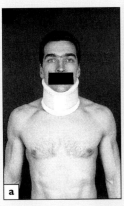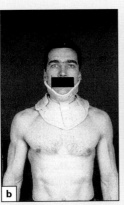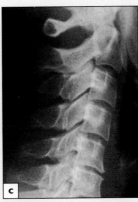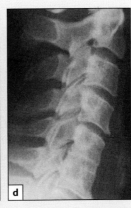

17.9 Cervical disc prolapse – treatment (a) Standard collar. (b) More rigid variety. (c, d) Operative treatment usually consists of anterior disc removal and bone grafting. In this case the intervertebral disc height at C5/6 has been restored but now, some years later, there are signs of disc degeneration above and below the fused segment.

Cervical spine infections Pain is unrelenting and local spasm severe. X-rays show erosion of the vertebral end-plates.

Cervical tumours Neurological signs are progressive and x-rays reveal bone destruction.

Rotator cuff lesions Although the distribution of pain may resemble that of a prolapsed cervical disc, tenderness is localized to the rotator cuff and shoulder movements are abnormal.

Treatment

Heat and analgesics are soothing but, as with lumbar disc prolapse, there are only three satisfactory ways of treating the prolapse itself.

Rest A collar will prevent unguarded movement; it may be made of felt, sponge-rubber or plastic. It seldom needs to be worn for more than a week or two.

Reduce Traction may enlarge the disc space, permitting the prolapse to subside. The head of the couch is raised and weights (up to 8kg) are tied to a harness fitting under the chin and occiput. Traction is applied intermittently for no more than 30 minutes at a time.

Remove If symptoms are refractory and severe enough, if there is a progressive neurological deficit or if there are signs of an acute myelopathy then surgery is indicated. The disc may be removed through an anterior approach; bone grafts are inserted to fuse the affected area and to restore the normal intervertebral height. If only one level is affected, and there is no bony encroachment on the intervertebral foramen, anterior decompression can be expected to give good long-term relief from radicular symptoms.

CERVICAL SPONDYLOSIS

This vague term is applied to a cluster of abnormalities arising from chronic intervertebral disc degeneration. Changes are most common in the lower two segments of the cervical spine (C5–C7), the area which is prone to intervertebral disc prolapse. The discs degenerate, flatten and become less elastic. The facet joints and the uncovertebral joints are slightly displaced and become arthritic, giving rise to pain and stiffness in the neck. Bony spurs, ridges or bars appear at the anterior and posterior margins of the vertebral bodies; those that develop posteriorly may encroach upon the spinal canal or the intervertebral foramena, causing pressure on the dura (which is pain sensitive) and the neural structures.

Clinical features

The patient, usually aged over 40 years, complains of *neck pain and stiffness*. The symptoms come on gradually and are often worse on first getting up. The pain may radiate widely: to the occiput, the back of the shoulders and down one or both arms; it is sometimes accompanied by paraesthesia, weakness and clumsiness in the arm and hand. Typically there are exacerbations of more acute discomfort, and long periods of relative quiescence.

The appearance is normal, but the muscles at the back of the neck and across the scapulae are tender. Neck movements are limited and painful.

Sometimes the clinical picture is dominated by features arising from narrowing of the intervertebral foramena and compression of the nerve roots (*radiculopathy*): these include changes in sensibility, muscle weakness and depressed reflexes in the arm or hand. In advanced cases there may be narrowing of the spinal canal and changes due to pressure on the cord (*myelopathy* – see below).

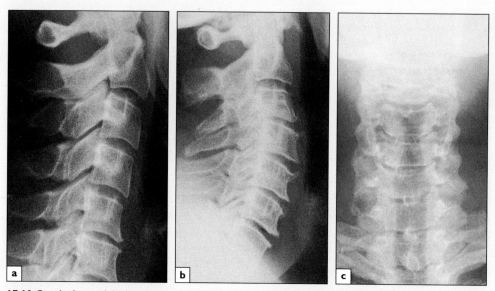

17.10 Cervical spondylosis – x-rays (a) Lateral view showing disc narrowing and slight lipping of the vertebral bodies at C5/6. (b) A more advanced case: several levels are involved and there is marked spur formation (erroneously called 'osteophytes') at both the anterior and posterior borders of the vertebral bodies. (c) The anteroposterior view shows narrowing of the uncovertebral joints (compare with Fig. 17.4).

Imaging

X-rays show narrowing of one or more intervertebral spaces, with spur formation (or lipping) at the anterior and posterior margins of the disc. These bony ridges (often referred to as 'osteophytes') may encroach upon the intervertebral foramina. *MRI* is more reliable for showing whether the nerve roots are compressed.

Diagnosis

Other disorders associated with neck and/or arm pain and sensory symptoms must be excluded. Cervical spine 'degenerative changes' are so common after the age of 40 years that they are likely to be seen in most middle-aged and elderly people who complain of pain, and it is easy to persuade oneself that they are the cause of the patient's symptoms.

Nerve entrapment syndromes Median or ulnar nerve entrapment may give rise to intermittent symptoms of pain and paraesthesia in the hand. Characteristically the symptoms are worse at night or are related to posture. Careful examination will show that the changes follow a peripheral nerve rather than a root distribution. In doubtful cases, nerve conduction studies and electromyography will help to establish the diagnosis. Remember, though, that the patient may have symptoms from both a peripheral and a central abnormality; indeed, there is some evidence to suggest

that long-standing cervical spondylosis may make the patient more vulnerable to the effects of peripheral nerve entrapment.

Rotator cuff lesions Pain may resemble that of cervical spondylosis, but shoulder movements are abnormal and there may be x-ray and MRI features of rotator cuff degeneration.

Cervical tumours Metastatic deposits in the cervical spine can cause misleading symptoms, but sooner or later bone destruction produces diagnostic x-ray changes. With tumours of the spinal cord, nerve roots or lymph nodes, symptoms are usually continuous, and the lesion may appear on imaging.

Thoracic outlet syndrome This condition is described in Chapter 11. Symptoms resemble those of cervical spondylosis; pain and sensory abnormalities appear mainly down the ulnar border of the forearm and may be aggravated by upper limb traction or by elevation and external rotation of the shoulder. Importantly, neck movements are neither painful nor restricted. X-rays may reveal a cervical rib, although the mere presence of this anomaly is not necessarily diagnostic.

Treatment

Analgesics are prescribed when necessary. Heat and massage are often soothing, but restricting neck movements in a collar is the most effective treatment during painful attacks. Physiotherapy is the mainstay of treatment, patients usually being maintained in relative comfort by various measures including exercises, gentle passive manipulation and intermittent traction.

Operation is seldom indicated, but if only one intervertebral level is affected and symptoms are relieved only by a rigid and irksome support, anterior fusion is appropriate. If there is definite evidence of foraminal narrowing and nerve root compression, foramenotomy may be indicated. For multiple level spondylosis, the long-term results of fusion are not significantly better than those following conservative treatment.

OSSIFICATION OF THE POSTERIOR LONGITUDINAL LIGAMENT

Reports on ossification of the posterior longitudinal ligament (OPLL) have appeared mainly from Japan (Ono *et al.*, 1977; Tsuyama, 1984). However, it is now recognized that this condition is quite common and widespread. It occurs mainly in the cervical spine and may be associated with bone-forming conditions such as diffuse idiopathic skeletal hyperostosis (DISH) and fluorosis. The cause is unknown. The significance of the disease is that it may give rise to spinal stenosis and cervical myelopathy.

The patient, usually a man between 50 and 70 years of age, may present with any combination of pain in the neck and upper limb(s), sensory symptoms and muscle weakness in the arms and upper motor neurone (cord) symptoms and signs in the lower limbs. The most disturbing features are motor abnormalities such as weakness, incoordination, clumsiness, muscle wasting and incontinence.

X-rays show dense ossification along the back of the vertebral bodies (and sometimes also the ligamentum flavum) in the mid-cervical spine.

Treatment is not always necessary; indeed people with typical x-ray features may be completely asymptomatic. If the symptoms and signs are disturbing or progressive, operative decompression will be needed.

The most successful method reported is some form of posterior laminoplasty; the laminae are split and the posterior elements are 'jacked open' to provide more room for the cord (Hirabayashi *et al.*, 1999).

SPINAL STENOSIS AND CERVICAL MYELOPATHY

The sagittal diameter of the mid-cervical spinal canal (the distance, on plain x-rays, from the posterior surface of the vertebral body to the base of the spinous process) varies considerably from one individual

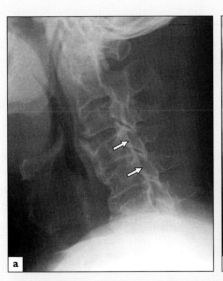
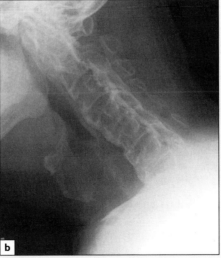

17.11 Ossification of the posterior longitudinal ligament (a) Lateral x-ray of the cervical spine showing the thin dense band running down the backs of the vertebral bodies (arrows); this appearance is typical of posterior longitudinal ligament ossification, which resulted in cervical spinal stenosis. (b) X-ray taken after posterior spinal decompression (laminoplasty): the spinous processes have been removed, the laminae split on one side of the mid-line and the posterior arch 'jacked' open. The sagittal diameter of the spinal canal is now considerably greater than before. (Courtesy of Mr HK Wong, Singapore.)

to another; anything less than 11mm is suggestive of stenosis. Abnormally small canals are seen in rare dysplasias, such as achondroplasia, and may give rise to cord compression. Many asymptomatic, and apparently normal, people also have small canals and they are at risk of developing the clinical symptoms of spinal stenosis if there is any further encroachment due to intervertebral disc degeneration, posterior 'osteophytosis', osteoarthritis of the facet joints, thickening of the ligamentum flavum, ossification of the posterior longitudinal ligament or vertebral displacement. If the changes are severe enough, the patient may develop neurological symptoms and signs (*cervical myelopathy*), which are thought to be due to both direct compression and ischaemia of the cord and nerve roots arising from impaired venous drainage and reduced arterial flow.

Clinical features

Patients usually have neck pain and brachialgia but also complain of paraesthesia, numbness, weakness and clumsiness in the arms and legs and an increasingly unsteady gait. Symptoms may be precipitated by acutely hyperextending the neck, and some patients present for the first time after a hyperextension injury. They may experience involuntary spasms in the legs and, occasionally, episodes of spontaneous clonus. In severe cases there may be urinary and rectal dysfunction or incontinence.

The 'classic' picture of weakness and spasticity in the legs and numbness in the hands is easy to recognize, but the features are not always as clear-cut as that. However, careful examination should reveal upper motor neurone signs in the lower limbs (increased muscle tone, brisk reflexes and clonus), while sensory signs depend on which part of the cord is compressed: there may be decreased sensibility to pain and temperature (spinothalamic tracts) or diminished vibration and position sense (posterior columns).

The condition is usually slowly progressive, but occasionally a patient with long-standing symptoms starts deteriorating rapidly and treatment becomes urgent.

IMAGING
A *plain lateral radiograph* which shows an anteroposterior diameter of the spinal canal of less than 11mm strongly supports the diagnosis of cervical spinal stenosis. A better measure is the Pavlov ratio (the anteroposterior diameter of the canal divided by the diameter of the vertebral body at the same level) because this is not affected by magnification error. A ratio of less than 0.8 is abnormal.

MRI demonstrates the spinal cord and soft tissue structures, and helps to exclude other causes of similar neurological dysfunction. *CT myelography* is superior to MRI in demonstrating osseous detail.

Differential diagnosis

Full neurological investigation and imaging studies are required to eliminate other diagnoses such as vertebral disease, multiple sclerosis (episodic symptoms), amyotrophic lateral sclerosis (purely motor dysfunction), syringomyelia and spinal cord tumours.

Treatment

Most patients can be treated conservatively with analgesics, a collar, isometric exercises and gait training. Manipulation and traction should be avoided.

Patients with progressive myelopathy or rapid deterioration should be considered for surgery. Acute, severe myelopathy is a surgical emergency, requiring immediate decompression.

Discogenic causes and osteophytosis limited to one or two levels can usually be dealt with by anterior discectomy and fusion, with good results in over 80% of cases. Ossification of the posterior longitudinal ligament and other bone disorders require posterior decompression.

PYOGENIC INFECTION

Pyogenic infection of the cervical spine is uncommon, and therefore often misdiagnosed in the early stages when antibiotic treatment is most effective.

The organism – usually a staphylococcus – reaches the spine via the blood stream. Initially, destructive changes are limited to the intervertebral disc space and the adjacent parts of the vertebral bodies. Later, abscess formation occurs and pus may extend into the spinal canal or into the soft-tissue planes of the neck.

Clinical features

Vertebral infection may occur at any age. The patient complains of pain in the neck, often severe and associated with muscle spasm and marked stiffness. However, systemic symptoms are often mild. On examination, neck movements are severely restricted.

Blood tests may show a leucocytosis and an increased ESR.

X-rays at first show either no abnormality or only slight narrowing of the disc space; later there may be more obvious signs of bone destruction.

Treatment

Treatment is by antibiotics and rest. The cervical spine is 'immobilized' by traction; once the acute phase subsides, a collar may suffice. Operation is seldom necessary; as the infection subsides the intervertebral space is obliterated and the adjacent vertebrae fuse. If there is frank abscess formation, this will require drainage.

TUBERCULOSIS

Cervical spine tuberculosis is very rare. As with other types of infection, the organism is blood-borne and the infection localizes in the intervertebral disc and the interior parts of the adjacent vertebral bodies. As the bone crumbles, the cervical spine collapses into kyphosis. A retropharyngeal abscess forms and points behind the sternomastoid muscle at the side of the neck. In late cases cord damage may cause neurological signs varying from mild weakness to tetraplegia.

Clinical features

The patient – usually a child – complains of neck pain and stiffness. In neglected cases a retropharyngeal abscess may cause difficulty in swallowing or swelling at the side of the neck. On examination the neck is extremely tender and all movements are restricted. In late cases there may be obvious kyphosis, a fluctuant abscess in the neck or a retropharyngeal swelling. The limbs should be examined for neurological defects.

X-rays show narrowing of the disc space and erosion of the adjacent vertebral bodies.

Treatment

Treatment is initially by *antituberculous drugs* and 'immobilization' of the neck in a cervical brace or plaster cast for 6–18 months. *Operative treatment* may become necessary (1) to drain a retropharyngeal abscess, (2) to decompress a threatened cord or (3) to fuse an unstable spine. Debridement of necrotic bone and anterior fusion with bone grafts may also be offered as an alternative to prolonged immobilization in a brace or cast.

RHEUMATOID ARTHRITIS

The cervical spine is severely affected in 30% of patients with rheumatoid arthritis (see also Chapter 3). Three types of lesion are common: (1) erosion of the atlantoaxial joints and the transverse ligament, with

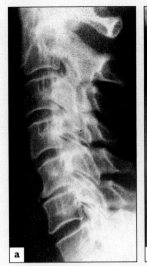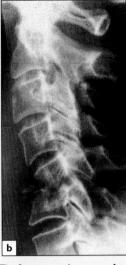

17.12 Pyogenic infection (a) The first x-ray, taken soon after the onset of symptoms, shows narrowing of the C5/6 disc space but no other abnormality. (b) Three weeks later there is dramatic destruction and collapse; the speed at which these have occurred distinguishes pyogenic from tuberculous infection.

resulting instability; (2) erosion of the atlanto-occipital articulations, allowing the odontoid peg to ride up into the foramen magnum (cranial sinkage); and (3) erosion of the facet joints in the mid-cervical region, sometimes ending in fusion but more often leading to subluxation. In addition, vertebral osteoporosis is common, due either to the disease or to the effect of corticosteroid therapy, or both.

Considering the amount of atlantoaxial displacement that occurs (often greater than 1cm), neurological complications are uncommon. However, they do occur – especially in long-standing cases – and are produced by mechanical compression of the cord, by local granulation tissue formation or (very rarely) by thrombosis of the vertebral arteries.

Clinical features

The patient is usually a woman with advanced rheumatoid arthritis. She has neck pain, and movements are markedly restricted. Symptoms and signs of root compression may be present in the upper limbs; less often there is lower limb weakness and upper motor neurone signs due to cord compression. There may be symptoms of vertebro-basilar insufficiency, such as vertigo, tinnitus and visual disturbance. Some patients, though completely unaware of any neurological deficit, are found on careful examination to have mild sensory disturbance or pyramidal tract signs (e.g. abnormally brisk reflexes).

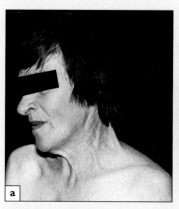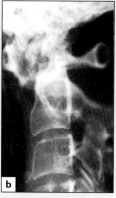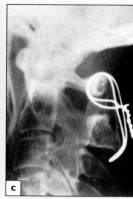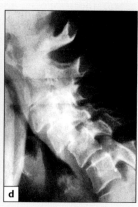

17.13 Rheumatoid arthritis (a) Movement is severely restricted; attempted rotation causes pain and muscle spasm. (b) Atlantoaxial subluxation is common; erosion of the joints and the transverse ligament has allowed the atlas to slip forward about 2cm; (c) reduction and posterior fusion with wire fixation. (d) This patient has subluxation, not only at the atlantoaxial joint but also at two levels in the mid-cervical region.

General debility and peripheral joint involvement can mask the signs of myelopathy. Lehrmitte's sign – paraesthesia in the legs on flexing the neck – may be present. Sudden death from catastrophic neurological compression is rare.

X-RAYS

X-rays show the features of an erosive arthritis, usually at several levels. *Atlantoaxial instability* is visible in lateral films taken in flexion and extension; in flexion the anterior arch of the atlas rides forwards, leaving a gap of 5mm or more between the back of the anterior arch and the odontoid process; on extension the subluxation is reduced. *Atlanto-occipital erosion* is more difficult to see, but a lateral tomograph shows the relationship of the odontoid to the foramen magnum. Normally the odontoid tip is less than 5mm above McGregor's line (a line from the posterior edge of the hard palate to the lowest point on the occiput); in erosive arthritis the odontoid tip may be 10–12mm above this line. Flexion views may also show *anterior subluxation in the mid-cervical region*.

CT AND MRI

These methods are useful for imaging 'difficult' areas such as the atlantoaxial and atlanto-occipital articulations, and for viewing the soft-tissue structures (especially the cord).

Treatment

Despite the startling x-ray appearances, serious neurological complications are uncommon. Pain can usually be relieved by wearing a collar.

The indications for operative stabilization of the cervical spine are (1) severe and unremitting pain, and (2) neurological signs of root or cord compression.

Arthrodesis is by bone grafting followed by a halo-body cast, or by internal fixation (posterior wiring or a rectangular fixator) and bone grafting. Postoperatively a cervical brace is worn for 3 months; however, if instability is marked and operative fixation insecure, a halo-jacket may be necessary. In patients with very advanced disease and severe erosive changes, postoperative morbidity and mortality are high. This is an argument for operating at an earlier stage for 'impending neurological deficit', as diagnosed from x-ray signs of severe atlantoaxial subluxation, upward migration of the odontoid or subaxial vertebral subluxation together with CT, myelographic or MR images of cord or brainstem compression.

ANKYLOSING SPONDYLITIS

Ankylosing spondylitis is the most common seronegative spondyloarthropathy to affect the cervical spine. Neck pain and stiffness tend to occur some years after the onset of backache. The neck becomes progressively stiff and kyphotic although some movement is usually preserved at the atlanto-occipital and atlantoaxial joints.

An unacceptable 'chin-on-chest' deformity, or inability to lift the head high enough to see more than ten paces ahead, are indications for cervical spine osteotomy.

The ankylosed spine is osteoporotic and prone to fracture. A patient with ankylosing spondylitis and an increase in neck pain must be assumed to have a fracture until proven otherwise (by bone scan or MRI if plain radiographs are normal). Neurological compromise is common. A displaced fracture needs careful closed reduction with halo traction then halo-vest immobilization. Surgery carries a high complication rate.

SPASMODIC TORTICOLLIS

This, the most common form of focal dystonia, is characterized by involuntary twisting or clonic movements of the neck. Spasms are sometimes triggered by emotional disturbance or attempts at correction. Even at rest the neck assumes an abnormal posture, the chin usually twisted to one side and upwards; the shoulder on that side may be elevated. In some cases involuntary muscle contractions spread to other areas and the condition is revealed as a more generalized form of dystonia.

The exact cause is unknown, but some cases are associated with lesions of the basal ganglia. Correction is extremely difficult; various drugs, including anticholinergics, have been used, though with little success. Some patients respond to local injections of botulinum toxin into the sternomastoid muscle.

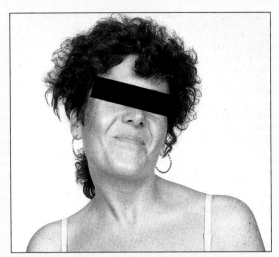

17.14 Spasmodic torticollis Attempted correction was forcibly resisted. The deformity can be very distressing.

NOTES ON APPLIED ANATOMY

In the upright posture the neck has a gentle anterior convexity; this natural lordosis may straighten but is never quite reversed, even in flexion, unless it is abnormal.

Eight pairs of nerve roots from the cervical cord pass through the relatively narrow intervertebral foramina, the first between the occiput and C1, and the eighth between C7 and the first thoracic (T1) vertebra. Thus each segmental root from the first to the seventh lies above the vertebra of the same number, so that a lesion between C5 and C6 might compress the sixth root.

The intervertebral discs lie close to the nerve roots as they emerge through the foramina; even a small herniation often causes root symptoms rather than neck pain. Moreover, disc degeneration is associated with spur formation on both the posterior aspect of the vertebral body and the associated facet joint; the resulting encroachment on the intervertebral foramen traps the nerve root. It is important to remember, however, that 'root pain' alone (i.e. pain in the shoulder and arm) does not necessarily signify nerve-root irritation; it may be referred from the facet joint or the soft structures around it. Only paraesthesiae and sensory or motor loss are unequivocal evidence of nerve root compression.

At the atlanto-occipital joint, the movements that occur are nodding and tilting (lateral flexion); there is no rotation, and when this movement takes place (at the atlantoaxial joint) the atlas and the skull move as one. In the rest of the cervical spine, movements are flexion, extension and tilting to either side; the facets permit subluxation or dislocation to occur without fracture, a displacement which is normally prevented by the strong posterior ligaments.

REFERENCES AND FURTHER READING

Agarwal AK, Peppelman WC, Kraus DR, Eisenbeis CH (1993) The cervical spine in rheumatoid arthritis. *British Medical Journal* **306**, 79-80

Copley LA, Dormans JP (1998) Cervical spine disorders in infants and children. *Journal of the American Academy of Orthopaedic Surgeons* **6**, 204-214

Garfin SR, Herkowitz HN (1992) The degenerative neck. *Orthopaedic Clinics of North America* **23**(3)

Hirabayashi K, Toyama Y, Chiba K (1999) Expansive laminoplasty in ossification of the posterior longitudinal ligament. *Clinical Orthopaedics and Related Research* **359**, 35–48

Hensinger RN (1991) Congenital anomalies of the cervical spine. *Clinical Orthopaedics and Related Research* **264**, 16-38

Law MD, Bernhardt M, White AA (1994) Evaluation and management of cervical spondylotic myelopathy. *Journal of Bone and Joint Surgery* **76**A, 1420-1433

Levine MJ, Albert TJ, Smith MD (1996) Cervical radiculopathy. *Journal of the American Academy of Orthopaedic Surgeons* **4**, 305-316

Ono K, Ota H, Tada K *et al* (1977) Ossified posterior longitudinal ligamanet. *Spine* **2**, 126

Tsuyama N (1984) Ossification of the posterior longitudinal ligament of the spine. *Clinical Orthopaedics and Related Research* **184**, 71-84

CLINICAL ASSESSMENT

SYMPTOMS

The usual symptoms of back disorders are pain, stiffness and deformity in the back, and pain, paraesthesia or weakness in the lower limbs. The mode of onset is very important: did it start suddenly, perhaps after a lifting strain; or gradually without any antecedent event? Are the symptoms constant, or are there periods of remission? Are they related to any particular posture? Has there been any associated illness or malaise?

Pain, either sharp and localized or chronic and diffuse, is the commonest presenting symptom. Backache is usually felt low down and on either side of the midline, often extending into the upper part of the buttock.

Sciatica is a term used to describe pain radiating from the buttock into the thigh and calf – more or less in the distribution of the sciatic nerve. However, it is rarely due to sciatic nerve pathology. It is a type of referred pain, usually from the dural sleeve of a lumbar or sacral nerve root or from an abnormal vertebral joint. Kellgren (1977), in a classic experiment, showed that almost any structure in a spinal segment can, if irritated sufficiently, give rise to pain spreading into the lower limbs. In practice, however, pain referred from the root dura is characteristically more intense, aggravated by coughing or straining, and often accompanied by symptoms of root pressure such as numbness or paraesthesia.

Stiffness may be sudden in onset and almost complete (after a disc prolapse) or continuous and predictably worse in the mornings (suggesting arthritis or ankylosing spondylitis).

Deformity is usually noticed by others, but the patient may become aware of shoulder asymmetry or of clothes not fitting well.

Numbness or paraesthesia is felt anywhere in the lower limb, but can usually be mapped fairly accurately over one of the dermatomes. It is important to ask if it is aggravated by standing or walking and relieved by sitting down – the classic symptom of spinal stenosis.

Urinary retention or incontinence can be due to pressure on the cauda equina. *Faecal incontinence* or urgency, and impotence, may also occur.

Other symptoms important in back disorders are *urethral discharge, diarrhoea* and *sore eyes* – the features of Reiter's disease.

Signs with the patient standing

Adequate exposure is essential; patients should strip to their underclothes

Look

Start by examining the skin. Scars, pigmentation or abnormal tufts of hair are important clues to underlying spinal disorders.

Look carefully at the patient's shape and posture, both from in front and from behind. Asymmetry of the chest, trunk or pelvis may be obvious, or may appear only when the patient bends forwards. Lateral deviation of the spinal column is described as a *list* to one or other side; lateral curvature is *scoliosis*.

Seen from the side, the back normally has a slight forwards curve, or *kyphosis*, in the thoracic region and a shorter backwards curve, or *lordosis*, in the lumbar segment (the 'hollow' of the back). Excessive thoracic kyphosis is sometimes called hyperkyphosis, to distinguish it from the normal; if the spine is sharply angulated the prominence is called a *kyphos* or *gibbus*. The lumbar spine may be excessively lordosed (hyperlordosis) or unusually flat (effectively a lumbar kyphosis).

Undue or asymmetrical prominence of the paravertebral muscles may be due to spasm, an important sign in acute back disorders.

If the patient consistently stands with one knee bent (even though his or her legs are equal in length) this suggests nerve root tension on that side; flexing the knee relaxes the sciatic nerve and reduces the pull on the nerve root.

Feel

The spinous processes and the interspinous ligaments are palpated, noting any prominence or a 'step'. *Tenderness* should be localized to (1) bony structures, (2) the intervertebral tissues or (3) the paravertebral muscles.

Move

Flexion is tested by asking the patient to try to touch his or her toes. Even with a stiff back they may be able to do this by flexing the hips; so watch the lumbar spine to see if it really moves, or, better still, measure the spinal

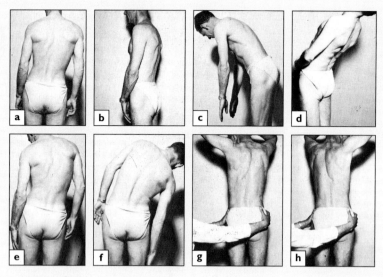

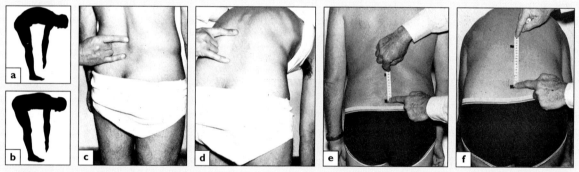

18.2 Examination (2) In both diagrams the hands nearly reach the toes; to distinguish spine flexion (**a**) from hip flexion (**b**), watch the lumbar lordosis undoing as the patient bends. Alternatively (**c**, **d**), note the separation of fingers placed on the spinous processes. Better still (**e**, **f**), measure the lumbar excursion; with the patient upright, two bony points 10cm apart are selected – in full flexion they should separate by at least a further 5cm.

excursion (Fig. 18.2 e, f). *The mode of flexion* (whether it is smooth or hesitant) and the way in which the patient comes back to the upright position are also important. In lumbar instability the patient tends to regain the upright position by pushing on the front of his thighs. To test *extension* ask the patient to lean backwards, but see that he or she doesn't cheat by bending the knees.

The *'wall test'* will unmask a minor flexion deformity; standing with the back flush against a wall, the heels, buttocks, shoulders and occiput should all make contact with the surface.

Lateral flexion is tested by asking the patient to bend sideways, sliding his or her hand down the outer side of his or her leg; the two sides are compared. *Rotation* is examined by asking the patient to twist the trunk to each side in turn while the pelvis is anchored by the examiner's hands; this is essentially a thoracic movement and should not be limited in lumbosacral disease.

Rib-cage excursion is assessed by measuring the *chest circumference* in full expiration and then in full inspiration; the normal difference is about 7cm.

While the patient is standing, you can test *muscle power* in the legs by asking him or her to stand up on the toes (plantarflexion) and then to rock back on the heels (dorsiflexion); small differences between the two sides are easily spotted.

SIGNS WITH THE PATIENT LYING FACE DOWNWARDS

Make sure that the patient is lying comfortably on the examination couch, and remove the pillow so that he or she is not forced to arch his or her back (or be smothered). Again, look for localized deformities and muscle spasm; and examine the buttocks for gluteal wasting.

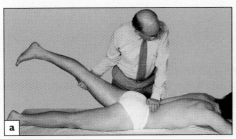

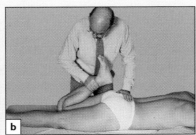

18.3 Femoral stretch test
Lumbar root sensitivity can be detected by applying tension to the femoral nerve. This is done either by (**a**) hyperextending the hip or (**b**) acutely flexing the knee with the hip held in the neutral position.

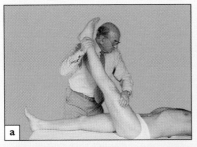

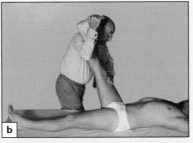

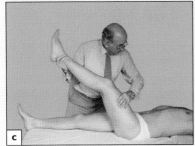

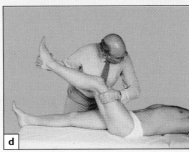

18.4 Sciatic stretch tests (**a**) Straight-leg raising. The knee is kept absolutely straight while the leg is slowly lifted; note where the patient complains of tightness and pain in the buttock – normally around 80 or 90°. (**b**) At that point, passive dorsiflexion of the foot causes an added stab of pain. (**c**) The 'bowstring sign' is a confirmatory test for sciatic tension. At the point where the patient experiences pain, relax the tension by bending the knee slightly; the pain should disappear. (**d**) Then apply firm pressure behind the lateral hamstrings to tighten the common peroneal nerve; the pain recurs with renewed intensity.

Feel the *bony outlines* (is there an unexpected 'step' or prominence?) and check for localized *tenderness*.

The popliteal and posterior tibial *pulses* are felt, hamstring *power* is tested and sensation on the back of the limbs assessed.

The *femoral stretch test* (for lumbar root sensitivity) is carried out by flexing the patient's knee or by lifting the hip into extension (or both in one movement); pain may be felt in the front of the thigh and in the back.

SIGNS WITH THE PATIENT LYING FACE UPWARDS

The patient is observed as he or she turns – is there pain or stiffness? A rapid appraisal of the thyroid, chest (and breasts), abdomen (and scrotum) is worthwhile, and essential if there is even a hint of generalized disease. Hip and knee mobility are assessed before testing for cord or root involvement.

The *straight leg raising test* discloses lumbosacral root tension. With the knee held absolutely straight, the leg is lifted from the couch until the patient expe-

riences pain – not merely in the lower back (which is common and not significant), but also in the buttock, thigh and calf (Lasegue's test); the angle at which this occurs is noted. Normally it should be possible to raise the limb to 80–90°; people with lax ligaments can go even further. In a full-blown disc prolapse, straight leg raising may be restricted to 20 or 30°. At the point where the patient experiences discomfort, passive dorsiflexion of the foot may cause an additional stab of pain.

The *'bowstring' sign* is even more specific. Raise the patient's leg to the point where pain is experienced; now, without reducing the amount of lift, bend the knee so as to relax the sciatic nerve – buttock pain is immediately relieved; pain may then be reinduced without extending the knee by simply pressing on the lateral popliteal (common peroneal) nerve, to tighten it like a bowstring.

Sometimes straight leg raising on the unaffected side produces pain on the affected side. This *'crossed sciatic tension'* is indicative of severe root irritation, usually due to a central prolapsed disc, and suggests risk to the sacral nerve roots that control bladder function.

A *full neurological examination* of the lower limbs is then carried out. The extremities are carefully examined for *trophic changes* and the *pulses* are felt in the groin and popliteal fossa and around the ankle.

Unless the signs point unequivocally to a spinal disorder, *rectal and vaginal examination* may also be necessary.

IMAGING

Plain x-rays begin with anteroposterior and lateral views of the spine; for the lumbar region, oblique views of the spine, an anteroposterior x-ray of the pelvis and a posteroanterior view of the sacroiliac joints may also be needed.

In the anteroposterior view the spine should look perfectly straight and the soft-tissue shadows should outline the normal muscle planes. Curvature (scoliosis) is obvious, and bulging of the psoas muscle plane may indicate a paravertebral abscess. Individual vertebrae may show alterations in structure, e.g. asymmetry or collapse. *Check if there is a missing pedicle, an important clue to metastatic disease.* The intervertebral spaces may be edged by bony spurs (suggesting disc degeneration) or bridged by fine bony syndesmophytes. The sacroiliac joints may show erosion or ankylosis.

In the lateral view the normal thoracic kyphosis and lumbar lordosis should be regular and uninterrupted. Anterior shift of an upper segment upon a lower (spondylolisthesis) may be associated with defects of the posterior arch which show best in oblique views. Vertebral bodies, which should be rectangular, may be wedged or biconcave. Bone density and trabecular markings also are best seen in lateral films.

Radioisotope scanning may pick up areas of increased activity, suggesting a fracture, a 'silent' metastasis or a local inflammatory lesion.

Computed tomography (CT) is helpful in the diagnosis of structural bone changes (e.g. vertebral fracture) and intervertebral disc prolapse. When combined with *myelography* it gives valuable information about the contents of the spinal canal.

Magnetic resonance imaging (MRI) has virtually done away with the need for myelography. The spinal canal and disc spaces are clearly outlined in various planes.

Discography and *facet joint arthrography* are sometimes performed in the investigation of chronic back pain. Remember, though, that disc degeneration and facet joint arthritis are common in older people and are not necessarily the cause of the patient's symptoms.

SPINAL DEFORMITIES

Variations and abnormalities of segmentation are common; they include anomalies such as lumbarization of the first sacral segment, 'sacralization' of one or both transverse processes of the fifth lumbar vertebra and asymmetry of the apophyseal joints, as well as such conditions as hemivertebra, which may give rise to severe spinal deformity (see below).

The most serious type of *congenital defect* is spina bifida, which is dealt with in Chapter 10.

'Spinal deformity' (as opposed to deformities of individual vertebrae) affects the entire shape of the back and manifests as abnormal curvature, in either the coronal plane (scoliosis) or the sagittal plane (hyperkyphosis and hyperlordosis).

SCOLIOSIS

Scoliosis is an apparent lateral (sideways) curvature of the spine. 'Apparent' because, although lateral curvature does occur, the commonest form of scoliosis is actually a triplanar deformity with lateral, anteroposterior and rotational components (Dickson *et al.*, 1984). Two broad types of deformity are defined: *postural* and *structural*.

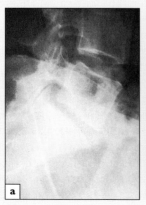 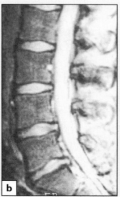 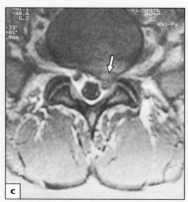

18.5 Lumbar spine imaging (a) Lateral x-ray of the lumbosacral junction. The L5/S1 disc is diminished in height. **(b)** T1-weighted lateral MRI showing a small posterior disc bulge at L4/5 and a more significant protrusion at L5/S1. **(c)** Axial MRI demonstrating the marked disc prolapse obscuring the intervertebral canal on the left side.

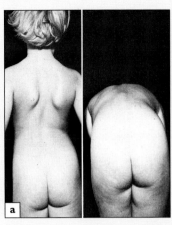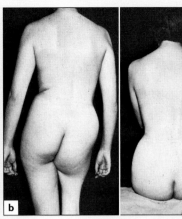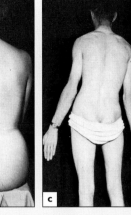

18.6 Postural or mobile scoliosis (a) Postural scoliosis disappears on flexion. (b) Short leg scoliosis disappears when the patient sits. (c) Sciatic scoliosis disappears when the underlying cause (a prolapsed disc) has been treated.

POSTURAL SCOLIOSIS

In postural scoliosis the deformity is secondary or compensatory to some condition outside the spine, such as a short leg, or pelvic tilt due to contracture of the hip; when the patient sits (thereby cancelling leg asymmetry) the curve disappears. Local muscle spasm associated with a prolapsed lumbar disc may cause a skew back; although sometimes called 'sciatic scoliosis' this, too, is a spurious deformity.

STRUCTURAL SCOLIOSIS

In structural scoliosis there is a non-correctable deformity of the affected spinal segment, an essential component of which is vertebral rotation. The spinous processes swing round towards the concavity of the curve and the transverse processes on the convexity rotate posteriorly; in the thoracic region the ribs on the convex side stand out prominently, producing the rib hump which is a characteristic part of the overall deformity. Dickson *et al.* (1984) pointed out that this is really a lordoscoliosis associated with rotational buckling of the spine. The initial deformity is probably correctable, but once it exceeds a certain point of mechanical stability the spine buckles and rotates into a fixed deformity which does not disappear with changes in posture. Secondary (compensatory) curves nearly always develop to counterbalance the primary deformity; they are usually less marked and more easily correctable, but with time they, too, become fixed.

Once fully established, the deformity is liable to increase throughout the growth period. Thereafter, further deterioration is slight, though curves greater than 50° may go on increasing by 1° per year. With very severe curves, chest deformity is marked and cardiopulmonary function is usually affected.

Most cases have no obvious cause (*idiopathic scoliosis*); other varieties are *congenital or osteopathic* (due to bony anomalies), *neuropathic, myopathic* (associated with some muscle dystrophies) and a *miscellaneous* group of connective-tissue disorders.

Clinical features

Deformity is usually the presenting symptom: an obvious skew back or a rib hump in thoracic curves, and asymmetrical prominence of one hip in thoracolumbar curves. Balanced curves sometimes pass unnoticed until an adult presents with *backache*. Where school screening programmes are conducted, children will be referred with very minor deformities.

Pain is a rare complaint and should alert the clinician to the possibility of a neural tumour and the need for MRI.

There may be a *family history* of scoliosis or a record of some *abnormality during pregnancy or childbirth*; the *early developmental milestones* should be noted.

The trunk should be completely exposed and the patient examined from in front, from the back and from the side. *Skin* pigmentation and congenital anomalies such as sacral dimples or hair tufts are sought.

The *spine* may be obviously deviated from the midline, or this may become apparent only when the patient bends forwards. The level and direction of the major curve convexity are noted (e.g. 'right thoracic' means a curve in the thoracic spine and convex to the right). The hip sticks out on the concave side and the scapula on the convex. The breasts and shoulders also may be asymmetrical. With thoracic scoliosis, rotation causes the rib angles to protrude, thus producing an asymmetrical rib hump on the convex side of the

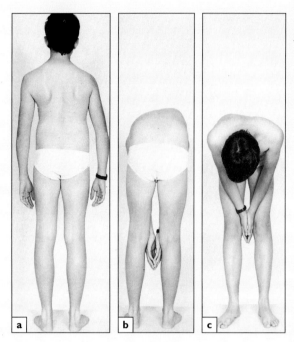

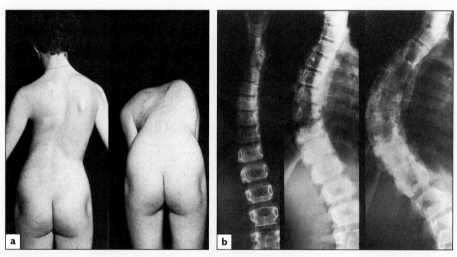

18.8 Structural scoliosis (**a**) A fixed (structural) curve is more obvious on flexion. (**b**) Over a period of 4 years this curve increased – most rapidly in the previous 12 months, during the prepubertal spurt of growth.

curve. In balanced deformities the occiput is over the midline; in unbalanced (or decompensated) curves it is not. This can be determined more accurately by dropping a plumb-line from the prominent spinous process of C7 and noting whether it falls along the gluteal cleft.

The diagnostic feature of fixed (as distinct from postural or mobile) scoliosis is that forwards bending makes the curve more obvious. Spinal mobility should be assessed and the effect of lateral bending on the curve noted; is there some flexibility in the curve and can it be passively corrected?

Side-on posture should also be observed. There may appear to be excessive kyphosis or lordosis.

Neurological examination is important. Any abnormality suggesting a spinal cord lesion calls for CT and/or MRI.

Leg length is measured. If one side is short, the pelvis is levelled by standing the patient on wooden blocks and the spine is re-examined.

General examination includes a search for the possible cause and an assessment of cardiopulmonary function (which is reduced in severe curves).

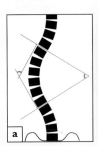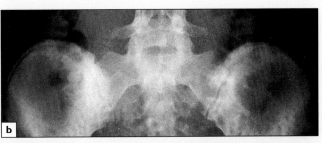

18.9 Scoliosis – measurement and maturity (a) Measuring the primary curve; the disc spaces are wider on the convex side – lines drawn at each end of the primary curve show the angle of deformity (Cobb's angle). (b) When the iliac apophyses are completely ossified, spinal maturity has been reached; there may be a further increase of curvature, but it will be slight.

Imaging

PLAIN X-RAYS Full length posteroanterior (PA) and lateral x-rays of the spine and iliac crests must be taken with the patient erect. Structural curves show vertebral rotation: in the PA x-ray, vertebrae towards the apex of the curve appear to be asymmetrical and the spinous processes are deviated towards the midline. Remember that PA in relation to the patient is not PA in relation to the rotated vertebrae! For this, additional oblique views (face-on to the rotated vertebrae) will be needed.

The upper and lower ends of the curve are identified as the levels where vertebral symmetry is regained. The degree of curvature is measured by drawing lines on the x-ray at the upper border of the uppermost vertebra and the lower border of the lowermost vertebra of the curve; the angle subtended by these lines is *the angle of curvature* (Cobb's angle).

The site of the curve apex should be noted. Right thoracic curves are the commonest; in adolescent idiopathic scoliosis, left thoracic curves are so unusual that if this is seen it should be further investigated by MRI. The primary structural curve is usually balanced by compensatory curves above and below, or by a second 'primary' curve, also with vertebral rotation (sometimes there are multiple 'primary' curves).

What is not readily appreciated from these films is the degree of lordosis in the primary curve(s) and kyphosis in the compensatory curves (Archer and Dickson, 1989); indeed, it is postulated that flattening or reversal of the normal thoracic kyphosis superimposed on coronal plane asymmetry leads, with growth, to progressive idiopathic scoliosis. Lateral bending views are taken to assess the degree of curve correctability.

Skeletal maturity is assessed in several ways (this is important because the curve often progresses most during the period of rapid skeletal growth and maturation). The iliac apophyses start ossifying shortly after puberty; ossification extends medially and, once the iliac crests are completely ossified, further progression of the scoliosis is minimal (Risser's sign). This stage of development usually coincides with fusion of the vertebral ring apophyses. 'Skeletal age' may also be estimated from x-rays of the wrist and hand.

SPECIAL IMAGING CT and MRI may be necessary to define a vertebral abnormality or cord compression.

Special investigations

Pulmonary function tests are performed in all cases of severe chest deformity. A marked reduction in vital capacity is associated with diminished life expectancy and carries obvious risks for surgery.

Patients with muscular dystrophies or connective tissue disorders require full *biochemical* and *neuromuscular* investigation of the underlying condition.

Prognosis and treatment

Prognosis is the key to treatment: the aim is to prevent severe deformity. Generally speaking, the younger the child and the higher the curve the worse is the prognosis. Management differs for the different types of scoliosis, which are considered below.

IDIOPATHIC SCOLIOSIS

This group constitutes about 80% of all cases of scoliosis. The deformity is often familial, and the population incidence of serious curves (over 30° and therefore needing treatment) is three per 1000; trivial curves are very much more common. The age at onset has been used to define three groups: *adolescent*, *juvenile* and *infantile*. A simpler division is *early onset (before puberty)* and *late onset (after puberty) scoliosis*.

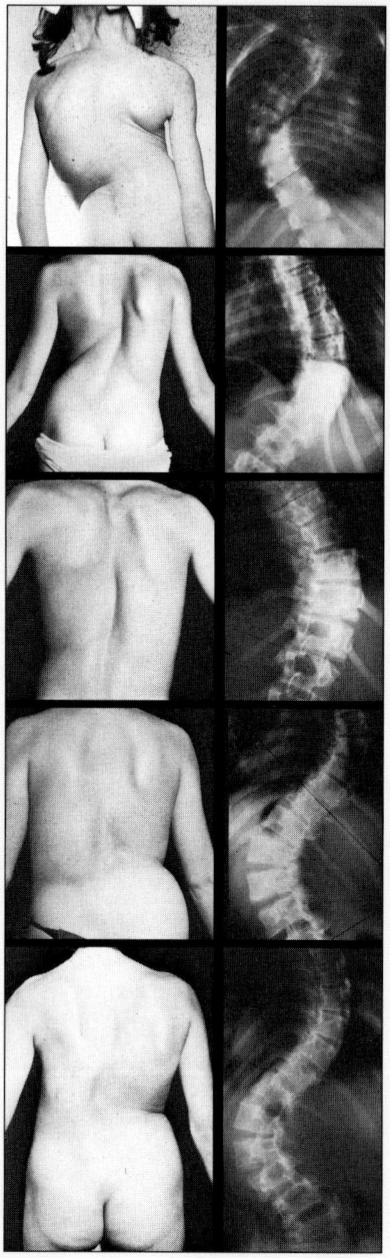

18.10 Structural scoliosis – idiopathic curve patterns

Infantile thoracic

60% male.
90% convex to left.
Associated with ipsilateral plagiocephaly. May be resolving or progressive.
Progressive variety becomes severe.

Adolescent thoracic

90% female.
90% convex to right.
Rib rotation exaggerates the deformity.
50% develop curves of greater than 70°.

Thoracolumbar

Slightly more common in females.
Slightly more common to right.
Features mid-way between adolescent thoracic and lumbar.

Lumbar

More common in females.
80% convex to left.
One hip prominent but no ribs to accentuate deformity.
Therefore not noticed early, but backache in adult life.

Combined

Two primary curves, one in each direction.
Even when radiologically severe, clinical deformity relatively slight because always well balanced.

ADOLESCENT IDIOPATHIC SCOLIOSIS (PRESENTING AT AGED 10 YEARS OR OVER)

This, the commonest type, occurs mostly (90%) in girls. Primary thoracic curves are usually convex to the right, lumbar curves to the left; intermediate (thoracolumbar) and combined (double primary) curves also occur. Progression is not inevitable; indeed, most curves under 20° either resolve spontaneously or remain unchanged. However, once a curve starts to progress, it usually goes on doing so throughout the remaining growth period (and, to a much lesser degree, beyond that). Reliable predictors of progression are (1) a very young age, (2) marked curvature and (3) an incomplete Risser sign at presen-

tation (Lonstein and Carlson, 1984). In prepubertal children, rapid progression is liable to occur during the growth spurt.

Treatment

The aims of treatment are (1) to prevent a mild deformity from becoming severe, and (2) to correct an existing deformity that is unacceptable to the patient. A period of preliminary observation may be needed before deciding between conservative and operative treatment. At four-monthly intervals the patient is examined, photographed and x-rayed so that curves can be measured and checked for progression.

NON-OPERATIVE TREATMENT

If the patient is approaching skeletal maturity and the deformity is acceptable (which usually means it is less than 30° and well balanced), treatment is probably unnecessary unless sequential x-rays show definite progression. *Exercises* are often prescribed; they have no effect on the curve but they do maintain muscle tone and may inspire confidence in a favourable outcome. If a curve between 20 and 30° is progressing, some form of *bracing* may, in addition, be needed. *The Milwaukee brace* is principally a thoracic support consisting of a pelvic corset connected by adjustable steel supports to a cervical ring carrying occipital and chin pads; its purpose is to reduce the lumbar lordosis and encourage active stretching and straightening of the thoracic spine. The *Boston brace* is a snug-fitting underarm brace which provides lumbar or low thoracolumbar support. Corrective pads may be added to these devices to apply pressure at a particular site. A well-made brace can be worn 23 hours out of 24 and does not preclude full daily activities, including sport and exercises. The patient (and the doctor) must appreciate that bracing will not improve the curve; at best it will stop it from getting worse.

OPERATIVE TREATMENT

Surgery is indicated (1) for curves of more than 30° that are cosmetically unacceptable, especially in pre-pubertal children who are liable to develop marked progression during the growth spurt, and (2) for milder deformity that deteriorates significantly despite conservative treatment. Balanced, double primary curves require operation only if they are greater than 60° and progressing (Kostuik, 1990).

The objectives are (a) to straighten the curve (including the rotational component) by some form of instrumentation, and (b) to arthrodese the entire primary curve.

The Harrington system In the original system a rod was applied posteriorly along the concave side of the curve; attached to the rod were movable hooks which were engaged in the uppermost and lowermost vertebrae so as to distract the curve. If the curve is flexible, it will passively correct and bone grafts are then applied to obtain fusion over the length of the curve. A major drawback of the original distraction instrumentation is that it does nor correct the rotational deformity at the apex of the curve and thus the rib prominence remains virtually unchanged.

Rod and sublaminar wiring (Luque) This is a modification of the Harrington system. Wires are passed under the vertebral laminae at multiple levels and fixed to the rod on the concave side of the curve, thus providing a more controlled and secure fixation. By bending the rod and arranging the mechanism so that the wires pull backwards rather than merely sideways, the rotational component of the deformity can also be substantially improved. However, the sublaminar wires are dangerously close to the dura and the risk of neurological damage is increased.

The Cotrel–Dubousset system This is again a posterior rod system, with multiple hooks which can be placed at various levels to produce either distraction or compression. With double rods one can distract on the concave and compress on the convex side of the curve; by appropriate manipulation of the implants one can obtain correction also in the sagittal plane. It has been claimed that this system can correct the rotational deformity. It is also sufficiently rigid to make postoperative bracing unnecessary.

Anterior instrumentation (Dwyer; Zielke) Rigid curves and thoracolumbar curves associated with lumbar lordosis can be corrected by approaching the spine from the

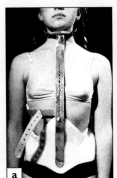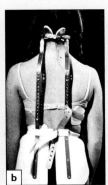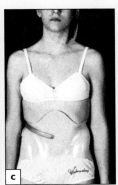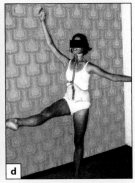

18.11 Structural scoliosis – conservative treatment (a, b) The Milwaukee brace fits snugly over the pelvis below; chin and head pads promote active postural correction; a thoracic pad presses on the ribs at the apex of the curve. **(c)** The Boston brace is used for low curves. All braces are cumbersome, but **(d)** if well made they need not interfere much with activity.

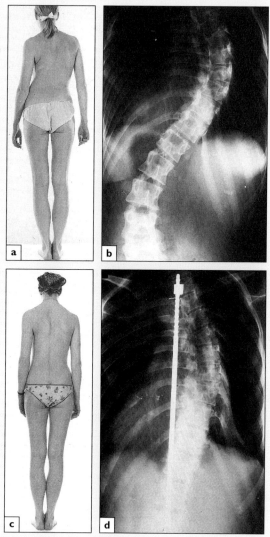

18.12 Structural scoliosis – operative treatment (**a**, **b**) Before, and (**c**, **d**) after correction and fusion using a Harrington rod.

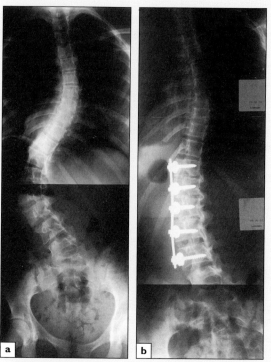

18.13 Scoliosis – anterior instrumentation (Zielke method) (**a**) This 14-year old girl had a very stiff lumbar curve. It was planned to correct this by two-stage anterior and posterior release and fusion. (**b**) X-ray taken after the anterior instrumentation. Through a trans-thoracic, trans-diaphragmatic approach the intervertebral discs and vertebral end-plates from T12 to L4 were excised and replaced with morselized bone grafts; screws were inserted into the five vertebral bodies along the convex side of the curve; a rod was inserted through the screw heads and fixed in position, progressively tightening the system and straightening the vertebral column. The post-operative x-ray shows that considerable correction has been achieved. Further correction is expected after the second-stage posterior instrumentation.

front, removing the discs throughout the curve and then applying a compression device (either a threaded rod and screws or a braided cable) along the convex side of the curve. Bone grafts are added to achieve fusion. In some cases combined anterior and posterior instrumentation is necessary.

Advantages of this system are (a) that it provides strong fixation with fewer vertebral segments having to be fused, and (b) that overall shortening of the involved segment (by disc excision and vertebral compression) lessens the risk of cord injury due to spinal distraction.

WARNING Whatever method is used, spinal cord function should be monitored during the operation. Ideally this is done by measuring somatosensory and motor-evoked potentials during spinal correction. If these facilities are not available, the 'wake-up test' is used:

anaesthesia is reduced to bring the patient to a semi-awake state, who is then instructed to move his or her feet. If there are signs of cord compromise, the instrumentation is relaxed or removed and re-applied with a lesser degree of correction.

The rib hump The best of the instrumentation systems cannot completely eliminate the rib hump. If the deformity is marked, it can be reduced by performing a costoplasty.

COMPLICATIONS OF SURGERY
Neurological compromise With modern techniques the incidence of permanent paralysis has been reduced to less than 1%. From the patient's point of view this is small comfort. Every effort should be made to provide adequate safeguards.

Spinal decompensation Over-correction may produce an unbalanced spine. This should be avoided by careful pre-operative planning and selection of the appropriate levels of fusion.

Pseudarthrosis Incomplete fusion occurs in about 2% of cases, and may require further operation and grafting.

Implant failure Hooks may cut out and rods may break. If this is associated with a symptomatic pseudarthrosis, operative treatment (compression fixation) will be needed.

JUVENILE IDIOPATHIC SCOLIOSIS (PRESENTING AT AGE 4–9 YEARS)

This is uncommon. The characteristics of this group are similar to those of the adolescent group, but the prognosis is worse and surgical correction may be necessary before puberty. However, if the child is very young, a brace may hold the curve stationary until he or she is about 10 years old, when fusion is more likely to succeed.

INFANTILE IDIOPATHIC SCOLIOSIS (PRESENTING AGE 3 YEARS OR UNDER)

This variety is rare in North America and is becoming uncommon elsewhere, perhaps because most babies nowadays are allowed to sleep prone. Boys predominate and most curves are thoracic with convexity to the left. Although 90% of infantile curves resolve spontaneously, progressive curves can become very severe; those in which the rib–vertebra angle at the apex of the curve differs on the two sides by more than 20° are likely to deteriorate (Mehta, 1972). And because this also influences the development of the lungs, there is a high incidence of cardiopulmonary dysfunction.

Curves assessed as being potentially progressive should be treated by applying serial elongation–derotation–flexion (EDF) plaster casts under general anaesthesia, until the deformity resolves or until the child is big enough to manage in a brace. From about 4 years onwards curve progression slows down or ceases and the child may not need further treatment. If the deformity continues to deteriorate, surgical correction may be required. This takes the form of anterior disc excision, possibly with the use of a rod to aid correction, but posterior fusion should be avoided.

OSTEOPATHIC (CONGENITAL) SCOLIOSIS

Although fractures and bone softening (as in rickets or osteogenesis imperfecta) may lead to scoliosis, the commonest bony cause is some type of vertebral anom-

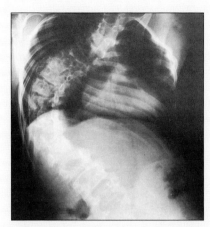

18.14 Infantile idiopathic scoliosis 'Idiopathic' curves in young children usually resolve, but some increase progressively and become very severe. Measurement of the rib–vertebra angles at the curve apex is a good prognostic indicator.

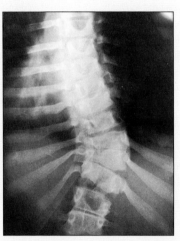

18.15 Congenital scoliosis Partial fusion of the vertebrae at T10, 11 and 12 has resulted in a localized scoliosis.

aly – *hemivertebra, wedged vertebra, fused vertebrae* and *absent or fused ribs*. Overlying tissues often show angiomas, naevi, excess hair, dimples or a pad of fat. Spina bifida may be associated and visceral anomalies are common. These children require painstaking clinical investigation and imaging (a) in order to discover any other congenital anomalies and (b) to assess the risk of spinal cord damage.

While congenital scoliosis is often mild, some cases progress to severe deformity, particularly those with unilateral fusion of vertebrae (unilateral unsegmented bar). Before any operation is undertaken, advanced imaging is needed to exclude an associated dysraphism, particularly diastematomyelia and cord tethering, which must be dealt with prior to curve correction.

Treatment is more difficult and specialized than that of idiopathic infantile scoliosis. Progressive deformities (usually involving rigid curves) will not respond to bracing alone, and surgical correction carries a significant risk of cord injury. These children should be treated in special units; the approach is to undertake staged resection of the curve apex, followed by instrumentation and spinal fusion. If multiple segments of the spine are involved, surgery may be too hazardous and should probably be withheld.

NEUROPATHIC AND MYOPATHIC SCOLIOSIS

Neuromuscular conditions associated with scoliosis include *poliomyelitis*, *cerebral palsy*, *syringomyelia*, *Friedreich's ataxia* and the rarer lower *motor neurone disorders* and *muscle dystrophies*; the curve may take some years to develop. The typical paralytic curve is long, convex towards the side with weaker muscles (spinal, abdominal or intercostal), and at first is mobile. In severe cases the greatest problem is loss of stability and balance, which may make even sitting difficult or impossible. Additional problems are generalized muscle weakness and (in some cases) loss of sensibility with the attendant risk of pressure ulceration.

X-ray with traction applied shows the extent to which the deformity is correctable.

Treatment depends upon the degree of functional disability. Mild curves may require no treatment at all. Moderate curves with spinal stability are managed as for idiopathic scoliosis. Severe curves, associated with pelvic obliquity and loss of sitting balance, can often be managed by fitting a suitable sitting support. If this does not suffice, operative treatment may be indicated. This involves stabilization of the entire paralysed segment by combined anterior and posterior instrumentation and fusion.

SCOLIOSIS AND NEUROFIBROMATOSIS

About one-third of patients with neurofibromatosis develop spinal deformity, the severity of which varies from very mild (and not requiring any form of treatment) to the most marked manifestations accompanied by skin lesions, multiple neurofibromata and bony dystrophy affecting the vertebrae and ribs. The scoliotic curve is typically 'short and sharp'. Other clues to the diagnosis lie in the appearance of the skin lesions and any associated skeletal abnormalities (see page 155).

Mild cases are treated as for idiopathic scoliosis. More severe deformities will usually need combined anterior and posterior instrumentation and fusion. As with other forms of skeletal neurofibromatosis, graft dissolution and pseudarthrosis are not uncommon.

KYPHOSIS

Rather confusingly, the term 'kyphosis' is used to describe both the normal (the gentle rounding of the thoracic spine) and the abnormal (excessive thoracic curvature or straightening out of the cervical or lumbar lordotic curves). Excessive thoracic curvature might be better described as 'hyperkyphosis'. *Kyphos*, or *gibbus*, is a sharp posterior angulation due to localized collapse or wedging of one or more vertebrae. This may be the result of a congenital defect, a fracture (sometimes pathological) or spinal tuberculosis.

POSTURAL KYPHOSIS

Postural kyphosis is usually associated with other postural defects such as flat feet. It is voluntarily

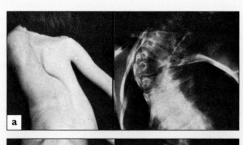
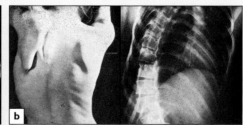
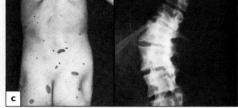

18.16 Structural scoliosis – non-idiopathic (a) Congenital – a curve as high as this is not 'idiopathic'; (b) paralytic – a characteristic long C curve, following polio; (c) with neurofibromatosis a short sharp curve is not uncommon.

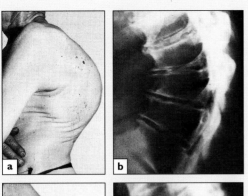

18.17 'Kyphosis' and 'kyphos' (**a, b**) Kyphosis – a generalized exaggeration of the normal thoracic 'rounding', in this case due to a combination of long-standing Scheuermann's disease and post-climacteric osteoporosis. (**c, d**) Kyphos – a localized spinal angulation, or gibbus, due to collapse of one or two spinal segments (in this case following spinal tuberculosis).

correctable. If treatment is needed, this consists of posture training and exercises.

Compensatory kyphosis is secondary to some other deformity, usually increased lumbosacral lordosis. This deformity, too, is correctable.

STRUCTURAL KYPHOSIS

Structural kyphosis is fixed and associated with changes in the shape of the vertebrae. *In children* this may be due to congenital vertebral defects; it is also seen in skeletal dysplasias such as achondroplasia and in osteogenesis imperfecta. Older children may develop severe deformity secondary to tuberculous spondylitis.

In adolescence the commonest cause is Scheuermann's disease (see below).

In adults kyphosis could be due to an old childhood disorder, tuberculous spondylitis, ankylosing spondylitis or spinal trauma.

In elderly people, osteoporosis may result in vertebral compression and an increase in a previously mild, asymptomatic deformity.

CONGENITAL KYPHOSIS

Vertebral anomalies leading to kyphosis may be due to failure of formation (type I), failure of segmentation (type II) or a combination of these.

Type I (failure of formation) is the commonest (and the worst). If the anterior part of the vertebral body fails to develop, progressive kyphosis and posterior displacement of the hemivertebra may lead to cord compression. In children under 6 years with curves of less than 40°, posterior spinal fusion alone may prevent further progression. Older children or more severe curves may need combined anterior and posterior fusion; and those with neurological complications will require cord decompression as well as fusion.

Type II (failure of segmentation) usually takes the form of an anterior intervertebral bar; as the posterior elements continue to grow, that segment of the spine gradually becomes kyphotic. The risk of neurological compression is much less, but if the curve is progressive a posterior fusion will be needed.

ADOLESCENT KYPHOSIS (SCHEUERMANN'S DISEASE)

Scheuermann, in 1920, described a condition which he called juvenile dorsal kyphosis, distinguishing it from the more common postural (correctable) kyphosis. The characteristic feature was a fixed round-back deformity associated with wedging of several thoracic vertebrae. The term 'vertebral osteochondritis' was adopted because the primary defect appeared to be in the ossification of the ring epiphyses which define the peripheral rims on the upper and lower surfaces of each vertebral body. The true nature of the disorder is still not known; the cartilaginous end-plates may be weaker than normal (perhaps due to a collagen defect) and are then damaged by pressure of the adjacent intervertebral discs during strenuous activity. The normal curve of the thoracic spine ensures that the anterior edges of the vertebrae are subjected to the greatest stress and this is where the damage is greatest. Similar changes may occur in the lumbar spine, but here wedging is unusual.

Clinical features

The condition starts at puberty and affects boys more often than girls. The parents notice that the child, an otherwise fit teenager, is becoming increasingly round-shouldered. The patient may complain of backache and fatigue; this sometimes increases after the end of growth and may become severe.

A smooth thoracic kyphosis is seen; it may produce a marked hump. Below it is a compensatory lumbar lordosis. The deformity cannot be corrected by changes in posture. Movements are normal but tight hamstrings often limit straight leg raising. A mild scoliosis is not uncommon. Rare complications are spastic paresis of the lower limbs and – with severe deformity of the thorax – cardiopulmonary dysfunction.

In later life patients with thoracic kyphosis may develop lumbar backache. This has been attributed to chronic low back strain or facet joint dysfunction due to compensatory hyperextension of the lumbar spine. In some cases, however, lumbar Scheuermann's disease itself may cause pain (see below).

X-RAY

In lateral radiographs of the spine the vertebral end-plates of several adjacent vertebrae (usually T6–T10) appear irregular or fragmented. The changes are more marked anteriorly and one or more vertebral bodies may become wedge shaped. There may also be small radiolucent defects in the subchondral bone (Schmorl's nodes), which are thought to be due to central (axial) disc protrusions.

The angle of deformity is measured in the same way as for scoliosis, except that here the lateral x-ray is used and the lines mark the uppermost and lowermost affected vertebrae. Wedging of more than 5° in three adjacent vertebrae and an overall kyphosis angle of more than 40° are abnormal. Mild scoliosis is not uncommon.

Differential diagnosis

Postural kyphosis Postural 'round back' is common in adolescence. It is painless, and the deformity is correctable by the patient's own effort if properly instructed. The curve is a long one and other postural defects are common. The x-ray appearance is normal.

Discitis, osteomyelitis and tuberculous spondylitis If the changes are restricted to one intervertebral level, they can be mistaken for an infective lesion. However, infection causes more severe pain, may be associated with systemic symptoms and signs, and produces more marked x-ray changes, including signs of bone erosion and paravertebral soft-tissue swelling.

Spondyloepiphyseal dysplasia In mild cases this can produce changes at multiple levels resembling those of Scheuermann's disease. Look for the characteristic defects in other joints.

Outcome

The condition is often quite painful during adolescence, but (except in the most severe cases) symptoms subside

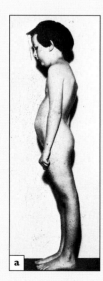
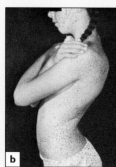
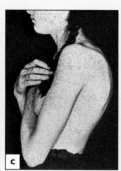
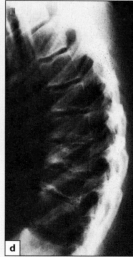

18.18 Kyphosis (a) Postural kyphosis and (b) kyphosis compensatory to a lumbar (sway-back). Unlike these two varieties, the deformity in Scheuermann's disease (c, d) is fixed.

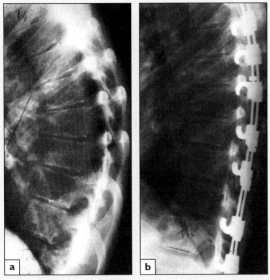

18.19 Scheuermann's disease – operative treatment A severe curve may need operation especially if, as in this girl (**a**), it is associated with chronic pain. (**b**) The same girl after operative correction and fixation with Harrington rods; bone grafts were added and can be expected to produce fusion after a year or two.

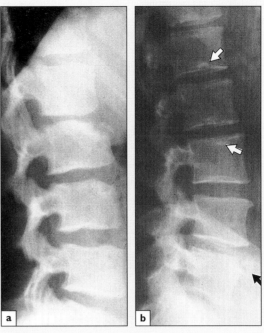

18.20 Lumbar Scheuermann's disease (**a**) The x-ray appearances of lumbar Scheuermann's disease are often mistaken for a fracture (or worse). The 'fragmentation' anteriorly is due to abnormal ossification of the ring epiphysis. (**b**) Schmorl's nodes (arrows) may also be seen.

after a few years. There may be a recurrence of backache in later life, though overall disability is seldom marked (Murray *et al.*, 1993).

Treatment

Curves of 40° or less require only back-strengthening exercises and postural training. More severe curvature in a child who still has some years of growth ahead responds well to a period of 12–24 months in a brace that holds the lumbar spine flat and the thoracic spine in 'extension' (decreased kyphosis). Check the position by x-ray to ensure that the brace is effective.

The older adolescent or young adult with a rigid curve of more than 60° may need operative correction and fusion using a hook-rod system (modified Harrington or Cotrel–Dubousset). In severe cases (kyphosis of more than 75°), an anterior release operation and fusion should precede the posterior fusion. Even then, the deformity is usually only partially corrected.

THORACOLUMBAR SCHEUERMANN'S DISEASE

Vertebral end-plate defects are sometimes limited to the lower thoracic and lumbar spine. In mild cases the condition is usually asymptomatic and discovered only incidentally when x-rays are obtained for other reasons. In some cases, however, the patient (usually a teenager at the end of growth or a young adult) complains of back pain and inability to undertake sustained bending, lifting and carrying activities. There is nothing striking to see on clinical examination and it may be difficult to determine whether the backache is due to the Scheuermann disorder or to some other condition such as spondylolysis or facet joint dysfunction.

Treatment consists of muscle strengthening exercises and avoidance of excessive bending and lifting.

KYPHOSIS IN THE ELDERLY

Degeneration of intervertebral discs probably produces the gradually increasing stoop characteristic of the aged. The disc spaces become narrowed and the vertebrae slightly wedged. There is little pain unless osteoarthritis of the facet joints is also present.

OSTEOPOROTIC KYPHOSIS

Postmenopausal osteoporosis may result in one or more compression fractures of the thoracic spine. Patients are usually in their 60s or 70s and may complain of pain. Kyphosis is seldom marked. Often the main complaint is of lumbosacral pain, which results from the compensatory lumbar lordosis in an ageing, osteoarthritic spine. Treatment is directed at the underlying condition and may include hormone replacement therapy.

Senile osteoporosis affects both men and women. Patients are usually over 75 years of age, often incapacitated by some other illness, and lacking exercise. They complain of back pain, and spinal deformity may be marked. X-rays reveal multiple vertebral fractures. It is important to exclude other conditions such as *metastatic disease* or *myelomatosis*.

Treatment is symptomatic. Bed rest and spinal bracing merely aggravate the osteoporosis.

SPINAL INFECTION

PYOGENIC OSTEOMYELITIS AND DISCITIS

Acute pyogenic infection of the spine is uncommon and, because the diagnosis is not considered, treatment is often unnecessarily delayed.

Pathology

Staphylococcus aureus is responsible in 50–60% of cases; Gram-negative organisms such as *E. coli*, *Pseudomonas* and *Proteus* are increasingly evident and opportunistic infections in immunosuppressed patients are no longer as rare as they used to be.

The common sources of infection are (a) direct innoculation during invasive procedures (spinal injections and disc operations) and (b) indirect haematogenous spread from a pelvic infection or a more remote site. The very old and very young, the chronically ill and the immunodeficient are at greatest risk.

The infection may appear to start in an intervertebral disc, but it is more likely that the initial site is the adjacent vertebra, with secondary spread to the disc. Further spread may occur along the anterior intervertebral ligament to an adjacent vertebra, and outwards into the paravertebral soft tissues. A paravertebral abscess occasionally tracks along the muscle planes to point in the groin, the buttock or the lumbar region. The spinal canal is rarely involved.

Clinical features

Localized pain is the cardinal symptom; it is often intense, unremitting and associated with muscle spasm and restricted movement. There may also be point tenderness over the affected vertebra. Sometimes, however, pain is referred to the chest or abdomen. The patient may give a history of some spinal procedure, or a distant infection, during the preceding few weeks. Systemic signs such as pyrexia and tachycardia are often present but not particularly marked.

The white cell count and ESR are usually elevated, but not markedly so. Antistaphylococcal antibodies may be present in high titre. Agglutination tests for salmonella and brucella should always be performed.

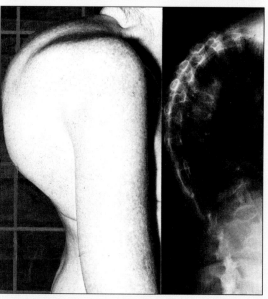

18.21 Senile kyphosis Progressive kyphosis in the elderly can occur because of collapse and wedging of osteoporotic vertebrae. Typically, the x-ray shows only faint bony outlines. In a case as severe as this, some pre-existing deformity or long-standing metabolic bone disease was probably present.

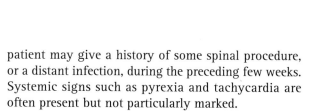

18.22 Pyogenic osteomyelitis and discitis Typical x-ray features are loss of disc height, irregularity of the disc 'space', endplate erosion and reactive sclerosis. It is impossible to tell (in this case) whether the infection began in the disc or in the bone.

IMAGING

X-rays may show no change for several weeks; if the diagnosis is delayed, the examination should be repeated. Early signs are loss of disc height, irregularity of the disc 'space', erosion of the vertebral end-plate and reactive new bone formation. Soft-tissue swelling may be visible.

Radionuclide scanning will show the site of increased activity, but this is non-specific.

MRI is the definitive diagnostic tool, showing characteristic changes in the vertebral end-plates, the intervertebral disc and the paravertebral tissues.

Bacteriological investigations

A biopsy is needed, not so much to confirm the diagnosis as to obtain material for bacteriological culture and tests for antibiotic sensitivity. Blood culture, during the early stages, is usually negative.

Treatment

Once all the tests have been set in train, treatment is begun on the assumed diagnosis of infection. This includes complete bed rest, pain relief and intravenous antibiotic administration using a 'best guess' preparation which can be changed once the laboratory results and sensitivities are known. Intravenous antibiotics are continued for 4–6 weeks; if there is a good response (clinical improvement, a falling ESR and a normal white cell count), oral antibiotics are then used for another 6–8 weeks and the patient is allowed up in a spinal brace.

Operative treatment is seldom needed. The indications are (1) failure to respond to conservative treatment; (2) the appearance of neurological signs; and (3) the need to drain a soft-tissue abscess. An anterior approach is preferred; dead and infected material is removed and, if necessary, the cord is decompressed. Bone defects are filled with suitable grafts. If the spine is unstable, posterior fixation may be necessary. Postoperatively the spine is supported in a firm brace until healing occurs.

DISCITIS

Infection limited to the intervertebral disc is rare and when it does occur it is usually due to direct inoculation during the course of some procedure such as discography, chemonucleolysis or discectomy. Blood-borne infection is said to occur, but most of these turn out to be cases of osteomyelitis. As in other types of spinal infection, the vertebral end-plates are rapidly attacked and from there infection spreads into the vertebral body.

Clinical features

With direct infection there is always a history of some invasive procedure. Acute back pain and muscle spasm following an injection into the disc should never be attributed merely to the irritant effect of the injection. Systemic features are usually mild, but the ESR is increased.

In children the infection is assumed to be blood-borne. There may be a history of a flu-like illness followed by back pain, local tenderness, muscle spasm and severe limitation of movement.

X-rays and *radioscintigraphy* show the same features as in pyogenic spondylitis.

Needle biopsy is advisable, but often no organism is found.

Treatment

Prevention is always better than cure. With injections into the disc, a broad-spectrum antibiotic should be given, either locally or intravenously.

Non-iatrogenic discitis is usually self-limiting, and symptoms and signs gradually settle down over a period of a few months. During the acute stage bed rest is prescribed, together with analgesics if necessary. If symptoms do not resolve rapidly, systemic antibiotics are given. Only if there are signs of abscess formation, or cord or nerve root pressure, is surgical evacuation necessary.

TUBERCULOSIS

The spine is the most common site of skeletal tuberculosis (see also Chapter 2), and the most dangerous. It is thought that there may be as many as 2 million people with active spinal tuberculosis in the world today.

Pathology

Blood-borne infection usually settles in a vertebral body adjacent to the intervertebral disc. Bone destruction and caseation follow, with infection spreading to the disc space and to the adjacent vertebrae. As the vertebral bodies collapse into each other, a sharp angulation (or kyphos) develops. Caseation and cold abscess formation may extend to neighbouring vertebrae or escape into the paravertebral soft tissues. There is a major risk of cord damage due to pressure by the abscess or displaced bone, or ischaemia from spinal artery thrombosis.

With healing, the vertebrae recalcify and bony fusion may occur between them. Nevertheless, if there

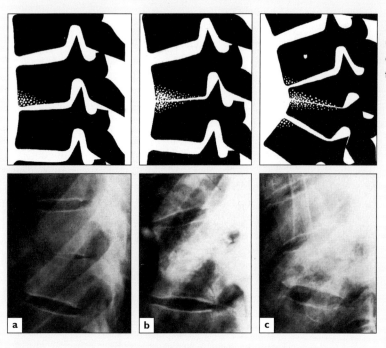

18.23 Spine tuberculosis – pathology
(**a**, **b**, **c**) Progressively increasing destruction of the front of the vertebral bodies leads to forwards collapse.

Clinical features

There is usually a long history of ill-health and backache. In some cases deformity is the dominant feature. Occasionally the patient presents with a cold abscess pointing in the groin, or with paraesthesia and weakness of the legs. There is local tenderness and spinal movements are restricted.

A characteristic feature in late cases is an angular thoracic kyphos, best seen from the side. In the lumbar spine the kyphos is scarcely visible but an abscess in the loin or groin may be obvious.

Neurological examination may show motor and/or sensory changes in the lower limbs.

POTT'S PARAPLEGIA Paraplegia is the most feared complication of spinal tuberculosis. *Early-onset paresis* is due to pressure by an abscess, caseous material or a bony sequestrum. The patient presents with lower limb weakness, upper motor neurone signs and sensory dysfunction, together with vertebral disease. CT and MRI may reveal cord compression and myelography demonstrates a block. *Late-onset paresis* is due to increasing deformity, or reactivation of disease or vascular insufficiency of the cord.

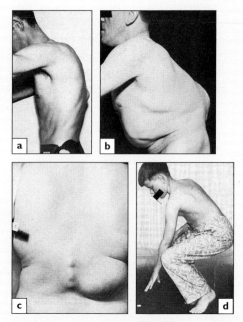

18.24 Spine tuberculosis – clinical features (**a**) This kyphos is slight but diagnostic. If collapse continues (**b**), kyphos becomes severe. (**c**) Large lumbar abscess. (**d**) The coin test – he bends his hips and knees rather than bending his back.

Imaging

X-ray The entire spine should be x-rayed, because vertebrae distant from the obvious site may also be affected. The earliest signs of infection are local osteo-

has been much forwards angulation, the spine is usually 'unsound', and flares are common, with further illness and further collapse. With progressive kyphosis there is again a risk of cord compression.

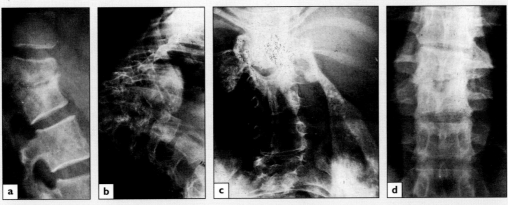

18.25 Spine tuberculosis – x-rays (a) Early disease with loss of the disc space. (b) If several vertebrae are involved, forwards collapse is severe – this patient did not, however, have any signs of paraplegia. (c) Psoas abscesses often calcify during the healing stage. (d) A paravertebral abscess is a fairly constant finding with thoracic disease.

porosis of two adjacent vertebrae and narrowing of the intervertebral disc space, sometimes with fuzziness of the end-plates. Later there are more obvious signs of bone destruction, and collapse of adjacent vertebral bodies into each other, producing an angular deformity of the spine. Paraspinal soft-tissue shadows may be due either to oedema and swelling or to a paravertebral abscess. This is a characteristic feature of thoracic disease. With healing, bone density increases and the ragged appearance disappears; paravertebral abscesses may calcify.

CT and MRI are useful in the investigation of cord compression.

Investigations

The Mantoux test is positive and in the acute stage the ESR is raised.

If there is serious doubt about the diagnosis, a needle biopsy is performed and material is obtained for histological and bacteriological examination.

Differential diagnosis

Spinal tuberculosis must be distinguished from other causes of vertebral destruction and kyphosis, particularly *pyogenic infection* and *malignant disease*. Disc space collapse is typical of infection; disc preservation is typical of metastatic disease. Metastases may cause vertebral body collapse but, in contrast to tuberculous spondylitis, the disc space is usually preserved.

If the patient presents with paraplegia, other causes of cord compression have to be excluded.

Treatment

The objectives are (1) to eradicate or at least arrest the disease, (2) to prevent or correct deformity and (3) to prevent or treat the major complication – paraplegia.

Antituberculous chemotherapy is as effective as any other method (including surgical debridement) in stemming the disease. However, conservative treatment alone carries the risk of progressive kyphosis if the infection is not quickly eradicated. A more radical school of surgeons argues that anterior resection of diseased tissue and anterior spinal fusion with a strut graft offers the double advantage of early and complete eradication of the infection and prevention of spinal deformity (Leong, 1990).

With modern antituberculous drugs, a reasonable compromise would be as follows:

Ambulant chemotherapy alone is appropriate for early or limited disease with no abscess formation. Treatment is continued for 6–12 months, or until the x-ray shows resolution of the bone changes. Compliance is sometimes a problem.

Continuous bed rest and chemotherapy may be used for more advanced disease when the necessary skills and facilities for radical anterior spinal surgery are not available, or where the technical problems are too daunting (e.g. in lumbosacral tuberculosis) – provided there is no abscess that needs draining.

Operative treatment is indicated (1) when there is an abscess that can readily be drained and (2) for advanced disease with marked bone destruction and threatened or actual severe kyphosis or paraparesis. Through an anterior approach, all infected and necrotic material is evacuated or excised and the gap is filled with rib grafts that act as a strut. If several levels are involved, posterior fixation and fusion may be needed for additional stability. Antituberculous chemotherapy is still necessary, of course.

NON-INFECTIVE INFLAMMATORY DISEASE

Ankylosing spondylitis and the seronegative spondyloarthropathies are dealt with in Chapter 3.

DISC DISORDERS, OSTEOARTHRITIS AND 'MECHANICAL' BACKACHE

DISC DEGENERATION AND PROLAPSE

Lumbar backache is one of the most common causes of chronic disability in North American and European societies, and in the majority of cases the backache is associated with some abnormality of the intervertebral discs at the lowest two levels of the spine (L4/5 and L5/S1).

Pathology

With normal ageing the disc gradually dries out: the nucleus pulposus changes from a turgid, gelatinous bulb to a brownish, desiccated structure, and the annulus fibrosus develops fissures parallel to the vertebral end-plates running mainly posteriorly. Small herniations of nuclear material squeeze through the annulus in all directions and frequently perforate the vertebral end-plates to produce the Schmorl's nodes that are found in over 75% of autopsies.

Disc degeneration is therefore a common expression of senescence. Chronic herniation causes reactive bone formation around the Schmorl's nodes and where the discs protrude at the vertebral margins. Flattening of the disc and marginal osteophytes are readily seen on x-ray and the overall picture is referred to as *spondylosis*.

Displacement of the facet joints is an inevitable consequence of disc space collapse, and this in turn leads to *osteoarthritis*; if this is severe, osteophytes may narrow the lateral recesses of the spinal canal and the intervertebral foramina. Encroachment on the spinal canal leads to *spinal stenosis*.

Acute disc herniation (prolapse, rupture) is less common, but more dramatic. Physical stress (a combination of flexion and compression) is the proximate cause but, even at L4/5 or L5/S1 (where stress is most severe), it seems unlikely that a disc would rupture unless there were also some disturbances of the hydrophilic properties of the nucleus. When rupture does occur, fibrocartilaginous material is extruded posteriorly and the annulus usually bulges to one side of the posterior longitudinal ligament. With a complete

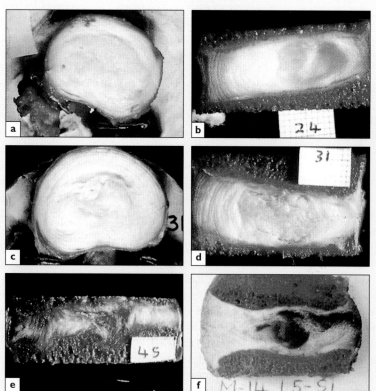

18.26 Disc lesions – pathology (1) (a, b) Transverse and sagittal sections through a young (teenage) intervertebral disc. The nucleus is soft, homogeneous and almost translucent. The annulus is composed of regular lamellae of fibrocartilage. (c, d) Mature (50-year-old) normal disc. The nucleus is more fibrous and less homogeneous. The annulus is thickened and the vertebral body end-plates are intact. (e) Degenerating disc, which is markedly flattened with break-up of the nucleus and disruption of the vertebral body end-plates. (f) Young disc stained with analine blue dye to demonstrate a fissure extending posteriorly through the annulus fibrosus.

rupture, part of the nucleus may sequestrate and lie free in the spinal canal or work its way into the intervertebral foramen. A large central rupture may cause compression of the cauda equina. A posterolateral rupture presses on the nerve root proximal to its point of exit through the intervertebral foramen; thus a herniation at L4/5 will compress the fifth lumbar nerve root, and a herniation at L5/S1 the first sacral root. Sometimes a local inflammatory response with oedema aggravates the symptoms.

The pain of acute disc herniation arises from disruption of the outermost layers of the annulus fibrosus, stretching or tearing of the posterior longitudinal ligament and pressure on the dura. If the disc protrudes to one side, it may irritate the dural covering of the adjacent nerve root causing pain in the buttock, posterior thigh and calf (*sciatica*). Pressure on the nerve root itself causes *paraesthesia* and/or *numbness* in the corresponding dermatome, as well as *weakness* and *depressed reflexes* in the muscles supplied by that nerve root.

Secondary effects of disc degeneration are loss of disc thickness, displacement of the posterior facet joints, vertebral instability and facet joint osteoarthritis. The cardinal symptom is chronic or recurrent backache, but any of these conditions may also cause referred pain in the buttock and thigh ('sciatica').

Acquired stenosis of the spinal canal, or the lateral recesses of the canal, may result from thickening of the facet joints and new bone formation ('osteophytosis') at the posterior edges of the vertebral body.

Clinical features

Acute disc prolapse may occur at any age, but is uncommon in the very young and the very old. The patient is usually a fit adult of 20–45 years, though sometimes there is a history of mild, recurrent backache in the past. Typically, while lifting or stooping he or she has severe back pain and is unable to straighten up. Either then or a day or two later pain is felt in the buttock and lower limb (sciatica). Both backache and sciatica are made worse by coughing or straining. Later there may be paraesthesia or numbness in the leg or foot, and occasionally muscle weakness. Cauda equina compression is rare but may cause urinary retention.

The patient usually stands with a slight list to one side ('sciatic scoliosis'). Sometimes the knee on the painful side is held slightly flexed to relax tension on the sciatic nerve; straightening the knee makes the skew back more obvious. All back movements are restricted, and during forwards flexion the list may increase.

There is often tenderness in the midline of the low back, and paravertebral muscle spasm. Straight leg raising is restricted and painful on the affected side; dorsiflexion of the foot and bowstringing of the lateral popliteal nerve may accentuate the pain. Sometimes raising the unaffected leg causes acute sciatic tension on the painful side ('crossed sciatic tension'). With a high or mid-lumbar prolapse the femoral stretch test may be positive.

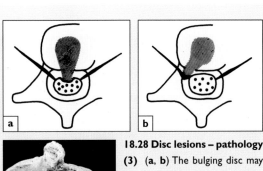

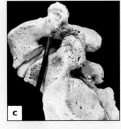

18.27 Disc lesions – pathology (2) From above, downwards: an abnormal increase in pressure within the nucleus causes splitting and bulging of the annulus; the posterior ligament may rupture, allowing disc material to extrude into the spinal canal; with chronic degeneration (lowest level) the disc space narrows and the posterior facet joints are displaced, giving rise to osteoarthritis.

Normal disc

Increased nuclear pressure causing bulging

Ruptured annulus and ligament

Degeneration + joint displacement

18.28 Disc lesions – pathology (3) **(a, b)** The bulging disc may press on the dura or on a nerve root. **(c)** The nerve is particularly vulnerable near the entrance to the intervertebral foramen.

a

b

c

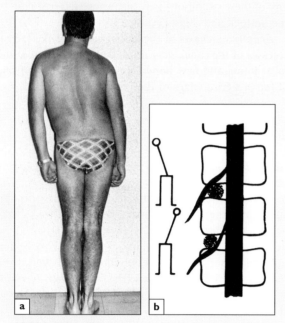

18.29 Lumbar disc – signs (a) The patient has a sideways list or tilt. (b) If the disc protrudes medial to the nerve root the tilt is towards the painful side (to relieve pressure on the root); with a far lateral prolapse (lower level) the tilt is away from the painful side.

NEUROLOGICAL EXAMINATION may show muscle weakness (and, later, wasting), diminished reflexes and sensory loss corresponding to the affected level. L5 impairment causes weakness of knee flexion and big toe extension, as well as sensory loss on the outer side of the leg and the dorsum of the foot. Paradoxically, the quadriceps reflex may appear to be *increased*, because of weakness of the antagonists (which are supplied by L5). S1 impairment causes weak plantarflexion and eversion of the foot, a depressed ankle jerk and sensory loss along the lateral border of the foot. Occasionally an L4/5 disc prolapse compresses both L5 and S1. Cauda equina compression causes urinary retention and sensory loss over the sacrum.

Imaging

X-rays are helpful, not to show an abnormal disc space but to exclude bone disease. After several attacks the disc space may be narrowed and small osteophytes appear.

Myelography (radiculography) using iopamidol (Niopam) is a fairly reliable method of confirming the disc protrusion, localizing it and excluding intrathecal tumours; however, it carries a significant risk of unpleasant side effects, such as headache (in over 30%), nausea and dizziness. Moreover, it is useless for showing a far lateral disc protrusion (lateral to the intervertebral foramen); if this is suspected CT or MRI is essential.

CT and *MRI* are more reliable than myelography and have none of its disadvantages. These are now the preferred methods of spinal imaging.

Differential diagnosis

The full-blown syndrome is unlikely to be misdiagnosed, but with repeated attacks and with lumbar spondylosis gradually supervening (see below), the features often become atypical. There are four diagnostic aphorisms:

- Sciatica is referred pain and can occur in other lumbar spine disorders.
- Disc rupture affects at most two neurological levels; if multiple levels are involved, suspect a neurological disorder.
- In disc rupture the episodes of pain are punctuated by intervals of normality. With severe, unrelenting pain suspect a tumour or infection.

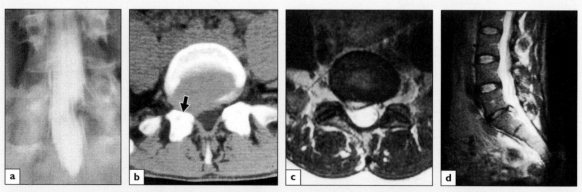

18.30 Lumbar disc – imaging (a) Radiculogram in which absence of the contrast medium shows where a disc has protruded. (b) CT scan showing how disc protrusion can obstruct the intervertebral foramen. (c, d) MRI showing the relationship of the disc protrusion to the dural sac and intervertebral foramen (axial and sagittal views).

- Very young and very old people seldom sustain acute ruptures. In adolescents, look for infection, a benign tumour or spondylolisthesis; in the elderly, look for a compression fracture or malignant disease.

Inflammatory disorders, such as infection or ankylosing spondylitis, cause severe stiffness, a raised ESR and erosive changes on x-ray.

Vertebral tumours cause severe pain and marked spasm. With metastases the patient is ill, the ESR raised and the x-rays show bone destruction or sclerosis.

Nerve tumours, such as a neurofibroma of the cauda equina, may cause 'sciatica' but pain is continuous and advanced imaging will confirm the diagnosis.

Treatment

Heat and analgesics soothe and exercises strengthen muscles; but there are only three ways of treating the prolapse itself – *rest, reduction* or *removal*; followed by *rehabilitation*.

REST With an acute attack the patient should be kept in bed, with hips and knees slightly flexed and 10kg traction to the pelvis. An anti-inflammatory drug such as indomethacin is useful.

REDUCTION Continuous bed rest and traction for 2 weeks will reduce the herniation in over 90% of cases. If the symptoms and signs have not improved significantly by then, an epidural injection of corticosteroid and local anaesthetic may help.

Chemonucleolysis – dissolution of the nucleus pulposus by percutaneous injection of a proteolytic enzyme (chymopapain) – is in theory an excellent way of reducing a disc prolapse. However, controlled studies have shown that it is less effective (and potentially more dangerous) than surgical removal of the disc material (Ejeskär *et al.*, 1982).

REMOVAL The indications for operative removal of a disc are: (1) a cauda equina compression syndrome that does not clear up within 6 hours of starting bed rest and traction – this is an emergency; (2) neurological deterioration while under conservative treatment; and (3) persistent pain and signs of sciatic tension (especially crossed sciatic tension) after 3 weeks of conservative treatment. The presence of a prolapsed disc, and the level, must be confirmed by CT, MRI or myelography before operating. Surgery in the absence of a clear preoperative diagnosis is usually unrewarding.

Partial laminectomy Part of the lamina and the ligamentum flavum on one side are removed, taking great care not to damage the facet joint. The dura and nerve root are then gently retracted towards the midline and the pea-like bulge is displayed. This is incised and the mushy disc material plucked out piecemeal with pituitary forceps. The nerve is traced to its point of exit in order to exclude other pathology.

A far lateral disc protrusion is very difficult to expose by the standard interlaminar approach without damaging the facet joint. An intertransverse approach may be more suitable for these cases.

The main intraoperative complication is bleeding from epidural veins. This is less likely to occur if the patient is placed on his or her side or in the kneeling position, thus minimizing the rise in venous pressure. The major postoperative complication is disc space infection, but fortunately this is rare.

Microdiscectomy This is essentially similar to the standard posterior operation, except that the exposure is very limited and the procedure is carried out with the aid of an operating microscope. Morbidity and length of hospitalization are certainly less than with open surgery, but there are drawbacks: careful x-ray control is needed to ensure that the correct level is entered; intraoperative bleeding may be difficult to control; there is a considerable 'learning curve' and the inexperienced operator risks injuring the dura or a stretched nerve root, or missing essential pathology; there is a slightly increased risk of disc space infection, and prophylactic antibiotics are advisable.

REHABILITATION After recovery from an acute disc rupture, or disc removal, the patient is taught isometric exercises and how to lie, sit, bend and lift with the least strain. Ideally this should be done as part of an education programme in a 'back school' (Zachrisson, 1981).

PERSISTENT POSTOPERATIVE BACKACHE AND SCIATICA

Persistent symptoms after operation may be due to: (1) residual disc material in the spinal canal; (2) disc prolapse at another level; or (3) nerve root pressure by a hypertrophic facet joint or a narrow lateral recess ('root canal stenosis'). After careful investigation, any of these may call for reoperation; but second procedures do not have a high success rate – third and fourth procedures still less.

ARACHNOIDITIS

Diffuse back pain and vague lower limb symptoms such as 'cramps', 'burning' or 'irritability' sometimes appear after myelography, epidural injections or disc operations. There may also be sphincter dysfunction and male impotence. Patients complain bitterly and many are labelled neurotic. However, in some cases there are electromyographic abnormalities, and dural scarring with obliteration of the subarachnoid space can be demonstrated by MRI or at operation.

Treatment is generally unrewarding. Corticosteroid injections at best give only temporary relief, and surgical 'neurolysis' may actually make matters worse. Sympathetic management in a pain clinic, psychological support and a graduated activity programme are the best that can be offered.

SEGMENTAL INSTABILITY AND FACET JOINT DYSFUNCTION

The concept of segmental instability has been elaborated during the last few decades (Kirkaldy-Willis and Farfan, 1982). However, the clinical syndrome was recognized long before that, even though the pathology was poorly understood. Patients with chronic backache may develop intermittent episodes of severe pain and 'sciatica' in the absence of any evidence of intervertebral disc prolapse. These attacks are usually triggered by fairly modest lifting strains, but they may also occur 'spontaneously'. Kirkaldy-Willis has suggested that the symptoms are due to abnormal movement and mechanical stress at the posterior facet joints, arising from local injury or non-specific dysfunction of the lower lumbar segment of the spine. The theory is controversial, partly because of differences about the meaning of the word 'instability' in this context and partly because some patients with demonstrably abnormal motion have no symptoms at all.

Facet joint abnormalities which have been demonstrated at operation or necropsy are: (1) anatomical variations which limit articular movement; (2) anatomical variations which permit excessive movement; (3) malapposition of the articular surfaces secondary to loss of disc height; (4) softening and fibrillation of the facet articular cartilage; (5) loose bodies in the facet joint; (6) synovial thickening; and (7) classic changes of osteoarthritis, progressing from fibrillation to complete loss of articular cartilage and osteophytic thickening of the facets. Some of these abnormalities are associated with demonstrable intervertebral instability; in others the abnormal movement is considered to be more subtle and it is not surprising that this has given rise to semantic argument.

Clinical features

The patient, usually a young adult engaged in bending and/or lifting activities, may have experienced mild backache from time to time. Typically this culminates in a particular episode of more severe back pain, possibly accompanied by 'sciatica' (i.e. referred pain in the buttock or the back of the thigh) but no true neurological symptoms. Pain is usually relieved by rest, mobilization exercises or chiropractic manipulation, only to recur a few weeks or months later after a similar episode of physical stress. In the established case, the patient gives a history of intermittent backache related to spells of hard work, standing or walking a lot or sitting in one position during a long journey. Some patients find relief by lying down, others feel better when up and moving about. As the condition modulates from instability to osteoarthritis of the facet joints, pain is more constant but can sometimes be temporarily relieved by manipulation, local warmth and anti-inflammatory drugs.

During a painful spell there may be muscle spasm and movements are restricted. Occasionally the patient presents with a 'locked back', which is suddenly and dramatically relieved by skilful manipulation. Between acute attacks, physical signs are less obvious and often unconvincing. The *range* of movement may not be much restricted, but the *pattern of movement* often is: characteristically the patient bends forwards quite easily but when asked to return to the upright position he or she does so with a noticeable 'heave' or 'catch' and may seek support by pushing with the hands on the front of the thighs.

Straight leg raising may be slightly restricted; neurological examination is normal, unless there has been a disc prolapse in the past.

Imaging

Signs of segmental instability are seen mainly at L4/5 or L5/S1. These are:

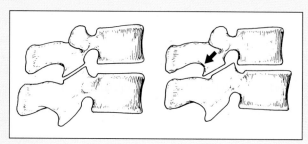

18.31 Facet joint dysfunction Diagrams showing how the sloping facet joints must inevitably be displaced in the direction of the arrow if the disc space collapses.

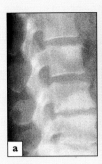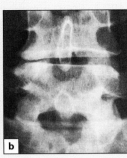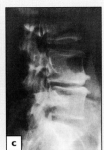

18.32 Segmental instability (a) One of the earliest signs of segmental instability is a wedge of sclerosis adjacent to the disc space – evidence of abnormal loading. Other features are (b) vertebral tilting and (c) small anterior traction spurs.

ON X-RAY

- Asymmetry of the disc space or facet joints in the anteroposterior view.
- Narrowing of the disc space, or a 'vacuum sign' (abnormal radiolucency in the disc space) on the lateral view.
- Localized sclerosis of the vertebral body adjacent to the disc space, a sign of abnormal loading.
- Traction spurs – bony spurs anteriorly away from the upper or lower rim of the vertebral body.
- Sagittal displacement of one vertebra upon another, either forwards (spondylolisthesis) or backwards (retrolisthesis); this may be become apparent only during flexion or extension.
- Abnormalities on discography and facetography; these investigations are not routinely available and there is some controversy about their reliability.

ON CT AND MRI

- Asymmetry of the facet joints.
- Early signs of facet joint osteoarthritis.
- A full thickness tear of the annulus fibrosus.
- Advanced disc degeneration and signs of previous herniation.

Diagnosis

Recurrent backache is often attributed to one particular abnormal feature, such as 'disc degeneration' or 'an annular tear'. It is difficult to prove a simple association of this kind, especially when the targetted structure is not itself pain-sensitive. The discovery of one abnormality should, however, prompt the clinician to look for others; it is the *set* of clinical and imaging features, rather than any single sign, that makes the diagnosis of segmental instability.

DISC DEGENERATION, INSTABILITY AND OSTEOARTHRITIS
Disc degeneration is one of the causes of instability, and abnormal motion and malalignment may eventually lead to osteoarthritis of the facet joints. The non-specific term *spondylosis* is often used to cover these changes, and particularly the associated x-ray features of disc space narrowing, marginal 'osteophyte' formation and distortion of the facet joints. Symptoms and signs are similar to those of chronic instability, but with time the intervals between painful attacks become shorter and shorter until the patient experiences more or less continuous backache and loss of lumbar movement. In the

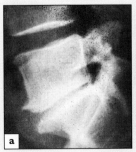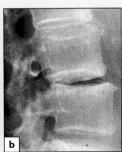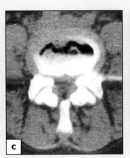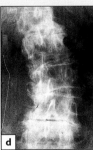

18.33 Spondylosis and osteoarthritis Typical x-ray features are (a) narrowing of the intervertebral space and anterior traction spurs, and (b) retrolisthesis and a vacant area in the disc space – the 'vacuum sign'. (c) CT showing the vacuum sign and hypertrophic osteoarthritis of the facet joints. (d) In advanced cases several levels are involved, with deformity of the spine.

most advanced stage, osteoarthritic hypertrophy of the facet joint may lead to nerve root entrapment in the lateral recess or intervertebral foramen, giving rise to neurological symptoms and signs.

A perennial puzzle is the poor correlation between the severity of x-ray changes and clinical symptoms. Advanced features, including disc collapse and 'osteophyte' formation, are sometimes discovered incidentally during x-ray investigation of other disorders in a patient who has never experienced backache.

Treatment

CONSERVATIVE MEASURES
Initially the symptoms of segmental instability are neither severe nor disabling; conservative measures should be encouraged for as long as possible.

General care and attention Poor understanding has led to the condition being neglected and, unless there is a very obvious abnormality which is amenable to surgery, patients soon come to feel that the doctor has lost interest in their complaints. Little wonder that many of them turn for help to 'alternative' practitioners. They should be given a clear explanation of the cause of their symptoms and an outline of the proposed treatment. In more enlightened (and better supported) centres patients are enrolled in a 'back school'.

Physiotherapy Conventional physiotherapy, including spinal 'mobilization', often relieves pain dramatically – at least for a while. In the longer term, weight control and strengthening of the vertebral and abdominal muscles will make for fewer recurrences. There is also no reason why orthopaedic surgeons and chiropractors or osteopaths should not be able to collaborate in designing treatment programmes.

Facet joint injections If clinical and x-ray signs point consistently to one or two facet levels, injection of local anaesthetic and corticosteroids may be carried out under fluoroscopic control. Most patients can be expected to obtain short-term benefit and some are relieved of symptoms for periods of more than a year.

Spinal support A soft lumbar support may give relief in some cases; obese patients benefit from having their centre of gravity pulled in close to the spine.

Drug treatment Mild analgesics may be needed for pain control. However, beware the patient who becomes dependent on increasing doses of medication.

Modification of activities One of the most important aspects of treatment is modification of daily activities (bending, lifting, climbing, etc.) and specific activities relating to work. The patient may need retraining for a different job. The co-operation of employers is essential.

Psychological support Chronic back pain can be psychologically as well as physically debilitating. Counselling and support are often welcomed by the patient.

SURGERY
Only after all the above measures have been tried and found to be ineffectual should a spinal fusion be considered. Even then very strict guidelines should be followed if one is to avoid embarking on a road already crowded with patients labelled 'failed back surgery'. (1) Repeated examination should ensure that there is no other treatable pathology. (2) There should have been at least some response to conservative treatment; patients who 'benefit from nothing' will not benefit from spinal fusion either. (3) There should be unequivocal evidence of facet joint instability or osteoarthritis at a specific level. (4) The patient should be emotionally stable and should not exaggerate his or her or symptoms, nor display inappropriate physical signs (see below). And (5) the patient should be warned that: (a) a 'fusion' doesn't always fuse (there is a 10–20% failure rate); and (b) a fusion at one level does not preclude further pathology developing at another level; Lehmann *et al.* (1987), in a long-term follow-up of patients who had undergone spinal fusion, found that after 10 years 40% had developed signs of instability elsewhere.

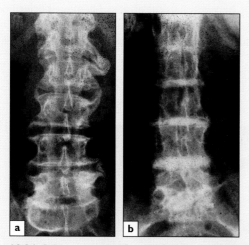

18.34 Other causes of 'spondylosis' (a) In Forestier's disease (see page 85) there are large spurs at multiple levels, often worse on the right side; (b) in ochronosis intervertebral calcification is characteristic.

SPONDYLOLISTHESIS

'Spondylolisthesis' means forwards shift of the spine. The shift is nearly always between L4 and L5, or between L5 and the sacrum. Normal laminae and facets constitute a locking mechanism which prevents each vertebra from moving forwards on the one below. Forwards shift (or slip) occurs only when this mechanism has failed.

Classification

Various classifications have been suggested. Basically there are six types of spondylolisthesis.

DYSPLASTIC (20%) The superior sacral facets are congenitally defective; slow but inexorable forwards slip leads to severe displacement. Associated anomalies (usually spina bifida occulta) are common.

LYTIC OR ISTHMIC (50%) In this, the commonest variety, there are defects in the pars interarticularis (spondylolysis); or repeated breaking and healing may lead to elongation of the pars. The defect (which occurs in about 5% of people) is usually present by the age of 7 years, but the slip may only appear some years later (Fredrickson *et al.*, 1984). It is difficult to exclude a genetic factor because spondylolisthesis often runs in families, and is more common in certain races, notably Eskimos; but the incidence increases with age, so an acquired factor probably supervenes to produce what is essentially a stress fracture. The condition is more common than usual in those whose spines are subjected to extraordinary stresses (e.g. competitive gymnasts and weightlifters).

DEGENERATIVE 25% Degenerative changes in the facet joints and the discs permit forwards slip (nearly always at L4/5) despite intact laminae. Many of these patients have generalized osteoarthritis and pyrophosphate crystal arthropathy.

POST-TRAUMATIC Unusual fractures may result in destabilization of the lumbar spine.

PATHOLOGICAL Bone destruction (e.g. due to tuberculosis or neoplasm) may lead to vertebral slipping.

POST-OPERATIVE Occasionally, operative removal of bone results in progressive instability.

Pathology

In the common lytic type of spondylolisthesis the pars interarticularis is in two pieces (spondylolysis) and the gap is occupied by fibrous tissue; behind the gap the spinous process, laminae and inferior articular facets remain as an isolated segment. With stress, the vertebral body and superior facets in front of the gap may subluxate or dislocate forwards, carrying the superimposed vertebral column; the isolated segment of neural arch maintains its normal relationship to the sacral facets. When there is no gap, the pars interarticularis is elongated or the facets are defective.

The degree of slip is measured by the amount of overlap of adjacent vertebral bodies and is usually expressed as a percentage.

With forwards slipping there may be pressure on the dura mater and cauda equina, or on the emerging nerve roots; these roots may also be compressed in the narrowed intervertebral foramina. Disc prolapse is liable to occur.

Clinical features

Spondylolysis, and even a well-marked spondylolisthesis, may be discovered incidentally during routine x-ray examination.

In children the condition is painless but the mother may notice the unduly protruding abdomen and peculiar stance.

In adolescents and *adults* backache is the usual presenting symptom; it is often intermittent, coming on after exercise or strain. Sciatica may occur in one or both legs.

Patients aged over 50 years are usually women with degenerative spondylolisthesis. They always have backache; some have sciatica; and some present because of pseudoclaudication due to spinal stenosis.

 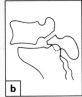 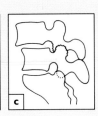

18.35 Spondylolisthesis – varieties (a) The pars interarticularis is long and attenuated, with forwards shift of the upper vertebra on the lower. (b) There is a break in the pars interarticularis – this is a kind of stress fracture. (c) Degeneration of the facet joints (usually at L4/5) has allowed forwards slipping to occur.

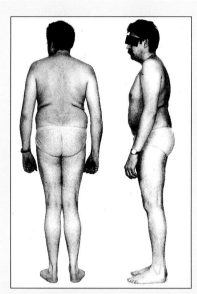

18.36 Spondylolisthesis – clinical appearance The transverse loin creases, forwards tilting of the pelvis and flattening of the lumbar spine are characteristic.

On examination the buttocks look curiously flat, the sacrum appears to extend to the waist and transverse loin creases are seen. The lumbar spine is on a plane in front of the sacrum and looks too short. Sometimes there is a scoliosis.

A 'step' can often be felt when the fingers are run down the spine. Movements are usually normal in the younger patients but there may be 'hamstring tightness'; in the degenerative group the spine is often stiff.

X-RAYS show the forwards shift of the upper part of the spinal column on the stable vertebra below; elongation of the arch or defective facets may be seen. The gap in the pars interarticularis is best seen in the oblique views. In doubtful cases, *CT* may be helpful.

Prognosis

Dysplastic spondylolisthesis appears at an early age, often goes on to a severe slip and carries a significant risk of neurological complications.

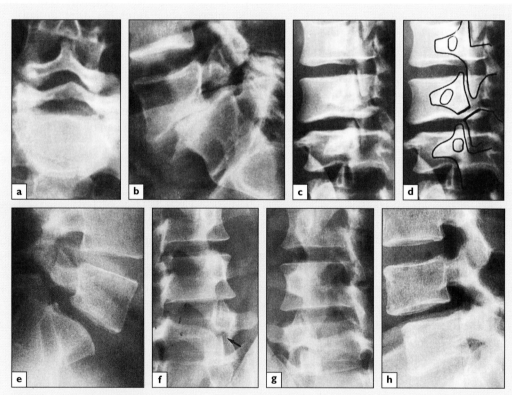

18.37 Spondylolisthesis – x-rays (**a**) In the anteroposterior x-ray the superior surface of the 'slipped' vertebral body may be seen almost end-on. In the lateral x-ray (**b**) the slip may be obvious, but the defect in the pars interarticularis is better seen in the oblique view (**c, d**) where it is likened to a 'collar' around the 'neck' of an illusory 'dog'. (**e, f, g**) In this case the break in the pars is seen in the lateral x-ray. Oblique views show that on one side there is a defect (arrow) but on the other the break has healed with elongation of the pars. In degenerative spondylolisthesis (**h**) there is no pars defect; the unstable facet joints permit slipping, usually at L4/5.

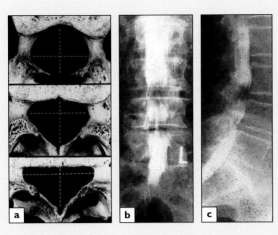

18.38 Spinal stenosis (a) The shape of the lumbar spinal canal varies from oval (with a large capacity) to trefoil (with narrow lateral recesses); further encroachment on an already narrow canal can cause an ischaemic neuropathy and 'spinal claudication'. (**b, c**) Myelogram showing marked narrowing of the radio-opaque column at the level of stenosis.

Lytic (isthmic) spondylolisthesis with less than 10% displacement is usually asymptomatic, does not progress after adulthood, does not predispose the patient to later back problems and is not a contraindication to strenuous work (Wiltse *et al.*, 1990). With slips of more than 25% there is an increased risk of backache in later life.

Degenerative spondylolisthesis is rare before the age of 50 years, progresses slowly and seldom exceeds 30% displacement.

Treatment

Conservative treatment, similar to that for segmental instability, is suitable for most patients.

Operative treatment is indicated: (1) if the symptoms are disabling and interfere significantly with work and recreational activities; (2) if the slip is more than 50% and progressing; and (3) if neurological compression is significant.

For children, posterior intertransverse fusion *in situ* is almost always successful; if neurological signs appear, decompression can be done later. For adults, either posterior or anterior fusion is suitable. However, in the 'degenerative' group, where neurological symptoms predominate, decompression without fusion may suffice.

Note on post-traumatic spondylolisthesis The patient found to have spondylolysis or spondylolisthesis after recent back injury (usually hyperextension) may have fractured the pars, or merely have strained the fibrous tissue of a pre-existing lesion. If doubt exists (and it usually does) a plaster jacket is worn for 3 months; the recent fracture may join spontaneously. If union does not occur, the assumption is that spondylolisthesis was present before injury and treatment is along the lines already indicated.

SPINAL STENOSIS

The lumbar spinal canal is normally round or oval in cross section; in a minority of cases the L5 canal is trefoil-shaped and the lateral recesses are narrower than usual, yet still wide enough to allow free passage of the nerve roots through the intervertebral foramena. The term *spinal stenosis* is used to describe abnormal narrowing of the central canal, the lateral recesses or the intervertebral foramena to the point where the neural elements are compromised. When this occurs the patient develops neurological symptoms and signs in the lower limbs.

The causes of spinal stenosis are: (1) congenital vertebral dysplasia (e.g. in achondroplasia or hypochondroplasia); (2) chronic disc protrusion and peri-discal fibrosis or ossification; (3) displacement and hypertrophy, or osteoarthritis, of the apophyseal (facet) joints; (4) hypertrophy or ossification of the ligamentum flavum; (5) bone thickening due to Paget's disease; and (6) spondylolisthesis. Unilateral narrowing of the intervertebral foramen (*root canal stenosis*) may result from an unresolved lateral disc herniation, post-discectomy fibrosis or unilateral facet joint osteoarthritis.

What constitutes abnormal narrowing, or stenosis? Two measurements are used: the mid-sagittal (anteroposterior) diameter and the interpedicular (transverse) diameter of the spinal canal. On plain x-rays the lower limits of normal are usually taken as 15mm for the anteroposterior and 20mm for the transverse diameters. However, the boundaries of the canal are sometimes difficult to define and more accurate measurements can be obtained from CT; anything less than 11mm for the anteroposterior diameter and 16 mm for the transverse diameter is considered abnormal.

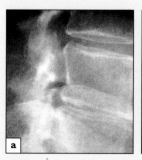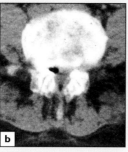

18.39 Spinal stenosis (**a**) A lateral film shows marked narrowing of the spinal canal, but (**b**) a CT scan provides even more convincing and dramatic evidence.

Clinical features

The patient, usually a man aged over 50 years, complains of aching, heaviness, numbness and paraesthesia in the thighs and legs; it comes on after standing upright or walking for 5–10 minutes, and is consistently relieved by sitting, squatting or leaning against a wall to flex the spine (hence the term 'spinal claudication'). The patient may prefer walking uphill, which flexes the spine, to downhill, which extends it. With root canal stenosis the symptoms may be unilateral. The patient sometimes has a previous history of disc prolapse, chronic backache or spinal operation.

Examination, especially after getting the patient to reproduce the symptoms by walking, may show neurological deficit in the lower limbs. Electromyography is helpful if the clinical findings are equivocal.

IMAGING
X-rays may show degenerative spondylolisthesis or advanced disc degeneration and osteoarthritis. Measurement of the spinal canal can be carried out on plain films, but more reliable information is obtained from *CT and MRI* (see above).

Treatment

Conservative measures, including instruction in spinal posture, may suffice. Most patients are prepared to put up with their symptoms and simply avoid uncomfortable postures. If discomfort is marked and activities are severely restricted, operative decompression is almost always successful. A wide laminectomy is performed, if necessary extending over several levels and outwards to clear the nerve root canals. This relieves the leg pain, but not the back pain, and occasionally it actually increases instability; consequently in patients under 60 years of age the operation is sometimes combined with spinal fusion.

APPROACH TO DIAGNOSIS IN PATIENTS WITH LOW BACK PAIN

Chronic backache is such a frequent cause of disability in the community that it has become almost a disease in itself. The following is a suggested approach to more specific diagnosis.

Careful history taking and examination will uncover one of five pain patterns.

TRANSIENT BACKACHE FOLLOWING MUSCULAR ACTIVITY This suggests a simple *back strain*, which will respond to a short period of rest followed by gradually increasing exercise. People with thoracic kyphosis (of whatever origin), or fixed flexion of the hip, are particularly prone to back strain because they tend to compensate for the deformity by holding the lumbosacral spine in hyperlordosis.

SUDDEN, ACUTE PAIN AND SCIATICA In young people (those under 20 years of age) it is important to exclude *infection* and *spondylolisthesis*; both produce recognizable x-ray changes. Patients aged 20–40 years are more likely to have an *acute disc prolapse*: diagnostic features are (1) a history of a lifting strain, (2) unequivocal sciatic tension and (3) neurological symptoms and signs. Elderly patients may have osteoporotic *compression fractures*, but *metastatic disease* and *myeloma* must be excluded.

INTERMITTENT LOW BACK PAIN AFTER EXERTION Patients of almost any age may complain of recurrent backache following exertion or lifting activities and relieved by rest. Features of disc prolapse are absent but there may be a history of acute sciatica in the past. In early cases x-rays usually show no abnormality; later there may be signs of *facet joint dysfunction, intervertebral disc degeneration and/or segmental instability*; in those over 50 years of age, *osteoarthritis* of the facet joints is common. These patients need painstaking examination (a) to uncover any features of segmental instability or facet joint osteoarthritis and (b) to determine whether those features are incidental or do indeed account for the patient's symptoms. In the process, disorders such as *ankylosing spondylitis, chronic infection, myelomatosis* and other *bone disease* must be excluded by appropriate imaging and blood investigations.

BACK PAIN PLUS PSEUDOCLAUDICATION These patients are usually aged over 50 years and may give a history of previous, long-standing, back trouble. The diagnosis of *spinal stenosis* should be confirmed by suitable imaging studies.

SEVERE AND CONSTANT PAIN LOCALIZED TO A PARTICULAR SITE This suggests local bone pathology, such as a *compression fracture, Paget's disease*, a *tumour* or

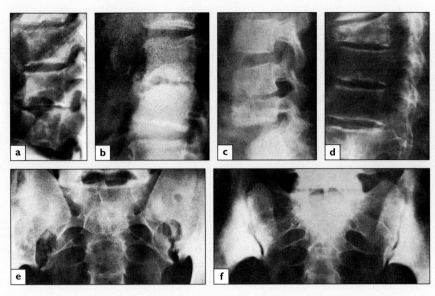

18.40 Some causes of chronic backache (**a**) Tuberculosis; (**b**) acute osteomyelitis – note the sclerosis which developed within a few weeks; (**c**) discitis. (**d**) Here, unlike the previous three, the disc spaces are normal – the bodies are not – these are secondary deposits. (**e**) Bilateral sacroiliac tuberculosis; (**f**) osteitis condensans ilii, which is probably not the cause of the backache.

infection. Spinal osteoporosis in middle-aged men is pathological and calls for a full battery of tests to exclude primary disorders such as *myelomatosis, carcinomatosis, hyperthyroidism, gonadal insufficiency, alcoholism* or *corticosteroid usage.*

THE 'CHRONIC BACK PAIN SYNDROME'

Patients with chronic backache may despair of finding a cure for their trouble (or, indeed, even a diagnosis that everyone agrees on), and they often develop affective and psychosomatic ailments which subsequently become the chief focus of attention. This 'illness behaviour' is both self-perpetuating and self-justifying. It is usually accompanied by '*non-organic*' (*inappropriate*) *physical signs* (Waddell *et al.,* 1980, 1984), such as: (1) pain and tenderness of bizarre degree or distribution; (2) pain on performing impressive but non-stressful manoeuvres such as pressing vertically on the spine or passively rotating the entire trunk; (3) variations in response to tests such as deliberate straight leg raising (which is apparently restricted) and the same test repeated later while distracting the patient's attention; (4) sensory and/or motor abnormalities which do not fit the known anatomical and physiological patterns; and (5) overdetermined behaviour during physical examination (trembling, sweating, hyperventilating, inability to move, a tendency to fall and exaggerated withdrawal) – usually accompanied by loud groaning and exclamations of discomfort. Patients with these features are unlikely to respond to surgery and they may require prolonged support and management in a special pain clinic – but only after every effort has been made to exclude organic pathology.

NOTES ON APPLIED ANATOMY

THE SPINE AS A WHOLE The spine has to be able to move, transmit weight and protect the spinal cord. In an upright human the lumbar segment is lordotic and the column acts like a crane; the paravertebral muscles are the cables that counterbalance any weight carried anteriorly. The resultant force, which passes through the nucleus pulposus of the lowest lumbar disc, is therefore much greater than if the column were loaded directly over its centre; even at rest, tonic contraction of the posterior muscles balances the trunk, so the lumbar spine is always loaded. Nachemson and Morris (1964) measured the intradiscal pressure in volunteers during various activities and found it as high as 10–15kg/cm^2 while sitting, about 30% less on standing upright and 50% less on lying down. Leaning forward or carrying a weight produces much higher pressures, though when a heavy weight is lifted breathing stops and the abdominal muscles contract, turning the trunk into a tightly inflated bag which cushions the force anteriorly against the pelvis. (Could it be that champion weightlifters benefit in this way from having voluminous bodies?)

Seen from the side, the dorsal spine is convex backwards (kyphosis); the cervical and lumbar regions are convex forwards (lordosis). In forwards flexion the lordotic curves straighten out. Lying supine with the legs straight tilts the pelvic brim forwards; the lumbar spine compensates by increasing its lordosis. If the hips are unable to extend fully (fixed-flexion deformity), the lumbar lordosis increases still more until the lower limbs lie flat and the flexion deformity is masked.

THE VERTEBRAL COMPONENTS Each segment of the vertebral column transmits weight through the vertebral body anteriorly and the facet joints posteriorly.

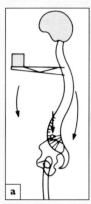
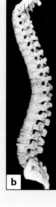
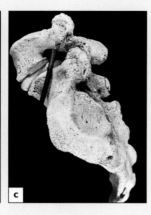

18.41 Anatomy (**a, b**) The vertebral column has a series of gentle curves which produce lordosis in the cervical and lumbar regions and kyphosis in the dorsal segment. The column functions like a crane, the weight in front of the spine being counterbalanced by contraction of the posterior muscles. (**c**) Relationship of nerve root to disc and facet joint.

Between adjacent bodies (and firmly attached to them) lie the intervertebral discs. These compressible 'cushions', and the surrounding ligaments and muscles, act as shock-absorbers; if they are degenerate or weak their ability to absorb some of the force is diminished and the bones and joints suffer the consequences.

The vertebral body is cancellous, but the upper and lower surfaces are condensed to form sclerotic endplates. In childhood these are covered by cartilage, which contributes to vertebral growth. Later the peripheral rim ossifies and fuses with the body, but the central area remains as a thin layer of cartilage adherent to the intervertebral disc. The epiphyseal end-plates may be damaged by disc pressure during childhood, giving rise to irregular ossification and abnormal vertebral growth (Scheuermann's disease).

THE INTERVERTEBRAL DISC   The disc consists of *a central avascular nucleus pulposus* – a hydrophilic gel made of protein-polysaccharide, collagen fibres, sparse chondroid cells and water (88%) – surrounded by concentric layers of fibrous tissue, the *annulus fibrosus*. If the physicochemical state of the nucleus pulposus is normal, the disc can withstand almost any load that the muscles can support; if it is abnormal, even small increases in force can produce sufficient stress to rupture the annulus.

MOVEMENTS   The axis of movements in the thoracocolumbar spine is the nucleus pulposus; the disposition of the facet joints determines which movements occur. In the lumbar spine these joints are in the anteroposterior plane, so flexion, extension and side-ways tilting are free but there is virtually no rotation. In the thoracic spine the facet joints face backwards and laterally, so rotation is relatively free; flexion, extension and tilting are possible but are grossly restricted by the ribs. The costovertebral joints are involved in respiration and their limitation is an early feature of ankylosing spondylitis.

THE SPINAL CANAL   The shape of the canal changes from ovoid in the upper part of the spine to triangular in the lower. Variations are common and include the trefoil canal whose shape is mainly due to thickening of the laminae (Eisenstein, 1980). This shape is harmless in itself, but further encroachment on the canal (e.g. by a bulging disc or hypertrophic facet joints) may cause compression of the spinal contents (spinal stenosis).

THE SPINAL CORD   The spinal cord ends at about L1 in the conus medullaris, but lumbosacral nerve roots continue in the spinal canal as the cauda equina and leave at appropriate levels lower down. The dural sac continues as far as S2, and whenever a nerve root leaves the spine it takes with it a dural sleeve as far as the exit from the intervertebral foramen. These dural sleeves can be outlined by contrast medium radiography (radiculography).

THE INTERVERTEBRAL FORAMINA AND NERVE ROOTS   Each intervertebral foramen is bounded anteriorly by the disc and adjoining vertebral bodies, posteriorly by the facet joint, and superiorly and inferiorly by the pedicles of adjacent vertebrae. It can therefore be narrowed by a bulging disc or by joint osteophytes. The segmental nerve roots leave the spinal canal through the intervertebral foramina, each pair below the vertebra of the same number (thus, the fourth lumbar root runs between L4 and L5). The segmental blood vessels to and from the cord also pass through the intervertebral foramen. Occlusion of this little passage may occasionally compress the nerve root directly or may cause nerve root ischaemia (especially when the spine is held in extension).

NERVE SUPPLY OF THE SPINE The spine and its contents (including the dural sleeves of the nerve roots themselves) are supplied by small branches from the anterior and posterior primary rami of the segmental nerve roots. Lesions of different structures (e.g. the posterior longitudinal ligament, the dural sleeve or the facet joint) may therefore cause pain of similar distribution. *Pain down the thigh and leg ('sciatica') does not necessarily signify root pressure; it may equally well be referred from a facet joint.*

BLOOD SUPPLY In addition to the spinal arteries, which run the length of the cord, segmental arteries from the aorta send branches through the intervertebral foramina at each level. Accompanying veins drain into the azygos system and inferior vena cava, and anastomose profusely with the extradural plexus which extends throughout the length of the spinal canal (Batson's plexus).

REFERENCES AND FURTHER READING

Archer IA, Dickson RA (1989) Spinal deformities. 1. Basic principles. *Current Orthopaedics* 3, 72-76

Cotrel Y, Dubousset J, Guillamet M (1988) New universal instrumentation in spinal surgery. *Clinical Orthopaedics and Related Research* **227**, 10-23

Dickson RA (1989) Idiopathic spinal deformities. *Current Orthopaedics* 3, 77-85

Dickson RA, Lawton JD, Archer IA, Butt WP (1984) The pathogenesis of idiopathic scoliosis. *Journal of Bone and Joint Surgery* **66B**, 8-15

Eisenstein S (1980) The trefoil configuration of the lumbar vertebral canal. *Journal of Bone and Joint Surgery* **62B**, 73-77

Ejeskär A, Nachemson A, Herberts P *et al* (1982) Surgery versus chemonucleolysis for herniated lumbar discs. *Clinical Orthopaedics and Related Research* **171**, 252-259

Fredrickson BE, Baker DR, McHolick WJ *et al* (1984) The natural history of spondylolysis and spondylolisthesis. *Journal of Bone and Joint Surgery* **66A**, 699-700

Kellgren JH (1977) The anatomical source of back pain. *Rheumatology and Rehabilitation* 16, 3-14

Kirkaldy-Willis WH, Farfan HF (1982) Instability of the lumbar spine. *Clinical Orthopaedics and Related Research* **165**, 110-123

Kostuik JP (1990) Operative treatment of idiopathic scoliosis. *Journal of Bone and Joint Surgery* **72A**, 1108-1113

Lehmann TR, Spratt KF, Tozzi JE *et al* (1987) Long-term follow-up of lower lumbar fusion patients. *Spine* 12, 97-104

Leong JCY (1990) Spinal infections. Pyogenic and tuberculous infections. In *The Lumbar Spine* (eds Weinstein JN, Weisel SW). WB Saunders, Philadelphia, pp699-723

Lonstein JE, Carlson JM (1984) The prediction of curve progression in untreated idiopathic scoliosis during growth. *Journal of Bone and Joint Surgery* **66A**, 1061-1071

McCulloch JA (1980) Chemonucleolysis: experience with 2000 cases. *Clinical Orthopaedics and Related Research* **146**, 128-135

Mehta MH (1972) The rib–vertebra angle in the early diagnosis between resolving and progressive infantile scoliosis. *Journal of Bone and Joint Surgery* **54B**, 230-243

Murray PM, Weinstein SL, Spratt KF (1993) The natural history and long-term follow-up of Scheuermann kyphosis. *Journal of Bone and Joint Surgery* **75A**, 236-248

Nachemson A, Morris JM (1964) In vivo measurements of intradiscal pressure. *Journal of Bone and Joint Surgery* **46A**, 1077-1092

Waddell G, McCulloch JA, Kummel E, Venner RM (1980) Nonorganic physical signs in low-back pain. *Spine* 5, 117-125

Waddell G, Birche, M, Finlayson D, Main CJ (1984) Symptoms and signs: physical disease or illness behaviour. *British Medical Journal* **289**, 739-741

Wiltse LL, Rothman SLG, Milanowska *et al.* (1980) Lumbar and lumbosacral spondylolisthesis. In *The Lumbar Spine* (eds. JN Weinstein and SW Wiesel), WB Saunders, Philadelphia, pp. 471–545

Zachrisson M (1981) The back school. *Spine* 6, 104-106

CLINICAL ASSESSMENT

SYMPTOMS

Pain arising in the hip joint is felt in the groin, down the front of the thigh and, sometimes, in the knee; occasionally knee pain is the only symptom! Pain at the back of the hip is seldom from the joint; it usually derives from the lumbar spine.

Limp is the next most common symptom. It may simply be a way of coping with pain, or it may be due to a change in limb length, weakness of the hip abductors or joint instability.

Snapping or clicking in the hip suggests a number of causes: slipping of the gluteus maximus tendon over the greater trochanter, detachment of the acetabular labrum or psoas bursitis.

Stiffness and deformity are late symptoms, and tend to be well compensated for by pelvic mobility.

Walking distance may be curtailed; or, reluctantly, the patient starts using a walking stick.

SIGNS WITH THE PATIENT UPRIGHT

Start by standing face-to-face with the patient and note his or her general build and the symmetry of the lower limbs. First impressions are important and can be put to the test as the examination proceeds. The patient in Fig. 19.1, for example, seems to have unusually short lower limbs in comparison to his trunk length. Is it a growth disorder, or are the hips dislocated?

While the patient is upright, take the opportunity to examine the spine for deformity or limitation of movement.

Trendelenburg's sign

This is a test for postural stability when the patient stands on one leg. In a normal two-legged stance the body's centre of gravity is placed midway between the two feet. Normally, in a one-legged stance, the pelvis is pulled up on the unsupported side and the centre of gravity is placed directly over the standing foot. If the weightbearing hip is unstable, the pelvis *drops* on the unsupported side; to avoid falling, the person has to throw his or her body towards the loaded side so that the centre of gravity is again over that foot (see Fig. 19.1b).

If the difference between the two hips is marked (as in Fig.19.1) you can detect it by simply looking at the patient's stance. However, small differences are not so obvious. In the classic Trendelenburg test the examiner stands behind the patient and looks at the buttock-folds. Normally, in a one-legged stance the buttock on the opposite side rises as the person lifts that leg; in a positive (abnormal) test the opposite buttock-fold drops.

The causes of a positive Trendelenburg sign are (1) pain on weightbearing; (2) weakness of the hip abductors; (3) shortening of the femoral neck; and (4) dislocation or subluxation of the hip.

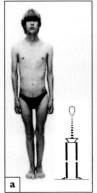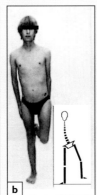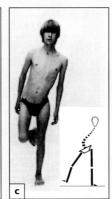

19.1 Trendelenburg's sign (a) Standing normally on two legs. (b) Standing on the right leg which has a normal hip whose abductor muscles ensure correct weight transference. (c) Standing on the left leg whose hip is faulty, and so abduction cannot be achieved; the pelvis drops on the unsupported side and the shoulder swings over to the left.

Gait

Now ask the patient to walk and observe each phase of the gait. The commonest abnormalities are a *short-leg limp* (a regular, even dip on the short side*), an antalgic gait* (an irregular limp, with the patient moving more quickly off the painful side) and a *Trendelenburg lurch* (a variant of Trendelenburg's sign).

SIGNS WITH THE PATIENT SITTING

This is the best way to test for iliopsoas function. The patient should be sitting on the edge of the examination couch. Place a hand firmly on his thigh and ask him to lift the thigh (flex the hip) against resistance. This is a predominantly psoas action; pain or weakness suggests a local disorder such as tendinitis or psoas bursitis.

SIGNS WITH THE PATIENT LYING

Look

Scars or sinuses may be seen (or they may be at the back of the hip). Compare the two sides for signs of muscle wasting or swelling.

Check that the pelvis is horizontal (both anterior superior iliac spines at the same level) and the legs placed symmetrically. Limb length can be gauged by looking at the ankles and heels, but measurement is more accurate. With the two legs in identical positions, measure the distance from the anterior superior iliac spine to the medial malleolus on each side. The limb may lie in an abnormal position; excessive rotation is

19.2 Trendelenburg's test This man has a positive Trendelenburg sign on the left, due to osteoarthritis of the hip. **(a)** He can steady himself perfectly well when balancing on the right hip; **(b)** when he attempts to stand on the left hip, his pelvis dips and the right buttock drops.

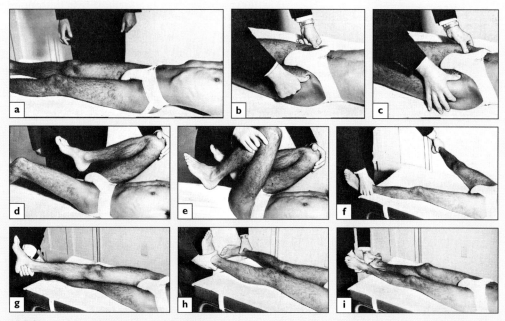

19.3 Signs with patient supine **(a)** Looking at the patient: his legs and pelvis are square with the couch; the lordosis indicates fixed flexion of the hip. **(b)** Feeling the anterior superior iliac spines. **(c)** Locating the top of the greater trochanter. **(d)** Flexing the right hip causes the left to lift off the couch (fixed flexion). The left hip also has limitation of **(e)** flexion, **(f)** abduction, **(g)** adduction, **(h)** internal rotation and **(i)** external rotation.

easy to detect but other deformities are often masked by tilting of the pelvis.

Sometimes the *real length*, as determined by measuring between two bony points, is quite different from the *apparent length* with the patient lying in repose. This happens when the pelvis is tilted and one limb is hitched upwards. Almost invariably this is due to an uncorrectable deformity at the hip: with fixed adduction on one side, the limbs would tend to be crossed; when the legs are placed side by side the pelvis has to

tilt upwards on the affected side, giving the impression of a shortened limb. The exact opposite occurs when there is fixed abduction, and the limb seems to be longer on the affected side.

If real shortening is present it is usually possible to establish where the fault lies. With the knees flexed and the heels together, it can be seen whether the discrepancy is below or above the knee. If it is above, the next question is whether the abnormality lies above the greater trochanter. The thumbs are pressed firmly against the anterior superior iliac spines and the middle fingers grope for the tops of the greater trochanters; any elevation of the trochanter on one side is readily appreciated.

Feel

Skin temperature and soft tissue contours can be felt, but are unhelpful unless the patient is very thin.

Bone contours are felt when levelling the pelvis and judging the height of the greater trochanters. *Tenderness* may be elicited in and around the joint.

Move

The assessment of hip movements is difficult because any limitation can easily be obscured by movement of the pelvis. Thus, even a gross limitation of extension, causing a *fixed-flexion deformity*, can be completely

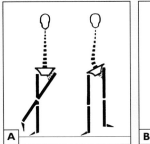
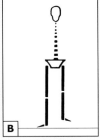

19.4 Shortening (1) – real or apparent? A leg may look short without actually being short. Thus A, with adduction of his left hip, has to hitch up his pelvis in order to uncross his legs; this makes the leg appear short. B has no hip deformity; unlike A he is able to stand (or lie) with his legs at right angles to his pelvis. His leg really is short.

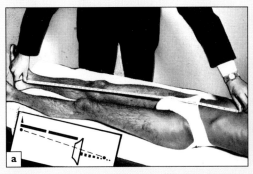
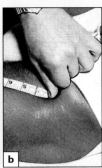
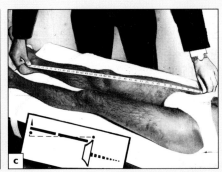

19.5 Shortening (2) – measurements *Apparent length* (**a**) is measured from a fixed point in the midline (e.g. the xiphisternum) to the bottom of the medial malleolus. *Real length* is measured from the anterior superior iliac spine; note how the thumb is pressed hard up against it (**b**) – also to the medial malleolus (**c**).

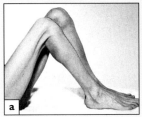
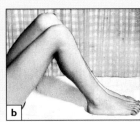

19.6 Shortening (3) Provided the backs of both heels are exactly level, bending the knees immediately shows whether the shortening is (**a**) above the knee or (**b**) below it.

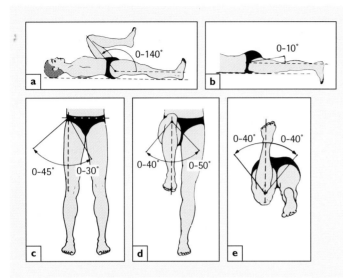

19.7 Normal range of movements (a) The hip should flex until the thigh meets the abdomen, but (b) extends only a few degrees. (c) Abduction is usually greater than adduction. The relative amounts of internal and external rotation may vary according to whether the hip is in (d) flexion or (e) extension.

masked simply by arching the back into excessive lordosis. Fortunately it can be just as easily unmasked by performing *Thomas' test*: both hips are flexed simultaneously to their limit, thus completely obliterating the lumbar lordosis; holding the 'sound' hip firmly in position (and thus keeping the pelvis still), the other limb is lowered gently; with any flexion deformity the knee will not rest on the couch. Meanwhile the full range of *flexion* will also have been noted; the normal range is about 130°.

Similarly, when testing *abduction* the pelvis must be prevented from tilting sideways. This is achieved by placing the 'sound' hip (the hip opposite to the one being examined) in full abduction and keeping it there. A hand is placed on one iliac crest to detect the slightest movement of the pelvis. Then, after checking that the anterior superior iliac spines are level, the affected joint is moved gently into abduction. The normal range is about 40°.

Adduction is tested by crossing one limb over the other; the pelvis must be watched and felt to determine the point at which it starts to tilt. The normal range of adduction is about 30°.

To test *rotation* both legs, lifted by the ankles, are rotated first internally and then externally; the patellae are watched to estimate the amount of rotation. Rotation in flexion is tested with the hip and knee each flexed 90°.

If internal rotation is full with the hip extended, but restricted in flexion, this suggests pathology in the anterosuperior portion of the femoral head, probably avascular necrosis (the so-called 'sectoral sign'). But in a young person pain on internal rotation with the hip flexed may indicate a torn acetabular labrum.

Abnormal movement is rarely elicited. Telescoping (excessive movement when the limb is alternately pulled and pushed in its long axis) is a sign of gross instability.

Don't forget the back of the hip. Ask the patient to roll over into the prone position. Check for scars and sinuses. Feel for tenderness and test the range of hip extension.

IMAGING

The minimum required is an anteroposterior *x-ray* of the pelvis showing both hips and a lateral view of each hip separately. The two sides can be compared: any difference in the size, shape or position of the femoral heads is important. With a normal hip Shenton's line, which continues from the inferior border of the femoral neck to the inferior border of the superior pubic ramus, looks continuous; any interruption in the line suggests an abnormal position of the femoral head. Narrowing of the joint 'space' is a sure sign of arthritis.

A lateral view is obligatory for assessing the shape, position and architecture of the femoral head; for example, when a slipped epiphysis or avascular necrosis is suspected.

Ultrasonography has a secure place in the early diagnosis of congenital hip dysplasia, when the joint is cartilaginous. It is also useful for demonstrating intra-articular effusions.

Arthrography may be used to show the outline of the cartilaginous femoral head in young children. It may also reveal loose bodies, a loose flap of articular cartilage or a tear of the acetabular labrum.

Computed tomography (CT) is ideal for demonstrating structural abnormalities of the joint, e.g. in the assessment of fracture-dislocations of the hip.

Radioscintigraphy is helpful in investigating the blood supply of the femoral head or cellular activity in the subchondral bone.

Magnetic resonance imaging (MRI) is the best method for detecting changes in the marrow and is the only certain way of diagnosing early avascular necrosis, in which the changes are confined to the marrow.

ARTHROSCOPY

Arthroscopy has come much later to the hip than to other joints such as the knee and shoulder. The procedure is

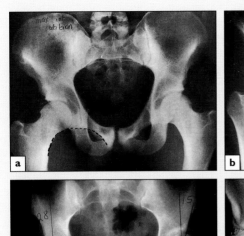
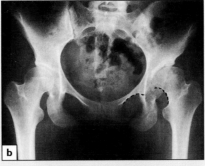
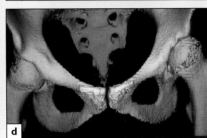

19.8 Imaging (a) Anteroposterior x-ray of normal hips, showing Shenton's line. **(b)** X-ray of a patient with secondary osteoarthritis of the left hip due to congenital subluxation. The joint 'space' is narrowed and Shenton's line is broken. **(c, d)** X-ray and three-dimensional CT showing how shallow the acetabula are, and how much of the femoral head is uncovered, especially in the left hip. (Courtesy of Professor KJeld Søballe, Århus Universitetshopital.)

technically difficult and the indications for its use are still being defined. In a recent review of 328 patients presenting with pain in the hip and subsequently undergoing arthroscopy, it is reported that in over half the cases the procedure contributed to the diagnosis beyond the information derived from clinical and imaging studies. In 172 cases some type of operation was performed as well, usually debridement of osteoarthritic tissue, extraction of loose bodies, removal of labral tears and biopsies (Baber *et al.*, 1999). Arthroscopy is now considered to be more reliable than MRI for the diagnosis of non-osseous loose bodies, labral tears and cartilage damage.

THE DIAGNOSTIC CALENDAR

Hip disorders are characteristically seen in certain well-defined age groups. Whilst there are exceptions to this rule, it is sufficiently true to allow the age at onset to serve as a guide to the probable diagnosis.

DEVELOPMENTAL DYSPLASIA OF THE HIP

The condition formerly known as congenital dislocation of the hip (CDH), and now called developmental dysplasia of the hip (DDH), comprises a spectrum of disorders: acetabular dysplasia without displacement; instability (subluxation or dislocation); and teratological forms of malarticulation. Whether the instability comes first and then affects acetabular development because of imperfect seating of the femoral head, or is a result of a

Table 19.1 The diagnostic calendar

Age at onset (years)	Probable diagnosis
0 (birth)	Congenital dislocation
0–5	Perthes' disease
10–20	Slipped epiphysis
Adult	Osteoarthritis
	Avascular necrosis
	Rheumatoid arthritis

primary acetabular dysplasia, is still not known for sure. Both mechanisms might be important.

The reported incidence of neonatal hip instability is 5–20 per 1000 live births; however, most of these hips stabilize spontaneously, and on re-examination 3 weeks after birth the incidence of instability is only 1 or 2 per 1000 infants. Girls are much more commonly affected than boys, the ratio being about 7:1. The left hip is more often affected than the right; in 1 in 5 cases the condition is bilateral.

Aetiology and pathogenesis

Genetic factors must play a part in the aetiology, for DDH tends to run in families and even in entire populations (e.g. in countries along the northern and eastern Mediterranean seaboard). Wynne-Davies (1970) identified two heritable features which could predispose to hip instability: generalized joint laxity (a dominant trait), and shallow acetabuli (a polygenic trait which is seen mainly in girls and their mothers). However, this cannot be the whole story because in 4 out of 5 cases only one hip is dislocated.

Hormonal factors (e.g. high levels of maternal oestrogen, progesterone and relaxin in the last few weeks of pregnancy) may aggravate ligamentous laxity in the infant. This could account for the rarity of instability in premature babies, born before the hormones reach their peak.

Intrauterine malposition (especially a breech position with extended legs) favours dislocation; this so-called 'packaging disorder' is linked with the higher incidence in first-born babies, among whom spontaneous version is less likely. Unilateral dislocation usually affects the left hip; this fits with the usual vertex presentation (left occiput anterior) in which the left hip is somewhat adducted.

Postnatal factors may contribute to persistence of neonatal instability and acetabular maldevelopment. Dislocation is very common in Lapps and North American Indians who swaddle their babies and carry them with legs together, hips and knees fully extended, and is rare in southern Chinese and black Africans who carry their babies astride their backs with legs widely abducted. There is also experimental evidence that simultaneous hip and knee extension leads to hip dislocation during early development (Yamamuro and Ishida, 1984).

Pathology

At birth the hip, though unstable, is probably normal in shape but the capsule is often stretched and redundant.

During infancy a number of changes develop, some of them perhaps reflecting a primary dysplasia of the acetabulum and/or the proximal femur, but most of them from adaptation to persistent instability and abnormal joint loading.

The femoral head dislocates posteriorly but, with extension of the hips, it comes to lie first posterolateral and then superolateral to the acetabulum. The cartilaginous socket is shallow and anteverted. The cartilaginous femoral head is normal in size but the bony nucleus appears late and its ossification is delayed throughout infancy.

The capsule is stretched and the ligamentum teres becomes elongated and hypertrophied. Superiorly the acetabular labrum and its capsular edge may be pushed into the socket by the dislocated femoral head; this fibrocartilaginous limbus may obstruct any attempt at closed reduction of the femoral head.

After weightbearing commences, these changes are intensified. Both the acetabulum and the femoral neck remain anteverted and the pressure of the femoral head induces a false socket to form above the shallow acetabulum. The capsule, squeezed between the edge of the acetabulum and the psoas muscle, develops an hourglass appearance. In time the surrounding muscles become adaptively shortened.

Clinical features

The ideal, still unrealized, is to diagnose every case at birth. For this reason, every newborn child should be examined for signs of hip instability. Where there is a family history of congenital instability, and with breech presentations or signs of other congenital abnormalities, extra care is taken and the infant may have to be examined more than once. Even then some cases are missed.

IN THE NEONATE

There are several ways of testing for instability. In *Ortolani's test,* the baby's thighs are held with the thumbs medially and the fingers resting on the greater trochanters; the hips are flexed to 90° and gently abducted. Normally there is smooth abduction to almost 90°. In congenital dislocation the movement is usually impeded, but if pressure is applied to the greater trochanter there is a soft 'clunk' as the dislocation reduces, and then the hip abducts fully (the 'jerk of entry'). If abduction stops half-way and there is no jerk of entry, there may be an irreducible dislocation.

Barlow's test is performed in a similar manner, but here the examiner's thumb is placed in the groin and, by grasping the upper thigh, an attempt is made to lever the femoral head in and out of the acetabulum during abduction and adduction. If the femoral head is normally in the reduced position, but can be made to

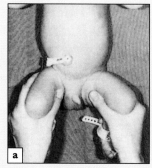 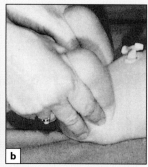 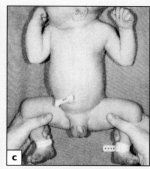

19.9 Congenital hip dislocation – early signs (a, b) Position of the hands for performing Ortolani's test. (c) The test has been performed – the right hip has not abducted fully; with a little more pressure there was a 'jerk of entry'.

slip out of the socket and back in again, the hip is classed as 'dislocatable' (i.e. unstable).

Every hip with signs of instability – however slight – should be examined by *ultrasonography*. This shows the shape of the cartilaginous socket and the position of the femoral head. If there is any abnormality, the infant is placed in a splint with the hips flexed and abducted (see under 'Management') and is recalled for re-examination – in the splint – at 2 weeks and at 6 weeks. By then it should be possible to assess whether the hip is reduced and stable, reduced but unstable (dislocatable by Barlow's test), subluxated or dislocated.

LATE FEATURES

An observant mother may spot asymmetry, a clicking hip or difficulty in applying the napkin (diaper) because of limited abduction.

With unilateral dislocation the skin creases look asymmetrical and the leg is slightly short and externally rotated; a thumb in the groin may feel that the femoral head is missing. With bilateral dislocation there is an abnormally wide perineal gap. Abduction is decreased.

Contrary to popular belief, late walking is not a marked feature; nevertheless, in children who do not walk by 18 months dislocation must be excluded. Likewise, a limp or Trendelenburg gait, or a waddling gait could be a sign of missed dislocation.

Approach to the limping child

1. Measure limb length
2. Check the foot
   Splinter? Injury?
   Swollen ankle: Infection? Arthritis?
3. Examine the knee
   Swelling: Infection? Arthritis? Tumour?
   Tenderness: Injury? Infection?
   Instability: Patellar subluxation?
4. Examine the hip
   Septic arthritis?
   Dislocation? Subluxation? Coxa vara? Transient synovitis?
   Perthes' disease? Arthritis? Tumour?
5. General assessment
   Exclude non-accidental injury

Imaging

Plain x-rays X-rays of infants are difficult to interpret and in the newborn they can be frankly misleading. This is because the acetabulum and femoral head are largely (or entirely) cartilaginous and therefore not visible on x-ray. As a consequence the relationship of the femoral head to the acetabular socket has to be gauged, indirectly, by observing the relative positions of the ossified femoral shaft and the visible margins of the hip. This exercise is helped by drawing lines on

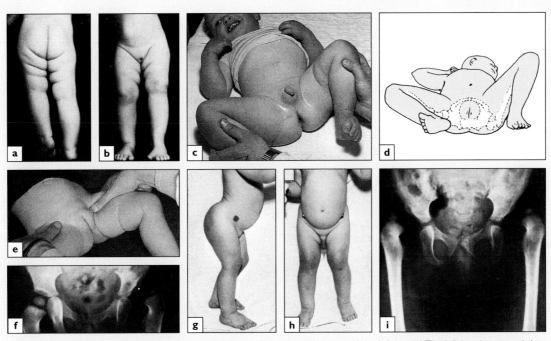

19.10 Congenital hip dislocation – late signs (**a, b**) Unilateral dislocation of the left hip. (**c**) The left hip does not abduct more than half way, and (**d**) the drawing shows why – the femoral head is caught up on the rim of the acetabulum. (**e**) The thumb sinks in too far on the left hip, because (**f**) the head is not in the socket. (**g–i**) The clinical appearance and x-rays of a bilateral dislocation.

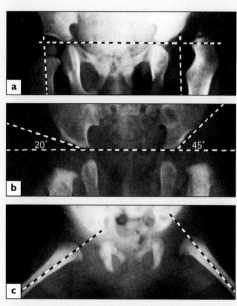

19.11 Congenital hip dislocation – x-rays (a) The epiphysis should lie medial to a vertical line which defines the outer edge of the acetabulum (Perkins' line) and below a horizontal line which passes through the triradiate cartilages (Hilgenreiner's line). (b) The acetabular roof angle should not exceed 30°. (c) Von Rosen's lines: with the hips abducted 45°, the femoral shafts should point into the acetabulum.

the x-ray plate to define various geometric indices (see Figure 19.11). At best x-rays offer only an approximation of the true anatomy and the image changes according to the position of the infant's legs and the tilt of the pelvis.

Ultrasonography Ultrasound scanning has largely replaced radiography for imaging hips in the newborn. The radiographically 'invisible' acetabulum and femoral head can, with practice, be displayed and real-time ultrasound gives an accurate picture of their relationship to each other (Harcke and Kumar, 1991).

Screening

Neonatal screening in dedicated centres has led to a marked reduction in missed cases of DDH. *Risk factors* such as family history, breech presentation, oligohydramnios and the presence of other congenital abnormalities are taken into account in selecting newborn infants for special examination and ultrasonography. Ideally all neonates should be examined, but if the programme is to be effective those doing the examining should receive special training (Harcke and Kumar, 1991; Jones, 1994).

Management

THE FIRST 3–6 MONTHS

The simplest policy is to regard all infants with a high-risk background, or a positive Ortolani or Barlow test, as 'suspect' and to nurse them in double napkins or an abduction pillow for the first 6 weeks. At that stage they are re-examined: those with stable hips are left free but kept under observation for at least 6 months; those with persistent instability are treated by more formal abduction splintage (see below) until the hip is stable and x-ray shows that the acetabular roof is developing satisfactorily (usually 3–6 months).

There are two drawbacks to this simple approach: the sensitivity of the clinical tests is not high enough to ensure that all cases will be spotted (Jones, 1994); and of those hips that are unstable at birth, 80–90% will stabilize spontaneously in 2–3 weeks. It therefore seems more sensible not to start splintage immediately unless the hip is already dislocated. This reduces the small (but significant) risk of epiphyseal necrosis that attends any form of restrictive splintage in the neonate. Thus, if a hip is dislocatable but not habitually dislocated, the baby is left untreated but re-examined weekly; if at 3 weeks the hip is still unstable, abduction splintage is applied (see below). If the hip is already dislocated at the first examination, it is gently placed in the reduced position and abduction splintage is applied from the outset. Reduction is maintained until the hip is stable; this may take only a few weeks, but the safest policy is to retain some sort of splintage until x-ray shows a good acetabular roof.

Where facilities for ultrasound scanning are available, a more refined protocol can be applied. All newborn infants with a high-risk background or a suggestion of hip instability are examined by ultrasonography. If this shows that the hip is reduced and has a normal cartilaginous outline, no treatment is required but the child is kept under observation for 3–6 months. If the anatomy is less than perfect, the hip is splinted in abduction and at 6 weeks ultrasound scanning is repeated. Some hips will now appear normal and these need no further treatment, apart from routine observation for 3–6 months. A few will show persistent abnormality and for these splintage in abduction is continued until a further scan at 3 months or an x-ray at 6 months shows a well-formed acetabular roof.

Splintage The object of splintage is to hold the hips somewhat flexed and abducted; extreme positions are avoided and the joints should be allowed some movement in the splint. For the newborn, double napkins or a soft abduction pillow may suffice. Von Rosen's splint is an H-shaped malleable splint that has the merit of being easy to apply (and the demerit of being equally easy to take off!). The Pavlik harness is more difficult to apply but gives the child more freedom while still maintaining position. The least complicated – and most

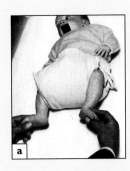
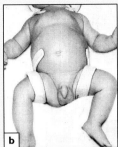
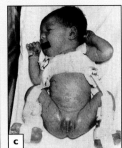

19.12 Congenital hip dislocation – treatment before weightbearing Reduction is usually easy and can be held by (**a**) an abduction pillow, (**b**) Von Rosen's malleable splint, or – best of all – (**c**) the Pavlik harness. The hips should not be more than about 60° abducted, though flexion sometimes needs to be well beyond a right angle.

resistant to the mother's attentions – is the application of 'knee plasters' with a cross-bar holding the hips in 90° of flexion and about 45° of abduction, or 10° more than the angle at which the 'jerk of entry' is felt. The three golden rules of splintage are: (1) the hip must be properly reduced before it is splinted; (2) extreme positions must be avoided; (3) the hips should be able to move.

Follow-up Whatever policy is adopted, follow-up is continued until the child is walking. Sometimes, even with the most careful treatment, the hip may later show some degree of acetabular dysplasia.

PERSISTENT DISLOCATION: 6–18 MONTHS

If, after early treatment, the hip is still incompletely reduced, or if the child presents late with a 'missed' dislocation, the hip must be reduced – preferably by closed methods but if necessary by operation – and held reduced until acetabular development is satisfactory.

Closed reduction This is the ideal but risks damaging the blood supply to the femoral head and causing necrosis. To minimize this risk reduction must be gradual; traction is applied to both legs, preferably on a vertical frame, and abduction is gradually increased until,

by 3 weeks, the legs are widely separated. This manoeuvre alone (aided if necessary by *adductor tenotomy*) may achieve stable concentric reduction. This should be checked by an examination under anaesthesia, x-ray and *arthrography*.

Splintage The concentrically reduced hip is held in a plaster spica at 60° of flexion, 40° of abduction and 20° of internal rotation. After 6 weeks the spica is replaced by a splint which prevents adduction but allows movement – a Pavlik harness (not so easy to apply at that age) or 'knee plasters' with a cross-bar. This is retained for another 3–6 months, checking by x-ray to ensure that the femoral head is concentrically reduced and the acetabular roof is developing normally. Splintage is then gradually abandoned by allowing the child longer and longer periods of freedom.

Operation If, at any stage, concentric reduction has not been achieved, open operation is needed. The psoas tendon is divided; obstructing tissues (redundant capsule, 'limbus', thickened ligamentum teres) are removed and the hip is reduced. It is usually stable in 60° of flexion, 40° of abduction and 20° of internal rotation. A spica is applied and the hip is splinted as described above.

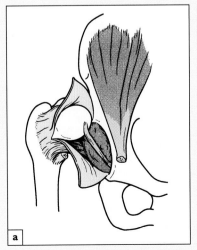
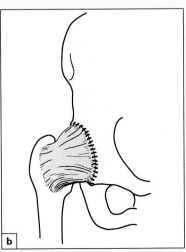

19.13 DDH – open reduction (**a**) The psoas is divided, redundant capsule is excised – and if necessary also a 'limbus' and ligamentum teres. (**b**) The hip is then reduced and the capsule securely closed.

If stability can be achieved only by markedly internally rotating the hip, a corrective subtrochanteric osteotomy of the femur is carried out, either at the time of open reduction or 6 weeks later. In young children this usually gives a good result.

PERSISTENT DISLOCATION: 18 MONTHS–4 YEARS
In the older child, closed reduction is less likely to succeed; many surgeons would proceed straight to arthrography and open reduction.

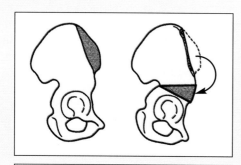

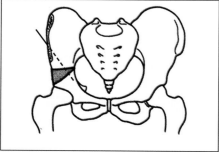

19.14 DDH – Salter osteotomy The osteotomy is performed through the innominate bone above the acetabulum; the acetabulum is then tilted downwards and anteriorly; the gap is filled by a bone graft taken from the ilium and secured with a Kirschner wire.

Traction Even if closed reduction is unsuccessful, a period of traction (if necessary combined with psoas and adductor tenotomy) will help to loosen the tissues and bring the femoral head down opposite the acetabulum.

Arthrography An arthrogram at this stage will clarify the anatomy of the hip and show whether there is an inturned limbus or any marked degree of acetabular dysplasia.

Operation The joint capsule is opened anteriorly, any inturned capsule or 'limbus' is removed and the femoral head is seated in the acetabulum. Usually a derotation femoral osteotomy held by a plate and screws will be required. At the same time a small segment can be removed from the proximal femur to reduce pressure on the hip (Klisic and Jankovic, 1976). If there is marked acetabular dysplasia, some form of acetabuloplasty will also be needed – either a pericapsular reconstruction of the acetabular roof (Pemberton's operation) or an innominate (Salter) osteotomy which repositions the entire innominate bone and acetabulum.

Splintage After operation, the hip is held in a plaster spica for 3 months and then in a splint which permits some hip movement for a further 1–3 months, checking by x-ray to ensure that the hip is reduced and developing satisfactorily.

DISLOCATION IN CHILDREN OVER 4 YEARS
Reduction and stabilization become increasingly difficult with advancing age. Nevertheless, in children between 4 and 8 years of age – especially if the dislocation is unilateral – it is still worth attempting, bearing in mind that the risk of avascular necrosis and hip stiffness is reported as being in excess of 25%. The principles of treatment are as described immediately above.

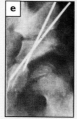
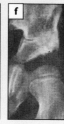
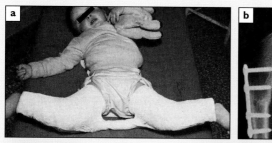
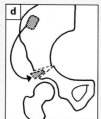
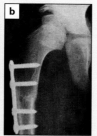
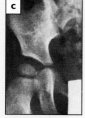

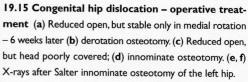

19.15 Congenital hip dislocation – operative treatment (a) Reduced open, but stable only in medial rotation – 6 weeks later (b) derotation osteotomy. (c) Reduced open, but head poorly covered; (d) innominate osteotomy. (e, f) X-rays after Salter innominate osteotomy of the left hip.

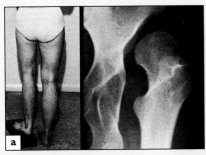
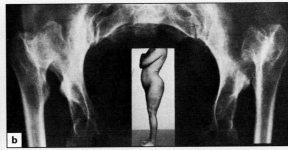

19.16 Congenital hip dislocation – above the age limit (a) Unilateral dislocation in a young adult. (b) Bilateral dislocation – this patient had no symptoms till 40 years of age when she presented with backache.

Unilateral dislocation in the child over 8 years of age often leaves the child with a mobile hip and little pain. This is the justification for non-intervention, though in that case the child must accept the fact that gait is distinctly abnormal. If reduction is attempted it will require an open operation and acetabular reconstruction. These procedures are best undertaken in centres specializing in this area.

With *bilateral dislocation* the deformity – and the waddling gait – is symmetrical and therefore not so noticeable; the risk of operative intervention is also greater because failure on one or other side turns this into an asymmetrical deformity. Therefore, in these cases, most surgeons avoid operation above the age of 4 years unless the hip is painful or deformity unusually severe. The untreated patient walks with a waddle but may be surprisingly uncomplaining.

Complications

Failed reduction Multiple attempts at treatment, with failure to achieve concentric reduction, may be worse than no treatment. The acetabulum remains undeveloped, the femoral head may be deformed, the neck is usually anteverted and the capsule is thickened and adherent. It is important to enquire also *why* reduction failed: is the dislocation part of a generalized condition, or a neuromuscular disorder associated with muscle imbalance? The principles of treatment for children over 8 years of age are the same as those discussed above.

Avascular necrosis A much feared complication of treatment is ischaemia of the immature femoral head. It may occur at any age and any stage of treatment and is probably due to vascular injury or obstruction resulting from forceful reduction and hip splintage in abduction. The effects vary considerably: in the mildest cases the changes are confined to the ossific nucleus, which appears to be slightly distorted and irregular on x-ray. The cartilaginous epiphysis retains its shape and physeal growth is normal. After 12–24 months the appearances return to normal. In more severe cases the epiphyseal and physeal

growth plates also suffer; the ossific nucleus looks fragmented, the epiphysis is distorted to a greater or lesser extent and metaphyseal changes lead to shortening and deformity of the femoral neck.

Prevention is the best cure: forced manipulative reduction should not be allowed; traction should be gentle and in the neutral position; positions of extreme abduction must be avoided; soft-tissue release (adductor tenotomy) should precede closed reduction; and if difficulty is anticipated open reduction is preferable.

Once the condition is established, there is no effective treatment except to avoid manipulation and weightbearing until the epiphysis has healed. In the mildest cases there will be no residual deformity, or at worst a femoral neck deformity which can be corrected by osteotomy. In severe cases the outcome may be flattening and mushrooming of the femoral head, shortening of the neck (with or without coxa vara), acetabular dysplasia and incongruency of the hip. Surgical correction of the proximal femur and pelvic osteotomy to reposition or deepen the acetabulum may be needed.

PERSISTENT DISLOCATION IN ADULTS

Adults who appear to have managed quite well for many years may present in their 30s or 40s with increasing discomfort due to an unreduced congenital dislocation. Walking becomes more and more tiring and backache is common. With bilateral dislocation, the loss of abduction may hamper sexual intercourse in women.

Disability may be severe enough to justify *total joint replacement*. The operation is difficult and should be undertaken only by those with experience of hip reconstructive surgery. The femoral head is seated above the acetabulum, which is shallow or completely obliterated. A new socket should be fashioned at the normal anatomical site; however, the pelvic wall is usually thin and it may be necessary to build up the roof of the socket with bone grafts. It is then difficult to bring the femoral head down to the level of the socket without risking damage to the sciatic nerve; if necessary, an osteotomy should be performed and a small segment of femoral bone removed to allow a safe fit. The proximal

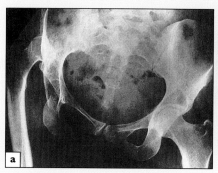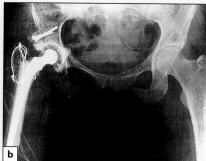

**19.17 Congenital hip disloca-
tion – hip replacement**
(**a**) This patient, aged 35 years, had
a very short leg, a severe limp and
back pain; she could walk only a
few hundred yards. (**b**) Hip
replacement restored her to near
normality – clearly the risk was
worth taking.

femur is usually very narrow and the neck may be
markedly anteverted; this also may need correction
when the osteotomy is performed, and special implants
are available to fit the small medullary canal.

ACETABULAR DYSPLASIA AND SUBLUXATION OF THE HIP

Acetabular dysplasia may be genetically determined or
may follow incomplete reduction of a congenital dislocation, damage to the lateral acetabular epiphysis or
maldevelopment of the femoral head (either congenital or, for example, after Perthes' disease). The socket
is unusually shallow, the roof is sloping and there is
deficient coverage of the femoral head superolaterally
and anteriorly; in some cases the hip subluxates. Faulty
load transmission in the lateral part of the joint may
lead to secondary osteoarthritis.

Clinical features

During infancy, limited abduction of the hip is suspicious
and ultrasonography may reveal a deficient acetabulum.

In children the condition is usually asymptomatic
and discovered only when the pelvis is x-rayed for some
other reason. Sometimes, however, the hip is painful –
especially after strenuous activity – and the child may
develop a limp. If there is subluxation the Trendelenburg
sign is positive, leg length may be asymmetrical and the
femoral head may be felt as a lump in the groin; movement – particularly abduction in flexion – is restricted.

Older adolescents and young adults may complain
of pain over the lateral side of the hip, probably due
to muscle fatigue and/or segmental overload towards
the edge of the acetabulum. Some experience episodes
of sharp pain in the groin, possibly the result of a
labral tear or detachment.

Older adults (predominantly in their 30s and 40s)
usually present with features of secondary osteoarthritis. Indeed, in Southern Europe dysplasia of the hip is
the commonest cause of symptomatic osteoarthritis.

NOTE It is worth emphazising that most people with
mild acetabular dysplasia go through life without
knowing that they are in any way abnormal and the
condition exists only as a 'x-ray diagnosis'.

Imaging

X-rays should be taken lying and standing (the latter
may show minor degrees of incongruity). The acetabulum looks shallow, the roof is sloping and the femoral
head is uncovered. Subtle abnormalities are revealed by
measuring the depth of the socket and the relationship
between the centre of the femoral head and the edge of
the acetabulum – Wiberg's centre-edge (CE) angle. With
subluxation, Shenton's line is broken. Congruity and
stability of the hip may be best assessed by examination
and arthrography under anaesthesia (Catterall, 1992).

CT and MRI are helpful in those who are considered
for operative treatment. Three dimensional CT reconstruction is particularly useful in providing an accurate
picture of the anatomy (see Fig 19.8).

Diagnosis

It is often difficult to be sure that the patient's symptoms
are due to the dysplastic acetabulum; other conditions
causing pain and limp must be excluded (see page 411).

Bilateral dysplasia is a feature of developmental
disorders, such as multiple epiphyseal dysplasia.

Treatment

Infants with subluxation are treated as for dislocation:
the hip is splinted in abduction until the acetabular roof
looks normal.

Older children and young adolescents, provided the
hip is reducible and congruent, often manage with no
more than muscle strengthening exercises. If symptoms persist, they may need an operation to augment
the acetabular roof, either a lateral shelf procedure or
a pelvic osteotomy, both of which may be combined
with a varus osteotomy of the proximal femur.

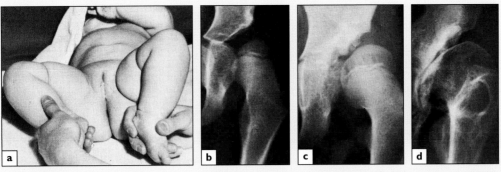

19.18 Congenital subluxation (**a**) The cardinal physical sign, restricted abduction; (**b**) x-ray in childhood; (**c**) in adolescence; (**d**) degeneration in early adult life.

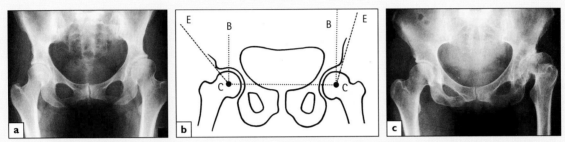

19.19 Acetabular dysplasia (**a**) X-ray showing a dysplastic left acetabulum. The socket is shallow and the roof sloping, leaving much of the femoral head uncovered. Note that the femoral neck–shaft angle is somewhat valgus on both sides. (**b**) Measuring Wiberg's centre-edge (CE) angle: the line C-C joins the centre of each femoral head; C–B is perpendicular to this and C–E cuts the superior edge of the acetabulum. The angle BCE should not be less than 30°; in this case the left hip is abnormal. (**c**) X-ray of another patient showing advanced secondary osteoarthritis in an untreated dysplastic left hip.

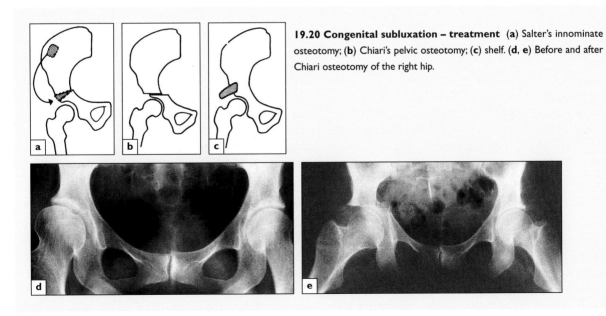

19.20 Congenital subluxation – treatment (**a**) Salter's innominate osteotomy; (**b**) Chiari's pelvic osteotomy; (**c**) shelf. (**d**, **e**) Before and after Chiari osteotomy of the right hip.

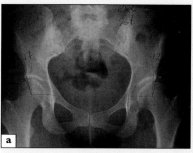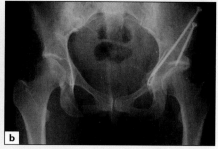

19.21 Acetabular dysplasia – periacetabular osteotomy (a) Bilateral acetabular dysplasia, symptomatic on the left. (b) X-ray after periacetabular osteotomy. Cuts were made through the innominate, the ischium and the lateral part of the superior pubic ramus; the entire segment containing the acetabulum was then rotated so as to cover the load-bearing part of the femoral head super-laterally and anteriorly. (Courtesy of Professor KJeld Søballe, Århus Universitetshopital.)

Older adolescents and young adults with pain, weakness, instability and subluxation of the hip are candidates for one of the newer types of periacetabular osteotomy and three dimensional re-orientation of the entire hip (Ganz *et al.*, 1998).

Patients with secondary osteoarthritis may need intertrochanteric osteotomy or total hip replacement.

ACQUIRED DISLOCATION OF THE HIP

Dislocation occurring after the first year of life is usually due to one of three causes: *pyogenic arthritis*, *muscle imbalance* or *trauma*. Rare causes of acquired dislocation include tuberculosis and Charcot's disease.

DISLOCATION FOLLOWING SEPSIS

In infancy the femur may be infected via the umbilicus or via femoral vein puncture; at this age the growth disc is no barrier and infection readily spreads from the metaphysis to involve the femoral head and the joint. In older children the metaphysis is intracapsular, so here again the joint is readily infected.

If the infection is unchecked, the proximal end of the femur may be destroyed and a pathological dislocation result. The pus may escape and, when the child recovers, the sinus heals. The hip signs then resemble those of a congenital dislocation, but the tell-tale scar remains.

On x-ray the femoral head appears to be completely absent; however, some part of it often survives, although it is too osteoporotic to be seen.

Treatment of the acute infection is discussed elsewhere. The dislocation should be managed by traction, followed, if necessary, by open reduction. In the absence of a femoral head, the greater trochanter can be placed in the acetabulum; varus osteotomy of the upper femur helps to achieve stability. In later life the patient will require further reconstructive surgery or total joint replacement.

DISLOCATION DUE TO MUSCLE IMBALANCE

Unbalanced paralysis in childhood may result in the hip abductors being weaker than the adductors. This is seen in *cerebral palsy*, in *myelomeningocele* and after *poliomyelitis* (see Chapter 10). The greater trochanter fails to develop properly, the femoral neck becomes valgus and the hip may subluxate or dislocate.

Treatment is similar to that of congenital dislocation, but in addition some muscle rebalancing operation is essential.

PERSISTENT TRAUMATIC DISLOCATION

Occasionally dislocation of the hip is missed while attention is focused on some more distal (and more obvious) injury. Reduction is essential, if necessary by open operation; even if avascular necrosis or hip stiffness supervenes, a hip in the anatomical position presents an easier prospect for reconstructive surgery than one that remains persistently dislocated.

FEMORAL ANTEVERSION (IN-TOE GAIT)

A familiar sight at every paediatric orthopaedic clinic is the child brought because of an in-toe gait. The child walks awkwardly and trips over his or her feet when running. The cause is rarely serious but a bland assurance that "he will grow out of it" may fail to convince the parents and certainly won't satisfy the grandparents.

Below the age of 3 years in-toeing is usually due to forefoot adduction or tibial torsion, both of which may correct spontaneously as the child grows.

Above the age of 3 years the commonest cause of in-toe gait is excessive anteversion (persistent fetal alignment) of the femoral neck, so that internal rotation of the hip is increased and external rotation diminished. The gait may look clumsy but this is no bar to athletic prowess and usually improves with growth. These children often sit on the floor in the 'television position' with the knees facing each other. With the child standing, the patellae are turned inwards ('squinting patellae') and there may be compensatory external torsion of the tibiae.

Femoral neck anteversion can be assessed by ultrasonography or by obtaining CT scans across the hips and the knees and measuring the angle between the axis of the femoral neck and the transverse axis across the femoral condyles.

Correction by femoral osteotomy is feasible but seldom indicated, and certainly not before the age of 8 years.

Other causes of in-toe gait include femoral shaft torsion, tibial torsion and forefoot adduction. To differentiate between these the child is examined first with hips and knees extended, then with both flexed to a right angle; finally the position of the foot is inspected.

PROTRUSIO ACETABULI (OTTO PELVIS)

In this condition the socket is too deep and bulges into the cavity of the pelvis. The *'primary' form* shows a slight familial tendency. It affects females much more often than males and develops soon after puberty; at this stage there are usually no symptoms although movements are limited. *X-rays* show the sunken acetabulum, with the inner wall bulging beyond the iliopectineal line. Secondary osteoarthritis may develop in later life, but until then the condition does not require treatment.

Protrusio may occur in later life secondary to bone 'softening' disorders, such as *osteomalacia* or *Paget's disease*, and in long-standing cases of *rheumatoid arthritis*. If pain is severe, or movements are markedly restricted, joint replacement is indicated.

COXA VARA

The normal femoral neck-shaft angle is 160° at birth, decreasing to 125° in adult life. An angle of less than 120° is called coxa vara. The deformity may be either congenital or acquired.

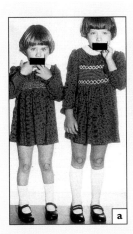
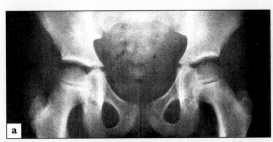

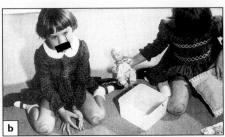

19.22 In-toe gait (**a**) These two sisters have excessive anteversion with an in-toe gait. (**b**) This explains their sitting posture when playing or watching television.

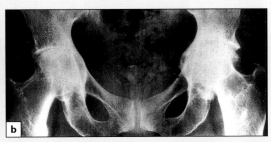

19.23 Protrusio acetabuli (**a**) The early stage in a child. (**b**) In this adult with protrusio, degenerative changes have developed in both hips.

CONGENITAL COXA VARA

This is a rare developmental disorder of infancy and early childhood. It is due to a defect of endochondral ossification in the medial part of the femoral neck. When the child starts to crawl or stand, the femoral neck bends or develops a stress fracture, and with continued weightbearing it collapses increasingly into varus and retroversion. Sometimes there is also shortening or bowing of the femoral shaft. The condition is bilateral in about one-third of cases.

Clinical features The abnormality is usually diagnosed when the child starts to walk. The leg is short and the thigh may be bowed. X-rays show that the femoral neck is in varus and abnormally short. Often there is a separate fragment of bone in a triangular notch on the inferomedial surface of the femoral neck. Because of the distorted anatomy, it is difficult to measure the neck–shaft angle. A helpful alternative is to measure Hilgenreiner's epiphyseal angle – the angle subtended by a horizontal line joining the centre (triradiate cartilage) of each hip and another parallel to the physeal line; the normal angle is about 30° (see Fig. 19.24).

With bilateral coxa vara the patient may not be seen until he or she presents as a young adult with osteoarthritis.

Treatment If the epiphyseal angle is more than 40° but less than 60°, the child should be kept under observation and re-examined at intervals for signs of progression. If it is more than 60°, or if shortening is progressive, the deformity should be corrected by a subtrochanteric valgus osteotomy, aiming to correct Hilgenreiner's angle to 30–40°. Varus does not recur, but there may be some permanent shortening.

ACQUIRED COXA VARA

Coxa vara can develop if the femoral neck bends or if it breaks. A 'mechanical' coxa vara sometimes results from severe shortening of the femoral neck and relative overgrowth of the greater trochanter; during weightbearing the abductor muscles are at a mechanical disadvantage and the patient walks with a severe Trendelenburg gait.

During childhood, coxa vara is seen in rickets and bone dystrophies, and sometimes after Perthes' disease. Deformity presenting in adolescence is more likely to be due to epiphysiolysis.

At any age bone 'softening' may result in coxa vara; causes include osteomalacia, fibrous dysplasia, pathological fracture or the aftermath of infection.

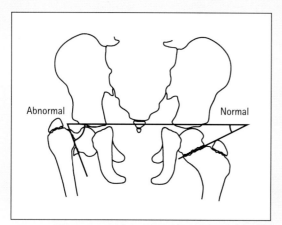

19.24 Congenital coxa vara Measurement of Hilgenreiner's epiphyseal angle: 25–35° is normal; 40–60° calls for careful follow-up and review; more than 60° is an indication for valgus osteotomy.

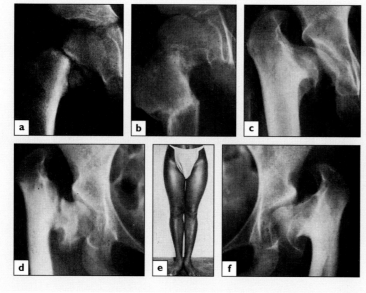

19.25 Infantile coxa vara (**a**) Physis too vertical and a triangle of bone on the undersurface of the neck; (**b**) abduction osteotomy should be performed early; otherwise (**c**) the shaft migrates upwards.

(**d, e, f**) Bilateral infantile coxa vara – untreated. The patient's hips look symmetrical but abduction was severely limited.

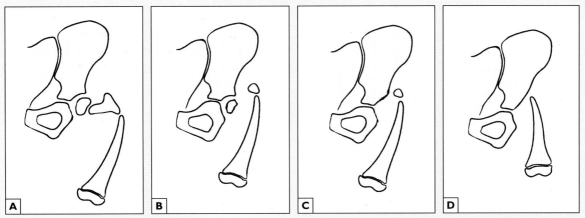

19.26 Proximal femoral focal deficiency – Aitkin's classification In types A and B the femoral head and acetabulum are present, though showing varying degrees of dysplasia. Coxa vara may be marked and shortening is significant. In types C and D there is no effective hip joint, shortening is severe and distal deficiencies may be present.

Other causes of deformity are malunited fractures and Paget's disease.

Treatment in the form of a corrective (valgus) osteotomy is needed only if there is marked shortening or intolerable discomfort. If the problem is due to a disproportionately high greater trochanter, distal transposition of the trochanter may suffice.

PROXIMAL FEMORAL FOCAL DEFICIENCY

This is a rare non-genetic (possibly teratogenic) anomaly in which part or all of the proximal femur is missing. The most useful classification is that of Aitken. In *type A* there appears to be a gap in the femoral neck or subtrochanteric region, which is in fact a segment of unossified cartilage. This does eventually ossify, but by then the proximal femur has developed a varus deformity and shortening. In *type B* the 'gap' persists, the femoral head and acetabulum are dysplastic and there is significant shortening. In *type C* the femoral head is missing and the acetabulum is undeveloped. In *type D* there is agenesis of the entire proximal femur and acetabulum. Both hips may be affected and in half the cases there are also distal anomalies.

Clinical features The hip is held flexed, abducted and externally rotated; in types C and D there may be bizarre shortening of the limb. MRI is helpful in defining the anatomical abnormalities.

Treatment In types A and B there is a mechanically functional hip joint (albeit that in type B the socket is often dysplastic); the neck angle and hip stability can

be improved by performing a subtrochanteric osteotomy, and bone grafts are added to promote ossification. If shortening is marked, limb lengthening can be performed.

In types C and D the choice lies between amputation (sometimes together with knee fusion) or a van Ness rotationplasty and distal prosthesis. In the latter operation the foot is turned 'back-to-front' by rotational osteotomy of the tibia, so that an acceptable prosthesis can be fitted; this is no small undertaking.

Patients with bilateral symmetrical anomalies are functionally better than those with unilateral deformity; were it not for the cosmetic problem, they are probably best left alone.

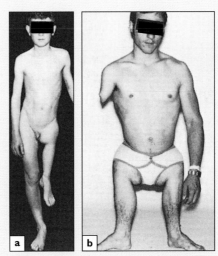

19.27 Proximal femoral focal deficiency Two patients with Type D proximal femoral focal deficiency: (**a**) unilateral and (**b**) bilateral.

THE IRRITABLE HIP

This vague term for what is thought to be a transient synovitis is attached to a well-recognized syndrome of transient hip pain and restriction of movement in an otherwise healthy child. It is the commonest cause of hip pain in children; boys are affected twice as often as girls.

Clinical features

The patient – typically between 6 and 12 years of age – presents with pain and a limp, often intermittent and following activity. Pain is felt in the groin or front of the thigh, sometimes reaching as far as the knee. Slight wasting may be detectable but the cardinal sign is restriction of all movements with pain at the extremes of the range in all directions. General examination, blood investigations and x-rays are normal, but ultrasonography may reveal a small joint effusion. Scintigraphy is usually normal during the acute phase.

Characteristically, symptoms last for 1–2 weeks and then subside spontaneously; hence the synonym 'transient synovitis'. The child may have more than one episode, with an interval of months between attacks of pain.

Diagnosis

The condition is important largely because it resembles a number of serious disorders which have to be excluded.

Perthes' disease is the main worry. Acute symptoms usually last longer than 2 weeks and x-rays may show an increased 'joint space'. Later, of course, the x-ray features of Perthes' disease are unmistakable.

Slipped epiphysis may present as an 'irritable hip'. Initially the x-ray looks normal and this may lead to complacency. If the age and general build are suggestive, or if the symptoms persist, the x-ray should be repeated.

Tuberculous synovitis produces a raised erythrocyte sedimentation rate (ESR) and the Heaf test is positive.

Juvenile chronic arthritis and ankylosing spondylitis may start with synovitis of one hip and it may take months before other joints are affected. Look for systemic features and a raised ESR. In doubtful cases, synovial biopsy may be helpful.

Treatment

If the child is otherwise completely healthy, the symptoms and signs are mild and the joint effusion is slight, the child can be treated by simple bed rest at home. In more severe cases – and particularly if the diagnosis is in doubt – the child should be admitted for continuous bed rest and traction. The hip should be kept slightly flexed and in some external rotation, as extension and internal rotation increase the intra-articular pressure and may predispose to ischaemia.

Ultrasonography is repeated at intervals and weight-bearing is allowed only when the symptoms disappear and the effusion resolves.

PERTHES' DISEASE

Perthes' disease – or rather Legg–Calvé–Perthes disease, for in 1910 the condition was described independently by three different people – is a painful disorder of childhood characterized by avascular necrosis of the femoral head. It is uncommon in any community – the quoted incidence is about one in 10,000 – but particularly rare in black Africans. Patients are usually 4–8 years old and boys are affected four times as often as girls.

The condition may be part of a general disorder of growth. Epidemiological studies in the UK have shown that there is a higher than usual incidence in underprivileged communities. Affected children and their siblings have slightly retarded growth of the trunk and limbs. As in other forms of non-traumatic osteonecrosis, inherited thrombophilia has been postulated as a contributary cause and antithrombotic factor deficiencies and hypofibrinolysis have been reported in children with Perthes' disease (Glueck *et al.*, 1996). This hypothesis has been questioned and all one can say is that the jury is still out on the answer (Liesner, 1999).

Pathogenesis

The precipitating cause of Perthes' disease is unknown but the cardinal step in the pathogenesis is ischaemia of the femoral head. Up to the age of 4 months, the femoral head is supplied by (1) metaphyseal vessels which penetrate the growth disc, (2) lateral epiphyseal vessels running in the retinacula and (3) scanty vessels in the ligamentum teres. The metaphyseal supply gradually declines until, by the age of 4 years, it has virtually disappeared; by the age of 7 years, however, the vessels in the ligamentum teres have developed. Between 4 and 7 years of age the femoral head may depend for its blood supply and venous drainage almost entirely on the lateral epiphyseal vessels whose situation in the retinacula makes them susceptible to stretching and to pressure from an effusion. Although such pressure may be insufficient to block off the arterial flow, it could easily cause venous stasis resulting in a rise in intraosseous pressure and consequent ischaemia (Lin and Ho, 1991). This may be enough to tip the balance towards infarction and necrosis in children who are constitutionally predisposed.

The immediate cause of capsular tamponade may be an effusion following trauma (of which there is a history in over half the cases) or a non-specific synovitis. Two or more such incidents may be needed to produce the typical bone changes.

19.28 Blood supply of the infant femoral head
1, Metaphyseal vessels; 2, lateral epiphyseal vessels; 3, vessels in the ligamentum teres.

Pathology

The pathological process takes 2–4 years to complete, passing through three stages.

STAGE 1: ISCHAEMIA AND BONE DEATH All or part of the bony nucleus of the femoral head is dead; it still looks normal on plain x-ray but stops enlarging. The cartilaginous part of the femoral head, being nourished by synovial fluid, remains viable and becomes thicker than normal. There may also be thickening and oedema of the synovium and capsule.

STAGE 2: REVASCULARIZATION AND REPAIR Within weeks (possibly even days) of infarction, a number of changes begin to appear. Dead marrow is replaced by granulation tissue, which sometimes calcifies. The bone is revascularized and new lamellae are laid down on the dead trabeculae, producing the appearance of increased density on x-ray. Some of the dead trabecular fragments are resorbed and replaced by fibrous tissue; when this happens, the alternating areas of sclerosis and fibrosis appear on the x-ray as 'fragmentation' of the epiphysis. The metaphysis may become hyperaemic and on x-ray looks rarefied or cystic. In older children, and more severe cases, morphological changes may also appear in the acetabulum.

STAGE 3: DISTORTION AND REMODELLING If the repair process is rapid and complete, the bony architecture may be restored before the femoral head loses its shape. If it is tardy, the bony epiphysis may collapse and subsequent growth of the head and neck will be distorted: the head becomes oval or flattened – like the head of a mushroom – and enlarged laterally, while the neck is often short and broad. Slowly the femoral head is displaced laterally in relation to the acetabulum.

Clinical features

The patient – typically a boy of 4–8 years – complains of pain and starts limping. Symptoms continue for weeks on end or may recur intermittently. The child appears to be well, though often somewhat undersized. In 4% there is an associated urogenital anomaly.

The hip looks deceptively normal, though there may be a little wasting. Early on, the joint is irritable so that all movements are diminished and their extremes painful. Often the child is not seen till later, when most movements are full; but abduction (especially in flexion) is nearly always limited and usually internal rotation also.

X-rays

Although the condition may be suspected from the clinical appearances, diagnosis hinges on the x-ray changes.

At first the x-rays may seem normal, though subtle changes such as widening of the 'joint space' and slight asymmetry of the ossific centres are usually present. Radionuclide scanning may show a 'void' in the anterolateral part of the femoral head. The classic feature of increased density of the ossific nucleus occurs somewhat later; this may be accompanied by fragmentation, or a crescentic subarticular fracture often best seen in the lateral view. At this stage scintigraphy shows increased activity.

Later still there is obvious increase in the joint space as well as flattening and lateral displacement of the epiphysis, with rarefaction and widening of the metaphysis.

The picture varies with the age of the child, the stage of the disease and the amount of head that is necrotic. Catterall (1982) described four groups, based on the appearances in both anteroposterior and lateral x-rays. In group 1 the epiphysis has retained its height and less than half the nucleus is sclerotic. In group 2 up to half the nucleus is sclerotic and there may be some collapse of the central portion. In group 3 most of the nucleus is involved, with sclerosis, fragmentation and collapse of the head. Metaphyseal resorption may be present. Group 4 is the worst: the whole head is involved, the ossific nucleus is flat and dense and metaphyseal resorption is marked.

With healing the femoral head may regain its normal (or near-normal) shape; however, in less fortunate cases the femoral head becomes mushroom shaped, larger than normal and laterally displaced in a dysplastic acetabular socket.

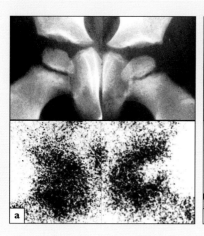 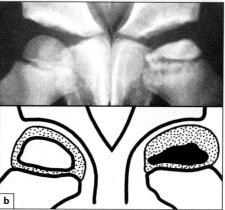

Differential diagnosis

The irritable hip of early Perthes' disease must be differentiated from other causes of irritability; the child's fitness, the increased joint space and the patchy bone density are characteristic. In transient synovitis the x-ray is normal.

Morquio's disease, cretinism, multiple epiphyseal dysplasia, sickle-cell disease and Gaucher's disease may resemble Perthes' disease radiologically, especially if they are bilateral; however, in bilateral Perthes' disease the two sides are always at different stages. Moreover, in the other conditions additional diagnostic features are usually apparent.

Prognostic features

The outlook for children with Perthes' disease, as a group, is well summarized by Herring (1994): "A small percentage of patients have a very difficult course, with recurrent loss of motion, pain, and an eventual poor outcome. However, most children have moderate problems in the active phase of the disease and then improve steadily, eventually having a satisfactory outcome."

This does not, of course, absolve one from undertaking careful analysis and planning in dealing with the individual case. *Age* is the most important prognostic factor: in children under 6 years the outlook is almost always excellent; thereafter, the older the child the less good is the prognosis. There is a poorer prognosis, too, for *girls* than for boys.

A widely used radiographic guide is the *Catterall classification* (see above). The greater the degree of femoral head involvement, the worse the outcome. This is recognized in the simpler *classification of Salter and Thompson*, into those with more than and those with less than half the head involved (Simmons

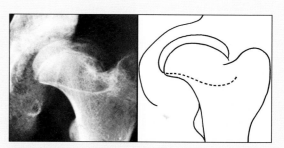

19.30 Perthes' disease – late features In those with favourable prognostic signs, healing results in a normal-looking femoral head. Others, however (as in this case), may end up with a mushroom-shaped femoral head and acetabular dysplasia. Here we also see the 'sagging rope sign' – a sclerotic line curving across the femoral neck, probably due to distortion and remodelling of the femoral head.

et al., 1990). There is also the concept of the *head at risk* – radiographic signs which presage increasing deformity and displacement of the femoral head: (1) progressive uncovering of the epiphysis; (2) calcification in the cartilage lateral to the ossific nucleus; (3) a radiolucent area at the lateral edge of the bony epiphysis (Gage's sign); and (4) severe metaphyseal resorption.

Common to all these predictive systems is the importance of the structural integrity of the superolateral (principal loadbearing) part of the femoral head. This is reflected in Herring's *lateral pillar classification*. In the anteroposterior x-ray, the femoral head is divided into three 'pillars' by lines at the medial and lateral edges of the central 'sequestrum'. Group A are those with normal height of the lateral pillar. Group B are patients with partial collapse (but still more than 50% height) of the lateral pillar; those under 9 years of age usually have a good outcome but older children are likely to develop flattening of the femoral head. Group C cases show more severe collapse of the lateral pillar (less than 50% of normal height); these take longer to heal and usually end up with significant distortion of the femoral head.

Management

As long as the hip is irritable the child should be in bed with skin traction applied to the affected leg and the hip in a little flexion and external rotation. Once irritability has subsided, which usually takes about 3 weeks, movement is encouraged – particularly abduction. The clinical and radiographic features are then reassessed and the bone age is determined from x-rays of the wrist. The choice of further management is between (a) symptomatic treatment and (b) containment.

Symptomatic treatment means pain control (if necessary by further spells of traction), gentle exercise to

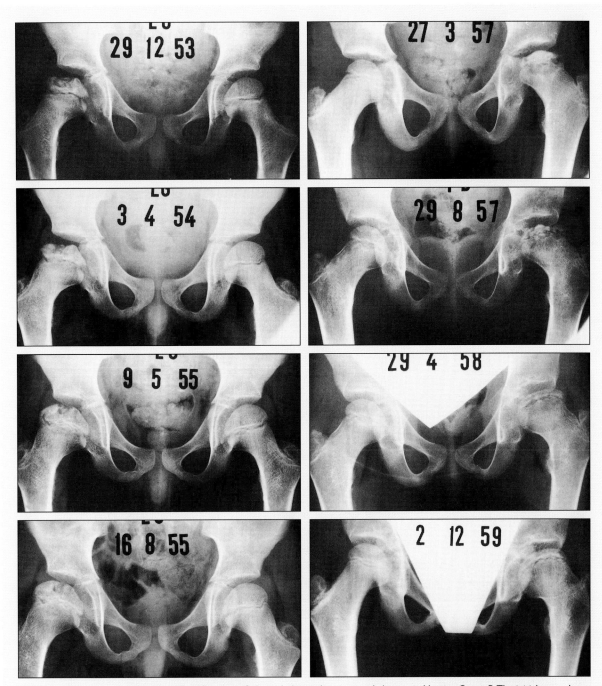

19.31 Perthes' disease – Herring classification Column 1 shows the sequential changes in Herring Group B. The initial x-ray shows that the lateral pillar has maintained more than 50% of its normal height; the outcome 2 years later is good. Column 2 shows the changes in Herring Group C. The lateral pillar is markedly flattened from the outset and the outcome is a distorted femoral head.

maintain movement and regular reassessment. During asymptomatic periods the child is allowed out and about but sport and strenuous activities are avoided.

Containment means taking active steps to seat the femoral head congruently and as fully as possible in the acetabular socket, so that it may retain its sphericity and not become displaced during the period of healing and remodelling. This is achieved (a) by holding the hips widely abducted, in plaster or in a removable brace (ambulation, though awkward, is just possible, but the position must be maintained for at least a year); or (b) by operation, either a varus osteotomy of the femur or an innominate osteotomy of the pelvis. There is no evidence that any of these methods is superior to the others.

Guidelines to treatment

There is no general agreement on the 'correct' course of treatment for all cases. Decisions are based on an assessment of the stage of the disease, the prognostic x-ray classifications and the age of the patient. The following guidelines are derived from the review by Herring (1994).

CHILDREN UNDER 6 YEARS OF AGE
No specific form of treatment has much influence on the outcome (which is usually good). Symptomatic treatment, including a period of traction and thereafter reduced activity, is appropriate.

CHILDREN AGED 6–8 YEARS
In this group the bone age is more important than the chronological age.

BONE AGE AT OR BELOW 6 YEARS
Lateral pillar groups A and B (or Catterall stages 1 and 2) – symptomatic treatment.
Lateral pillar group C (or Catterall stages 3 and 4) – abduction brace.

BONE AGE OVER 6 YEARS
Lateral pillar groups A and B (Catterall stages 1 and 2) – abduction brace or osteotomy.
Lateral pillar group C (Catterall stages 3 and 4) – outcome probably unaffected by treatment, but some would operate.

CHILDREN 9 YEARS AND OLDER
Except in very mild cases (which is rare), operative containment is the treatment of choice.

SLIPPED CAPITAL FEMORAL EPIPHYSIS

Displacement of the proximal femoral epiphysis – also known as *epiphysiolysis* – is uncommon and virtually confined to children going through the pubertal growth spurt. Boys (usually between 14 and 16 years old) are affected more often than girls (who are, on average, 2–3 years younger). The left hip is affected more commonly than the right and if one side slips there is a considerable risk of the other side also slipping.

Aetiology

The slip occurs through the hypertrophic zone of the cartilaginous growth plate. Why should the physis give way during a period of accelerated growth? Many of the patients are either fat and sexually immature or excessively tall and thin. It is tempting to formulate a theory of *hormonal imbalance* as the underlying cause of physeal disruption. Normally, pituitary hormone activity, which stimulates rapid growth and increased physeal hypertrophy during puberty, is balanced by increasing gonadal hormone activity, which promotes physeal maturation and epiphyseal fusion. A disparity between these two processes may result in the physis being

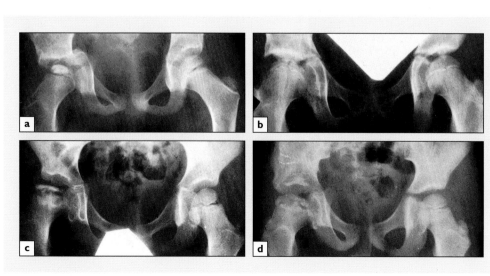

19.32 Perthes' disease – treatment Containment by pelvic osteotomy: (**a, b**) shows the effect of a Chiari osteotomy, and (**c, d**) of an innominate osteotomy.

unable to resist the shearing stresses imposed by the increase in body weight. This occurs most obviously in the hypogonadal 'Frohlich type' of child, and it may be a factor in cases associated with juvenile hypothyroidism. There are also instances of epiphysiolysis occurring in children with craniopharyngioma after successful treatment and sudden reactivation of pituitary activity.

Trauma plays a part, especially in the 30% of cases with an 'acute' slip. In the other 70% there is a slow, progressive displacement – or a series of slight displacements – sometimes culminating in a major slip after relatively mild mechanical stress (the 'acute-on-chronic' slip).

Pathology

In slipped epiphysis the femoral shaft rolls into external rotation and the femoral neck is displaced forwards while the epiphysis remains seated in the acetabulum. Disruption occurs through the hypertrophic zone of the physis and, relatively speaking, the epiphysis slips posteriorly on the femoral neck. If the slip is severe, the anterior retinacular vessels are torn. At the back of the femoral neck the periosteum is lifted from the bone with the vessels intact; this may be the main – or the only – source of blood supply to the femoral head, and damage to these vessels by manipulation or operation may result in avascular necrosis.

Physeal disruption leads to premature fusion of the epiphysis – usually within 2 years of the onset of symptoms. This is accompanied by considerable bone modelling and, although there may be a permanent external rotation deformity and apparent coxa vara, adaptive changes often ensure good joint function even without treatment.

Clinical features

Slipping usually occurs as a series of minor episodes rather than a sudden, acute event; or there may be a protracted history leading to a severe climax – the 'acute-on-chronic' slip. In over 50% of cases there is a history of injury.

The patient is usually a child around puberty, typically overweight or very tall and thin. Pain, sometimes in the groin, but often only in the thigh or knee, is the presenting symptom. It may be called a 'sprain'; often, and unfortunately, it is disregarded. It soon disappears only to recur with further exercise. Limp also occurs early and is more constant. Sometimes the child becomes aware that the leg is 'turning out'.

On examination the leg is externally rotated and is 1–2cm short. Characteristically there is limitation of flexion, abduction and medial rotation. A classic sign is the tendency to increasing external rotation as the hip is flexed.

Following an acute slip, the hip is irritable and all movements are accompanied by pain.

X-ray

In very early cases the x-ray may be reported as 'normal'; changes can be extremely subtle. This should not be taken as a signal to forego further examination if symptoms persist! In most cases, even trivial slipping can be diagnosed. In the anteroposterior view the epiphyseal plate seems to be too wide and too 'woolly'. A line drawn along the superior surface of the neck remains superior to the head instead of passing through it (Trethowan's sign). In the lateral view the femoral epiphysis is tilted backwards; this is the most reliable x-ray sign and minor

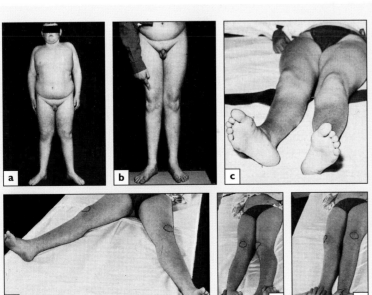

19.33 Slipped epiphysis – clinical features (a) The build is unmistakable; (b) this boy complained of pain only in the knee; (c) the right leg lies in external rotation. Another patient, showing (d) diminished abduction of the right hip; (e) diminished internal rotation; and (f) increased external rotation on the right side.

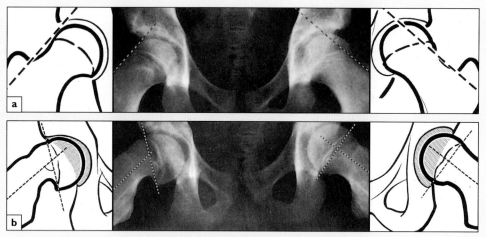

19.34 Slipped epiphysis – x-rays (a) Anteroposterior and (b) lateral views of early slipped epiphysis of the right hip. The upper diagrams show Trethowan's line passing just above the head on the affected side, but cutting through it on the normal side. The lateral view is diagnostically more reliable; even minor degrees of slip can be shown by drawing lines through the base of the epiphysis and up the middle of the femoral neck – if the angle indicated is less than 90°, the epiphysis has slipped posteriorly.

abnormalities can be detected by measuring the angle of the epiphyseal base to the femoral neck; this is normally a right angle and anything less than 87° means that the epiphysis is tilted posteriorly.

Treatment

The aims of treatment are (1) to preserve the epiphyseal blood supply, (2) to stabilize the physis and (3) to correct any residual deformity. Manipulative reduction of the slip carries a high risk of avascular necrosis and should be avoided. The choice of treatment depends on the degree of slip.

MINOR SLIPS Here the slippage is less than one-third the width of the epiphysis on the anteroposterior x-ray with less than 20° tilt in the lateral view. Deformity is minimal and needs no correction. The position is accepted and the physis is stabilized by inserting one or two screws or threaded pins along the femoral neck and into the epiphysis.

MODERATE SLIPS Slippage is between one-third and two-thirds of the width of the epiphysis on the anteroposterior x-ray with 20–40° of tilt in the lateral view. Deformity resulting from this degree of slip, though noticeable, is often tempered by gradual bone modelling and may in the end cause little disability. One can therefore accept the position, fix the epiphysis *in situ* and then wait: if, after a year or two, there is a noticeable deformity, a corrective osteotomy is performed below the femoral neck (see below). This approach is safe – but 'fixing' the epiphysis is easier said than done: because the head is tilted backwards, pins

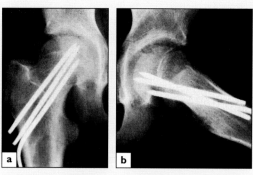

19.35 Treatment – minor slip Slipping was minimal so no reduction was attempted, but further slipping was prevented by pinning the epiphysis.

driven up the femoral neck will either enter the most anterior segment of the epiphysis (and be very insecure) or will penetrate the posterior cortex of the femoral neck and damage the retinacular vessels. Therefore, short threaded pins are inserted on the anterior femoral neck and directed posteromedially into the centre of the epiphysis. Alternatively – and probably with less risk of complications – fusion can be achieved by bone graft epiphyseodesis. At the same time any protruding bump on the anterosuperior metaphysis can be trimmed to prevent impingement on the lip of the acetabulum.

SEVERE SLIPS These are slips of more than two-thirds the width of the epiphysis on the anteroposterior x-ray and more than 40 degrees of tilt in the lateral view. A sever slip, the 'unacceptable slip', causes marked deformity which, untreated, will predispose to secondary

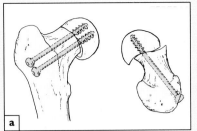
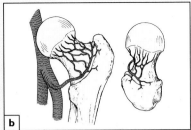
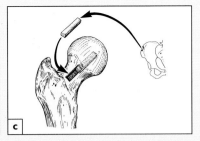

19.36 Moderate slip – treatment (**a**) A moderate slip can be accepted and fixed internally; it is essential that the threaded pins or screws enter the femur anteriorly so as not to risk damaging the retinacular vessels on the back of the femoral neck. (**b**) The femoral neck seen from behind and from above, showing the position of the vessels posterosuperiorly. (**c**) An alternative method of fixation – the Heyman and Herndon epiphyseodesis.

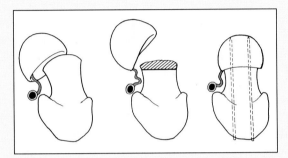

19.37 Severe slip – open reduction Dunn's operation for a severe slip. A small segment of the femoral neck is removed so that the epiphysis can be reduced and pinned without placing tension on the posterior vessels.

osteoarthritis. Closed reduction by manipulation is dangerous. Open reduction by Dunn's method (Dunn and Angel, 1978) gives good results, but should be reserved for the specialist. The greater trochanter is elevated and the femoral neck exposed. By gentle subperiosteal dissection, the posterior retinacular vessels are preserved whilst mobilizing the epiphysis (which is usually stuck down by young callus). A small segment of the femoral neck is then removed, so that the epiphysis can be repositioned without tension on the posterior structures; once reduced, it is held by two or three pins. In all but the most experienced hands, this still carries a 5–10% risk of avascular necrosis or chondrolysis. The alternative – and the method recommended for the less experienced surgeon – is to fix the epiphysis as for a 'moderate slip' and then, as soon as fusion is complete, to perform a compensatory intertrochanteric osteotomy: the easiest is a triplane osteotomy with simultaneous repositioning of the proximal femur in valgus, flexion and medial rotation; more anatomical is the geometric flexion osteotomy described by Griffith (1976). However, the patient should be told that this may result in 2–3cm of shortening.

GENERAL NOTE Most of the complications of slipped epiphysis are related to treatment – injudicious attempts at manipulative reduction of the slip, or failure to recognize the hazards of internal fixation (Riley *et al.*, 1990). The first rule of surgical treatment is 'thou shalt do no harm'.

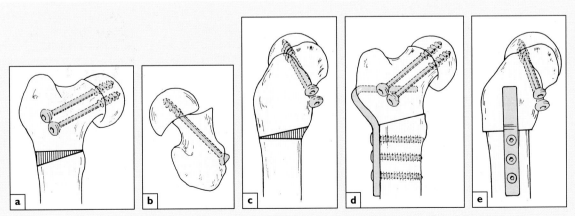

19.38 Severe slip – fixation and osteotomy (**a, b, c**) A severe slip can be treated by fixing it and then performing a compensatory osteotomy. Wedges are cut based laterally and anteriorly so as to permit valgus, flexion and rotation at the osteotomy. (**d, e**) The position after osteotomy and internal fixation.

Complications

SLIPPING AT THE OPPOSITE HIP In at least 20% of cases slipping occurs at the other hip – sometimes while the patient is still in bed. Forewarned is forearmed: the asymptomatic hip should be checked by x-ray and at the least sign of abnormality the epiphysis should be pinned.

AVASCULAR NECROSIS Death of the epiphysis used to be common. It is now recognized that it hardly ever occurs in the absence of treatment. This iatrogenic complication is minimized by avoiding forceful manipulation and operations which might damage the posterior retinacular vessels.

ARTICULAR CHONDROLYSIS Cartilage necrosis probably results from vascular damage (often iatrogenic), but in these cases bone changes are minimal. There is progressive narrowing of the joint space and the hip becomes stiff.

COXA VARA A slipped epiphysis that goes unnoticed – or is inadequately treated – may result in coxa vara. Except in the most severe cases, this is more apparent than real; the head slips backwards rather than downwards and the deformity is essentially one of *femoral neck retroversion*. Secondary effects are *external rotation deformity* of the hip, possibly *shortening* of the femur and (still a point of contention) *secondary osteoarthritis*.

SLIPPED EPIPHYSIS IN ADULTS

Epiphysiolysis is occasionally seen in young adults with endocrine disorders (hypogonadism, hypopituitarism or hypothyroidism). This is a risk to be borne in mind in all patients with open physes in the proximal femur, and especially those who are then treated with growth hormone and suddenly increase in stature before the physes stabilize. Treatment is the same as in children.

PYOGENIC ARTHRITIS

Pyogenic arthritis of the hip is usually seen in children under 2 years of age (see also Chapter 2). The organism (usually a staphylococcus) reaches the joint either directly from a distant focus or by local spread from osteomyelitis of the femur. Unless the infection is rapidly aborted, the femoral head, which is largely cartilaginous at this age, is liable to be destroyed by the proteolytic enzymes of bacteria and pus.

Adults, also, may develop pyogenic hip infection, either as a primary event in states of debilitation or (more often) secondary to invasive procedures around the hip.

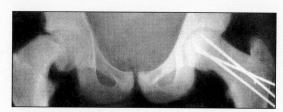

19.39 Slipped epiphysis – complications The left side has been pinned; now the right epiphysis has slipped – the patient should be warned of this possibility.

Clinical features

The child is ill and in pain, but it is often difficult to tell exactly where the pain is! The affected limb may be held absolutely still and all attempts at moving the hip are resisted. With care and patience it may be possible to localize a point of maximum tenderness over the hip; the diagnosis is confirmed by aspirating pus or fluid from the joint and submitting it for laboratory examination and bacteriological culture.

In the acute stage x-rays are of little value but sometimes they show soft-tissue swelling, displacement of the femoral head and a vacuum sign in the joint. Ultrasonography will reveal the joint effusion.

Diagnosis can be difficult, especially in neonates who may be almost asymptomatic. If the baby looks ill and no cause is apparent, think of *deep sepsis* and look for a possible source (e.g. an intravascular line). A high index of suspicion is the best aid.

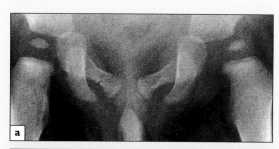

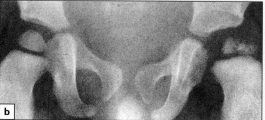

19.40 Pyogenic arthritis in children (a) In this infant, with early pyogenic arthritis of the left hip, the joint is distended and the head displaced laterally. (b) A later x-ray shows that the epiphysis has been partly destroyed and part of it is avascular. Treatment was delayed too long.

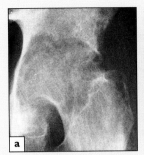
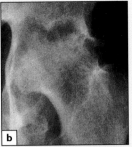

19.41 Pyogenic arthritis in adults Untreated, staphylococcal arthritis may cause rapid bone destruction: (**a**) 1 month after onset of symptoms; (**b**) 3 weeks later.

Treatment

Intravenous antibiotics should be given as soon as the diagnosis is reasonably certain. The joint is aspirated under general anaesthesia and, if pus is withdrawn, anterior arthrotomy is performed; the joint is washed out, antibiotics are instilled locally and the wound is closed without drainage. Systemic antibiotics are essential, and the hip is kept on traction or splinted in abduction until all evidence of disease activity has disappeared.

Complications

If the infection is unchecked the head and neck of the femur may be destroyed and a pathological dislocation result. The pus may escape and, when the child recovers, the sinus heals. The hip signs then resemble those of a congenital dislocation, but the tell-tale scar remains and on x-ray the femoral head is completely absent.

TUBERCULOSIS

The disease may start as a synovitis, or as an osteomyelitis in one of the adjacent bones (see also Chapter 2). Once arthritis develops, destruction is rapid and may result in pathological dislocation. Healing usually leaves a fibrous ankylosis with considerable limb shortening and deformity.

Clinical features

The condition starts insidiously with aching in the groin and thigh, and a slight limp; later, pain is more severe and may wake the patient from sleep.

With early disease (synovitis or osteomyelitis) the joint is held slightly flexed and abducted, and extremes of movement are restricted and painful; but until x-ray changes appear the hip is merely 'irritable' and diagnosis is difficult. If arthritis supervenes the hip becomes flexed, adducted and medially rotated, muscle wasting becomes obvious, and all movements are grossly limited by pain and spasm.

X-RAY
The earliest change is general rarefaction but with a normal joint space and outline; the femoral epiphysis may be enlarged or a bone abscess visible; with arthritis, in addition to the general rarefaction, there is destruction of the acetabular roof (wandering

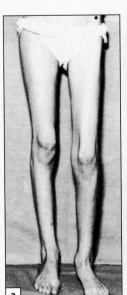
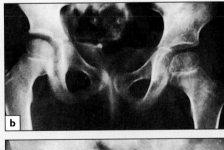
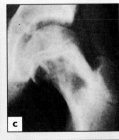
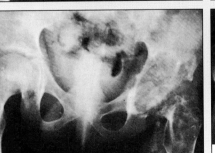
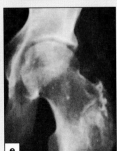

19.42 Hip tuberculosis – active (**a**) Apparent lengthening in early disease of the left hip. (**b**) Synovitis of left hip. (**c**) Bone infection in the femoral neck. (**d**) Florid arthritis. (**e**) Trochanteric infection – this rarely extends to the joint. Note the osteoporosis of the left hip in (**b**) and (**d**).

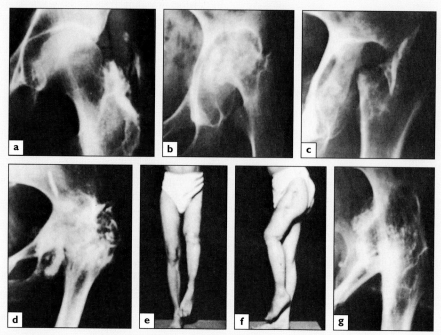

19.43 Hip tuberculosis – healing and aftermath (**a**) Healed trochanteric disease with the hip joint still normal. (**b**) Healing arthritis with gross enlargement of the acetabulum. (**c**) Healing arthritis with large acetabulum and destruction of the head. (**d**) Joint destruction with considerable calcification in the aftermath stage; and (**e, f**) appearance of the hip in this patient – note the gross shortening. (**g**) A patient in whom secondary infection was followed by bony ankylosis.

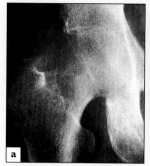
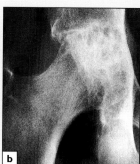
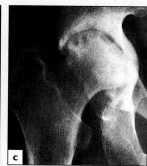

19.44 Hip tuberculosis – drug treatment In this patient antituberculous drugs alone resulted in healing – though of course hip movements were still limited.

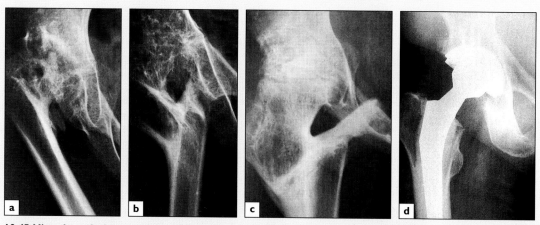

19.45 Hip tuberculosis – operative treatment (**a, b**) Before and after osteotomy in the late healing stage. (**c**) Combined osteotomy and arthrodesis. (**d**) This patient's disease had been quiescent for 2 years; hip replacement under cover of antituberculous drugs was successful.

acetabulum) or the femoral head, and usually both; the joint may be subluxed or even dislocated. With healing the bones recalcify.

Early disease, if properly treated, may heal leaving a normal or almost normal hip; but once the articular surface is destroyed the usual result is an unsound fibrous joint. In untreated cases, the leg becomes scarred and thin; shortening is often severe because of bone destruction, adduction and flexion deformity of the hip and (in children) damage to the upper femoral epiphysis and occasionally premature fusion of the lower femoral epiphysis.

Treatment

Antituberculous drugs are essential, and these alone may result in healing. Skin traction is applied and, for a child, an abduction frame may be used. An abscess in the femoral neck is best evacuated; if the arthritis does not settle, joint 'debridement' is performed. As the disease subsides, traction is discontinued and movement is encouraged.

If the joint has been destroyed, arthrodesis may be necessary once all signs of activity have disappeared, but usually not before the age of 14 years.

In older patients with residual pain and deformity, if the disease has clearly been inactive for a considerable time, total joint replacement is feasible and often successful; with antituberculous drugs, which are essential, the chances of recurrence are not great.

RHEUMATOID ARTHRITIS

The hip joint is frequently affected in rheumatoid arthritis (see also Chapter 3); occasionally the disease remains monarticular for several years, but eventually other sites are affected. Persistent synovitis in a weight-bearing joint soon leads to the destruction of cartilage and bone; the acetabulum is eroded and eventually the femoral head may perforate its floor. The hallmark of the disease is progressive bone destruction on both sides of the joint without any reactive osteophyte formation.

Clinical features

Usually the patient already has rheumatoid disease affecting many joints. Pain in the groin comes on insidiously; limp, though common, may be ascribed to pre-existing arthritis of the foot or knee. With advancing disease the patient has difficulty getting into or out of a chair, and even movements in bed may be painful. Occasionally the slow symptomatic progression is punctuated by acute flares with intense pain in the hip.

Wasting of the buttock and thigh is often marked, and the limb is usually held in external rotation and fixed flexion. All movements are restricted and painful.

X-RAYS
During the early stages there is osteoporosis and diminution of the joint space; later, the acetabulum and femoral head are eroded. Protrusio acetabuli is common. In the worst cases (and especially in patients on corticosteroids) there is gross bone destruction and the floor of the acetabulum may be perforated.

Treatment

If the disease can be arrested by general treatment, hip deterioration may be slowed down. But once cartilage and bone are eroded, no treatment will influence the progression to joint destruction. Total joint replacement is then the best answer. It relieves pain and restores a useful range of movement. It is advocated even in younger patients, because the polyarthritis so limits activity that the implants are not unduly stressed.

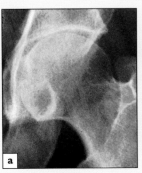
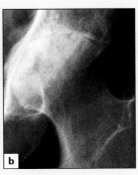
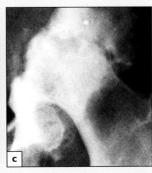

19.46 Rheumatoid arthritis Three stages in the development of rheumatoid arthritis: (**a**) loss of joint space; (**b**) erosion of bone after cartilage has disappeared; (**c**) perforation of the acetabular floor – such marked destruction is more likely to occur if the patient is having corticosteroids.

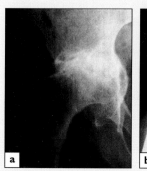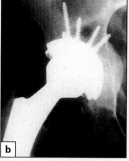

19.47 Rheumatoid arthritis – treatment Severe erosive arthritis treated by hip replacement with an uncemented socket and bone grafting of the acetabulum.

Care should be taken during operation to prevent fracture or perforation of the osteoporotic bone. If the acetabular floor is deficient, a supportive cage and bone grafting will be needed.

Children with juvenile chronic arthritis may need custom-made prostheses for their small and often delicate bones.

Postoperative infection poses a greater risk in rheumatoid patients than in others – more particularly if the patient is on corticosteroid therapy. Prophylaxis is even more important than usual.

OSTEOARTHRITIS

The hip joint is one of the commonest sites of osteoarthritis (see also Chapter 5), though in some populations (e.g. black Africans and southern Chinese) this joint seems peculiarly immune to the disease. This may simply be because certain predisposing conditions (acetabular dysplasia, Perthes' disease, slipped epiphysis) show a similar differential incidence in these populations.

Where there is an obvious underlying cause the term *'secondary osteoarthritis'* is applied (Table 19.2); these patients are often in their third or fourth decade and the appearance of the joint reflects the preceding abnormality. Thus in regions where congenital dislocation and acetabular dysplasia are common (e.g. in southern Europe), women are more often affected than men, the hips may be the only joints affected and lateral subluxation is common.

When no underlying cause is apparent, the term *'primary osteoarthritis'* is used. Patients are somewhat older – usually in their sixth or seventh decade – with a slight predominance of women, and often other areas (knees or spine) also are affected. There may be evidence of chondrocalcinosis.

Pathology

The articular cartilage becomes soft and fibrillated whilst the underlying bone shows cyst formation and sclerosis. These changes are most marked in the area of maximal loading (chiefly the top of the joint); at the margins of the joint there are the characteristic osteophytes. Synovial hypertrophy is common and capsular fibrosis may account for joint stiffness.

Sometimes – and for no obvious reason – articular destruction progresses very rapidly, with erosion of the femoral head or acetabulum (or both), occasionally going on to perforation of the pelvis.

Clinical features

Pain is felt in the groin but may radiate to the knee. Typically it occurs after periods of activity but later it is more constant and sometimes disturbs sleep. Stiffness at first is noticed chiefly after rest; later it increases progressively until putting on socks and shoes becomes difficult. Limp is often noticed early and the patient may think the leg is getting shorter.

The patient is usually fit and over 50 years of age, but secondary osteoarthritis can occur at 30 or even 20 years of age. There may be an obvious limp and, except in early cases, a positive Trendelenburg sign. The affected leg usually lies in external rotation and adduction, so it appears short; there is nearly always some fixed flexion, although this may only be revealed by Thomas' test. Muscle wasting is detectable but rarely severe. Deep pressure may elicit tenderness, and the greater trochanter is somewhat high and posterior. Movements, though often painless within a limited range, are restricted; internal rotation, abduction and extension are usually affected first and most severely.

X-RAY

The earliest sign is a decreased joint space, usually maximal in the superior weightbearing region but sometimes affecting the entire joint. Later signs are subarticular sclerosis, cyst formation and osteophytes. The shape of the femoral head or acetabulum may give

Table 19.2 Causes of osteoarthritis of the hip

Abnormal stress	Defective cartilage	Abnormal bone
Subluxation	Infection	Fracture
Coxa magna	Rheumatoid	Necrosis
Coxa vara	Calcinosis	Paget's
Minor deformities		Other causes
Protrusio		of sclerosis

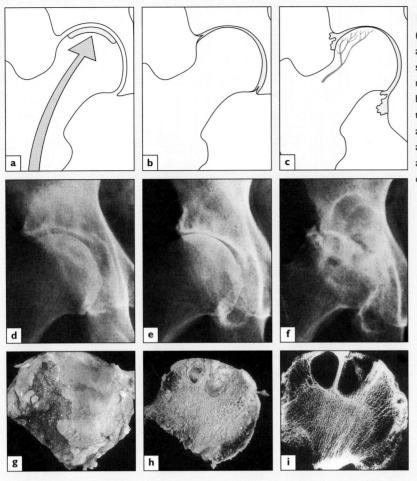

19.48 Osteoarthritis – pathology
(**a**, **b**, **c**) Cartilage softening and thinning are greatest in the zone of maximal stress. There is a vascular reaction and new-bone formation in the subchondral bone as well as osteophytic growth at the margins of the joint. These changes, as well as subchondral cyst formation, are reflected in the sequential x-ray appearances (**d**, **e**, **f**) and in the morphology of the excised femoral head (**g**, **h**, **i**).

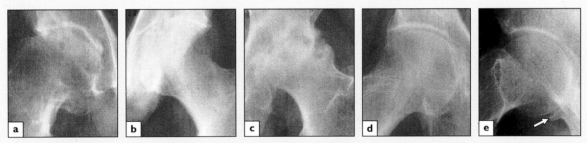

19.49 Osteoarthritis – x-rays X-ray features of (**a**) hypertrophic osteoarthritis, (**b**) atrophic osteoarthritis, (**c**) rapidly destructive osteoarthritis and (**d**, **e**) posterior marginal osteoarthritis.

a clue to an underlying condition (e.g. old Perthes' disease). Bilateral cases occasionally show features of a generalized dysplasia.

Treatment

Analgesics and anti-inflammatory drugs may be helpful, and warmth is soothing. The patient is encouraged to use a walking-stick and to try to preserve movement and stability by non-weightbearing exercises. In early cases physiotherapy (including manipulation) may relieve pain for long periods. Activities are adjusted so as to reduce stress on the hip.

OPERATIVE TREATMENT The indications for operation are (1) progressive increase in pain, (2) severe restriction of activities, (3) marked deformity and (4) progressive loss

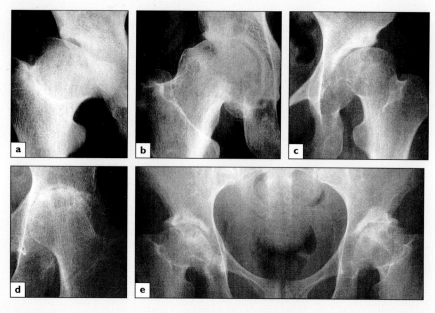

19.50 Secondary osteoarthritis (a) After Perthes' disease. (b) After slipped upper femoral epiphysis. (c) After congenital subluxation. (d) After rheumatoid disease. (e) Bilateral in a patient with multiple epiphyseal dysplasia.

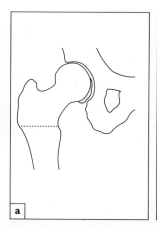 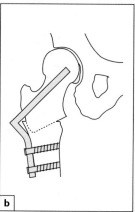 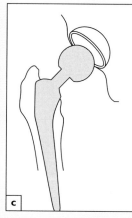

19.51 Osteoarthritis – treatment (a) When only part of the joint is damaged, a realignment osteotomy may allow redistribution of stress to a less damaged part of the articular surface (b). In older patients, and when articular destruction is marked, joint replacement (c) is indicated.

of movement (especially abduction), together with (5) x-ray signs of joint destruction.

In the usual case – a patient aged over 60 years with a long history of pain and increasing disability – the preferred operation is *total joint replacement*. In those between 40 and 60 years this may still be the best operation if joint destruction is severe.

In younger patients, particularly those with some preservation of articular cartilage, an *intertrochanteric realignment osteotomy* may be considered. If performed early, it can arrest or delay further cartilage destruction, and if the operation is well planned it does not preclude later replacement arthroplasty.

Arthrodesis of the hip is a practical solution for young adults with marked destruction of a single joint, and particularly when the conditions for advanced reconstructive surgery are less than ideal. If well executed, the operation guarantees freedom from pain and permanent stability, though it has the disadvantages of restricted mobility and a significant incidence of later backache, as well as deformity and discomfort in other nearby joints (Solomon, 1998).

OSTEONECROSIS

The femoral head is the commonest site of symptomatic osteonecrosis (see also Chapter 6), mainly because of its peculiar blood supply which renders it vulnerable to ischaemia from *arterial cut-off, venous stasis, intravascular thrombosis, intraosseous sinusoidal compression,* or a *combination of several of these.*

Post-traumatic osteonecrosis usually follows a displaced fracture of the femoral neck or dislocation of the hip. The main cause is interruption of the arterial blood supply, but contributory factors are venous stasis and thrombosis of intramedullary arterioles and capillaries.

Non-traumatic osteonecrosis is seen in association with infiltrative disorders of the marrow, Gaucher's disease, sickle-cell disease, coagulopathies, caisson disease, systemic lupus erythematosus and – more commonly – high-dosage corticosteroid administration and alcohol abuse. Perthes' disease is a special example which is dealt with elsewhere in this chapter.

The pathogenesis and pathological anatomy of the bone changes are discussed in Chapter 6.

Clinical features

Post-traumatic osteonecrosis develops soon after injury to the hip, but symptoms and signs may take months to appear.

Non-traumatic osteonecrosis is more insidious. Children are affected in conditions such as Perthes' disease, sickle-cell disease and Gaucher's disease. Adult patients come from both sexes and all ages.

The presenting complaint is usually pain in the hip (or, in over 50% of cases, both hips), which progresses over a period of 2–3 years to become quite severe. However, in over 10% of cases the condition is asymptomatic and discovered incidentally after x-ray or MRI during investigation of a systemic disorder or long-standing symptoms in the other hip.

On examination, the patient walks with a limp and may have a positive Trendelenburg sign. The thigh is wasted and the limb may be 1 or 2cm short. Movements are restricted, particularly abduction and internal rotation. A characteristic sign is a tendency for the hip to twist into external rotation during passive flexion; this corresponds to the 'sectoral sign' in which, with the hip extended, internal rotation is almost full, but with the hip flexed it is grossly restricted.

Imaging

X-rays, during the early stages, are normal. The first signs probably appear only 6–9 months after the occurrence of bone death and are due mainly to reactive changes in the surrounding (live) bone. Thus, the classic feature of increased density (or sclerosis) is a sign of repair rather than necrosis. With time, destructive changes do appear in the necrotic segment: a thin subchondral fracture line (the 'crescent sign'), slight

flattening of the weightbearing zone and then increasing distortion, with eventual collapse, of the articular surface of the femoral head.

MRI shows characteristic changes in the marrow long before the appearance of x-ray signs – a mean of 3.6 months after the initiation of corticosteroid treatment in one published study (Sakamoto *et al.*, 1997). The diagnostic feature is a band of altered signal intensity running through the femoral head (diminished intensity in the T1-weighted SE image and increased intensity in the STIR image). This 'band' represents the reactive zone between living and dead bone and thus demarcates the ischaemic segment, the extent and location of which are important in staging the lesion.

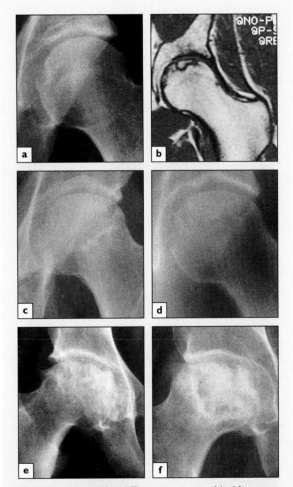

19.52 Osteonecrosis (**a**) This patient in stage I had few symptoms and virtually normal x-rays, but (**b**) the MRI shows a small segment of osteonecrosis in the dome of the femoral head. (**c, d**) X-ray and tomogram of stage 2, with increased density but preservation of the spherical shape of the head. (**e, f**) Stages 3 and 4 – increasing distortion of the femoral head and secondary osteoarthritis.

Diagnosis

X-ray features of destructive or sclerotic forms of *osteoarthritis* are sometimes mistaken for those of advanced osteonecrosis. There may, indeed, be elements of bone necrosis in some types of osteoarthritis, but there is an important point of distinction between these two conditions: in osteoarthritis the articular 'space' diminishes before the bone breaks up, whereas in osteonecrosis the articular 'space' is preserved to the last (because it is not primarily a disease of articular cartilage).

Transient osteoporosis of the hip is sometimes confused with avascular necrosis. The condition is described below.

The causative disorder

Diagnosis should include elucidation of the causative disorder. There may be a history of trauma, a familial condition such as sickle-cell disease or Gaucher's disease, an occupational background suggesting dysbaric ischaemia, an underlying disease such as systemic lupus erythematosus, or a known background of corticosteroid

administration or alcohol abuse. If there is no such history, the patient should be fully investigated for these associated conditions (see Chapter 6).

It is important to recognize that pathogenic factors are cumulative, so a patient with systemic lupus or a moderately severe alcohol habit may develop osteonecrosis following comparatively low doses of cortisone, and occasionally even after prolonged or excessive use of topical corticosteroids (Solomon and Pearse, 1994).

Staging

Ficat and Arlet's radiographic staging of femoral head necrosis is widely used (see Chapter 6). In *Stage 1* the patient has little or no pain and the plain x-ray shows no abnormality. However, there are typical changes on MRI (see Figure 19.52). In *Stage 2* there are early x-ray signs but no distortion of the femoral head. *Stage 3 is* more advanced, with increasing signs of bone destruction and femoral head distortion. *Stage 4* is characterized by collapse of the articular surface and joint disorganization. This is a useful descriptive classification of the current state of affairs, but it does not provide a guide to prognosis (and therefore treatment) in the early stages of the condition.

Shimuzu *et al.* (1994) proposed a classification based on MR images which define the extent, location and intensity of the abnormal segment in the femoral head. The risk of femoral head collapse (at least over a period of 2–3 years) was related mainly to the *extent* (the area of the coronal femoral head image involved) and *location* (the portion of the weightbearing surface) in the initial MRI. In general terms, their findings suggested that: (1) the extent of the ischaemic segment is determined at the outset and does not increase over time; (2) lesions occupying less than one-quarter of the femoral head coronal diameter and involving only the medial third of the weightbearing surface rarely go on to collapse; (3) lesions occupying up to one-half of the femoral head diameter and involving between one-third and two-thirds of the weightbearing surface are likely to collapse in about 30% of cases; and (4) lesions occupying more than one-quarter of the femoral head diameter and involving more than

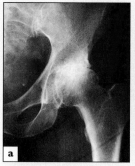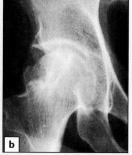

19.53 Diagnosis **(a)** Osteoarthritis sometimes shows marked segmental sclerosis on x-ray. These features are often mistaken for those of osteonecrosis. The clue lies in the absent joint 'space', a cardinal sign in osteoarthritis. Compare this with **(b)**, an x-ray of severe osteonecrosis in which the joint 'space' is preserved in the face of bone collapse.

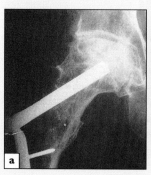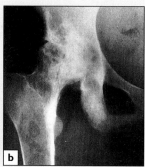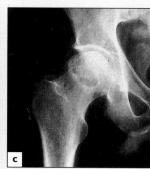

19.54 Osteonecrosis
Femoral head necrosis due to **(a)** femoral neck fracture, **(b)** Gaucher's disease and **(c)** chronic alcohol abuse.

two-thirds of the weightbearing surface will collapse within 3 years in over 70% of cases. When discussing treatment, we shall refer to these three degrees of severity as *Grade I, Grade II* and *Grade III.*

[Note that although this classification is useful for predicting outcome and planning treatment, *extent* (in this context) is not synonymous with *volume*; the true volume of the necrotic segment is very difficult to determine (Kim *et al.*, 1998).]

Treatment of post-traumatic osteonecorsis

Femoral head necrosis following fracture or dislocation of the hip usually ends in collapse of the femoral head. Very young patients (those under 40 years), in whom one is reluctant to perform hip replacement, can be treated by realignment osteotomy, with or without bone-grafting of the necrotic segment. Older patients will almost invariably opt for partial or total joint replacement.

Treatment of non-traumatic osteonecrosis

EARLY

Grade I lesions (those restricted to the medial part of the femoral head) progress very slowly or not at all. Almost any treatment for this group is therefore liable to be assessed as 'beneficial'. All that is needed is symptomatic treatment and reassurance, but it is wise to observe the patient over several years in case there should be a change.

Grade II lesions (those occupying up to one-half of the femoral head and between one- and two-thirds of the weightbearing surface) are liable to progress. If they are seen before there is any distortion of the femoral head, it would therefore be justifiable to advise conservative surgery (core decompression or decompression and bone grafting of the femoral head). Coring of the femoral head was introduced by Ficat (1985) as a means of reducing the intraosseous pressure in patients with early non-traumatic osteonecrosis. The intraosseous pressure is measured and, if it is raised, a 7mm core of bone is removed by drilling up the femoral neck under image intensification fluoroscopy. It is impossible to say which cases will respond favourably, but the attempt is worthwhile and sustained symptomatic improvement is seen in 30–50% of patients. The alternative is realignment osteotomy in younger patients and partial or total hip replacement in patients over 45 years old with increasing symptoms.

Grade III lesions (those occupying a large part of the femoral head and more than two-thirds of the weight-bearing surface) have a poor prognosis. Decompression is unlikely to have a lasting effect. For younger patients, therefore, realignment osteotomy is the treatment of choice. X-rays and CT will show exactly where the necrotic segment is and the angulation osteotomy can be planned so as to displace the necrotic segment

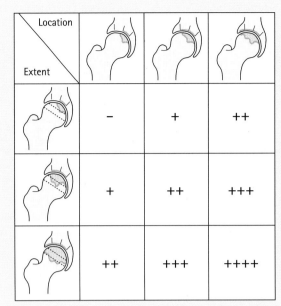

19.55 Predictive staging The likelihood of progression to collapse depends on the *location* and *extent* of the boundary changes on MRI. In this figure the risk of progression is represented by + signs. The general scheme is based on findings published by Shimuzu *et al.* (1994).

away from the maximal loadbearing trajectory. A flexion osteotomy will be needed for most cases. The more radical transtrochanteric rotational osteotomy of Sugioka (Sugioka and Mohtai, 1998)) is difficult to perform and the results in most hands are no better than those of the more conventional osteotomies. Older patients with intrusive symptoms will be better served by partial or total joint replacement.

LATE

Patients with advanced osteonecrosis and bone collapse (Ficat stage 3 or 4) will need reconstructive surgery: osteotomy, with or without bone grafting, or joint replacement.

There is a limited place for arthrodesis in young men who are willing to accept the limitations of a 'stiff' hip in return for pain relief (Solomon, 1998).

TRANSIENT OSTEOPOROSIS OF THE HIP (MARROW OEDEMA SYNDROME)

This is a well-recognized, though uncommon, syndrome characterized by pain and rapidly emerging osteoporosis of the femoral head and adjacent pelvis (see Chapter 6). Radionuclide scanning shows increased activity on both sides of the hip but not in the soft tissues. The condition was originally described in women in the last trimester of pregnancy, but it is now seen in patients of both sexes

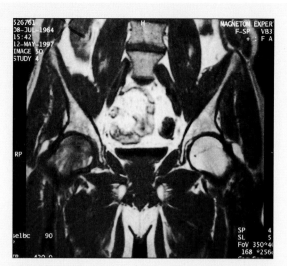

19.56 Marrow oedema syndrome This patient complained of pain in the right hip. X-ray showed no obvious abnormality, although the area around the hip looked somewhat osteoporotic. The MRI disclosed the typical picture of diffuse signal reduction (in the right femoral head) in the T1-weighted scans. This contrasts sharply with the localized bands which are characteristic of osteonecrosis.

and all ages from early adulthood onwards. Typically the changes last for 6–12 months, after which the symptoms subside and the x-ray gradually returns to normal.

The cause is unknown, but *MRI features* are characteristic of marrow oedema. It has been suggested that the condition is a precursor (or *forme fruste*) of avascular necrosis, but there is little evidence to support this (see page 100).

Treatment The condition almost always resolves spontaneously and most patients require no more than symptomatic treatment. However, pain can be rapidly abolished by operative decompression of the femoral head (drilling up the femoral neck), and some would prefer this to the long wait for a natural 'cure'. If there is any doubt about whether the MRI changes are due to osteonecrosis or marrow oedema, operative decompression is recommended.

BURSITIS AND TENDINITIS AROUND THE HIP

TROCHANTERIC BURSITIS

Pain over the lateral aspect of the hip and thigh may be due to local trauma or overuse, resulting in inflammation of the trochanteric bursa which lies deep to the tensor fascia lata. There is local tenderness and sometimes crepitus on flexing and extending the hip. Swelling is unusual but post-traumatic bleeding can produce a bursal haematoma.

X-rays may show evidence of a previous fracture, or a protruding metal implant or trochanteric wires dating from some former operation. There may also be calcification or shadows suggesting swelling of the soft tissues. It is important to exclude underlying disorders such as gout, rheumatoid disease and infection (including tuberculosis).

Pain around the hip	
Anteriorly (groin)	**Laterally**
Synovitis and arthritis	Referred from spine
Perthes' disease	Slipped epiphysis
Labral tear or detachment	Trochanteric bursitis
Loose bodies in the joint	Stress fracture
Stress fracture	Trochanteric tuberculosis
Osteitis pubis	
Other bone lesions	
Inguinal hernia	
Inguinal lymphadenopathy	**Posteriorly**
Iliopsoas tendinitis or bursitis	Refereed from spine
Iliopsoas abscess	Gluteus medius tendinitis
Adductor longus strain or tendinitis	

Other causes of pain and tenderness over the greater trochanter are stress fractures (in athletes and elderly patients), slipped epiphysis (in adolescents) and bone infection (in children). The commonest cause of misdiagnosis is referred pain from the lumbar spine.

The usual treatment of trochanteric bursitis is rest, administration of non-steroidal anti-inflammatory drugs and (provided infection is excluded) injection of local anaesthetic and corticosteroid. If a haematoma is present it should be drained.

GLUTEUS MEDIUS TENDINITIS

Acute tendinitis may cause pain and localized tenderness just behind the greater trochanter. This is seen particularly in dancers and athletes. The clinical and x-ray features are similar to those of trochanteric bursitis, and the differential diagnosis is the same. Treatment is by rest and injection of local anaesthetic and corticosteroid.

ADDUCTOR LONGUS STRAIN OR TENDINITIS

This overuse injury is often seen in footballers and athletes. The patient complains of pain in the groin and tenderness can be localized to the adductor longus origin, close to the pubis. Swelling below this site may signify an adductor longus tear.

Acute strains are treated by rest and heat. Chronic strains may need prolonged physiotherapy.

ILIOPSOAS BURSITIS

Pain in the groin and anterior thigh may be due to an iliopsoas bursitis. The site of tenderness is difficult to define and there may be guarding of the muscles overlying the lesser trochanter. Hip movements are sometimes restricted; indeed, the condition may arise from synovitis of the hip since there is often a potential communication between the bursa and the joint. The most typical feature is a sharp increase in pain on adduction and internal rotation of the hip. Pain can also be elicited by testing psoas contraction against resistance (see page 406).

The differential diagnosis of anterior hip pain includes inguinal lymphadenopathy, hernia, a psoas abscess, fracture of the lesser trochanter, slipped epiphysis, local infection and arthritis.

Treatment is by non-steroidal anti-inflammatory drugs and injection of local anaesthetic and corticosteroid; the injection is best performed under fluoroscopic control.

SNAPPING HIP

'Snapping hip' is a disorder in which the patient (usually a young woman) complains of the hip 'jumping out of place, or 'catching', during walking. The snapping is caused by a thickened band in the gluteus maximus aponeurosis flipping over the greater trochanter. In the swing phase of walking the band moves anteriorly; then, in the stance phase, as the gluteus maximus contracts and pulls the hip into extension, the band flips back across the trochanter, causing an audible 'snap'. This is usually painless but it can be quite distressing, especially if the hip gives way. Sometimes there is tenderness around the hip, and it may be possible to reproduce the peculiar sensation by flexing and extending the hip while the patient contracts the abductors.

The condition must be distinguished from other causes of painful clicking, particularly a *tear of the acetabular labrum* or an *osteocartilaginous flap* on the femoral head (similar to osteochondritis dissecans). Contrast arthrography, or arthroscopy if this is available, will exclude these entities.

Treatment of the snapping tendon is usually unnecessary; the patient merely needs an explanation and reassurance. Occasionally, though, if discomfort is marked the band can be either divided or lengthened by a Z-plasty.

PRINCIPLES OF HIP OPERATIONS

Exposure of the hip

Operative approaches to the hip can be broadly divided into anterior, anterolateral, lateral and posterior.

The anterior (Smith–Petersen) approach starts in the plane between sartorius and rectus femoris medially and tensor fascia femoris laterally and remains anterior to the gluteus medius. The hip capsule is exposed by detaching the origins of rectus femoris. This provides adequate exposure for many operations, including open reduction of the dislocated hip in infants and the various types of pelvic osteotomy. However, it is not ideal for major reconstructive surgery in adults.

The anterolateral (Watson–Jones) approach is also anterior to the gluteus medius, but behind the tensor fascia femoris. It provides reasonable exposure of the hip joint, with minimal detachment of muscles, but the gluteus medius is in the way and this makes hip replacement difficult.

Lateral approaches suffer from the fact that the gluteus medius and minimus obstruct the view of the acetabulum. The abductors are dealt with by (1) retracting them posterosuperiorly (a limited solution), or (2) splitting them and raising the anterior portion intact from the greater trochanter (Hardinge's direct lateral approach), or (3) osteotomizing the greater trochanter and retracting it upwards with the attached abductors (as in the Charnley approach for total joint replacement). This provides excellent exposure; however, there may be problems with reattachment of the trochanteric fragment.

The posterior approach is the most direct. By splitting the anterior part of gluteus maximus, the rotators at the back of the hip are exposed and the sciatic nerve is retracted safely beneath the bulk of the posterior portion of gluteus maximus. Once the short rotators are detached, the hip is entered directly. Many surgeons prefer this approach for joint replacement. It has two minor disadvantages: orientation is more difficult, especially for placing the acetabular cup; and it is associated with an increased incidence of postoperative dislocation.

Planning

Reconstructive surgery of the hip needs careful preoperative planning. Tracings of plain x-rays are useful for taking measurements and working out repositioning angles. For the most difficult cases, three-dimensional imaging studies should be obtained.

INTERTROCHANTERIC OSTEOTOMY

RATIONALE Intertrochanteric osteotomy has three objectives: (1) to change the orientation of the femoral head in the socket so as to reduce mechanical stress in a damaged segment; (2) by realigning the proximal femur, to improve joint congruity; and (3) by transecting the bone, to reduce intraosseous hypertension and

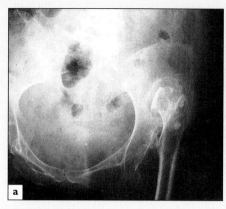
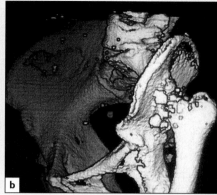

19.57 Planning (a) Plain x-rays showing an old unreduced congenital dislocation. (b) The three-dimensional MRI reveals more clearly the problems of reconstructive surgery.

relieve pain. An unintentional, and poorly understood, consequence is (4) fibrocartilaginous repair of the articular surface.

INDICATIONS In children osteotomy is used to correct angular or rotational deformities of the proximal femur (e.g. in congenital dislocation, coxa vara or severe slips of the capital epiphysis), or to produce 'containment' of the femoral head in Perthes' disease.

In adults, the main indication is osteoarthritis associated with joint dysplasia, particularly in patients who are younger than 50 years. Pain is often relieved immediately (probably due to reduced vascular congestion) and sometimes the articular space is gradually restored. The other prime indication is in localized avascular necrosis of the femoral head; if only a small segment is involved, realignment can rotate this segment out of the path of maximum stress.

CONTRAINDICATIONS Osteotomy is unsuitable in elderly patients and in those with severe stiffness; movement may be even further decreased afterwards. It is also contraindicated in rheumatoid arthritis, and even in osteoarthritis if there is widespread loss of articular substance; repositioning is useless if other parts of the femoral head are equally damaged.

TECHNICAL CONSIDERATIONS The osteotomy allows repositioning of the femoral head in valgus, varus or different degrees of rotation. Exact placement and angulation can be ensured only by meticulous preoperative planning and painstaking execution of the bone cuts. The fragments are fixed with suitably angled plates and screws. Postoperatively the patient is permitted only partial weightbearing for 3–6 months. About 15% of patients will require some assistance (a walking stick) for the rest of their lives.

Sugioka (Sugioka and Mohtai, 1998) devised a transtrochanteric rotational osteotomy which allows the femoral neck to be rotated on its long axis, thus turning the femoral head through an arc of 90° or more. The operation is used mainly for segmental necrosis of the femoral head.

COMPLICATIONS The main complication is malposition of the bone. Only careful planning can prevent this. Non-union of the osteotomy is rare.

RESULTS Provided the indications are strictly observed, the results are moderately good. In one series of 368 osteotomies, survivorship analysis showed that 10 years after osteotomy 47% of patients had required no further surgery (Werners *et al.*, 1990).

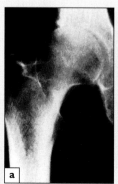
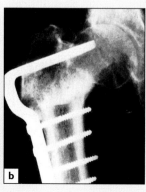
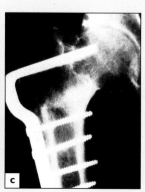

19.58 Osteoarthritis – treatment by osteotomy Following a varus type of osteotomy this patient lost most of her pain, and the x-rays suggest articular cartilage regeneration (would 'rejuvenation' be too strong a word?).

ARTHRODESIS

RATIONALE Fusion of the hip is guaranteed to relieve pain and provide stability for a lifetime. But at what cost? Surprisingly, though the joint is fused the patient retains a great deal of 'mobility' because lumbosacral tilting and rotation are preserved and often increased. Nevertheless, there are restrictions: for sitting comfortably the hip needs 60° of flexion; for climbing stairs, 45°; and for walking, 20°. In the stance phase of walking the normal hip is in slight abduction, but in the swing phase it is carried in slight adduction. No position of fusion can satisfy all these demands, so one aims at a compromise. And sometimes it is wrong, with the result that function is seriously impaired.

INDICATIONS Arthrodesis should be considered for any destructive condition of the hip when there are serious contraindications to osteotomy or arthroplasty: for example, a patient who is too young, a hip that is already stiff but painful and previous infection. Young patients adapt well; those aged over 30–40 years respond unpredictably.

CONTRAINDICATIONS Elderly patients, and any patient with a good range of movement, will resent a 'stiff hip'. Other contraindications are lack of bone stock and abnormalities in the 'compensating joints' (lumbar spine, knees and opposite hip).

TECHNICAL CONSIDERATIONS The recommended position for arthrodesis is 20° of flexion, 10° of adduction (unless the leg is short) and neutral or slight external rotation. However, in young people there is a tendency for the 'joint' to drift into further flexion and by the age of 40 years this may be as much as 40°. Some form of internal fixation is used to secure the bones in the desired position. It is important to ensure that these implants do not destroy the abductors; though they are not needed while the hip is arthrodesed, they will be essential if ever the fusion is converted to an arthroplasty.

COMPLICATIONS The major complications are (1) failure to fuse and (2) malposition, which hampers function and puts unwanted strain on other joints. Late complications are (3) compensatory deformities in other joints (knees and opposite hip) and (4) low backache, which occurs in over 60% of patients 20 years after fusion. Women may complain of (5) difficulty with sexual intercourse. And (6) squatting is, of course, impossible. However, it should be remembered that total replacement is still possible after a hip has been arthrodesed.

RESULTS Provided the 'compensating joints' (lumbar spine, knee and opposite hip) are completely normal, young patients in particular may derive great benefit from arthrodesis, with many years of comfort, a well-disguised limp and the ability to walk long distances and play games. Older patients fare less well: they find walking more difficult, tend to develop backache and seem more prone to degenerative changes in other joints.

TOTAL HIP REPLACEMENT

RATIONALE Total replacement of the articular surfaces seems the ideal way of treating any disorder causing joint destruction (Charnley, 1979). However, there are several problems to be overcome: (1) the prosthetic

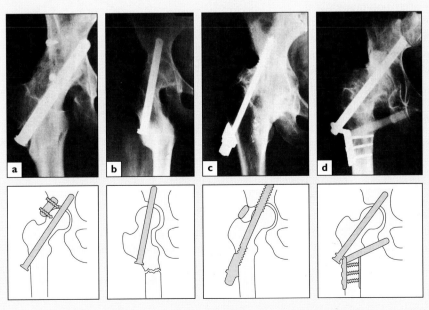

19.59 Arthrodesis (a) Watson–Jones' method. **(b)** Pyrford arthrodesis – the hip is pinned in its deformed position and the deformity corrected by an osteotomy; the patient is kept on traction for 6 weeks, then in a short hip spica for a further 6 weeks. **(c)** Compression arthrodesis. **(d)** Norwich V arthrodesis.

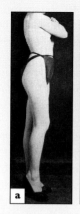
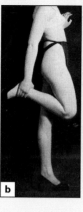
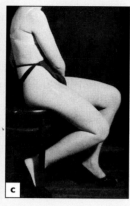

19.60 Arthrodesis Stiffness of the hip is largely disguised by mobility of the spine and knee.

implants must be durable; (2) they must permit slippery movement at the articulation; (3) they must be firmly fixed to the skeleton; and (4) they must be inert and not provoke any unwanted reaction in the tissues. The usual combination is a metal femoral component (stainless steel, titanium or cobalt–chrome alloy) articulating with a polyethylene socket. Ceramic components have better frictional characteristics but are more easily broken. Fixation is either by embedding the implant in methylmethacrylate cement, which acts as a grouting material filling the interstices, or by fitting the implant closely to the bone bed without cement. The 'bond' between bone and the implant surface, or cement, is never perfect. The best that can be hoped for is ingrowth of trabecular bone on the implant or cement (osseointegration). There are various ways of enhancing this process: (1) if cement is used, it is applied under pressure and allowed to cure without movement or extrusion after the implant has been inserted; (2) Ling and his co-workers have shown that a smooth, tapered and collarless femoral prosthesis will continue settling within the cement mantle even after polymerization, thereby maintaining expansile pressure between cement and bone (Fowler *et al.*, 1988); (3) uncemented implants may be covered with a mesh or porous coating that encourages bone ingrowth (Engh *et al.*, 1987); (4) the implant may be coated with hydroxyapatite, an excellent substrate for osteoblastic new-bone formation and osseointegration (Geesink, 1990).

INDICATIONS Because of the tendency for implants to loosen with time, joint replacement is usually reserved for patients over 60 years. However, with improved cementing techniques and rapid advances in the design of uncemented prostheses, the operation is being offered to younger patients with destructive hip disorders, and occasionally even to children severely crippled with rheumatoid disease.

CONTRAINDICATIONS Overt or latent sepsis is the chief contraindication to joint replacement. An infected

arthroplasty spells disaster. Patients under 60 years of age are considered only if other operations are unsuitable.

TECHNICAL CONSIDERATIONS The fear of infection dictates a host of prophylactic measures, including the use of special ultra-clean air operating theatres, occlusive theatre clothing and perioperative antibiotic cover (Lidwell *et al.*, 1984; Marotte *et al.*, 1987). In addition, some surgeons routinely use antibiotic-laden cement. A variety of joint exposures is recommended: none has any significant advantages over the others. The choice of implant should depend on sound biomechanical and biological testing, but seems to be determined as much

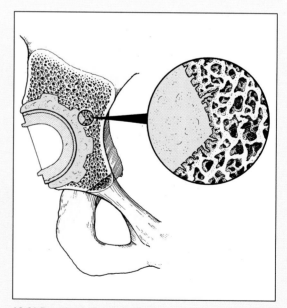

19.61 Prosthetic fixation Fixation between cement and bone is by (**a**) interlock (interdigitation of large irregularities in cement and bone) and, more completely, by (**b**) osseointegration (intimate penetration of cement between endosteal trabeculae).

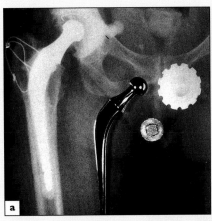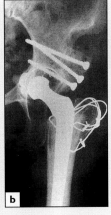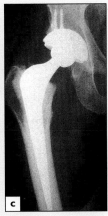

19.62 Total hip replacement (**a**) The Charnley hip replacement system, forerunner of all the modern methods of total arthroplasty. The small wire-mesh disc is used as a plug to prevent cement extrusion into the pelvis. (**b**) In this patient with untreated congenital dislocation a small off-set cup has been used, and the dysplastic acetabulum has been augmented with a bone graft. (**c**) 'Hybrid' arthroplasty, using an uncemented cup and a cemented collarless femoral prosthesis.

by personal prejudice. The array of over 300 different mechanisms currently on the market represents the triumph of hope over reason. The argument of 'cemented versus cementless' goes on. In the end, sound technique is probably more important than anything else.

Postoperatively the implant should be protected from full loading until osseointegration is advanced; 6–10 weeks on crutches is not unreasonable.

COMPLICATIONS Hip replacements are often performed on patients who are somewhat elderly; some are rheumatoid and may be having corticosteroid therapy. Consequently the general complication rate is by no means trivial; deep vein thrombosis in particular is common.

There are a number of complications which are peculiar to total hip replacement. Factors that may contribute to their development include previous hip operations, severe deformity, lack of pre-operative planning, inadequate 'bone stock', an insufficiently sterile operating environment and lack of experience or expertise on the part of the surgeon or his or her team.

Intra-operative complications include perforation or even fracture of the femur or acetabulum. Special care should be taken in patients who are very old or osteoporotic and in those who have had previous hip operations.

Sciatic nerve palsy (usually due to traction but occasionally caused by direct injury) may occur with any type of arthroplasty but is more common with a posterior approach. Most cases recover spontaneously but if there is reason to suspect nerve damage the area should be explored.

Postoperative dislocation is rare if the prosthetic components are correctly placed. Reduction is easy and traction in abduction usually allows the hip to stabi-

lize. If malposition of the femoral or acetabular component is severe, revision may be needed, or possibly augmentation of the socket.

Heterotopic bone formation around the hip is seen in about 20% of patients 5 years after joint replacement. The cause is unknown, but patients with skeletal hyperostosis and ankylosing spondylitis are particularly at risk. In severe cases this is associated with pain and stiffness. Ossification can be prevented in high-risk patients by giving either a course of non-steroidal anti-inflammatory drugs for 3–6 weeks postoperatively or a single dose of irradiation to the hip.

Aseptic loosening of either the acetabular socket or the femoral stem is the commonest cause of long-term failure. Figures for its incidence vary widely, depending on the criteria used. With modern methods of implant fixation, there is likely to be radiographic evidence of loosening in about 10–20% of patients 10 years after operation; at microscopic level many stable implants show cellular reaction and membrane formation at the bone–cement interface (Linder and Carlsson, 1986). Fortunately, only a fraction of these are symptomatic. Pain may be a feature, especially when first taking weight on the leg after sitting or lying, but the diagnosis usually rests on x-ray signs of progressively increasing radiolucency around the implant, fracturing of cement, movement of the implant or bone resorption (Gruen *et al.*, 1979). Radionuclide scanning shows increased activity, and it is claimed that the pattern of ^{99}Tc-HDP and ^{67}Ga uptake can differentiate between aseptic loosening and infection (Taylor *et al.*, 1989). If symptoms are marked, and particularly if there is evidence of progressive bone resorption, the implant and cement should be painstakingly removed and a new prosthesis

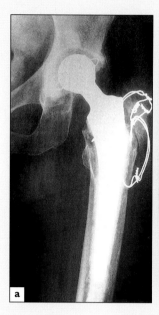
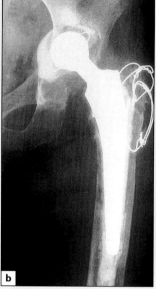
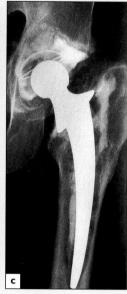

19.63 Hip replacement – loosening (a) Five years after hip replacement there is a distinct radiolucent line around the femoral implant and resorption of the calcar. (b) A year later the x-ray shows fracturing of the cement mantle, tilting of the femoral prosthesis and migration of the acetabular cup. (c) Another case, showing aggressive osteolysis around a cemented femoral stem.

inserted – either cemented or uncemented, depending on the condition of the bone.

Aggressive osteolysis, with or without implant loosening, is sometimes seen. It is associated with granuloma formation at the interface between cement (or implant) and bone. This may be due to a severe histiocyte reaction stimulated by cement, polyethylene or metal particles that find their way into the boundary zone. Revision is usually necessary and this may have to be accompanied by impaction grafting with morsellized bone.

Infection is the most serious postoperative complication. With adequate prophylaxis the risk should be less than 1%, but it is higher in the very old, in patients with rheumatoid disease or psoriasis, and in those on immunosuppressive therapy (including corticosteroids).

The large bulk of foreign material restricts the access of the body's normal defence mechanisms; consequently, even slight wound contamination may be serious. Organisms may multiply in the postoperative haematoma to cause early infection, and, even many years later, haematogenous spread from a distant site may cause late infection.

Early wound infection sometimes responds to antibiotics. Later infection does so less often and may need operative 'debridement' followed by irrigation with antibiotic solution for 3–4 weeks. Once the infection has cleared, a new prosthesis can be inserted, preferably without cement. An alternative, more applicable to 'mild' or 'dubious' infection, is a one-stage exchange arthroplasty using gentamicin-impregnated cement. The results of revision arthroplasty for infection are only moderately good (Goodman and Schurman, 1988). If all else fails the prosthesis and cement may have to be removed, leaving an excisional (Girdlestone) arthroplasty.

RESULTS The success rate of primary total hip replacement is now so high that only with a prolonged follow-up of a large number of cases can we evaluate the relative merits of different models (Johnston *et al.*, 1990). It is important to compare like with like; present-day cementing (and non-cementing) techniques are far superior to those of only a decade ago and implant survival rates of more than 95% at 10 years are being reported.

NOTES ON APPLIED ANATOMY

The ball-and-socket arrangement of the hip combines stability for weightbearing with freedom of movement for locomotion. A deeper acetabulum would confer greater stability, but would limit the range of movement. Even with the fibrocartilaginous labrum the socket is not deep enough to accommodate the whole of the femoral head, whose articular surface extends considerably beyond a hemisphere.

The opening of the acetabulum faces downwards and forwards (about 30° in each direction); the neck of the femur points upwards and forwards. Consequently, in the neutral position, the anterior portion of the head is not 'contained'. The amount of forward inclination of the neck relative to the shaft (the angle of anteversion) varies from 10 to 30° in the adult. The upward inclination of the neck is such that the neck–shaft angle is 125°.

A neck–shaft angle of less than 125° is referred to as 'coxa vara' because, were the neck normally aligned relative to the pelvis, the limb would be deviated towards the midline of the body – in varus; a neck–shaft angle greater than 125° (i.e. with the neck unduly vertical) is coxa valga. The angle is mechanically important because the further away the abductor muscles are from the hip, the greater is their leverage and their efficiency.

During standing and walking, the femoral neck acts as a cantilever; the line of body weight passes medial to the hip joint and is balanced laterally by the abductors (especially gluteus medius). The combination of body weight, leverage effect and muscle action means that the resultant force transmitted through the femoral head can be very great - about five times the body weight when walking slowly and much more when running or jumping. It is easy to see why the hip is so liable to suffer from cartilage failure – the essential feature of osteoarthritis.

The ligaments of the hip, though very strong in front, are weak posteriorly; consequently, posterior dislocation is much more common than anterior. When the hip is adducted and medially rotated it is particularly vulnerable, and when this position results from unbalanced paralysis the hip can slip unobtrusively out of position.

During the swing phase of walking not only does the hip flex, it also rotates; this is because the pelvis swivels forwards. As weight comes onto the leg, the abductor muscles contract, causing the pelvis to tilt downwards on the weightbearing side; it is failure of this abductor mechanism which causes the Trendelenburg lurch.

The femoral head receives its arterial blood supply from three sources: (1) intraosseous vessels running up the neck, which are inevitably damaged with a displaced cervical fracture; (2) vessels in the retinacula reflected from capsule to neck, which may be damaged in a fracture or compressed by an effusion; and (3) vessels in the ligamentum teres, which are undeveloped in the early years of life and even later convey only a meagre blood supply. The relative importance of these vessels varies with age, but at all ages avascular necrosis is a potential hazard.

The nerve supply of the hip, unlike the blood supply, is plentiful. Sensory fibres, conveying proprioception as well as pain, abound in the capsule and ligaments. But the venous sinusoids of the bones also are supplied with sensory fibres; a rise in the intraosseous venous pressure accounts for some of the pain in osteoarthritis, and a reduction of this pressure for some of the relief which may follow osteotomy.

The tensor fascia femoris, though a relatively small muscle, has, through its action in tightening the iliotibial tract, a surprisingly large range of functions. This tract is anterior to the axis of knee flexion when the knee is straight, so its tension helps to hold the knee slightly hyperextended while standing. It is also important in getting up from the sitting position, as well as during the phases of walking and running when weight is being taken on the slightly flexed knee.

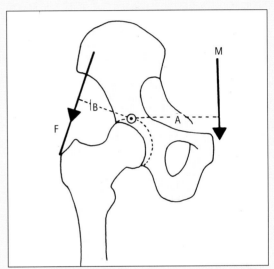

19.64 Forces around the hip When standing on one leg the pelvis is balanced on the femoral head. The vertical force due to the body weight (M) is counterbalanced by contraction of the lateral muscles (F). The force borne by the femoral head is produced by the combined moments M × A and F × B.

REFERENCES AND FURTHER READING

Baber YF, Robinson AHN, Villar RN (1999) Is diagnostic arthroscopy of the hip worthwhile? *Journal of Bone and Joint Surgery* **81B**, 600-603

Catterall A (1982) *Legg-Calve-Perthes Disease.* Churchill Livingstone, Edinburgh

Catterall A (1992) Assessment of adolescent acetabular dysplasia. In *Recent Advances in Orthopaedics – 6* (ed Catterall A). Churchill Livingstone, Edinburgh

Charnley Sir J (1979) *Low Friction Arthroplasty of the Hip.* Springer, Berlin, Heidelberg and New York

Dunn DM, Angel JC (1978) Replacement of the femoral head by open operation in severe adolescent slipping of the upper femoral epiphysis. *Journal of Bone and Joint Surgery* **60B**, 394-403

Engh CA, Bobyn JD, Glassman AH (1987) Porous-coated hip replacement: the factors governing bone ingrowth, stress shielding and clinical results. *Journal of Bone and Joint Surgery* **69B**, 45-55

Fowler JL, Gie GA, Lee AJC, Ling RSM (1988) Experience with the Exeter total hip since 1970. *Orthopedic Clinics of North America* **19**, 477-489

Ganz R, Klaue K, Mast J *et al* (1998) Periacetabular osteotomy. In *Hip Surgery – Materials and Developments* (eds Sedel L, Cabanela ME). Martin Dunitz, London

Geesink RGT (1990) Hydroxy-apatite-coated total hip prostheses. *Clinical Orthopaedics and Related Research* **261**, 39–58

Glueck CJ, Crawford A, Roy D *et al* (1996) Association by antithrombotic factor deficiencies and hypofibrinolysis with Legg–Perthes disease. *Journal of Bone and Joint Surgery* **78A**, 3–13

Goodman SB, Schurman DJ (1988) Outcome of infected total hip arthroplasty: an inclusive, consecutive series. *Journal of Arthroplasty* **3**, 97–102

Griffith MJ (1976) Slipping of the capital femoral epiphysis. *Annals of the Royal College of Surgeons of England* **58**, 34–42

Gruen TA, McNeice GM, Amstutz HC (1979) 'Modes of failure' of cemented stem-type femoral components. *Clinical Orthopaedics and Related Research* **141**, 17–27

Harcke T, Kumar J (1991) The role of ultrasound in the diagnosis and management of congenital dislocation and dysplasia of the hip. *Journal of Bone and Joint Surgery* **73A**, 622–628

Herring JA (1994) The treatment of Legg–Calve–Perthes' disease. *Journal of Bone and Joint Surgery* **76A**, 448–458

Johnston RC, Fitzgerald RH, Harris WH *et al* (1990) Clinical and radiographic evaluation of total hip replacement. *Journal of Bone and Joint Surgery* **72A**, 161–168

Jones DA (1994) Principles of screening and congenital dislocation of the hip. *Annals of the Royal College of Surgeons of England* **76**, 245–250

Kim Y-M, Ahn JH, Kang HS *et al* (1998) Estimation of the extent of osteonecrosis of the femoral head using MRI. *Journal of Bone and Joint Surgery* **80B**, 954–958

Klisic P, Jankovic L (1976) Combined procedure of open reduction and shortening of the femur in treatment of congenital dislocation of the hip in older children. *Clinical Orthopaedics and Related Research* **119**, 60–69

Lidwell OM, Lowbury EJL, Whyte W *et al* (1984) Infection and sepsis after operations for total hip or knee joint replacement: influence of ultraclean air, prophylactic antibiotics and other factors. *Journal of Hygiene (Camb)* **83**, 505–529

Liesner RJ (1999) Editorial: Does thrombophilia cause Perthes' disease in children? *Journal of Bone and Joint Surgery* **81B**, 565–566

Lin S-L, Ho T-C (1991) The role of venous hypertension in the pathogenesis of Legg–Perthes disease. *Journal of Bone and Joint Surgery* **73A**, 194–200

Linder L, Carlsson AS (1986) The bone–cement interface in hip arthroplasty: a histologic and enzyme study of stable components. *Acta Orthopaedica Scandinavica* **57**, 495–500

Marotte JH, Lord GA, Blanchard JP *et al* (1987) Infection rate in total hip arthroplasty as a function of air cleanliness and antibiotic prophylaxis. *Journal of Arthroplasty* **2**, 77–82

Riley PM, Weiner DS, Akron RG (1990) Hazards of internal fixation in the treatment of slipped capital femoral epiphysis. *Journal of Bone and Joint Surgery* **72A**, 1500–1509

Sakamoto M, Shimuzu K, Iida S *et al* (1997) Osteonecrosis of the femoral head. A prospective study with MRI. *Journal of Bone and Joint Surgery* **79B**, 213–219

Shimuzu K, Moriya H, Akita T *et al* (1994) Prediction of collapse with magnetic resonance imaging of avascular necrosis of the femoral head. *Journal of Bone and Joint Surgery* **76A**, 215–223

Simmons ED, Graham HK, Szalai JP (1990) Interobserver variability in grading Perthes' disease. *Journal of Bone and Joint Surgery* **72B**, 202–204

Solomon L (1998) Arthrodesis – is there still an indication? In *Hip Surgery – Materials and Developments* (eds Sedel L, Cabanela ME). Martin Dunitz, London

Solomon L, Pearse MF (1994) Osteonecrosis following low-dose short-course corticosteroids. *Journal of Orthopaedic Rheumatology* **7**, 203–205

Sugioka Y, Mohtai M (1998) Osteonecrosis of the femoral head: a conservative surgical solution. In *Hip Surgery – Materials and Developments* (eds Sedel L, Cabanela ME). Martin Dunitz, London

Taylor DN, Maughan J, Patel MP, Clegg J (1989) A simple method of identifying loosening or infection of hip prostheses in nuclear medicine. *Nuclear Medicine Communications* **10**, 551–556

Tooke SMT, Amstutz HC, Hedley AK (1987) Results of transtrochanteric rotational osteotomy for femoral head osteonecrosis. *Clinical Orthopaedics and Related Research* **224**, 150–157

Werners R, Vincent B, Bulstrode C (1990) Osteotomy for osteoarthritis of the hip. *Journal of Bone and Joint Surgery* **72B**, 1010–1013

Wynne-Davies R (1970) Acetabular dysplasia and familial joint laxity: two aetiological factors in congenital dislocation of the hip. *Journal of Bone and Joint Surgery* **52B**, 704–716

Yamamuro T, Ishida. (1984) Recent advances in the prevention, early diagnosis and treatment of congenital dislocation of the hip in Japan. *Clinical Orthopaedics and Related Research* **184**, 34–40

The knee

CLINICAL ASSESSMENT

SYMPTOMS

Pain is the most common knee symptom. With inflammatory or degenerative disorders it is usually diffuse, but with mechanical disorders and especially after injury it is often localized – the patient can, and should, point to the painful spot. If the patient can describe the mechanism of the injury, this is extremely useful: a direct blow to the front of the knee may damage the patellofemoral joint; a blow to the side may rupture the collateral ligament; twisting injuries are more likely to cause a torn meniscus or a cruciate ligament rupture.

Stiffness must be distinguished from inhibition of movement due to pain. Post-inactivity stiffness suggests arthritis.

Locking is different from stiffness. The knee, quite suddenly, cannot be straightened fully, although flexion is still possible. This happens when a torn meniscus or loose body is caught between the articular surfaces. By wiggling the knee around, the patient may be able to 'unlock' it; sudden unlocking is reliable evidence that something mobile had previously obstructed full extension.

Deformity (knock knees or bandy legs) is common but, in itself, seldom troublesome. Unilateral deformity, especially if it is progressive, is more significant.

Swelling may be localized or diffuse. If there was an injury, it is important to ask whether the swelling appeared immediately (suggesting a haemarthrosis) or only after some hours (typical of a torn meniscus).

Giving way suggests a mechanical disorder, although it can result from muscle weakness; when it occurs particularly on stairs, the patellofemoral joint is suspect.

Limp may be due to either pain or instability.

SIGNS WITH THE PATIENT UPRIGHT

Valgus or varus deformity is best seen with the patient standing and bearing weight. Then he or she should be observed walking: in the stance phase note whether the knee extends fully and if there is any lateral instability; in the swing phase note whether the knee moves freely or is held rigid (usually because of patellofemoral pain).

SIGNS WITH THE PATIENT LYING SUPINE

Look

The colour of the *skin* and any sinuses or scars are noted.

Wasting of the quadriceps is a sure sign of joint disorder. The visual impression can be checked by measuring the girth of the thigh at the same level (e.g. a certain distance above the joint line) in each limb.

Swelling of the knee and *lumps* around the joint are observed; the shape of the patella is compared with that of the opposite knee.

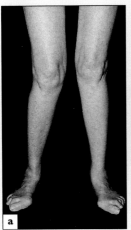
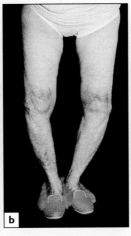
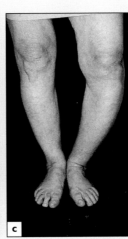

20.1 Examination – standing (a) Valgus deformity in a patient with rheumatoid arthritis. (b) Bilateral varus deformities due to osteoarthritis. (c) Is the deformity in the joint or in the tibia? This patient has Paget's disease of the left tibia.

Note the *position* of the knee; it may lie in valgus or varus, partially flexed or hyperextended. The position of the patella should also be noted.

Feel

Increased *warmth* is detected by comparing the two knees. The 'temperature gradient' is assessed by running a hand down the length of the limb; normally there is a linear decrease in warmth from proximal to distal.

Check for *intra-articular fluid*. There are four useful tests. (1) Cross-fluctuation: the left hand compresses and empties the suprapatellar pouch while the right hand straddles the front of the joint below the patella; by squeezing with each hand alternately, a fluid impulse is transmitted across the joint. (2) The patellar tap: again the suprapatellar pouch is compressed with the left hand, while the index finger of the right pushes the patella sharply backwards; with a positive test the patella can be felt striking the femur and bouncing off again. (3) The bulge test: this is useful when very little fluid is present. The medial compartment is emptied by pressing on that side of the joint; the hand is then lifted away and the lateral side is sharply compressed; a distinct ripple is seen on the flattened medial surface. (4) The patellar hollow test: when the normal knee is flexed, a hollow appears lateral to the patellar ligament and disappears with further flexion; with excess fluid the hollow fills and disappears at a lesser angle of flexion (Mann *et al.*, 1991).

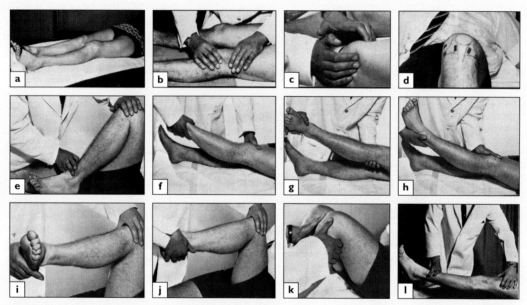

20.2 Examination – supine (**a**) Looking at both knees – the left is swollen and the thigh wasted; (**b**) testing for fluid by cross-fluctuation; (**c**) feeling for synovial thickening; (**d**) the points which should be palpated for tenderness. Testing movements: (**e**) flexion, (**f**) extension, (**g**) abduction, (**h**) adduction. Lateral rotation (**i**), medial rotation (**j**) and anteroposterior glide (**k**) are tested with the knee bent; (**l**) testing quadriceps power.

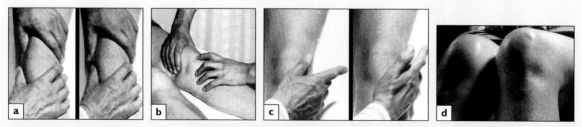

20.3 Tests for fluid (**a**) Cross-fluctuation, the easiest test for large quantities of fluid. (**b**) The patellar tap, most likely to be positive with a moderate amount of fluid. (**c**) The bulge test detects small quantities of fluid. (**d**) The patellar hollow test – noting at what angle the hollow lateral to the patellar ligament disappears, as compared with the normal side – a very reliable test of even very small quantities of fluid.

The soft tissues and bony outlines are then palpated systematically, feeling for thickening and localized tenderness. This is done first with the knee in extension and then flexed to 90°; in flexion the joint line can be felt more easily. The undersurface of the patella is also accessible if the bone is pushed first to one side and then to the other. Synovial thickening is best appreciated as follows: placing the knee in extension, the examiner grasps the edges of the patella in a pincer made of the thumb and middle finger, and tries to lift the patella forwards; normally the bone can be grasped quite firmly, but if the synovium is thickened the fingers simply slip off the edges of the patella.

Move

Flexion and extension Full extension is assessed by pressing the thigh against the couch and trying to lift the leg. Then flexion is tested. Normally the knee flexes until the calf meets the ham, and extends completely with a snap; even slight loss of extension or 'springiness' on attempting it, is important. The range of flexion is recorded in degrees and any hyperextension as a minus quantity.

Crepitus during movement may be felt with a hand placed on the front of the knee. It usually signifies patellofemoral roughness.

Movement with compartmental loading The medial or lateral compartment of the knee can be loaded separately during movement by applying varus or valgus stress during flexion. Pain with this manoeuvre suggests articular cartilage softening in one or other compartment. Cartilage is, of course, insensitive and the pain is probably due to pressure on the subarticular bone.

Rotation The patient's hip and knee are flexed to 90°; one hand steadies and feels the knee, the other rotates the foot. The normal range of internal and external rotation is about 10°.

TESTS FOR STABILITY

In testing for stability it is essential to compare the normal with the abnormal knee.

The collateral ligaments The medial and lateral ligaments are tested by stressing the knee into valgus and varus: this is best done by tucking the patient's foot under your arm and holding the extended knee firmly with one hand on each side of the joint; the leg is then angulated alternately towards abduction and adduction. The test is performed at full extension and again at 30° of flexion. There is normally some mediolateral movement at 30°, but if this is excessive

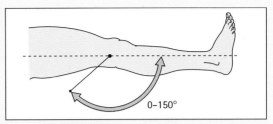

20.4 Normal range of movements Full extension is recorded as 0°. Flexion is usually from 0 to about 150°.

(compared to the normal side) it suggests a torn or stretched collateral ligament. Sideways movement in full extension is always abnormal; it may be due to either (1) torn or stretched ligaments and capsule or (2) loss of articular cartilage or bone, which allows the affected compartment to collapse.

The cruciate ligaments Routine tests for cruciate ligament stability are based on examining for abnormal gliding movements in the sagittal plane. With both knees flexed 90° and the feet resting on the couch, the upper tibia is inspected from the side; if its upper end has dropped back, or can be gently pushed back, this indicates a tear of the posterior cruciate ligament (the 'sag sign'). With the knee in the same position, the foot is anchored by the examiner sitting on it (provided this is not painful); then, using both hands, the upper end of the tibia is grasped firmly and rocked backwards and forwards to see if there is any anteroposterior glide (the *'drawer test'*). Excessive anterior movement (a positive anterior drawer sign) denotes anterior cruciate laxity; excessive posterior movements (a positive posterior drawer sign) signifies posterior cruciate laxity.

More sensitive is the *Lachman test* – but this is difficult if the patient has big thighs (or the examiner has small hands). The patient's knee is flexed 20 degrees; with one hand grasping the lower thigh and the other the upper part of the leg, the joint surfaces are shifted backwards and forwards upon each other. If the knee is stable, there should be no gliding.

In both the drawer test and Lachman test, note whether the end-point of abnormal movement is 'soft' or 'hard'.

Special tests for stability When only a collateral or cruciate ligament is damaged the diagnosis is relatively easy: the direction of unstable movement is either sideways or front-to-back. With combined injuries the direction of instability may be oblique or rotational. Special clinical tests have been developed to detect these abnormalities; they are described in the section on chronic post-traumatic instability on page 706.

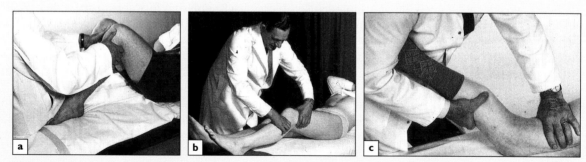

20.5 Tests for sideways instability Two ways of testing for collateral ligament laxity. (**a, b**) By stressing first the lateral, then the medial side of the knee, it was easy to see that this patient had medial laxity. (**c**) If the surgeon holds the leg between his arm and his chest he can impart valgus and varus stresses and, with his hands, detect any knee laxity with precision.

20.6 Testing for anteroposterior instability Cruciate laxity can be tested with the knee at 90° as shown in (**a**); the leg can be stabilized by sitting on the patient's foot, and the fingers ensure that the hamstrings are relaxed. The leg is alternately tugged forwards and pushed backwards. (**b**) More reliable is Lachman's test: with the knee at 20–30° the leg and thigh are grasped firmly and moved in opposite directions. (**c**) The Lachman test is sometimes better performed with the patient prone; one hand stabilizes the thigh, the other moves the tibia.

McMurray's test

This is the classic test for a torn meniscus and is based on the fact that the loose tag can sometimes be trapped between the articular surfaces and then induced to snap free with a palpable and audible click. The knee is flexed as far as possible; one hand steadies the joint and the other rotates the leg medially and laterally while the knee is slowly extended. The test is repeated several times, with the knee stressed in valgus or varus, feeling and listening for the click.

A positive test is helpful but not pathognomonic; a negative test does not exclude a tear.

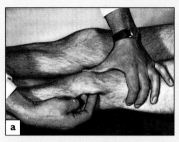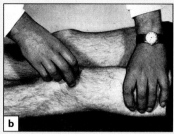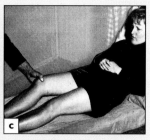

20.7 Examination of patella (**a**) Feeling for tenderness behind the patella; (**b**) the patellar friction test; (**c**) the apprehension test.

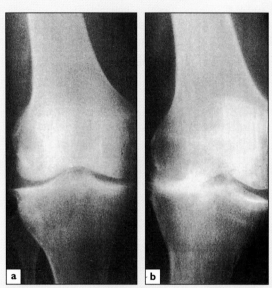

20.8 X-rays These films are of the same knee: (**a**) with the patient lying on the x-ray table, and (**b**) with the patient taking weight on the leg.

THE PATELLOFEMORAL JOINT

The size, shape and position of the patella are noted. The bone is felt, first on its anterior surface and then along its edges and at the attachments of the quadriceps tendon and the patellar ligament. Much of the posterior surface, too, is accessible to palpation if the patella is pushed first to one side and then to the other; tenderness suggests synovial irritation or articular cartilage softening.

Moving the patella up and down while pressing it lightly against the femur (the 'friction test') causes painful grating if the central portion of the articular cartilage is damaged. Pressing the patella laterally with the thumb while flexing the knee slightly may induce anxiety and resistance to further movement; this, the 'apprehension test', is diagnostic of recurrent patellar subluxation or dislocation.

SIGNS WITH THE PATIENT LYING PRONE

Scars or lumps in the popliteal fossa are noted. If there is a swelling, is it in the midline (most likely a bulging capsule) or to one side (possibly a bursa)? A semi-membranous bursa is usually just above the joint line, a Baker's cyst below it.

The popliteal fossa is carefully palpated. If there is a lump, where does it originate? Does it pulsate? Can it be emptied into the joint?

Apley's test The knee is flexed to 90° and rotated while a compression force is applied; this, the grinding test, reproduces symptoms if a meniscus is torn. Rotation is then repeated while the leg is pulled upwards with the surgeon's knee holding the thigh down; this, the distraction test, produces increased pain only if there is ligament damage (Apley, 1947).

Lachman's test can be readily performed with the patient prone.

X-RAYS

Anteroposterior and lateral views are routine; it is often useful also to obtain tangential ('skyline') patellofemoral views and intercondylar (or 'tunnel') views. The anteroposterior view should be taken with the patient standing; unless the femorotibial compartment is loaded, narrowing of the articular space may be missed. Both knees should be x-rayed, so as to compare the abnormal with the normal side.

Tibiofemoral alignment can be measured on full-length standing views. Normal indices have also been established for patellar height and patellofemoral congruence. These features are discussed in the relevant sections of the chapter.

OTHER FORMS OF IMAGING

Radioscintigraphy may show increased activity in the subarticular bone in early osteoarthritis. It is also helpful in showing 'hot spots' due to infection after joint replacement.

Computed tomography (CT) is useful for showing patellofemoral congruence at various angles of flexion.

Magnetic resonance imaging (MRI) is the most helpful method for detecting meniscal and cruciate ligament injuries, or osteochondral lesions.

ARTHROSCOPY

Diagnostic arthroscopy is a useful tool, especially in the knee which, of all the joints, is most accessible. However, a direct 'look inside' is not a substitute for clinical examination; a detailed history and meticulous assessment of the physical signs are indispensable preliminaries and remain the sheet anchor of diagnosis. It is not that arthroscopy fails to disclose what is there; the problem is that it shows too much, and the clinician will still have to decide which of the abnormalities detected (if any!) are the cause of the patient's complaints.

THE DIAGNOSTIC CALENDAR

Depending on the patient's age and the likely diagnosis, different aspects of the examination need to be emphasized.

Adolescents with anterior knee pain are usually found to have chondromalacia patellae, patellar instability, osteochondritis or a plica syndrome. But remember – knee pain may be referred from the hip!

Young adults engaged in sports are the most frequent victims of meniscal tears and ligament injuries. Examination should include a variety of tests for ligamentous instability.

Patients above middle age with chronic pain and stiffness probably have osteoarthritis. With primary osteoarthritis of the knees, other joints also are often affected; polyarthritis does not necessarily (nor even most commonly) mean rheumatoid arthritis.

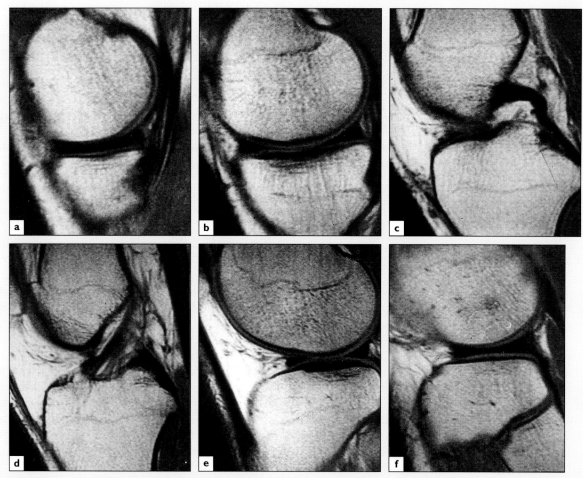

20.9 MRI A series of sagittal T1-weighted images proceeding from medial to lateral to show the normal appearances of (**a, b**) the medial meniscus, (**c**) the posterior cruciate ligament, (**d**) the somewhat fan-shaped anterior cruciate ligament and (**e, f**) the lateral meniscus.

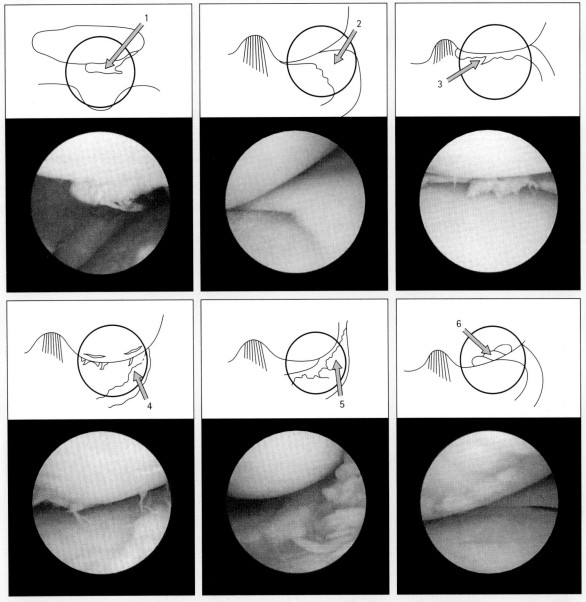

20.10 Arthroscopy In each case the view is of the right knee from the lateral side. (1) Chondromalacia patellae; (2) normal medial meniscus; (3) torn medial meniscus; (4) degenerate medial meniscus and osteoarthritic femoral condyle; (5) rheumatoid synovium; (6) osteochondritis dissecans of medial femoral condyle.

DEFORMITIES OF THE KNEE

By the end of growth the knees are normally in 5–7° of valgus. Any deviation from this may be regarded as 'deformity', though often it bothers no one – least of all the possessor of the knees. The three common deformities are bow leg (genu varum), knock knee (genu valgum) and hyperextension (genu recurvatum).

BOW LEGS AND KNOCK KNEES IN CHILDREN

Deformity is usually gauged from simple observation. Bilateral bow leg can be recorded by measuring the distance between the knees with the child standing and the heels touching; it should be less than 6cm. Similarly, knock knee can be estimated by measuring the distance between the medial malleoli when the knees are touching with the patellae facing forwards; it is usually less than 8cm.

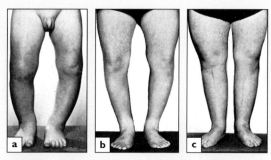

20.11 Bow legs (**a**) Infantile, which usually recovers spontaneously. (**b**) In this older child, deformity persisted and osteotomy was performed (**c**).

Physiological bow legs and knock knees

Bow legs in babies and knock knees in 4-year-olds are so common that they are considered to be *normal stages of development*. Other postural abnormalities such as 'pigeon toes' and flat feet may coexist but these children are normal in all other respects; the parents should be reassured and the child should be seen at intervals of 6 months to record progress.

In the occasional case where, by the age of 10 years, the deformity is still marked (i.e. the intercondylar distance is more than 6cm or the intermalleolar distance more than 8cm), operative correction should be advised. Stapling of the physes on one or other side of the knee can be done to restrict growth on that side and allow correction of the deformity (the staples are removed once the knee has over-corrected slightly); there is a risk, however, that normal growth will not resume when the staples are removed. Similar correction can be obtained by performing a hemi-epiphysodesis (fusion of one-half of the growth plate) on the 'convex' side of the deformity; this requires careful timing guided by charting the child's bone age and estimating the corrective effect of arresting further growth on one side of the bone (Bowen *et al.*, 1985). The alternative is to encourage the child (and the parents) to put up with the 'deformity' until growth is complete and then undergo a corrective osteotomy (supracondylar osteotomy for valgus knees and high tibial osteotomy for varus knees).

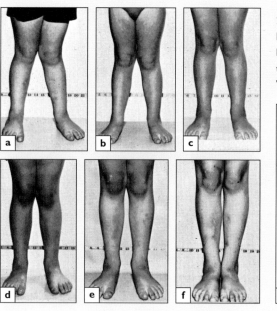

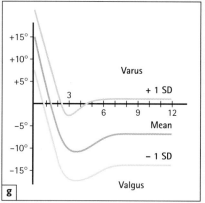

20.12 Genu valgum Idiopathic knock knee – natural history without treatment. Same child at various stages between 3 and 7 years. The graph shows the normal variation in tibiofemoral angle at different ages (after Salenius and Vankka, 1975).

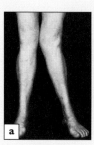
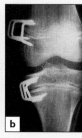
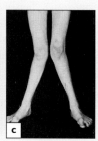
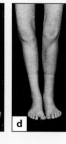

20.13 Persistent genu valgum Only rarely does knock knee persist: (**a, b**) an adolescent treated by stapling; (**c, d**) before and after bilateral osteotomy for severe deformity.

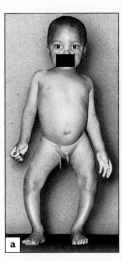
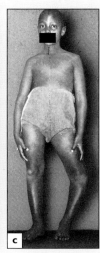
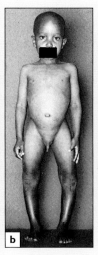
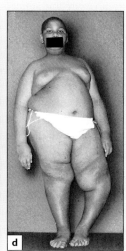

20.14 Bow legs (a) Blount's disease; (b) healed rickets; (c) trauma has damaged the upper tibial epiphysis; (d) this patient has an endocrine disorder and her upper tibial epiphysis has slipped.

Compensatory deformities

Varus, valgus and rotational deformities of the proximal femur may give rise to complex compensatory deformities of the knees and legs once the child starts to walk. Thus persistent anteversion of the femoral neck may come to be associated with 'squinting knees' (the patellae face inwards when the hips are fully located), genu valgum, tibial torsion and valgus heels. It is essential to analyse all components of these deformities before focusing on the knees. Often they correct spontaneously by the end of growth, or if some elements persist, they cause little or no problem; only in severe cases – and after the most meticulous preoperative planning – are osteotomies undertaken.

Pathological bow leg and knock knee

Disorders which cause distorted epiphyseal and/or physeal growth may give rise to bow leg or knock knee; these include some of the skeletal dysplasias and the various types of rickets, as well as injuries of the epiphyseal and physeal growth cartilage. A unilateral deformity is likely to be pathological, but it is essential in all cases to look for signs of injury or generalized skeletal disorder. If angulation is severe, operative correction will be necessary, but it should be deferred until near the end of growth lest the deformity recur with further growth.

BLOUNT'S DISEASE

This is a progressive bow-leg deformity associated with abnormal growth of the posteromedial part of the proximal tibia. The children are usually overweight and start walking early; the condition is bilateral in 80% of

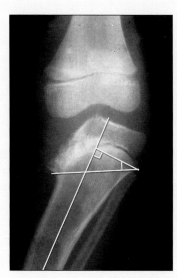

20.15 Blount's disease X-ray showing the typical features of Blount's disease. The metaphyseo-diaphyseal angle is found by drawing one line perpendicular to the axis of the tibia and another across the metaphyseal flare as shown on the x-ray; if it exceeds 11° it is probably abnormal.

cases. Children of negroid descent appear to be affected more frequently than others. Deformity is noticeably worse than in physiological bow legs and may include internal rotation of the tibia (see Fig. 20.14a). The child walks with an outwards thrust of the knee; in the worst cases there may be lateral subluxation of the tibia.

On x-ray the proximal tibial epiphysis is flattened medially and the adjacent metaphysis is beak-shaped. The medial cortex of the proximal tibia appears thickened; this is an illusory effect produced by internal rotation of the tibia. The tibial epiphysis sometimes looks 'fragmented'; occasionally the femoral epiphysis also is affected. In the late stages a bony bar forms across the medial half of the tibial physis, preventing further growth on that side. The degree of proximal tibia vara can be quantified by measuring the metaphyseo-diaphyseal angle (see Fig. 20.15).

Treatment Spontaneous resolution is rare and, once it is clear that the deformity is progressing, a corrective osteotomy should be performed, addressing both the varus and the rotational components. A pre-operative (or per-operative) arthrogram, to outline the misshapen epiphysis, will help in planning the operation. Slight over-correction should be aimed for as some recurrence is inevitable. In severe cases it may be necessary also to elevate the depressed medial tibial plateau. If a bony bar has formed, it may be possible to excise the bar and replace it with a free fat graft. In older children operative correction of the deformity can be combined with an epiphysiodesis, followed (if necessary) by lengthening of the tibia at a later stage. Corrective osteotomies in the proximal tibia should be accompanied by fasciotomy to reduce the risk of a post-operative compartment syndrome.

GENU VARUM AND VALGUM IN ADULTS

Angular deformities are common in adults (usually bow legs in men and knock knees in women). They may be the *sequel to childhood deformity* and if so usually cause no problems. However, if the deformity is associated with joint instability, this can lead to osteoarthritis – of the medial compartment in varus knees and the lateral compartment in valgus knees. Genu valgum may also cause abnormal tracking of the patella and predispose to patellofemoral osteoarthritis. Even in the absence of overt osteoarthritis, if the patient complains of pain, or if there are clinical or radiological signs of joint damage, a 'prophylactic' osteotomy is justified: above the knee for valgus deformity and below the knee for varus.

Deformity may be *secondary to arthritis* – usually varus in osteoarthritis and valgus in rheumatoid arthritis. In these cases the joint is often unstable and corrective osteotomy less predictable in its effect. Stress x-rays are essential in the assessment of these cases.

Other causes of varus or valgus deformity *are ligament injuries, malunited fractures* and *Paget's disease*. Where possible, the underlying disorder should be dealt with; provided the joint is stable, corrective osteotomy may be all that is necessary.

HYPEREXTENSION OF THE KNEE (GENU RECURVATUM)

Congenital recurvatum This may be due to abnormal intra-uterine posture; it usually recovers spontaneously. Rarely, gross hyperextension is the precursor of true congenital dislocation of the knee.

Lax ligaments Normal people with generalized joint laxity tend to stand with their knees back-set. Prolonged traction, especially on a frame, or holding the knee hyperextended in plaster, may overstretch ligaments, leading to permanent hyperextension deformity.

Ligaments may also become overstretched following chronic or recurrent synovitis (especially in rheumatoid arthritis), the hypotonia of rickets, the flailness of poliomyelitis or the insensitivity of Charcot's disease.

In paralytic conditions such as poliomyelitis, recurvatum is often seen in association with fixed equinus of the ankle and foot: in order to set the foot flat on the ground, the knee is forced into hyperextension. In moderate degrees, this may actually be helpful (e.g. in stabilizing a knee with weak extensors). However, if excessive and prolonged, it may give rise to a permanent deformity. If bony correction is undertaken, the knee should be left with some hyperextension to preserve the stabilizing mechanism. If quadriceps power is poor, the patient may need a caliper. Severe paralytic hyperextension can be treated by fixing the patella into the tibial plateau, where it acts as a bone block (Hong-Xue Men *et al.,* 1991).

Other causes of recurvatum are *growth plate injuries* and *malunited fractures*. These can be safely corrected by osteotomy.

MENISCUS LESIONS

The menisci have an important role in (1) improving articular congruency and increasing the stability of the knee, (2) controlling the complex rolling and gliding actions of the joint and (3) distributing load during movement. During weightbearing, at least 50% of the contact stresses are taken by the menisci when the knee is loaded in extension, rising to almost 90% with the knee in flexion. If the menisci are removed, articular stresses are markedly increased; even a partial meniscectomy of one-third of the width of the meniscus will produce a three-fold increase in contact stress in that area.

The medial meniscus is much less mobile than the lateral, and it cannot as easily accommodate to abnormal stresses. This may be why meniscal lesions are more common on the medial side than on the lateral.

Even in the absence of injury, there is gradual stiffening and degeneration of the menisci with age, so splits and tears are more likely in later life – particularly if there is any associated arthritis or chondrocalcinosis. In young people, meniscal tears are usually the result of trauma.

TEARS OF THE MENISCUS

The meniscus consists mainly of circumferential fibres held by a few radial strands. It is, therefore, more likely to tear along its length than across its width. The split is usually initiated by a rotational grinding force, which occurs (for example) when the knee is flexed and twisted while taking weight; hence the frequency in footballers. In middle life, when fibrosis has restricted mobility of the meniscus, tears occur with relatively little force.

Pathology

The medial meniscus is affected far more frequently than the lateral, partly because its attachments to the capsule make it less mobile. Tears of both menisci may occur with severe ligament injuries.

In 75% of cases the split *is vertical* in the length of the meniscus. If the separated fragment remains attached front and back, the lesion is called a *bucket-handle tear*. The torn portion sometimes displaces towards the centre of the joint and becomes jammed between femur and tibia, causing a block to extension ('locking'). If the tear emerges at the free edge of the meniscus, it leaves a tongue based anteriorly (*an anterior horn tear)* or posteriorly (a *posterior horn tear*).

Horizontal tears are usually 'degenerative' or due to repetitive minor trauma. Some are associated with meniscal cysts (see below).

Most of the meniscus is avascular and spontaneous repair does not occur unless the tear is in the outer third, which is vascularized from the attached synovium and capsule. The loose tag acts as a mechanical irritant, giving rise to recurrent synovial effusion and, in some cases, secondary osteoarthritis.

Clinical features

The patient is usually a young person who sustains a twisting injury to the knee on the sports field. Pain (usually on the medial side) is often severe and further activity is avoided; occasionally the knee is 'locked' in partial flexion. Almost invariably, swelling appears some hours later, or perhaps the following day.

With rest the initial symptoms subside, only to recur periodically after trivial twists or strains. Sometimes the knee gives way spontaneously and this is again followed by pain and swelling.

It is important to remember that in patients aged over 40 years the initial injury may be unremarkable and the main complaint is of recurrent 'giving way' or 'locking'.

'Locking' – that is, the sudden inability to extend the knee fully – suggests a bucket-handle tear. The patient sometimes learns to 'unlock' the knee by bending it fully or by twisting it from side to side.

On examination the joint may be held slightly flexed and there is often an effusion. In long-standing cases the quadriceps will be wasted. Tenderness is localized to the joint line, in the vast majority of cases on the medial side. Flexion is usually full but extension is often slightly limited.

Between attacks of pain and effusion there is a disconcerting paucity of signs. The history is helpful, and McMurray's test or Apley's grinding test may be positive.

Investigations

Plain x-rays are usually normal. *MRI* is the most reliable method of confirming the diagnosis, and may even reveal tears that are missed by arthroscopy (Fig. 20.18).

Arthroscopy has the advantage that, if a lesion is identified, it can be treated at the same time.

Differential diagnosis

Loose bodies in the joint may cause true locking. The history is much more insidious than with meniscal tears and the attacks are variable in character and intensity. A loose body may be palpable and is often visible on x-ray.

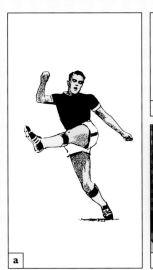
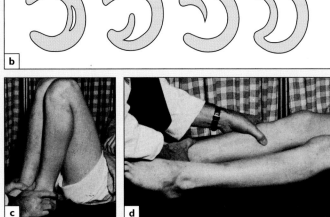

20.16 Torn medial meniscus (a) The meniscus is torn by a twisting force with the knee bent and taking weight; **(b)** the initial split may extend anteriorly and posteriorly; **(c)** a locked knee flexes fully but **(d)** lacks full extension.

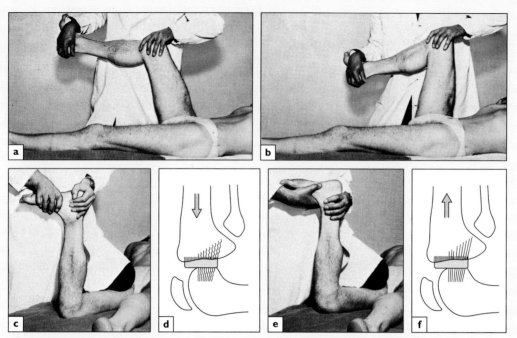

20.17 Torn medial meniscus – tests (**a, b**) McMurray's test is performed at varying angles of flexion. (**c, d**) The grinding test relaxes the ligaments but compresses the meniscus – it causes pain with meniscus lesions. (**e, f**) The distraction test releases the meniscus but stretches the ligaments and causes pain if these are injured.

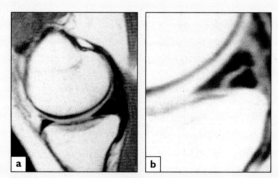

20.18 Torn meniscus – MRI (**a**) Sagittal proton density sequence showing a horizontal tear of the posterior horn of the medial meniscus. (**b**) Enlarged image on 'meniscal window' setting. This type of tear is easily missed on arthroscopy.

meniscus, so that the meniscus loses mobility. The patient complains of recurrent attacks of pain and giving way, followed by tenderness on the medial side. Sleep may be disturbed if the medial side rests upon the other knee or the bed. As with a meniscus injury, rotation is painful; but unlike a meniscus lesion, the grinding test gives less pain and the distraction test more pain.

A torn anterior cruciate ligament can cause chronic instability, with a sense of the knee 'giving way' or buckling when the patient turns sharply towards the side of the affected knee. Careful examination should reveal signs of rotational instability, a positive Lachman test or a positive anterior drawer sign. MRI or arthroscopy will settle any doubts.

Treatment

Recurrent dislocation of the patella causes the knee to give way; typically the patient is caught unawares and collapses to the ground. Tenderness is localized to the medial edge of the patella and the apprehension test is positive.

Fracture of the tibial spine follows an acute injury and may cause a block to full extension. However, swelling is immediate and the fluid is blood-stained. X-ray may show the fracture.

A partial tear of the medial collateral ligament may heal with adhesions where it is attached to the medial

Dealing with the locked knee Usually the knee 'unlocks' spontaneously; if not, gentle passive flexion and rotation may do the trick. Forceful manipulation is unwise (it may do more damage) and is usually unnecessary; after a few days' rest the knee may well unlock itself. However, if the knee does not unlock, or if attempts to unlock it cause severe pain, arthroscopy is indicated. If symptoms are not marked, it may be better to wait a week or two and let the synovitis settle down, thus making the operation easier; if the tear is confirmed, the offending fragment is removed.

Conservative treatment If the joint is not locked, it is reasonable to hope that the tear is peripheral and can therefore heal spontaneously. After an acute episode, the joint is held straight in a plaster backslab for 3–4 weeks; the patient uses crutches and quadriceps exercises are encouraged. Operation can be put off as long as attacks are infrequent and not disabling and the patient is willing to abandon those activities that provoke them. MRI will show if the meniscus has healed.

Operative treatment Surgery is indicated (1) if the joint cannot be unlocked and (2) if symptoms are recurrent. For practical purposes, the lesion is usually dealt with as part of the 'diagnostic' arthroscopy. Tears close to the periphery, which have the capacity to heal, can be sutured; at least one edge of the tear should be red (i.e. vascularized). In appropriate cases the success rate for both open and arthroscopic repair is almost 90%.

Tears other than those in the peripheral third are dealt with by excising the torn portion (or the bucket handle). Total meniscectomy is thought to cause more instability and so predispose to late secondary osteoarthritis; certainly in the short term it causes greater morbidity than partial meniscectomy and has no obvious advantages.

Arthroscopic meniscectomy has distinct advantages over open meniscectomy: shorter hospital stay, lower costs and more rapid return to function. However, it is by no means free of complications (Sherman *et al.*, 1986).

Post-operative pain and stiffness are reduced by prophylactic non-steroidal anti-inflammatory drugs. Quadriceps-strengthening exercises are important.

Outcome

Neither a meniscal tear by itself nor removal of the meniscus necessarily leads to secondary osteoarthritis. The likelihood is increased if the patient has a tendency to generalized osteoarthritis and even more so if, because of associated injuries or as a consequence of any operation, the knee becomes unstable.

MENISCAL DEGENERATION

Patients over 45 years old may present with symptoms and signs of a meniscal tear. Often, though, they can recall no preceding injury. At arthroscopy there may be a horizontal cleavage in the medial meniscus – the characteristic 'degenerative' lesion – or detachment of the anterior or posterior horn without an obvious tear. Associated osteoarthritis or chrondrocalcinosis is common.

A detached anterior or posterior horn can be sutured firmly in place. Meniscectomy is indicated only if symptoms are marked or if, at arthroscopy, there is a major tear.

DISCOID LATERAL MENISCUS

In the fetus the meniscus is not semilunar but disc-like; if this shape persists, symptoms are likely. A young patient complains that, without any history of injury, the knee gives way and 'thuds' loudly. A characteristic clunk may be felt at 110° as the knee is bent and at 10° as it is being straightened. The diagnosis is easily confirmed by MRI.

If there is only a clunk, treatment is not essential. If pain is disturbing, the meniscus may be excised, though a more attractive procedure is arthroscopic partial excision leaving a normally shaped meniscus (Dimakopoulos and Patel, 1990).

MENISCAL CYSTS

Cysts of the menisci are probably traumatic in origin, arising from either a small horizontal cleavage tear or repeated squashing of the peripheral part of the meniscus.

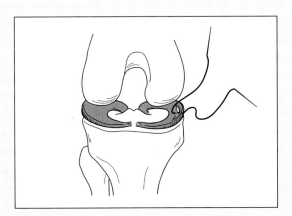

20.19 Meniscal repair Repair is appropriate if at least one edge of the tear is vascularized. This can be done arthroscopically.

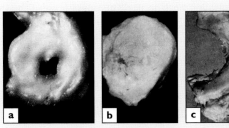

20.20 Other meniscus lesions Whereas tears are much more common on the medial side, discoid meniscus and cysts are much more common on the lateral. **(a)** Partial and **(b)** complete discoid lateral meniscus. **(c)** Cyst of lateral meniscus.

It is also suggested that synovial cells infiltrate into the vascular area between meniscus and capsule and there multiply. The multilocular cyst contains gelatinous fluid and is surrounded by thick fibrous tissue.

Clinical features

The lateral meniscus is affected much more frequently than the medial. The patient complains of an ache or a small lump at the side of the joint. Symptoms may be intermittent, or worse after activity.

On examination the lump is situated at or slightly below the joint line, usually anterior to the collateral ligament. It is seen most easily with the knee slightly flexed; in some positions it may disappear altogether. Lateral cysts are often so firm that they are mistaken for a solid swelling. Medial cysts are usually larger and softer.

Differential diagnosis

Apart from cysts, various conditions may present with a small lump along the joint line.

A *ganglion* is quite superficial, usually not as 'hard' as a cyst, and unconnected with the joint.

Calcific deposits in the collateral ligament usually appear on the medial side, are intensely painful and tender, and often show on the x-ray.

A *prolapsed, torn meniscus* occasionally presents as a rubbery, irregular lump at the joint line. In some cases the distinction from a 'cyst' is largely academic.

Various tumours, both of soft tissue (lipoma, fibroma) and of bone (osteochondroma), may produce a medial or lateral joint lump. Careful examination will show that the lump does not arise from the joint itself.

Treatment

If the symptoms warrant operation, the cyst may be removed. In the past this was usually combined with total meniscectomy, in order to prevent an inevitable recurrence of the cyst. However, it is quite feasible to examine the meniscus by arthroscopy, remove only the torn or damaged portion and then decompress the cyst from within the joint. The recurrence rate following such arthroscopic surgery is negligible (Parisien, 1990).

CHRONIC LIGAMENTOUS INSTABILITY

The knee is a complex hinge which depends heavily on its ligaments for mediolateral, anteroposterior and rotational stability. Ligament injuries, from minor strains through partial ruptures to complete tears, are common

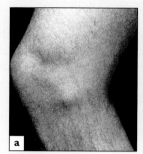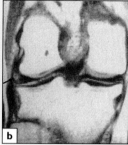

20.21 Meniscal cyst (a) The tense swelling just below the midline. **(b)** MRI showing the cyst arising from the edge of the lateral meniscus.

in sportsmen, athletes and dancers. Whatever the nature of the acute injury, the victim may be left with chronic instability of the knee – a sense of the joint wanting to give way, or actually giving way, during unguarded activity. Sometimes this is accompanied by pain and recurrent episodes of swelling. There may be a meniscal tear, but meniscectomy is likely to make matters worse; sometimes patients present with meniscectomy scars on both sides of the knee!

Examination should include special tests for ligamentous instability as well as radiological investigation and arthroscopy. It is important not only to establish the nature of the lesion but also to measure the level of functional impairment against the needs and demands of the individual patient before advocating treatment.

The subject is dealt with in detail in Chapter 30.

RECURRENT DISLOCATION OF THE PATELLA

Acute dislocation of the patella is dealt with on page 717. In 15–20% of cases (mostly children) the first episode is followed by recurrent dislocation or subluxation after minimal stress. This is due, in some measure, to disruption or stretching of the ligamentous structures which normally stabilize the extensor mechanism. However, in a significant proportion of cases there is no history of an acute strain and the initial episode is thought to have occurred 'spontaneously'. It is now recognized that in all cases of recurrent dislocation, but particularly in the latter group, one or more *predisposing factors* are often present: (1) generalized ligamentous laxity; (2) underdevelopment of the lateral femoral condyle and flattening of the intercondylar groove; (3) maldevelopment of the patella, which may be too high or too small; (4) valgus deformity of the knee; (5) external tibial torsion; or (6) a primary muscle defect.

Repeated dislocation damages the contiguous articular surfaces of the patella and femoral condyle; this may result in further flattening of the condyle, so facilitating further dislocations.

Dislocation is almost always towards the lateral side; medial dislocation is seen only in rare iatrogenic cases following overzealous lateral release or medial transposition of the patellar tendon.

Clinical features

Girls are affected more commonly than boys and the condition may be bilateral. Dislocation occurs unexpectedly when the quadriceps muscle is contracted with the knee in flexion. There is acute pain, the knee is stuck in flexion and the patient may fall to the ground.

Although the patella always dislocates laterally, the patient may think it has displaced medially because the uncovered medial femoral condyle stands out prominently. If the knee is seen while the patella is dislocated, the diagnosis is obvious. There is a lump on the lateral side, while the front of the knee (where the patella ought to be) is flat. The tissues on the medial side are tender, the joint may be swollen and aspiration may reveal a blood-stained effusion.

More often the patella has reduced by the time the patient is seen. Tenderness and swelling may still be present and *the apprehension test* is positive: if the

patella is pushed laterally with the knee slightly flexed, the patient resists and becomes anxious, fearing another dislocation The patient will normally volunteer a history of previous dislocation.

Between attacks the patient should be carefully examined for features that are known to predispose to patellar instability (see above).

IMAGING
X-rays may reveal loose bodies in the knee, derived from old osteochondral fragments. A lateral view with the knee in slight flexion may show a high-riding patella and tangential views can be used to measure the sulcus angle and the congruence angle.

MRI is helpful and may show signs of the previous patellofemoral soft-tissue disruption.

Treatment

If the patella is still dislocated, it is pushed back into place while the knee is gently extended. The only indications for immediate surgery are (1) inability to reduce the patella (e.g. with a rare 'intra-articular' dislocation), and (2) the presence of a large, displaced osteochondral fragment.

A plaster cylinder or splint is applied and retained for 2–3 weeks; isometric quadriceps strengthening exercises are encouraged and the patient is allowed to walk with the aid of crutches.

Exercises should be continued for at least 3 months, concentrating on strengthening the vastus medialis muscle. If recurrences are few and far between, conservative treatment may suffice; as the child grows older the patellar mechanism tends to stabilize. However, about 15% of children with patellar instability suffer repeated and distressing episodes of dislocation and for these patients surgical reconstruction is indicated.

OPERATIVE TREATMENT
The principles of operative treatment are (a) to repair or strengthen the medial patellofemoral ligaments and (b) to realign the extensor mechanism so as to produce

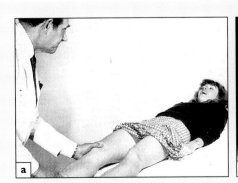

20.22 Dislocated patella (a) Clinical picture and (b) x-ray showing dislocation of the right patella.

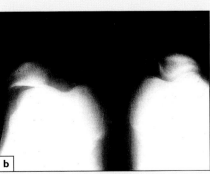

20.23 Patellar instability
(a) The apprehension test – the patient's facial expression shows that she is apprehensive that the patella may dislocate.
(b) Subluxation of the patella.

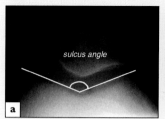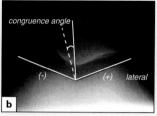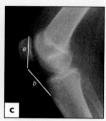

20.24 Clues to the causes of patellar instability (a) Tangential ('skyline') views of the patella allow an assessment of how well it 'sits' in the femoral trochlea – the sulcus angle is about 137° if the x-ray is taken at 30° to 45° of knee flexion. (b) The congruence angle, which is measured between a bisector of the sulcus angle and a line drawn to the lowest point of the patella, averages 8°; it is given a negative value if the lowest point is lateral to the bisector of the sulcus angle (Merchant *et al.*, 1974). (c) The position of the patella on a lateral x-ray can also be assessed; if the ratio of a:b (length of patella:length of patellar ligament) is less than 1, the patella is abnormally high – *patella alta* (Insall and Salvati, 1971).

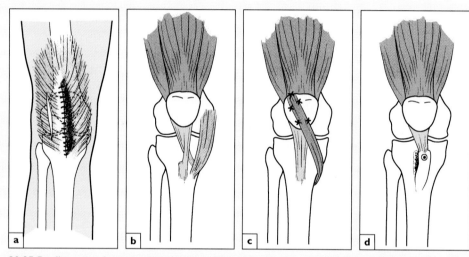

20.25 Realignment for recurrent patellar dislocation There are several methods popularly used. Most involve a lateral release of the capsule and some form of 'tether' medially. This check-rein may be created from (a) vastus medialis *(Insall)*, (b) the semitendinosus tendon *(Galleazzi)* or by (c) transposing the lateral half of the patellar ligament medially *(Roux–Goldthwait)*. In adults, bony operations which shift the position of the patellar tubercle may be tried *(Elmslie–Trillat)*.

a mechanically more favourable angle of pull. This can be achieved in several ways (see Fig. 20.25).

Suprapatellar realignment (Insall) The lateral retinaculum and capsule are divided. The quadriceps tendon adjacent to the vastus medialis is split longitudinally to the level of the tibial tubercle; the free edge is then sutured over the middle of the patella, thus bringing vastus medialis distally and closer to the midline.

Infrapatellar soft-tissue realignment (Goldthwait) The lateral half of the patellar ligament is detached, threaded under the medial half and reattached more medially and distally. This operation is seldom used by itself, but may be combined with suprapatellar realignment.

Infrapatellar bony realignment (Elmslie–Trillat) The tibial tubercle is osteotomized and moved medially, thus improving the angle of pull on the patella. This procedure is only appropriate after closure of the proximal tibial physis; if growth is incomplete, damage to the physis may result in a progressive recurvatum deformity.

NOTE All these procedures can be combined with repair or tightening of the medial patellofemoral ligament. At the end of the operation it is essential to check that the patella moves smoothly to at least 60° of knee flexion; excessive tightening or uneven tension may cause maltracking (and, occasionally, even medial subluxation!) of the patella.

Patellectomy Occasionally the patellofemoral cartilage is so damaged that patellectomy is indicated, but this operation should be avoided if possible. There is a small risk that after patellectomy the patellar tendon may continue to dislocate and require realignment by the tibial tubercle transfer.

RECURRENT SUBLUXATION

Patellar dislocation is sometimes followed by recurrent subluxation rather than further episodes of complete displacement. This is the borderline between frank instability and maltracking of the patella (see below).

OTHER TYPES OF NON-TRAUMATIC DISLOCATION

Congenital dislocation, in which the patella is permanently displaced, is fortunately very rare. Reconstructive procedures, such as semitendinosus tenodesis, have been tried but the results are unpredictable.

Habitual dislocation differs from recurrent dislocation in that the patella dislocates every time the knee is bent and reduces each time it is straightened. In long-standing cases the patella may be permanently dislocated.

The probable cause is *contracture of the quadriceps,* which may be congenital or may result from repeated injections (usually antibiotics) into the muscle.

Treatment requires lengthening of the quadriceps. Additionally a lateral capsular release and medial plication may be needed to hold the patella in the intercondylar groove.

PATELLOFEMORAL OVERLOAD SYNDROME (CHONDROMALACIA OF THE PATELLA; PATELLAR PAIN SYNDROME)

The syndrome of anterior knee pain and patellofemoral tenderness is common among active adolescents and young adults. It is often (but not invariably) associated with softening and fibrillation of the articular surface of the patella – *chondromalacia patellae.* Having no other pathological label, orthopaedic surgeons have tended to regard chondromalacia as the cause (rather than one of the effects) of the disorder. Against this are the facts that (1) chondromalacia is commonly found at arthroscopy in young adults who have no anterior knee pain, and (2) some patients with the typical clinical syndrome have no cartilage softening.

Pathogenesis and pathology

The basic disorder is probably mechanical overload of the patellofemoral joint. Rarely, a single injury (sudden impact on the front of the knee) may damage the articular surfaces. Much more common is repetitive overload due to either (1) *malcongruence* of the patellofemoral surfaces because of some abnormal shape of the patella or intercondylar groove or (2) *malalignment* of the extensor mechanism, or relative weakness of the vastus medialis, which causes the patella to tilt, or subluxate, or bear more heavily on one facet than the other during flexion and extension. 'Overload' as used here means either direct stress on a load-bearing facet or sheer stresses in the depths of the articular cartilage at the boundary between high-contact and low-contact areas (Goodfellow *et al.,* 1976).

Patellofemoral overload leads to changes in both the articular cartilage and the subchondral bone, not necessarily of parallel degree. Thus, the cartilage may look normal and show only biochemical changes such as overhydration or loss of proteoglycans, while the underlying bone shows reactive vascular congestion (a potent cause of pain). Or there may be obvious cartilage softening and fibrillation, with or without subarticular intraosseous hypertension. This would account for the variable relationship between (1) malalignment syndrome, (2) cartilage softening, (3) subchondral vascular congestion and (4) anterior knee pain.

Cartilage fibrillation usually occurs on the medial patellar facet or the median ridge, remains confined to the superficial zones and generally heals spontaneously (Bentley, 1985). Thus it is not a precursor of osteoarthritis in later life. Occasionally the lateral facet is involved – Ficat's 'hyperpression zone' syndrome – and this may well be progressive (Ficat and Hungerford, 1977).

Clinical features

The patient, often a teenage girl or an athletic young adult, complains of pain over the front of the knee or 'underneath the knee-cap'. Occasionally there is a history of injury or recurrent displacement. Symptoms are aggravated by activity or climbing stairs, or when standing up after prolonged sitting. The knee may give way and occasionally swells. It sometimes 'catches' but this is not true locking. Often both knees are affected.

At first sight the knee looks normal but careful examination may reveal malalignment or tilting of the patellae. Other signs include quadriceps wasting, fluid in the knee, tenderness under the edge of the patella and crepitus on moving the knee.

Patellofemoral pain is elicited by pressing the patella against the femur and asking the patient to contract the quadriceps – first with central pressure, then compressing the medial facet and then the lateral. If, in addition, the apprehension test is positive, this suggests previous subluxation or dislocation.

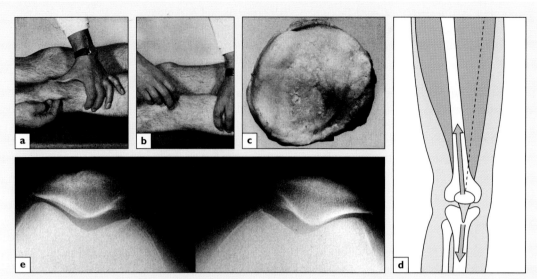

20.26 Patellofemoral overload and chondromalacia (**a–c**) Chondromalacia, with (**a**) tenderness of the posterior aspect of the patella, (**b**) pain on patellar friction and (**c**) softening and irregularity of the articular surface. (**d**) The Q-angle, between the line of the patellar ligament and the line of pull of the quadriceps. (**e**) The skyline view shows lateral tilting of the patella, worse on the left than the right.

Patellar tracking can be observed with the patient seated on the edge of the couch, flexing and extending the knee against resistance; in some cases subluxation is obvious.

With the patient lying supine, patellar alignment can be gauged by measuring the quadriceps angle, or Q-angle – the angle subtended by the line of quadriceps pull (a line running from the anterior superior iliac spine to the middle of the patella) and the line of the patellar ligament; this should not exceed 20°.

Lastly, the structures around the knee are carefully examined for other sources of pain, and the hip is examined to exclude referred pain.

IMAGING

X-ray examination should include skyline views of the patella, which may show abnormal tilting or subluxation, and a lateral view with the knee half-flexed to see if the patella is high or small.

The most accurate way of showing and measuring patellofemoral malposition is *by CT or MRI* with the knees in full extension and varying degrees of flexion.

ARTHROSCOPY

Cartilage softening is common in asymptomatic knees, and painful knees may show no abnormality. However, arthroscopy is useful in excluding other causes of anterior knee pain; it can also serve to gauge patellofemoral congruence, alignment and tracking.

Differential diagnosis

Other causes of anterior knee pain must be excluded before finally accepting the diagnosis of patellofemoral overload (see box). Even then, the cause of 'overload'

must be established: is it abnormal posture, overuse, patellar malalignment, subluxation or some abnormality in the shape of the bones?

Causes of anterior knee pain
Patellofemoral overload
Maltracking
Overuse
Patellar instability
Patellar subluxation
Patellar tilt
Intra-articular pathology
Plica syndrome
Meniscal disorders
Osteochondritis dissecans
Patellofemoral arthritis
Peri-patellar disorders
Bursitis
Tendinitis
Apophysitis
Disorders of the patella
Bipartite patella
Bone tumours
Referred pain
Hip disorders, e.g slipped femoral epiphysis

Treatment

CONSERVATIVE MANAGEMENT

In the vast majority of cases the patient will be helped by adjustment of stressful activities and physiotherapy, combined with reassurance that most patients recover. Exercises are directed specifically at strengthening the medial quadriceps so as to counterbalance the tendency to lateral tilting or subluxation of the patella. Some patients respond to simple measures such as providing support for a valgus foot. Aspirin does no more than reduce pain, and corticosteroid injections should be avoided.

OPERATIVE TREATMENT

Surgery should be considered only if (1) there is a demonstrable abnormality that is correctable by operation, or (2) conservative treatment has been tried for at least 6 months and (3) the patient is genuinely incapacitated. Operation is intended to improve patellar alignment and patellofemoral congruence and to reduce patellofemoral pressure. Various measures are employed: lateral release, with or without one of the re-alignment procedures illustrated in Figure 20.25, may be needed if there is any sign of patellar instability; other operations are the patellar ligament elevation procedure of Maquet and – as a last resort – patellectomy.

Lateral release The lateral knee capsule and extensor retinaculum are divided longitudinally, either open or arthroscopically. This sometimes succeeds on its own (particularly if significant patellar tilting can be demonstrated on x-ray or MRI), but more often patellofemoral realignment will be needed as well.

Proximal realignment This is achieved by a combined open release of the lateral retinaculum and reefing of the oblique part of the vastus medialis.

Distal realignment The distal soft-tissue and bony realignment procedures are described on page 464. They will improve the tracking angle but run the risk of increasing patellofemoral contact pressures and thus aggravating the patient's symptoms.

Distal elevation of the patellar ligament In Maquet's (1976) tibial tubercle advancement operation, the tubercle, with the attached patellar ligament, is hinged forwards and held there with a bone-block. This has the effect of reducing patellofemoral contact pressures. Some patients resent the bump on the front part of the tibia and the operation may substitute a new set of complaints for the old.

Chondroplasty Shaving of the patellar articular surface is usually performed arthroscopically using a power tool. Soft and fibrillated cartilage is removed, in severe cases down to the level of subchondral bone; the hope is that it will be replaced by fibrocartilage. The operation should be followed by lavage and can be combined with any of the realignment procedures.

Patellectomy This is a last resort, but patients with severe discomfort are grateful for the relief it brings after other operations have failed.

OSTEOCHONDRITIS DISSECANS

A small, well-demarcated, avascular fragment of bone and overlying cartilage sometimes separates from one of the femoral condyles and appears as a loose body in the joint (see also Chapter 6). The most likely cause is trauma, either a single impact with the edge of the patella or repeated microtrauma from contact with an adjacent tibial ridge. The fact that over 80% of lesions occur on the lateral part of the medial femoral condyle, exactly where the patella makes contact in full flexion, supports the first of these. There may also be some general predisposing factor, because several joints can be affected, or several members of one family. Lesions are bilateral in 25% of cases.

Pathology

The lower or lateral part of the medial femoral condyle is usually affected, rarely the lateral condyle, and still more rarely the patella. An area of subchondral bone becomes avascular and within this area an ovoid osteo-cartilaginous segment is demarcated from the surrounding bone. At first the overlying cartilage is intact and the fragment is stable; over a period of months the fragment separates but remains in position; finally the fragment breaks free to become a loose body in the joint. The small crater is slowly filled with fibrocartilage, leaving a depression on the articular surface.

Clinical features

The patient, usually a male aged 15–20 years, presents with intermittent ache or swelling. Later, there are attacks of giving way such that the knee feels unreliable, and locking may occur.

The quadriceps muscle is wasted and there may be a small effusion. Soon after an attack there are two signs that are almost diagnostic: (1) tenderness localized to one femoral condyle; and (2) Wilson's sign: if the knee is flexed to 90°, rotated medially and then gradually straightened, pain is felt; repeating the test with the knee rotated laterally is painless.

IMAGING

Plain x-rays may show a line of demarcation around a lesion *in situ*, usually in the lateral part of the medial femoral condyle. This site is best displayed in special intercondylar (tunnel) views, but even then a small lesion or one situated far back may be missed. Once the fragment has become detached, the empty hollow may be seen – and possibly a loose body elsewhere in the joint.

Radionuclide scans show increased activity around the lesion, and *MRI* consistently shows an area of low signal intensity in the T1-weighted images; the adjacent

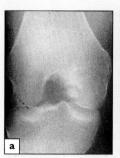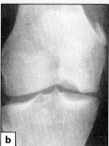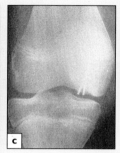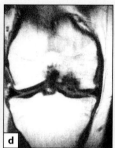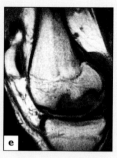

20.27 Osteochondritis dissecans At first the affected area separates ('dissects') but still remains in position. **(a)** The 'tunnel' view may be the most helpful. **(b)** The anteroposterior view shows the loose fragment and the crater on the medial femoral condyle from which it came. **(c)** Pinning the fragment back is one method of treatment. **(d, e)** MRI shows that the surrounding bone, too, is abnormal.

bone may also appear abnormal, probably due to oedema. These investigations usually indicate whether the fragment is 'stable' or 'loose'.

ARTHROSCOPY

With early lesions the articular surface looks intact, but probing may reveal that the cartilage is soft. Loose segments are easily visualized.

Differential diagnosis

Avascular necrosis of the femoral condyle – usually associated with corticosteroid therapy or alcohol abuse – may result in separation of a localized osteocartilaginous fragment. However, on x-ray the lesion is always on the dome of the femoral condyle, and this distinguishes it clearly from osteochondritis dissecans.

Treatment

For the purposes of management, it is useful to 'stage' the lesion; hence the importance of radionuclide scanning, MRI and arthroscopy.

In the earliest stage, when the cartilage is intact and the lesion 'stable', no treatment is needed but activities are curtailed for 6–12 months. Small lesions often heal spontaneously.

If the fragment is 'unstable' – i.e. surrounded by a clear boundary with sclerosis of the underlying bone, or showing MRI features of separation – treatment depends on the size of the lesion: a small fragment should be removed by arthroscopy and the base drilled; the bed will eventually be covered by fibrocartilage, leaving only a small defect. A large fragment (say more than 1cm in diameter) should be fixed *in situ* with pins or Herbert screws. In addition, it may help to drill the underlying sclerotic bone to promote union of the necrotic fragment. For drilling, the area is approached from a point some distance away, beyond the articular cartilage.

If the fragment is completely detached but in one piece and shown to fit nicely in its bed, the crater is cleaned and the floor drilled before replacing the loose fragment and fixing it with Herbert screws. If the fragment is in pieces or ill-shaped, it is best discarded; the crater is drilled and allowed to fill with fibrocartilage.

In recent years attempts have been made to fill the residual defects by articular cartilage transplantation: either the insertion of osteochondral plugs harvested from another part of the knee or the application of sheets of cultured chondrocytes.

After any of the above operations the knee is held in a cast for 6 weeks; thereafter movement is encouraged but weightbearing is deferred until x-rays show signs of healing.

LOOSE BODIES

The knee – relatively capacious, with large synovial folds – is a common haven for loose bodies. These may be produced by: (1) injury (a chip of bone or cartilage); (2) osteochondritis dissecans (which may produce one or two fragments); (3) osteoarthritis (pieces of cartilage or osteophyte); (4) Charcot's disease (large osteocartilaginous bodies); and (5) synovial chondromatosis (cartilage metaplasia in the synovium, sometimes producing hundreds of loose bodies).

Clinical features

Loose bodies may be symptomless. The usual complaint is attacks of sudden locking without injury. The joint gets stuck in a position which varies from one attack to another. Sometimes the locking is only momentary and usually the patient can wriggle the knee until it suddenly unlocks. The patient may be aware of something 'popping in and out of the joint'.

In adolescents, a loose body is usually due to osteo-chondritis dissecans, rarely to injury. In adults osteo-arthritis is the most frequent cause.

Only rarely is the patient seen with the knee still locked. Sometimes, especially after the first attack, there is synovitis or there may be evidence of the underlying cause. A pedunculated loose body may be felt; one that is truly loose tends to slip away during palpation (the well-named 'joint mouse').

X-Ray Most loose bodies are radio-opaque. The films also show an underlying joint abnormality.

Treatment

A loose body causing symptoms should be removed unless the joint is severely osteoarthritic. This can usually be done with the aid of arthroscopy, but finding the loose body may be difficult; it may be concealed in a synovial pouch or sulcus and a small body may even slip under the edge of one of the menisci.

SYNOVIAL CHONDROMATOSIS

This is a rare disorder in which the joint comes to contain multiple loose bodies, often in pearly clumps resembling sago ('snowstorm knee'). The usual explanation is that myriad tiny fronds undergo cartilage metaplasia at their tips; these tips break free and may ossify. It has, however, been suggested that chondrocytes may be cultured in the synovial fluid and that some of the products are then deposited onto previously normal synovium, so producing the familiar appearance (Kay *et al.*, 1989). X-rays reveal multiple loose bodies; on arthrography they show as negative defects.

Treatment The loose bodies should be removed. At the same time any patch of abnormal synovium should be carefully excised.

THE PLICA SYNDROME

A plica is the remnant of an embryonic synovial partition which persists into adult life. During development of the embryo, the knee is divided into three cavities – a large suprapatellar pouch and beneath this the medial and lateral compartments – separated from each other by membranous septa. Later these partitions disappear, leaving a single cavity. But part of a septum may persist as a synovial pleat or plica (from the Latin *plicare* =

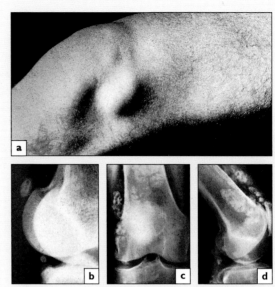

20.28 Loose bodies (**a**) This loose body slipped away from the fingers when touched; the term 'joint mouse' seems appropriate. (**b**) Which is the loose body here? – not the large one (which is a fabella), but the small lower one opposite the joint line. (**c**, **d**) Synovial chondromatosis – the multiple loose bodies are characteristic.

fold). This is found in over 20% of people, usually *as a median infrapatellar fold* (the ligamentum mucosum), less often as a *suprapatellar curtain* draped across the opening of the suprapatellar pouch or a *mediopatellar plica* sweeping down the medial wall of the joint.

Pathology

The plica in itself is not pathological. But if acute trauma, repetitive strain or some underlying disorder (e.g. a meniscal tear) causes inflammation, the plica may become oedematous, thickened and eventually fibrosed; it then acts as a tight bowstring impinging on other structures in the joint and causing further synovial irritation.

Clinical features

An adolescent or young adult complains of an ache in the front of the knee (occasionally both knees), with intermittent episodes of clicking or 'giving way'. There may be a history of trauma or markedly increased activity. Symptoms are aggravated by exercise or climbing stairs, especially if this follows a long period of sitting.

On examination there may be muscle wasting and a small effusion. The most characteristic feature is tenderness near the upper pole of the patella and over the femoral condyle. Occasionally the thickened band can be felt. Movement of the knee may cause catching or snapping.

Diagnosis

There is still controversy as to whether 'plica syndrome' constitutes a real and distinct clinical entity. In some quarters, however, it is regarded as a significant cause of anterior knee pain. It may closely resemble other conditions such as patellar overload or subluxation; indeed, the plica may become troublesome only when those other conditions are present. The diagnosis is often not made until arthroscopy is undertaken.

Treatment

The first line of treatment is rest, anti-inflammatory drugs and adjustment of activities. If symptoms persist, the plica can be divided or excised by arthroscopy.

TUBERCULOSIS

Tuberculosis of the knee may appear at any age, but it is more common in children than in adults (see also Chapter 2).

Clinical features

Pain and limp are early symptoms; or the child may present with a swollen joint and a low-grade fever. The thigh muscles are wasted, thus accentuating the joint swelling. The knee feels warm and there is synovial thickening. Movements are restricted and often painful. The Mantoux test is positive and the erythrocyte sedimentation rate (ESR) may be increased.

X-rays show marked osteoporosis and, in children, enlargement of the bony epiphyses. Unlike pyogenic arthritis, joint space narrowing is a late sign; this is because cartilage lysis is prevented by the presence of a plasmin inhibitor in the synovial exudate. In late cases the joint surfaces are eroded.

Diagnosis

Monarticular rheumatoid synovitis, or juvenile chronic arthritis, may closely resemble tuberculosis. A synovial biopsy may be necessary to establish the diagnosis.

Treatment

General antituberculous chemotherapy should be given for 6–9 months (see Chapter 2).

In the active stage the knee is rested in a bed splint. The synovitis usually subsides, but if it does not do so after a few weeks' treatment, then surgical debridement will be needed. All diseased and necrotic tissue is removed and bone abscesses are evacuated.

In the healing stage the patient is allowed up wearing a weight-relieving caliper. Gradually this is left off, but the patient is kept under observation for any sign of recurrent inflammation. If the articular cartilage has been spared, movement can be encouraged and weight-bearing is slowly resumed. However, if the articular surface is destroyed, immobilization is continued until the joint stiffens.

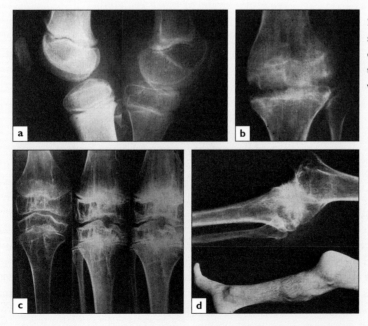

20.29 Tuberculosis – clinical and x-rays In synovitis (**a**) the bones are porotic and the epiphyses enlarged compared with the normal side; (**b**) arthritis. (**c**) Series showing healing with recalcification, but with joint destruction. (**d**) The aftermath of arthritis.

In the aftermath the joint may be painful; it is then best arthrodesed, but in children this is usually postponed until growth is almost completed. The ideal position for fusion is 15° of flexion and 7° of valgus.

In some cases, once it is certain that the disease is quiescent, joint replacement may be feasible.

RHEUMATOID ARTHRITIS

Occasionally, rheumatoid arthritis starts in the knee as a chronic monarticular synovitis (see also Chapter 3).

Sooner or later, however, other joints become involved.

Clinical features

The general features of rheumatoid disease are described in Chapter 3.

During stage 1 (synovitis) the patient complains of pain and chronic swelling. There is some wasting, there may be a large effusion and the thickened synovium is easily palpable. At this stage, while the joint is still stable and the muscles are reasonably strong, there is a danger of rupturing the posterior capsule; the joint contents are extruded into a large posterior bursa or between the muscle planes of the calf, causing sudden pain and swelling which closely mimic the features of calf vein thrombosis.

In stage 2 there is increasing instability of the joint, muscle wasting is marked and there is some loss of flexion and extension. X-rays may show loss of joint space and marginal erosions; the condition is easily distinguishable from osteoarthritis by the complete absence of osteophytes, but in the monarticular variety biopsy may be needed to exclude tuberculosis.

In stage 3 pain and disability are usually severe. In some patients stiffness is so marked that the patient has to be helped to stand and the joint has only a jog of painful movement. In others, cartilage and bone destruction predominate and the joint becomes increasingly unstable and deformed. The commonest deformities are fixed flexion and valgus; abnormal mobility (increased anteroposterior glide and lateral wobble) is present. X-rays reveal the bone destruction characteristic of advanced disease.

Treatment

The majority of patients can be managed by conservative measures. In addition to general treatment with anti-inflammatory and disease-modifying drugs, local splintage and injection of triamcinolone usually reduce the synovitis. A more prolonged effect may be obtained by injecting radiocolloids such as yttrium-90 (^{90}Y). Even those with posterior joint rupture will usually settle down after a period of splintage, and symptoms will not recur as long as the synovitis is kept under control.

OPERATIVE TREATMENT

Synovectomy and debridement Only if other measures fail to control the synovitis (which nowadays is rare) is synovectomy indicated. This can be done very effectively by arthroscopy. Articular pannus and cartilage tags are removed at the same time. Postoperatively, any haematoma must be drained and movements are commenced as soon as pain has subsided.

Supracondylar osteotomy Realignment osteotomy is unlikely to have any protective effect in a disease which is marked by generalized cartilage erosion. However, if the knee is stable and pain-free but troublesome because of valgus and flexion deformity, a corrective supracondylar osteotomy is useful.

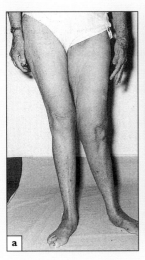 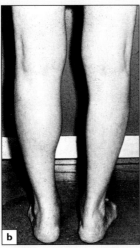 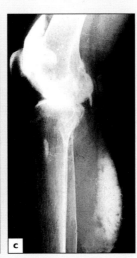

20.30 Rheumatoid arthritis
(**a**) The typical deformity: slight flexion, valgus and external rotation.
(**b, c**) Sometimes the patient presents with pain and swelling in the calf ('pseudothrombosis'); the arthrogram shows that the capsule has ruptured and fluid has extruded into the calf.

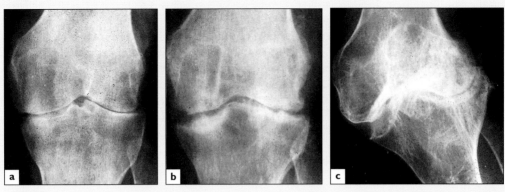

20.31 Rheumatoid arthritis (a) Early changes are cartilage erosion (giving a narrow joint space) and osteoporosis. (b) Later, joint destruction becomes more obvious, and (c) in severe cases gross deformity may result.

Arthroplasty Total joint replacement is useful when joint destruction is advanced. However, it is less successful if the knee has been allowed to become very unstable or very stiff; timing of the operation is important.

OSTEOARTHRITIS

The knee is the commonest of the large joints to be affected by osteoarthritis (see also Chapter 5). Often there is a predisposing factor: injury to the articular surface, a torn meniscus and ligamentous instability or pre-existing deformity of the hip or knee, to mention a few. However, in many cases no obvious cause can be found.

Osteoarthritis is often bilateral and there is a strong association with Heberden's nodes.

Pathology

Cartilage breakdown usually starts in an area of excessive loading. Thus, with long-standing varus the changes are most marked in the medial compartment. The characteristic features of cartilage fibrillation, sclerosis of the subchondral bone and peripheral osteophyte formation are usually present; in advanced cases the articular surface may be denuded of cartilage and underlying bone may eventually crumble.

Chondrocalcinosis is common, but whether this is cause or effect – or quite unrelated – remains unknown.

Clinical features

Patients are usually over 50 years old; they tend to be overweight and may have long-standing bow-leg deformity.

Pain is the leading symptom, worse after use, or (if the patellofemoral joint is affected) on stairs. After rest, the joint feels stiff and it hurts to 'get going' after sitting for any length of time. Swelling is common, and giving way or locking may occur.

On examination there may be an obvious deformity (usually varus) or the scar of a previous operation. The quadriceps muscle is usually wasted.

Except during an exacerbation, there is little fluid and no warmth; nor is the synovial membrane thickened. Movement is somewhat limited and is often accompanied by patellofemoral crepitus.

It is useful to test movement applying first a varus and then a valgus force to the knee; pain indicates which tibiofemoral compartment is involved. Pressure on the patella may elicit pain.

The natural history of osteoarthritis is one of alternating 'bad spells' and 'good spells'. Patients may experience long periods of lesser discomfort and only moderate loss of function, followed by exacerbations of pain and stiffness (perhaps after unaccustomed activity).

X-RAY

The anteroposterior x-ray *must* be obtained with the patient standing and bearing weight; only in this way can small degrees of articular cartilage thinning be revealed. The tibiofemoral joint space is diminished (often only in one compartment) and there is subchondral sclerosis. Osteophytes and subchondral cysts are usually present and sometimes there is soft-tissue calcification in the suprapatellar region or in the joint itself (chrondrocalcinosis).

If only the patellofemoral joint is affected, suspect a pyrophosphate arthropathy.

Treatment

If symptoms are not severe, treatment is conservative. Joint loading is lessened by using a walking stick.

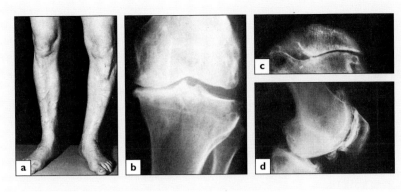

20.32 Osteoarthritis of the knee
(**a, b**) Varus deformity and degeneration on the medial side. (**c, d**) Sometimes it is the patellofemoral joint that is mainly affected.

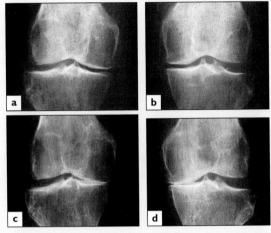

20.33 Osteoarthritis – x-rays The upper films, taken with the patient lying on the x-ray couch, show only slight narrowing of the medial joint space; but with weightbearing, as in the lower films, it is clear that the changes are considerable.

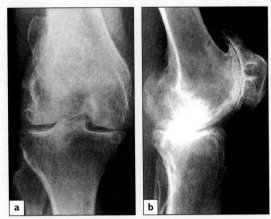

20.34 Patellofemoral osteoarthritis Osteoarthritis mainly in the patellofemoral joint suggests pyrophosphate arthropathy. This patient had other characteristic features: (**a**) chondrocalcinosis and periarticular ossification; and (**b**) large trailing osteophytes around the patella.

Quadriceps exercises are important. Analgesics are prescribed for pain, and warmth (e.g. radiant heat or shortwave diathermy) is soothing. A simple elastic support may do wonders, probably by improving proprioception in an unstable knee.

Intra-articular corticosteroid injections will often relieve pain, but this is a stopgap – and not a very good one, because repeated injections may permit (or even predispose to) progressive cartilage and bone destruction.

OPERATIVE TREATMENT
Persistent pain unresponsive to conservative treatment, progressive deformity and instability are the usual indications for operative treatment.

Arthroscopic washouts, with trimming of degenerate meniscal tissue and osteophytes, may give temporary relief; this is a useful measure when there are contraindications to reconstructive surgery.

Patellectomy is indicated only in those rare cases where osteoarthritis is strictly confined to the patellofemoral joint. However, bear in mind that extensor power will be reduced and if a total joint replacement is later needed pain relief will be less predictable than usual (Paletta and Laskin, 1995).

Realignment osteotomy is often successful in relieving symptoms and staving off the need for 'end-stage' surgery. The ideal indication is a 'young' patient (under 50 years) with a varus knee and osteoarthritis confined to the medial compartment: a high tibial valgus osteotomy will redistribute weight to the lateral side of the joint.

Replacement arthroplasty is indicated in older patients with progressive joint destruction. This is usually a 'resurfacing' procedure, with a metal femoral condylar component and a metal-backed polyethylene table on the tibial side. If the disease is largely confined to one compartment, a unicompartmental replacement can be done as an alternative to osteotomy. With modern techniques, and meticulous attention to anatomical alignment of the knee, the results of replacement arthroplasty are excellent.

Arthrodesis is indicated only if there is a strong contraindication to arthroplasty (e.g. previous sepsis) or to salvage a failed arthroplasty.

OSTEONECROSIS

Non-traumatic osteonecrosis of the knee, though not as common as femoral head necrosis, has the same aetiological and pathogenetic background (see Chapter 6). The bone changes are usually seen in the femoral condyles, but sometimes the tibial condylar surface also is affected. Corticosteroid therapy and alcohol abuse are the commonest precipitating agents, but in some cases (especially in elderly people) no specific cause is discovered.

Clinical features

Patients are usually 30-50 years old and women are affected more often than men. There may be a background of systemic lupus erythematosus, sickle-cell disease or one of the other conditions associated with non-traumatic osteonecrosis; by far the commonest risk factors, however, are high-dosage corticosteroid administration and excessive alcohol consumption. Other joints may already have been affected in the same way.

Typically the patient complains of pain around the knee, which may suddenly have increased in severity during recent weeks. Sometimes both knees are affected. On examination there is often an effusion, and movements may be restricted and painful; the classic feature, however, is tenderness on pressure upon the medial or lateral femoral or tibial condyle.

IMAGING
The x-ray appearances are often unimpressive at the beginning, but MRI will show the typical changes of marrow necrosis and a radionuclide scan may show increased activity in the subchondral bone. Later the classic radiographic features of osteonecrosis appear (see Chapter 6). On the femoral side, it is almost always the dome of the condyle that is affected, unlike the picture in osteochondritis dissecans. In about 20% of cases bone changes are seen also in the adjacent tibial condyle.

Elderly women sometimes present with similar changes only in one of the tibial condyles; it may be impossible to tell from the x-ray whether this is due to osteonecrosis or an osteoporotic insufficiency fracture.

Clinical progress

Symptoms and signs may stabilize and the patient be left with no more than slight distortion of the articular surface; or one of the condyles may collapse, leading to secondary osteoarthritis and instability of the knee.

Treatment

Treatment is *conservative* in the first instance and consists of analgesics for pain long-term measures to reduce loading of the joint. If symptoms or signs increase, however, operative treatment should be considered.

Core decompression has been advocated for early lesions (Mont *et al.*, 2000). However, if the articular surface has collapsed, further measures may be needed. If only one compartment is involved, a *realignment osteotomy* will redistribute load from this area to an intact part of the joint (e.g. a valgus osteotomy for medial femoral condyle necrosis). With advanced bone collapse, *replacement arthroplasty* (unicompartmental or bicompartmental) will be required.

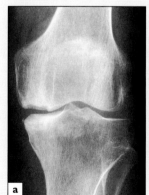 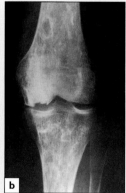 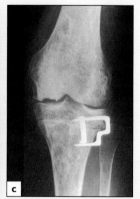

20.35 Osteonecrosis (a) X-ray showing the typical features of subarticular bone fragmentation and surrounding sclerosis situated in the highest part (the dome) of the medial femoral condyle; the adjacent tibial condyle also is affected. (Compare this with the appearance in osteochondritis dissecans, where the necrotic segment is almost always on the inner surface of the medial femoral condyle). (**b, c**) In this case the medial compartment was 'unloaded' by performing a high tibial valgus osteotomy. The patient remained pain-free for 6 years before dying of leukaemia.

CHARCOT'S DISEASE

Charcot's disease (neuropathic arthritis) is a rare cause of joint destruction (see also Chapter 5). Because of loss of pain sensibility and proprioception, the articular surface breaks down and the underlying bone crumbles. Fragments of bone and cartilage are deposited in the hypertrophic synovium and may grow into large masses. The capsule is stretched and lax, and the joint becomes progressively unstable.

Clinical features

The patient chiefly complains of instability; pain (other than tabetic lightning pains) is unusual. The joint is swollen and often grossly deformed. It feels like a bag of bones and fluid but is neither warm nor tender. Movements beyond the normal limits, without pain, are a notable feature. Radiologically the joint is subluxated, bone destruction is obvious and irregular calcified masses can be seen.

Treatment

Patients often seem to manage quite well despite the bizarre appearances. However, marked instability may demand treatment – usually a moulded splint or caliper will do – and occasionally pain becomes intolerable. Arthrodesis is feasible but fixation is difficult and fusion is very slow.

HAEMOPHILIC ARTHRITIS

The knee is the joint most commonly involved in bleeding disorders (see also Chapter 5). Repeated haemorrhage leads to chronic synovitis and articular cartilage erosion. Movement is progressively restricted and the joint may end up deformed and stiff.

Clinical features

Fresh bleeds cause pain and swelling of the knee, with the typical clinical signs of a haemarthrosis. Between episodes of bleeding the knee often continues to be painful and somewhat swollen, with restricted mobility. There is a tendency to hold the knee in flexion and this may become a fixed deformity.

X-rays may show little abnormality, apart from local osteoporosis. In more advanced cases the joint space is narrowed and large 'cysts' or erosions may appear in the subchondral bone.

Treatment

Both the haematologist and the orthopaedic surgeon should participate in treatment. The acute bleed may need aspiration, but only if this can be 'covered' by giving the appropriate clotting factor; otherwise it is better treated by splintage until the acute symptoms settle down.

Flexion deformity must be prevented by gentle physiotherapy and intermittent splintage. If the joint is painful and eroded, operative treatment may be considered. However, although replacement arthroplasty is feasible, this should be done only after the most searching discussion with the patient, in which all the risks are considered, and only if a full haematological service is available.

SWELLINGS OF THE KNEE

The knee is prone to a number of disorders which present essentially as 'swelling'; and, because it is such a large joint with a number of synovial recesses, the swelling is often painless until the tissues become tense. Conditions to be considered can be divided into four groups: *swelling of the entire joint; swellings in front of the joint; swellings behind the joint; and bony swellings.*

ACUTE SWELLING OF THE ENTIRE JOINT

Post-traumatic haemarthrosis

Swelling immediately after injury means blood in the joint. The knee is very painful and it feels warm, tense and tender. Later there may be a 'doughy' feel. Movements are restricted. X-rays are essential to see if there is a fracture; if there is not, then suspect a tear of the anterior cruciate ligament.

The joint should be aspirated under aseptic conditions. If a ligament injury is suspected, examination under anaesthesia is helpful and may indicate the need for operation; otherwise a crepe bandage is applied and the leg cradled in a back-splint. Quadriceps exercises are practised from the start. The patient may get up when comfortable, retaining the back-splint until muscle control returns.

Bleeding disorders

In patients with clotting disorders, the knee is the most common site for acute bleeds. If the appropriate clotting factor is available, the joint should be aspirated and treated as for a traumatic haemarthrosis. If the factor is not available, aspiration is best avoided; the knee is splinted in slight flexion until the swelling subsides.

Acute septic arthritis

Acute pyogenic infection of the knee is not uncommon. The organism is usually *Staphylococcus aureus*, but in adults gonococcal infection is almost as common.

The joint is swollen, painful and inflamed; the white cell count and ESR are elevated. Aspiration reveals pus in the joint; fluid should be sent for bacteriological investigation, including anaerobic culture.

Treatment consists of systemic antibiotics and drainage of the joint – either open or by arthroscopy and irrigation; if fluid reaccumulates, it can be aspirated through a wide-bore needle. As the inflammation subsides, movement is begun, but weightbearing is deferred for 4–6 weeks.

Traumatic synovitis

Injury stimulates a reactive synovitis; typically the swelling appears only after some hours, and subsides spontaneously over a period of days. There is inhibition of quadriceps action and the thigh wastes. The knee may need to be splinted for several days but movement should be encouraged and quadriceps exercise is essential. If the amount of fluid is considerable, its aspiration hastens muscle recovery. In addition, any internal injury will need treatment.

Aseptic non-traumatic synovitis

Acute swelling, without a history of trauma or signs of infection, suggests *gout* or *pseudogout*. Aspiration will provide fluid which may look turbid, resembling pus, but it is sterile and microscopy (using polarized light)

reveals the crystals. Treatment with anti-inflammatory drugs is usually effective.

CHRONIC SWELLING OF THE JOINT

The diagnosis can usually be made on clinical and x-ray examination. The more elusive disorders should be fully instigated by joint aspiration, synovial fluid examination, arthroscopy and synovial biopsy.

Arthritis

The commonest causes of chronic swelling are *osteoarthritis* and *rheumatoid arthritis*. Other signs, such as deformity, loss of movement or instability, may be present and x-ray examination will usually show characteristic features.

Synovial disorders

Chronic swelling and synovial effusion without articular destruction should suggest conditions such as *synovial chondromatosis* and *pigmented villondular synovitis*. The diagnosis will usually be obvious on arthroscopy and can be confirmed by synovial biopsy.

The most important condition to exclude is *tuberculosis*. There has been a resurgence of cases during the past 10 years and the condition should be seriously considered whenever there is no obvious alternative diagnosis. Investigations should include Mantoux testing, synovial biopsy and microbiological investigations. The ideal is to start antituberculous chemotherapy before joint destruction occurs.

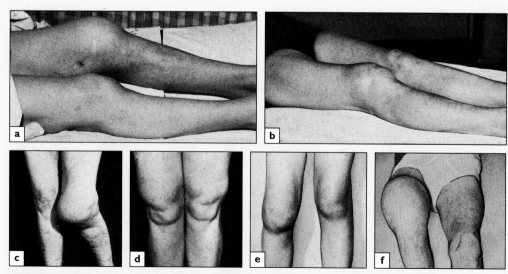

20.36 Swollen knees Some causes of chronic swelling in the absence of trauma: (**a**) tuberculous arthritis; (**b**) rheumatoid arthritis; (**c**) Charcot's disease; (**d**) villous synovitis; (**e**) haemophilia; (**f**) malignant synovioma.

SWELLINGS IN FRONT OF THE JOINT

Prepatellar bursitis ('housemaid's knee')

The fluctuant swelling is confined to the front of the patella and the joint itself is normal. This is an uninfected bursitis due not to pressure but to constant friction between skin and bone. It is seen mainly in carpet layers, paving workers, floor cleaners and miners who do not use protective knee pads. Treatment consists of firm bandaging, and kneeling is avoided; occasionally aspiration is needed. In chronic cases the lump is best excised.

Infection (possibly due to foreign body implantation) results in a warm, tender swelling. Treatment is by rest, antibiotics and, if necessary, aspiration or incision.

Infrapatellar bursitis ('clergyman's knee')

The swelling is below the patella and superficial to the patellar ligament, being more distally placed than prepatellar bursitis; it used to be said that one who prays kneels more uprightly than one who scrubs! Treatment is similar to that for prepatellar bursitis. Occasionally the bursa is affected in gout.

Other bursae

Occasionally a bursa deep to the patellar tendon or the pes anserinus becomes inflamed and painful. Treatment is non-operative.

SWELLINGS AT THE BACK OF THE KNEE

Semimembranosus bursa

The bursa between the semimembranosus and the medial head of gastrocnemius may become enlarged in children or adults. It presents usually as a painless lump behind the knee, slightly to the medial side of the midline and most conspicuous with the knee straight. The lump is fluctuant but the fluid cannot be pushed into the joint, presumably because the muscles compress and obstruct the normal communication. The knee joint is normal. Occasionally the lump aches, and if so it may be excised through a transverse incision. However, recurrence is common and, as the bursa normally disappears in time, a waiting policy is perhaps wiser.

Popliteal 'cyst'

Bulging of the posterior capsule and synovial herniation may produce a swelling in the popliteal fossa. The lump, which is usually seen in older people, is in the midline of the limb and at or below the level of the joint. It fluctuates but is not tender. Injection of radio-opaque medium into the joint, and x-ray, will show that the 'cyst' communicates with the joint.

The condition was originally described by Baker, whose patients were probably suffering from tuberculous synovitis. Nowadays it is more likely to be caused by rheumatoid or osteoarthritis, but it is still often called a 'Baker's cyst'. Occasionally the 'cyst' ruptures and the synovial contents spill into the muscle planes causing

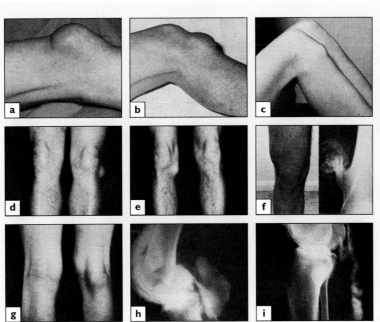

20.37 Lumps around the knee In front: (a) prepatellar bursa; (b) infrapatellar bursa; (c) Osgood–Schlatter's disease. On either side: (d) cyst of lateral meniscus; (e) cyst of medial meniscus; (f) cartilage-capped exostosis. Behind: (g) semimembranosus bursa; (h) arthrogram of popliteal cyst; (i) leaking cyst.

pain and swelling in the calf – a combination which can easily be mistaken for deep vein thrombosis.

The swelling may diminish following aspiration and injection of hydrocortisone; excision is not advised, because recurrence is common unless the underlying condition is treated.

Popliteal aneurysm

This is the commonest limb aneurysm and is sometimes bilateral. Pain and stiffness of the knee may precede the symptoms of peripheral arterial disease, so it is essential to examine any lump behind the knee for pulsation. A thrombosed popliteal aneurysm does not pulsate, but it feels almost solid.

BONY SWELLINGS AROUND THE KNEE

Because the knee is a relatively superficial joint, bony swellings of the distal femur and proximal tibia are often visible and almost always palpable. Common examples are cartilage-capped exostoses (osteochondromata) and the characteristic painful swelling of Osgood–Schlatter's disease of the tibial tubercle (see below).

RUPTURES OF THE EXTENSOR APPARATUS

Resisted extension of the knee may tear the extensor mechanism. The patient stumbles on a stair, catches his or her foot while walking or running, or may be kicking a muddy football. In all these incidents, active knee extension is prevented by an obstacle. The precise location of the lesion varies with the patient's age. In the elderly the injury is usually above the patella; in middle life the patella fractures; in young adults the patellar ligament can rupture. In adolescents the upper tibial apophysis is occasionally avulsed; much more often it is merely 'strained'.

Tendon rupture sometimes occurs with minimal strain; this is seen in patients with connective tissue disorders (e.g. systemic lupus erythematosus) and advanced rheumatoid disease, especially if they are also being treated with corticosteroids.

Rupture above the patella

Rupture may occur in the belly of the rectus femoris. The patient is usually elderly, or on long-term corticosteroid treatment. The torn muscle retracts and forms a characteristic lump in the thigh. Function is usually good, so no treatment is required.

Avulsion of the quadriceps tendon from the upper pole of the patella is seen in the same group of people. Sometimes it is bilateral. Operative repair is essential.

Rupture below the patella

This occurs mainly in young people. The ligament may rupture or may be avulsed from the lower pole of the patella. Operative repair is necessary.

Osgood–Schlatter's disease ('apophysitis' of the tibial tubercle)

In this common disorder of adolescence the tibial tubercle becomes painful and 'swollen'. Although often called osteochondritis or apophysitis, it is nothing more than a traction injury of the apophysis into which part of the patellar tendon is inserted (the remainder is inserted on each side of the apophysis and prevents complete separation).

There is no history of injury and sometimes the condition is bilateral. A young adolescent complains of pain after activity, and of a lump. The lump is tender and its situation over the tibial tuberosity is diagnostic. Sometimes active extension of the knee against resistance is painful and x-rays may reveal fragmentation of the apophysis.

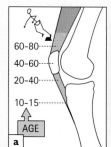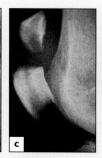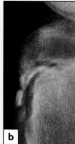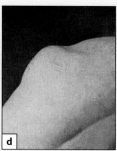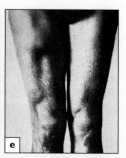

20.38 Extensor mechanism lesions These follow resisted action of the quadriceps; they usually occur at a progressively higher level with increasing age (**a**). (**b**) Schlatter's disease – the only one that usually does not follow a definite accident; (**c**) gap fracture of patella; (**d**) ruptured quadriceps tendon (note the suprapatellar depression); (**e**) ruptured rectus femoris causing a lump with a hollow below.

Spontaneous recovery is usual but takes time, and it is wise to restrict such activities as cycling and soccer. Occasionally, symptoms persist and, if patience or wearing a back-splint during the day are unavailing, a separate ossicle in the tendon is usually responsible; its removal is then worthwhile.

CALCIFICATION AND OSSIFICATION AROUND THE KNEE

Calcification in the medial ligament

Acute pain in the medial collateral ligament may be due to a soft calcific deposit among the fibres of the ligament. There may be a small, exquisitely tender lump in the line of the ligament. Pain is dramatically relieved by operative evacuation of the deposit.

Pellegrini—Stieda's disease

X-rays sometimes show a plaque of bone lying next to the femoral condyle under the medial collateral ligament. Occasionally this is a source of pain. It is generally ascribed to ossification of a haematoma following a tear of the medial ligament, though a history of injury is not always forthcoming. Treatment is rarely needed.

Patellar 'tendinopathy'

In Sinding–Johansson–Larsen's disease the patellar ligament is partially avulsed from the lower pole of the patella; a traction 'tendinitis' develops, usually with calcification. The condition is comparable to Osgood–Schlatter's disease and usually recovers with rest. A similar condition has been described at the proximal pole of the patella.

Pain and tenderness in the middle portion of the patellar ligament may occur in athletes; CT or ultrasonography will reveal an abnormal area. If rest fails to provide relief, the abnormal area is removed and the paratenon stripped (King *et al.*, 1990; Khan *et al.*, 1998).

PRINCIPLES OF KNEE OPERATIONS

ARTHROSCOPY

Arthroscopy is useful: (1) to establish or refine the accuracy of diagnosis; (2) to help in deciding whether to operate and (3) to perform certain operative procedures.

TECHNIQUE   Full asepsis in an operating theatre is essential. The patient is anaesthetized (though local anaesthesia may suffice for short procedures) and a thigh tourniquet applied. Through a tiny incision, a trocar and cannula are introduced; sometimes, saline is injected to distend the joint before it is punctured. Entry into the joint is confirmed when saline flows easily into it or, if the joint was distended previously, by the outflow when the trocar is withdrawn. A fibre-optic viewer, light source and irrigation system are attached; a small television camera and monitor make it much easier for the operator to concentrate on manipulating the instruments with both hands ('triangulation'). All compartments of the joint are now systematically inspected; with special instruments and, if necessary, through multiple portals, biopsy, partial meniscectomy, patellar shaving, removal of loose bodies, synovectomy, ligament replacement and many other procedures are possible. Before withdrawing the instrument, saline is squeezed out. A firm bandage is applied; the arthroscopic portals are often small enough not to require sutures. Post-operative recovery is remarkably rapid.

COMPLICATIONS   Intra-articular effusions and small haemarthroses are fairly common but seldom troublesome.

Reflex sympathetic dystrophy (which may resemble a low-grade infection during the weeks following arthroscopy) is sometimes troublesome. It usually settles down with physiotherapy and treatment with non-steroidal anti-inflammatory drugs; occasionally it requires more radical treatment (see page 226).

LIGAMENT RECONSTRUCTION

The collateral and cruciate ligaments and the knee capsule are important constraints which allow normal knee function; laxity or rupture of these structures, either singly or in combination, is often the source of recurrent episodes of 'giving way'. Although a significant proportion of such injuries (usually grade 1 or 2 sprains) are treated non-operatively, complete ruptures may require surgery in 'high-demand' individuals.

Surgery for ligament reconstruction includes: (1) *repair*, usually for collateral ligament mid-substance ruptures when they are found in combination with cruciate ligament injuries: this repair can be a simple end-to-end suture; (2) *substitution*, usually for anterior cruciate ruptures: the semitendonosus can be carefully anchored to the femur and tibia ensuring that stability is restored without loss of knee movement; another method is to use an autologous graft from the patellar tendon; (3) *tenodesis*, using a variety of tendons which are passed either through bony or soft tissue tunnels to 'check' the abnormal movement resulting from ligament rupture.

OSTEOTOMY

Osteotomy may be carried out either above or below the knee. As a general rule, and for sound biomechanical reasons, a valgus osteotomy (i.e. to correct a varus deformity) is best done through the proximal end of the tibia whereas a varus osteotomy (to correct a valgus deformity) is more effective at the femoral supracondylar level.

RATIONALE Osteotomy aims to divide the bone and reposition the fragments, either in order to correct an existing deformity or to alter the load-bearing mechanics of the joint. It may also relieve intraosseous venous congestion.

INDICATIONS Varus or valgus deformity, hyperextension or fixed flexion may result from a variety of conditions; growth defects, epiphyseal injuries, malunited fractures, articular destruction due to arthritis or stretched ligaments. In these cases the operation is indicated primarily for the correction of deformity, though it may also prevent or delay the development of osteoarthritis.

Osteoarthritis is often associated with varus deformity, and medial compartment overload causes localized pain and progressive destruction of the articular surfaces in one-half of the joint. When this occurs in a relatively young patient, and provided the joint has a reasonable range of movement and is still stable, a high tibial valgus osteotomy offers a reasonable alternative to a unicompartmental arthroplasty. By realigning the joint, load is transferred from the medial compartment to the centre or towards the lateral side. Slight over-correction may further offload the medial compartment but marked valgus should be avoided as this will rapidly lead to cartilage loss in the lateral compartment. The reduction of pain may, to some extent, be due to decompression of the hypervascular subchondral bone.

TECHNIQUE Angles must be accurately measured and the position of correction carefully calculated before starting the operation. In a high tibial osteotomy the fibula must be released either by dividing it lower down or by disrupting the proximal tibiofibular joint. The tibia is divided and fixed in one of two ways. (1) A wedge of bone, based laterally, is cut out at a level above the attachment of the patellar ligament; the gap is closed and the fragments are fixed with staples in the corrected position; the limb is then immobilized in plaster for 4–6 weeks (Coventry, 1985). (2) Alternatively, the tibia is divided in a dome-shaped fashion just above the tibial tubercle, the desired position is obtained and the fragments are held by compression pins until union occurs (Maquet, 1976).

An alternative technique is *hemicallotasis*: here, rather than a closing wedge laterally, an opening wedge is gradually created on the medial side. The osteotomy is usually above the insertion of the patellar ligament and often only two-thirds of the width of the proximal tibia needs to be divided. A gradual distraction force is applied by an external fixator fixed to the medial

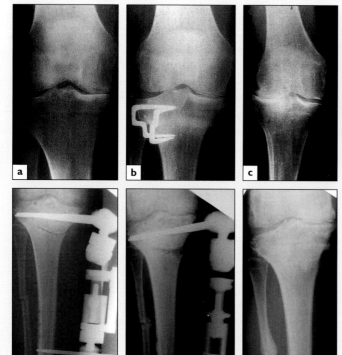
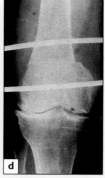

20.39 Osteotomy (a, b) For varus deformity, a high tibial osteotomy is the most effective. **(c, d)** For valgus deformity, the osteotomy should be on the femoral side of the joint. **(e, f, g)** An alternative method for treating a varus deformity is hemicallotasis, where a partial division of the tibial plateau proximal to the tibial tubercle is combined with gradual correction in an external fixator.

surface of the tibia after an initial delay of 5 days; this creates an opening wedge which is quickly filled with callus. The advantages of this technique are (a) the ability to 'titrate' the correction and (b) the avoidance of plaster immobilization. The external fixator usually remains on the patient for 10–12 weeks.

RESULTS High tibial valgus osteotomy, when done for osteoarthritis, gives good results provided (1) the disease is confined to the medial compartment and (2) the knee has a good range of movement and is stable. Relief of pain is good in 85% of cases in the first year but drops to approximately 60% after 5 years. In most cases osteotomy is seen as an alternative to a (medial) unicompartmental arthroplasty.

COMPLICATIONS The most important early complication of tibial osteotomy is a *compartment syndrome* of the leg. Careful and repeated checks should be carried out during the early postoperative period to ensure that there are no symptoms or signs of impending ischaemia.

The main late complication is *failure to correct the deformity*, which is really a defect in technique. With medial compartment osteoarthritis, unless a slight valgus position is obtained (about 5° more than in the opposite, normal knee), the result is liable to be unsatisfactory.

ARTHRODESIS

A stiff knee is a considerable disability; it makes climbing difficult and sitting in crowded areas distinctly awkward. Consequently, arthrodesis is not often performed. Nevertheless, it remains the only certain way of relieving pain permanently, and it may particularly be indicated for a failed knee replacement. A short period in plaster before operation enables the patient to decide if the inconvenience is tolerable.

TECHNIQUE A vertical midline incision is used. If the operation is for tuberculosis the diseased synovium is excised; otherwise it is disregarded. The posterior vessels and nerves are protected and the ends of the tibia and femur removed by means of straight saw cuts, aiming to end with 15° of flexion and 7° of valgus as the position of fusion. Charnley's method, using thick Steinman pins inserted parallel through the distal femur and proximal tibia, and connecting these with compression clamps, was a standard method. Nowadays, multiplanar external fixation is used.

KNEE REPLACEMENT

INDICATIONS
The main indication for knee replacement is pain, especially when combined with deformity and instability. Most replacements are performed for rheumatoid arthritis or osteoarthritis.

TYPES OF OPERATION
Partial replacement The role of unicompartmental replacement has yet to be firmly established. Early results for medial osteoarthritis were promising but longer-term studies have suggested the need for meticulous and exacting surgical technique to avoid high revision rates. When successful, relief of pain and restoration of function can

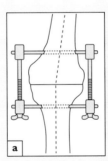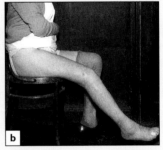

20.40 Arthrodesis (a) Compression arthrodesis with the joint in slight flexion and valgus. (**b**) The patient with a stiff knee has some difficulty sitting comfortably – and keeping the leg out of the way of passers-by.

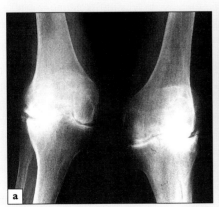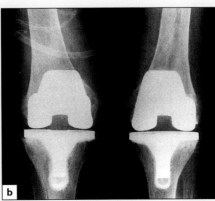

20.41 Total joint replacement X-rays (**a**) before and (**b**) after resurfacing of the femur, tibia and patella.

be impressive, but for the present it is reserved for older patients; tibial and femoral osteotomies are used in the younger population.

Patellar resurfacing, a kind of partial replacement, is rarely performed alone; usually it is combined with surface replacement of the condyles.

Minimally constrained total replacement The term 'minimally constrained' is used for prostheses where some of the stability after replacement is provided by the prosthesis and some through preservation of the knee ligaments. Most modern minimally constrained designs allow sacrifice of the anterior cruciate ligament; some even allow both cruciates to be removed without detriment to the long-term survival of the prosthesis. Totally unconstrained devices, where both cruciates are preserved, are rarely used as results were poor compared to the minimally constrained group.

At operation all the articular surfaces are replaced – metal on the femoral side, polyethylene on a metal tray on the tibial side and polyethylene alone on the patella. It is important to ensure correct placement of the implants so as to reproduce the normal mechanics of the knee as closely as possible.

The tibial and patellar components are fixed with cement, whereas the femoral component may be press-fitted. Bone defects may be filled either with bone graft, metal augmentation wedges or cement. The development of suitable prostheses and instrumentation in recent years has led to vast improvements in technique, so the results are now similar to those of hip replacement.

Constrained joints Joints with fixed hinges are used when there is marked bone loss and severe instability. Their main value nowadays is to provide a mobile joint following resection of tumours at the bone ends. The lack of rotation in these implants places severe stresses on the bone–implant interfaces and they are liable to loosen, to break or to erode the tibial or femoral shafts unless inactivity severely limits their use. Moreover, a considerable amount of bone has to be removed, and this makes subsequent arthrodesis difficult.

COMPLICATIONS

General As with all knee operations (except arthroscopy) in which a tourniquet is used, there is a high incidence of deep vein thrombosis. Prophylaxis, either pharmacological (anticoagulants) or mechanical (foot pumps, compression stockings), is recommended.

Infection The methods of preventing and treating infection are similar to those used in hip replacement. Treatment by debridement and antibiotics, or by exchange replacement in one or two stages, are obvious possibilities, though probably the safest salvage operation is arthrodesis.

Loosening This results from faulty prosthetic design or inaccurate bone shaping and placement of the implants. It is important: (1) to overcome deformity (the knee should finally be about 7° valgus); (2) to promote stability (by tailoring the bone cuts so that the collateral ligaments are equally tense in both flexion and extension); and (3) to permit rotation (otherwise cemented prostheses are liable to loosen). Revision surgery for loose prostheses must deal with the cause, be it malposition of the prosthesis, wear debris or infection. A loose prosthesis can be re-cemented, but unless the cause is dealt with loosening will recur.

Patellar problems Though relatively uncommon, these can be very disabling. They include (1) recurrent patellar subluxation or dislocation, which may need realignment, and (2) complications associated with patellar resurfacing, such as loosening of the prosthetic component, fracture of the remaining bony patella and catching of soft tissues between the patella and the femur. Patella tracking as assessed on the operating table after implantation of the prosthesis is important; any tendency to sublux must be corrected – often the cause is unequal soft tissue tension (for which a lateral release will be needed) or a tibial component placed in internal rotation. The risk of patellar fracture post-operatively can also be lessened if care is taken not to divide the geniculate vessels when performing a lateral release.

NOTES ON APPLIED ANATOMY

The knee joint combines two articulations – tibiofemoral and patellofemoral. The bones of the tibiofemoral joint have little or no inherent stability; this depends largely upon strong ligaments and muscles. The patellofemoral joint is so shaped that the patella moves in a shallow path (or track) between the femoral condyles; if this track is too shallow the patella readily dislocates, and if its line is faulty the patellar articular cartilage is subject to excessive wear. One important function of the patella is to increase the power of extension; it lifts the quadriceps forwards, thereby increasing its moment arm.

The patellar tendon is inserted into the upper pole of the patella. It is in line with the shaft of the femur, whereas the patellar ligament is in line with the shaft of the tibia. Because of the angle between them (the Q-angle) quadriceps contraction would pull the patella laterally were it not for the fibres of vastus medialis, which are transverse. This muscle is therefore important and it is essential to try to prevent the otherwise rapid wasting that is liable to follow any effusion.

The shaft of the femur is inclined medially, while the tibia is vertical; thus the normal knee is slightly valgus (average 7°). This amount is physiological and the term 'genu valgum' is used only when the angle exceeds 7°; significantly less than this amount is genu varum.

During walking, weight is necessarily taken alternately on each leg. The line of body weight falls medial to the knee and must be counterbalanced by muscle action lateral to the joint (chiefly the tensor fascia femoris). To calculate the force transmitted across the knee, that due to muscle action must be added to that imposed by gravity; moreover, since with each step the knee is braced by the quadriceps, the force that this imposes also must be added.

Clearly the stresses on the articular cartilage are (as they also are at the hip) much greater than consideration only of body weight would lead one to suppose. It is also obvious that a varus deformity can easily overload the medial compartment, leading to cartilage breakdown; similarly, a valgus deformity may overload the lateral compartment.

As the knee bends, the axis of the tibiofemoral 'hinge' moves further and further backwards, so that the rolling movement of the femoral condyles is accompanied by backwards gliding of the tibia. As the knee straightens, these are reversed; in addition, during the final stages of extension the tibia rotates laterally (hence the differing shapes of the two femoral condyles). The complex combination of a rolling, gliding and rotating movement is difficult to analyse; it is even more difficult to reproduce in a prosthesis.

Situated as they are between these complexly moving surfaces, the fibrocartilaginous menisci are prone to injury, particularly during unguarded movements of extension and rotation on the weightbearing leg. The medial meniscus is especially vulnerable because, in addition to its loose attachments via the coronary ligaments, it is firmly attached at three widely separated points: the anterior horn, the posterior horn and the medial collateral ligament. The lateral meniscus more readily escapes damage because it is attached only at its anterior and posterior horns and these are close to each other.

The function of the menisci is not known for certain, but they certainly increase the contact area between femur and tibia. They play a significant part in weight transmission and this applies at all angles of flexion and extension; as the knee bends they glide backwards, and as it straightens they are pushed forwards.

The deep portion of the medial collateral ligament, to which the meniscus is attached, is fan-shaped and blends with the posteromedial capsule. It is, therefore, not surprising that medial ligament tears are often associated with tears of the medial meniscus and of the posteromedial capsule. The lateral collateral ligament is situated more posteriorly and does not blend with the capsule; nor is it attached to the meniscus, from which it is separated by the tendon of popliteus.

The two collateral ligaments resist sideways tilting of the extended knee. In addition, the medial ligament prevents the medial tibial condyle from subluxating forwards. Forwards subluxation of the lateral tibial condyle, however, is prevented, not by the lateral collateral ligament but by the anterior cruciate. Only when the medial ligament and the anterior cruciate are both torn can the whole tibia subluxate forwards (giving a marked positive anterior drawer sign). Backwards subluxation of the tibia is prevented by the powerful posterior cruciate ligament in combination with the arcuate ligament on its lateral side and the posterior oblique ligament on its medial side.

The cruciate ligaments are crucial, in the sense that they are essential for stability of the knee. The anterior cruciate ligament prevents forwards displacement of the tibia on the femur and, in particular, it prevents forwards subluxation of the lateral tibial condyle, a movement that tends to occur if a person who is running twists suddenly. The posterior cruciate ligament prevents backwards displacement of the tibia on the femur and its integrity is therefore important when progressing downhill.

REFERENCES AND FURTHER READING

Apley AG (1947) The diagnosis of meniscus injuries: some new clinical methods. *Journal of Bone and Joint Surgery* **29**, 78-84

Bentley G (1985) Articular cartilage changes in chondromalacia patellae. *Journal of Bone and Joint Surgery* **67B**, 769-774

Bowen JR, Leahy JL, Zhang Z, MacEwen GD (1985) Partial epiphyseodesis at the knee to correct angular deformity. *Clinical Orthopaedics* **198**, 184-190

Coventry MB (1985) Upper tibial osteotomy for osteoarthritis. *Journal of Bone and Joint Surgery* **67A**, 1136-1140

Crotty JM, Monu JU, Pope TL Jr (1996) Magnetic resonance imaging of the musculoskeletal system. Part 4. The knee. *Clinical Orthopaedics and Related Research* **330**, 288-303

Dandy DJ (1995) Chronic patellofemoral instability. *Journal of Bone and Joint Surgery* **78B**, 328-35

Dimakopoulos P, Patel D (1990) Partial excision of discoid meniscus. *Acta Orthopaedica Scandinavica* **61**, 1-40

Ficat RP, Hungerford DS (1977) *Disorders of the Patello-femoral Joint*. Williams & Wilkins,. Baltimore

Goodfellow J, Hungerford DS, Zindel M (1976a) Patello-femoral joint mechanics and pathology. 1. Functional anatomy of the patello-femoral joint. *Journal of Bone and Joint Surgery* **58B**, 287-90

Goodfellow J, Hungerford DS, Woods C (1976b) Patello-femoral joint mechanics and pathology. 2. Chondromalacia patellae. *Journal of Bone and Joint Surgery* **58B**, 291-9

Goodfellow JW, Kershaw CJ, Benson MKD'A, O'Connor JJ (1988) The Oxford knee for unicompartmental osteoarthritis. *Journal of Bone and Joint Surgery* **70**B, 692-701

Grelsamer RP (1995) Unicompartmental osteoarthrosis of the knee. *Journal of Bone and Joint Surgery* **77**A, 278-92

Hong-Xue Men, Chan-Hua Bian, Chan-Dou Yang *et al* (1991) Surgical treatment of the flail knee after poliomyelitis. *Journal of Bone and Joint Surgery* **73**B, 195-198

Inone M, Shino K, Hirose H *et al* (1988) Subluxation of the patella. Computed tomography analysis of patellofemoral congruence. *Journal of Bone and Joint Surgery* **70**A, 1331-1337

Insall JN, Salvati E (1971) Patella position in the normal knee joint. *Radiology* **101**, 101

Kay PR, Freemont AJ, Davies DRA (1989) The aetiology of multiple loose bodies. *Journal of Bone and Joint Surgery* **71**B, 501-504

Khan KM, Maffulli N, Coleman BD *et al* (1998) Patellar tendinopathy: some aspects of basic science and clinical management. *British Journal of Sports Medicine* **32**, 346-55

King JB, Perry DJ, Mourad K, Kumar SJ (1990) Lesions of the patellar ligament. *Journal of Bone and Joint Surgery* **72**B, 46-48

Liu SH, Mirzayan R (1995) Current review. Functional knee bracing. *Clinical Orthopaedics and Related Research* **317**, 273-81

Mann G, Finsterbush A, Franfkl U *et al* (1991) A method of diagnosing small amounts of fluid in the knee. *Journal of Bone and Joint Surgery* **73**B, 346-347.

Maquet PGJ (1976) *Biomechanics of the Knee*. Springer, Berlin, Heidelberg and New York

Merchant AC, Mercer RL, Jacobsen RH, Cool CR (1974) Roentgenographic analysis of patellofemoral congruence. *Journal of Bone and Joint Surgery* **56**A, 1391-1396

Mont MA, Baumgarten KM, Rifai A et al. (2000) Atraumatic osteonecrosis of the knee. *Journal of Bone and Joint Surgery* **82**A, 1279–1290

Paletta GA Jr, Laskin RS (1995) Total knee arthroplasty after a previous patellectomy. *Journal of Bone and Joint Surgery* **77**A, 1708-1712

Parisien JS (1990) Arthroscopic treatment of cysts of the menisci. *Clinical Orthopaedics and Related Research* **257**, 154-158

Salenius P, Vankka E (1975) The development of the tibiofemoral angle in children. *Journal of Bone and Joint Surgery* **57**A, 259-261

Schenck RC Jr, Goodnight JM (1996) Osteochondritis dissecans. *Journal of Bone and Joint Surgery* **78**A, 439-456

Sherman OH, Fox JM, Snyder SJ et al. (1986) Arthroscopy – 'No-problem surgery'. An analysis of complications in two thousand six hundred and forty cases. *Journal of Bone and Joint Surgery* **68**A, 256–265

CLINICAL ASSESSMENT

SYMPTOMS

The most common presenting symptoms are pain, deformity, swelling and giving way. It is important to know whether standing or walking provokes the symptoms and whether shoe pressure is a factor.

Pain over a bony prominence or a joint is probably due to some local disorder. Pain across the forefoot (*metatarsalgia*) is less specific and is often associated with uneven loading and muscle fatigue.

Deformity may be in the ankle, the foot or the toes. Parents often worry about their children who are 'flat-footed' or 'pigeon-toed'. Elderly patients may complain chiefly of having difficulty fitting shoes.

Swelling may be diffuse and bilateral, or localized; unilateral swelling nearly always has a surgical cause, bilateral swelling is more often 'medical' in origin. Swelling over the medial side of the first metatarsal head (a *bunion*) is common in older women.

Corns and callosities may give rise to shoe pressure and acute tenderness over prominent joints or under the metatarsal heads.

Instability of the ankle or subtalar joint produces repeated episodes of the joint 'giving way'.

Numbness and paraesthesia may be felt in all the toes or in a circumscribed field served by a single nerve or one of the nerve roots from the spine.

SIGNS WITH THE PATIENT UPRIGHT

The patient, whose lower limbs should be exposed from the knees down, stands first facing the surgeon, then with his or her back to the surgeon. Ask the patient to rise up on tiptoes and then settle back on the heels. Note the posture of the feet throughout this movement. Normally the heels are in slight valgus while standing and inverted on tiptoes; the degree of inversion should be equal on the two sides, showing that the subtalar joint is mobile and the tibialis posterior functioning. Viewed from behind, if there is excessive eversion of one foot, the lateral toes are more easily visible on that side (the *'too-many-toes' sign*).

Gait The patient is then asked to walk normally. Note whether the gait is smooth or halting and whether the feet are well balanced. Gait is easier to analyse if one concentrates on the sequence of movements that make up the walking cycle. It begins with heel-strike, then moves into stance, then push-off and finally swing-through before making the next heel-strike. The stance phase itself can be further divided into three intervals: from heel-strike to flat foot; progressive ankle dorsiflexion as the body passes over the foot; and ankle plantarflexion leading to toe-off.

Gait may be disturbed by pain, muscle weakness, deformity or stiffness. The position and mobility of the ankle is of prime importance. A fixed equinus deformity results in the heel failing to strike the ground at the beginning of the walking cycle; sometimes the patient forces heel contact by hyperextending the knee.

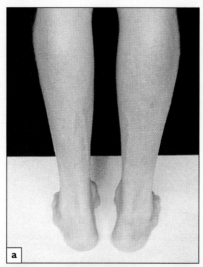

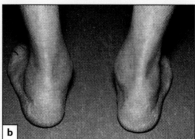

21.1 Examination Look – from behind. (**a**) In this patient the heels are turned inwards (varus) and the longitudinal arches are higher than normal (cavus). (**b**) This is the opposite: the left foot is in valgus, due to rupture of the tibialis posterior tendon; note the 'too-many-toes' sign.

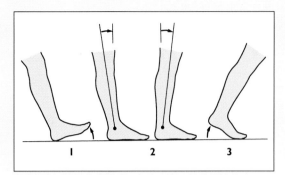

21.2 Gait – the three rockers of ankle-stance phase The first rocker begins with heel strike – if the anterior compartment muscles are weak, a 'foot slap' is noticeable; or if the ankle is in fixed equinus, this rocker may be absent altogether. In mid-stance, the centre of gravity of the body (and ground reaction force) moves from a position posterior to the ankle joint to anterior (second rocker). The third rocker produces an acceleration force which shifts the fulcrum of the pivot forwards to the metatarsal heads, just prior to toe-off (Gage, 1991).

If the ankle dorsiflexors are weak, the forefoot may hit the ground prematurely, causing a 'slap'; this is referred to as foot-drop (or drop-foot). During swing-through the leg is lifted higher than usual so that the foot can clear the ground; this is known as a high-stepping gait.

Hindfoot and midfoot deformities may interfere with level ground-contact in the second interval of stance; the patient walks on the inner or outer border of the foot.

Toe contact, especially of the great toe, is also important; pain or stiffness in the first metatarsophalangeal joint may prevent normal push-off.

SIGNS WITH THE PATIENT SITTING OR LYING

The patient is next examined lying on a couch, or it may be more convenient if he or she sits opposite the examiner and places each foot in turn on the examiner's lap.

Look

The heel is held square so that any foot deformity can be assessed. The toes and sole should be inspected for skin changes. Thickening and keratosis may be seen over the proximal toe joints (corns); or on the soles (callosities).

Look for signs of skin breakdown or ulcers: those near the ends of the toes are usually ischaemic; those overlying bony prominences may be neuropathic.

Feel

The skin temperature is assessed and the pulses are felt. Remember that one in every six normal people do not have a dorsalis pedis artery. If all the foot pulses are absent, feel for the popliteal and femoral pulses; the patient may need further evaluation by Doppler ultrasound.

If there is tenderness in the foot it must be precisely localized, for its site is often diagnostic. Any swelling, oedema or lumps must be examined.

Sensation may be abnormal; the precise distribution of any change is important. If a neuropathy is suspected (e.g. in a diabetic patient) test also for vibration sense, protective sensation and sense of position in the toes.

Move

The foot comprises a series of joints which should be examined methodically.

Ankle joint With the heel grasped in the left hand and the midfoot in the right, the ranges of plantarflexion (flexion) and dorsiflexion (extension) are estimated. Beware not to let the foot go into valgus during passive dorsiflexion as this will give an erroneous idea of the range of movement.

Subtalar joint It is important to 'lock' the ankle joint when assessing subtalar inversion and eversion. This is done simply by ensuring that the ankle is plantigrade when the heel is moved. It is often easier to record the amount of subtalar movement if the patient is examined prone. Inversion is normally greater than eversion.

Midtarsal joint One hand grips the heel firmly to stabilize the hindfoot while the other hand moves the forefront up and down and from side to side.

Toes The metatarsophalangeal and interphalangeal joints are tested separately. Extension (dorsiflexion) of the great toe at the metatarsophalangeal joint should normally exceed 70° and flexion 10°.

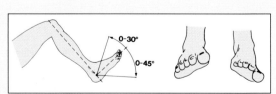

21.3 Normal range of movement All movements are measured from zero with the foot in the 'neutral' or 'anatomical' position: thus, dorsiflexion is 0–30° and plantarflexion 0–45°. Inversion is normally greater than eversion.

Stability

Stability is assessed by moving the joints across the normal physiological planes and noting any abnormal 'clunks'. Ankle stability should be tested in both coronal and sagittal planes, always comparing the two joints. Patients with recent ligament injury may have to be examined under anaesthesia.

Medial and lateral stability are checked by stressing the ankle first in valgus and then in varus. *Anteroposterior stability* is assesed by performing an anterior 'drawer test': the patient lies on the examination couch with hips and knees flexed and the feet resting on the couch surface; the examiner grasps the distal tibia with both hands and pushes firmly backwards, feeling for abnormal translation of the tibia upon the talus. Another way of doing this is to stabilize the distal tibia with one hand while the other grasps the heel and tries to shift the hindfoot forwards and backwards.

The same tests can be performed under x-ray and the positions of the two ankles measured and compared (see below).

Muscle power

Power is tested by resisting active movement in each direction. The patient will be more cooperative if you demonstrate precisely what movement is required. While the movement is held, feel the muscle belly and tendon to establish whether they are intact and functioning.

Shoes

Don't forget to examine the shoes; they also can provide valuable information about faulty stance or gait.

General examination

If there are any symptoms or signs of vascular or neurological impairment, or if multiple joints are affected, a more general examination is essential.

IMAGING

There are practical problems with imaging in children, and babies in particular, because of the need for the child's cooperation. Interpretation is often difficult owing to the incompletely ossified skeleton.

X-rays In the adult, the standard views of the ankle are anteroposterior, mortise (an anteroposterior view with the ankle internally rotated 15–20°) and lateral. Although the subtalar joint can be seen in a lateral view of the foot, medial and lateral oblique projections allow better assessment of the joint. These views are often used to check articular congruity after treatment of calcaneal fractures. The calcaneum itself is usually x-rayed in axial and lateral views, but a weight-bearing view is helpful in defining its relationship to the talus and tibia (Cobey, 1976). The foot, toes and the intertarsal joints are well displayed in standing anteroposterior and medial oblique views, but occasionally a true lateral view is needed.

Stress x-rays These complement the clinical tests for ankle stability. The patient should be completely relaxed; if the ankle is too painful, stress x-rays can be performed under regional or general anaesthesia. Both ankles should be examined, for comparison.

Computed tomography (CT) CT provides excellent coronal views and is important in assessing fractures and congenital bony coalitions.

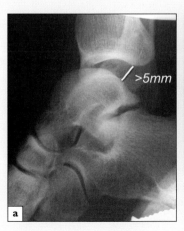
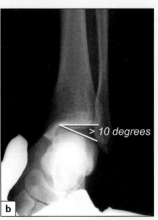

21.4 X-rays – stress views The ankle is held in approximately 10° of plantarflexion when carrying out the anterior drawer or talar tilt test. Comparisons are made with the normal side. **(a)** The anterior drawer tests the integrity of the anterior talofibular ligament; a difference of more than 5mm between the two sides signifies rupture of the ligament. **(b)** Inversion stress tests the integrity of both the anterior talofibular and calcaneofibular ligaments; a difference of greater than 10° of talar tilt between the two sides suggests ligament rupture (Mardner, 1994; Colville, 1994).

Radioscintigraphy Radioisotope scanning, though non-specific, is excellent for localizing areas of abnormal blood flow or bone remodelling activity; it is useful in the diagnosis of covert infection.

Magnetic resonance imaging (MRI) and ultrasound These methods are used to demonstrate soft-tissue problems, such as tendon and ligament injuries.

PEDOBAROGRAPHY

A record of pressures beneath the foot can be obtained by having the patient stand or walk over a force plate; sensors in the plate produce a dynamic map of the peak pressures and the time over which these are recorded can be obtained. Although this is sometimes helpful in clinical decision-making, or for comparing pre- and post-operative function, the investigation is used mainly as a research tool.

CONGENITAL DEFORMITIES

Congenital deformities of the foot are common. Many appear as part of a more widespread genetic disorder; only those in which the foot is the main (or only) problem are considered in this section. Isolated abnormalities of the toes, also, are dealt with elsewhere.

TALIPES EQUINOVARUS (IDIOPATHIC CLUB-FOOT)

The term *'talipes'* is derived from *talus* (L = ankle bone) and *pes* (L = foot). Equinovarus is one of several different *talipes* deformities; others are talipes calcaneus and talipes valgus (see below)

In the full-blown equinovarus deformity the heel is in equinus, the entire hindfoot in varus and the mid- and forefoot adducted and supinated. The abnormality is relatively common, the incidence ranging from 1–2 per thousand births; boys are affected twice as often as girls and the condition is bilateral in one-third of cases.

The exact cause is not known, although the resemblance to other disorders suggests several possible mechanisms. It could be a genetic defect, or a form of arrested development. Its occurrence in neurological disorders and neural tube defects (e.g. myelomeningocele and spinal dysraphism) points to a neuromuscular disorder. Severe examples of club-foot are seen in association with arthrogryposis, tibial deficiency and constriction rings. In some cases it is no more than a postural deformity caused by tight packing in an overcrowded uterus.

Pathological anatomy

The neck of the talus points downwards and deviates medially, whereas the body is rotated slightly outwards in relation to both the calcaneum and the ankle mortise (Herzenberg *et al.*, 1988). The posterior part of the calcaneum is held close to the fibula by a tight calcaneo-fibular ligament, and is tilted into equinus and varus; it is also medially rotated beneath the ankle. The navicular and the entire forefoot are shifted medially and rotated into supination (the composite varus deformity).

The skin and soft tissues of the calf and the medial side of the foot are short and underdeveloped. If the condition is not corrected early, secondary growth changes occur in the bones; these are permanent. Even with treatment the foot is liable to be short and the calf may remain thin.

Clinical features

The deformity is usually obvious at birth; the foot is both turned and twisted inwards so that the sole faces posteromedially. More precisely, the ankle is in equinus, the heel is inverted and the forefoot is adducted and supinated; sometimes the foot also has a high medial arch (cavus), and the talus may protrude on the dorsolateral surface of the foot. The heel is usually small and high, and deep creases appear posteriorly and medially; some of these creases are incomplete constriction bands. In some cases the calf is abnormally thin.

In a normal baby the foot can be dorsiflexed and everted until the toes touch the front of the leg. In club foot this manoeuvre meets with varying degrees of resistance and in severe cases the deformity is fixed.

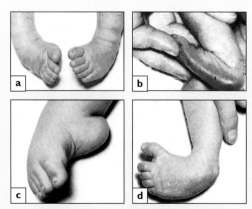

21.5 Talipes equinovarus (club foot) (**a**) True club foot is a fixed deformity, unlike (**b**) 'postural' talipes, which is easily correctable by gentle passive movement. (**c**) With true club foot the poorly developed heel is higher than the forefoot, which is also (**d**) varus.

The infant must always be examined for associated disorders such as congenital hip dislocation and spina bifida. The absence of creases suggests arthrogryposis; look to see if other joints are affected.

X-rays

X-rays are used mainly to assess progress after treatment. The *anteroposterior film* is taken with the foot 30° plantarflexed and the tube likewise angled 30° to the perpendicular. Lines can be drawn through the long axis of the talus parallel to its medial border and through that of the calcaneum parallel to its lateral border; they normally cross at an angle of 20–40° (Kite's angle) but in club foot the two lines may be almost parallel. Incomplete ossification makes it difficult to decide exactly where to draw these lines and this means that there is a considerable degree of inter-observer variation.

The *lateral film* is taken with the foot in forced dorsiflexion. Lines drawn through the mid-longitudinal axis of the talus and the lower border of the calcaneum should meet at an angle of about 40°. Anything less than 20° shows that the calcaneum cannot be tilted up into true dorsiflexion; the foot may *seem* to be dorsiflexed but it may actually have 'broken' at the midtarsal level, producing the so-called *rocker-bottom deformity.*

Treatment

The aim of treatment is to produce and maintain a plantigrade, supple foot that will function well. There are several methods of treatment but relapse is common, especially in babies with associated neuromuscular disorders.

CONSERVATIVE TREATMENT

Treatment should begin early, preferably within a day or two of birth. This consists of repeated manipulation and adhesive strapping which maintains the correction; the manipulations are taught to the child's parents who are then able to carry out gentle stretches on a regular basis with the strapping still in place. Treatment is supervised by a physiotherapist who alters the strapping as correction is gradually obtained. If this level of care is not available, it may be better to hold position by applying a light plaster cast (over a protective layer of strapping) which is soaked off and changed every week.

The three main components of the deformity are always corrected in the following order. First the forefoot must be brought into rotational alignment with the hindfoot; paradoxically this is done by increasing the supination deformity of the forefoot so that it corresponds with the relatively more supinated hindfoot. Next, both hindfoot and forefoot are together gradually brought out of varus and supination; correction is assisted by keeping the fulcrum on the lateral side of the head of the talus. Finally, equinus is corrected by bringing the heel down and dorsiflexing the ankle. It may be necessary, *en route*, to perform percutaneous tendo Achillis lengthening in order to overcome the equinus (Ponseti, 1992).

The objective (ideally) is to achieve not only correction but *overcorrection*. The position should be checked by x-ray in order to ensure that there is no 'rocker-bottom' defect; attempts to overcome equinus before the other deformities are corrected may 'break' the foot in the midtarsal region.

Resistant cases will usually declare themselves after 8–12 weeks of serial manipulations and strapping. The surgeon then faces a choice of early surgery or continued conservative treatment. The results of early operation, in particular neonatal surgery, have not been

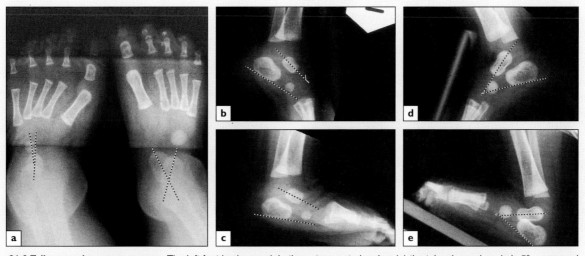

21.6 Talipes equinovarus – x-rays The left foot is abnormal. In the anteroposterior view (**a**) the talocalcaneal angle is 5°, compared to 42° on the right. In the lateral views, the left talocalcaneal angle is 10° in plantarflexion (**b**) and 14° in dorsiflexion (**c**); in the normal foot the angle is unchanged at 44°, whatever the position of the foot (**d, e**).

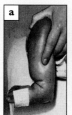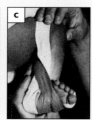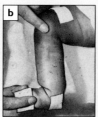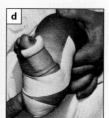

21.7 Treatment of club foot – strapping (**a–d**) Manipulation and strapping for talipes equinovarus.

shown to be better than those of late surgery. Delaying surgery until the child is near walking age has the advantages of operating on a larger foot (making surgery easier) and using the forces in normal walking to help maintain the correction obtained at surgery.

This delayed operative approach is suitable for severe, rigid deformities; however, for less severe cases it may be preferable to operate at around 6 months of age, but manipulation and splintage must still be continued until the child is walking.

OPERATIVE TREATMENT

The objectives of club foot surgery are (a) the complete release of joint 'tethers' (capsular and ligamentous contractures and fibrotic bands) and (b) lengthening of tendons so that the foot can be positioned normally without undue tension. A detailed knowledge of the pathological anatomy is a *sine qua non*.

Access to the involved structures is through either an extended posteromedial incision (Turco), a posterior curved transverse incision extended anteriorly on both medial and lateral sides ('Cincinatti' – Crawford), or a posterolateral incision combined with a separate curved medial incision (Caroll). The tendo Achillis and tibialis posterior tendons are lengthened through Z-divisions; the posterior capsules of the ankle and subtalar joints often have to be divided to allow adequate correction of hindfoot equinus. Sometimes flexor digitorum longus and flexor hallucis longus also require attention. The calcaneo-fibular ligament, a key structure in keeping the calcaneum malrotated, is then released. A complete subtalar release is performed to allow the hindfoot to be corrected. The superficial deltoid ligament is freed on the medial side but the deep part is preserved to prevent ankle instability.

Correction of the forefoot deformity is carried out by releasing the contractures around the talonavicular and calcaneocuboid joints. The interosseous ligament in the sinus canal should be preserved, especially in children with ligamentous laxity, as division may lead to overcorrection. Finally, the origin of the intrinsic muscles and plantar fascia from the calcaneum may need to be divided to reduce any cavus or plantaris.

The foot, in its corrected position, is immobilized in a plaster cast. Kirschner wires are sometimes inserted across the talonavicular and subtalar joints to augment the hold. The wires and cast are removed at 6–8 weeks,

after which hobble boots (Dennis Browne) or a custom ankle–foot orthosis is used, depending on whether the child has started walking. Stretching exercises which were performed prior to surgery are continued. The period of splintage varies: some surgeons wait until active dorsiflexion and eversion are established whereas others recommend some form of splintage until skeletal maturity.

LATE OR RELAPSED CLUB FOOT

Late presenters often have severe deformities with secondary bony changes, and the relapsed clubfoot is complicated by scarring from previous surgery. If the child is young (aged 4–7 years), a revision of the soft tissue releases may be considered together with a shortening of the lateral side of the foot by calcaneo-cuboid fusion or cuboid enucleation (Dilwyn Evans). Calcaneal osteotomies, in the form of lateral closing wedges or lateral translations, improve heel varus. Tendon transfers, once popular, now have a more limited role; a split tibialis anterior tendon transfer to the dorsum of the base of the fourth metatarsal may help balance weak evertors, whereas a transfer of tibialis posterior through the interosseous membrane to the dorsum will act as a dorsiflexor in neurological cases. However, tendon transfers work well only if the joints are mobile, and this is seldom the case in these patients.

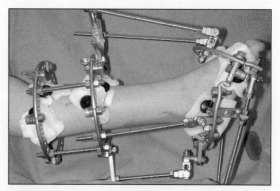

21.8 Treatment of club foot – the Ilizarov method This is used principally for those deformities which have relapsed despite multiple attempts at soft tissue surgery. By gradually modifying the shape of the external fixator, the joint contractures are progressively corrected.

Gradual correction by means of a circular external fixator (the Ilizarov method) has gained popularity in treating difficult relapsed cases and severe deformities; the early results are encouraging. Full corrections can be achieved even in feet severely scarred from previous surgery, and there is often an increase in the size of the foot, which is thought to be due to an increase in the blood supply during distraction. However, the procedure can be painful and long and, for the time being, it is best reserved for these very difficult cases.

Despite initially successful surgery, deformities do still recur. A deformed, stiff and painful foot in an adolescent is best salvaged by corrective osteotomies and fusions. The distorted anatomy makes triple arthrodesis a real challenge, but it is possible to end up with a plantigrade, stable and pain-free foot.

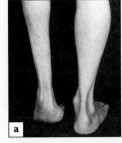
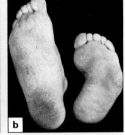

21.9 Late uncorrected club foot Adult appearance when club foot has not been adequately corrected. Note the thin calf and underdeveloped heel (**a**) as well as the persistent equino-varus deformity (**b**).

METATARSUS ADDUCTUS

Metatarsus adductus varies from a slightly curved fore-foot to something resembling a mild club foot. The majority (90%) either improve spontaneously or can be managed non-operatively using serial corrective casts followed by straight-last shoes. The more severe examples need operation. Extensive capsulectomies of the tarsometatarsal joints followed by prolonged splintage have fallen out of favour because of the risk of early degenerative arthritis in the repositioned joints. Variations of the Dilwyn Evans procedure (which aims to balance the lengths of the medial and lateral columns of the foot), often in combination with basal metatarsal osteotomies, are suitable for the small percentage of children who require surgical treatment.

TALIPES CALCANEOVALGUS

Calcaneovalgus is a common deformity which presents in the newborn as an acutely dorsiflexed foot. There is a deep crease (or several wrinkles) on the front of the ankle, and the calcaneum juts out posteriorly. Unlike congenital vertical talus (which also presents as an acutely dorsiflexed foot) this deformity is flexible. In addition, the anterior creases in congenital vertical talus are located over the midfoot.

Calcaneovalgus is usually bilateral. There is an association with hip dysplasia, especially if it presents on one side only; examination of the hips followed by ultrasound or x-rays is therefore recommended.

This is a postural deformity, probably due to abnormal intrauterine positioning, and it often corrects spontaneously in the neonatal period. Severe deformities occasionally require serial casts for correction.

FLAT-FOOT (PES PLANUS AND PES VALGUS)

'Our feet are no more alike than our faces.' This truism from a *British Medical Journal* Editorial sums up the

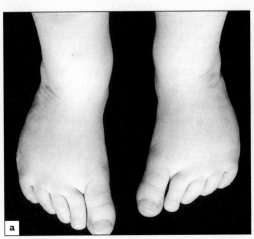
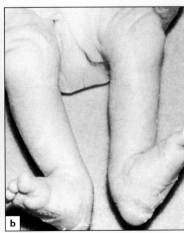

21.10 Other varieties of 'talipes' (**a**) Bilateral metatarsus adductus (which may improve, but seldom corrects completely). (**b**) Bilateral calcaneovalgus (which usually corrects spontaneously).

problem of 'normally abnormal' feet. The medial arch may be normally high or normally low. The term 'flat-foot' applies when the apex of the arch has collapsed and the medial border of the foot is in contact (or nearly in contact) with the ground; the heel becomes valgus and the foot pronates at the subtalar–midtarsal complex. The problems associated with flat-foot differ in babies, children and adults and these three categories will therefore be considered separately.

CONGENITAL CONVEX PES VALGUS (CONGENITAL VERTICAL TALUS)

This rare condition is seen in infants, usually affecting both feet. Superficially it resembles other types of valgus foot, but the deformity is more severe; the medial arch is not only flat, it is the most prominent part of the sole, producing the appearance of a 'rocker-bottom' foot. The hindfoot is in equinus and valgus and the talus points almost vertically towards the sole; the forefoot is abducted, pronated and dorsiflexed, with subluxation of the talonavicular joint. Passive correction is impossible; by the time the child is seen, the tendons and ligaments on the dorsolateral side of the foot are usually shortened.

X-ray features are characteristic: the calcaneum is in equinus and the talus points into the sole of the foot, with the navicular dislocated dorsally onto the neck of the talus. It is important to repeat the lateral x-ray with the foot maximally plantarflexed; in congenital vertical talus the appearance will be unchanged, whereas in flexible flat-foot the dorsally subluxated navicular returns to the normal position.

The only effective *treatment* is by operation, ideally before the age of 2 years. Correction is done in one stage through separate incisions. The tendo Achillis is lengthened, with capsulotomies of the ankle and subtalar joints; via a medial approach the talonavicular joint is reduced and the tibialis anterior tendon is transferred to the neck of the talus; if necessary, the lateral structures are lengthened or released. The reduced position is held with a Kirschner wire transfixing the talonavicular joint and plaster immobilization for 8–12 weeks (the wire can be removed at 6 weeks). Reasonably good results have been reported with this method (Duncan and Fixsen, 1999).

FLAT-FOOT IN CHILDREN AND ADOLESCENTS

Flat-foot is a common complaint among children. Or rather their parents – the children themselves usually don't seem to notice it!

FLEXIBLE FLAT-FOOT Flexible pes valgus appears in toddlers as a normal stage in development, and it usually disappears after a few years when medial arch development is complete; occasionally, though, it persists into adult life. The arch can often be restored by simply dorsiflexing the great toe (the jack, or great toe extension, test), and during this manoeuvre the tibia rotates externally (Rose *et al.*, 1985). Many of these children have ligamentous laxity and there may be a family history of both flat feet and joint hypermobility.

STIFF (OR 'RIGID') FLAT-FOOT A deformity which cannot be corrected passively should alert the examiner to an underlying abnormality. *Congenital vertical talus* is dealt with above. In older children, conditions to be considered are *tarsal coalition*, an *inflammatory joint disorder* or a *neurological disorder*. These conditions are dealt with in later sections.

COMPENSATORY FLAT-FOOT This is a spurious deformity which occurs in order to accommodate some other postural defect. For example, a tight tendo Achillis (or a mild fixed equinus) may be accommodated by everting the foot; or if the lower limbs are externally rotated the body weight falls anteromedial to the ankle and the feet go into valgus – the Charlie Chaplin look.

Clinical assessment

Although there is usually nothing to worry about, the parents' concern should not be dismissed without a proper assessment of the child. Enquire about neonatal problems and a family history.

Watch the child stand and note the position of the heels from behind. Are they in neutral or valgus, and do they invert when the child stands on tiptoe? The tiptoe test will confirm a mobile subtalar joint and functioning tibialis posterior tendon. Let the child walk: is the gait normal for that age? Are the heels set flat

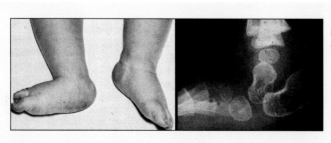

21.11 Flat-foot – congenital Note the 'rocker-bottom' foot and the vertical talus.

during the stance phase, or does the child have tight Achilles tendons?

Examine the foot and note its shape. In the neonate, the rare congenital vertical talus presents as a stiff, acutely dorsiflexed and very flat (almost rocker-bottom) foot. Palpate for tenderness: are there signs of arthritis or infection? Test the movements in the ankle as well as the subtalar and midtarsal joints: a tight Achilles tendon may be 'constitutional' or part of a neuromuscular problem.

Try to correct the flat foot by gentle passive manipulation. Perform the great toe extension test (see above) to distinguish between a flexible and a stiff ('rigid') deformity.

The spine, hips and knees also should be examined. The clinical assessment is completed by a swift general examination for joint hypermobility and signs of neuromuscular abnormalities.

Imaging

X-rays are unnecessary for asymptomatic, flexible flat feet. For pathological flat feet (which are usually painful or stiff) standing anteroposterior, lateral and oblique views may help to identify underlying disorders. On the lateral view, 'beaking' of the head of the talus suggests the presence of a tarsal coalition. Narrowing of the talocalcaneal joint, which is sometimes seen in talocalcaneal coalition, is easily mistaken for 'arthritis'. Calcaneonavicular bars, if ossified, can be seen in oblique views of the foot.

CT scanning is the most reliable way of demonstrating tarsal coalitions.

Radioscintigraphy is occasionally used if a covert infection or osteoid osteoma is suspected. It may also help to identify a 'hot' accessory navicular before advocating its removal.

Treatment

Physiological flat-foot Young children with flexible flat feet require no treatment. Parents need to be reassured and told that the 'deformity' will probably correct itself in time; even if it does not fully correct, function is unlikely to be impaired. Some parents will cite examples of other children who were helped by insoles or moulded heel-cups. These appliances serve mainly to alter the pattern of weight-bearing and hence that of shoe wear; simply put, they are more effective in treating the shoes than the feet.

Tight tendo Achillis Flat-foot associated with a tight tendo Achillis and restricted dorsiflexion at the ankle may benefit from tendon stretching exercises.

Accessory navicular Sometimes the main complaint (with a flexible flat-foot) is tenderness over an unusually prominent navicular on the medial border of the midfoot. X-rays may show an extra ossicle at this site – the accessory navicular. Symptoms are due to pressure (and possibly a 'bursitis') over the bony prominence, or repetitive strain at the synchondrosis between the accessory ossicle and the navicular proper. If symptoms warrant it, the accessory bone can be shelled out from within the tibialis posterior tendon. If the medial arch has 'dropped' significantly, the tibialis posterior tendon can be used as a 'hitch' by reinserting it through a hole drilled in the navicular and suturing the loop with the foot held in maximum inversion (Kidner's operation).

PERONEAL SPASTIC FLAT-FOOT (TARSAL COALITION)

Older children and teenagers sometimes present with a painful, rigid flat-foot in which the peroneal and

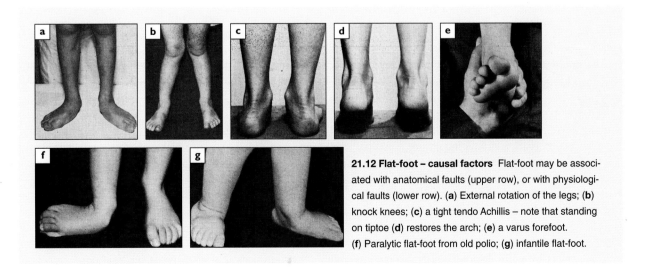

21.12 Flat-foot – causal factors Flat-foot may be associated with anatomical faults (upper row), or with physiological faults (lower row). **(a)** External rotation of the legs; **(b)** knock knees; **(c)** a tight tendo Achillis – note that standing on tiptoe **(d)** restores the arch; **(e)** a varus forefoot. **(f)** Paralytic flat-foot from old polio; **(g)** infantile flat-foot.

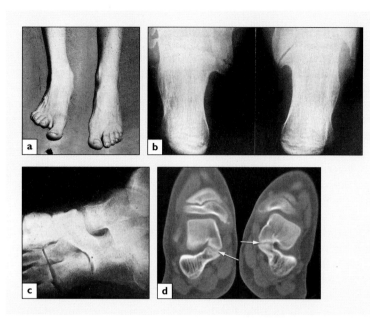

21.13 Tarsal coalition (**a**) Peroneal spasm causing a rigid flat foot. (**b**) An axial view x-ray shows talocalcaneal coalition on the left; this is more difficult to see than (**c**) a calcaneonavicular bar. (**d**) CT image showing incompletely ossified talocalcaneal bars bilaterally (arrows).

extensor tendons are in spasm. X-rays and CT may show one or several of a variety of unions or partial unions between adjacent tarsal bones; the commonest are talocalcaneal, calcaneonavicular and talonavicular coalitions. The anomaly is inherited as an autosomal dominant and is present at birth but it becomes symptomatic only when the abnormal fibrous syndesmosis matures into a stiffer, cartilaginous synchondrosis which later still ossifies to become a rigid bar. The child, usually at puberty or during early adolescence, develops an increasingly stiff flat-foot deformity. Pain may be due to abnormal tarsal stress or even fracture of an ossified bar. The picture differs from that of the more common 'idiopathic' flat-foot in that the deformity is more or less rigid, with spasm of the peroneal muscles. The diagnosis is confirmed by x-ray and/or CT, but other causes of rigid flat-foot must be excluded (e.g. inflammatory arthritis and infection of the hind- or mid-foot).

Treatment

One of the problems with treatment of this condition is that the presence of a tarsal coalition is not necessarily the cause of the patient's symptoms; the anomaly is sometimes discovered as an incidental finding in asymptomatic feet. For this reason the initial treatment should always be conservative. A walking plaster is applied with the foot plantigrade and is retained for 6 weeks; splintage with an outside iron and inside T-strap may have to be continued for another 3–6 months. Obviously if an inflammatory joint disorder is discovered, this will have to be treated. If symptoms do not settle, operative treatment is needed. A calcaneonavicular bar can be resected without much difficulty through a lateral approach, and the operation may be performed before puberty; a

portion of the bar is removed and the gap filled with fat or a piece of muscle (e.g. extensor digitorum brevis) to prevent recurrence. Talocalcaneal coalitions are more difficult to deal with and it may be wiser to wait till after puberty and then perform a triple arthrodesis.

FLAT–FOOT IN ADULTS

As in children, the usual picture is of a flexible flat-foot with no obvious cause. However, underlying disorders are common enough always to warrant a careful search for abnormal ligamentous laxity, tarsal coalitions, disorders of the tibialis posterior tendon, post-traumatic deformity, degenerative arthritis, neuropathy and conditions resulting in muscular imbalance.

Clinical features

Although most adults with *flexible flat feet* are asymptomatic, some do complain of aching after long periods of standing or walking. When the patient is weight-bearing, the flattened arch is obvious; the heel is valgus and the forefoot abducted and pronated. As the patient rises on his or her toes, the heel inverts quite normally.

Acquired and rigid flat feet are often painful. The heel does not invert when the patient goes on tiptoe and the flat-foot may not be passively correctable. In these cases a careful examination for underlying disorders is essential.

Treatment

Asymptomatic flat-foot needs no treatment and there is no reason to restrict activities.

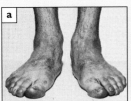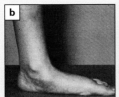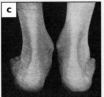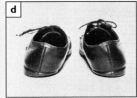

21.14 Flat-foot in adults – clinical features (**a**) The feet appear pronated; (**b**) the arch is flat and the tuberosity of the navicular looks prominent; (**c**) the heels are in valgus and in severe cases, 'too many toes' are seen lateral to the outer edge of the heel, as seen in the left foot here. If this sign is found in adults who present with an acute flat-foot deformity, suspect a rupture of the tibialis posterior tendon; (**d**) faulty shoe wear, a common reason for prescribing heel cups which do little to the underlying condition.

Symptomatic flexible flat-foot should be treated conservatively, by adapting the shoes, fitting arch supports and encouraging muscle strengthening exercises.

Symptomatic stiff flat-foot may be due to tarsal coalition, subtalar injury, gout or inflammatory arthritis. When these disorders have been excluded there remains a residue of patients in whom no pathology can be demonstrated; some of the most intractable cases fall into this group. Some patients respond to non-steroidal anti-inflammatory medication; others are helped by immobilization in a walking cast for 6 or 8 weeks. If a calcaneonavicular bar is discovered, it can be excised (even though it is not always certain that this is the cause). Post-traumatic lesions and tarsal osteoarthritis may warrant arthrodesis. For the remainder, attention to comfortable footwear and analgesic medication is all that can be offered.

Flat-foot associated with tibialis posterior synovitis can be treated by anti-inflammatory medication, intrasynovial injection of corticosteroids and splintage with a lateral iron and medial T-strap (see Fig. 3.9).

Rupture of the tibialis posterior tendon is not always obvious; it should be carefully tested for, especially in those cases where the deformity develops rapidly in one foot (see page 485). In young and physically active patients, operative repair or tendon transfer (using flexor digitorum longus) is worthwhile. In elderly or poorly mobile patients, splintage may be adequate; if this fails, and symptoms are sufficiently marked, then triple arthrodesis should be considered.

HIGH-ARCHED FEET (PES CAVUS)

In pes cavus the arch is higher than normal, and often there is also clawing of the toes. The close resemblance to deformities seen in neurological disorders where the intrinsic muscles are weak or paralysed suggests that all forms of pes cavus are due to some type of muscle imbalance. There are rare congenital causes, such as arthrogryposis, but in the majority of cases pes cavus

Neuromuscular causes of high-arched feet

Level	Cause	Example
Muscle	Muscle dystrophies	Duchenne, Becker
Peripheral nerve	Hereditary neuropathy	HMSN I, II
Spinal cord	Viral disease	Polio
	Structural abnormality	Diastematomyelia
		Tethered cord
		Syringomelia
Brain	Congenital	Friedreich's ataxia
		Cerebral palsy

results from an acquired neuromuscular disorder. A specific abnormality can often be identified; hereditary motor and sensory neuropathies and spinal cord abnormalities (tethered cord syndrome, diastematomyelia) are the commonest in North America and Europe, but poliomyelitis is the most common cause worldwide. Occasionally the deformity follows trauma – burns or a compartment syndrome resulting in Volkmann's contracture of the sole.

Pathology

The toes are drawn up into a 'clawed' position, the metatarsal heads are forced down into the sole and the arch at the mid-foot is accentuated. Often the heel is inverted and the soft tissues in the sole are tight. Under the prominent metatarsal heads callosities may form.

Clinical features

Patients usually present at the age of 8–10 years. Deformity may be noticed by the parents or the school doctor before there are any symptoms. There may be a past history of a spinal disorder or a family history of neuromuscular defects. As a rule both feet are affected.

Pain may be felt under the metatarsal heads or over the toes where shoe pressure is most marked. Callosities

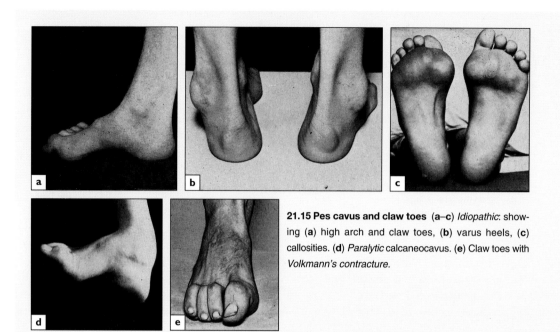

21.15 Pes cavus and claw toes (**a–c**) *Idiopathic*: showing (**a**) high arch and claw toes, (**b**) varus heels, (**c**) callosities. (**d**) *Paralytic* calcaneocavus. (**e**) Claw toes with *Volkmann's contracture*.

appear at the same sites and walking tolerance is reduced. Enquire about symptoms of neurological disorders, such as muscle weakness and joint instability.

The overall cavus deformity is usually obvious; in addition the toes are often clawed and the heel may be varus. Closer inspection will show what are the components of the high arch; this is important because it leads to an understanding of the responsible deforming forces. Rang (1993) has presented a tripod analogy which simplifies the problem (see Fig. 21.16). The foot is likened to a tripod of which the calcaneum, fifth metatarsal and first metatarsal form the legs. Combinations of deformities affecting one or more of these 'legs' produce the common types of high arch, namely plantaris, cavo-varus, calcaneus and calcaneo-cavus.

The toes are held cocked up, with hyperextension at the metatarsophalangeal joints and flexion at the interphalangeal joints. There may be callosities under the metatarsal heads and corns on the toes. Early on the toe deformities are 'mobile' and can be corrected passively by pressure under the metatarsal heads; as the forefoot lifts, the toes flatten out automatically. Later the deformities become fixed, with the metatarsophalangeal joints permanently dislocated.

Mobility in the ankle and foot joints is important. In the cavo-varus foot, the heel is inverted. The block test (Coleman) is useful to check if the deformity is reversible (Fig. 21.17); if it is, this signifies that the subtalar joint is mobile. If the cavus deformity has been present for a long time, then movements of the ankle, subtalar and midtarsal joints are usually limited.

A neurological examination is important to try to identify a reason for the deformity. Disorders such as hereditary sensory and motor neuropathy and Friedreich's ataxia must always be excluded, and the spine should be examined for signs of dysraphism.

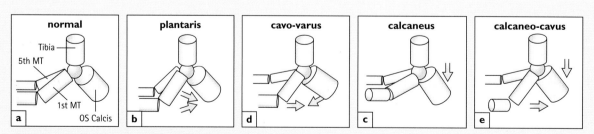

21.16 The tripod analogy for high arched feet This simplifies understanding of the various types of 'pes cavus'. (**a**) The calcaneum, first and fifth metatarsals of the foot are likened to the spokes of a tripod. (**b**) When the first and fifth rays are drawn closer to the heel, a plantaris deformity is present. In a cavo-varus deformity (**c**), the first ray alone is drawn towards the heel which itself is in varus. In calcaneus (**d**), the heel is pushed plantarwards; finally, a calcaneo-cavus deformity is present (**e**) when the heel is in calcaneus and the first ray is drawn in.

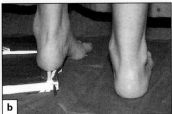

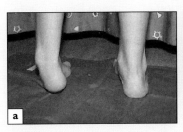

21.17 Coleman's block test This simple test is used on a high arched foot to see if the heel is flexible. **(a)** Normal stance showing the varus position of the heel. **(b)** With the patient standing on a low block to permit the depressed first metatarsal to hang free, the heel varus is automatically corrected if the subtalar joint is mobile.

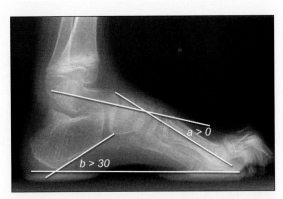

21.18 Weight-bearing x-rays in foot deformities Non-weight-bearing films are notorious for 'hiding' the true components of foot deformities. In standing lateral views, some measurements are useful in describing the type of high arched foot: **(a)** the axes of the talus and first metatarsal are parallel in normal feet but cross each other in a plantaris deformity (Meary's angle); **(b)** the calcaneal pitch is greater than 30° in calcaneus deformities.

Imaging

Weight-bearing x-rays of the foot contribute further to the assessment of the deformity and the state of the individual joints. On the lateral view, measurement of the calcaneal pitch and Meary's angle help to determine the components of the high arch. In a normal foot the *calcaneal pitch* is between 10 and 30°, whereas *Meary's angle*, formed by the axes of the talus and first metatarsal, is 0°, i.e. these axes are parallel. In a calcaneus deformity, the calcaneal pitch is increased; in a plantaris deformity, Meary's lines meet at an angle.

MRI scans of the spine will exclude a structural disorder, especially if this is more common than polio as a cause of high arched feet in the region.

Treatment

Often no treatment is required; apart from the difficulty of fitting shoes, the patient has no complaints.

The foot deformity In general, patients need treatment only if they have symptoms. However, the problem with high arched feet is that it is often a progressive disorder which becomes more difficult to treat when the deformities are fixed; therefore treatment should start before the feet become stiff. Non-operative treatment in the form of custom-made shoes with moulded inserts may provide some relief but does not alter the deformity or influence its progression. Surgery is often needed and the type of procedure will depend on the child's age, the underlying cause, the site and flexibility of the individual deformities and the type of muscle imbalance.

The aim of surgery is to provide a pain-free, plantigrade, supple but stable foot. The methods available are soft tissue releases, osteotomies and tendon transfers. However, the deformity first needs to be corrected before a tendon transfer is considered; additionally, the transfer only works if the joints are mobile.

An equinus contracture is dealt with by lengthening of the tendo Achillis and posterior capsulotomies of the ankle and subtalar joints. The varus hindfoot, if shown to be reversible by Coleman's block test, may benefit from a release of the plantar fascia (the tight fascia acts as a contracted windlass on weight-bearing, accentuating the deformity). However, if the subtalar joint is stiff, then calcaneal osteotomy will be needed; two types are commonly used: the lateral closing wedge (an opening wedge on the medial side is a comparable operation but is fraught with wound problems) or a lateral translation osteotomy.

Treatment of a calcaneo-cavus deformity (which is the least common type of high arch) differs according to the age of the child. In young children (who usually have a neurological problem) tendon transfers – e.g. transferring tibialis anterior through the interosseous membrane to the calcaneum – may be combined with tenodesis of the ankle using tendo Achilles (Banta *et al.*, 1981). Older children may need crescentic calcaneal osteotomies which will correct both varus and calcaneus deformities (Samilson, 1976) or variations of a triple arthrodesis (Cholmeley, 1953).

Midfoot deformities are usually cavus (plantarflexed first metatarsal) or plantaris (plantarflexed first and fifth metatarsals). The Jones tendon transfer helps elevate the depressed first metatarsal by using extensor hallucis longus tendon as a sling through the neck of the metatarsal. Often peroneus longus is overactive and is partly responsible for pulling the first metatarsal down; some balance is restored by dividing this tendon on the lateral side of the foot and attaching the proximal end to peroneus brevis, thereby removing the deforming force and improving the power of eversion simultaneously. Occasionally the deformity affecting the first metatarsal is fixed, in which case a dorsal closing wedge osteotomy at the base of the metatarsal is needed. A plantaris deformity is treated along similar lines for the first ray, and combined with a plantar fascia release if the deformity is mobile, but basal metatarsal osteotomies or even a wedge resection and arthrodesis across the midfoot are needed for rigid deformities.

In severe examples and in those patients who have either relapsed or who have responded poorly with soft tissue releases and osteotomies, salvage surgery in the form of a triple arthrodesis is recommended; it produces a stiff but plantigrade and pain-free foot.

Clawed toes Correction of a clawed first toe is by the Jones tendon transfer which involves either a tenodesis or fusion of the interphalangeal joint. Clawing of the lesser toes is treated with a flexor tendon transfer to the extensor hood (Girdlestone) of each toe, and metatarsophalangeal joint capsulotomies if the toes are still passively correctable; however, if the deformities are fixed, proximal interphalangeal fusion is needed.

HALLUX VALGUS

Hallux valgus is the commonest of the foot deformities (and probably of all musculoskeletal deformities). In people who have never worn shoes the big toe is in line with the first metatarsal, retaining the slightly fan-shaped appearance of the forefoot. In people who habitually wear shoes the hallux assumes a valgus

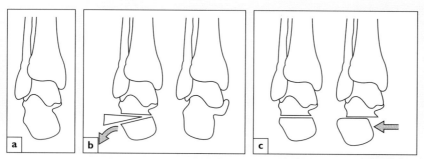

21.19 Treatment of pes cavus 1 In a normal foot, the point of contact of the heel is slightly lateral to the centre of the ankle, producing an eversion lever when weight is borne (Perry, 1983). In a varus heel (**a**) the point of heel contact is too far medial. Restoring the eversion lever can be accomplished in two ways: by (**b**) excising a wedge of bone from the lateral side, or (**c**) a lateral translation osteotomy.

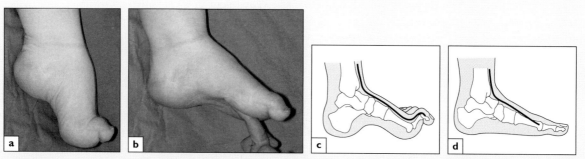

21.20 Treatment of pes cavus 2 (**a**, **b**) If the great toe is clawed and the first metatarsal depressed, reducing the subluxation at the metatarsophalangeal joint by simply elevating the neck of the metatarsal often reduces the severity of the cavus deformity. The surgical equivalent of this effect is (**c**, **d**) the Robert Jones tendon transfer: the extensor hallucis longus tendon is detached distally and transferred to the neck of the first metatarsal; the interphalangeal joint is then either fused or tenodesed.

position; but only if the angulation is excessive is it referred to as 'hallux valgus'.

Splaying of the forefoot, with varus angulation of the first metatarsal, predisposes to lateral angulation of the big toe in people who wear shoes. *Metatarsus primus varus* may be congenital, or it may result from loss of muscle tone in the forefoot in elderly people. Hallux valgus is also common in rheumatoid arthritis.

A family history is obtained in about 60% of cases.

Pathological anatomy

The elements of the deformity are lateral deviation and rotation of the hallux, together with a prominence of the medial side of the head of the first metatarsal (a bunion). Lateral deviation of the hallux may lead to overcrowding of the lateral toes and sometimes overriding. When the valgus deformity exceeds 30 or 40°, the great toe rotates into pronation so that the nail faces medially and the sessamoid bones of flexor hallucis brevis are displaced laterally; in severe deformities the tendons of flexor and extensor hallucis longus bowstring on the lateral side, thus adding to the deforming forces.

Prominence of the first metatarsal head is due to subluxation of the metatarsophalangeal joint; there may also be an overlying bursa and thickened soft tissue. The capsule of the joint is stretched medially but contracted laterally. When exposed at operation, the medial prominence looks like an exostosis (because of a deep sagittal sulcus on the head of the metatarsal), but there is no true exostosis.

In long-standing cases the metatarsophalangeal joint becomes osteoarthritic and osteophytes may then add to the prominence of the metatarsal head.

Clinical features

Hallux valgus is most commonly seen in women between 50 and 70 years, and is usually bilateral. An important sub-group, which has a strong familial tendency, appears during late adolescence.

Often there are no symptoms apart from the deformity. Pain, if present, may be due to (1) shoe pressure on a large or an inflamed bunion, (2) splaying of the forefoot with metatarsalgia and pain under the metatarsal heads, (3) associated deformities of the lesser toes and (4) secondary osteoarthritis of the first metatarsophalangeal joint. There are often bitter complaints about the difficulty of purchasing comfortable shoes.

The deformity is obvious and the bunion is often swollen and inflamed. The forefoot is too wide and the great toe is in valgus and often rotated. The second toe is crowded and hammer toe deformities are common. Old shoes will show the traces of long-standing pressure.

The site of tenderness is important and must be accurately localized, for it will influence treatment: it may be (1) over the bunion, (2) in the joint or (3) between the metatarsals.

Unless osteoarthritis has supervened, the metatarsophalangeal joint has a good range of movement.

X-RAYS

X-rays should be taken with the patient standing, to show the degree of metatarsal and hallux angulation. Lines are drawn along the middle of the first and second metatarsals and the proximal phalanx of the great toe; normally the intermetatarsal angle is less than 9° and the valgus angle at the metatarsophalangeal joint less than 15°. Any greater degree of angulation should be regarded as 'hallux valgus'.

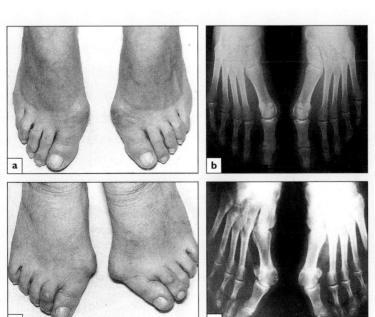

21.21 Hallux valgus (**a**, **b**) This girl's feet are well on the way to becoming as deformed as (**c**, **d**) those of her mother. Hallux valgus is not uncommonly familial.

However, not all types of valgus deformity are equally progressive and troublesome. Based on the x-ray appearances, patients can be divided into three groups (Piggott, 1960). If the articular surfaces of the first metatarsophalangeal joint are marked by two lines drawn across their width, the relationship of these lines can define three types: (1) a congruous joint in which the articular surfaces are parallel and centred; (2) a deviated joint in which the surfaces are still centred but not parallel and therefore not congruous; and (3) a subluxated joint in which the surfaces are neither centred nor congruous. Type 1 is a stable joint and any deformity is likely to progress very slowly or not at all. Type 2 is somewhat unstable and likely to progress. Type 3 is even more unstable and almost certain to progress.

Treatment

ADOLESCENTS

Many young patients are asymptomatic, but worry over the shape of the toe and an anxious mother keen not to let the condition become as severe as her own will bring the patient to the clinic. It is wise to try conservative measures first, mainly because surgical correction in this age group carries a 20–40% recurrence rate. This consists essentially of encouraging the patient to wear shoes with wide and deep toe-boxes, soft uppers and low heels – 'trainers' are a good choice. If x-rays show a Type 1 (congruous) deformity, the patient can be reassured that it will progress only very slowly if at all. If there is an incongruous deformity, surgical correction will sooner or later be required.

In mild deformities, where the hallux valgus angle is less than 25°, correction can be obtained by either a soft-tissue rebalancing operation or by a metatarsal osteotomy. If the x-ray shows a congruent articulation, the deformity is largely bony and therefore amenable to correction by a distal osteotomy, either Mitchell's or a chevron osteotomy. A drawback of the Mitchell's procedure is that it shortens the metatarsal and may cause excessive loading and pain under the lesser metatarsals; this can be alleviated if the distal fragment of the osteotomy is plantarflexed slightly before fixation. In comparison, the chevron osteotomy keeps the length of the metatarsal, but the amount of correction possible with this operation is less than 10°; also, there is a risk of avascular necrosis of the metatarsal head – this is more likely to happen if a lateral soft-tissue release is combined with the distal metatarsal osteotomy. If the metatarsophalangeal articulation is incongruent the deformity is in the joint and soft-tissue realignment is indicated. The tight structures on the lateral side (adductor hallucis, transverse metatarsal ligament and lateral capsule) are released and the capsule on the medial side reefed.

In moderate and severe deformities the hallux valgus angle may be greater than 30° and intermetatarsal angle wider than 15°. If the metatarsophalangeal joint is congruent, either Mitchell's operation or a chevron osteotomy combined with a corrective osteotomy of the base of the proximal phalanx (Aikin's osteotomy) is recommended. If the joint is

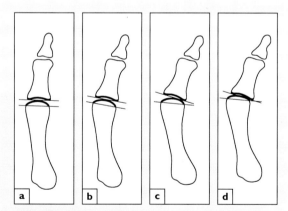

21.23 Hallux valgus – the three groups X-ray outlines of (**a**) a normal first ray and (**b**, **c**, **d**) the three types of hallux valgus. The margins of the articular surfaces of the metatarsophalangeal joint are joined by lines. In normal feet (**a**) these lines are parallel and the opposing articular surfaces are centred upon each other. In (**b**), the congruent type of hallux valgus, the articular surfaces are set more obliquely to the long axes of their respective bones but the lines are still parallel and the joint is centred. In (**c**) the deviated type, the lines are not parallel and the articular surfaces are not congruent. In the subluxated type (**d**) the surfaces are neither parallel nor centred (Piggott, 1960).

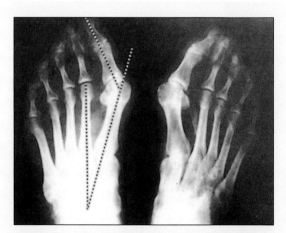

21.22 Hallux valgus – measurements The intermetatarsal angle (between the first and second metatarsals) as well as the metatarsophalangeal angle of the hallux are recorded.

subluxed, a soft tissue adjustment is needed as well as a proximal metatarsal osteotomy. This basal osteotomy, with a closing wedge laterally, is done to reduce a wide intermetatarsal angle; care is needed not to injure the open physis or else growth of the metatarsal will be stunted.

ADULTS

The general approach to surgical treatment is similar to that described above. In addition, however, there may be osteoarthritis in the metatarsophalangeal joint; in that case, the patient may be better off with an arthrodesis of the joint.

Hallux valgus in the elderly is best treated by shoe modifications; where this fails, and in those whose functional demands are low, treatment by excision arthroplasty is usually successful. In the classic Keller's operation the proximal third of the proximal phalanx is removed; relief of pain is good but the toe is floppy and this can sometimes give rise to other problems.

HALLUX RIGIDUS

'Rigidity' (or stiffness) of the first metatarsophalangeal joint occurs at almost any age from adolescence onwards. In young people it may be due to local trauma or osteochrondritis dissecans of the first metatarsal head. In older people it is usually caused by long-standing joint disorders such as gout, pseudogout or osteoarthritis. In contrast to hallux valgus, men and women are affected with equal frequency.

Clinical features

Pain on walking, especially on slopes or rough ground, is the predominant symptom. The hallux is straight and often has a callosity under the medial side of the distal phalanx. The metatarsophalangeal joint feels knobbly; a tender dorsal 'bunion' (actually a large osteophyte) is

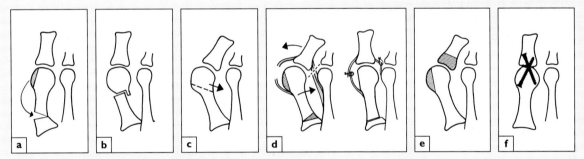

21.24 Hallux valgus – treatment (a) Basal osteotomy with bone graft inserted. (b) Mitchell's osteotomy. (c) Wilson's osteotomy. (d) Before and after basal osteotomy and capsulorrhaphy. (e) Keller's operation. (f) Arthrodesis.

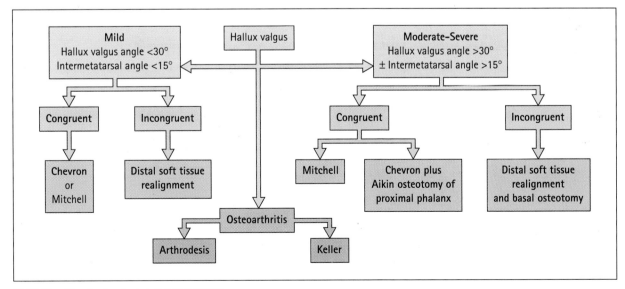

21.25 Algorithm for treatment of hallux valgus.

diagnostic. Dorsiflexion is restricted and painful, and there may be compensatory hyperextension at the interphalangeal joint. The outer side of the sole of the shoe may be unduly worn – the result of rolling the foot outwards to avoid pressing on the big toe.

It is important to check the state of the other joints in the foot in order to rule out a polyarthropathy.

X-RAYS The features are essentially those of osteoarthritis; the joint space is narrowed, there is bone sclerosis and, often, large osteophytes. There may be signs of recent or old osteochondritis ('squaring' of the metatarsal head).

Treatment

A rocker-soled shoe may abolish pain by allowing the foot to 'roll' without the necessity for dorsiflexion at the metatarsophalangeal joint. Nowadays few young people are willing to wear such shoes.

If walking is painful despite this type of shoe adjustment, an operation is advised. For young patients the best procedure is a simple *extension osteotomy* of the proximal phalanx, to mimic dorsiflexion at the interphalangeal joint. Check that there is reasonable plantarflexion before doing this.

In older patients, *cheilectomy* is the procedure of choice: the dorsal osteophytes and the dorsal edge of the metatarsal head are removed in an attempt to restore extension (dorsiflexion) at the metatarsophalangeal joint; even 30° can make a difference to the discomfort that the patient experiences each time the toe is forced into extension at the end of the stance phase in walking.

Joint replacement, using a Silastic prosthesis, may likewise increase movement and relieve pain; however, Silastic synovitis, fracture of the implant and osteolysis are complications which make later salvage difficult.

Arthrodesis of the metatarsophalangeal joint gives a more predictable result, especially in patients engaged in strenuous activities. The joint should be fused in 10° of valgus and 10–15° of dorsiflexion in relation to the sole of the foot; too little dorsiflexion will cause pain during toe-off and too much will result in the toe pressing against the shoe upper.

DEFORMITIES OF THE LESSER TOES

The commonest deformities of the lesser toes are 'claw', 'hammer' and 'mallet'. These terms are often used interchangeably, leading to confusion.

Claw toe is characterized by hyperextension at the metatarsophalangeal joint and flexion at both interphalangeal joints.

Hammer toe is an acute flexion deformity of the proximal interphalangeal joint only; in severe examples there may be some extension at the metatarsophalangeal joint. The distal interphalangeal joint is either straight or hyperextended.

Mallet toe is a flexion deformity of the distal interphalangeal joint.

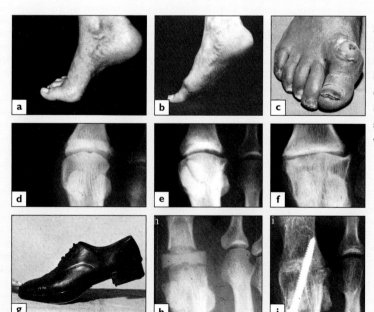

21.26 Hallux rigidus (a) In normal walking the hallux dorsiflexes (extends) considerably. With rigidus (b), dorsiflexion is limited; a dorsal callosity (c) may develop. (d) Splitting osteochondritis or (e) a bipartite sesamoid may be precursors of (f) joint degeneration. (g) A rocker-sole relieves symptoms; operations include joint replacement with a Silastic spacer (h) and arthrodesis (i).

CLAW TOES

The interphalangeal joints are flexed and the metatarsophalangeal joints hyperextended. This is an 'intrinsic-minus' deformity which is seen in neurological disorders (e.g. peroneal muscular atrophy, poliomyelitis and peripheral neuropathies) and in rheumatoid arthritis. Usually, however, no cause is found. The condition may also be associated with pes cavus.

Clinical features

The patient complains of pain in the forefoot and under the metatarsal heads. Usually the condition is bilateral and walking may be severely restricted. At first the joints are mobile and can be passively corrected; later the deformities become fixed and the metatarsophalangeal joints subluxed or dislocated. Painful corns may develop on the dorsum of the toes and callosities under the metatarsal heads. In the most severe cases the skin ulcerates at the pressure sites.

Treatment

FLEXIBLE DEFORMITY

So long as the toes can be passively straightened the patient may obtain relief by wearing a metatarsal support or by having a transverse metatarsal bar fitted to the shoe. If these measures fail to relieve discomfort, an operation is indicated. 'Dynamic' correction is achieved by transferring the long toe flexors to the extensors. The operation at one stroke removes a powerful interphalangeal flexor and converts it to a metatarsophalangeal flexor and interphalangeal extensor.

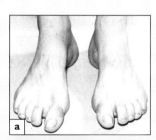

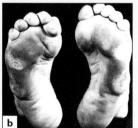

21.27 Claw toes Claw-toe deformity suggests muscle imbalance, with relative weakness of the intrinsics. Only occasionally, however (as in these examples of peroneal muscular atrophy), is a definite neurological defect found.

FIXED DEFORMITY

When the deformity is fixed, it may either be accepted and accommodated by special footwear or treated by one of the following operations.

Interphalangeal arthrodesis If there is no joint disease, proximal interphalangeal arthrodesis and dorsal capsulotomy of the metatarsophalangeal joints permits active flexion of the metatarsophalangeal joints by the long flexors. This is sometimes combined with transfer of the extensor hallucis longus to the first metatarsal, thus removing a deforming force while retaining the muscle as a forefoot stabilizer.

Joint excision Fixed claw deformities, usually associated with destruction of the metatarsophalangeal joints (e.g. in rheumatoid arthritis), can be dealt with by excision arthroplasties of the metatarsophalangeal joints – preferably removal of only the bases of the proximal phalanges and trimming of the metatarsal heads. This can usually be achieved through two longitudinal incisions on the dorsum of the foot. The base of the proximal phalanx is excised and the plantar pad (which is often displaced in these deformities) is returned to its normal position beneath the metatarsal head; the space between the metatarsal and phalanx is then filled by suturing the long extensor tendon to the flexor. If the great toe is affected, a modified Keller's operation or arthrodesis is performed.

HAMMER TOE

The proximal joint is fixed in flexion, while the distal joint and the metatarsophalangeal joint are extended. The second toe of one or both feet is commonly affected. Shoe pressure may produce painful corns or callosities on the dorsum of the toe and under the prominent metatarsal head.

The cause is obscure: the similarity to boutonnière deformity of a finger suggests an extensor dysfunction, a view supported by the frequent association with a dropped metatarsal head, flat anterior arch and hallux valgus. A simpler explanation is that the toe was too long or the shoe too short.

Treatment Operative correction is indicated for pain or for difficulty with shoes. The toe is shortened and straightened by excising the joint. An ellipse of tissue (including the corn and the underlying extensor tendon) is removed and the proximal interphalangeal joint is entered; the articular surfaces are nibbled away and the raw ends of the proximal and middle phalanges are brought together with the toe almost straight. The position is held by a longitudinally placed Kirschner wire which is retained for 6 weeks. An alternative (and some would say preferable) operation is simple excision of the head of the proximal phalanx, or excision of both articular surfaces, without formal arthrodesis; the toe is splinted for 3 weeks to allow healing in the corrected position.

Occasionally, a dorsal capsulotomy of the metatarosphalangeal joint is needed to allow the toe to lie in line with its neighbours.

MALLET TOE

In mallet toe it is the distal interphalangeal joint that is flexed. The toenail or the tip of the toe presses into the shoe, resulting in a painful callosity.

If conservative treatment (chiropody and padding) does not help, operation is indicated. The distal interphalangeal joint is exposed, the articular surfaces excised and the toe straightened; flexor tenotomy may be needed. A thin Kirschner wire is inserted across the joint and left in position for 6 weeks.

FIFTH TOE DEFORMITIES

OVERLAPPING FIFTH TOE
This is a common congenital anomaly. If symptoms warrant, the toe may be straightened by a dorsal V/Y-plasty, reinforced by transferring the flexor to the extensor tendon. Tight dorsal and medial structures may have to be released. The toe is held in the over-corrected position with tape or Kirschner wire for 6 weeks. Severe deformities or relapses may need a transfer of the long extensor tendon beneath the proximal phalanx to the abductor digiti minimi (Lapidus).

COCK-UP DEFORMITY
The metatarsophalangeal joint is dislocated and the little toe sits on the dorsum of the metatarsal head. Operative treatment is usually successful: through a longitudinal plantar incision, the proximal phalanx is winkled out and removed; the wound is closed transversely, thus pulling the toe out of the hyperextended position.

TAILOR'S BUNION
An irritating or painful bunionette may form over an abnormally prominent fifth metatarsal head. If the shoe cannot be adjusted to fit the bump, the bony prominence can be trimmed, taking care not to sever the tendon of the fifth toe abductor. If the metatarsal shaft is bowed laterally (as is often the case), it can be straightened by performing either a distal osteotomy or a varus correction at the base of the metatarsal.

TUBERCULOUS ARTHRITIS

Tuberculous infection of the ankle joint begins as a synovitis or as an osteomyelitis (see also Chapter 2) and, because walking is painful, may present before true arthritis supervenes. The ankle is swollen and the calf markedly wasted; the skin feels warm and movements are restricted. Sinus formation occurs early.

X-rays show generalized rarefaction, sometimes a bone abscess and, with late disease, narrowing and irregularity of the joint space.

TREATMENT In addition to general treatment (Chapter 2) a removable splint is used to rest the foot in neutral position. If the disease is arrested early, the patient is allowed up non-weight-bearing in a calliper; gradually he or she takes more weight, then discards the calliper. Following arthritis, weight-bearing is harmless, but stiffness is inevitable and usually arthrodesis is the best treatment.

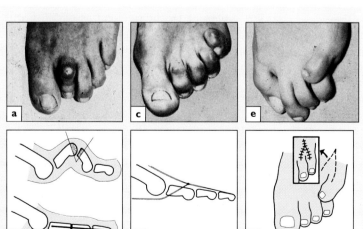

21.28 Toe disorders (**a**) Hammer toe, and (**b**) treatment by excision–arthrodesis. (**c**) Curly toes and (**d**) treatment by flexor-to-extensor transfer. (**e**) Overlapping fifth toe, and (**f**) treatment by V/Y-plasty.

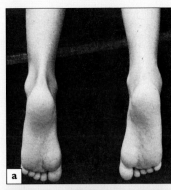

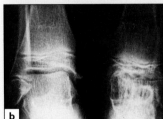

21.29 Tuberculous arthritis of the ankle (a) The swelling is best seen from behind; (b) shows rarefaction and joint destruction.

RHEUMATOID ARTHRITIS

The ankle and foot are affected almost as often as the wrist and hand (see also Chapter 3). During *stage 1* there is synovitis of the metatarsophalangeal, intertarsal and ankle joints, as well as of the sheathed tendons (usually the peronei and tibialis posterior). In *stage 2*, joint erosion and tendon dysfunction prepare the ground for the progressive deformities of *stage 3*.

THE FOREFOOT

Pain and swelling of the metatarsophalangeal joints are among the earliest features of rheumatoid arthritis. Shoes feel uncomfortable and the patient walks less and less. Tenderness is at first localized to the metatarsophalangeal joints; later the entire forefoot is painful on pressing or squeezing. With increasing weakness of the intrinsic muscles and joint destruction, the characteristic deformities appear: a flattened anterior arch, hallux valgus, claw toes and prominence of the metatarsal heads in the sole (patients say it feels like walking on pebbles). Subcutaneous nodules are common and may ulcerate. Dorsal corns and plantar callosities also may break down and become infected. In the worst cases the toes are dislocated, inflamed, ulcerated and useless.

X-rays show osteoporosis and periarticular erosion at the metatarsophalangeal joints. Curiously – in contrast to the hand - the smaller digits (fourth and fifth toes) are affected first.

TREATMENT During the stage of synovitis, corticosteroid injections and attention to footwear may relieve symptoms; operative synovectomy is occasionally needed. Once deformity is advanced, treatment is that of the claw toes and hallux valgus. Sometimes specially made shoes will accommodate the toes in relative comfort. If this does not help, the most effective operation is excision arthroplasty in order to relieve pressure in the sole and to correct the toe deformities (see page 503). For the hallux, an alternative is metatarsophalangeal fusion.

Forefoot surgery is more likely to succeed if the hindfoot is held in the anatomical position. It is important, therefore, to treat the foot as a whole and attend also to the proximal joints.

THE ANKLE AND HINDFOOT

The earliest symptoms are pain and swelling around the ankle. Walking becomes increasingly difficult and, later, deformities appear. On examination, swelling and tenderness are usually localized to the back of the medial malleolus (tenosynovitis of tibialis posterior) or the lateral malleolus (tenosynovitis of the peronei). Less often the ankle swells (joint synovitis) and its movements are restricted. Inversion and eversion may be painful and limited; subtalar erosion is common. In the late stages the tibialis posterior may rupture (all too often this is missed), or become ineffectual with progressive erosion of the tarsal joints, and the foot gradually drifts into severe valgus deformity. X-rays show osteoporosis and, later, erosion of the tarsal and ankle joints. Soft-tissue swelling may be marked.

TREATMENT In the stage of synovitis, splintage is helpful (to allow inflammation to subside and to prevent deformity) while waiting for systemic treatment to control the disease. Initially, tendon sheaths and joints may be injected with methylprednisolone, but this should not be repeated more than two or three times. A lightweight below-knee calliper with an inside supporting strap restores stability and may be worn almost indefinitely.

If the synovitis does not subside, operative synovectomy is advisable. Frayed tendons cannot be repaired and, although tendon replacement is technically feasible, progressive erosion of the hindfoot joints will countervail any improvement this might achieve.

In the very late stage, arthrodesis of the ankle and tarsal joints can still restore modest function and abolish pain. The place of arthroplasty is not yet firmly established.

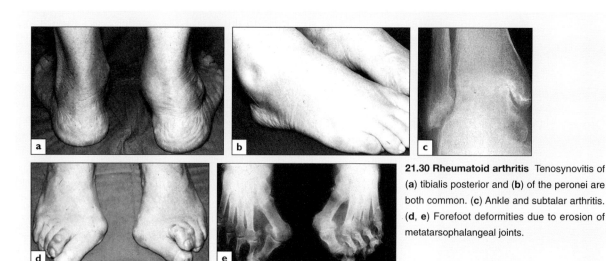

21.30 Rheumatoid arthritis Tenosynovitis of (**a**) tibialis posterior and (**b**) of the peronei are both common. (**c**) Ankle and subtalar arthritis. (**d**, **e**) Forefoot deformities due to erosion of metatarsophalangeal joints.

SERONEGATIVE ARTHROPATHIES

The seronegative arthropathies are dealt with in Chapter 3. These conditions are similar to rheumatoid arthritis, but there are differences in the pattern of joint involvement, the severity of the changes and the soft tissue features.

The clinical features are often asymmetrical and the ankle and hindfoot tend to be more severely affected than the forefoot. However, in psoriatic arthritis the toe joints are sometimes completely destroyed.

An inflammatory reaction around the insertions of tendons and ligaments is a feature of the spondyloarthropathies. This appears in the foot as plantar fasciitis and Achilles tendinitis. Splintage and local injection of triamcinolone are helpful.

GOUT

Swelling, redness, heat and exquisite tenderness of the metatarsophalangeal joint of the big toe ('podagra') is the epitome of gout (see also Chapter 4). The ankle joint, or one of the toes, may be similarly affected – especially following a minor injury. The condition may closely resemble septic arthritis, but the systemic features of infection are absent. The serum uric acid level may be raised.

Treatment with anti-inflammatory drugs will abort the acute attack of gout; until the pain subsides the foot should be rested and protected from injury.

Chronic tophaceous gout Tophi may appear around any of the joints. The diagnosis is suggested by the characteristic x-ray features and confirmed by identifying the typical crystals in the tophus. Treatment may require local curettage of the bone lesions.

Plantar fasciitis Pain under the heel due to plantar fasciitis is another manifestation of gout, though the association may be hard to prove in any particular case.

OSTEOCHONDRITIS DISSECANS OF THE TALUS

Unexplained pain and slight limitation of movement in the ankle of a young person may be due to a small osteochondral fracture of the upper surface of the talus, though the injury may have been forgotten.

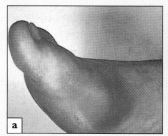
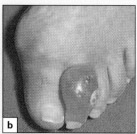
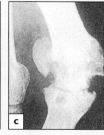

21.31 Gout (**a**) The classic picture – acute inflammation of the big toe metatarsophalangeal joint. (**b**) Tophaceous gout of the second toe. (**c**) X-ray of the first metatarsophalangeal joint; the large excavations are occupied by crystalline tophi.

X-rays taken at appropriate angles to produce tangential views of the talar surface show the small bony separation (no more than a few millimetres in diameter) at either the anteromedial or the posterolateral part of the superior surface of the talus. MRI is also helpful and the lesion may be visualized directly by arthroscopy.

Treatment depends on the degree of cartilage damage. As long as the articular cartilage is intact, it is sufficient to restrict activities. Once it is softened, arthroscopic drilling may be helpful. A loose fragment may need removal, but often the symptoms are insufficient to warrant intervention.

ATRAUMATIC OSTEONECROSIS OF THE TALUS

Osteonecrosis of the talus (see also Chapter 6) is a well-recognized complication of trauma (dislocation or fracture of the neck of the talus). Atraumatic osteonecrosis, though less common than its counterpart in the femoral head, is associated with the same group of systemic disorders as the latter (hypercortisonism, alcoholism, systemic lupus erythematosus, Gaucher's disease, sickle-cell disease, etc.) and is often one of multiple sites affected.

Patients complain of pain, which is often aggravated by weight-bearing, and gradually increasing restriction of movement. X-rays and MRI show the typical features of osteonecrosis, almost always involving the posterolateral part of the talar dome. Lesions can be staged according to Ficat's radiographic classification (see Chapter 6). For purposes of treatment, it is important to distinguish between 'pre-collapse' and 'collapse' of the talar dome.

Conservative treatment is sometimes effective; the ankle is more forgiving than the hip and patients may cope for some years on simple analgesics and restricted weight-bearing. If symptoms persist and interfere significantly with function, operative treatment may be needed. During the pre-collapse phase,

core decompression is worth trying as a first approach. If this fails, ankle arthrodesis is indicated (Delanois *et al.*, 1998).

OSTEOARTHRITIS

Osteoarthritis of the ankle is almost always secondary to some underlying disorder (see also Chapter 5): a malunited fracture, recurrent instability, osteochondritis dissecans of the talus, avascular necrosis of the talus or repeated bleeding with haemophilia. Sometimes, however, the ankle is involved in generalized osteoarthritis and crystal arthropathy.

Symptoms are often quite tolerable, because extremes of range are not required with normal use.

Treatment, in the first instance, is conservative: anti-inflammatory drugs and, sometimes, splintage or simply wearing a strong boot.

If operation is required, an arthrodesis is usually the best option. The ideal position for fusion is at 0° in the sagittal plane (the foot therefore plantigrade) and 5° of valgus. Using rigid internal fixation, or an efficient circular external fixator, the non-union rate is low.

Joint replacement is sometimes used for patients with low functional demands.

THE DIABETIC FOOT

The complications of long-standing diabetes mellitus often appear in the foot, causing chronic disability. Over 30% of patients attending diabetic clinics have

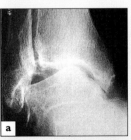
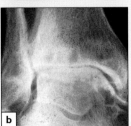

21.33 Osteoarthritis (a) The obvious malalignment which followed an old injury has led to osteoarthritis. (b) In this ankle the narrowed joint space and subarticular cysts are characteristic of osteoarthritis; the cause is not clear, though it may have been trauma.

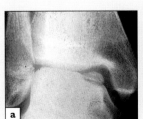
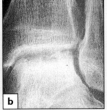

21.32 Osteochondritis dissecans (a) Osteochondritis dissecans at the common site, the anteromedial segment of the articular surface. (b) Sometimes an extensive part of the dome of the talus is affected; secondary osteoarthritis is inevitable.

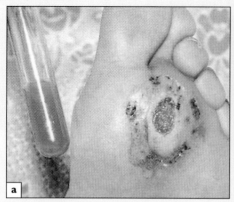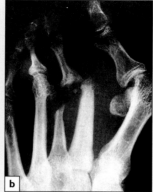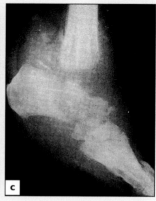

21.34 The diabetic foot 1 (a) Ulceration in a patient with poorly controlled diabetes. (b, c) Despite the severe changes in these two patients with diabetic neuropathy, the feet were relatively painless.

evidence of peripheral neuropathy or vascular disease and about 40% of non-trauma-related amputations in British hospitals are for complications of diabetes.

Factors affecting the foot are (1) a predisposition to peripheral vascular disease, (2) damage to peripheral nerves, (3) reduced resistance to infection and (4) osteoporosis.

PERIPHERAL VASCULAR DISEASE Atherosclerosis affects mainly the medium-sized vessels below the knee. The patient may complain of claudication or ischaemic changes and ulceration in the foot. The skin feels smooth and cold, the nails show trophic changes and the pulses are weak or absent. Doppler studies should corroborate the clinical findings. Superficial ulceration occurs on the toes, deep ulceration typically under the heel; unlike neuropathic ulcers, these are painful and tender. Digital vessel occlusion may cause dry gangrene of one or more toes; proximal vascular occlusion is less common but more serious, sometimes resulting in extensive wet gangrene.

PERIPHERAL NEUROPATHY Early on, patients are usually unaware of the abnormality but clinical tests will discover loss of vibration and joint position sense and diminished temperature discrimination in the feet. Symptoms, when they occur, are mainly due to sensory impairment: symmetrical numbness, dryness and blistering of the skin, superficial burns and skin cracks or ulceration due to shoe scuffing or localized pressure. Motor loss usually manifests as claw toes with high arches and this, in turn, may predispose to plantar ulceration.

NEUROPATHIC JOINT DISEASE 'Charcot joints' occur in less than 1% of diabetic patients, yet diabetes is the commonest cause of a neuropathic joint in North America, Europe and other industrialized countries (leprosy and tertiary syphilis being the other common causes worldwide). The midtarsal joints are the most commonly affected, followed by the metatarsophalangeal and ankle joints. There is usually a provocative incident, such as a twisting injury or a fracture, following which the joint collapses relatively painlessly. X-rays show marked and fairly rapid destruction of the articular surfaces. These changes are easily mistaken for infection but the simultaneous involvement of several small joints and the lack of systemic signs point to a neuropathic disorder. Joint aspiration and microbiological investigation will also help to exclude infection.

In late cases there may be severe deformity and loss of function. A 'rocker-bottom' deformity from collapse of the midfoot is diagnostic.

OSTEOPOROSIS There is a generalized loss of bone density in diabetes. In the foot the changes may be severe enough to result in insufficiency fractures around the ankle or in the metatarsals.

INFECTION Diabetes, if not controlled, is known to have a deleterious effect on white cell function. This, combined with local ischaemia, insensitivity to skin injury and localized pressure due to deformity, makes sepsis an ever-recurring hazard.

Management

The orthopaedic surgeon will usually be one member of a multidisciplinary team comprising a physician (or endocrinologist), surgeon, chiropodist and orthotist. The best way of preventing complications is to insist on regular attendance at a diabetic clinic, full compliance with medication, examination for early signs of vascular or neurological abnormality, advice on foot care and footwear and a high level of skin hygiene.

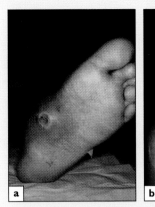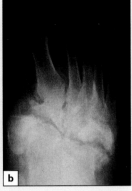

21.35 The diabetic foot 2 (a) This patient presented with midfoot collapse and intractable medial ulceration, a picture which is typical of diabetic neuropathy. (b) The x-ray shows destruction of the midtarsal joints.

Examination for early signs of neuropathy should include the use of Semmes-Weinstein hairs (for testing skin sensibility) and a biothesiometer (for testing vibration sense). Peripheral vascular examination is enhanced by using a Doppler ultrasound probe. Ulcers must be swabbed for infecting organisms; frequently, multiple bacterial types are isolated (anaerobes make a regular appearance). X-ray examination may reveal periosteal reactions, osteoporosis, cortical defects near the articular margins and osteolysis – often collectively described as 'diabetic osteopathy'.

Great care is needed with nail trimming; skin cracks should be kept clean and covered; ulcers should be treated with local dressings and antibiotics if necessary. Occasionally, septicaemia calls for admission to hospital and treatment with intravenous antibiotics.

Ischaemic changes need the attention of a vascular surgeon who can advise on ways of improving the local blood supply. Arteriography may show that bypass surgery is feasible. Dry gangrene of the toe can be allowed to demarcate before local amputation; severe occlusive disease with wet gangrene may call for immediate amputation.

Indolent neuropathic ulcers require patient dressing and – if infected – antibiotic treatment. Total contact casts may avoid the need for prolonged in-patient stays or bed-rest (Coleman *et al.*, 1984). If a bony 'high spot' is identified, it should be trimmed or excised. Custom-made shoes with total contact insoles must follow the successful healing of these ulcers to avoid recurrence.

Insufficiency fractures should be treated, if possible, without immobilizing the limb; or, if a cast is essential, it should be retained for the shortest possible period.

Neuropathic joint disease is a major challenge. Arthrodesis is fraught with difficulties, not least a very poor union rate, and sometimes is simply not feasible. 'Containment' of the problem in a weight-relieving orthosis may be the best option.

Bone or joint infection is an ever-present risk and should be borne in mind in the differential diagnosis of insufficiency fractures and neuropathic joint erosion. This will require urgent treatment.

DISORDERS OF THE TENDO ACHILLIS

PERITENDINITIS

Athletes, joggers and hikers often develop pain and swelling around the tendo Achillis. This is due to local irritation of the paratenon; sometimes there is also degeneration within the tendon, and a small, tender lump can be felt just above the heel.

Treatment is conservative: rest, ultrasound and a heel raise usually bring relief. Corticosteroid injections are sometimes preferred; they certainly relieve pain but it is feared that they may precipitate tendon rupture.

For intractable cases, an operation to excise inflamed and degenerate tissue may be successful. However, if much of the tendon has to be removed, a formal reconstruction will be needed.

RUPTURE

Probably rupture occurs only if the tendon is degenerate. Consequently most patients are aged over 40 years. While pushing off (running or jumping), the calf muscle contracts; but the contraction is resisted by body weight and the tendon ruptures. The patient feels as if he or she has been struck just above the heel, and is unable to tiptoe. Soon after the tear occurs, a gap can be seen and felt 5cm above the insertion of the tendon. Plantarflexion of the foot is weak and is not accompanied by tautening of the tendon. Where doubt exists, Simmonds' test is helpful: with the patient prone, the calf is squeezed; if the tendon is intact the foot is seen to plantarflex; if the tendon is ruptured the foot remains still.

Differential diagnosis

Incomplete tear A complete rupture is often mistaken for a partial tear; in fact, partial tears are very uncommon. The mistake arises because, if a complete rupture is not seen within 24 hours, the gap is difficult to feel; moreover, the patient may by then be able to stand on tiptoe (just), by using his or her long toe flexors.

Tear of soleus muscle A tear at the musculotendinous junction causes pain and tenderness halfway up the calf. This recovers with the aid of physiotherapy and raising the heel of the shoe.

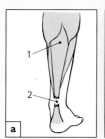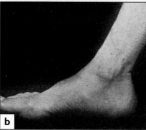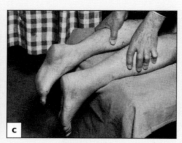

21.36 Tendo Achillis (a) The soleus may tear at its musculotendinous junction (1), but the tendo Achillis itself ruptures about 5cm above its insertion (2). (b) The depression seen in this picture at the site of rupture later fills with blood. (c) Simmonds' test: both calves are being squeezed but only the left foot plantarflexes – the right tendon is ruptured.

Treatment

If the patient is seen early, the ends of the tendon may approximate when the foot is passively plantarflexed. If so, plaster is applied with the foot in equinus and is worn for 8 weeks. A shoe with a raised heel is worn for a further 6 weeks. The 're-rupture rate' is about 10%.

Operative repair is probably safer, but immobilization in equinus for 8 weeks and a heel raise for a further 6 weeks are still needed for walking. This may be provided by a plaster cast, but a more sophisticated alternative is a lockable brace which permits early ankle movement yet blocks tension on the newly repaired tendon.

If repair is performed through a vertical incision, wound breakdown is not uncommon. A small transverse incision is often adequate and it is even possible to use an entirely percutaneous method.

For ruptures that present late, reconstruction using local tendon substitutes (e.g. flexor digitorum longus tendon) or strips of fascia lata is still possible.

THE PARALYSED FOOT

Weakness or paralysis of the foot may be symptomless, or may present in one of three characteristic ways: the patient may complain of difficulty in walking; he or she may 'catch his or her toe' on climbing stairs (due to weak dorsiflexion); or the patient may stumble and fall (due to instability).

Clinical features

UPPER MOTOR NEURONE LESIONS Spastic paralysis may occur in children with cerebral palsy or in adults following a stroke. Muscle imbalance usually leads to equinus or equinovarus deformity. The reflexes are brisk but sensation is normal. The entire limb (or both lower limbs) is usually abnormal.

LOWER MOTOR NEURONE LESIONS Poliomyelitis was (and in some parts of the world still is) a common cause of foot paralysis. If all muscle groups are affected, the foot is flail and dangles from the ankle; if knee extension also is weak, the patient cannot walk without a calliper. With unbalanced weakness, the foot develops fixed deformity; it may also be smaller and colder than normal, but sensation is normal. Other lower motor neurone disorders such as spinal cord tumours, peroneal muscular atrophy and severe nerve root compression are rare causes of foot weakness or deformity.

PERIPHERAL NERVE INJURIES The sciatic, lateral popliteal or peroneal nerve may be affected. The commonest abnormalities are drop foot and weakness of peroneal action. Post-operative or post-immobilization drop-foot may be due to pressure on the lateral popliteal or on the peroneal nerve as the leg rolls into external rotation. In addition to motor weakness there is an area of sensory loss. Unless the nerve is divided, recovery is possible but may take many months.

Treatment

The weakness may need no treatment at all, or only a splint.

The drop-foot following nerve palsy can be treated by transferring the tibialis posterior through the interosseous membrane to the midtarsal region.

Spastic paralysis can be treated by tendon release and transfer, but great care is needed to prevent overaction in the new direction. Thus, a spastic equinovarus deformity may be converted to a severe valgus deformity by transferring tibialis anterior to the lateral side; this is avoided if only half the tendon is transferred.

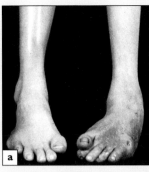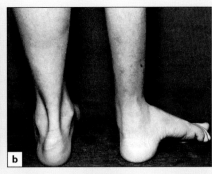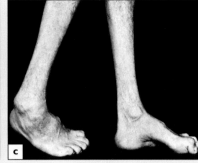

21.37 The paralysed foot (**a**) In spina bifida – the small ulcer is an indication of insensitive skin. (**b**) Poliomyelitis and (**c**) peroneal muscular atrophy, in both of which sensation is normal.

Fixed deformities must be corrected first before doing tendon transfers. If no adequate tendon is available to permit dynamic correction, the joint may be reshaped and arthrodesed; at the same time muscle rebalancing (even of weak muscles) is necessary, otherwise the deformity will recur.

PAINFUL FEET

'My feet are killing me!' The complaint is common but the cause is often elusive. Pain may be due to: (1) mechanical pressure (which is more likely if the foot is deformed); (2) joint inflammation or stiffness; (3) a localized bone lesion; (4) peripheral ischaemia; or (5) muscular strain – usually secondary to some other abnormality. Remember, too, that local disorders may be part of a generalized disease (e.g. diabetes or rheumatoid arthritis), so examination of the entire patient may be indicated.

Specific foot disorders that cause pain are considered below.

POSTERIOR HEEL PAIN

Two common causes of heel pain are traction 'apophysitis' and calcaneal bursitis.

Traction 'apophysitis' (Sever's disease) This condition usually occurs in boys of about 10 years. It is not a 'disease', but a mild traction injury. Pain and tenderness are localized to the tendo Achillis insertion. The x-ray report usually refers to increased density and fragmentation of the apophysis, but often the painless heel looks similar. The heel of the shoe should be raised a little and strenuous activities restricted for a few weeks.

Calcaneal bursitis Older girls and young women often complain of painful bumps on the backs of their heels. The posterolateral portion of the calcaneum is prominent and shoe friction causes retrocalcaneal bursitis. Symptoms are worse in cold weather and when wearing high-heeled shoes (hence the use of colloquial labels such as 'winter heels' and 'pump-bumps'). Treatment should be conservative – attention to footwear (open-back shoes are best) and padding of the heel. Operative treatment – removal of the bump or dorsal wedge osteotomy of the calcaneum – is feasible but the results are unpredictable (Taylor, 1986); despite the reduction in the size of the bumps, patients often continue to experience discomfort, now added to by an operation scar.

INFERIOR HEEL PAIN

Calcaneal bone lesions Any bone disorder in the calcaneum can present as heel pain: a stress fracture, osteomyelitis, osteoid osteoma, cyst-like lesions and Paget's disease are the most likely. X-rays usually provide the diagnosis.

Plantar fasciitis Pain under the ball of the heel, or slightly forwards of this, is a fairly common complaint in people (mainly men) aged 30–60 years. Characteristically the first step after a period of inactivity is the worst, but pain on weight-bearing is present throughout the day. There is marked tenderness along the distal edge of the heel contact area, corresponding to the attachment of the long plantar ligament; a lateral x-ray often shows a bone spur extending distally from this site.

The term 'plantar fasciitis' seems apt as the condition is sometimes associated with inflammatory disorders such as gout, ankylosing spondylitis and Reiter's disease, in which enthesopathy is one of the defining pathological lesions. Often, however, there is no obvious associated abnormality, or maybe only something

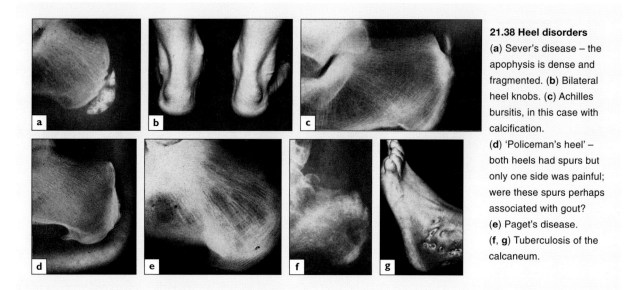

21.38 Heel disorders
(a) Sever's disease – the apophysis is dense and fragmented. (b) Bilateral heel knobs. (c) Achilles bursitis, in this case with calcification. (d) 'Policeman's heel' – both heels had spurs but only one side was painful; were these spurs perhaps associated with gout? (e) Paget's disease. (f, g) Tuberculosis of the calcaneum.

like flat-foot or pes cavus which is so common that a causative relationship is difficult to establish. The calcaneal spur sometimes seen on x-ray is not a 'cause' but some regard it as a type of traction lesion in the plantar ligament or flexor digitorum brevis muscle.

Treatment is conservative: anti-inflammatory drugs or local injection of corticosteroids, and a pad under the heel to off-load the painful area. Pain usually subsides after 6–12 months.

Painful fat pad Chronic pain and tenderness directly over the fat pad under the heel sometimes follows a direct blow to the area, e.g. in a fall from a height. The condition is also seen in athletes and has been attributed variously to separation of the fat pad from the bone, loss of its normal shock-absorbing effect and atrophy. Non-specific 'inflammation' has also been blamed. Treatment is palliative: wearing soft-soled shoes or shock-absorbing heel cups, foot baths and anti-inflammatory agents.

Nerve entrapment Entrapment of the first branch of the lateral plantar nerve has been reported as a cause of heel pain (Baxter and Pfeffer, 1992). The commonest complaint is pain after sporting activities. Characteristically, tenderness is maximal on the medial aspect of the heel where the small nerve branch is compressed between the deep fascia of abductor hallucis and the edge of the quadratus plantae muscle. Diagnosis is not easy, because the symptoms and signs may mimic those of plantar fasciitis.

Treatment, in the first instance, is conservative: a long trial (6–8 months) of shock-absorbing orthoses, foot baths, anti-inflammatory preparations and one or two corticosteriod injections. Only if these measures fail to give relief should surgical decompression of the nerve be considered.

PAIN OVER THE MIDFOOT

In children, pain in the midtarsal region is rare: one cause is *Köhler's disease* (osteochondritis of the navicular). The bony nucleus of the navicular becomes dense and fragmented. The child, under the age of 5 years, has a painful limp, and a tender warm thickening over the navicular. Usually no treatment is needed as the condition resolves spontaneously. If symptoms are severe, a short period in a below-knee plaster helps.

A comparable condition occasionally affects middle-aged women *(Brailsford's disease)*; the navicular becomes dense, then altered in shape, and later the midtarsal joint may degenerate.

In adults, especially if the arch is high, a ridge of bone sometimes develops on the adjacent dorsal surfaces of the medial cuneiform and the first metatarsal (the *'overbone'*). A lump can be seen which feels bony and may become bigger and tender if the shoe presses on it. If shoe adjustment fails to provide relief the lump may be bevelled off.

GENERALIZED PAIN IN THE FOREFOOT

METATARSALGIA Generalized ache in the forefoot is a common expression of foot strain, which may be due to a variety of conditions that give rise to faulty weight distribution (e.g. flattening of the metatarsal arch, or undue shortening of the first metatarsal), or merely the result of prolonged or unaccustomed walking, marching, climbing or standing. These conditions have this in common: they give rise to a mismatch between the loads applied to the foot, the structure on which those loads are acting, and the muscular effort required to maintain the structure so that it can

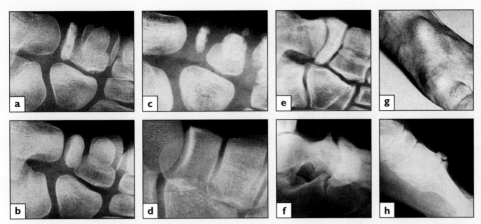

21.39 Painful tarsus (a) Köhler's disease compared with (b) the normal foot. (c) Another example of Köhler's disease, and (d) the same foot fully grown – it has become normal. (e) Brailsford's disease, the adult equivalent of Köhler's disease. (f) Degeneration of the talonavicular joint. (g, h) The 'overbone' at the first cuneiform–metatarsal joint.

support those loads. Treatment, therefore, involves (a) dealing with the mechanical disorder (correcting a deformity if it is correctable, supplying an orthosis which will redistribute the load, fitting a shoe which will accommodate the foot) and/or (b) doing muscle strengthening exercises, especially for the intrinsic muscles which maintain the anterior (metatarsal) arch of the foot.

PAIN IN THE METATARSOPHALANGEAL JOINTS Inflammatory arthritis (e.g. rheumatoid disease) may start in the foot with synovitis of the metatarsophalangeal joints. Pain in these cases is associated with swelling and tenderness of the forefoot joints and the features are almost always bilateral and symmetrical.

LOCALIZED PAIN IN THE FOREFOOT

Pain and tenderness at a specific site could be due to a variety of local bone or soft-tissue disorders; those peculiar to the foot are 'sessamoiditis', osteochondritis of a metatarsal head (Freiberg's disease), a metatarsal stress fracture and digital nerve entrapment (Morton's metatarsalgia).

'SESSAMOIDITIS' Pain and tenderness directly under the first metatarsal head, typically aggravated by walking or passive dorsiflexion of the great toe, may be due to 'sessamoiditis'. This term is a misnomer: symptoms usually arise from irritation or inflamation of the peritendinous tissues around the sessamoids – more often the medial sessamoid, which is subjected to most stress during weight-bearing on the ball of the foot.

Acute 'sessamoiditis' may be initiated by direct trauma (jumping from a height) or unaccustomed stress (e.g. in new athletes and dancers). *Chronic sessamoid*

pain and tenderness should alert one to the possibility of sessamoid displacement, local infection (particularly in a diabetic patient) or avascular necrosis.

Sesamoid chondromalacia is a term coined by Apley (1966) to explain changes such as fragmentation and cartilage fibrillation of the medial sessamoid. X-rays in these cases may show a bipartite or multipartite medial sessamoid, which is often mistaken for a fracture.

Treatment, in the usual case, consists of reduced weight-bearing and a pressure pad in the shoe. In resistant cases, a local injection of methylprednisolone and local anaesthetic often helps; otherwise the sessamoid should be shaved down or removed, taking great care not to interrupt the flexor hallucis brevis tendon.

FREIBERG'S DISEASE This is a crushing type of osteochondritis of the second metatarsal head (rarely the third). It usually affects young adults, mostly women. A bony lump (the enlarged head) is palpable and tender and the metatarsophalangeal joint is irritable. X-rays show the head to be too wide and flat, the neck thick and the joint space increased.

If discomfort is marked, a walking plaster or moulded sandal will help to reduce pressure on the metatarsal head. If pain and stiffness persist, operative synovectomy, debridement and trimming of the metatarsal head should be considered. Pain relief is usually good and the range of dorsiflexion is improved.

STRESS FRACTURE Stress fracture, usually of the second or third metatarsal, occurs in young adults after unaccustomed activity or in women with postmenopausal osteoporosis. The dorsum of the foot may be slightly oedematous and the affected shaft feels thick and tender. The x-ray appearance is at first normal, but later shows fusiform callus around a fine transverse fracture.

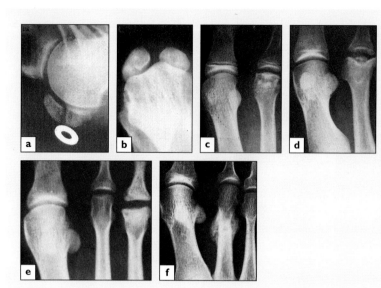

21.40 Localized pain in the forefoot (a, b) Sesamoid 'chondromalacia'. Lateral and sky-line x-ray views showing a bipartite medial sesamoid. The patient complained of localized pain and the site of tenderness is pinpointed by a metal marker. The sesamoid was removed through a plantar incision, with complete relief of symptoms. (c, d) Stages in the development of Freiberg's disease. (e) The comparable disorder in the third metatarsal (Köhler's second disease). (f) Stress fracture of the second metatarsal; the facture is difficult to see but, a week or two later, callus and periosteal new bone can be made out in the x-ray.

Long before x-ray signs appear, a radioisotope scan will show increased activity. Treatment is either unnecessary or consists simply of rest.

INTERDIGITAL NERVE COMPRESSION (MORTON'S METATARSALGIA) The patient, usually a woman of around 50 years, complains of pain in the forefoot, and sometimes burning and tingling radiating to the toes (usually the third and fourth). Symptoms are aggravated by wearing tight shoes and relieved by removing the shoes. Tenderness is localized to one of the intermetatarsal spaces – usually the third – and pressure just proximal to the interdigital web may elicit both the pain and the tingling previously experienced by the patient. Sometimes sensation is diminished the affected toes. If the diagnosis is in doubt, a diagnostic 'blocking' test can be performed: an injection of local anaesthetic beneath the transverse intermetatarsal ligament will relieve the pain.

This is essentially an entrapment or compression syndrome affecting one of the digital nerves, but secondary thickening of the nerve creates the impression of a 'neuroma'. If symptoms do not respond to the use of protective padding and wearing wider shoes, the nerve should be released by dividing the tight transverse intermetatarsal ligament; this can be done through either a dorsal longitudinal or a plantar incision. In intractable cases it may be necessary to excise the thickened portion of the nerve.

'NEUROLOGICAL PAIN' (TARSAL TUNNEL SYNDROME)

Pain and sensory disturbance in the medial part of the forefoot, unrelated to weight-bearing, may be due to compression of the posterior tibial nerve behind and below the medial malleolus. Sometimes this is due to a space-occupying lesion, e.g. a ganglion, haemangioma or varicosity. The pain is often worse at night and the patient may seek relief by walking around or stamping his or her foot. Paraesthesia and numbness may follow the characteristic sensory distribution, but these symptoms are not as well defined as in other entrapment syndromes. The diagnosis is difficult to establish as nerve conduction studies are often normal.

Treatment To decompress the nerve it is exposed behind the medial malleolus and followed into the sole; sometimes it is trapped by the belly of adductor hallucis arising more proximally than usual.

SKIN DISORDERS

Painful skin lesions are important for two reasons: (a) they demand attention in their own right, and (b) postural adjustments to relieve pressure may give rise to secondary problems and metatarsalgia.

Corns and calluses These are hyperkeratotic lesions which develop as a reaction to localized pressure or friction. Corns are fairly small and situated at 'high spots' in contact with the shoe upper: the dorsal knuckle of a claw toe or hammer toe, or the tip of the toe if it impinges against the shoe. Soft corns also appear on adjacent surfaces of toes which rub against each other. Treatment consists of paring the hyperkeratotic skin, applying felt pads which will prevent shoe or toe pressure, correcting any significant deformity (if necessary by operation) and attending to footwear.

Calluses are more diffuse keratotic plaques on the soles – either under prominent metatarsal heads or under the heel. They are seen mainly in people with 'dropped' metatarsal arches and claw toes, or varus or valgus heels.

Treatment is much the same as for corns; it is important to redistribute foot pressure by altering the shoes, fitting pressure-relieving orthoses and ensuring that the shoes can accommodate the malshaped feet. Surgical treatment for claw toes may be needed.

Plantar warts Plantar warts resemble calluses but they tend to be more painful and tender, especially if squeezed. They can be distinguished from calluses by paring down the hyperkeratotic skin to expose the characteristic papillomatous 'core' which is seen to be dotted with fine blood vessels. These are viral lesions but it is usually local pressure which renders them painful. Treatment is frustrating as they are difficult to eradicate. Salicylic acid plasters are applied at regular intervals, and smaller lesions may respond to cryosurgery. Surgical excision is avoided as this usually leaves a painful scar at the pressure site.

Foreign body 'granuloma' The sole is particularly at risk of penetration by small foreign bodies (usually a thorn, a splinter or a piece of glass) which may give rise to a painful lump resembling a wart or callus. This diagnosis should always be considered if the 'callosity' is situated in a non-pressure area. X-rays may help to detect the foreign body. Treatment consists of removing the object; the reactive lesion quickly heals.

TOENAIL DISORDERS

The toenail of the hallux may be ingrown, overgrown or undergrown.

INGROWN The nail burrows into the nail groove; this ulcerates and its wall grows over the nail, so the term 'embedded toenail' would be better. The patient is taught to cut the nail square, to insert pledgets of wool under the ingrowing edges and always to keep the feet clean and dry.

If these measures fail, the portion of germinal matrix which is responsible for the 'ingrow' should be ablated, either by operative excision or by chemical ablation with phenol; the phenol is applied to the exposed matrix with a cotton bud for 1 minute and then washed off with alcohol which neutralizes the caustic effect. Rarely is it necessary to remove the entire nail or completely ablate the nail bed.

OVERGROWN (ONYCHOGRYPOSIS) The nail is hard, thick and curved. A chiropodist can usually make the patient comfortable, but occasionally the nail may need excision.

UNDERGROWN A subungual exostosis grows on the dorsum of the terminal phalanx and pushes the nail upwards. The exostosis should be removed.

NOTES ON APPLIED ANATOMY

The ankle and foot function as an integrated unit, and together provide stable support, proprioception, balance and mobility.

THE ANKLE

The ankle fits together like a tenon and mortise; the tibial and fibular parts of the mortise are bound together by the inferior tibiofibular ligament, and stability is augmented by the collateral ligaments. The medial ligament fans out from the tibial malleolus to the talus, the superficial fibres forming the deltoid

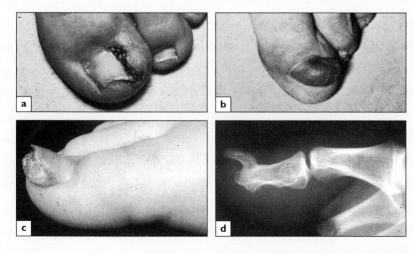

21.41 Toenail disorders (a) Ingrown toenail. (b) Overgrown toenail (onychogryposis). (c) Undergrown toenail, caused by (d) a subungual exostosis.

ligament. The lateral ligament has three thickened bands: the anterior and posterior talofibular ligaments and, between them, the calcaneofibular ligament. Tears of these ligaments may cause tilting of the talus in its mortise. Forced abduction or adduction may disrupt the mortise altogether by (1) forcing the tibia and fibula apart (diastasis of the tibiofibular joint), (2) tearing the collateral ligaments or (3) fracturing the malleoli.

THE FOOT

The footprint gives some idea of the arched structure of the foot. This derives from the tripodial bony framework between the calcaneum posteriorly and the first and fifth metatarsal heads. The medial arch is high, with the navicular as its keystone; the lateral arch is flatter. The anterior arch, formed by the metatarsal bones, thrusts maximally upon the first and fifth metatarsal heads and flattens out (spreading the foot) during weight-bearing; it can be pulled up by contraction of the intrinsic muscles, which flex the metatarsophalangeal joints.

MOVEMENTS

The ankle allows movement in the sagittal plane only – plantarflexion and dorsiflexion. Adduction and abduction (turning the toes towards or away from the midline) are produced by rotation of the entire leg below the knee; if either is forced at the ankle, the mortise fractures. Pronation and supination occur at the intertarsal and tarsometatarsal joints; the foot rotates about an axis running through the second metatarsal, the sole turning laterally (pronation) or medially (supination) – movements analogous to those of the forearm. The combination of plantarflexion, adduction and supination is called inversion; the opposite movement of dorsiflexion, abduction and pronation is eversion.

Inversion and eversion are necessary for walking on rough ground or across a slope. If the joints at which they occur are arthrodesed in childhood, a compensatory change may occur at the ankle so that it becomes a ball-and-socket joint.

FOOT POSITIONS AND DEFORMITIES

A downward-pointing foot is said to be in equinus; the opposite is calcaneus. If only the forefoot points downwards the term 'plantaris' is used. Supination with adduction produces a varus deformity; pronation with abduction causes pes valgus. An unusually high arch is called pes cavus. Many of these terms are used as if they were definitive diagnoses when, in fact, they are nothing more than Latin translations of descriptive anatomy.

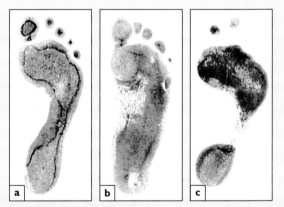

21.42 Footprints (**a**) The normal foot, (**b**) flat-foot (the medial arch touches the ground), and (**c**) cavus foot (even the lateral arch barely makes contact).

REFERENCES AND FURTHER READING

Aldham CH (1989) Repair of calcaneal tendon ruptures. A safe technique. *Journal of Bone and Joint Surgery* **71B**, 486-488

Apley AG (1966) Open sessamoid. *Proceedings of the Royal Society of Medicine* **59**, 120

Banta J, Sutherland DH, Wyatt M (1981) Anterior tibialis transfer to os calcis with Achilles tenodesis for calcaneal deformity in myelomeningocoele. *Journal of Paediatric Orthopaedics* **1**, 125-130

Baxter DE, Pfeffer GB (1992) Treatment of chronic heel pain by surgical release of the first branch of the lateral plantar nerve. *Clinical Orthopaedics and Related Research* **279**, 229-236

Caroll NC (1994) Technique of plantar fascia release and calcaneocuboid joint release in clubfoot surgery. In *The Clubfoot* (ed Simons GW) pp 246-252. Springer-Verlag, New York

Cholmeley JA (1953) Elmslie's operation for the calcaneus foot. *Journal of Bone and Joint Surgery* **35B**, 46-49

Cobey JC (1976) Posterior roentgenogram of the foot. *Clinical Orthopaedics and Related Research* **118**, 202-207

Coleman WC, Brand PW, Birke JA (1984) The total contact cast. A therapy for plantar ulceration on insensitive feet. *Journal of the American Podiatry Association* **74**, 548-552

Colville MR (1994) Reconstruction of the lateral ankle ligaments. *Journal of Bone and Joint Surgery* **76A**, 1092-1102

Crawford A, Marxen J, Osterfield D (1982) The Cincinatti incision: a comprehensive approach for surgical procedures of the foot and ankle in childhood. *Journal of Bone and Joint Surgery* **64A**, 1355-1388

Delanois RE, Mont MA, Yoon TR *et al* (1998) Atraumatic osteonecrosis of the talus. *Journal of Bone and Joint Surgery* **80A**, 529-536

Duncan RDD, Fixsen JA (1999) Congenital convex pes valgus. *Journal of Bone and Joint Surgery* **81B**, 250-254

Evans D (1961) Relapsed clubfoot. *Journal of Bone and Joint Surgery* **43B**, 722-733

Gage JR (1991) Normal gait. In *Gait Analysis in Cerebral Palsy*. Mac Keith Press, London, pp 61-100

Herzenberg JE, Carroll NC, Christofersen MR *et al* (1988) Clubfoot analysis with three-dimensional computer modeling. *Journal of Pediatric Orthopedics*. **8**, 257-62

Lapidus PW (1942) Transplantation of the extensor tendon for correction of the overlapping fifth toe. *Journal of Bone and Joint Surgery* **24**, 555-559

Maffulli N (1999) Current concepts review: Rupture of the Achilles tendon. *Journal of Bone and Joint Surgery* **81A**, 1019-1036

Mann RA (1993) Biomechanics of the foot and ankle. In *Surgery of the Foot and Ankle* (eds Mann RA, Couglin MJ), Chapter 1, pp 4-43. Mosby–Year Book, St. Louis

Mardner RA (1994) Current methods for the evaluation of ankle ligament injuries. *Journal of Bone and Joint Surgery* **76A**, 1103-1111

Perry J (1983) Anatomy and biomechanics of the hindfoot. *Clinical Orthopaedics and Related Research* **177**, 9-15

Piggott H (1960) The natural history of hallux valgus in adolescence and early adult life. *Journal of Bone and Joint Surgery* **42B**, 749-760

Ponseti IV (1992).Treatment of congenital club foot. *Journal of Bone and Joint Surgery* **74A**, 448-454

Rang M (1993) High arches. In *The Art and Practice of Children's Orthopaedics* (eds Wenger DR, Rang M) pp 168-179. Raven Press, New York

Rose GK, Welton EA, Marshall T (1985) The diagnosis of flat foot in the child. *Journal of Bone and Joint Surgery* **67B**, 71-78

Samilson RL (1976) Proscentic osteotomy of the os calcis for calcaneocavus feet. In *Foot Science* (ed Bateman JE) 18. WB Saunders, Philadelphia

Taylor GJ (1986) Prominence of the calcaneus: is operation justified? *Journal of Bone and Joint Surgery* **68B**, 467-470

Turco V (1971) Surgical correction of the resistant clubfoot. One stage posteromedial release with internal fixation; a preliminary report. *Journal of Bone and Joint Surgery* **53A**, 477-497

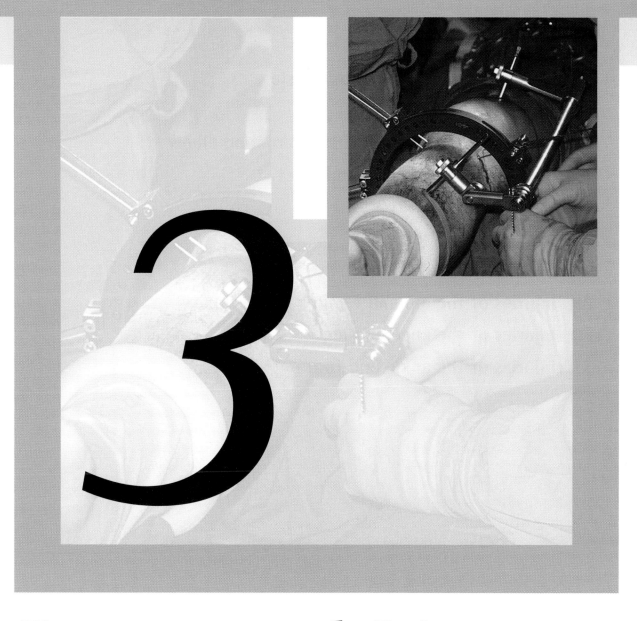

Fractures and Joint Injuries

In This Section

22 **The management of major injuries**   521

23 **Principles of fractures**   539

24 **Injuries of the shoulder, upper arm and elbow**   583

25 **Injuries of the forearm and wrist**   611

26 **Hand injuries**   629

27 **Injuries of the spine**   643

28 **Injuries of the pelvis**   667

29 **Injuries of the hip and femur**   681

30 **Injuries of the knee and leg**   705

31 **Injuries of the ankle and foot**   733

22

The management of major injuries

Trauma is the commonest cause of death in people under 40 years of age. In the industrial world, road accidents alone claim 1 in 10,000 lives each year. Most deaths occur within the first hour of injury, often before the patient arrives at hospital; the cause of death in these cases is usually severe brain or cardiovascular injury for which countermeasures are of limited value. Death can also occur rapidly from airway obstruction and external bleeding, both of which are preventable by simple first-aid measures. A second (much lower) peak in trauma deaths occurs between 1 and 4 hours after injury; these usually result from hypoxia or uncompensated blood loss and, with a competent accident system, most are preventable. This period during which lives can be saved by prompt and efficient treatment has been called *the golden hour*. A third peak in the cumulative mortality rate appears days or weeks later when patients die of the late complications of trauma and multiple organ failure.

For most severe injuries, management proceeds in several well-defined stages: emergency treatment at the scene of the accident and during transit to hospital; resuscitation and evaluation in the accident department; early treatment of visceral injuries and cardiorespiratory complications; provisional fixation followed by definitive treatment of musculoskeletal injuries; and, finally, long-term rehabilitation of the patient.

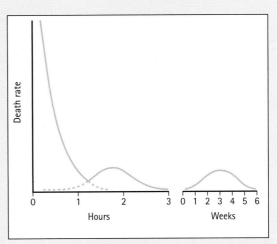

22.1 Death following trauma The trimodal pattern of mortality following severe trauma.

MANAGEMENT AT THE SCENE OF AN ACCIDENT

MULTIPLE ACCIDENTS

The first duty of a doctor arriving at the scene of a major accident is to introduce calm and order into the prevailing chaos and to avoid injury to him or herself and others. The doctor's actions should be swift yet unhurried, cautious yet purposeful. Until the police or other authorities arrive he or she should assume control and, after rapidly assessing the situation, decide on priorities. If unskilled help is at hand, messages are sent to the emergency services (ambulance, police and fire); the nearest accident centre is alerted and, where mobile operating theatres and surgical teams are available, they may need to be summoned. Bystanders can be taught how to maintain an airway with a jaw thrust or chin lift, maintain in-line immobilization of the neck and compress external bleeding points.

THE INDIVIDUAL PATIENT

Treatment of the individual patient begins at once. The usual sequence (modified to suit the circumstances) is: *obtain access; establish an airway but protect the cervical spine, ensure ventilation; arrest haemorrhage and combat shock; give analgesia; extricate; splint fractures; and transport.*

Access

When a patient is trapped or buried, the objects covering him should be moved, rather than pulling him out from beneath them. Priority is given to freeing the head and trunk. If the patient is conscious he will need immediate reassurance.

Airway, protection of the cervical spine and breathing

If the patient is breathing stertorously the angle of the jaw is pulled forwards and the mouth opened; should the difficulty persist a finger is inserted into the mouth to ensure that breathing is not being obstructed by the tongue, false teeth, vomit, blood clot or any other foreign material. The cervical spine may have been injured; the neck should be immobilized manually or with a hard collar if available. *The neck must not be extended to gain an airway.* If, despite clearing the upper airway, the patient still cannot ventilate freely, he or she may have a pneumothorax,

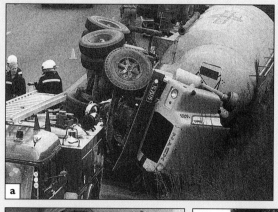
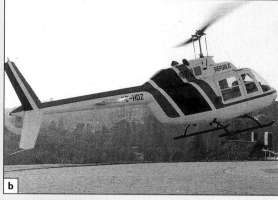
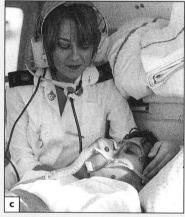
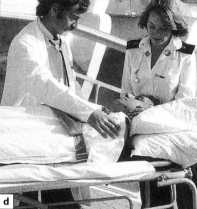

22.2 The major accident Major accidents call for a rapid response, expert care during transport and a 24-hour medical service in the accident centre.

haemothorax, flail chest or sucking wound of the chest wall. A tension pneumothorax should be drained with a hollow needle, even a ball-pen tube. A sucking chest wound should be covered with a dressing strapped firmly in position. If suitable equipment is available, endotracheal intubation or chest drain insertion can be carried out as an emergency measure and oxygen administered.

Haemorrhage

External bleeding can usually be stopped by pressure with a finger or a firm pad. Tourniquets are rarely necessary; if one must be used, a label stating the time of its application is attached to the patient in a prominent position.

Where facilities are available, intravenous fluids may be given. *No food or fluids should be given by mouth;* if the patient is unconscious these may enter the trachea, and even if he or she is conscious their presence in the stomach increases the hazards of anaesthesia during the next few hours.

Examination

A detailed examination is neither practicable nor essential, but the pulse is felt, capillary return measured, the respirations are observed, and the head, chest, abdomen and limbs, if accessible, are quickly palpated.

Analgesia

Morphine is useful but should not be given to patients with abdominal or head injuries. Entonox (nitrous oxide and oxygen) is a useful analgesic agent. Ketamine is a useful anaesthetic agent which can be administered for emergency amputation.

Extrication

A patient with fractures should not be dragged forcibly from overlying impedimenta. When obstructions have been lifted he or she can be gently moved, though injured limbs may need to be splinted before this is done. Twisting and flexion must be avoided if there is the possibility of spinal injury; special equipment is available, to which the patient can be strapped for protection of the spine.

Splintage

A broken limb should be gently straightened by traction; splintage reduces pain, blood loss, ischaemic necrosis of tented skin and injury to nerves and blood vessels. A fractured arm is easily splinted by bandaging it to the trunk, and a leg by tying it to the other leg if this is intact. Ambulances should carry inflatable splints, and only occasionally are improvised splints needed; an umbrella, walking stick, piece of wood or tubular steel is nearly always available. Open wounds are covered with a clean dressing.

Transport

To move a severely injured patient onto a stretcher at least four people are required, so that he or she is transferred 'in one piece'; this is particularly important with spinal fractures. The airway, breathing and circulation should be checked again before the ambulance departs, with the crew continuing this during the journey.

Ambulances should be equipped with splints, dressings, airways, oxygen and transfusion apparatus. They should be in two-way radio communication with the accident unit. In difficult terrain, helicopter ambulances are almost essential. Ambulance attendants are usually highly trained but every effort should be made by the staff of the accident unit to keep them continually informed, up to date and interested in their work. Their observations on the circumstances of the accident, the patient's state of consciousness and general condition are invaluable.

MANAGEMENT IN HOSPITAL

Patients who arrive in hospital after a major accident are at risk of falling into the second 'mortality peak' with death from either hypoxia or hypovolaemic shock. They are also at risk of further damage to their cervical spine, thoraco-lumbar spine and brain. This is *'the golden hour'*, during which effective resuscitation can save lives. The Advanced Trauma Life Support Programme, supervised by the American College of Surgeons, has become the standard of emergency care, consisting of four inter-related stages:

- a rapid *primary survey with simultaneous resuscitation*;
- a detailed *secondary survey*;
- constant *re-evaluation*;
- Initiation of *definitive care*.

THE PRIMARY SURVEY

A simple pnemonic for remembering the elements of the primary survey is based on the first five letters of the alphabet.

A = Airway maintenance with control of cervical spine
B = Breathing and oxygenation
C = Circulation and control of bleeding
D = Disability
E = Exposure and avoidance of hypothermia.

Airway and cervical spine control

A clear airway must be established as an absolute priority. However, this may endanger the cervical spine which must, therefore, be controlled with either manual support in the neutral position or immobilization by sandbags, forehead tape or collar until the attendant has satisfied him or herself that the airway is secure and a there is no cervical spine injury. A systematic sequence is followed: *chin lift – jaw thrust – finger sweep – suction – oropharyngeal tube – orotracheal tube – and, if necessary, surgical cricothyroidotomy.*

Breathing and oxygenation

Even if the airway is clear, the peripheral tissues will not be adequately oxygenated unless the patient can breathe. The patient's chest should be exposed and inspected for respiratory rate, open injuries, equilateral chest movements and bruising. Deviation of the trachea from the midline is noted. The chest is percussed for either dullness or hyper-resonance and is auscultated for normal/abnormal or absent breath sounds. Life-threatening injuries such as tension pneumothorax, sucking chest wound, massive haemothorax and flail chest must be considered. Most chest injuries can be managed with a cannula or chest tube. If necessary, the patient is ventilated artificially. All severely injured patients should receive high doses of oxygen, best provided through a reservoir bag. A blood sample should be taken for measurement of PCO_2 and PO_2.

Circulation and control of bleeding

Major external haemorrhage is controlled by direct pressure. Protruding weapons or other penetrating objects should be left alone and removed only when operating facilities are available and ready. The extremities are examined for coolness and delayed capillary return; the pulse rate and blood pressure are measured. Two large intravenous cannulae are inserted, if necessary by venous cut-down. Blood is sent to the laboratory for cross-matching. If fluid replacement is required, then warmed crystalloid is infused. An initial bolus of 2 litres is appropriate; if the patient fails to respond, then blood transfusion is necessary. Look for possible sources of bleeding, such as open wounds, pelvic fracture, intra-abdominal injury, intrathoracic injury or multiple long-bone fractures.

Cardiac tamponade should be suspected if there is a significant chest injury or penetrating wound, if the blood pressure cannot be maintained by rapid infusion of intravenous fluids, or if there are clinical features

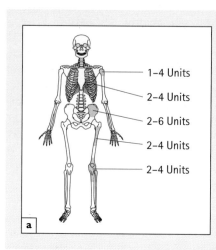

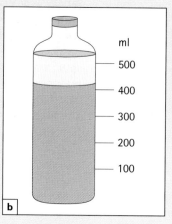

22.3 Severe injuries – blood loss (**a**) Range of probable blood loss in closed fractures. (**b**) From a 540ml container the patient receives only 400–420ml of actual blood – the rest is anticoagulant and space. *Moral* – The severely injured patient may lose more blood than you think, and receive less.

such as distended neck veins and a paradoxical pulse. Tamponade is a life-threatening condition and should be treated by immediate decompression with a needle or catheter inserted below the xiphisternum.

Disability

The *Glasgow Coma Score (GCS)* is recorded, the pupil size assessed and each extremity examined, if possible, for equality of movement. Although alcohol and other drugs might affect the level of consciousness, their presence should not be assumed until hypoxia, hypovolaemia and a head injury have been excluded.

Exposure and avoidance of hypothermia

On the one hand it is essential that the patient is fully undressed early on so that he or she can be thoroughly examined; even a small stab wound can be the cause of profound blood loss. On the other hand, the patient may lose body warmth and become increasingly hypothermic while waiting in the Emergency Department. Resuscitation fluids should be warmed and the patient should be covered immediately before and after the full examination. Children are particularly prone to hypothermia.

CONSTANT RE–EVALUATION

The patient must be re-evaluated frequently to assess the response to resuscitation and to detect any deterioration at the earliest moment.

A urethral catheter should be passed, provided there is no evidence of urethral injury following inspection of the meatus and a rectal examination.

A nasogastric tube is inserted, to reduce the risk of acute gastric dilatation and aspiration of fluid;

Table 22.1 Glasgow coma scale	
	Score
Eye-opening	
Spontaneous	4
On command	3
On pain	2
Nil	1
Best motor response	
Obeys	6
Localizes pain	5
Normal flexor	4
Abnormal flexor	3
Extensor	2
Nil	1
Verbal response	
Orientated	5
Confused	4
Words	3
Sounds	2
Nil	1

however, if there is a possibility of a basal skull fracture the tube should be passed by mouth so as to avoid the risk of entering the brain through the roof of the nose. Blood in the aspirate suggests a gastrointestinal injury.

Electrocardiograophy (ECG) monitoring may show electro-mechanical dissociation tension pneumothorax, cardiac tamponade or severe blood loss; cardiac arrhythmias may follow direct contusion of the heart muscle.

Blood pressure, arterial blood gases, oxygen saturation, expired carbon dioxide concentration and *central venous pressure* are all useful guides to the patient's condition.

SECONDARY SURVEY

Once the patient has been resuscitated, he or she is examined thoroughly from head to toe. In the Emergency Room, anteroposterior x-rays of the chest and pelvis and a lateral x-ray of the spine are obtained; these may show major injuries requiring further treatment. Other investigations may be needed, depending on the findings of the secondary survey. However, the patient should not leave the Emergency Department for these investigations unless his or her condition is absolutely stable.

DEFINITIVE TREATMENT

This is decided by the findings during the primary and secondary surveys. Other specialist assistance may be required and the patient may need transfer. Regular re-assessment is essential; *no patient should be transferred unless his or her condition is stable or unless he or she is being taken to the operating theatre for the control of haemorrhage.* Proper communication between hospital departments is important!

Once the golden hour has passed, the patient still risks suffering lethal complications such as the respiratory distress syndrome, fat embolism, infection and multiple organ failure (see below). Priority is given at all times to preventive measures such as blood volume replacement and oxygenation. There is also good evidence that the risk of acute pulmonary dysfunction is lessened by immediate external fixation of unstable fractures.

AIRWAY PROBLEMS

The first and most important priority in managing the severely traumatized patient is to ensure a clear airway. The airway may be compromised because of a decreased level of consciousness, facial trauma, neck trauma or inhalation of vomit or teeth.

Clinical assessment

A patient who is able to respond clearly to questions can be assumed, at that time, to have a patent airway. Patients who are unconscious, agitated, obtunded or cyanosed may have airway obstruction. The sound of an obstructed airway – stridor – is unmistakable.

Management

A free airway must be secured, *but remember that manoeuvres to achieve an airway may put the cervical spine at risk.* For this reason, the head and neck should be immobilized in a neutral position, either by in-line manual traction or by sandbags, collar and a tape across the forehead.

A gloved finger is an effective instrument for removing vomitus, blood or teeth from the mouth. Suction is used if it is available. Simple manoeuvres, such as a chin lift and jaw thrust, will open the mouth and a short oropharyngeal airway will maintain the channel.

If these measures fail to secure a safe airway, then an orotracheal tube should be inserted. Paralysing agents to assist this are used only if the necessary expertise, drugs and equipment are immediately available.

If the trachea cannot be intubated directly through the mouth, then a surgical airway must be created. As a temporary measure, a high flow of oxygen can be provided via a needle passed through the cricothyroid membrane, with 1 second of insufflation and 3 seconds deflation. This buys time for some 30 minutes until the carbon dioxide levels begin to rise. A more definitive procedure is surgical cricothyrotomy. Under direct vision, a hole is made in the cricothyroid membrane and an endotracheal tube is inserted. *This procedure is potentially dangerous in children in whom there is risk of subsequent laryngeal stenosis.*

Severely injured patients require 100% oxygen immediately. This is best provided with a reservoir bag and a high flow of oxygen (15l/min). The reservoir bag is required because the peak inspiratory flow rate (about 40l/min) otherwise exceeds the available flow from the oxygen supply. A nasal catheter or a non-rebreathing mask can be used if a reservoir bag is not available.

The airway must be checked frequently throughout the resuscitation phase; one that appears initially to be safe may not remain so. Pulse oxymetry and end-tidal carbon dioxide monitoring show whether an adequate airway is being maintained.

CHEST INJURIES

IMMEDIATELY LIFE-THREATENING CHEST INJURIES

As soon as the airway and neck are safe, and a high dose of oxygen supplied, the patient must be assessed for chest injuries, because these can kill – and rapidly. The most dangerous are *tension pneumothorax, sucking chest wounds, flail chest, cardiac tamponade* and *massive haemothorax.* The great majority of chest injuries can be managed, in an emergency, with a needle or a tube.

Tension pneumothorax

This occurs when air leaks either from the lung or the chest wall into the pleural space but then cannot escape. The pressure within the pleural space gradually

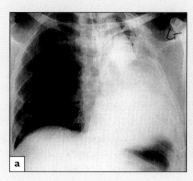
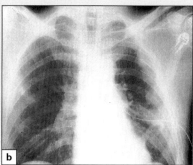

22.4 Tension pneumothorax (a) This patient with rib fractures became distressed. The x-ray shows a 'black-out' of the right side of the chest, with the mediastinal contents shifted to the left. (b) The situation after intercostal drainage.

rises, displacing the mediastinum (and thus the trachea) in the opposite direction. The high intrathoracic pressure obstructs venous return to the heart and as a result cardiac output falls.

The diagnosis should always be made clinically; if one waits to confirm this on an x-ray the patient can die. The patient is in extreme respiratory distress, tachycardic and hypotensive; the trachea is pushed away to one side; on the side of the pneumothorax breath sounds are absent and the chest is hyper-resonant to percussion. Then the neck veins distend and cyanosis develops.

Tension pneumothorax calls for immediate decompression, initially by inserting a large-bore needle into the second intercostal space in the mid-clavicular line. Once the emergency is over, the needle is replaced by a thoracostomy tube which is inserted through the fourth intercostal space in the mid-axillary line and connected to an underwater seal; this is retained until the lung re-expands.

Sucking chest wound

If there is an open wound in the chest wall, air is sucked preferentially through this wound rather than through the trachea. Sucking wounds should be covered immediately with a sterile occlusive dressing, taped on three sides. The fourth side is left open so that it can act as a 'flutter valve' to drain the associated pneumothorax. A chest drain is then passed and definitive surgical closure of the wound arranged.

Large haemothorax

The chest is a huge potential space into which the patient can exsanguinate following penetrating trauma (and, occasionally, closed trauma). Breath sounds are absent and there is dullness on percussion on that side of the chest. There may be signs of hypovolaemic shock.

A large haemothorax is managed by passing a chest tube. At the same time blood volume must be restored.

An early thoracotomy is needed if the initial drainage exceeds 1500ml or if blood continues to drain from the chest tube at more than 200ml/h.

Cardiac tamponade

This usually results from a penetrating injury which causes bleeding into the pericardial sac. The sac has a relatively small volume and cannot expand, so even a small amount of blood dramatically inhibits cardiac function.

The physical signs include the classic *Beck's triad*: distended neck veins, reduced arterial blood pressure and muffled heart sounds. The patient may also display *Kussmaul's sign*: a rise in the jugular venous pressure on inspiration. In the terminal stage, the ECG shows electro-mechanical dissociation.

This is a difficult clinical diagnosis to make because a shocked patient may not have distended neck veins and muffled heart sounds are very difficult to detect in a noisy Emergency Department. Therefore, any patient with a penetrating chest or abdominal injury who remains shocked despite appropriate replacement of blood volume, should be suspected of developing a cardiac tamponade. Treatment is urgent; a needle is inserted into the pericardial space and the haematoma is relieved. This is usually only a temporary measure because the blood can reaccumulate; a definitive thoracotomy is almost always required.

Stove-in chest (flail chest)

A crushing blow to the chest may cause multiple, bilateral rib fractures, often together with a haemothorax or pneumothorax and/or lung damage. Sometimes an entire section of the chest wall is isolated as a flail segment which is sucked inwards during inspiration and blown outwards during expiration. This so-called *paradoxical respiration* is useless for ventilating the lung and it may lead to respiratory failure, particularly if the lung is also damaged or if a pneumothorax or haemothorax develops. If unrecognized or untreated this condition may be fatal.

Treatment is initially by oxygenation and adequate, but not overenthusiastic, fluid transfusion. If the patient remains hypoxic, then endotracheal intubation and positive pressure ventilation are necessary. It is not essential to fix the fractures, provided positive pressure respiration is continued. If for some reason this cannot be done, the ribs should be stabilized with Kirschner wires.

CHEST INJURIES FOUND DURING THE SECONDARY SURVEY

Other chest injuries, which also are potentially lethal, should be looked for during the secondary survey.

Pulmonary contusion

Pulmonary contusion is common. The patient becomes progressively hypoxic as the damaged lung becomes oedematous and further mis-matching between ventilation and perfusion occurs. The initial chest x-ray often underestimates the severity of the injury

Treatment calls for prompt and aggressive oxygenation; if the patient is still hypoxic, then intubation and ventilation are required.

Myocardial contusion

This is suspected from the mechanism of injury, usually a direct blow to the front of the chest. On examination, the patient may have bruising over the front of the chest and painful crepitus from a sternal fracture. The ECG may show various arrhythmias. The patient should be admitted and monitored closely with continuous ECG.

Ruptured aorta

Rupture of the aorta is a common cause of sudden death in a car accident or a fall from a height. The vessel is usually torn where the relatively mobile arch becomes secured to the thoracic wall near the ligamentum arteriosum. Some patients survive when the adventitial layer of the aorta contains the haematoma. Sooner or later, though, this may rupture with catastrophic consequences.

Physical signs are usually absent but a high index of suspicion should be prompted by a knowledge of the type of injury. The chest x-ray may show a widened mediastinum although this is difficult to interpret on the typical antero-posterior view taken in the Emergency Department. Other radiological signs include fractures of the upper ribs, deviation of the trachea to the right, loss of the aortic knuckle or a pleural cap. If the injury is suspected, an angiogram or a contrast-enhanced computed tomography (CT) is required. If this confirms the diagnosis, urgent operation is needed.

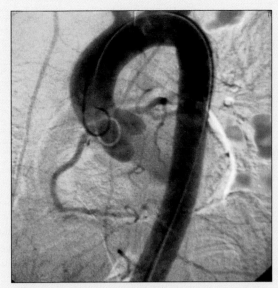

22.5 Arch aortogram In this case the aortogram was normal, thus excluding an aortic intimal tear.

Ruptured diaphragm

This is usually associated with blunt trauma to the abdomen and occurs on the left side, because on the right the diaphragm is protected by the liver. The diagnosis can be elusive and the patient sometimes presents days, months or even years after injury.

The chest x-ray may show an indistinct hemidiaphragm, bowel gas or a coiled gastric tube in the chest. Occasionally, bowel may be felt when a finger is passed to clear the way for a chest drain. A barium swallow confirms the diagnosis. The patient should be referred for surgical treatment.

Isolated rib fractures

Rib fractures are almost always due to direct injury. However, in osteoporotic patients ribs may fracture with minor stresses such as coughing or sneezing. Fractures of the first and second ribs are ominous as they suggest a very significant transfer of energy and are associated with, for example, transection of the thoracic aorta or damage to the adjacent brachial plexus or subclavian vein. In children, the ribs are flexible and it takes great force to break them. Severe underlying injury must be suspected.

The patient complains of a sharp pain in the chest. This is aggravated by deep breathing or coughing, or by antero-posterior compression of the chest wall. Fractures are easily overlooked on a chest x-ray. However, a week or two after injury they can be detected by radioscintigraphy.

In most cases treatment is needed only for pain; an injection of local anaesthetic will bring immediate relief. Breathing exercises are then encouraged.

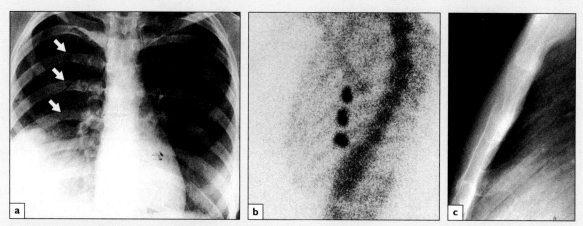

22.6 Thoracic cage fractures (**a**) Rib fractures are usually obvious on plain x-ray. (**b**) Undisplaced fractures are sometimes difficult to see; a week later they show up clearly on the radionuclide scan. (**c**) Sternal fracture with minimal displacement.

COMPLICATIONS A threatening problem with isolated rib fractures is that while the bone injury may appear to be trivial the potential complications can be very serious. *Haemothorax* can result from damage to an intercostal vessel and *pneumothorax* may occur if the pleura is punctured by a jagged bone fragment. Worst of all is a *tension pneumothorax*; this should always be suspected if the patient starts feeling increasingly uncomfortable after being sent home with a 'minor' rib fracture. Treatment is described on page 525.

Pulmonary contusion may give rise to hypoxaemia. This usually occurs only after multiple rib fractures.

Visceral injury is occasionally produced by a sharp rib spike which damages the intrathoracic abdominal organs (liver or spleen). Beware the patient with a rib fracture and signs of excessive bleeding.

Surgical emphysema is produced by air leaking into the soft tissues of the chest wall. Despite the sometimes dramatic appearance, treatment is not usually required.

Fracture of the sternum

The sternum may be fractured by a direct blow to the chest, or indirectly during a flexion injury of the spine; in the latter case there may be an associated thoracic vertebral crush fracture. Occasionally the underlying myocardium is damaged and patients with a significant injury should be monitored for cardiac arrhythmias.

If displacement is minimal, no treatment is needed. If the fragments are severely displaced, they can be lifted forwards (under general anaesthesia) with the aid of a bone hook.

Patients may continue to complain of chest pain and/or thoracic back pain for months afterwards. A severe vertebral fracture will, of course, need treatment in its own right.

SHOCK

Shock is defined as 'inadequate perfusion and oxygenation of tissues'. Various types of shock are encountered in the severely injured patient:

- hypovolaemic shock;
- cardiogenic shock;
- neurogenic shock;
- septic shock.

HYPOVOLAEMIC SHOCK

This is the most common cause of shock following injury. During the primary survey, it must be clearly established whether there has been external or internal bleeding. If there has, then resuscitation and efforts to stop the bleeding should go hand in hand.

Clinical features

An adult's blood volume comprises about 7% of body weight. This represents about 5 litres in a 70kg man. In a child, the blood volume is about 8%. In modest blood loss (e.g. 15% or less of blood volume), there are few reliable clinical signs. There may be a mild tachycardia and slightly reduced capillary return in the fingertips. Blood pressure is not reduced; indeed the diastolic blood pressure is often raised due to peripheral vasoconstriction from the release of catecholamines

With blood loss of 20–30%, the heart rate and respiratory rate begin to rise. The systolic blood pressure remains steady but the diastolic pressure begins to fall and the pulse pressure is widened. The patient seems a little anxious and the urine output is slightly reduced.

When about a third of the blood volume has been lost, the classic signs of hypovolaemia appear. The patient is cool, clammy, tachycardic, tachypnoeic and hypotensive.

When more than 40% of the blood volume has been lost, the patient's life is in danger. There is a rapid tachycardia, a greatly reduced systolic blood pressure, no urine output and marked confusion.

Management

There is little point in re-establishing blood volume if the blood is not being oxygenated. Therefore, management of the airway and breathing must take priority. Any obvious bleeding sites should be directly compressed to avoid continuing blood loss. Venous access is established. If possible, a peripheral vein should be cannulated. This is sometimes difficult and one must not hesitate to resort to a venous cut-down. Subclavian central venous cannulation is inappropriate in the early stages after trauma: it is difficult to locate a central vein in a hypovolaemic patient and there is a real risk of penetrating the pleural cavity.

Initially, isotonic electrolyte solution (saline, Ringer's lactate or Hartmann's solution) is infused in a bolus of 1–2 litres for an adult and 20ml/kg for a child. If the patient's shock promptly responds, then there should be a period of further observation. If the shock only transiently responds or responds not at all, then blood transfusion is essential and surgery highly likely. Three types of blood are generally available for transfusion. Ideally, one should use fully cross-matched blood; this may take up to an hour to receive. In more urgent circumstances, use type specific blood; this has not been fully checked for minor antigens, but is available far more quickly. In dire circumstances, use O Rh-negative blood.

With resuscitative measures in progress, a close search is made for hidden sources of bleeding in the thorax, abdomen and pelvis. *Intrathoracic bleeding* may be apparent from clinical examination, the chest X-ray or drainage from a chest tube; *intra-abdominal bleeding* from clinical examination, diagnostic peritoneal lavage, ultrasound or CT scanning; and *pelvic bleeding* from clinical and x-ray signs of a major pelvic fracture.

Continuing haemorrhage may necessitate immediate surgical intervention – thoracotomy, laparotomy or pelvic external fixation. A pelvic external fixator can be life-saving for a hypovolaemic patient with an unstable pelvic fracture. If bleeding still persists, then angiographic embolization may be required. It must be remembered that the pelvic fracture may not be the only source of blood loss; abdominal injuries, multiple fractures and chest injuries often coincide.

CARDIOGENIC SHOCK

This happens when the heart does not pump adequately, for example after severe *myocardial contusion* (which either directly damages the heart or sets off dysrhythmias), in *cardiac tamponade* (where cardiac contraction is inhibited) or with a *tension pneumothorax* (where intrathoracic pressure is so high that venous return is impeded). Management must include prompt treatment of the underlying condition.

NEUROGENIC SHOCK

Transection of the spinal cord interrupts the sympathetic innervation to the heart and blood vessels. The peripheral vessels dilate and the heart rate slows, resulting in a drop in blood pressure. This is initially treated with volume expanders; central venous pressure measurement and vasopressors are helpful in managing this difficult problem.

SEPTIC SHOCK

Widespread infection is unusual in the first few days after major trauma. However, it may develop several days later in patients who have had open injuries to the abdomen, thorax or limbs. It may also be seen as part of the multi-organ failure syndrome. On examination the patient typically has a mild tachycardia, a raised temperature, warm extremities, a slightly reduced systolic pressure and a greatly reduced diastolic pressure (i.e. a wider pulse pressure).

ABDOMINAL INJURIES

There is a real danger that abdominal injuries may be overlooked, either because an unconscious patient can give no history or because the initial physical signs are subtle. It can take quite some time for a ruptured viscus or intra-abdominal bleeding to become apparent. The patient must therefore be re-assessed at regular intervals.

The abdomen is inspected for bruising and perforating wounds. The size of a wound is no guide to the amount of damage; a sharp bicycle spoke may perforate bowel, spleen, diaphragm and heart in a single blow. The posterior abdominal wall must also be inspected; otherwise a stab to the back could be overlooked. However, if the back is inspected, precautions must be taken to protect the spine by log rolling. Local tenderness, rigidity and absence of bowel sounds suggest visceral damage. A ruptured spleen or liver can be deceptively 'silent' and the diagnosis must never await the appearance of gross signs.

A *rectal examination* is important to feel for sphincter tone, fragments of bone and the presence of blood. A high-riding prostate suggests a urethral injury. Bleeding from the urethral meatus suggests a urethral or bladder injury. Bruising around the genitalia suggests a urethral or pelvic injury.

Plain x-rays are useful only insofar as they can show free air beneath the diaphragm in a patient who can be sat up for this purpose. In experienced hands, *ultrasound* shows blood and injury to major organs such as the spleen, liver and pancreas. A *CT scan* readily demonstrates injury to the liver, spleen or pancreas. However, a patient must never be transferred from the relative safety of the Emergency Department to the depths of a Radiology Department unless the airway, ventilation and circulation are secure.

Diagnostic peritoneal lavage may reveal blood or bowel contents in the abdominal cavity but it does not show its source.

Management

A gastric tube should be passed in all patients with multiple injuries. It should be introduced through the mouth rather than the nose if there is any chance of a basal skull fracture. A bladder catheter should be inserted during resuscitation in order to monitor urinary output and the response to fluid replacement. However, the patient should not be catheterized if there is the possibility of a urethral injury (look for blood at the tip of the urethra, bruising around the genitalia or a high-riding prostate).

At laparotomy, bleeding is dealt with by packing followd by ligatures or diathermy. The viscera are examined. Small ruptures of the spleen and liver can often be managed without the need for resection. However, severe injuries may require either splenectomy or (in the case of the liver) vascular ligation, oversewing or partial resection. Bowel injuries can usually be repaired; prophylactic antibiotics are essential and colonic diversion may be required

HEAD INJURIES

Applied anatomy

The anatomy of the *scalp* is readily remembered by the mnemonic SCALP (Skin, subCutis, Aponeurosis, Loose areolar tissue, Periosteum).

The *skull* comprises the vault and the base. The vault has an inner and outer table of bone and is particularly thin in the temporo-parietal regions.

The *meninges* consist of the *dura* (a thick, fibrous membrane firmly attached to the inner surface of the skull), the *arachnoid* (a thin, transparent layer) and the

pia (a vascular layer attached to the surface of the brain itself). Blood vessels lie between the dura and the inner table of the skull. Rupture of these vessels, particularly the middle meningeal, causes an extradural haematoma. Small vessels pass between the arachnoid and the dura and rupture of these causes a subdural haematoma. Bleeding into the space between the arachnoid and the pia produces a subarachnoid haemorrhage.

The *brain* itself is divided into the *cerebral hemispheres* and the *brain stem*. The brain stem comprises the *midbrain,* the *pons* and the *medulla*. The mid brain passes through a large opening in the *tentorium* (a fibrous membrane separating the *middle fossa* and *posterior fossa* of the skull). The *third cranial nerve* also passes through this opening. If pressure is increased above the tentorium, usually from a haematoma or brain swelling, part of the temporal lobe of the cerebral hemisphere may be forced through the opening. This compresses the third cranial nerve (causing a dilated pupil) and the cerebral peduncle (causing spastic weakness of the opposite arm and leg)

Pathophysiology of brain injury

Intracranial pressure is determined by the combined volume of cerebrospinal fluid (CSF), brain and blood. The mean systemic blood pressure must exceed the intracranial pressure if the brain is to be adequately perfused. Therefore anything which raises the intracranial pressure (especially an intracranial haematoma or brain swelling) will reduce the cerebral perfusion pressure. The patients's level of consciousness falls. The brain compensates by reducing the volume of CSF or venous blood through local autoregulatory mechanisms; also reduced perfusion to the vasomotor part of the medulla causes a sympathetic discharge, which increases the systemic arterial pressure. As blood pressure rises, systemic arterial pressure receptors cause a reflex reduction in heart rate.

Primary and secondary brain injury

Primary brain injury is caused by mechanisms such as a *direct blow, contra-coup* (sudden compression against the other side of the skull), *penetration by a hard object* or *shear* on the brain from acceleration forces. The severity of the injury is determined at the moment of impact and (generally) cannot be influenced directly by medical management. Brain cells cannot regenerate or heal themselves. Some will have been irreversibly damaged at the time of primary brain injury; others will be in a critical state, but may recover in ideal conditions; and yet other cells, not damaged at the time of the primary injury, later suffer secondary injury. The first group cannot be helped; the second and third groups must be protected from secondary injury.

Secondary brain injury usually arises from cerebral hypoxia due to a failed airway, inadequate breathing or poor circulation. Cerebral hypoxia will spell the demise of critically injured brain cells and cause other brain cells to swell: this leads to a viscious circle of further oedema, further rise in intracranial pressure, further reduction in cerebral perfusion pressure and therefore further ischaemia.

Other causes of secondary brain injury include impaired cerebrovascular autoregulation, disruption of the blood-brain barrier with consequent vascular fluid shifts, and focal contusions which are associated with swelling and oozing of blood into the surrounding brain tissue.

Initial assessment

It is crucial to realize that, however appalling a head injury may appear, the airway, cervical spine, breathing and circulation all take priority. Prior to examination of the head, the neck must be immobilized or a neck injury conclusively excluded. During the primary survey one establishes whether there is a major intracranial haematoma which might require urgent operation and sets a base-line against which to judge further deterioration. To do this, the GCS is calculated, the pupils are examined for equality and the arms and legs are assessed for one-sided weakness.

The *GCS* (see page 524) is the most widely used and validated system. This is based on descending levels of eye opening, verbal response and motor response. The maximum score is 15. A score of eight or less defines coma. The most important aspect of the GCS is that it represents the patient's level of consciousness at that moment in time. A deterioration in the coma scale is extremely significant and usually justifies immediate senior help and a CT scan.

The pupils are examined for asymmetric dilatation and the light reflexes tested on each side. With increased intracranial pressure, compression of the third nerve results in dilatation of the pupil and a failure to react to light. A unilateral fixed and dilated pupil indicates that the medial temporal lobe has herniated (unless the orbit has been damaged). Bilateral fixed dilated pupils may be due to inadequate cerebral perfusion or to herniation of the entire mid-brain through the tentorium. This is a very grave prognostic sign.

The limbs are examined in conscious patients for spontaneous movement; one-sided weakness suggests a space-occupying lesion in the opposite cortex or compression of the cerebral peduncles as they pass through the tentorium.

Secondary survey

The head injury is assessed further during the secondary survey. The history of injury, as usual, is most important. What was the precise mechanism of injury? Did

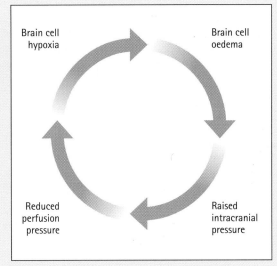

22.7 The vicious circle of secondary brain injury

the patient lose consciousness? If so, for how long? Was there a period of amnesia? Did the patient take drugs or alcohol? Is there a previous history of fits or neurological disorder? What other injuries are present?

The head should be systematically examined. The scalp and face should be inspected for lacerations; the nose and ears are examined for CSF leakage. Other signs of a basal skull fracture are subconjunctival haemorrhage without a posterior margin, racoon eyes (periorbital bruising) and bruising behind the mastoid (Battle's sign). The skull is palpated systematically; in a conscious patient a tender area may suggest an underlying fracture. Scalp lacerations are carefully inspected for depressed skull fractures, brain tissue, dirt and CSF.

Imaging

Plain x-rays are routine in patients who have had significant head or facial injuries, and especially in those who have lost consciousness (however briefly). Fractures of the vault and around the orbit can be detected, but detail is often poor and intracranial damage cannot be assessed at all. If a fracture is seen the patient should be admitted to hospital and kept under observation, whatever the level of consciousness. However, basal fractures are not reliably shown on plain x-rays; if the clinical features are suggestive, the diagnosis should be confirmed by CT.

CT is far more useful than a skull x-ray in the management of head injuries. It will define the position and extent of intracranial haemorrhage and can indicate the severity of brain swelling. Ideally, therefore, a CT scan should be obtained in every patient with a skull fracture, but particularly those who have open or depressed fractures or penetrating wounds of the head or face. Other

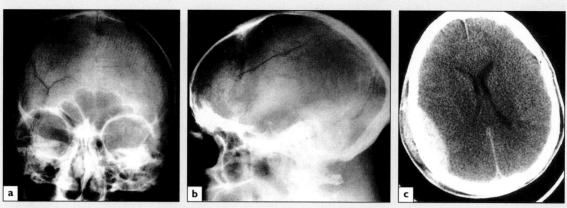

22.8 Head injuries – imaging (**a, b**) X-rays showing a fracture of the parietal bone. (**c**) This CT scan shows an extradural haematoma with distortion of the lateral ventricle on that side.

indications are the presence of focal neurological signs, an epileptic fit, a reduced level of consciousness or a fixed, dilated pupil. Remember, though, that the scan records the situation only at one moment in time and there should be no hesitation in repeating it if there is any change in the patient's condition.

Management

GENERAL PRINCIPLES

1. *A safe airway* is crucial. A patient in coma cannot control his or her own airway; coughing and choking raise intracranial pressure, thus decreasing brain perfusion.
2. *The cervical spine must be protected* because associated neck injuries are common.
3. *Ventilation must be adequate*; if there is any doubt then controlled ventilation is required. Modest hyperventilation to maintain a slightly reduced PCO_2 improves cerebral perfusion; however, a low PCO_2 causes vasoconstriction and hypoxia.
4. *Blood volume must be carefully regulated.* Low blood pressure almost never results from a head injury; indeed, as intracranial pressure rises, systemic blood pressure tends also to rise. Blood loss from other injuries must be sought. Hypotension reduces cerebral perfusion pressure and thus causes secondary brain injury; on the other hand, care must be taken not to overtransfuse a patient, since this itself can cause brain oedema.

SCALP WOUNDS

In children, bleeding from scalp wounds can be life-threatening. In both adults and children, the presence of an underlying skull fracture should be excluded. The wound should be thoroughly washed and any debris removed. Larger vessels may need to be clamped and tied.

MINOR HEAD INJURIES

Most head injuries are rather trivial and require no more than careful examination and reassurance. In patients who appear comatosed, drowsy, restless or merely confused, it is difficult to distinguish the effects of a head injury from those of alcohol, drugs, hypoxia or shock. All such patients should be kept under observation until the diagnosis is clear. If there is any doubt, a CT scan is necessary.

Patients with no history of loss of consciousness and a normal examination can be safely discharged to the care of a responsible adult. Patients with a history of loss of consciousness should have a skull x-ray performed. If this is normal, the period of loss of consciousness less than 5 minutes and the patient fully conscious on assessment, he or she can be discharged as long as there is a sensible adult to look after the patient. Those with either a skull fracture or an impaired level of consciousness should be admitted for further observation; a CT scan is often necessary.

SKULL FRACTURES

Linear skull fractures, especially in the temporo-parietal region, carry a high risk of an intracranial haemorrhage, which should be sought by a CT scan.

Basal fractures are managed by avoiding secondary brain injury. Persistent CSF leaks from the nose or ear occasionally need surgery. A gastric tube should not be passed through the nose lest it enters the brain through the base of the skull.

Depressed fractures may need elevation to reduce the longer term risk of epilepsy.

Open fractures, like any open fracture, must be surgically cleaned as soon as possible.

DIFFUSE BRAIN INJURY

Concussion Concussion is effectively a diffuse neurapraxia. Following a blow there is a temporary loss of consciousness, often associated with amnesia. The period of loss of consciousness is broadly related to the severity of concussion. A period greater than 5 minutes usually warrants hospital admission.

Diffuse axonal injury This is more common than an intracranial haematoma. There is widespread microscopic damage throughout the brain. A patient may be deeply comatose, sometimes with a decerebrate or decorticate posture. The CT scan shows no intracranial haematoma, but it may show widespread haemorrhages and oedema.

The condition is managed essentially by avoiding secondary brain injury. Hypoxia and hypovolaemia must be corrected. The patient is intubated and ventilated; a modest reduction in PCO_2 is achieved. Central venous pressure is monitored. With appropriate neurosurgical facilities an intracranial pressure monitor can be inserted. This allows the early detection of an evolving intracranial haematoma. The patient is nursed in the head-up position and monitored for other complications, particularly cardiac arrhythmias (from unregulated sympathetic outflow), neurogenic pulmonary oedema (precise cause unknown) and disseminated intravascular coagulation (thromboplastins are released from injured brain tissue).

In the longer term, as these patients recover they will need specialized rehabilitation.

FOCAL BRAIN INJURIES

Contusions These vary in severity. They can be identified on the CT scan and are managed by avoiding secondary brain injury. Contusions can bleed, thus further increasing the intracranial pressure.

Acute subdural haematoma Subdural haematoma is at least three times more common than an extradural haematoma. It is also far more serious because it usually reflects considerable underlying brain damage. It is due either to rupture of veins which cross between the cerebral cortex and the dura or from lacerations to the brain. A skull fracture is not always present. Evacuation of an acute subdural haematoma requires a large craniotomy. This is very difficult surgery and should be performed only by someone with neurosurgical experience.

Acute extradural haematoma This usually occurs from a tear of the middle meningeal artery and occasionally from a tear in a dural sinus. This type of haemorrhage is rare, but important because it is treatable with prompt surgery. Typically a head-injured patient seems to be perfectly well, but then rapidly becomes unconscious. A fixed dilated pupil develops on the side of the haematoma and limb weakness on the opposite side. An urgent CT scan will demonstrate the site of the haematoma which is then drained through a burr-hole. This is best undertaken by a neurosurgeon, unless in dire circumstances. While surgery is being arranged, a mannitol infusion should be considered after consultation with a neurosurgeon.

BURNS

The ABC of managing burn injuries is to attend to the Airway, Breathing, Circulation and Dermis – in that order.

The airway Airway injury is the most important consideration for a burned patient; fire probably kills more people by asphyxia than by burning. The airway damage is often insidious, caused by progressive swelling in the heat-damaged tissues. It becomes increasingly difficult to maintain an airway in these circumstances; a high dose of oxygen should be provided immediately and the airway secured as soon as possible. With burns of the face or neck, immediate intubation or tracheostomy may be necessary.

Breathing Difficulty with breathing is the next threat. The lungs may have been directly damaged by hot gases. Carbon monoxide displaces oxygen from the haemoglobin molecule and causes profound hypoxia. Circumferential full-thickness burns to the chest restrict ventilation and may require escharotomy.

The circulation Burnt tissue exudes protein-rich fluid. If the patient has burns over more than 10% of the body area, then fluid replacement is essential. Large diameter short catheters should be inserted. Transfusion is begun initially with warmed crystalloid fluids and then with plasma and blood. The fluid volume required depends on the patient's body weight, the percentage of surface area which has been burnt and the time elapsed since the burn.

Skin damage A full-thickness circumferential burn may cause ischaemia to the extremity needing escharotomy. Wound infection is a risk. The burned area should be covered with clean sterile dressings or a sterile polythene-type dressing. Prophylactic antibiotics are avoided, as they may lead to infection with multiply-resistant bacteria.

Electricity burns Patients with electrical burns are a special case. The entry and exit wounds may be very small, but there can be substantial damage to the intervening tissues. Patients are also at risk of cardiac arrhythmias. Myoglobin from widespread muscle damage can block the kidneys. In this case, an alkaline diuresis should be achieved with mannitol and sodium bicarbonate.

Maintenance Patients with full thickness burns greater than 5% of body surface area, those with burns to the hands and face or genitalia, and children should all be considered for transfer to a special Burns Unit. If this is impossible or if transfer is unavoidably delayed, general supportive treatment must be continued. Fluid losses must continually be made good with blood, plasma, or plasma and saline solution as required. Sedation is continued. Metabolic requirements are met by oral feeding or, in children, intravenously. At least every 4 hours the patient is examined; the skin colour, pulse, blood pressure and urine output are noted. An indwelling catheter is useful in assessing the all-important fluid balance. In severe cases the blood haemoglobin, electrolytes and urea are examined 4-hourly and used as a guide to further treatment.

THE METABOLIC RESPONSE TO TRAUMA

The general effects of trauma are profound and widespread; they involve a host of hormonal and cellular mechanisms designed to counteract the acute effects of tissue damage, blood loss, shock and cardiopulmonary dysfunction, as well as an inflammatory response which initiates the process of repair. Energy requirements for these vital processes are secured at the expense of less dependent tissues such as muscle and fat.

The metabolic adjustments occur in two phases: an early post-traumatic phase, or 'ebb', covering the first 24–48 hours, followed by a more prolonged 'flow' phase which is dominated first by tissue breakdown (the catabolic period) and later by tissue repair (the anabolic period).

The *early response* (or *'ebb' phase)* is concerned with the body's defence mechanisms. The fluid shifts that occur during shock trigger a number of humoral mechanisms (mainly increased secretion of renin, aldosterone, cortisol and pituitary antidiuretic hormone) which ensure more effective conservation of sodium and water. At a local level, the inflammatory response to tissue damage is mediated by cytokines such as interleukin 1 (IL-1) and tumour necrosis factor (TNF), arachidonic acid derivatives (prostaglandins), and other vasoactive chemicals.

Ready energy for these processes comes from a number of sources. The classic reaction to stress involves increased hypothalamic–pituitary and sympathetic–adrenal activity. There is increased secretion of adrenocorticotropic hormone (ACTH), cortisol, catecholamines (adrenalin, dopamine) and glucagon; among the effects of these hormones are increased glycogenolysis and gluconeogenesis in the liver, reduced glucose utilization by muscle and stimulation of free fatty acid and glycerol release from the fat stores. Within the first 24 hours after injury the blood sugar rises and there is an increase in metabolic rate, oxygen uptake and body temperature.

As the initial 'fight or flight' reaction subsides, the patient enters *the 'flow' phase*. In the early recovery period there is still a need for energy supplies. Blood sugar levels may return to near normal but glucose turnover is increased and gluconeogenesis in the liver continues at an enhanced level. Free fatty acid turnover, likewise, is increased and this is probably the major source of energy

in patients who do not receive glucose supplements. One of the most important effects during the catabolic phase is the loss of body protein, resulting in muscle wasting. Amino acids are needed by the liver both for gluconeogenesis and for replenishment of the acute phase proteins required by the inflammatory response. Thus, C-reactive protein levels are at first diminished but, provided the liver is not damaged, the serum levels return to normal or may be increased. These changes are reflected in the continued elevation of the metabolic rate and increased excretion of nitrogen in the urine.

As healing proceeds, the need for increased energy supplies subsides and the patient moves into the *anabolic phase* of recovery. The metabolic parameters return to normal, body weight increases and muscle bulk is slowly restored.

Nutritional supplementation

With minor or even moderately severe injuries the patient usually adjusts to the metabolic changes quite well, provided the patient is well-oxygenated, blood loss is restored and there is no supervening complication such as sepsis or pulmonary dysfunction. However, in all cases of severe trauma it is important to assess the patient's nutritional status and to ensure that the necessary protein, lipid and energy requirements are being met. If there are major complications such as prolonged bleeding, pulmonary dysfunction or sepsis, enteral or parenteral supplementation will almost certainly be necessary.

COMPLICATIONS OF MAJOR TRAUMA

TETANUS

The tetanus organism flourishes only in dead tissue. It produces an exotoxin which passes to the central nervous system via the blood and the perineural lymphatics from the infected region. The toxin is fixed in the anterior horn cells and therefore cannot be neutralized by antitoxin.

Established tetanus is characterized by tonic, and later clonic, contractions, especially of the muscles of the jaw and face (trismus, risus sardonicus), those near the wound itself and later of the neck and trunk. Ultimately, the diaphragm and intercostal muscles may be fixed in spasm and the patient dies of asphyxia.

Prophylaxis

Active immunization of the whole population by tetanus toxoid is an attainable ideal. To the patient so immunized, booster doses of toxoid are given after all but trivial skin wounding. In non-immunized patients prompt and thorough wound toilet together with antibiotics may be adequate, but if the wound is contaminated, and particularly with delay before operation, antitoxin is advisable. Horse serum carries a considerable risk of anaphylaxis, and human antitoxin (tetanus immunoglobulin) should be used. The opportunity is taken to initiate active immunization with toxoid at the same time.

Treatment

With established tetanus, intravenous antitoxin (again, human for choice) is advisable. Heavy sedation and muscle relaxant drugs may help; tracheal intubation and controlled respiration are employed for the patient with respiratory and swallowing embarrassment.

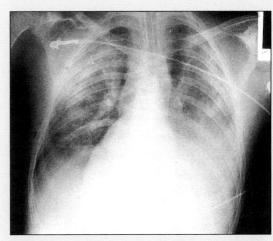

22.9 Adult respiratory distress syndrome X-ray showing diffuse pulmonary infiltrates in both lungs.

ADULT RESPIRATORY DISTRESS SYNDROME (ARDS)

During the later stages of shock and septicaemia, endothelial cell damage and increased small-vessel permeability cause haemorrhagic, protein-rich fluid to leak into the pulmonary interstitial tissue and alveoli. Capillary fat emboli and perivascular inflammatory exudates appear; the alveoli become distorted and increasingly awash with fluid, and ventilation is impaired. Over a period of about 10 days the picture changes from a predominantly exudative phase, with pulmonary oedema, to one of pneumocyte proliferation, interstitial fibrosis, microvascular occlusion and alveolar destruction. The early changes are reversible, but once diffuse alveolar damage occurs there is usually an inexorable progression to severe hypoxaemia, multiple organ failure and death.

Clinical features

About 36 hours after injury and (usually) a period of hypovolaemic shock, the patient develops mild dyspnoea. Even before this, if blood gases are measured they may show a diminished PO_2. These changes are common after long-bone fractures, and fat embolism is often suspected. By the second or third day the clinical features are more obvious; the patient is restless, mildly cyanosed and shows signs of respiratory distress. Blood gases remain abnormal, with PO_2 often below 8kPa (60mmHg). X-rays may now show diffuse pulmonary infiltrates. Special tests will show features such as reduced lung compliance and tidal volume, increased shunt, increased dead space and increased pulmonary artery pressure. Once the condition reaches this stage the prognosis is poor; deterioration proceeds despite treatment and the outcome is often fatal, due to multiple organ failure and hypoxaemia precipitating cardiac failure and, finally, cardiac arrest.

Treatment

The most important aspect of management is the early and effective treatment of hypoxia and shock. There is also good evidence that, in patients with multiple injuries, the incidence of pulmonary dysfunction is reduced by early stabilization of fractures.

The treatment of established ARDS is supportive and aims to minimize further lung damage until recovery occurs, whilst optimizing oxygen delivery to the tissues. A high dependency unit or intensive care unit is needed.

Mild ARDS can be managed by continuous positive airway pressure (CPAP) supplied by a close-fitting mask. CPAP increases functional residual volume and reduces shunt, thereby increasing arterial oxygen tension. Usually, however, endotracheal intubation is required, with positive pressure ventilation using minimum airway pressure and the lowest inspired oxygen concentration that will provide adequate arterial oxygenation.

FAT EMBOLISM SYNDROME

Fat embolism is a common phenomenon. Circulating fat globules larger than 10μm in diameter occur in most adults after closed fractures of long bones and histological traces of fat can be found in the lungs and other internal organs. A small percentage of these patients develop clinical features similar to those of ARDS; this was recognized as the *fat embolism syndrome* long before ARDS entered the medical literature. Whether the fat embolism syndrome is an expression of the same condition or whether it is an entirely separate entity is still uncertain.

The source of the fat emboli is probably the bone marrow, and the condition is more common in patients with multiple fractures.

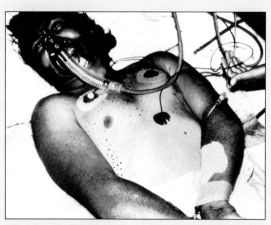

22.10 Fat embolism This man with bilateral femoral shaft fractures (closed) sustained fat embolism. When this photograph was taken he was unconscious, his face was congested and he was on continuous oxygen with cardiac monitoring. The petechiae were smaller and fainter than shown here; they have been accentuated for clarity and to show their distribution.

Clinical features

The patient is usually a young adult with a lower-limb fracture. Early warning signs (within 72 hours of injury) are a slight rise of temperature and pulse rate. In more pronounced cases there is breathlessness and mild mental confusion or restlessness; petechiae should be sought on the front and back of the chest, in the axillae and in the conjunctival folds and retinae. In the most severe cases there may be marked respiratory distress and coma, due partly to brain emboli and partly to hypoxia from involvement of the lungs. In fact, the features at this stage are essentially those of ARDS. The blood PO_2 will be low and a chest x-ray may show changes in the lungs.

Management

Severe fat embolism syndrome can probably be avoided by the use of high doses of oxygen immediately after injury and by the prompt stabilization of long-bone fractures. Intramedullary nailing is not thought to increase the risk of developing the syndrome. Fixation of fractures also allows the patient to be nursed in the sitting position, which optimizes the ventilation–perfusion match in the lungs.

There is no infallible test for fat embolism; however, the blood PO_2 should always be monitored during the first 72 hours of any major injury and values below 8kPa (60mmHg) must be regarded with grave suspicion.

In mild cases, treatment is supportive with high inspired oxygen tensions supplemented if necessary by mechanical ventilation. In severe cases recovery is unpredictable and the mortality rate is high.

DISSEMINATED INTRAVASCULAR COAGULATION

An insidious complication of severe injury and blood loss is a widespread disorder of coagulation and haemostasis. This is due, at least in part, to the release of tissue thromboplastins into the circulation, endothelial damage and platelet activation. The result is a complex mixture of intravascular coagulation, depletion of clotting factors, fibrinolysis and thrombocytopenia. Microvascular occlusion causes haemorrhagic infarctions and tissue necrosis, while deficient haemostasis leads to abnormal bleeding.

Clinical features

The patient, usually after a period of severe blood loss and transfusion and sometimes sepsis, develops symptoms and signs suggesting diffuse microvascular thrombosis: restlessness, confusion, neurological dysfunction, skin infarcts, oliguria and renal failure. Abnormal haemostasis causes excessive bleeding at operation, oozing drip sites and wounds, spontaneous bruising, gastrointestinal bleeding and haematuria. The diagnosis is confirmed by finding a low haemoglobin concentration, prolonged prothrombin and thrombin times, thrombocytopenia, hypofibrinogenaemia and raised levels of fibrinogen degradation products.

Treatment The best 'treatment' is the prevention or early correction of hypovolaemic shock. If the bleeding is marked, it may help to replace clotting factors and platelets. However, this is a complex problem and it is wise to seek the advice of a haematologist.

CRUSH SYNDROME

This is seen when a limb is compressed for many hours. The patient may have been trapped in a vehicle or rubble; the condition can also occur after prolonged use of a pneumatic anti-shock garment.

The crushed limb is deprived of blood flow; tissues begin to die and toxic metabolites accumulate. When the limb is freed, a *reperfusion injury* occurs. Reactive oxygen metabolites are formed which further damage the tissues. The ion-pumps in the capillary and muscle cells fail, leading to fluid shifts which cause swelling; this leads to a compartment syndrome which in turn causes further ischaemia. Meanwhile, toxic metabolites are released into the circulation. The resultant hyperkalemia, metabolic acidosis and hypocalcaemia can arrest the heart. The kidneys try to excrete the large load of myoglobin from muscle breakdown but they may be overwhelmed and renal failure results.

Clinical features

In a full-blown case shock is profound. The released limb is pulseless and later becomes red, swollen and blistered; sensation and muscle power may be lost. Renal secretion diminishes and a low-output uraemia with acidosis develops. If renal secretion returns within a week the patient will survive; most patients, unless treated by renal dialysis, become increasingly drowsy and die within 14 days.

Management

The most important measure is prevention. During prolonged extrication from a crush injury, a high urine flow must be ensured by giving large volumes of intravenous crystalloid. When urine is flowing, a forced mannitol–alkaline diuresis is maintained until myoglobin is no longer detected in the urine.

If there is a compartment syndrome, confirmed by pressure measurement, then a fasciotomy is performed. Excision of dead muscle must be radical to avoid sepsis. Similarly, if there is an open wound then this should be aggressively managed. If there is no open wound and the compartment pressures are not high, then the risk of infection is probably lower if early surgery is avoided.

Occasionally a limb crushed severely and for several hours has to be amputated above the site of compression and before compression is released.

If oliguria persists, renal dialysis will be needed.

MULTISYSTEM ORGAN FAILURE

Multisystem organ failure (MSOF) is defined as the progressive and sometimes sequential dysfunction of physiological systems following trauma, surgery or infection. Once systems begin to fail, treatment becomes increasingly ineffective and death becomes increasingly likely.

Pathophysiology

Direct cell trauma (from multiple injuries) or cell ischaemia (from hypovolaemic shock or prolonged hypoxia) triggers an inflammatory response which, in general, is potentially helpful since it initiates healing and reinforces the immune responses. In MSOF, the inflammatory response becomes generalized and uncontrolled, mediated in particular by cytokines.

The lungs are usually the first organs to fail, followed by the liver, gut mucosa and kidneys. Furthermore, the central nervous system, clotting system and immune system all begin to fail. The patient is hypermetabolic; protein stores in skeletal muscle are raided for energy. This further reduces the capacity to heal tissues and fight off infection. The patient usually appears septicaemic, either as a cause or as a result of the MSOF.

Management

The key word is *PREVENTION*. The objectives are:

- prompt stabilization of fractures;
- treatment for shock;
- prevention of hypoxia;
- excision of all dirty and dead tissue;
- early diagnosis and treatment of infection;
- nutritional support.

Established MSOF needs intensive care; treatment is essentially an extension of these same objectives, with expert monitoring of the patient's progress and frequent re-assessment of needs.

TRAUMA SCORING METHODS

Scoring methods are used in trauma for triage, prediction of outcome and assessment of illness. *Triage* is defined as the process by which patients are prioritized. When there are many casualties, the severity of injury must be promptly established so that priorities can be established and resources allocated on a rational basis. In the longer term, scores are necessary for both *audit* (finding out if one's practice matches established standards) and *research* (finding out what the established standard should be).

The scoring methods can be broadly divided into those based on the patient's *physiological status* and those based on the degree of *anatomical damage*. Examples of each are given.

PHYSIOLOGICAL SCORES

The Glasgow Coma Scale

The GCS is a simple, reliable way of recording the patient's level of consciousness and it correlates well with outcome after head injury (see page 524).

The Revised Trauma Score

The Revised Trauma Score (RTS) is a more general form of assessment which reflects the patient's overall physiological status. It combines the GCS, systolic blood pressure and respiratory rate, using a weighted score for each. Diminishing score values indicate a progressively diminishing probability of survival. This type of functional (or 'dynamic') evaluation can be used for pre-hospital and emergency room triage, or for comparative reassessment during and after resuscitation, without the need for accurate diagnosis of structural damage. However, it lacks predictive value in patients with well-compensated physiological reactions whose condition may suddenly deteriorate from one time-point to the next.

ANATOMICAL SCORES

The Abbreviated Injury Scale

Using a special dictionary, in the Abbreviated Injury Scale (AIS) every injury is assigned a code according to its anatomical site, nature and severity. The severity is graded from 1 to 6:

1 minor;
2 moderate;
3 serious, not life-threatening;
4 severe, life-threatening;
5 critical, survival uncertain;
6 fatal.

The Injury Severity Score

The Injury Severity Score (ISS) provides a measure of severity in multiply injured patients. The body is divided into six regions: head and neck, thorax, face, abdomen and pelvic contents, extremities and pelvic girdle, burns.

The ISS is the sum of the squares of the highest AIS score from three of the six regions. The highest ISS score is 75; major trauma is defined as a score greater than 16. The score has been validated for use with both blunt and penetrating injuries, giving a correlation between ISS and mortality.

AUDIT

The Major Trauma Outcome Study, devised in the USA, allows one to compare the probability of survival for an individual patient between centres (TRISS methodology, or Trauma Score-Injury Severity Score). The probability is calculated from the RTS, ISS, mechanism of injury and age.

REFERENCES AND FURTHER READING

Advanced Trauma Life Support for Doctors (1997). American College of Surgeons, Chicago

Champion HR, Copes WR, Sacco WJ *et al* (1990) A new characterization of injury severity. *Journal of Trauma* 30, 539-546

Chandle CL, Cummins B (1995) Initial assessment and management of the severely head-injured patient. *British Journal of Hospital Medicine* 53, 102-108

Saadia R, Lipman J (1996) Multiple organ failure after trauma. *British Medical Journal* 313, 573-574

Smith EJ, Ward AJ, Smith D (1990) Trauma scoring methods. *British Journal of Hospital Medicine* 44, 114-117

Teasedale G, Gennett B (1974) Assessment of coma and impaired consciousness: a practical scale. *Lancet* 2, 81-84

Teasdale GM, Mendelow AD, Anderson B *et al* (1990) Risks of acute traumatic intracranial haematoma in children and adults: implications for managing head injuries. *British Medical Journal* 300, 365-367

A fracture is a break in the structural continuity of bone. It may be no more than a crack, a crumpling or a splintering of the cortex; more often the break is complete and the bone fragments are displaced. If the overlying skin remains intact it is a *closed* (or *simple*) *fracture;* if the skin or one of the body cavities is breached it is an *open* (or *compound*) *fracture*, liable to contamination and infection.

HOW FRACTURES HAPPEN

Bone is relatively brittle, yet it has sufficient strength and resilience to withstand considerable stress. Fractures result from: (1) a single traumatic incident; (2) repetitive stress; or (3) abnormal weakening of the bone (a 'pathological' fracture).

Fractures due to a traumatic incident

Most fractures are caused by sudden and excessive force, which may be direct or indirect.

With a direct force the bone breaks at the point of impact; the soft tissues also must be damaged. A direct blow usually causes a transverse fracture and damage to the overlying skin; crushing is more likely to cause a comminuted fracture with extensive soft-tissue damage.

With an indirect force the bone breaks at a distance from where the force is applied; soft-tissue damage at the fracture site is not inevitable. Although most fractures are due to a combination of forces (twisting, compression, bending, tension), the x-ray pattern may suggest the dominant mechanism:

- twisting causes a spiral fracture;
- compression causes a short oblique fracture;
- bending results in fracture with a triangular 'butterfly' fragment;
- tension tends to break the bone transversely; however, in some situations it may simply result in avulsion of a small fragment of bone at the point of ligament or tendon insertion.

NOTE: The above description applies mainly to the long bones. A cancellous bone, such as a vertebra or the calcaneum, when subjected to sufficient force, sustains a comminuted crush fracture. At the knee or elbow resisted extension may cause an avulsion fracture of the patella or olecranon; and in a number of situations resisted muscle action may pull off the bony attachment of the muscle.

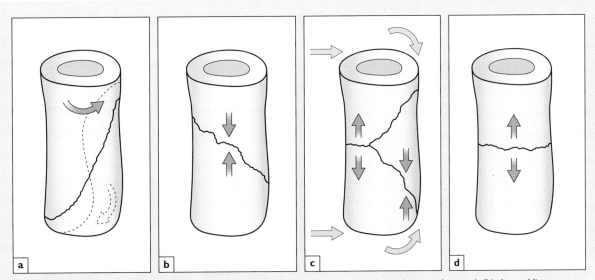

23.1 Mechanisms of injury Some fracture patterns suggest the causal mechanism: (**a**) spiral pattern (twisting); (**b**) short oblique pattern (compression); (**c**) triangular 'butterfly' fragment (bending); and (**d**) transverse pattern (tension). Spiral and some (long) oblique patterns are usually due to low energy indirect injuries; bending and transverse patterns are caused by high energy direct trauma.

Fatigue or stress fractures

Cracks can occur in bone, as in metal and other materials, due to repetitive stress. This is most often seen in the tibia, fibula or metatarsals, especially in athletes, dancers and army recruits who go on long route marches.

Pathological fractures

Fractures may occur even with normal stresses if the bone has been weakened by a change in its structure (e.g. in osteoporosis and Paget's disease) or the presence of a lytic lesion (e.g. a bone cyst or a metastasis).

TYPES OF FRACTURE

Fractures are infinitely variable in appearance but for practical reasons they are divided into a few well-defined groups.

Complete fractures

The bone is completely broken into two or more fragments. If the fracture is *transverse*, the fragments usually remain in place after reduction; if it is *oblique* or *spiral*, they tend to slip and redisplace even if the bone is splinted. In an *impacted fracture* the fragments are jammed tightly together and the fracture line is indistinct. A *comminuted fracture* is one in which there are more than two fragments; because there is poor interlocking of the fracture surfaces, these lesions are often unstable.

Incomplete fractures

Here the bone is incompletely divided and the periosteum remains in continuity. In a *greenstick fracture* the bone is buckled or bent (like snapping a green twig); this is seen in children, whose bones are more springy than those of adults. Reduction is usually easy and healing is quick. *Compression fractures* occur when cancellous bone is crumpled. This happens in adults, especially in the vertebral bodies. Unless operated upon, reduction is impossible and some residual deformity is inevitable.

Classification of fractures

An alphanumeric classification of fractures, which can be used for computer storage and retrieval, has been developed (Müller *et al.*, 1990). The first digit specifies the bone (1 = humerus, 2 = radius/ulna, 3 = femur, 4 = tibia/fibula) and the second digit the segment (1 = proximal, 2 = diaphyseal, 3 = distal, 4 = malleolar). A letter specifies the type of fracture (diaphysis: A = simple, B = wedge, C = complex; proximal and distal: A = extra-articular, B = partial articular, C = complete articular). Two further numbers specify the detailed morphology of the fracture. Although this classification is comprehensive, there are reservations about its complexity and its reproducibility. 'Tailored' classifications for specific fractures are more useful for assessing prognosis and planning treatment.

HOW FRACTURES ARE DISPLACED

After a complete fracture the fragments usually become displaced, partly by the force of the injury, partly by

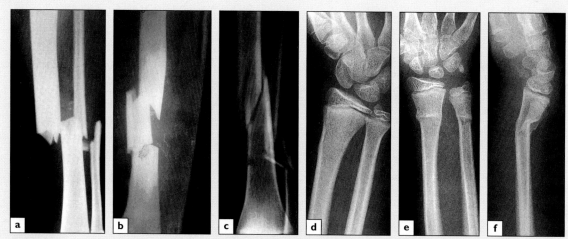

23.2 Varieties of fracture *Complete fractures*: (**a**) transverse; (**b**) segmental; (**c**) spiral. *Incomplete fractures*: (**d**) buckle or torus; (**e, f**) greenstick.

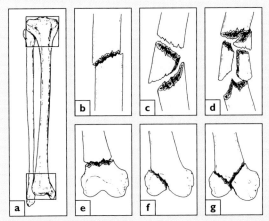

23.3 Müller's classification (a) Each long bone has three segments – proximal, diaphyseal and distal; the proximal and distal segments are each defined by a square based on the widest part of the bone. (b, c, d). Diaphyseal fractures may be simple, wedge or complex. (e, f, g) Proximal and distal fractures may be extra-articular, partial articular or complete articular.

gravity and partly by the pull of muscles attached to them. Displacement is usually described in terms of translation, alignment, rotation and altered length.

Translation (shift) The fragments may be shifted sideways, backwards or forwards in relation to each other, such that the fracture surfaces lose contact. The fracture will usually unite even if apposition is imperfect, or indeed even if the bone ends lie side by side with the fracture surfaces making no contact at all.

Alignment (angulation) The fragments may be tilted or angulated in relation to each other. Malalignment, if uncorrected, may lead to deformity of the limb.

Rotation (twist) One of the fragments may be rotated on its longitudinal axis; the bone looks straight but the limb ends up with a rotational deformity.

Length The fragments may be distracted and separated, or they may overlap, due to muscle spasm, causing shortening of the bone.

HOW FRACTURES HEAL

It is commonly supposed that, in order to unite, a fracture must be immobilized. This cannot be so since, with few exceptions, fractures unite whether they are splinted or not; indeed, without a built-in mechanism for union, land animals could scarcely have evolved. It is, however, naive to suppose that union would occur if a fracture were kept moving indefinitely; the bone ends must, at some stage, be brought to rest relative to one another. But it is not mandatory for the surgeon to impose this immobility artificially – Nature can do it, with callus; and callus forms in response to movement, not to splintage. *We splint most fractures, not to ensure union but (1) to alleviate pain, (2) to ensure that union takes place in good position and (3) to permit early movement and return of function.*

The process of fracture repair varies according to the type of bone involved and the amount of movement at the fracture site. In a tubular bone, and in the absence of rigid fixation, healing proceeds in five stages.

TISSUE DESTRUCTION AND HAEMATOMA FORMATION Vessels are torn and a haematoma forms around and within the fracture. Bone at the fracture surfaces, deprived of a blood supply, dies back for a millimetre or two.

INFLAMMATION AND CELLULAR PROLIFERATION Within 8 hours of the fracture there is an acute inflammatory reaction with proliferation of cells under the periosteum and within the breached medullary canal. The fragment ends are surrounded by cellular tissue, which bridges the fracture site. The clotted haematoma is slowly absorbed and fine new capillaries grow into the area.

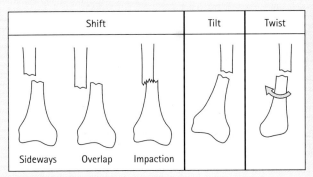

Shift			Tilt	Twist
Sideways	Overlap	Impaction		

23.4 Fracture displacements The different types of fracture displacement.

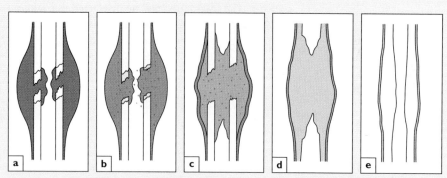

23.5 Fracture healing Five stages of healing. **(a)** *Haematoma*: there is tissue damage and bleeding at the fracture site; the bone ends die back for a few millimetres. **(b)** *Inflammation*: inflammatory cells appear in the haematoma. **(c)** *Callus*: the cell population changes to osteoblasts and osteoclasts; dead bone is mopped up and woven bone appears in the fracture callus. **(d)** *Consolidation*: woven bone is replaced by lamellar bone and the fracture is solidly united. **(e)** *Remodelling*: the new-formed bone is remodelled to resemble the normal structure.

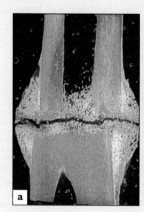
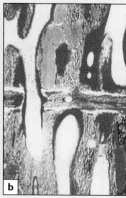

23.6 Fracture healing – histology Experimental fracture healing: **(a)** by bridging callus and **(b)** by direct penetration of the fracture gap by a cutting cone.

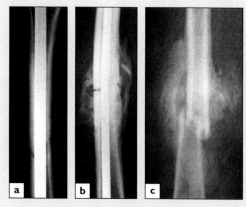

23.7 Callus and movement Three patients with femoral shaft fractures. **(a)** and **(b)** are both 6 weeks after fixation: in **(a)** the Kuntscher nail fitted tightly, preventing any movement, and there is no callus; in **(b)** the nail fitted loosely, permitting some movement, so there is callus. **(c)** This patient had cerebral irritation and thrashed around wildly; at 3 weeks callus is excessive.

CALLUS FORMATION   The proliferating cells are potentially chrondrogenic and osteogenic; given the right conditions, they will start forming bone and, in some cases, also cartilage. The cell population now also includes osteoclasts (probably derived from the new blood vessels) which begin to mop up dead bone. The thick cellular mass, with its islands of immature bone and cartilage, forms the callus or splint on the periosteal

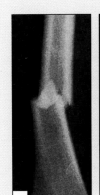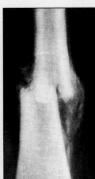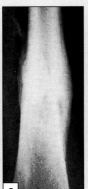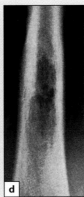

23.8 Fracture repair (a) Fracture; (b) union; (c) consolidation; (d) bone remodelling. The fracture must be protected until consolidated.

and endosteal surfaces. As the immature fibre bone (or 'woven' bone) becomes more densely mineralized, movement at the fracture site decreases progressively and ceases when the fracture 'unites'. The entire process is driven by inductive proteins, which include fibroblast growth factors, transforming growth factor-beta and bone morphogenic proteins.

CONSOLIDATION With continuing osteoclastic and osteoblastic activity the woven bone is transformed into lamellar bone. The system is now rigid enough to allow osteoclasts to burrow through the debris at the fracture line, and close behind them osteoblasts fill in the remaining gaps between the fragments with new bone. This is a slow process and it may be several months before the bone is strong enough to carry normal loads.

REMODELLING The fracture has been bridged by a cuff of solid bone. Over a period of months, or even years, this crude 'weld' is reshaped by a continuous process of alternating bone resorption and formation. Thicker lamellae are laid down where the stresses are high; unwanted buttresses are carved away; the medullary cavity is reformed. Eventually, and especially in children, the bone reassumes something like its normal shape.

Clinical and experimental studies have shown that callus is the response to movement at the fracture site. It serves to stabilize the fragments as rapidly as possible – a necessary precondition for bridging by bone. If the fracture site is absolutely immobile – for example, an impacted fracture in cancellous bone, or a fracture rigidly immobilized by a metal plate – there is no need for callus. Instead, osteoblastic new bone formation occurs directly between the fragments. Gaps between the fracture surfaces are invaded by new capillaries and osteoprogenitor cells growing in from the edges and new bone is laid down on the exposed surface (*gap healing*). Where the crevices are very narrow (less than 200μm), osteogenesis produces lamellar bone; wider gaps are filled first by woven bone which is then

remodelled to lamellar bone. By 3–4 weeks the fracture is solid enough to allow penetration and bridging of the area by bone remodelling units – i.e. osteoclastic 'cutting cones' followed by osteoblasts. Where the exposed fracture surfaces are in intimate contact and held rigidly from the outset, internal bridging may occasionally occur without any intermediate stages (*contact healing*).

Healing by callus, though less direct (the term 'indirect' could be used) has distinct advantages: it ensures mechanical strength while the bone ends heal; and, with increasing stress, the callus grows stronger and stronger (an example of Wolff's law). With rigid metal fixation, on the other hand, the absence of callus means that there is a long period during which the bone depends entirely upon the metal implant for its integrity. Moreover, the implant diverts stress away from the bone, which may become osteoporotic and not recover fully until the metal is removed. Flexible implants are now being tried in the hope of overcoming these drawbacks.

UNION, CONSOLIDATION AND NON-UNION

Repair of a fracture is a continuous process: any stages into which it is divided are necessarily arbitrary. In this book the terms 'union' and 'consolidation' are used, and they are defined as follows.

UNION

Union is incomplete repair; the ensheathing callus is calcified. Clinically the fracture site is still a little tender and, though the bone moves in one piece (and in that sense is united), attempted angulation is painful. X-rays show the fracture line still clearly visible, with fluffy callus around it. Repair is incomplete and it is not safe to subject the unprotected bone to stress.

CONSOLIDATION

Consolidation is complete repair; the calcified callus is ossified. Clinically the fracture site is not tender, no movement can be obtained and attempted angulation is painless. X-rays show the fracture line to be almost obliterated and crossed by bone trabeculae, with well-defined callus around it. Repair is complete and further protection is unnecessary.

TIMETABLE

How long does a fracture take to unite and to consolidate? No precise answer is possible because age, constitution, blood supply, type of fracture and other factors all influence the time taken.

Approximate prediction is possible and Perkins' timetable is delightfully simple. A spiral fracture in the upper limb unites in 3 weeks; for consolidation multiply by two; for the lower limb multiply by two again; for transverse fractures multiply again by two. A more sophisticated formula is as follows. A spiral fracture in the upper limb takes 6–8 weeks to consolidate; the lower limb needs twice as long. Add 25% if the fracture is not spiral or if it involves the femur. Children's fractures, of course, join more quickly. These figures are only a rough guide; there must be clinical and radiological evidence of consolidation before full stress is permitted without splintage.

NON-UNION

Sometimes the normal process of fracture repair is thwarted and the bone fails to unite. Causes of non-union are: (1) distraction and separation of the fragments, sometimes the result of interposition of soft tissues between the fragments; (2) excessive movement at the fracture line; (3) a severe injury which renders the local tissues non-viable or nearly so; and (4) poor local blood supply. Of course surgical intervention, if ill-judged, is another cause!

If local conditions are adversely affected by any of the factors listed above, cell proliferation may alter and become predominantly fibroblastic; the fracture gap is filled by fibrous tissue and the bone fragments remain mobile, at times creating a false joint or pseudarthrosis. The fibrous tissue is invisible on x-ray and this creates the impression that bone formation or any healing activity has petered out; the description *atrophic non-union* is therefore apt though not strictly accurate. In other instances periosteal bone formation is florid – usually as a result of excessive movement at the fracture site – but union fails because stability is insufficient to allow bridging of the gap. The fragment ends may then be thickened or widened; this *hypertrophic non-union* will ultimately proceed to union provided stability is ensured.

CLINICAL FEATURES

History

There is usually a history of *injury,* followed by *inability to use the injured limb.* But beware! The fracture is not always at the site of the injury: a blow to the knee may fracture the patella, the femoral condyles, the shaft of the femur or even the acetabulum. The patient's age and the mechanism of injury are important. If a fracture occurs with trivial trauma, suspect a pathological lesion. *Pain, bruising and swelling* are common symptoms, but they do not distinguish a fracture from a soft-tissue injury. *Deformity* is much more suggestive.

Always enquire about symptoms of *associated injuries*: numbness or loss of movement, skin pallor or cyanosis, blood in the urine, abdominal pain, difficulty with breathing or transient loss of consciousness.

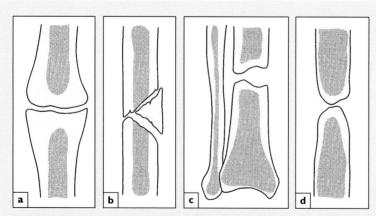

23.9 Non-unions These are generally divided into hypertrophic and atrophic types. Hypertrophic non-unions often have florid streams of callus around the fracture gap – the result of insufficient stability. They are sometimes given colourful names, like (**a**) elephant's foot. In contrast, atrophic non-unions usually arise from an impaired repair process; they are classified, according to the x-ray appearance, as (**b**) necrotic, (**c**) gap and (**d**) atrophic.

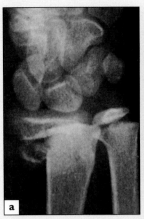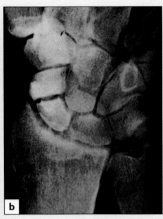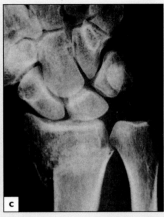

23.10 The patient's age Many fractures occur in typical age periods. Each of these patients fell on the outstretched hand: (**a**) aged 8 years sustained a fracture-separation of lower radial epiphysis; (**b**) aged 30 years suffered a fractured scaphoid; (**c**) aged 60 years has a Colles' fracture.

Once the acute emergency has been dealt with, ask about *previous injuries, or any other musculoskeletal abnormality* that might cause confusion when the x-ray is seen. Finally, a *general medical history* is important, in preparation for anaesthesia or operation.

General signs

Unless it is obvious from the history that the patient has sustained a localized and fairly modest injury, *priority must be given to dealing with the general effects of trauma* (see Chapter 22). Follow the ABC: look for, and if necessary attend to, Airway obstruction, Breathing problems, Circulatory problems and Cervical spine injury. During the secondary survey it will be necessary also to exclude other previously unsuspected injuries and to be alert to any possible predisposing cause (such as Paget's disease or a metastasis).

Local signs

Injured tissues must be handled gently. To elicit crepitus or abnormal movement is unnecessarily painful; x-ray diagnosis is more reliable. Nevertheless the familiar headings of clinical examination should always be considered, or damage to arteries, nerves and ligaments may be overlooked. A systematic approach is always helpful:

- examine the most obviously injured part;
- test for artery and nerve damage;
- look for associated injuries in the region;
- look for associated injuries in distant parts.

LOOK Swelling, bruising and deformity may be obvious, but the important point is whether the skin is intact; if the skin is broken and the wound communicates with the fracture, the injury is 'open' ('compound'). Note also the posture of the distal extremity and the colour of the skin (for tell-tale signs of nerve of vessel damage).

FEEL The injured part is gently palpated for localized tenderness. Some fractures would be missed if not specifically looked for; for example the classic sign (indeed the only clinical sign!) of a fractured scaphoid is tenderness on pressure precisely in the anatomical snuff-box. The common and characteristic associated injuries also should be felt for even if the patient does not complain of them; for example an isolated fracture of the proximal fibula should always alert one to the likelihood of an associated fracture or ligament injury of the ankle; and in high-energy injuries always examine the spine and pelvis. Vascular and peripheral nerve abnormalities should be tested for both before and after treatment.

MOVE Crepitus and abnormal movement may be present, but why inflict pain when x-rays are available? It is more important to ask if the patient can move the joints distal to the injury.

X-ray

X-ray examination is mandatory. *Remember the rule of twos:*

- *Two views* A fracture or a dislocation may not be seen on a single x-ray film, and at least two views (anteroposterior and lateral) must be taken.

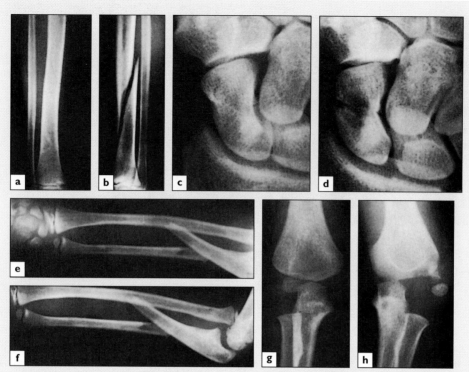

23.11 X-ray examination must be 'adequate' (**a, b**) *Two films of the same tibia*: the fracture may be 'invisible' in one view and perfectly plain in a view at right angles to that. (**c, d**) *More than one occasion*: A fractured scaphoid may not be obvious on the day of injury, but clearly seen 2 weeks later. (**e, f**) *Two joints*: The first x-ray (**e**) did not include the elbow. This was, in fact, a Monteggia fracture-dislocation; (**e**) shows the dislocated radiohumeral joint. (**g, h**) *Two limbs*: Sometimes the abnormality can be appreciated only by comparison with the normal side; in this case there is a fracture of the lateral condyle on the left side (**h**).

- *Two joints* In the forearm or leg, one bone may be fractured and angulated. Angulation, however, is impossible unless the other bone also is broken, or a joint dislocated. The joints above and below the fracture must both be included on the x-ray films.
- *Two limbs* In children, the appearance of immature epiphyses may confuse the diagnosis of a fracture; x-rays of the uninjured limb are needed for comparison.
- *Two injuries* Severe force often causes injuries at more than one level. Thus, with fractures of the calcaneum or femur it is important also to x-ray the pelvis and spine.
- *Two occasions* Some fractures are notoriously difficult to detect soon after injury, but another x-ray examination a week or two later may show the lesion. Common examples are undisplaced fractures of the distal end of the clavicle, the scaphoid, the femoral neck and the lateral malleolus, and also stress fractures and physeal injuries wherever they occur.

Special imaging

Sometimes the fracture – or the full extent of the fracture – is not apparent on the plain x-ray. *Tomography* may be helpful in lesions of the spine or fractures of the tibial condyles; *computed tomography (CT)* or *magnetic resonance imaging (MRI)* may be the only way of showing whether a fractured vertebra is threatening to compress the spinal cord; indeed, transectional images are essential for accurate visualization of fractures in 'difficult' sites such as the calcaneum or acetabulum, and three-dimensional reconstructed images are even better. *Radioisotope scanning* is helpful in diagnosing a suspected stress fracture or other undisplaced fractures.

Description

Diagnosing a fracture is not enough; the surgeon should picture it (and describe it) in all its complexity. (1) Is it open or closed? (2) Which bone is broken, and where? (3) Has it involved a joint surface? (4) What is the shape of the break? (5) Is it stable or unstable? (6) Is it a high-energy or a low-energy injury? And last but not least, (7) who is the person with the injury? In short, we must learn to recognize what has been aptly described as the 'personality' of the fracture.

THE SHAPE OF THE FRACTURE A *transverse fracture* is slow to join because the area of contact is small; if the broken surfaces are accurately apposed, however, the fracture is stable on compression. A *spiral fracture* joins more rapidly (because the contact area is large) but is not stable on compression. *Comminuted fractures* are often slow to join (a) because they are associated with more severe soft-tissue damage and (b) because they are likely to be unstable.

DISPLACEMENT For every fracture, three components must be assessed:

- *Shift or translation* – backwards, forwards, sideways, or longitudinally with impaction or overlap.
- *Tilt or angulation* – sideways, backwards or forwards.
- *Twist or rotation* – in any direction.

NOTE A problem often arises in the description of angulation. 'Anterior angulation' could mean that the apex of the angle points anteriorly or that the distal fragment is tilted anteriorly: in this text it is always the latter meaning which is intended ('anterior tilt of the distal fragment' is probably clearer).

Secondary injuries

Certain fractures are apt to cause secondary injuries and these should always be assumed to have occurred until proved otherwise.

THORACIC INJURIES Fractured ribs or sternum may be associated with injury to the lungs or heart. It is essential to check cardiorespiratory function.

SPINAL CORD INJURY With any fracture of the spine, neurological examination is essential – (1) to establish whether the spinal cord or nerve roots have been damaged and (2) to obtain a baseline for later comparison if neurological signs should change.

PELVIC AND ABDOMINAL INJURIES Fractures of the pelvis may be associated with visceral injury. It is especially important to enquire about urinary function; if a urethral or bladder injury is suspected, diagnostic urethrograms or cystograms may be necessary.

PECTORAL GIRDLE INJURIES Fractures and dislocations around the pectoral girdle may damage the brachial plexus or the large vessels at the base of the neck. Neurological and vascular examination are essential.

TREATMENT OF CLOSED FRACTURES

General treatment is the first consideration: *treat the patient, not only the fracture.* The principles are discussed in Chapter 22.

Treatment of the fracture consists of *manipulation* to improve the position of the fragments, followed by *splintage* to hold them together until they unite; meanwhile, joint *movement* and function must be preserved. Fracture healing is promoted by physiological loading of the bone, so muscle activity and early *weight-bearing* are encouraged. These objectives are covered by three simple injunctions:

- reduce;
- hold;
- exercise.

The problem is how to hold a fracture adequately and yet use the limb sufficiently: this is a conflict (*hold versus move*) which the surgeon seeks to resolve as rapidly as possible (e.g. by internal fixation); but he or she also wants to avoid unnecessary risks – here is a second conflict (*speed versus safety*). This dual conflict epitomizes the four factors that dominate fracture management (the term 'fracture quartet' was coined by Alan Apley).

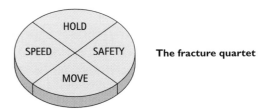

The fracture quartet

The fact that the fracture is closed (and not open) is no cause for complacency. *The most important factor in determining the 'natural' tendency to heal is the state of the surrounding soft tissues and the local blood supply.* Low-energy (or low-velocity) fractures cause only moderate soft-tissue damage; high-energy (velocity) fractures cause severe soft-tissue damage, no matter whether the fracture is open or closed.

Tscherne (1984) has devised a helpful classification of closed injuries:

- *Grade 0* is a simple fracture with little or no soft-tissue injury.
- *Grade 1* is a fracture with superficial abrasion or bruising of the skin and subcutaneous tissue.
- *Grade 2* is a more severe fracture with deep soft-tissue contusion and swelling.
- *Grade 3* is a severe injury with marked soft-tissue damage and a threatened compartment syndrome.

The more severe grades of injury are more likely to require some form of mechanical fixation; good skeletal stability aids soft-tissue recovery.

REDUCE

Although general treatment and resuscitation must always take precedence, there should be no undue delay in attending to the fracture; swelling of the soft parts during the first 12 hours makes reduction increasingly difficult. However, there are some situations in which reduction is unnecessary: (1) when there is little or no displacement; (2) when displacement does not matter (e.g. in fractures of the clavicle); and (3) when reduction is unlikely to succeed (e.g. with compression fractures of the vertebrae).

Reduction should aim for *adequate apposition* and *normal alignment* of the bone fragments. The greater the contact surface area between fragments the more likely is healing to occur. A gap between the fragment ends is a common cause of delayed union or non-union. On the other hand, so long as there is contact and the fragments are properly aligned, some overlap at the fracture surfaces is permissible. The exception is a fracture involving an articular surface; this should be reduced as near to perfection as possible because any irregularity may predispose to degenerative arthritis.

There are two methods of reduction: closed and open.

CLOSED REDUCTION

Under appropriate anaesthesia and muscle relaxation, the fracture is reduced by a threefold manoeuvre: (1) the distal part of the limb is pulled in the line of the bone; (2) as the fragments disengage, they are repositioned (by reversing the original direction of force if this can be deduced); and (3) alignment is adjusted in each plane. This is most effective when the periosteum and muscles on one side of the fracture remain intact; the soft-tissue strap prevents over-reduction and stabilizes the fracture after it has been reduced (Charnley, 1961).

Some fractures (e.g. of the femoral shaft) are difficult to reduce by manipulation because of powerful muscle pull and may need prolonged traction.

In general, closed reduction is used for all minimally displaced fractures, for most fractures in children and for fractures that are not unstable after reduction and can be held in some form of splint or cast. Unstable fractures also can be reduced 'closed', prior to external or internal fixation.

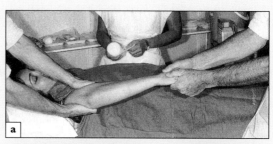
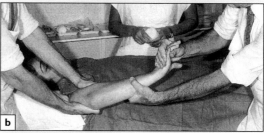
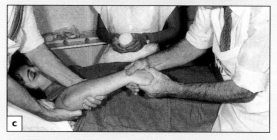

23.12 Closed reduction (a) Traction in the line of the bone. (b) Disimpaction. (c) Pressing fragment into reduced position.

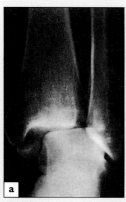
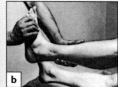
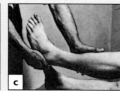
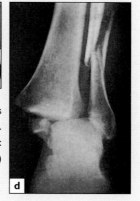

23.13 Closed reduction These two ankle fractures look somewhat similar but are caused by different forces. The causal force must be reversed to achieve reduction: (a) requires internal rotation (b); an adduction force (c) is needed for (d).

OPEN REDUCTION

Operative reduction of the fracture under direct vision is indicated: (1) when closed reduction fails, either because of difficulty in controlling the fragments or because soft tissues are interposed between them; (2) when there is a large articular fragment that needs accurate positioning; or (3) for traction fractures in which the fragments are held apart. As a rule, however, open reduction is merely the first step to internal fixation.

HOLD REDUCTION

The word 'immobilization' has been deliberately avoided because the objective is seldom complete immobility; usually it is the prevention of displacement. Nevertheless, some restriction of movement is needed to promote soft-tissue healing and to allow free movement of the unaffected parts.

The available methods of holding reduction are: (1) continuous traction; (2) cast splintage; (3) functional bracing; (4) internal fixation; and (5) external fixation.

In the modern technological age, 'closed' methods are often scorned – an attitude arising from ignorance more than from experience. The muscles surrounding a fracture, if they are intact, act as a fluid compartment; traction or compression creates a hydraulic effect which is capable of splinting the fracture. Therefore closed methods are most suitable for fractures with intact soft tissues, and are liable to fail if they are used as the primary method of treatment for fractures with severe soft-tissue damage. Other contraindications to non-operative methods are inherently unstable fractures, multiple fractures and fractures in confused or uncooperative patients. If these constraints are borne in mind, closed methods can be sensibly considered in choosing the most suitable method of fracture splintage. Remember, too, that the objective is to splint the fracture, not the entire limb!

CONTINUOUS TRACTION

Traction is applied to the limb distal to the fracture, so as to exert a continuous pull in the long axis of the bone with a counterforce in the opposite direction (to prevent the patient being merely dragged along the bed). This is particularly useful for spiral fractures of the shaft which are easily displaced by muscle contraction.

Traction cannot *hold* a fracture still; it can pull a long bone straight and hold it out to length but to maintain accurate reduction is sometimes difficult. And meanwhile the patient can *move* his or her joints and exercise his or her muscles.

Traction *is safe* enough, provided it is not excessive and care is taken when inserting the traction pin. The problem is *speed:* not because the fracture unites slowly (it does not) but because lower limb traction keeps the patient in hospital. Consequently, as soon as the fracture is 'sticky' (deformable but not displaceable), traction should be replaced by bracing, if this method is feasible.

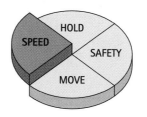

Continuous traction
'Speed' is the weak member of this quartet

TRACTION BY GRAVITY

This applies only to upper limb injuries. Thus, with a wrist sling the weight of the arm provides continuous traction to the humerus; for comfort and stability, especially with a transverse fracture, a U-slab of plaster may be bandaged on or, better, a removable plastic sleeve from the axilla to just above the elbow is held on with Velcro.

SKIN TRACTION

Skin traction will sustain a pull of no more than 4 or 5kg. Holland strapping or one-way-stretch Elastoplast is stuck to the shaved skin and held on with a bandage. The malleoli are protected by Gamgee tissue and cords or tapes are used for traction.

SKELETAL TRACTION

A stiff wire or pin is inserted – usually behind the tibial tubercle for hip, thigh and knee injuries, lower in the tibia or through the calcaneum for tibial fractures – and cords are attached for applying traction.

Whether by skin or skeletal traction, the fracture is reduced and held in one of three ways: fixed traction, balanced traction or a combination of the two.

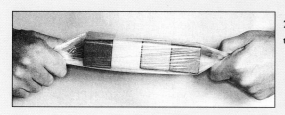

23.14 Hold reduction Showing how, if the soft tissues around a fracture are intact, traction will align the bony fragments.

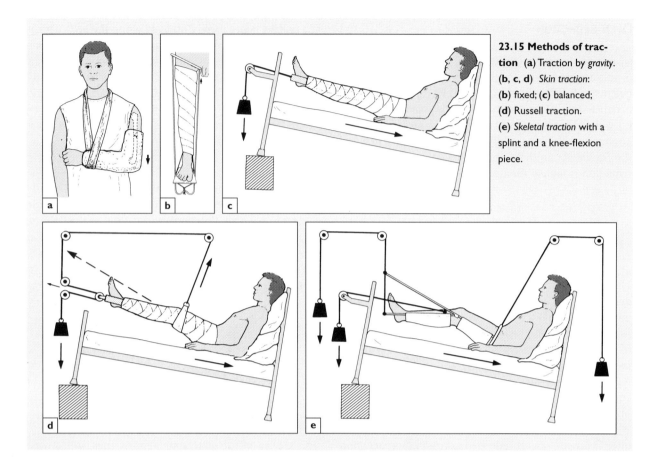

23.15 Methods of traction (a) Traction by *gravity*. (b, c, d) *Skin traction*: (b) fixed; (c) balanced; (d) Russell traction. (e) *Skeletal traction* with a splint and a knee-flexion piece.

Fixed traction The pull is exerted against a fixed point. The usual method is to tie the traction cords to the distal end of a Thomas' splint and pull the leg down until the proximal, padded ring of the splint abuts firmly against the pelvis.

Balanced traction Here the traction cords are guided over pulleys at the foot of the bed and loaded with weights; counter-traction is provided by the weight of the body when the foot of the bed is raised.

Combined traction If a Thomas' splint is used, the tapes can be tied to the end of the splint and the entire splint is then suspended, as in balanced traction.

Complications of traction

Circulatory embarrassment In children especially, traction tapes and circular bandages may constrict the circulation; for this reason 'gallows traction', in which the baby's legs are suspended from an overhead beam, should never be used for children over 12kg in weight.

Nerve injury In older people, leg traction may predispose to peroneal nerve injury and a resultant drop-foot; the limb should be checked repeatedly to see that it does not roll into external rotation during traction.

Pin-site infection Pin sites must be kept clean and should be checked daily.

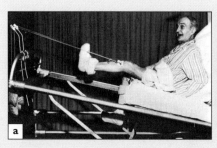
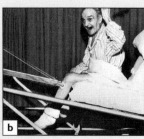

23.16 Continuous traction Balanced skeletal traction. The patient can move his joints while traction holds position; people imagine that without a splint the patient must be uncomfortable – but look at his face!

CAST SPLINTAGE

Plaster of Paris is still widely used as a splint, especially for distal limb fractures and for most children's fractures. It is *safe* enough, so long as one is alert to the danger of a tight cast and provided pressure sores are prevented. The *speed* of union is neither greater nor less than with traction, but the patient can go home sooner. *Holding* reduction is usually no problem and patients with tibial fractures can bear weight on the cast. However, joints encased in plaster cannot *move* and are liable to stiffen; stiffness, which has earned the sobriquet 'fracture disease', is the problem with conventional plasters. While the swelling and haematoma resolve, adhesions may form which bind muscle fibres to each other and to the bone; with articular fractures, plaster perpetuates surface irregularities (closed reduction is seldom perfect) and lack of movement inhibits the healing of cartilage defects. Newer substitutes have some advantages over plaster (they are impervious to water, and also lighter) but as long as they are used as full casts the basic drawback is the same.

Stiffness can be minimized by: (1) delayed splintage – that is, by using traction until movement has been regained, and only then applying plaster; or (2) starting with a conventional cast but, after a few days, when the limb can be handled without too much discomfort, replacing the cast by a functional brace which permits joint movement.

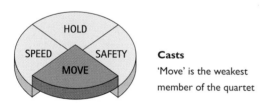

Casts
'Move' is the weakest member of the quartet

Technique

After the fracture has been reduced, stockinette is threaded over the limb and the bony points are protected with wool. Plaster is then applied. While it is setting the surgeon moulds it away from bony prominences; with shaft fractures three-point pressure can be applied to keep the intact periosteal hinge under tension and thereby maintain reduction.

If the fracture is recent, further swelling is likely; the plaster and stockinette are therefore split from top to bottom, exposing the skin. Check x-rays are essential and the plaster can be wedged if further correction of angulation is necessary.

With fractures of the shafts of long bones, rotation is controlled only if the plaster includes the joints above and below the fracture. In the lower limb, the knee is usually held slightly flexed, the ankle at a right angle and the tarsus and forefoot neutral (this 'plantigrade' position is essential for normal walking). In the upper limb the position of the splinted joints varies with the fracture. Splintage must not be discontinued (though a functional brace may be substituted) until the fracture is consolidated; if plaster changes are needed, check x-rays are essential.

Complications

Plaster immobilization is safe, but only if care is taken to prevent certain complications. These are tight cast, pressure sores and abrasion or laceration of the skin.

Tight cast The cast may be put on too tightly, or it may become tight if the limb swells. The patient complains of diffuse pain; only later – sometimes much later – do the signs of vascular compression appear. The limb should be elevated, but if the pain persists the only safe course is to split the cast and ease it open (1) throughout its length and (2) through all the padding down to skin. Whenever swelling is anticipated the cast should be applied over thick padding and the plaster should be split before it sets, so as to provide a firm but not absolutely rigid splint.

Pressure sores Even a well-fitting cast may press upon the skin over a bony prominence (the patella, the heel, the elbow or the head of the ulna). The patient complains of localized pain precisely over the pressure spot. Such localized pain demands immediate inspection through a window in the cast.

Skin abrasion or laceration This is really a complication of removing plasters, especially if an electric saw is used. Complaints of nipping or pinching during plaster removal should never be ignored; a ripped forearm is a good reason for litigation.

Loose cast Once the swelling has subsided, the cast may no longer hold the fracture securely. If it is loose, the cast should be replaced.

FUNCTIONAL BRACING

Functional bracing, using either plaster of Paris or one of the lighter materials, is one way of preventing joint stiffness while still permitting fracture splintage and loading. Segments of a cast are applied only over the shafts of the bones, leaving the joints free; the cast segments are connected by metal or plastic hinges which allow movements in one plane. The splints are 'functional' in that joint movements are much less restricted than with conventional casts.

Functional bracing is used most widely for fractures of the femur or tibia, but, since the brace is not very rigid, it is usually applied only when the fracture is beginning to unite, that is after 3–6 weeks of traction or conventional plaster. Used in this way, it

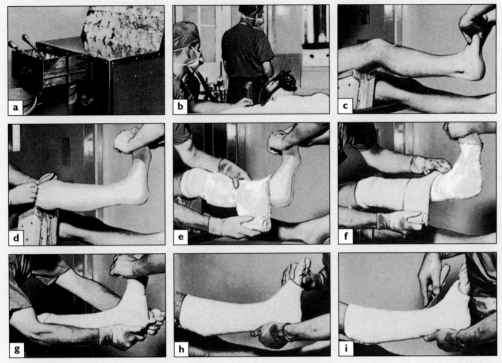

23.17 Plaster technique Applying a well-fitting and effective plaster needs experience and attention to detail. (**a**) A well-equipped plaster trolley is invaluable. (**b**) Adequate anaesthesia and careful study of the x-ray films are both indispensable. (**c**) For a below-knee plaster the thigh is best supported on a padded block. (**d**) Stockinette is threaded smoothly onto the leg. (**e**) For a padded plaster the wool is rolled on and it must be even. (**f**) Plaster is next applied smoothly, taking a tuck with each turn, and (**g**) smoothing each layer firmly onto the one beneath. (**h**) While still wet the cast is moulded away from the bony points. (**i**) With a recent injury the plaster is then split.

comes out well on all four of the basic requirements: the fracture can be *held* reasonably well; the joints can be *moved*; the fracture joins at normal *speed* without keeping the patient in hospital and the method is *safe*. However, except in experienced hands there is a greater risk of fracture malunion than with the use of full-length casts.

Technique

Considerable skill is needed to apply an effective brace. First the fracture is 'stabilized': by a few days on traction or in a conventional plaster for tibial fractures; and by a few weeks on traction for femoral fractures (till the fracture is sticky, i.e. deformable but not displace-

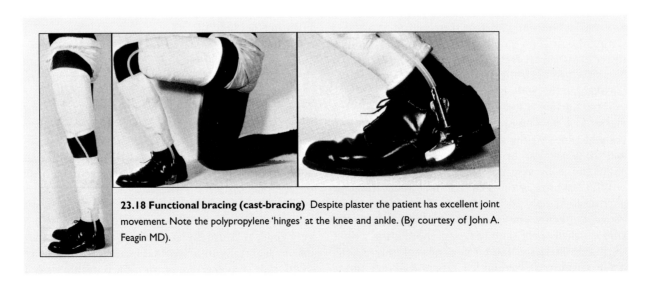

23.18 Functional bracing (cast-bracing) Despite plaster the patient has excellent joint movement. Note the polypropylene 'hinges' at the knee and ankle. (By courtesy of John A. Feagin MD).

able). Then a hinged cast or splint is applied which holds the fracture snugly but permits joint movement; functional activity, including weight-bearing, is encouraged. Details of technique and applications are given by Sarmiento and Latta (1981).

INTERNAL FIXATION

Bone fragments may be fixed with screws, transfixing pins or nails, a metal plate held by screws, a long intramedullary nail (with or without locking screws), circumferential bands or a combination of these methods.

Properly applied, internal fixation *holds* a fracture securely so that *movements* can begin at once; with early movement the 'fracture disease' (stiffness and oedema) is abolished. As far as *speed* is concerned, the patient can leave hospital as soon as the wound is healed, but he or she must remember that, even though the bone moves in one piece, the fracture is not united – it is merely held by a metal bridge; unprotected weight-bearing is, for some time, unsafe. The greatest *danger*, however, is sepsis; if infection supervenes, all the manifest advantages of internal fixation (precise reduction, immediate stability and early movement) may be lost. The risk of infection depends upon: (1) the patient – devitalized tissues, a dirty wound and an unfit patient are all dangerous; (2) the surgeon - thorough training, a high degree of surgical dexterity and adequate assistance are all essential; and (3) the facilities – a guaranteed aseptic routine, a full range of implants and staff familiar with their use are all indispensable.

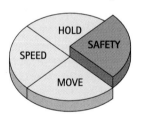

Internal fixation
'Safety' is the weak member of the quartet

Indications for internal fixation

Internal fixation is often the most desirable form of treatment. The chief indications are:

1. Fractures that cannot be reduced except by operation.
2. Fractures that are inherently unstable and prone to redisplacement after reduction (e.g. mid-shaft fractures of the forearm and displaced ankle fractures); also, those liable to be pulled apart by muscle action (e.g. transverse fracture of the patella or olecranon).
3. Fractures that unite poorly and slowly, principally fractures of the femoral neck.
4. Pathological fractures, in which bone disease may prevent healing.
5. Multiple fractures, in which early fixation (by either internal or external fixation) reduces the risk of

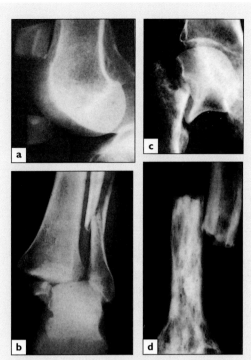

23.19 Indications for internal fixation (a) This patella has been pulled apart and can be held together only by internal fixation. (b) Fracture-dislocation of the ankle is often unstable after reduction and usually requires fixation. (c) This patient was considered to be too ill for operation; her femoral neck fracture has failed to unite without rigid fixation. (d) Pathological fracture in Paget bone; without fixation, union may not occur.

general complications and late multisystem organ failure (Phillips and Contreras, 1990).
6. Fractures in patients who present nursing difficulties (paraplegics, those with multiple injuries and the very elderly).

Types of internal fixation

Interfragmentary screws Screws which are only partially threaded (a similar effect is achieved by over-drilling the 'near' cortex of bone) exert a compression or 'lag' effect when inserted across two fragments. The technique is useful for reducing single fragments onto the main shaft of a tubular bone or fitting together fragments of a metaphyseal fracture.

Wires (transfixing, cerclage and tension-band) Transfixing wires, often passed percutaneously, can hold major fracture fragments together. They are used in situations in which fracture healing is predictably quick (e.g. in children or for distal radius fractures), and some form of external splintage (usually a cast) is applied as supplementary support.

Cerclage and tension-band wires are essentially loops of wire passed around two bone fragments and then tightened to compress the fragments together.

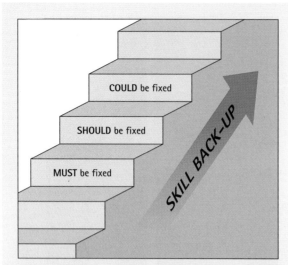

23.20 The indications staircase The indications for fixation are not immutable; thus, if the surgical skill or back-up facilities (staff, sterility and equipment) are of a low order, internal fixation is indicated only when the alternative is unacceptable (e.g. with femoral neck fractures). With average skill and facilities, fixation is indicated when alternative methods are possible but very difficult or unwise (e.g. multiple injuries). With the highest levels of skill and facilities, fixation is reasonable if it saves time, money or beds.

Both techniques are used for patellar fractures: the tension-band wire is placed such that the maximum compressive force is over the tensile surface, which is usually the convex side of the bone.

Plates and screws This form of fixation is useful for treating metaphyseal fractures of long bones and diaphyseal fractures of the radius and ulna. Plates have five different functions:

1. Neutralization – when used to bridge a fracture and supplement the effect of interfragmentary lag screws; the plate is to resist torque and shortening.
2. Compression – often used in metaphyseal fractures in which healing across the cancellous fracture gap may occur directly, without periosteal callus. This technique is less appropriate for diaphyseal fractures and there has been a move to the use of long plates which span the fracture, thus achieving some stability without totally sacrificing the biological effect of movement, which is a stimulus to periosteal callus formation.
3. Buttressing – here the plate props up the 'overhang' of the expanded metaphyses of long bones (e.g. in treating fractures of the proximal tibial plateau).

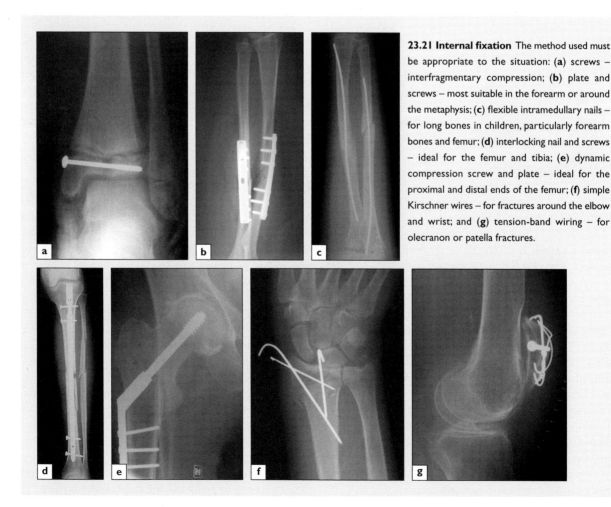

23.21 Internal fixation The method used must be appropriate to the situation: (**a**) screws – interfragmentary compression; (**b**) plate and screws – most suitable in the forearm or around the metaphysis; (**c**) flexible intramedullary nails – for long bones in children, particularly forearm bones and femur; (**d**) interlocking nail and screws – ideal for the femur and tibia; (**e**) dynamic compression screw and plate – ideal for the proximal and distal ends of the femur; (**f**) simple Kirschner wires – for fractures around the elbow and wrist; and (**g**) tension-band wiring – for olecranon or patella fractures.

4. Tension-band – using a plate in this manner, again on the tensile surface of the bone, allows compression to be applied to the biomechanically more advantageous side of the fracture.
5. Anti-glide – by fixing a plate over the apex of an angulated fracture and then using the plate as a reduction aid, the anatomy is restored with minimal stripping of soft tissues. The position of the plate acts to prevent shortening and recurrent displacement of the fragments.

Intramedullary nails These are suitable for long bones. A nail (or long rod) is inserted into the medullary canal to splint the fracture; rotational forces are resisted by introducing transverse *interlocking screws* which transfix the bone cortices and the nail proximal and distal to the fracture. Nails are used with or without prior reaming of the medullary canal; reamed nails achieve an interference fit in addition to the added stability from interlocking screws, but at the expense of temporary loss of the intramedullary blood supply.

Complications of internal fixation

Most of the complications of internal fixation are due to poor technique, poor equipment or poor operating conditions.

Infection Iatrogenic infection is now the most common cause of chronic osteomyelitis; the metal does not predispose to infection but the operation and the quality of the patient's tissues do.

Non-union If the bones have been fixed rigidly with a gap between the ends, the fracture may fail to unite. This is more likely in the leg or the forearm if one bone is fractured and the other remains intact. Other causes of non-union are stripping of the soft tissues and damage to the blood supply in the course of operative fixation.

Implant failure Metal is subject to fatigue, and until some union of the fracture has occurred metal implants are precarious. Stress must therefore be avoided and a patient with a plated tibia should walk with crutches and minimal weight-bearing for the first 3 months. Pain at the fracture site is a danger signal and must be investigated.

Intramedullary nails, owing to their location in the centre of the bone shaft, are spared some of the bending forces that occur during weight-bearing; even so, weight-bearing should be delayed if the fracture is comminuted or unstable and the bone therefore unable to share in carrying the load.

Refracture It is important not to remove metal implants too soon, or the bone may refracture. A year is the minimum and 18 or 24 months safer; for several weeks after removal the bone is weak, and care or protection is needed.

EXTERNAL FIXATION

A fracture may be held by transfixing screws or tensioned wires which pass through the bone above and below the fracture and are attached to an external frame. This is especially applicable to the tibia and the pelvis, but the method is also used for fractures of the femur, the humerus, the lower radius and even the bones of the hand.

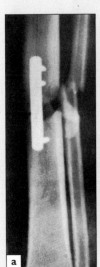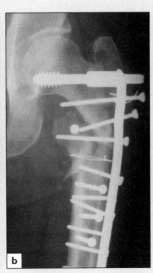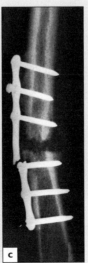

23.22 Bad fixation (how not to do it)
(a) Too little.
(b) Too much.
(c) Too weak.

Indications

External fixation is particularly useful for:

1. Fractures associated with severe soft-tissue damage for which the wound can be left open for inspection, dressing or skin grafting.
2. Fractures associated with nerve or vessel damage.
3. Severely comminuted and unstable fractures, which can be held out to length until healing commences.
4. Ununited fractures, which can be excised and compressed; sometimes this is combined with elongation.
5. Fractures of the pelvis, which often cannot be controlled by any other method.
6. Infected fractures, for which internal fixation might not be suitable.
7. Severe multiple injuries, in which early stabilization reduces the risk of serious complications (Phillips and Contreras, 1990).

Technique

The principle of external fixation is simple: the bone is transfixed above and below the fracture with screws or pins or tensioned wires and these are then connected to each other by rigid bars. There are numerous variations in fixation devices and techniques of applying these devices, providing varying degrees of rigidity and stability. All of them permit adjustment of length and angulation, and some allow reduction of the fracture in all three planes.

The fractured bone can be thought of as broken into segments – a simple fracture has two segments whereas a two-level (segmental) fracture has three and so on. Each segment should be held securely, ideally with the half-pins or tensioned wires straddling the length of that segment.

The wires and half-pins must be inserted with care. Knowledge of 'safe corridors' is essential so as to avoid injuring nerves or vessels; in addition, the entry sites should be irrigated during drilling to prevent burning of the bone (a temperature of 50°C can cause bone death).

The fracture is then reduced by connecting the various groups of pins and wires by rods.

Depending on the stability of fixation and the underlying fracture pattern, weight-bearing is started as early as possible to 'stimulate' fracture healing. Some fixators incorporate a telescopic unit that allows 'dynamization'; this will convert the forces of weight-bearing into axial micromovement at the fracture site, thus promoting callus formation and accelerating bone union (Kenwright et al., 1991).

Complications

Damage to soft-tissue structures Transfixing pins or wires may injure nerves or vessels, or may tether ligaments and inhibit joint movement. The surgeon must be thoroughly familiar with the cross-sectional anatomy before operating.

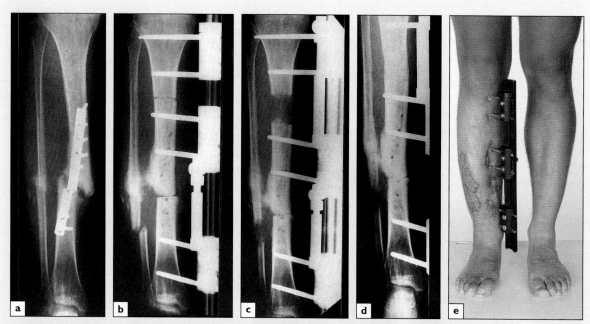

23.23 External fixation This young man broke his leg in a skiing accident. Despite internal fixation (**a**), the fracture went on to non-union. Osteotomy and callotasis in the proximal half of the bone permitted simultaneous lengthening of the tibia and compression fixation of the ununited fracture (**b, c, d**). The patient meanwhile was able to get about with his external fixation (**e**). 3 months later the fracture was united and the external fixator could be removed.

Overdistraction If there is no contact between the fragments, union is unlikely.

Pin-track infection This is less likely with good operative technique. Nevertheless, meticulous pin-site care is essential, and antibiotics should be administered immediately if infection occurs.

EXERCISE

More correctly, 'restore function' – not only to the injured parts but also to the patient as a whole. The objectives are to reduce oedema, preserve joint movement, restore muscle power and guide the patient back to normal activity.

Prevention of oedema Swelling is almost inevitable after a fracture and may cause skin stretching and blisters. Persistent oedema is an important cause of joint stiffness, especially in the hand; it should be prevented if possible, and treated energetically if it is already present, by a combination of elevation and exercise. Not every patient needs admission to hospital, and less severe injuries of the upper limb are successfully managed by placing the arm in a sling; but it is then essential to insist on active use, with movement of all the joints that are free. With most closed fractures, all open fractures and all fractures treated by internal fixation it must be assumed that swelling will occur; the limb should be elevated and active exercises begun as soon as the patient will tolerate this. The essence of soft-tissue care may be summed up thus: elevate and exercise; never dangle, never force.

Elevation An injured limb usually needs to be elevated; after reduction of a leg fracture the foot of the bed is raised and exercises are begun. If the leg is in plaster the limb must, at first, be dependent for only short periods; between these periods, the leg is elevated on a chair. The patient is allowed, and encouraged, to exercise the limb actively, but not to let it dangle. When the plaster is finally removed, a similar routine of activity punctuated by elevation is practised until circulatory control is fully restored.

Injuries of the upper limb also need elevation. A sling must not be a permanent passive arm-holder; the limb must be elevated intermittently or, if need be, continuously.

Active exercise Active movement helps to pump away oedema fluid, stimulates the circulation, prevents soft-tissue adhesion and promotes fracture healing. A limb encased in plaster is still capable of static muscle contraction and the patient should be taught how to do this. When splintage is removed the joints are mobilized and muscle-building exercises are steadily increased. Remember that the unaffected joints need exercising, too; it is all too easy to neglect a stiffening shoulder while caring for an injured wrist or hand.

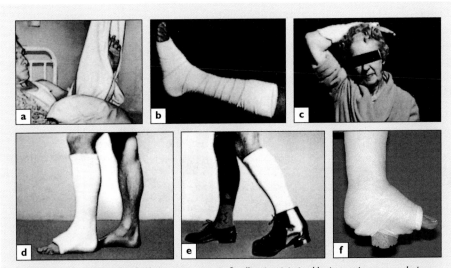

23.24 Some aspects of soft-tissue treatment Swelling is minimized by improving venous drainage. This can be accomplished by (**a**) elevation and (**b**) firm support. Stiffness is minimized by exercises: this patient (**c**) with a Colles' fracture is in no danger of a stiff shoulder. To exercise muscles under a plaster is less easy – a walking plaster should be plantigrade (**d**); an over-boot with rocker action (**e**) or a rocker applied directly to the sole of the cast (**f**) facilitates normal walking and muscle activity. Note that the point of the rocker should be placed in line with the anterior border of the tibia.

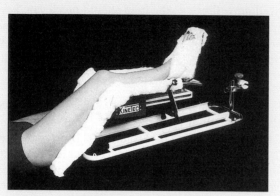

23.25 Continuous passive motion The motorized frame provides continuous flexion and extension to pre-set limits.

Assisted movement It has long been taught that passive movement can be deleterious, especially with injuries around the elbow where there is a high risk of developing myositis ossificans. Certainly forced movements should never be permitted, but gentle assistance during active exercises may help to retain function or regain movement after fractures involving the articular surfaces. Nowadays this is done with machines that can be set to provide a specified range and rate of movement ('continuous passive motion').

Functional activity As the patient's mobility improves, an increasing amount of directed activity is included in the programme. He or she may need to be taught again how to perform everyday tasks such as walking, getting in and out of bed, bathing, dressing or handling eating utensils. Experience is the best teacher and the patient is encouraged to use the injured limb as much as possible. Those with very severe or extensive injuries may benefit from spending time in a special rehabilitation unit. But the best incentive to full recovery is the promise of re-entry into family life, recreational pursuits and meaningful work.

TREATMENT OF OPEN FRACTURES

Initial management

Many patients with open fractures have multiple injuries and severe shock; for them, appropriate treatment at the scene of the accident is essential. The wound should be covered with a sterile dressing or clean material and left undisturbed until the patient reaches the accident department. In hospital a rapid general assessment is the first step, and any life-threatening conditions are addressed (see Chapter 22).

Tetanus prophylaxis is administered: toxoid for those previously immunized, human antiserum if not.

The wound is carefully inspected; ideally it should be photographed with a Polaroid camera, so that it can again be covered and left undisturbed until the patient is in the operating theatre. Four questions need to be answered:

- What is the nature of the wound?
- What is the state of the skin around the wound?
- Is the circulation satisfactory?
- Are the nerves intact?

Classifying the injury

Treatment is determined by the type of injury and the nature of the wound. Gustilo's classification of open fractures is widely used (Gustilo *et al.*, 1990).

Type I The wound is usually a small, clean puncture through which a bone spike has protruded. There is little soft-tissue damage with no crushing and the fracture is not comminuted (i.e. a low-energy fracture).

Type II The wound is more than 1cm long, but there is no skin flap. There is not much soft-tissue damage, and no more than moderate crushing or comminution of the fracture (also a low-energy fracture).

Type III There is extensive damage to skin, soft tissue and neurovascular structures, with considerable contamination of the wound. The injury is severe and involves high-energy transfer to the bone and soft tissues.

There are three grades of severity. In *type IIIA* the fractured bone can be adequately covered by soft tissue; in *type IIIB* it cannot and there is also periosteal stripping, as well as severe comminution of the fracture; the fracture is classified as *type IIIC* if there is an arterial injury which needs to be repaired, regardless of the amount of other soft-tissue damage.

NOTE: The incidence of wound infection correlates directly with the extent of soft-tissue damage, rising from less than 2% in type I to over 10% in type III fractures.

Principles of treatment

All open fractures, no matter how trivial they may seem, must be assumed to be contaminated; it is important to try to prevent them from becoming infected. The four essentials are:

- wound debridement;
- antibiotic prophylaxis;
- stabilization of the fracture;
- early wound cover.

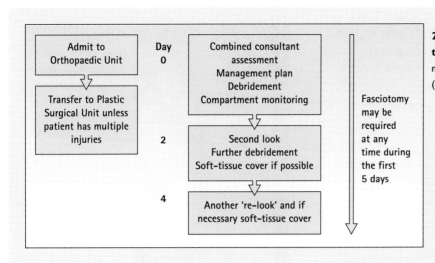

23.26 Management of open fractures Flow chart showing the management of open fractures of the tibia (Court-Brown *et al.*, 1997).

Sterility and antibiotic cover

The wound should be kept covered until the patient reaches the operating theatre. Antibiotics are given as soon as possible, no matter how small the laceration, and are continued until the danger of infection has passed. In most cases a combination of benzylpenicillin and flucloxacillin, or better still a second generation cephalosporin, given 6-hourly for 48 hours, will suffice; if the wound is heavily contaminated, it is prudent to cover also for Gram-negative organisms and anaerobes by adding gentamicin or metronidazole and to continue treatment for 4 or 5 days.

Debridement

The operation aims to render the wound devoid of foreign material and of dead tissue, leaving a good blood supply throughout. Under general anaesthesia the patient's clothing is removed, while an assistant maintains traction on the injured limb and holds it still. The dressing previously applied to the wound is replaced by a sterile pad and the surrounding skin is cleaned and shaved. The pad is then taken off and the wound is irrigated thoroughly with copious amounts of physiological saline. A tourniquet is not used because it would endanger the circulation still further and make it difficult to recognize which structures are devitalized.

As open fractures are often high-energy injuries with severe tissue damage, the operation should be performed by someone skilled in dealing with both skeletal and soft tissues; ideally this will be a joint effort by orthopaedic and plastic surgeons. The following principles must be observed:

- *Wound excision* The wound margins are excised, but only enough to leave healthy skin edges.

- *Wound extension* Thorough cleansing necessitates adequate exposure; poking around in a small wound to remove debris can be dangerous. If extensions are needed they should be planned so as not to jeopardize the creation of skin flaps for wound cover if this should be needed. If in doubt, consult a plastic surgeon.
- *Wound cleansing* All foreign material and tissue debris must be carefully removed. The wound is then washed out with copious quantities of saline. A common mistake is to inject syringefuls of fluid through a small aperture – this only serves to push contaminants further in; 6–12 litres of saline may be needed to irrigate and clean an open fracture of a long bone.
- *Removal of devitalized tissue* Devitalized tissue provides a nutrient medium for bacteria. Dead muscle can be recognized by its purplish colour, its mushy consistency, its failure to contract when stimulated and its failure to bleed when cut. All doubtfully viable tissue, whether soft or bony, should be removed; the only (debatable) exception would be a significant segment of an articular surface.
- *Nerves and tendons* As a general rule it is best to leave cut nerves and tendons alone, though if the wound is absolutely clean and no dissection is required – and provided the necessary expertise is available – they can be sutured.

Wound closure

A small, uncontaminated Type I wound may (after debridement) be sutured, provided this can be done without tension. All other wounds must be left open until the dangers of tension and infection have passed. The wound is lightly packed with sterile gauze and is inspected after 2 days: if it is clean, it is sutured or skin grafted (delayed primary closure).

Type III wounds may have to be debrided more than once and skin closure may call for advanced plastic surgery and the use of vascularized muscle flaps.

Ideally wound cover should be obtained within 72 hours; otherwise, as soon as possible after that. This almost always involves split skin grafting or flap cover (free flaps, fasciocutaneous flaps or muscle flaps).

Stabilization of the fracture

It is now recognized that stability of the fracture is important in reducing the likelihood of infection and assisting in recovery of the soft tissues. The method of fixation depends on the degree of contamination, the length of time from injury to operation and the amount of soft tissue damage. If there is no obvious contamination and the time lapse is less than 8 hours, open fractures of all grades up to type IIIA (Gustilo classification) can be treated as for closed injuries: cast splintage, intramedullary nailing or external fixation may be appropriate depending on the individual characteristics of the fracture and wound. More severe injuries will almost certainly require a joint approach by experienced plastic and orthopaedic surgeons; the precise method of stabilization depends to a large extent on the type of soft-tissue cover which may need to be employed, although external fixation (if properly planned) can probably accommodate to most problems. In specialized units, where the staff have a large experience of dealing with severe open fractures, even grade IIIB injuries have been treated successfully by locked nailing (Keating *et al.*, 2000). Plates and screws can be used for metaphyseal or articular fractures and for fractures of the smaller tubular bones, but only if the surgeon is experienced in their use and the circumstances are ideal.

Aftercare

In the ward, the limb is elevated and its circulation carefully watched. Shock may still require treatment. Antibiotic cover is continued; if the wound is open, cultures are obtained and, if necessary, a different antibiotic is substituted.

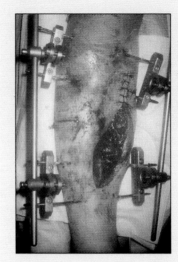

23.27 Open fractures – treatment Stabilization of the fracture is crucial and this is usually best achieved by external fixation.

If the wound has been left open, it is inspected at 2–3 days. Delayed primary suture is then often safe, or, if there has been much skin loss, split-skin grafts or skin flaps are applied. If, in spite of chemotherapy, the patient develops toxaemia or septicaemia, the wound should be drained (this is the only safe treatment if an infected fracture is not seen until 24 hours after injury).

Sequels to open fractures

SKIN If there has been skin loss or contracture, grafting may be necessary. When reparative or reconstructive surgery to deeper tissues is required, a local or distant flap is desirable.

BONE Infection may lead to sequestra and to sinuses. All avascular pieces of bone should be removed. If the resulting defect is too large for bone grafting at a later stage, the patient should be referred to a centre with the necessary experience and facilities for limb reconstruction.

Delayed union is inevitable after an infected fracture, but union will occur if infection is controlled and fracture stability maintained for sufficient time.

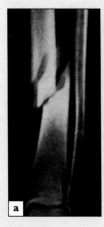
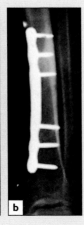
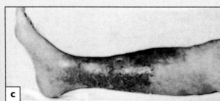
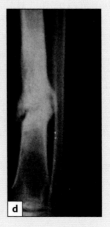

23.28 Open fractures – infection (a) The upper tibial fragment had punctured the skin; nevertheless the fracture was plated without adequate debridement **(b)**. The wound healed rapidly, the fracture did not; months later **(c)** signs of infection appeared. The plate was removed at 1 year **(d)**, by which time the bone was still infected and the fracture still ununited.

JOINTS When an infected fracture communicates with a joint, the principles of treatment are the same as with bone infection; namely, drugs, drainage and splintage. The joint should be splinted in the optimum position for ankylosis, lest this should occur.

With any open fracture, even if not communicating with a joint, some stiffness is almost inevitable. It can be minimized by slowly increasing active exercises, or by continuous passive motion, once it is certain that infection has been overcome.

Aphorisms of fracture management	
Think before you start	Are you treating the patient?
	Or merely the x-ray?
Think before you reduce	Have you worked out how to
	reduce it?
	And how to hold your reduction?
Think before you hold	Is your splint necessary?
	Is it harmful?
Think before you operate	Are your facilities good enough?
	Are you good enough?

GUNSHOT INJURIES

Missile wounds are looked upon as a special type of open injury. Tissue damage is produced by: (1) direct injury in the immediate path of the missile; (2) contusion of muscles around the missile track; and (3) bruising and congestion of soft tissues at a greater distance from the primary track. The exit wound (if any) is usually larger than the entry wound.

With high-velocity missiles (bullets, usually from rifles, travelling at speeds above 600m/s) there is marked cavitation and tissue destruction over a wide area. The splintering of bone resulting from the transfer of large quantities of energy creates secondary missiles, causing greater damage. With low-velocity missiles (bullets from civilian hand-guns travelling at speeds of 300–600m/s) cavitation is much less, and with smaller weapons tissue damage may be virtually confined to the bullet track. However, with all gunshot injuries debris is sucked into the wound, which is therefore contaminated from the outset.

Emergency treatment

As always, the arrest of bleeding and general resuscitation take priority. The wounds should each be covered with a sterile dressing and the area examined for artery or nerve damage. Antibiotics should be given immediately.

Definitive treatment

Traditionally, all missile injuries were treated as severe open injuries, by exploration of the missile track and formal debridement. However, it has been shown that low-velocity wounds with relatively clean entry and exit wounds can be treated as Gustilo type I injuries, by superficial debridement, splintage of the limb and antibiotic cover; the fracture is then treated as for similar open fractures.

High-velocity injuries demand thorough cleansing of the wound and debridement, with excision of deep damaged tissues and, if necessary, splitting of fascial compartments to prevent ischaemia; the wound is left open (covered only with gauze dressings) and the limb is elevated and splinted. The safest plan, if contamination is considerable, and if anatomical considerations permit, is to join the entry and exit wounds and leave the entire track open. If there are comminuted fractures, these are best managed by external fixation. The

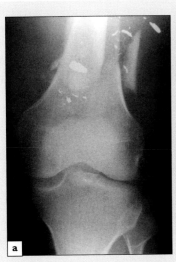
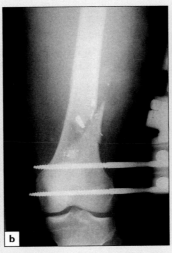
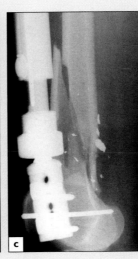

23.29 Gun shot injuries (a) Close-range shotgun blasts, although technically low velocity, transfer large quantities of destructive force to the tissues owing to the mass of shot. They should be treated like high-energy open fractures (**b, c**).

method of wound closure will depend on the state of tissues after several days; in some cases delayed primary suture is possible (Bowyer *et al.*, 1997).

Close-range shotgun injuries, although the missiles may be technically 'low velocity', are treated as high-velocity wounds because the mass of shot transfers large quantities of energy to the tissues.

COMPLICATIONS OF FRACTURES

The general complications of fractures (blood loss, shock, fat embolism, cardiorespiratory failure, etc.) are dealt with in Chapter 22.

Local complications can be divided into *early* (those that arise during the first few weeks following injury) and *late*.

Local complications of fractures		
Urgent	**Less urgent**	**Late**
Local visceral injury	Fracture blisters	Delayed union
Vascular injury	Plaster sores	Malunion
Nerve injury	Pressure sores	Non-union
Compartment syndrome	Nerve entrapment	Avascular necrosis
Haemarthrosis	Myositis ossificans	Muscle contracture
Infection	Ligament injury	Joint instability
Gas gangrene	Tendon lesions	Osteoarthriris
	Joint stiffness	
	Algodystrophy	

EARLY COMPLICATIONS

Early complications may present as part of the primary injury or may appear only after a few days or weeks.

VISCERAL INJURY

Fractures around the trunk are often complicated by injuries to adjacent viscera, the most important being penetration of the lung with life-threatening pneumothorax following rib fractures and rupture of the bladder or urethra in pelvic fractures. These injuries require emergency treatment.

VASCULAR INJURY

The fractures most often associated with damage to a major artery are those around the knee and elbow, and those of the humeral and femoral shafts. The artery may be cut, torn, compressed or contused, either by the initial injury or subsequently by jagged bone fragments. Even if its outward appearance is normal, the intima may be detached and the vessel blocked by thrombus, or a segment of artery may be in spasm. The effects vary from transient diminution of blood flow to profound ischaemia, tissue death and peripheral gangrene.

Common vascular injuries	
Injury	**Vessel**
First rib fracture	Subclavian
Shoulder dislocation	Axillary
Humeral supracondylar fracture	Brachial
Elbow dislocation	Brachial
Pelvic fracture	Presacral and internal iliac
Femoral supracondylar fracture	Femoral
Knee dislocation	Popliteal
Proximal tibial	Popliteal or its branches

Clinical features

The patient may complain of paraesthesia or numbness in the toes or the fingers. The injured limb is cold and pale, or slightly cyanosed, and the pulse is weak or absent. Plain x-rays will confirm the presence of a fracture. If a vascular injury is suspected an angiogram should be performed immediately; if it is positive, emergency treatment must be started without further delay.

Treatment

All bandages and splints should be removed. The fracture is x-rayed again and, if the position of the bones suggests that the artery is being compressed or kinked, prompt reduction is necessary. The circulation is then reassessed repeatedly over the next half hour. If there is no improvement, the vessels must be explored by operation – preferably with the benefit of preoperative or peroperative angiography. A torn vessel can be sutured, or a segment may be replaced by a vein graft; if it is thrombosed, endarterectomy may restore the blood flow. If vessel repair is undertaken, stable fixation is imperative; where it is practicable, the fracture should be fixed internally.

NERVE INJURY

Nerve injury is particularly common with fractures of the humerus or injuries around the elbow or the knee (see also Chapter 11). The tell-tale signs should be looked for (*and documented*) during the initial examination and again after reduction of the fracture.

In closed injuries the nerve is seldom severed, and spontaneous recovery should be awaited – it occurs in 90% of cases within 4 months. If recovery has not

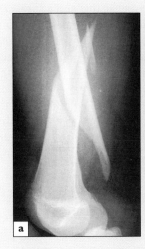
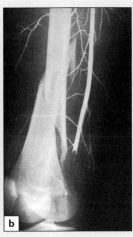
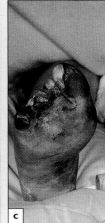

23.30 Vascular injury This patient was brought into hospital with a fractured femur and early signs of vascular insufficiency. The plain x-ray (**a**) looked as if the proximal bone fragment might have speared the popliteal artery. The angiogram (**b**) confirmed these fears. Despite vein grafting, he ended up with peripheral gangrene (**c**).

occurred by the expected time, and if nerve conduction studies fail to show evidence of recovery, the nerve should be explored.

Common nerve injuries	
Injury	**Vessel**
Shoulder dislocation	Axillary
Humeral shaft fracture	Radial
Humeral supracondylar fracture	Radial or median
Elbow medial condyle	Ulnar
Monteggia fracture-dislocation	Posterior interosseous
Hip dislocation	Sciatic
Knee dislocation	Peroneal

In open fractures any nerve lesion is more likely to be complete; the nerve is explored during wound debridement and repaired, either then or as a 'secondary' procedure 3 weeks later. A similar approach is used if there is a *concomitant vascular injury*.

Early exploration should also be considered if signs of a nerve injury appear *after manipulation of the fracture* (Siegel and Gelberman, 1991).

Acute nerve compression (as distinct from a direct injury) sometimes occurs with fractures or dislocations around the wrist. Complaints of numbness or paraesthesia in the distribution of the median or ulnar nerve should be taken seriously and the patient kept under observation. If there is no improvement within 48 hours after fracture reduction, the nerve should be explored and decompressed.

COMPARTMENT SYNDROME

Fractures of the arm or leg can give rise to severe ischaemia even if there is no damage to a major vessel. Bleeding, oedema or inflammation (infection) may increase the pressure within one of the osteofascial compartments; there is reduced capillary flow which results in muscle ischaemia, further oedema, still greater pressure and yet more profound ischaemia – a vicious circle that ends, after 12 hours or less, in necrosis of nerve and muscle within the compartment. Nerve is capable of regeneration but muscle, once infarcted, can never recover and is replaced by inelastic fibrous tissue (*Volkmann's ischaemic contracture*). A similar cascade of events may be caused by swelling of a limb inside a tight plaster cast.

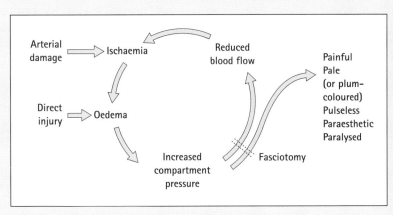

23.31 The vicious cycle of Volkmann's ischaemia (Modified from the *Journal of Bone and Joint Surgery*, 1979, **61B**, 298, by kind permission of Mr CE Holden and the Editor.)

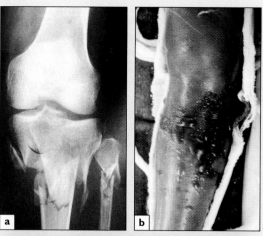

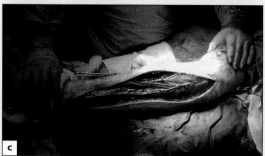

23.32 Compartment syndrome (**a**) A fracture at this level is always dangerous. This man was treated in plaster. Pain become intense and when the plaster was split (which should have been done immediately after its application), the leg was swollen and blistered (**b**). Tibial compartment decompression (**c**) requires fasciotomies of *all* the compartments in the leg.

Clinical features

High-risk injuries are fractures of the elbow, the forearm bones and the proximal third of the tibia; also multiple fractures of the foot or hand, crush injuries and circumferential burns. Other precipitating factors are operation (usually for internal fixation) or infection.

The classic features of ischaemia are the five Ps: pain, paraesthesia, pallor, paralysis and pulselessness. But it is criminal to wait until they are all present; the diagnosis can be made long before that. The earliest of the 'classic' features are pain (or a 'bursting' sensation) and altered sensibility. Skin sensation should be carefully and repeatedly checked.

Ischaemic muscle is highly sensitive to stretch. If the limb is unduly painful, swollen or tense, the muscles (which may be tender) should be tested by stretching them – when the toes or fingers are passively hyperextended there is increased pain in the calf or forearm.

The presence of a pulse does not exclude the diagnosis.

In doubtful cases the diagnosis can be confirmed by measuring the intracompartmental pressures. So impor-

tant is the need for early diagnosis that some surgeons advocate the use of continuous compartment pressure monitoring for high-risk injuries (e.g. fractures of the tibia and fibula) and especially for forearm or leg fractures in patients who are unconscious. A split catheter is introduced into the compartment and the pressure is measured close to the level of the fracture. A differential pressure (ΔP) – the difference between diastolic pressure and compartment pressure – of less than 30mmHg (4.00kPa) is an indication for immediate compartment decompression.

Treatment

The threatened compartment (or compartments) must be promptly decompressed. Casts, bandages and dressings must be completely removed – merely splitting the plaster is utterly useless – and the limb should be nursed flat (elevating the limb causes a further decrease in end capillary pressure and aggravates the muscle ischaemia). The ΔP should be carefully monitored; if it falls below 30mmHg, immediate open fasciotomy is performed. In the case of the leg, 'fasciotomy' means opening all four compartments through medial and lateral incisions. The wounds should be left open and inspected 2 days later: if there is muscle necrosis, debridement can be done; if the tissues are healthy, the wound can be sutured (without tension), or skin-grafted or simply allowed to heal by secondary intention.

NOTE: If facilities for measuring compartmental pressures are not available, the decision to operate will have to be made on clinical grounds. The limb should be examined at 15 minute intervals and if there is no improvement within 2 hours of removing the dressings, fasciotomy should be performed. Muscle will be dead after 4–6 hours of total ischaemia – there is no time to lose!

HAEMARTHROSIS

Fractures involving a joint may cause acute haemarthrosis. The joint is swollen and tense and the patient resists any attempt at moving it. The blood should be aspirated before dealing with the fracture.

INFECTION

Open fractures may become infected; closed fractures hardly ever do unless they are opened by operation.

Post-traumatic wound infection is now the most common cause of chronic osteitis. This does not necessarily prevent the fracture from uniting, but union will be slow and the chance of refracturing is increased.

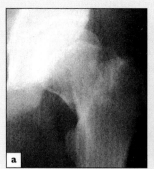
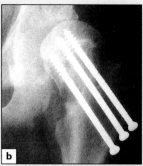
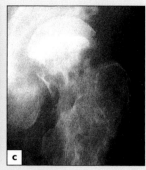

23.33 Infection (**a**) This fracture of the femoral neck was treated by internal fixation. 2 weeks later the patient was in pain and x-rays (**b**) showed the femoral head being displaced laterally, probably by fluid or pus in the joint. The outcome (**c**) was a chronic osteomyelitis with necrosis of the entire femoral head.

Clinical features

The history is of an open fracture or an operation on a closed fracture. The wound becomes inflamed and starts draining seropurulent fluid, a sample of which may yield a growth of staphylococci or mixed bacteria. Even if the bacteriological examination is negative, if the clinical features are suggestive the patient should be kept under observation continuously and treatment with intravenous antibiotics begun.

Treatment

All open fractures should be regarded as potentially infected and treated by giving antibiotics and meticulously excising all devitalized tissue.

If there are signs of acute infection and pus formation, the tissues around the fracture should be opened and drained; the choice of antibiotic is dictated by bacterial sensitivity.

If chronic osteitis supervenes the discharging sinus should be dressed daily and the fracture immobilized in an attempt to achieve union. External fixation is useful in such cases, but if an intramedullary nail has already been inserted and fixation is stable, this should not be removed; even worse than an infected fracture is one that is both infected and unstable.

The further treatment of chronic osteitis is discussed in Chapter 2.

GAS GANGRENE

This terrifying condition is produced by clostridial infection (especially *Clostridium welchii*). These are anaerobic organisms that can survive and multiply only in tissues with low oxygen tension; the prime site for infection, therefore, is a dirty wound with dead muscle

that has been closed without adequate debridement. Toxins produced by the organisms destroy the cell wall and rapidly lead to tissue necrosis, thus promoting the spread of the disease.

Clinical features appear within 24 hours of the injury: the patient complains of intense pain and swelling around the wound and a brownish discharge may be seen; gas formation is usually not very marked. There is little or no pyrexia but the pulse rate is increased and a characteristic smell becomes evident (once experienced this is never forgotten). Rapidly the patient becomes toxaemic and may lapse into coma and death.

It is essential to distinguish gas gangrene, which is characterized by myonecrosis, from anaerobic cellulitis, in which superficial gas formation is abundant but toxaemia usually slight. Failure to recognize the difference may lead to unnecessary amputation for the non-lethal cellulitis.

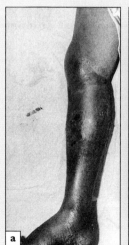
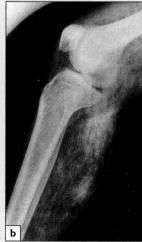

23.34 Gas gangrene (a) Clinical picture of gas gangrene. (b) X-rays show diffuse gas in the muscles of the calf.

Prevention

Deep, penetrating wounds in muscular tissue are dangerous; they should be explored, all dead tissue should be completely excised and, if there is the slightest doubt about tissue viability, the wound should be left open. Unhappily there is no effective antitoxin against *C. welchii*.

Treatment

The key to life-saving treatment is early diagnosis. General measures, such as fluid replacement and intravenous antibiotics, are started immediately. Hyperbaric oxygen has been used as a means of limiting the spread of gangrene. However, the mainstay of treatment is prompt decompression of the wound and removal of all dead tissue. In advanced cases, amputation may be essential.

FRACTURE BLISTERS

These are due to elevation of the superficial layers of skin by oedema, and can sometimes be prevented by firm bandaging. They should be covered with a sterile dry dressing.

PLASTER SORES AND PRESSURE SORES

Plaster sores occur where skin presses directly onto bone. They should be prevented by padding the bony points and by moulding the wet plaster so that pressure is distributed to the soft tissues around the bony points. While a plaster sore is developing the patient feels localized burning pain. A window must immediately be cut in the plaster, or warning pain quickly abates and skin necrosis proceeds unnoticed.

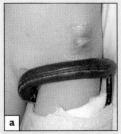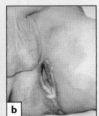

23.35 Pressure sores from fixed traction It is a mistake to think of non-operative treatment as 'simple' or 'easy'! It requires constant care and supervision. These pressure sores from the ring of a Thomas' splint kept the patient in hospital for months.

Traction on a Thomas' splint also poses problems and requires skill in nursing care; careless selection of ring size, or excessive traction on a 'fixed' (as opposed to a 'balanced') splint, can lead to pressure sores around the groin and iliac crest.

LATE COMPLICATIONS

DELAYED UNION

The timetable on page 544 is no more than a rough guide to the period in which a fracture may be expected to unite and consolidate. It must never be relied upon in deciding when treatment may be discontinued. If the time is unduly prolonged, the term 'delayed union' is used.

Causes

Factors causing delayed union can be summarized as *biological*, *biomechanical* or *patient-related*.

BIOLOGICAL
Inadequate blood supply A badly displaced fracture of a long bone will cause tearing of both the periosteum and interruption of the intramedullary blood supply. The fracture edges will become necrotic and depend on the formation of an ensheathing callus mass to bridge the break. If the zone of necrosis is extensive, as might occur in highly comminuted fractures, union may be hampered.

Severe soft tissue damage Severe damage to the soft tissues affects fracture healing by (a) reducing the effectiveness of muscle splintage, (b) damaging the local blood supply and (c) diminishing or eliminating the osteogenic stimulus of muscle pull on bone.

Periosteal stripping Overenthusiastic stripping of periosteum during internal fixation is an avoidable cause of delayed union and non-union.

BIOMECHANICAL
Imperfect splintage Excessive traction (creating a fracture gap) or excessive movement at the fracture site will delay ossification in the callus. In forearm or leg fractures, an intact fellow bone may also serve to splint a fracture apart.

Over-rigid fixation Contrary to popular belief, rigid fixation delays rather than promotes fracture union. It is only because the fixation device holds the fragments so securely that the fracture seems to 'unite'. However, union by primary bone healing is slow, and provided the stability is maintained throughout, the fracture does eventually unite.

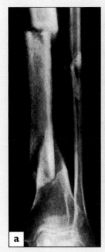
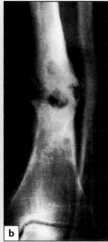
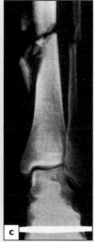
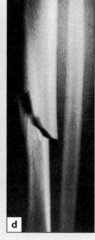

23.36 Delayed union Causes of delay include (**a**) a severe injury with marked soft-tissue damage; (**b**) infection; or a gap at the fracture site from (**c**) excessive traction or (**d**) an intact fibula which splints the tibial fragments apart.

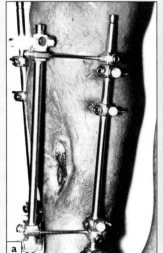
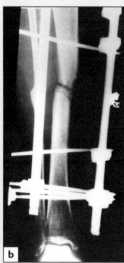
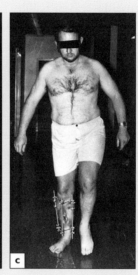
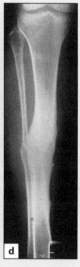

23.37 Infection and delayed union (**a**) Infected fracture of the tibia treated by wound excision and external fixation; (**b**) the x-ray after 6 weeks; (**c**) he was able to walk around with his apparatus, and gradually the wound healed; at 1 year (**d**) the fracture was completely solid.

Infection Both biology and stability are hampered by active infection: not only is there bone lysis, necrosis and pus formation, but also implants which are used to hold the fracture tend to loosen.

PATIENT FACTORS
In a less than ideal world, we may encounter patients who are:

- immense;
- immoderate;
- immovable;
- impossible.

Clinical features

Fracture tenderness persists and if the bone is subjected to stress, pain may be acute.

X-ray The fracture line remains visible and there is very little callus formation or periosteal reaction. However, the bone ends are not sclerosed or atrophic. The appearances suggest that, although the fracture has not united, it eventually will.

Treatment

CONSERVATIVE The two important principles are (1) to eliminate any possible cause of delayed union, and (2) to promote healing by providing the most appropriate biological environment. Immobilization (whether by cast or by internal fixation) should be sufficient to prevent shearing movement at the fracture site; but fracture loading is an important stimulus to union and this can be enhanced (a) by encouraging muscular exercise and (b) by weightbearing in the cast or brace. The watchword is patience; however, there comes a point with every fracture at which the ill-effects of prolonged immobilization outweigh the advantages of non-operative treatment, or where the risk of implant breakage begins to loom.

OPERATIVE Each case should be treated on its merits; however, if union is delayed for more than 6 months and there is no sign of callus formation, fixation and bone grafting are indicated. The operation should be planned in such a way as to cause the least possible damage to the soft tissues.

NON-UNION

In a minority of cases delayed union gradually turns into non-union; that is it becomes apparent that the fracture will never unite without intervention. Movement can be elicited at the fracture site and pain diminishes; the fracture gap becomes a type of pseudarthrosis.

On x-ray the fracture is clearly visible and the bone on either side of it may be either exuberant or rounded off. This contrasting appearance has led to non-unions being divided into hypertrophic and atrophic types.

In hypertrophic non-union the bone ends are enlarged, suggesting that osteogenesis is still active but not quite capable of bridging the gap.

Causes of non-union			
The injury		**The bone**	
Soft-tissue loss		Poor blood supply	
Bone loss		Poor haematoma	
Intact fellow bone		Infection	
Soft-tissue interposition		Pathological lesion	
The surgeon		**The patient**	
Distraction		Immense	
Poor splintage		Immoderate	
Poor fixation		Immovable	
Impatience		Impossible	

In atrophic non-union osteogenesis seems to have ceased. The bone ends are often tapered or rounded with no suggestion of new bone formation.

Treatment

CONSERVATIVE Non-union is occasionally symptomless, needing no treatment or, at most, a removable splint. Even if symptoms are present, operation is not the only answer; with hypertrophic non-union, functional bracing may be sufficient to induce union, but treatment often needs to be prolonged. Pulsed electromagnetic fields and low frequency pulsed ultrasound can also be used to stimulate union.

OPERATIVE With *hypertrophic non-union* and in the absence of deformity, very rigid fixation alone (internal or external) may lead to union. Often, though, bone grafts are added. With *atrophic non-union*, fixation alone is not enough. Fibrous tissue in the

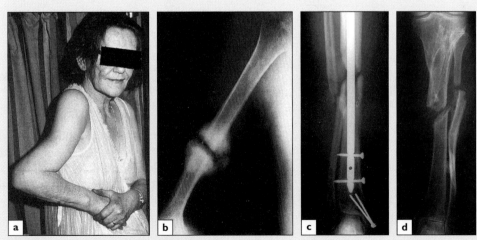

23.38 Non-union (**a**) This patient has an obvious pseudarthrosis of the humerus. The x-ray (**b**) shows a typical hypertrophic non-union. (**c, d**) Examples of atrophic non-union.

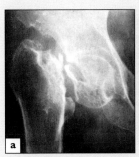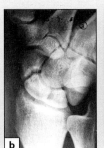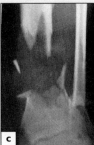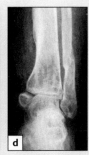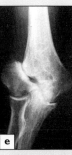

23.39 Non-union The femoral neck (**a**) and the carpal scaphoid (**b**) are two common sites of non-union. The tibia in (**c**) could hardly be expected to unite – so much bone had been left at the scene of the accident. (**d**) This medial malleolus failed to unite because a flap of periosteum was interposed. (**e**) This lateral condylar fragment has rotated, so that the articular surface faces into the fracture gap.

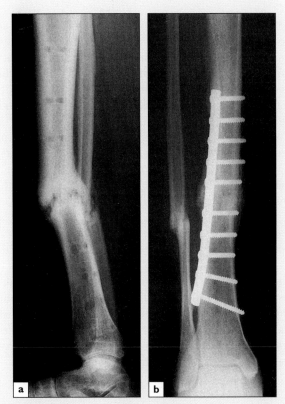

23.40 Non-union – treatment (**a**) Hypertrophic non-union after internal fixation. The metal was removed and the intervening fibrous tissue excised. (**b**) Rigid fixation has resulted in bony union.

MALUNION

When the fragments join in an unsatisfactory position (unacceptable angulation, rotation or shortening) the fracture is said to be malunited. Causes are failure to reduce a fracture adequately, failure to hold reduction while healing proceeds or gradual collapse of comminuted or osteoporotic bone.

Clinical features

The deformity is usually obvious, but sometimes the true extent of malunion is apparent only on x-ray. Rotational deformity of the femur, tibia, humerus or forearm may be missed unless the limb is compared with its opposite fellow. Rotational deformity of a metacarpal fracture is detected by asking the patient to flatten the fingers onto the palm and seeing whether the normal regular fan-shaped appearance is reproduced (see page 630).

X-rays are essential to check the position of the fracture while it is uniting. This is particularly important during the first 3 weeks when the situation may change without warning. At this stage it is sometimes difficult to decide what constitutes 'malunion'; acceptable norms differ from one site to another and these are discussed under the individual fractures.

Treatment

Incipient malunion may call for treatment even before the fracture has fully united; the decision on the need for re-manipulation or correction may be extremely difficult. A few guidelines are offered.

fracture gap, as well as the hard, sclerotic bone ends, are excised and bone grafts are packed around the fracture. If there is significant 'die-back', this will require more extensive excision and the gap is then dealt with by bone advancement using the Ilizarov technique (Ilizarov, 1992).

1. In adults, fractures should be reduced as near to the anatomical position as possible. However, apposition is less important than alignment and rotation.

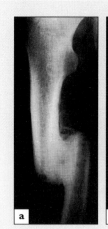
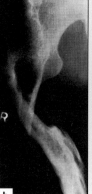
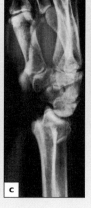
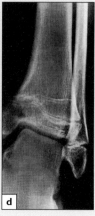

23.41 Malunion Primary malunion (**a**) with overlap, (**b**) with angulation. (**c**) Secondary malunion – this Colles' fracture was reduced satisfactorily, but displaced in plaster. (**d**) Secondary malunion following damage to the lower tibial physis.

Angulation of more than 10–15° in a long bone, or a noticeable rotational deformity, may need correction by remanipulation, or by osteotomy and internal fixation.

2. In children, angular deformities near the bone ends will usually remodel with time; rotational deformities will not.

3. In the lower limb, shortening of more than 2.0cm is seldom acceptable to the patient and a limb lengthening procedure may be indicated.

4. The patient's expectations (often prompted by cosmesis) may be quite different from the surgeon's; they are not to be ignored.

5. Early discussion with the patient, and a guided view of the x-rays, will help in deciding on the need for treatment and may prevent later misunderstanding.

6. Very little is known of the long-term effects of small angular deformities on joint function. However, it seems likely that malalignment of more than 15° in any plane may cause asymmetrical loading of the joint above or below and the late development of secondary osteoarthritis; this applies particularly to the large weightbearing joints.

AVASCULAR NECROSIS

Certain regions are notorious for their propensity to develop ischaemia and bone necrosis after injury (see also Chapter 6). They are (1) the head of the femur (after fracture of the femoral neck or dislocation of the hip); (2) the proximal part of the scaphoid (after fracture through its waist); (3) the lunate (following dislocation); and (4) the body of the talus (after fracture of its neck).

Accurately speaking, this is an early complication of bone injury, because ischaemia occurs during the first few hours following fracture or dislocation. However, the clinical and radiological effects are not seen until weeks or even months later.

Clinical features

There are no symptoms associated with avascular necrosis, but if the fracture fails to unite or if the bone collapses the patient may complain of pain. X-ray shows the characteristic increase in bone density (the consequence of new bone ingrowth in the necrotic segment and disuse osteoporosis in the surrounding parts).

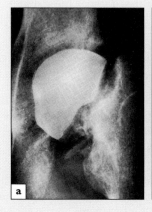
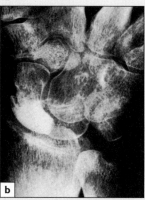
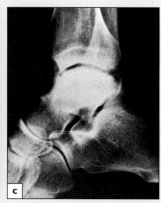

23.42 Avascular necrosis Injury to the blood supply may result in ischaemia and segmental necrosis of the bone furthest from the blood supply. The sites most commonly affected in traumatic osteonecrosis are: (**a**) the head of the femur, (**b**) the proximal portion of the scaphoid, and (**c**) the posterior half of the talus.

Treatment

Treatment usually becomes necessary when joint function is threatened. In old people with necrosis of the femoral head an arthroplasty is the obvious choice; in younger people, realignment osteotomy (or even arthrodesis) may be wiser. Avascular necrosis in the scaphoid or talus may need no more than symptomatic treatment, but vascularized bone-grafting, or arthrodesis of the wrist or ankle, is sometimes needed.

GROWTH DISTURBANCE

In children, damage to the physis may lead to abnormal or arrested growth. A transverse fracture through the growth plate is not disastrous; the fracture runs through the hypertrophic and calcified layers and not through the germinal zone so, provided it is accurately reduced, there is seldom any disturbance of growth. But fractures that split the epiphysis inevitably traverse the growing portion of the physis, and so further growth may be asymmetrical and the bone end characteristically angulated; if the entire physis is damaged, there may be slowing or complete cessation of growth.

The subject is dealt with in more detail on page 578.

BED SORES

Bed sores occur in elderly or paralysed patients. The skin over the sacrum and heels is especially vulnerable. Careful nursing and early activity can usually prevent bed sores; once they have developed, treatment is difficult; it may be necessary to excise the necrotic tissue and apply skin grafts.

MYOSITIS OSSIFICANS

Heterotopic ossification in the muscles sometimes occurs after an injury, particularly dislocation of the elbow or a blow to the brachialis, the deltoid or the quadriceps. It is thought to be due to muscle damage, but it also occurs without a local injury in unconscious or paraplegic patients.

Clinical features

Soon after the injury, the patient (usually a fit young man) complains of pain; there is local swelling and soft-tissue tenderness. X-ray is normal but a bone scan may show increased activity. Over the next 2–3 weeks the pain gradually subsides, but joint movement is limited; x-ray may show fluffy calcification in the soft tissues. By 8 weeks the bony mass is easily palpable and is clearly defined in the x-ray.

Treatment

The worst treatment is to attack an injured and stiffish elbow with vigorous muscle-stretching exercises; this is liable to precipitate or aggravate the condition. The joint should be rested in the position of function until pain subsides; gentle active movements are then begun.

Months later, when the condition has stabilized, it may be helpful to excise the bony mass. Indomethacin or radiotherapy should be given to help prevent a recurrence.

TENDON LESIONS

Tendinitis may affect the tibialis posterior tendon following medial malleolar fractures. It should be prevented by accurate reduction, if necessary at open operation.

Rupture of the extensor pollicis longus tendon may occur 6–12 weeks after a fracture of the lower radius. Direct suture is seldom possible and the resulting disability is treated by transferring the extensor indicis proprius tendon to the distal stump of the ruptured thumb tendon. Late rupture of the long head of biceps after a fractured neck of humerus usually requires no treatment.

NERVE COMPRESSION

Nerve compression may damage the lateral popliteal nerve if an elderly or emaciated patient lies with the leg in full external rotation. Radial palsy may follow the faulty use of crutches. Both conditions are due to lack of supervision.

Bone or joint deformity may result in local nerve entrapment with typical features such as numbness or paraesthesia, loss of power and muscle wasting in the distribution of the affected nerve. Common sites are: (1) the ulnar nerve, due to a valgus elbow following an un-united lateral condyle fracture; (2) the median nerve, following injuries around the wrist; (3) the posterior tibial nerve, following fractures around the

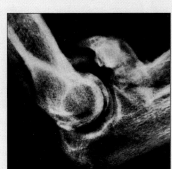

23.43 Myositis ossificans Myositis ossificans following a fractured head of radius.

ankle. Treatment is by early decompression of the nerve; in the case of the ulnar nerve this may require anterior transposition.

MUSCLE CONTRACTURE

Following arterial injury or a compartmental syndrome, the patient may develop ischaemic contractures of the affected muscles (*Volkmann's ischaemic contracture*). Nerves injured by ischaemia sometimes recover, at least partially; thus the patient presents with deformity and stiffness, but numbness is inconstant. The sites most commonly affected are the forearm and hand, the leg and the foot.

In a severe case affecting the forearm, there will be wasting of the forearm and hand and clawing of the fingers; if the wrist is passively flexed, the patient can extend the fingers, showing that the deformity is largely due to contracture of the forearm muscles. Detachment of the flexors at their origin and along the interosseous membrane in the forearm may improve the deformity, but function is no better if sensation and active movement are not restored. A pedicle nerve graft, using the proximal segments of the median and ulnar nerves may restore protective sensation in the hand, and tendon transfers (wrist extensors to finger and thumb flexors) will allow active grasp. In less severe cases, median nerve sensibility may be quite good and, with appropriate tendon releases and transfers, the patient regains a considerable degree of function.

Ischaemia of the hand may follow forearm injuries, or swelling of the fingers associated with a tight forearm bandage or plaster. The intrinsic hand muscles fibrose and shorten, pulling the fingers into flexion at the metacarpophalangeal joints, but the interphalangeal joints remain straight. The thumb is adducted across the palm (Bunnell's 'intrinsic-plus' position).

Ischaemia of the calf muscles may follow injuries or operations involving the popliteal artery or its divisions. This is more common than is usually supposed. The symptoms, signs and subsequent contracture are similar to those following ischaemia of the forearm. One of the causes of late claw-toe deformity is an undiagnosed compartment syndrome.

JOINT INSTABILITY

Following injury a joint may give way. Causes include the following.

Ligamentous laxity, especially at the knee, the ankle and the metacarpophalangeal joint of the thumb.

Muscle weakness, particularly if splintage has been excessive or prolonged, and exercises have been inadequate (again the knee and ankle are most often affected).

Bone loss, for example after a gunshot fracture, a severe compound injury or crushing of metaphyseal bone in a joint depression fracture.

Injury may also lead to *recurrent dislocation.* The commonest sites are the shoulder and the patella.

A more subtle form of instability is seen after fractures around the wrist. Patients complaining of persistent discomfort or weakness after wrist injury should be fully investigated for *chronic carpal instability* (see page 621).

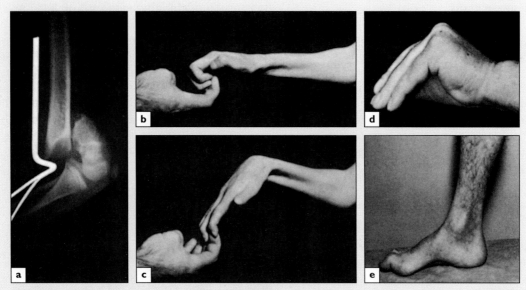

23.44 Volkmann's ischaemia (a) Kinking of the main artery is an important cause, but intimal tears may also lead to blockage from thrombosis. A delayed diagnosis of compartment syndrome carries the same sorry fate. (b, c) Volkmann's contracture of the forearm; the fingers can be straightened only when the wrist is flexed (the constant-length phenomenon). (d) Ischaemic contracture of the small muscles of the hand. (e) Ischaemic contracture of the calf muscles with clawing of the toes.

JOINT STIFFNESS

Joint stiffness after a fracture commonly occurs in the knee, the elbow, the shoulder and (worst of all) the small joints of the hand. Sometimes the joint itself has been injured; a haemarthrosis forms and leads to synovial adhesions. More often the stiffness is due to oedema and fibrosis of the capsule, the ligaments and the muscles around the joint, or adhesions of the soft tissues to each other or to the underlying bone. All these conditions are made worse by prolonged immobilization; moreover, if the joint has been held in a position where the ligaments are at their shortest, no amount of exercise will afterwards succeed in stretching these tissues and restoring the lost movement completely.

In a small percentage of patients with fractures of the forearm or leg, early post-traumatic swelling is accompanied by tenderness and progressive stiffness of the distal joints. These patients are at great risk of developing reflex sympathetic dystrophy (algodystrophy or complex regional pain syndrome); whether this is an entirely separate entity or merely an extension of the 'normal' post-traumatic soft-tissue reaction is uncertain. What is important is to recognize this type of 'stiffness' when it occurs and to insist on skilled physiotherapy until normal function is restored.

Treatment

The best treatment is prevention – by exercises that keep the joints mobile from the outset. If a joint has to be splinted, make sure that it is held in the 'position of safety' (see Fig. 26.1). Joints that are already stiff take time to mobilize, but prolonged and patient physiotherapy can work wonders. If the situation is due to intra-articular adhesions, gentle manipulation under anaesthesia may free the joint sufficiently to permit a more pliant response to further exercise.

Occasionally, adherent or contracted tissues need to be released by operation (e.g. when knee flexion is prevented by adhesions in and around the quadriceps).

ALGODYSTROPHY (COMPLEX REGIONAL PAIN SYNDROME)

Sudeck, in 1900, described a condition characterized by painful osteoporosis of the hand. The same condition sometimes occurs after fractures of the extremities and for many years it was called *Sudeck's atrophy*. It is now recognized that this advanced atrophic disorder is the late stage of a post-traumatic *reflex sympathetic dystrophy* (also known as *algodystrophy*), that it is much more common than originally believed (Atkins *et al.*, 1990) and that it may follow relatively trivial

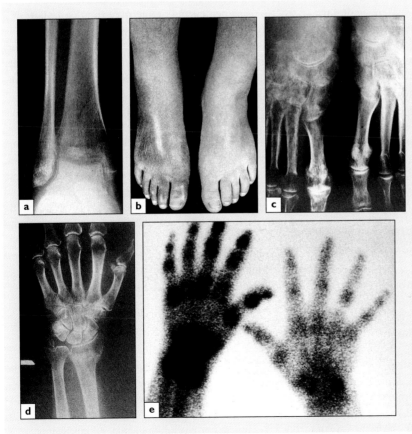

23.45 Osteoporosis and algodystrophy (a) Regional osteoporosis is common after fractures of the extremities. The radiolucent bands seen here are typical. (b) In algodystrophy the picture is exaggerated and the soft tissues also are involved: here the right foot is somewhat swollen and the skin has become dusky, smooth and shiny. (c) In the full-blown case, x-rays show a typical patchy osteoporosis. (d) Similar changes may occur in the wrist and hand; they are always accompanied by (e) increased activity in the radionuclide scan.

injury. Because of continuing uncertainty about its nature, the term *complex regional pain syndrome* has been introduced (see page 226).

The patient complains of continuous pain, often described as 'burning' in character. At first there is local swelling, redness and warmth, as well as tenderness and moderate stiffness of the nearby joints. As the weeks go by the skin becomes pale and atrophic, movements are increasingly restricted and the patient may develop fixed deformities. X-rays characteristically show patchy rarefaction of the bone.

The earlier the condition is recognized and treatment begun, the better the prognosis. Elevation and active exercises are important after all injuries, but in algodystrophy they are essential. In the early stage of the condition anti-inflammatory drugs are helpful. If this does not produce improvement, amitriptyline may help to control the pain.

Sympathetic block or sympatholytic drugs such as intravenous guanethidine have been advocated for this condition. They do sometimes appear to help but their effect is unpredictable. Prolonged and dedicated physiotherapy will usually be needed.

OSTEOARTHRITIS

A fracture involving a joint may severely damage the articular cartilage and give rise to post-traumatic osteoarthritis within a period of months. Even if the cartilage heals, irregularity of the joint surface may cause localized stress and so predispose to secondary osteoarthritis years later. Little can be done to prevent this once the fracture has united.

Malunion of a metaphyseal fracture may radically alter the mechanics of a nearby joint and this, too, can give rise to secondary osteoarthritis. It is often asserted that malunion in the shaft of a long bone (e.g. the tibia) may act in a similar manner; however, there is little evidence to show that residual angulation of less than 15° can cause proximal or distal osteoarthritis (see page 729).

STRESS FRACTURES

A stress or fatigue fracture is one occurring in the normal bone of a healthy patient. It is caused not by a specific traumatic incident but by repetitive stresses, which are of two main kinds – bending and compression.

Bending stress causes breaching of one cortex; healing begins, but with repeated stress the breach may extend across the bone. This variety affects young adults and is probably due to muscular action, which tends to deform bone; the athlete in training builds up muscle power quickly but bone strength only slowly, and a stress fracture may result; this accounts for the high incidence of stress fractures in military recruits.

Compression stress acts on soft cancellous bone; with frequent repetition an impacted fracture may follow.

NOTE It has been suggested that a stress fracture is the initial lesion in some of the osteochondritides; for example, Freiberg's disease.

Sites affected

Least rare are the following: shaft of humerus (adolescent cricketers); pars interarticularis of fifth lumbar vertebra (causing spondylolysis); pubic rami (inferior in children, both in adults); femoral neck (at any age); femoral shaft (chiefly lower third); patella (children and young adults); tibial shaft (proximal third in children, middle third in athletes and trainee paratroopers, distal third in the elderly); distal shaft of fibula (the 'runner's fracture'); calcaneum (adults); navicular (athletes); and metatarsals (especially the second).

Clinical features

There may be a history of unaccustomed and repeated activity. A common sequence of events is: pain after exercise – pain during exercise – pain without exercise. Occasionally the patient presents only after the fracture has healed; he or she may then complain of a lump (the callus).

The patient is usually healthy. The affected site may be swollen or red. It is sometimes warm and usually tender; the callus may be palpable. 'Springing' the bone (attempting to bend it) is often painful.

X-RAY
Early on, the fracture is difficult to detect, but a bone scan will show increased activity at the painful spot. A few weeks later one may see a small transverse defect in the cortex and, later still, localized periosteal new-bone formation. These appearances can be mistaken for those of an osteosarcoma, a horrifying trap for the unwary.

Compression stress fractures (especially of the femoral neck and upper tibia) may show as a hazy transverse band of sclerosis with (in the tibia) peripheral callus.

Diagnosis

Many disorders, including osteomyelitis, scurvy and the battered baby syndrome, may be confused with stress fractures. The great danger, however, is a mistaken diagnosis of osteosarcoma; scanning shows increased uptake in both conditions and even biopsy may be misleading.

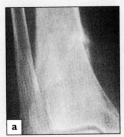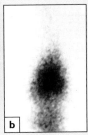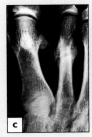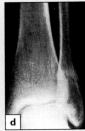

23.46 Stress fractures (**a**) The stress fracture of this tibia is only just visible, but it had already been diagnosed 2 weeks earlier when the scan (**b**) showed a 'hot' area above the ankle. (**c, d**) Stress fractures of the second metatarsal and the fibula.

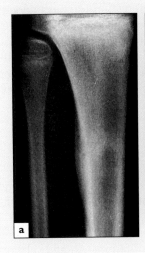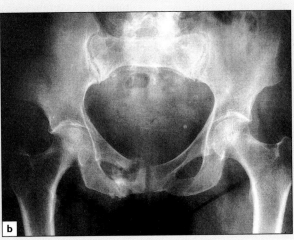

23.47 Stress fractures Stress-fractures are often missed or wrongly diagnosed. (**a**) This tibial fracture was at first thought to be an osteosarcoma. (**b**) Stress fractures of the pubic rami in elderly women can be mistaken for metastases.

Treatment

Most stress fractures need no treatment other than an elastic bandage and avoidance of the painful activity until the lesion heals; surprisingly, this can take many months and the forced inactivity is not easily accepted by the hard-driving athlete or dancer.

An important exception is stress fracture of the femoral neck. This should be suspected in all elderly people who complain of pain in the hip for which no obvious cause can be found. If the diagnosis is confirmed by bone scan, the femoral neck should be pinned as a prophylactic measure.

PATHOLOGICAL FRACTURES

When abnormal bone gives way this is referred to as a pathological fracture. The causes are numerous and varied; often the diagnosis is not made until a biopsy is examined (see the boxed summary).

Causes of Pathological Fracture

Generalized bone disease

1. Osteogenesis imperfecta
2. Postmenopausal osteoporosis
3. Metabolic bone disease
4. Myelomatosis
5. Polyostotic fibrous dysplasia
6. Paget's disease

Local benign conditions

1. Chronic infection
2. Solitary bone cyst
3. Fibrous cortical defect
4. Chondromyxoid fibroma
5. Aneurysmal bone cyst
6. Chondroma
7. Monostotic fibrous dysplasia

Primary malignant tumours

1. Chondrosarcoma
2. Osteosarcoma
3. Ewing's tumour

Metastatic tumours

Carcinoma from breast, lung, kidney, thyroid, colon and prostate

The history

Bone that fractures spontaneously, or after trivial injury, must be regarded as abnormal until proved otherwise. In older patients one should always ask about previous illnesses or operations; a malignant tumour, no matter how long ago it occurred, may be the source of a late metastatic lesion; a history of gastrectomy, intestinal malabsorption, chronic alcoholism or prolonged drug therapy should suggest a metabolic bone disorder.

Symptoms such as loss of weight, pain, a lump, cough or haematuria suggest that the fracture may be through a secondary deposit.

In younger patients, a history of several previous fractures may suggest a diagnosis of osteogenesis imperfecta, even if the patient does not show the classic features of the disorder.

Examination

Local signs of bone disease (an infected sinus, an old scar, swelling or deformity) should not be missed. The site of the fracture may suggest the diagnosis: patients with involutional osteoporosis develop fractures of the vertebral bodies and the corticocancellous junctions of long bones; a fracture through the shaft of the bone in an elderly patient is a pathological fracture until proved otherwise.

General examination may be informative. Congenital dysplasias, fibrous dysplasia, Cushing' syndrome and Paget' disease all produce characteristic appearances. The patient may be wasted (possibly due to malignant disease). The lymph nodes or liver may be enlarged. Is there a mass in the abdomen or pelvis? Old scars should not be overlooked. And rectal and vaginal examinations are mandatory.

Under the age of 20 years the common causes of pathological fracture are benign bone tumours and cysts. Over the age of 40 years the common causes are myelomatosis, secondary carcinoma and Paget' disease.

X-rays Understandably, the fracture itself attracts most attention. But the surrounding bone must also be examined, and features such as cyst formation, cortical erosion, abnormal trabeculation and periosteal thickening should be sought. The type of fracture, too, is important: vertebral compression fractures may be due to severe osteoporosis or osteomalacia, but they can also be caused by skeletal metastases or myeloma. Middle-aged men, unlike women, do not normally become osteoporotic: x-ray signs of bone loss and vertebral compression in a male under 75 years should be regarded as 'pathological' until proved otherwise.

Additional investigations

X-RAY EXAMINATION X-ray of other bones, the lungs and the urogenital tract may be necessary to exclude malignant disease.

BLOOD INVESTIGATION Investigations should always include a full blood count, erythrocyte sedimentation rate (ESR), protein electrophoresis, and tests for syphilis and metabolic bone disorders.

URINE EXAMINATION Urine examination may reveal blood from a tumour, or Bence-Jones protein in myelomatosis.

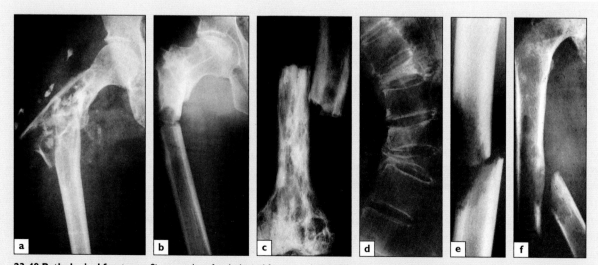

23.48 Pathological fractures Six examples of pathological fractures, due to: **(a)** primary chondrosarcoma; **(b)** post-operative bone infection at a screw-hole following plating of an intertrochanteric fracture; **(c)** Paget's disease; **(d)** vertebral metastases; **(e)** metastasis from carcinoma of the breast; and **(f)** myelomatosis.

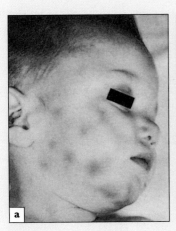
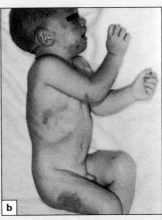
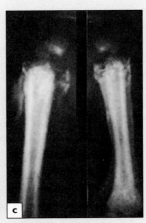

23.49 The battered baby syndrome. The fractures are not pathological but the family is. The metaphyseal lesions in each humerus are characteristic.

SCANNING Local radionuclide imaging may help elucidate the diagnosis, and whole body scanning is important in revealing or excluding other deposits.

Biopsy

Some lesions are so typical that a biopsy is unnecessary (solitary cyst, fibrous cortical defect, Paget's disease). Others are more obscure and a biopsy is essential for diagnosis. If open reduction of the fracture is indicated, the biopsy can be done at the same time; otherwise a definitive procedure should be arranged.

Treatment

The principles of fracture treatment remain the same: REDUCE, HOLD, EXERCISE. But the choice of method is influenced by the condition of the bone; and the underlying pathological disorder may need treatment in its own right (see Chapter 9).

GENERALIZED BONE DISEASE In most of these conditions (including Paget's disease) the bones fracture more easily, but they heal quite well provided the fracture is properly immobilized. Internal fixation is therefore advisable (and for Paget's disease almost essential). Patients with osteomalacia, hyperparathyroidism, renal osteodystrophy and Paget's disease may need systemic treatment as well.

LOCAL BENIGN CONDITIONS Fractures through benign cyst-like lesions usually heal quite well and they should be allowed to do so before tackling the local lesion. Treatment is therefore the same as for simple fractures in the same area, although in some cases it will be necessary to take a biopsy before immobilizing the

fracture. When the bone has healed, the tumour can be dealt with by curettage or local excision.

PRIMARY MALIGNANT TUMOUR The fracture may need splinting but this is merely a prelude to definitive treatment of the tumour, which by now will have spread to the surrounding soft tissues. The prognosis is almost always very poor.

METASTATIC TUMOURS Metastasis is a frequent cause of pathological fracture in older people. Breast cancer is the commonest source and the femur the commonest site. Nowadays cancer patients (even those with metastases) often live for several years and effective treatment of the fracture will vastly improve their quality of life.

Fracture of a long-bone shaft should be treated by internal fixation; if necessary the site is also packed with acrylic cement. Bear in mind that the implant will function as a load-*bearing* and not a load-*sharing* device; intramedullary nails are more suitable than plates and screws.

Fractures near a bone end can often be treated by excision and prosthetic replacement; this is especially true of femoral neck fractures.

Pre-operatively, imaging studies should be performed to detect other bone lesions; these may be amenable to prophylactic fixation. Once the wound has healed, local irradiation should be applied to reduce the risk of progressive osteolysis.

Pathological compression fractures of the spine cause severe pain. This is due largely to spinal instability and treatment should include operative stabilization (Hosono *et al.*, 1995). If there are either clinical or imaging features of actual or threatened spinal cord or cauda equina compression, the segment should also be decompressed. Post-operative irradiation is given as usual.

With all types of metastatic lesion, the primary tumour should be investigated and treated as well.

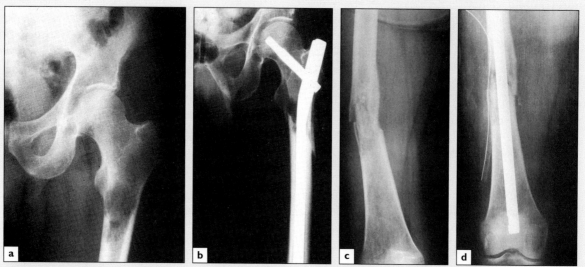

23.50 Pathological fractures – treatment (a) This patient with a secondary deposit below the lesser trochanter was advised to have prophylactic nailing. While she was being prepared she sustained an undisplaced fracture. This was securely fixed (b) and was followed by radiotherapy. (c, d) Fracture through a metastasis in the mid-shaft of the femur, fixed with an intramedullary nail.

INJURIES OF THE PHYSIS

In children over 10% of fractures involve injury to the growth plate (or physis). Because the physis is a relatively weak part of the bone, joint strains that might cause ligament injuries in adults are liable to result in separation of the physis in children. The fracture usually runs transversely through the hypertrophic or the calcified layer of the growth plate, often veering off into the metaphysis at one of the edges to include a triangular lip of bone. This has little effect on longitudinal growth, which takes place in the germinal and proliferating layers of the physis. However, if the fracture traverses the cellular 'reproductive' layers of the plate, it may result in premature ossification of the injured part and serious disturbances of bone growth.

Classification

The most widely used classification of physeal injuries is that of Salter and Harris (1963), which distinguishes five basic types of injury:

- *Type 1* A transverse fracture through the hypertrophic or calcified zone of the plate. Even if the fracture is quite alarmingly displaced, the growing zone of the physis is usually not injured and growth disturbance is uncommon.
- *Type 2* This is essentially similar to type 1, but towards the edge the fracture deviates away from the physis and splits off a triangular metaphyseal fragment of bone.
- *Type 3* A fracture that splits the epiphysis and then veers off transversely to one or the other side,

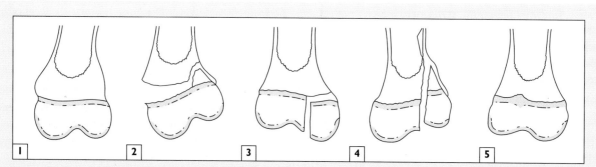

23.51 Physeal injuries *Type 1* – separation of the epiphysis – which usually occurs in infants but is also seen at puberty as a slipped femoral epiphysis. *Type 2* – fracture through the physis and metaphysis – is the commonest; it occurs in older children and seldom results in abnormal growth. *Type 3* – an intra-articular fracture of the epiphysis – needs accurate reduction to restore the joint surface. *Type 4* – splitting of the physis and epiphysis – damages the articular surface and may also cause abnormal growth; if it is displaced it needs open reduction. *Type 5* – crushing of the physis – may look benign but ends in arrested growth.

through the hypertrophic layer of the physis. Inevitably it damages the 'reproductive' layers of the physis and may result in growth disturbance.

- *Type 4* As with type 3, the fracture splits the epiphysis, but it extends into the metaphysis. These fractures are liable to displacement and a consequent misfit between the separated parts of the physis, resulting in asymmetrical growth.
- *Type 5* A longitudinal compression injury of the physis. There is no visible fracture but the growth plate is crushed and this may result in growth arrest.

Rang (1969) added *Type 6*, injury of the perichondrial ring (the peripheral zone of Ranvier), which carries a significant risk of growth disturbance. The diagnosis is usually made in retrospect after development of deformity.

Mechanism of injury

Physeal fractures usually result from falls or traction injuries. They occur mostly in road accidents and during sporting activities or playground tumbles.

Clinical features

These fractures are more common in boys than in girls and are usually seen either in infancy or between the ages of 10 and 12 years. Deformity is usually minimal, but any injury in a child followed by pain and tenderness near the joint should arouse suspicion, and x-ray examination is essential.

X-rays The physis itself is radiolucent and the epiphysis may be incompletely ossified; this makes it hard to tell whether the bone end is damaged or deformed. The younger the child, the smaller the 'visible' part of the epiphysis and thus the more difficult it is to make the diagnosis; comparison with the normal side is a great help. Tell-tale features are widening of the physeal 'gap', incongruity of the joint or tilting of the epiphyseal axis. If there is marked displacement the diagnosis is obvious, but even type 4 fracture may at first be so little displaced that the fracture line is hard to see; if there is the faintest suspicion of a physeal fracture, another x-ray after 4 or 5 days is essential. Type 5 injuries are usually diagnosed only in retrospect.

Treatment

Undisplaced fractures may be treated by splinting the part in a cast or a close-fitting plaster slab for 2–4 weeks (depending on the site of injury and the age of the child). However, with undisplaced type 3 and 4 fractures, a check x-ray after 4 days and again at

about 10 days is mandatory in order not to miss late displacement.

Displaced fractures should be reduced as soon as possible. With types 1 and 2 this can usually be done closed; the part is then splinted securely for 3–6 weeks. Type 3 and 4 fractures demand perfect anatomical reduction. An attempt can be made to achieve this by gentle manipulation under general anaesthesia; if this is successful, the limb is held in a cast for 4–8 weeks (the longer periods for type 4 injuries). If a type 3 or 4 fracture cannot be reduced accurately by closed manipulation, immediate open reduction and internal fixation with smooth Kirschner wires is essential. The limb is then splinted for 4–6 weeks, but it takes that long again before the child is ready to resume unrestricted activities.

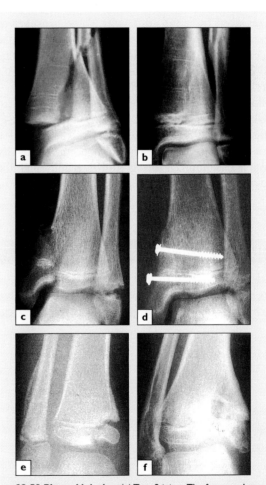

23.52 Physeal injuries (a) Type 2 injury. The fracture does not traverse the width of the physis; after reduction (b) bone growth is not distorted. (c, d) This Type 4 fracture of the tibial physis was treated immediately by open reduction and internal fixation and a good result was obtained. (e, f) In this case accurate reduction was not achieved and the physeal fragment remained displaced; the end result was partial fusion of the physis and severe deformity of the ankle.

Complications

Type 1 and 2 injuries, if properly reduced, usually have an excellent prognosis and bone growth is not adversely affected. Exceptions to this rule are injuries around the knee involving the distal femoral or proximal tibial physis; both are undulating in shape, so a transverse fracture may pass through more than just the hypertrophic zone and could damage also the proliferative zone. Elsewhere, complications such as malunion or non-union may occur if the diagnosis is missed and the fracture remains unreduced (e.g. fracture-separation of the medial humeral epicondyle).

Type 3 and 4 injuries may result in premature fusion of part of the growth plate or asymmetrical growth of the bone end. Type 5 fractures cause premature fusion and retardation of growth. The size and position of the bony bridge across the physis can be assessed by tomography or MRI. If the bridge is relatively small (less than half the width of the physis) it can be excised and replaced by a fat graft, with some prospect of preventing or diminishing the growth disturbance (Langenskiold, 1975, 1981). However, if the bone bridge is more extensive the operation is contraindicated as it can result in more harm than good.

Established deformity, whether from asymmetrical growth or from malunion of a displaced fracture (e.g. a valgus elbow due to proximal displacement of a lateral humeral condylar fracture) should be treated by corrective osteotomy. If further growth is abnormal, the osteotomy may have to be repeated.

INJURIES TO JOINTS

Joints are usually injured by twisting or tilting forces that stretch the ligaments and capsule. If the force is great enough the ligaments may tear, or the bone to which they are attached may be pulled apart. The articular cartilage, too, may be damaged if the joint surfaces are compressed or if there is a fracture into the joint.

As a general principle, forceful angulation will tear the ligaments rather than crush the bone, but in older people with porotic bone the ligaments may hold and the bone on the opposite side of the joint is crushed instead, while in children there may be a fracture-separation of the physis.

SPRAINS, STRAINS AND RUPTURES

There is much confusion about the use of the terms 'sprain', 'strain' and 'rupture'. Strictly speaking, a *sprain* is any painful wrenching (twisting or pulling) movement of a joint, but the term is generally reserved for joint injuries less severe than actual tearing of the capsule or ligaments. *Strain* is a physical effect of stress, in this case tensile stress associated with some stretching of the ligaments; in colloquial usage, 'strained ligament' is often meant to denote an injury somewhat more severe than a 'sprain', which possibly involves tearing of some fibres. If the stretching or twisting force is severe enough, the ligament may be strained to the point of partial or complete *rupture*.

STRAINED LIGAMENT

Only some of the fibres in the ligament are torn and the joint remains stable. The injury is one in which the joint is momentarily twisted or bent into an abnormal position. The joint is painful and swollen and the tissues may be bruised. Tenderness is localized to the injured ligament and tensing the tissues on that side causes a sharp increase in pain.

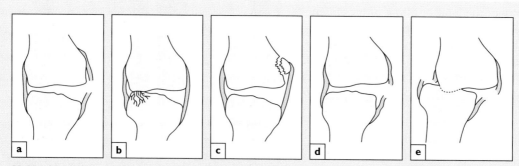

23.53 Joint injuries Severe stress may cause various types of injury. (**a**) A ligament may rupture, leaving the bone intact. If the soft tissues hold, the bone on the opposite side may be crushed (**b**), or a fragment may be pulled off by the taut ligament (**c**). Subluxation (**d**) means the articular surfaces are partially displaced; dislocation (**e**) refers to complete displacement of the joint.

Treatment The joint should be firmly strapped and rested until the acute pain subsides. Thereafter, active movements are encouraged, and exercises practised to strengthen the muscles.

RUPTURED LIGAMENT

The ligament is completely torn and the joint is unstable. Sometimes the ligament holds and the bone to which it is attached is avulsed; this is effectively the same lesion but easier to deal with because the bone fragment can be securely reattached.

As with a strain, the joint is suddenly forced into an abnormal position; sometimes the patient actually hears a snap. The joints most likely to be affected are the ones that are insecure by virtue of their shape or least well protected by surrounding muscles: the knee, the ankle and the finger joints.

Pain is severe and there may be considerable bleeding under the skin; if the joint is swollen, this is probably due to a haemarthrosis. The patient is unlikely to permit a searching examination, but under general anaesthesia the instability can be demonstrated; it is this that distinguishes the lesion from a strain. X-ray may show a detached flake of bone where the ligament is inserted.

Treatment

Torn ligaments heal by fibrous scarring. Previously this was thought inevitable and the surgeon's task was to ensure that the torn ends were securely sutured so as to restore the ligament to its normal length. In some injuries, for example rupture of the ulnar collateral ligament of the metacarpophalangeal joint of the thumb, this approach is still valid. In others, however, it has changed; thus, solitary collateral ligament injuries of the knee, even complete ruptures, are often treated non-operatively in the first instance. The joint is splinted and local measures are taken to reduce swelling. After 1–2 weeks, the splint is exchanged for a functional brace that allows joint movement but at the same time prevents repeated injury to the ligament, especially if some instability is also present. Physiotherapy is applied to maintain muscle strength and later proprioceptive exercises are added. This non-operative approach has shown better results not only in the strength of the healed ligament but also in the nature of healing – there is less fibrosis (Indelicato, 1983; Weiss *et al.*, 1991). An exception to this non-operative approach is when the ligament is avulsed with an attached fragment of bone; reattachment of the fragment is indicated if the piece is large enough. Occasionally non-operative treatment may result in some residual instability which is clinically detectable; often this is not symptomatic, but if it is then surgical reconstruction should be considered.

DISLOCATION AND SUBLUXATION

'Dislocation' means that the joint surfaces are completely displaced and are no longer in contact; 'subluxation' implies a lesser degree of displacement, such that the articular surfaces are still partly apposed.

Clinical features

Following an injury the joint is painful and the patient tries at all costs to avoid moving it. The shape of the joint is abnormal and the bony landmarks may be displaced. The limb is often held in a characteristic position; movement is painful and restricted. X-rays will usually clinch the diagnosis; they will also show whether there is an associated bony injury affecting joint stability – for example a fracture-dislocation.

The apprehension test If the dislocation is reduced by the time the patient is seen, the joint can be tested by stressing it as if almost to reproduce the suspected dislocation: the patient develops a sense of impending disaster and violently resists further manipulation.

Recurrent dislocation If the ligaments and joint margins are damaged, repeated dislocation may occur. This is seen especially in the shoulder and the patellofemoral joint.

Habitual (voluntary) dislocation Some patients acquire the knack of dislocating (or subluxating) the joint by voluntary muscle contraction. Ligamentous laxity may make this easier, but the habit often betrays a manipulative and neurotic personality. It is important to recognize this because such patients are seldom helped by operation.

Treatment

The dislocation must be reduced as soon as possible; usually a general anaesthetic is required, and sometimes a muscle relaxant as well. The joint is then rested or immobilized until soft-tissue healing occurs – usually after 3–4 weeks. If ligaments have been torn, they may have to be repaired.

Complications

Many of the complications of fractures are seen also after dislocations: vascular injury, nerve injury, avascular necrosis of bone, heterotopic ossification, joint stiffness and secondary osteoarthritis. The principles of diagnosis and management of these conditions have been discussed above.

REFERENCES AND FURTHER READING

Atkins RM, Duckworth T, Kanis JA (1990) Features of algodystrophy after Colles' fracture. *Journal of Bone and Joint Surgery* **72**B, 105-110

Bowyer GW, Rossiter ND (1997) Management of gunshot wounds of the limbs. *Journal of Bone and Joint Surgery* **79**B, 1031-1036

Browner BD, Jupiter JB, Levine AM, Trafton PG (1998) *Skeletal Trauma: Fractures, dislocations, ligamentous injuries* 2nd edition. WB Saunders Company, Philadelphia

Charnley J (1961) *The Closed Treatment of Common Fractures* 3rd edition. Churchill Livingstone, Edinburgh

Court-Brown CM, Cross AT, Hahn DM *et al* (1997) *A Report of the BOA/BAPS Working Party on the Management of Open Tibial Fractures*

Gustilo RB, Merkow RL, Templeman D (1990) Current concepts: the management of open fractures. *Journal of Bone and Joint Surgery* **72**A, 299-304

Hosono N, Yonenobu K, Fuji T (1995) Orthopaedic management of spinal metastases. *Clinical Orthopaedics* **312**, 148-159

Ilizarov GA. (1992) *Transosseous Osteosynthesis*. Springer Verlag, Berlin, Heidelberg and New York

Indelicato PA (1983) Non-operative treatment of complete tears of the medial collateral ligament of the knee. *Journal of Bone and Joint Surgery* **65**A, 323-329

Keating JF, Blatchut PA, O'Brien PJ, Court-Brown CM (2000) Reamed nailing of Gustilo grade-IIIB tibial fractures. *Journal of Bone and Joint Injury.* **82**B, 1113–1116

Kenwright J, Richardson JB, Cunningham JL *et al* (1991) Axial micromovement and tibial fractures. *Journal of Bone and Joint Surgery* **73**B, 654-659

Langenskiold A (1975) An operation for partial closure of an epiphyseal plate in children and its experimental basis. *Journal of Bone and Joint Surgery* **57**B, 325-330

Langenskiold A (1981) Surgical treatment of partial closure of the growth plate. *Journal of Paediatric Orthopaedics* **1**, 3-11

Leyvraz PF, Bachmann F, Hoek J *et al* (1991) Prevention of deep vein thrombosis after hip replacement: randomised comparison between unfractionated heparin and low molecular weight heparin. *British Medical Journal* **303**, 543-548

McKibbin B (1978) The biology of fracture healing in long bones. *Journal of Bone and Joint Surgery* **60**B, 150-162

Müller ME, Allgower M, Schneider R, Willeneger H (1991) *Manual of Internal Fixation* 3rd edition. Springer Verlag, Berlin, Heidelberg and New York

Müller ME, Nazarian S, Koch P, Schatzker J (1990) *The Comprehensive Classification of Fractures of Long Bones.* Springer Verlag, Berlin, Heidelberg and New York

Phillips TF, Contreras DM (1990) Timing of operative treatment of fractures in patients who have multiple injuries. *Journal of Bone and Joint Surgery* **72**B, 620-621

Rang M (1969) *The Growth Plate and its Disorders*. Churchill Livingstone, Edinburgh

Salter RB, Harris WR (1963) Injuries involving the epiphyseal plate. *Journal of Bone and Joint Surgery* **45**A, 587-622

Sarmiento A, Latta LL (1981) *Closed Functional Treatment of Fractures*. Springer Verlag, Berlin, Heidelberg and New York

Siegel D, Gelberman RH (1991) Peripheral nerve injuries associated with fractures and dislocations. In *Operative Nerve Repair and Reconstruction* (ed. Gelberman RH). JB Lippincott, Philadelphia

Tscherne H (1984) The management of open fractures. In *Fractures with Soft Tissue Injuries* (eds Tscherne H, Gotzen L). Springer, Berlin

Weiss JA, Woo SL-Y, Ohland KJ *et al* (1991) Evaluation of a new injury model to study medial collateral ligament healing: Primary repair versus non-operative treatment. *Journal of Orthopaedic Research* **9**, 516-528

Injuries of the shoulder, upper arm and elbow

The great bugbear of upper limb injuries is stiffness – particularly of the shoulder but sometimes of the elbow and hand as well. Two points should be constantly borne in mind:

- Whatever the injury, and however it is treated, all the joints that are not actually immobilized – and especially the finger joints – should be exercised from the start.
- In elderly patients it is sometimes best to disregard the fracture and concentrate on regaining movement.

FRACTURES OF THE CLAVICLE

In children the clavicle fractures easily, but it almost invariably unites rapidly and without complications. In adults this can be a much more troublesome injury.

Mechanism of injury

A fall on the shoulder or the outstretched hand may break the clavicle. In the common mid-shaft fracture, the outer fragment is pulled down by the weight of the arm and the inner half is held up by the sternomastoid muscle. In fractures of the outer end, if the ligaments are intact there is little displacement; but if the coracoclavicular ligaments are torn, or if the fracture is just medial to these ligaments, displacement may be severe and closed reduction impossible.

Clinical features

The arm is clasped to the chest to prevent movement. A subcutaneous lump may be obvious and occasionally a sharp fragment threatens the skin. Though vascular complications are rare, it is prudent to feel the pulse and gently to palpate the root of the neck. Outer third fractures are easily missed or mistaken for acromio-clavicular joint injuries.

X RAY

The fracture is usually in the middle third of the bone, and the outer fragment lies below the inner. A fracture of the outer third may be missed, or the degree of displacement underestimated, unless additional views of the shoulder are obtained. Clinical union usually precedes radiological union by some weeks.

Treatment

MIDDLE THIRD FRACTURES

Accurate reduction is neither possible nor essential. All that is needed is to support the arm in a sling until the pain subsides (usually 2–3 weeks). Thereafter active shoulder exercises should be encouraged; this is particularly important in older patients. In those for whom a gross deformity would be unacceptable, closed reduction by passively bracing back the shoulders and then applying a figure of eight bandage can be attempted. Internal fixation is rarely required – it may even

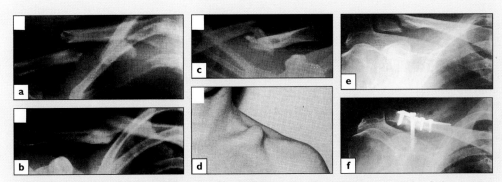

24.1 Fractured clavicle (a) The common site and displacement. (b) Uniting in a somewhat faulty position. (c) Comminuted fracture which united in this position leaving (d) a large lump. (e) Fracture of the outer (lateral) third with elevation of the shaft of the clavicle due to rupture of the medial part of the coracoclavicular ligament. This was treated by open reduction and internal fixation (f), using a long screw to fix the clavicle to the coracoid process.

increase the chance of non-union. Indications for internal fixation include open fractures and those with neurovascular compromise that fails to recover.

OUTER THIRD FRACTURES

Undisplaced outer third fractures, with ligaments intact, need no more than a sling for 2 or 3 weeks.

Displaced outer third fractures are associated with tears or detachment of the coracoclavicular ligament and usually cannot be reduced closed; the end of the medial fragment may be buried in the trapezius muscle. Left untreated, they cause deformity and often result in non-union with discomfort and weakness of the shoulder. Operative treatment is therefore indicated. Through a supraclavicular incision the fragments are reduced; if displacement is not marked and the apposed fragments seem stable, they can be held with two smooth pins which are passed laterally through the outer fragment and the acromion, and then back into the clavicular shaft; if necessary this can be reinforced with a tension band wire. The arm is held in a sling for 6 weeks and thereafter the pins are removed and full movement is encouraged. If displacement is marked and the fragments unstable, the clavicular shaft can be drawn downwards and fixed to the coracoid process with strong sutures or a screw (see Fig. 24.1f).

Complications

EARLY
Despite the close proximity of the clavicle to vital structures, a pneumothorax, damage to the subclavian vessels and brachial plexus injuries are all very rare.

LATE
Non-union A midshaft fracture rarely fails to unite unless someone has been unwise enough to operate on it. Displaced outer third fractures carry a significant risk of non-union; if this occurs, it can be treated by internal fixation and bone grafting.

Malunion A healed clavicular fracture often leaves a lump; in a child this always disappears in time, and in an adult it usually does. Someone anxious to obtain a good cosmetic result quickly may be willing to undergo more drastic treatment: the fracture is manually reduced under anaesthesia and held reduced by a plaster cuirass. Patients should be dissuaded from surgery because there is a risk of neurovascular damage and the bump can be replaced by non-union; furthermore, the operation may leave an unsightly scar.

Stiffness of the shoulder This is common but temporary; it results from fear of moving a fracture. Unless the fingers are exercised, they also may become stiff and take months to regain movement.

FRACTURES OF THE SCAPULA

MECHANISMS OF INJURY

The *body of the scapula* is fractured by a crushing force, which usually also fractures ribs and may dislocate the sternoclavicular joint. The *neck of the scapula* may be fractured by a blow or by a fall on the shoulder. The *coracoid process* may fracture across its base or be avulsed at the tip. *Fracture of the acromion* is due to direct force. *Fracture of the glenoid* may occur with dislocation of the shoulder.

Clinical features

The arm is held immobile and there may be severe bruising over the scapula or the chest wall. Because of the energy required to damage the scapula, fractures of the body of the scapula are often associated with severe injuries to the chest, brachial plexus, spine, abdomen and head.

X RAY
Fractures can be difficult to define on plain x-rays because of the surrounding soft tissues. The films may reveal a comminuted fracture of the body of the scapula, or a fractured scapular neck with the outer fragment pulled downwards by the weight of the arm. Occasionally a crack is seen in the acromion or the coracoid process. CT is useful for demonstrating glenoid fractures or body fractures.

Treatment

Neck fractures The fracture is usually impacted and the glenoid surface is intact. A sling is worn for comfort and early exercises begun.

Glenoid fractures If there is a fragment greater than 25% of the glenoid surface, particularly if dislocation was

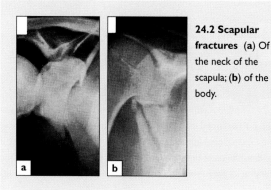

24.2 Scapular fractures (a) Of the neck of the scapula; **(b)** of the body.

the mechanism of injury, then internal fixation should be considered.

Body fractures Surgery is not necessary. The patient wears a sling for comfort, and from the start practises active exercises to the shoulder, elbow and fingers.

Acromion fractures Here again, non-operative treatment and early mobilization is usually appropriate.

SCAPULOTHORACIC DISSOCIATION

This is a high-energy injury. The scapula and arm are wrenched away from the chest, rupturing the subclavian vessels and brachial plexus. Many patients die.

Clinical features

The limb is flail and ischaemic. The diagnosis is usually made on the chest x-ray There is swelling above the clavicle from an expanding haematoma.

Treatment

The patient is resuscitated. The outcome for the upper limb is very poor. Neither vascular reconstruction nor brachial plexus exploration and repair are likely to give a functional limb.

ACROMIOCLAVICULAR JOINT INJURIES

Acute injury of the acromioclavicular joint is common and usually follows direct trauma. *Chronic sprains*, often associated with degenerative changes, are seen in people engaged in athletic activities like weightlifting or occupations such as working with jack-hammers and other heavy vibrating tools.

Mechanism of injury

A fall on the shoulder with the arm adducted may strain or tear the acromioclavicular ligaments and upwards subluxation of the clavicle may occur; if the force is severe enough, the coracoclavicular ligaments also may be torn, resulting in complete dislocation of the joint.

Pathological anatomy and classification

The injury is graded according to the type of ligament injury and the amount of displacement of the joint. *Type I* is an acute sprain of the acromioclavicular ligaments; the joint is undisplaced. In *type II* the acromioclavicular ligaments are torn and the joint is subluxated with slight elevation of the clavicle. In *type III* the acromioclavicular and coracoclavicular ligaments are torn and the joint is dislocated; the clavicle is elevated (or the acromion depressed) creating a visible and palpable 'step'. Other types of displacement are less common, but occasionally the clavicle is displaced posteriorly (*type IV)*, very markedly upwards (*type V*) or inferiorly beneath the coracoid process (*type VI*).

Clinical features

The patient can usually point to the site of injury and the area may be bruised. If there is tenderness but no deformity, the injury is probably a sprain or a subluxation. With dislocation the patient is in severe pain and a prominent 'step' can be seen and felt. Shoulder movements are limited.

X-RAY
The acromioclavicular joint is not always easily visualized; anteroposterior, cephalic tilt and axillary views

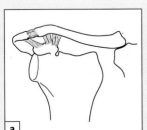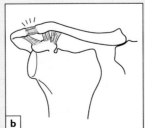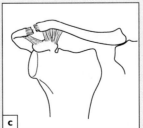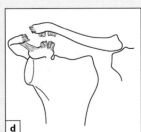

24.3 Acromioclavicular joint injuries (**a**) Normal joint. (**b**) Sprained acromioclavicular joint; no displacement. (**c**) Torn capsule and subluxation but coracoclavicular ligaments intact. (**d**) Dislocation with torn coracoclavicular ligaments.

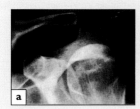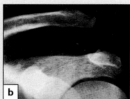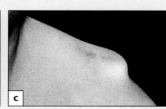

24.4 Acromioclavicular joint
(a) With subluxation, deformity is slight. (b, c) With complete dislocation, displacement is marked.

are advisable. In addition, a stress view is sometimes helpful in distinguishing between a type II and type III injury: this is an anteroposterior x-ray including both shoulders with the patient standing upright, arms by the side and holding a 5kg weight in each hand. The distance between the coracoid process and the inferior border of the clavicle is measured on each side; a difference of more than 50% is diagnostic of acromioclavicular dislocation.

Treatment

Sprains and subluxations do not affect function and do not require any special treatment; the arm is rested in a sling until pain subsides (usually no more than a week) and shoulder exercises are then begun.

Dislocations are poorly controlled by padding and bandaging, yet the role of surgery is controversial. The large variety of operations suggests that none is ideal. There is no convincing evidence that surgery provides a better functional result than conservative treatment for a straightforward type III injury. Operative repair should be considered only for patients with extreme prominence of the clavicle, those with posterior or inferior dislocation of the clavicle and those who aim to resume strenuous overarm or overhead activities. A well-tried technique is to repair the coracoclavicular ligaments and hold the reduction with a temporary coracoclavicular screw. The shoulder is rested for 2 weeks and exercises are then encouraged. The screw is removed after 8 weeks.

Complications

Rotator cuff syndrome An acute strain of the acromioclavicular joint is sometimes followed by supraspinatus tendinitis. Whether this is directly due to the primary injury or whether it results from post-traumatic oedema or inflammation of the overlying acromioclavicular joint is unclear. Treatment with anti-inflammatory preparations may help.

Unreduced dislocation An unreduced dislocation is ugly and sometimes affects function. Simple excision of the distal clavicle will only make matters worse. An attempt should be made to reconstruct the coraco-clavicular ligament. In the Weaver Dunn procedure, the coracoacromial ligament is detached from the acromion and fixed into the distal end of the clavicle; the acromioclavicular joint is fully reduced and held temporarily by an acromioclavicular screw.

Ossification of the ligaments The more severe injuries are quite often followed by ossification of the coracoclavicular ligaments. Bony spurs may predispose to later rotator cuff dysfunction, which may require operative treatment.

Secondary osteoarthritis A late complication of type I and II injuries is osteoarthritis of the acromioclavicular joint. This can usually be managed conservatively, but if pain is marked the outer 2cm of the clavicle can be excised. The patient will be aware of some weakness during strenuous overarm activities and pain is often not completely abolished.

STERNOCLAVICULAR DISLOCATIONS

Mechanism of injury

This uncommon injury is usually caused by lateral compression of the shoulders; for example, when someone is pinned to the ground following a road accident or an underground rock-fall. Rarely, it follows a direct blow to the front of the joint. Anterior dislocation is much more common than posterior. The joint can be sprained, subluxed or dislocated.

Clinical features

Anterior dislocation is easily diagnosed; the dislocated medial end of the clavicle forms a prominent bump over the sternoclavicular joint. The condition is painful but there are usually no cardiothoracic complications.

Posterior dislocation, though rare, is much more serious. Discomfort is marked; there may be pressure on the trachea or large vessels, causing venous congestion of the neck and arm, and circulation to the arm may be decreased.

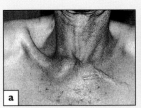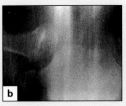

24.5 Sternoclavicular joint (a) Anterior dislocation is clinically obvious though difficult to demonstrate on plain x-rays. A tomogram shows the displacement well, though a CT would have been even better.

X-RAY
Because of overlapping shadows, plain x-rays are difficult to interpret. Special oblique views are helpful and CT is the ideal method.

Treatment

Sprains and subluxations do not require specific treatment.

Anterior dislocation can usually be reduced by exerting pressure over the clavicle and pulling on the arm with the shoulder abducted. However, the joint usually redislocates. Not that this matters much; full function will be regained, though this may take several months.

Internal fixation is unnecessary and very dangerous (because of the large vessels behind the sternum).

Posterior dislocation should be reduced as soon as possible. This can usually be done closed (if necessary under general anaesthesia) by positioning the patient supine with a sandbag between the scapulae and then pulling on the arm with the shoulder abducted and extended. The joint reduces with a snap and stays reduced. If this manoeuvre fails, the medial end of the clavicle is grasped with bone forceps and pulled forwards. If this, too, fails (a very rare occurrence) open reduction is justified, but great care must be taken not to damage the mediastinal structures. After reduction, the shoulders are braced back with a figure-of-eight bandage, which is worn for 3 weeks.

DISLOCATION OF THE SHOULDER

Of the large joints, the shoulder is the one that most commonly dislocates. This is due to a number of factors: the shallowness of the glenoid socket; the extraordinary range of movement; underlying conditions such as ligamentous laxity or glenoid dysplasia; and the sheer vulnerability of the joint during stressful activities of the upper limb.

In this chapter, acute anterior and posterior dislocations are described. Chronic instability is described in Chapter 13.

ANTERIOR DISLOCATION

Mechanism of injury

Dislocation is usually caused by a fall on the hand. The humerus is driven forwards, tearing the capsule or avulsing the glenoid labrum. Occasionally the posterolateral part of the head is crushed. Rarely, the acromion process levers the head downwards and *luxatio erecta* (with the arm pointing upwards) results; nearly always the arm then drops, bringing the head to its subcoracoid position.

Clinical features

Pain is severe. The patient supports the arm with the opposite hand and is loath to permit any kind of examination. The lateral outline of the shoulder may be flattened and, if the patient is not too muscular, a bulge may be felt just below the clavicle. The arm must always be examined for nerve and vessel injury before reduction is attempted.

X-RAY
The anteroposterior x-ray will show the overlapping shadows of the humeral head and glenoid fossa, with the head usually lying below and medial to the socket. A lateral view aimed along the blade of the scapula will show the humeral head out of line with the socket.

If the joint has dislocated before, special views may show flattening or an excavation of the posterolateral contour of the humeral head, where it has been indented by the anterior edge of the glenoid socket.

Treatment

Various methods of reduction have been described, some of them now of no more than historical interest. In a patient who has had previous dislocations, simple traction on the arm may be successful. Usually, sedation and occasionally general anaesthesia is required.

With *Stimson's technique*, the patient is left prone with the arm hanging over the side of the bed. After 15 or 20 minutes the shoulder may reduce.

In the *Hippocratic method*, gently increasing traction is applied to the arm with the shoulder in slight abduction, while an assistant applies firm counter-traction to the body (a towel slung around the patient's chest, under the axilla, is helpful).

With *Kocher's method*, the elbow is bent to 90° and held close to the body; no traction should be applied.

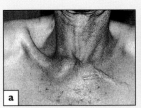

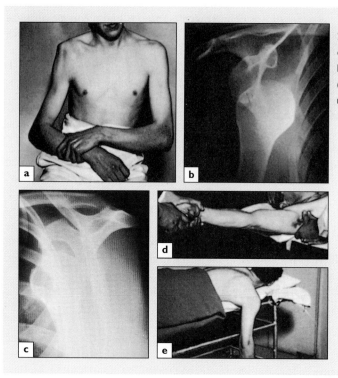

24.6 Anterior dislocation of the shoulder (a) The typical clinical picture. (b) Anteroposterior x-ray showing the humeral head lying below and medial to the glenoid socket. (c) Lateral trans-scapular view showing the humeral head anterior to the socket. (d, e) Two methods of reduction.

The arm is slowly rotated 75° laterally, then the point of the elbow is lifted forwards and finally the arm is rotated medially. This technique carries the risk of nerve, vessel and bone injury and is not recommended.

An x-ray is taken to confirm reduction and exclude a fracture. When the patient is fully awake, active abduction is gently tested to exclude an axillary nerve injury and rotator cuff tear. The median, radial, ulnar and musculocutaneous nerves are also tested and the pulse is felt.

The arm is rested in a sling for about 3 weeks in those under 30 years of age (who are most prone to recurrence) and for only a week in those over 30 (who are most prone to stiffness). Then movements are begun, but combined abduction and lateral rotation must be avoided for at least 3 weeks. Throughout this period, elbow and finger movements are practised every day.

Complications

EARLY

Rotator cuff tear This commonly accompanies anterior dislocation, particularly in older people. The patient may have difficulty abducting the arm after reduction; palpable contraction of the deltoid muscle excludes an axillary nerve palsy. Most do not require surgical attention, but young active individuals with large tears will benefit from early repair.

Nerve injury The axillary nerve is most commonly injured; the patient is unable to contract the deltoid muscle and there may be a small patch of anaesthesia over the muscle. The inability to abduct must be distinguished from a rotator cuff tear. The nerve lesion is usually a neuropraxia which recovers spontaneously after a few weeks; if it does not, then surgery should be considered as the results of repair are less satisfactory if the delay is more than a few months.

Occasionally the radial nerve, musculocutaneous nerve, median nerve or ulnar nerve can be injured. Rarely there is a complete infraclavicular brachial plexus palsy. This is somewhat alarming, but fortunately it usually recovers with time.

Vascular injury The axillary artery may be damaged, particularly in old patients with fragile vessels. This can occur either at the time of injury or during overzealous reduction. The limb should always be examined for signs of ischaemia both before and after reduction.

Fracture-dislocation If there is an associated fracture of the proximal humerus, open reduction and internal fixation may be necessary. The greater tuberosity may be sheared off during dislocation. It usually falls into place during reduction, and no special treatment is then required. If it remains displaced, surgical reattachment is recommended to avoid later subacromial impingement.

LATE

Shoulder stiffness Prolonged immobilization may lead to stiffness of the shoulder, especially in patients over the age of 40 years. There is loss of lateral rotation, which automatically limits abduction. Active exercises will usually loosen the joint. They are practised vigorously, bearing in mind that full abduction is not possible until lateral rotation has been regained. Manipulation under anaesthesia is advised only if progress has halted and at least 6 months have elapsed since injury. Lateral rotation should be restored before abduction, and the manipulation should be gentle and repeated rather than forceful.

Unreduced dislocation Surprisingly, a dislocation of the shoulder sometimes remains undiagnosed. This is more likely if the patient is either unconscious or very old. Closed reduction is worth attempting up to 6 weeks after injury; manipulation later may fracture the bone or tear vessels or nerves. Operative reduction is indicated after 6 weeks only in the young, because it is difficult, dangerous and followed by prolonged stiffness. An anterior approach is used, and the vessels and nerves are carefully identified before the dislocation is reduced. 'Active neglect' summarizes the treatment of unreduced dislocation in the elderly. The dislocation is disregarded and gentle active movements are encouraged. Moderately good function is often regained.

Recurrent dislocation If an anterior dislocation tears the shoulder capsule, repair occurs spontaneously following reduction and the dislocation does not recur; but if, instead, the glenoid labrum is detached, or the capsule

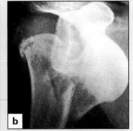

24.7 Anterior fracture-dislocation Anterior dislocation of the shoulder may be complicated by fracture of (**a**) the greater tuberosity or (**b**) the neck of the humerus – this often needs open reduction and internal fixation.

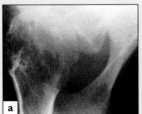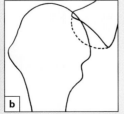

24.8 Recurrent subluxation X-ray showing anterior subluxation; the humeral head is riding on the lip of the glenoid.

is stripped off the front of the neck of the glenoid, repair is less likely and recurrence common. Detachment of the labrum occurs particularly in young patients, and, if at injury a bony defect has been gouged out of the posterolateral aspect of the humeral head, recurrence is even more likely. In older patients, especially if there is a rotator cuff tear or greater tuberosity fracture, recurrent dislocation is unlikely. The period of post-operative immobilization makes no difference.

The history is diagnostic. The patient complains that the shoulder dislocates with relatively trivial everyday actions. Often he can reduce the dislocation himself. Any doubt as to diagnosis is quickly resolved by the apprehension test: if the patient's arm is passively placed behind the coronal plane in a position of abduction and lateral rotation, his or her immediate resistance and apprehension are pathognomonic.

Even more common, but less readily diagnosed, is *recurrent subluxation*. The management of both types of instability is dealt with in Chapter 13.

POSTERIOR DISLOCATION OF THE SHOULDER

Posterior dislocation is rare, accounting for less than 2% of all dislocations around the shoulder.

Mechanism of injury

Indirect force producing marked internal rotation and adduction needs be very severe to cause a dislocation. This happens most commonly during a fit or convulsion, or with an electric shock. Posterior dislocation can also follow a fall on to the flexed, adducted arm, a direct blow to the front of the shoulder or a fall on the outstretched hand.

Clinical features

The diagnosis is frequently missed – partly because reliance is placed on a single anteroposterior x-ray (which may look almost normal) and partly because those attending to the patient failed to think of it. There are, in fact, several well-marked clinical features. The arm is held in medial rotation and is locked in that position. The front of the shoulder looks flat with a prominent coracoid, but swelling may obscure this deformity; seen from above, however, the posterior displacement is usually apparent.

X-RAY

In the anteroposterior film the humeral head, because it is medially rotated, looks abnormal in shape (like an electric light bulb) and it stands away somewhat from the glenoid fossa (the 'empty glenoid' sign). A lateral film is essential; it shows posterior subluxation or dislocation and sometimes a deep indentation on the anterior aspect of the humeral head. Posterior dislocation is sometimes complicated by fractures of the humeral neck, posterior glenoid rim or lesser tuberosity.

In difficult cases CT is helpful.

Treatment

The acute dislocation is reduced (usually under general anaesthesia) by pulling on the arm with the shoulder in adduction; a few minutes are allowed for the head of the humerus to disengage and the arm is then gently rotated laterally while the humeral head is pushed forwards. If reduction feels stable the arm is immobilized in a sling; otherwise the shoulder is held widely abducted and laterally rotated in a plaster spica for 3 weeks to allow the posterior capsule to heal in the shortest position. Shoulder movement is regained by active exercises.

Complications

Unreduced dislocation At least half the patients with posterior dislocation have 'unreduced' lesions when first seen. Sometimes weeks or months elapse before the diagnosis is made. Typically the patient holds the arm internally rotated; he or she cannot abduct the arm more than 70–80°, and if he lifts the extended arm forwards he cannot then turn the palm upwards. If the patient is young, or is uncomfortable and the dislocation fairly recent (say up to 8 weeks old), open reduction is indicated. Through a posterior approach, capsular repair and reefing are performed. Late dislocations, especially in the elderly, are best left, but movement is encouraged.

Recurrent dislocation or subluxation Chronic posterior instability of the shoulder is discussed in Chapter 13.

INFERIOR DISLOCATION OF THE SHOULDER (*LUXATIO ERECTA*)

Inferior dislocation is rare but it demands early recognition because the consequences are potentially very serious. Dislocation occurs with the arm in nearly full abduction/elevation. The humeral head is levered out of its socket and pokes into the axilla; the arm remains fixed in abduction.

Mechanism of injury and pathology

The injury is caused by a severe hyperabduction force. With the humerus as the lever and the acromion as the fulcrum, the humeral head is lifted across the infe-

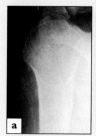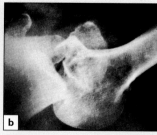

24.9 Posterior dislocation of the shoulder (a) The antero-posterior view may look almost normal, but the humeral head is globe-shaped; (b) the lateral view shows obvious dislocation.

rior rim of the glenoid socket; it remains in the sub-glenoid position, with the humeral shaft pointing upwards. Soft-tissue injury may be severe and includes avulsion of the capsule and surrounding tendons, rupture of muscles, fractures of the glenoid or proximal humerus and damage to the brachial plexus and axillary artery.

Clinical features

The startling picture of a patient with his or her arm locked in almost full abduction should make diagnosis quite easy. The head of the humerus may be felt in or below the axilla. *Always examine for neurovascular damage.*

X-RAY

The humeral shaft is shown in the abducted position with the head sitting below the glenoid. It is important to search for associated fractures of the glenoid or proximal humerus.

NOTE: True inferior dislocation must not be confused with postural downwards displacement of the humerus, which results quite commonly from weakness and laxity of the muscles around the shoulder, especially after trauma and shoulder splintage; here the shaft of

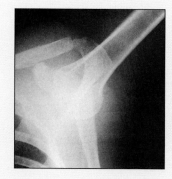

24.10 Inferior dislocation of the shoulder You can see why the condition is called *luxatio erecta*. The shaft of the humerus points upwards and the humeral head is displaced downwards.

the humerus lies in the normal anatomical position at the side of the chest. The condition is harmless and resolves as muscle tone is regained.

Treatment

Inferior dislocation can usually be reduced by pulling upwards in the line of the abducted arm, with counter-traction downwards over the top of the shoulder. If the humeral head is stuck in the soft tissues, open reduction is needed. *It is important to examine again, after reduction, for evidence of neurovascular injury.*

The arm is rested in a sling until pain subsides and movement is then allowed, but avoiding abduction for 3 weeks to allow the soft tissues to heal.

SHOULDER DISLOCATIONS IN CHILDREN

Traumatic dislocation of the shoulder is exceedingly rare in children. Children who give a history of the shoulder 'slipping out' almost invariably have either voluntary or involuntary (atraumatic) dislocation or subluxation. With *voluntary dislocation,* the child can demonstrate the instability at will. With *involuntary dislocation,* the shoulder slips out unexpectedly during everyday activities. Most of these children have gener-alized joint laxity and some have glenoid dysplasia. Examination may show that the shoulder subluxates in almost any direction (multidirectional instability). X-rays may confirm the diagnosis.

Treatment

Atraumatic dislocation should be viewed with great caution. Some of these children have behavioral prob-lems and this is where treatment should be directed. A prolonged exercise programme may also help. Only if the child is genuinely distressed by the disorder, and provided psychological factors have been excluded, should one consider reconstructive surgery – usually a meticulous reefing procedure

FRACTURES OF THE PROXIMAL HUMERUS

Fractures of the proximal humerus usually occur after middle age and are most common in osteoporotic, post-menopausal women. In the majority of cases displace-ment is not marked and treatment presents few problems. However, in about 20% there is considerable displacement of one or more fragments and a signifi-cant risk of complications.

Mechanism of injury

Fracture usually follows a fall on the out-stretched arm – the type of injury which, in younger people, might cause dislocation of the shoulder. Sometimes, indeed, there is both a fracture and a dislocation.

Pathological anatomy and classification

The most widely accepted classification is that of Neer (1970), who drew attention to the four major segments involved in these injuries: the head of the humerus, the lesser tuberosity, the greater tuberosity and the shaft. Neer's classification distinguishes between the number of displaced fragments, with displacement defined as greater than 45° of angulation or 1cm of separation. Thus, however many fracture lines there are, if the fragments are undisplaced it is regarded as a *one-part fracture;* if one segment is separated from the others, it is a *two-part fracture;* if two fragments are displaced, that is a *three-part fracture;* if all the major parts are displaced, it is *a four-part fracture.* Furthermore, a *fracture-dislocation* exists when the head is dislocated and there are two, three or four parts. The grading is based on x-ray appearances, although observers do not always agree with each other on which class a particular fracture falls into.

Neer's classification is helpful because it correlates fairly well with the outcome and gives a guide to treat-ment. Minimally displaced fractures cause few prob-lems; two-part fractures can usually be managed by closed reduction; three-part fractures are difficult to reduce and may need internal fixation; and four-part fractures, which generally have a poor outcome, are usually best treated by prosthetic replacement.

Clinical features

As the fracture is often firmly impacted, pain may not be severe. However, the appearance of a large bruise on the upper part of the arm is suspicious. Signs of axillary nerve or brachial plexus injury should be sought.

X-RAY

In *elderly* patients there often appears to be a single, impacted fracture extending across the surgical neck. However, with good x-rays, several undisplaced frag-ments may be seen. In *younger* patients, the fragments are usually more clearly separated.

Axillary and scapular-lateral views should always be obtained, to exclude dislocation of the shoulder. A CT scan is helpful in difficult cases.

As the fracture heals, the humeral head is sometimes seen to be subluxed downwards (inferiorly); this is due to muscle atony and it usually recovers once exercises are begun.

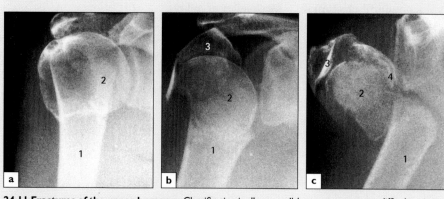

24.11 Fractures of the upper humerus Classification is all very well, but x-rays are more difficult to interpret than line drawings. **(a)** Two-part fracture. **(b)** Three-part fracture involving the neck and the greater tuberosity. **(c)** Four-part fracture. (1 = shaft of humerus; 2 = head of humerus; 3 = greater tuberosity; 4 = lesser tuberosity).

Treatment

MINIMALLY DISPLACED FRACTURES

These comprise the vast majority. They need no treatment apart from a week or two period of rest with the arm in a sling until the pain subsides, and then gentle passive movements of the shoulder. Once the fracture has united (usually after 6 weeks), active exercises are encouraged; the hand is, of course, actively exercised from the start.

TWO-PART FRACTURES

Surgical neck fractures The fragments are gently manipulated into alignment and the arm is immobilized in a sling for about 4 weeks or until the fracture feels stable and the x-ray shows some signs of healing. Elbow and hand exercises are encouraged throughout this period; shoulder exercises are commenced at about 4 weeks. The results of conservative treatment are generally satisfactory, considering that most of these patients are over 65 years of age and do not demand perfect function. However, if the fracture cannot be reduced closed or if the fracture is very unstable after closed reduction, then fixation is required. Options include percutaneous pins, bone sutures, intramedullary pins with tension-band wiring or a locked intramedullary nail. Plate fixation requires a wide exposure and often fails because of the soft bone; it is not widely recommended.

Greater tuberosity fractures Fracture of the greater tuberosity is often associated with anterior dislocation and it reduces to a good position when the shoulder is relocated. If it does not reduce, the fragment can be re-attached through a small incision with interosseous sutures or, in young hard bone, cancellous screws.

Anatomical neck fractures These are very rare. In young patients the fracture should be fixed with a screw. In older patients prosthetic repacement (hemi-arthroplasty) is preferable because of the high risk of avascular necrosis of the humeral head.

THREE-PART FRACTURES

These usually involve displacement of the surgical neck and the greater tuberosity; they are extremely difficult to reduce closed. In active individuals this injury is best managed by open reduction and internal fixation. A plate can be used but this is technically demanding and liable to fail, particularly in older, soft bone. An alternative is multiple interosseous sutures.

FOUR-PART FRACTURES

The surgical neck and both tuberosities are displaced. These are severe injuries with a high risk of complications such as vascular injury, brachial plexus damage, injuries of the chest wall and (later) avascular necrosis of the humeral head. The x-ray diagnosis is difficult (how many fragments are there, and are they displaced?). Often the most one can say is that there are 'multiple displaced fragments', sometimes together with glenohumeral dislocation. In young patients an attempt may be made at reconstruction with multiple wires and interosseous sutures; the outcome is generally poor. In older patients, closed treatment and attempts at open reduction and fixation usually result in continuing pain and stiffness; the treatment of choice is prosthetic replacement of the proximal humerus.

FRACTURE-DISLOCATION

Two-part fracture-dislocations (greater tuberosity with anterior dislocation and lesser tuberosity with posterior) can usually be reduced by closed means.

Three-part fracture-dislocations, when the surgical neck is also broken, usually require open reduction and fixation; the brachial plexus is at particular risk during this operation.

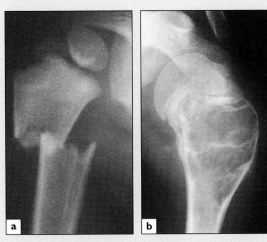

24.12 Fractures of the proximal humerus in children
(**a**) The typical metaphyseal fracture. Reduction need not be perfect as remodelling will compensate for malunion. (**b**) Fracture through a benign cyst.

Four-part fracture-dislocations have a poor prognosis; prosthetic replacement is recommended in all but young and very active patients.

Complications

Vascular injuries and nerve injuries should be sought at the initial examination. The axillary nerve is at particular risk, both from the injury and from surgery.

Stiffness of the shoulder is common; it can be prevented, or at least minimized, by starting exercises early. Unlike a frozen shoulder, the stiffness is maximal at the outset.

Malunion is not uncommon. It usually causes little disability, but loss of rotation may make it difficult to reach behind the neck or up the back.

Avascular necrosis of the head of the humerus occurs in about 10% of three-part fractures and 20% of four-part fractures. The extensive soft-tissue dissection needed to internally fix these fractures will increase the risk, particularly if the arcuate artery is damaged as it runs up alongside the bicipital groove.

SPECIAL FEATURES IN CHILDREN

At birth, the shoulder is sometimes dislocated or the proximal humerus fractured. Diagnosis is difficult and a clavicular fracture or brachial plexus injury should also be considered.

In infancy, the physis can separate (Salter–Harris I); reduction does not have to be perfect and a good outcome is usual.

In older children, metaphyseal fractures or type II physeal fractures occur. Considerable displacement and

angulation can be accepted; because of the marked growth and remodelling potential of the proximal humerus, malunion is readily compensated for during the remaining growth period.

Pathological fractures are not unusual, as the proximal humerus is a common site of bone cysts and tumours in children. Fracture through a simple cyst usually unites and the cyst often heals spontaneously; all that is needed is to rest the arm in a sling for 4–6 weeks. Other lesions require treatment in their own right.

FRACTURED SHAFT OF HUMERUS

Mechanism of injury

A fall on the hand may twist the humerus, causing a spiral fracture. A fall on the elbow with the arm abducted exerts a bending force, resulting in an oblique or transverse fracture. A direct blow to the arm causes a fracture which is either transverse or comminuted. Fracture of the shaft in an elderly patient may be due to a metastasis.

Pathological anatomy

With fractures above the deltoid insertion, the proximal fragment is adducted by pectoralis major. With fractures lower down, the proximal fragment is abducted by the deltoid. Injury to the radial nerve is common, though fortunately recovery is usual.

Clinical features

The arm is painful, bruised and swollen. It is important to test for radial nerve function *before and after treatment*. This is best done by assessing active extension of the metacarpophalangeal joints; active extension of the wrist can be misleading because extensor carpi radialis longus is sometimes supplied by a branch arising proximal to the injury.

X-RAY
The site of the fracture, its line (transverse, spiral or comminuted) and any displacement are readily seen. The possibility that the fracture may be pathological should be remembered.

Treatment

Fractures of the humerus heal readily. They require neither perfect reduction nor immobilization; the weight of the arm with an external cast is usually enough to pull the fragments into alignment. A 'hanging cast' is

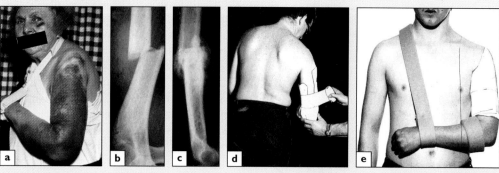

24.13 Fractured shaft of humerus (a) The tell-tale bruise. (b, c) Transverse fracture with only moderate displacement. (d) A U-slab of plaster (after a few days in a shoulder-to-wrist hanging cast) is usually adequate. (e) A ready-made functional brace is simpler and more comfortable, though it is not suitable for all cases.

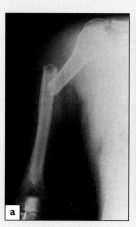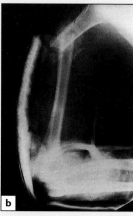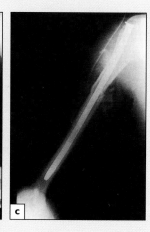

24.14 Fractured shaft of humerus – treatment (a, b) Most shaft fractures can be treated in a hanging cast or functional brace, but beware the upper third fracture which tends to angulate at the proximal border of a short cast. This fracture would have been better managed by (c) intramedullary nailing (and better still with a locking nail).

applied from shoulder to wrist with the elbow flexed 90°, and the forearm section is suspended by a sling around the patient's neck. This cast may be replaced after 2–3 weeks by a short (shoulder to elbow) cast or a functional polypropylene brace which is worn for a further 6 weeks.

The wrist and fingers are exercised from the start. Pendulum exercises of the shoulder are begun within a week, but active abduction is postponed until the fracture has united. Spiral fractures unite in about 6 weeks; the other varieties take 4–6 weeks longer. Once united, only a sling is needed until the fracture is consolidated.

OPERATIVE TREATMENT
Patients often find the hanging cast uncomfortable, tedious and frustrating; they can feel the fragments moving and this is sometimes quite distressing. The temptation is to 'do something', and the 'something' usually means an operation. It is well to remember (a) that the complication rate after internal fixation of the humerus is high and (b) that the great majority of humeral fractures unite with non-operative treatment.

There are, nevertheless, some well-defined *indications for surgery*:

- severe multiple injuries;
- an open fracture;
- segmental fractures;
- displaced intra-articular extension of the fracture;
- a pathological fracture;
- a 'floating elbow' – simultaneous unstable humeral and forearm fractures;
- radial nerve palsy after manipulation;
- non-union.

Fixation can be achieved with either (1) a compression plate and screws, (2) an interlocking intramedullary nail or semi-flexible pins or (3) an external fixator.

Plating permits excellent reduction and fixation, and has the added advantage that it does not interfere with shoulder or elbow function. However, it requires wide dissection and the radial nerve must be protected.

Antegrade nailing is performed with a rigid interlocking nail inserted through the rotator cuff under fluoroscopic control. It requires minimal dissection but has the

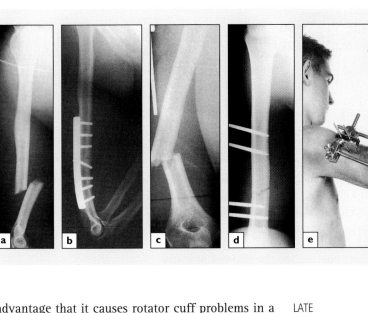

24.15 Fractured humerus – other methods of fixation **(a, b)** Compression plating, and **(c, d, e)** external fixation.

disadvantage that it causes rotator cuff problems in a significant proportion of cases (the reported incidence ranges from 5–40%!). If this happens, or if the nail backs out and the fracture has not yet united, exchange nailing and bone grafting of the fracture may be needed; alternatively, the nail can be replaced by an external fixator. *Retrograde nailing* with multiple flexible rods avoids these problems, but it is more difficult, less widely applicable and less secure in controlling rotation at the fracture site.

External fixation may be the best option for high-energy segmental fractures and open fractures. It is also a useful salvage procedure after failed intra-medullary nailing.

Complications

EARLY

Vascular injury If there are signs of vascular insufficiency in the limb, brachial artery damage must be excluded. Angiography will show the level of the injury. This is an emergency, requiring exploration and either direct repair or grafting of the vessel. In these circumstances, internal fixation is advisable.

Nerve injury Radial nerve palsy (wrist drop and paralysis of the metacarpophalangeal extensors) may occur with shaft fractures, particularly oblique fractures at the junction of the middle and distal thirds of the bone. In closed injuries the nerve is very seldom divided, so there is no hurry to operate. The wrist and hand must be regularly moved through a full passive range of movement to preserve joint motion until the nerve recovers. If there is no sign of recovery by 12 weeks, the nerve should be explored. In complete lesions (neurotmesis), nerve suture is often unsatisfactory, but function can be largely restored by tendon transfers. If nerve function was intact before manipulation but is defective afterwards, it must be assumed that the nerve has been snagged and surgical exploration is necessary.

LATE

Delayed union and non-union Transverse fractures sometimes take months to unite, especially if excessive traction has been used (a hanging cast must not be too heavy). Simple adjustments in technique may solve the problem; as long as there are signs of callus formation it is worth persevering with non-operative treatment, but remember to keep the shoulder moving. The rate of non-union in conservatively treated low-energy fractures is less than 3%. Segmental high energy fractures and open fractures are more prone to both delayed union and non-union.

Intramedullary nailing is likely to cause delayed union, but if rigid fixation can be maintained (if necessary by exchange nailing) the rate of non-union can probably be kept below 10%.

A particularly vicious combination is incomplete union and a stiff joint. If elbow or shoulder movements are forced before consolidation, or if an intramedullary nail is removed too soon (e.g. because of shoulder problems), the humerus may re-fracture and non-union is then more likely.

The treatment of established non-union is operative. The bone ends are freshened, bone chips are packed around them and the reduction is held with an intramedullary nail, a compression plate or an external fixator.

Joint stiffness Joint stiffness is common. It can be minimized by early activity, but transverse fractures (in which shoulder abduction is ill-advised) may limit shoulder movement for several weeks.

SPECIAL FEATURES IN CHILDREN

Fractures of the humerus are uncommon; in children under 3 years of age the possibility of child abuse should be considered. The fracture is treated by simply bandaging the arm to the body for 2–3 weeks. Older children require a short plaster splint.

FRACTURES AROUND THE ELBOW IN CHILDREN

The elbow is second only to the distal forearm for frequency of fractures in children. Most of these injuries are supracondylar fractures, the remainder being divided between condylar, epicondylar and proximal radial and ulnar fractures. Boys are injured more often than girls and more than half the patients are under 10 years old.

The usual accident is a fall directly on the point of the elbow or – more often – onto the outstretched hand with the elbow forced into valgus or varus. Pain and swelling are often marked and examination is difficult. X-ray interpretation also has its problems. The bone ends are largely cartilaginous and therefore radiographically incompletely visualized. A good knowledge of the normal anatomy is essential if fracture displacements are to be recognized.

Points of anatomy

The elbow is a complex hinge, providing sufficient mobility to permit the upper limb to reach through wide ranges of flexion, extension and rotation, yet also enough stability to support the necessary gripping, pushing, pulling and carrying activities of daily life. Its stability is due largely to the shape and fit of the bones that make up the joint – especially the humero-ulnar component – and this is liable to be compromised by any break in the articulating structures. The surrounding soft-tissue structures also are important, especially the capsular and collateral ligaments and, to a lesser extent, the muscles. Ligament disruption is also, therefore, a destabilizing factor.

The forearm is normally in slight valgus in relation to the upper arm, the average carrying angle in children being about 15°. (Published measurements range from 5 to 25 degrees!) When the elbow is flexed, the forearm comes to lie directly upon the upper arm. Doubts about the normality of these features can usually be resolved by comparing the injured with the normal arm.

With the elbow flexed, the tips of the medial and lateral epicondyles and the olecranon prominence form an isosceles triangle; with the elbow extended, they lie transversely in line with each other.

Though all the epiphyses are in some part cartilaginous, the secondary ossific centres can be seen on x-ray; they should not be mistaken for fracture fragments! The average ages at which the ossific centres appear are easily remembered by the mnemonic CRITOE: Capitulum – 2 years. Radial head – 4 years. Internal (medial) epicondyle – 6 years. Trochlea – 8 years. Olecranon – 10 years. External (lateral) epicondyle – 12 years. Obviously epiphyseal displace-ments will not be detectable on x-ray before these ages. Fracture displacement and accuracy of reduction can be inferred from radiographic indices such as Baumann's angle (see Fig. 24.17).

SUPRACONDYLAR FRACTURES

These are among the commonest fractures in children. The distal fragment may be displaced either *posteriorly* or *anteriorly*.

Mechanism of injury

Posterior angulation or displacement (95% of all cases) suggests a hyperextension injury, usually due to a fall on the outstretched hand. The humerus breaks just above the condyles. The distal fragment is pushed backwards and (because the forearm is usually in pronation) twisted inwards. The jagged end of the proximal fragment pokes into the soft tissues anteriorly, sometimes injuring the brachial artery or median nerve.

Anterior displacement is rare; it is thought to be due to direct violence (e.g. a fall on the point of the elbow) with the joint in flexion.

Classification

Supracondylar fractures may be classified according to severity and the degree of displacement (Wilkins, 1984). *Type I* is an undisplaced fracture. *Type II* is an angulated fracture with the posterior cortex still in continuity, *IIA* being less severe and merely angulated and *IIB* being more severe and both angulated and malrotated. *Type III* is a completely displaced fracture.

Clinical features

Following a fall, the child is in pain and the elbow is swollen; with a posteriorly displaced fracture the S-deformity of the elbow is usually obvious and the bony landmarks are abnormal. It is essential to feel the pulse and check the capillary return; passive extension of the flexor muscles should be pain-free. The wrist and the hand should be examined for evidence of nerve injury.

X-RAY

The fracture is seen most clearly in the lateral view. In an *undisplaced fracture* the 'fat pad sign' should raise suspicions: there is a triangular lucency in front of the distal humerus, due to the fat pad being pushed forwards by a haematoma.

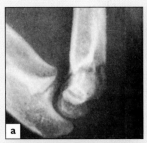
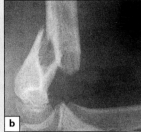
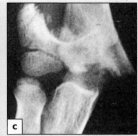
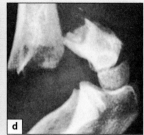
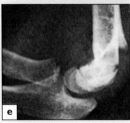

24.16 Supracondylar fractures X-rays showing supracondylar fractures of increasing severity. **(a)** Undisplaced. **(b)** Distal fragment posteriorly angulated and rotated. **(c, d)** Distal fragment completely separated and displaced posteriorly. **(e)** A rarer variety, with anterior displacement.

In the common *posteriorly displaced fracture* the fracture line runs obliquely downwards and forwards and the distal fragment is tilted backwards and/or shifted backwards. In the *anteriorly displaced fracture* the crack runs downwards and backwards and the fragment is tilted forwards.

An anteroposterior view is often difficult to obtain without causing pain and may need to be postponed until the child has been anaesthetized. It may show that the distal fragment is shifted or tilted sideways, and rotated (usually medially). Measurement of Baumann's angle is useful in assessing the degree of medial angulation before and after reduction.

Treatment

If there is even a suspicion of a fracture, the elbow is gently splinted in 30° of flexion to prevent movement and possible neurovascular injury during the x-ray examination. The definitive treatment recommended here is based on the guidelines suggested by O'Hara, *et al.* (2000).

TYPE I: UNDISPLACED FRACTURE
The elbow is immobilized at 90° and neutral rotation in a light-weight splint or cast and the arm is supported by a sling. *It is essential to obtain an x-ray 5–7 days later to check that there has been no displacement.* The splint is retained for 3 weeks and supervised movement is then allowed.

TYPE II A: POSTERIORLY ANGULATED FRACTURE – MILD
In these cases swelling is usually not severe and the risk of vascular injury is low. If the posterior cortices are in continuity, the fracture can be reduced under general

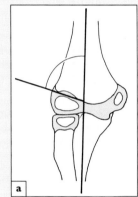
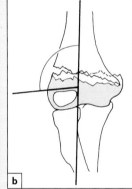

24.17 Baumann's angle In a child it is sometimes difficult to be sure that the distal fragment is reduced. Baumann's angle is subtended by the longitudinal axis of the humeral shaft and a line through the coronal axis of the capitellar physis. This is normally less than 80 degrees **(a)**. If the distal fragment is tilted in varus, the increased angle is readily detected **(b)**.

anaesthesia by the following step-wise manoeuvre: (1) traction for 2–3 minutes in the length of the arm with counter-traction above the elbow; (2) correction of any sideways tilt or shift and rotation (in comparison with the other arm); (3) gradual flexion of the elbow to 120°, and pronation of the forearm, while maintaining traction and exerting finger pressure behind the distal fragment to correct posterior tilt. *Then feel the pulse and check the capillary return* – if the distal circulation is suspect, immediately relax the amount of elbow flexion until it improves.

X-rays are taken to confirm reduction, checking carefully to see that there is no varus or valgus angulation and no rotational deformity. The anteroposterior

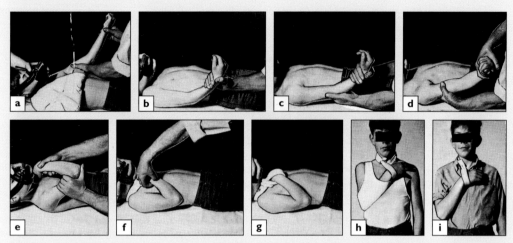

24.18 Supracondylar fractures – treatment (a) The uninjured arm is examined first; (b) traction of the fractured arm; (c) correcting lateral shift and tilt; (d) correctiing rotation; (e) correcting backwards shift and tilt; (f) feeling the pulse; (g) the elbow is kept well flexed while x-ray films are taken. (h) For the first 3 weeks the arm is kept under the clothes; after this (i) it is outside the clothes.

view is confusing and unreliable with the elbow flexed, but the important features can be inferred by noting Baumann's angle.

Following reduction, the arm is held in a collar and cuff; the circulation should be checked repeatedly during the first 24 hours. An x-ray is obtained after 3–5 days to confirm that the fracture has not slipped. The splint is retained for 3 weeks, after which movements are begun.

If the acutely flexed position cannot be maintained without disturbing the circulation, or if the reduction is unstable, the fracture should be fixed with percutaneous crossed Kirschner wires (take care not to skewer the ulnar nerve!).

TYPES IIB AND III: ANGULATED AND MALROTATED OR POSTERIORLY DISPLACED

These are usually associated with severe swelling, are difficult to reduce and are often unstable; moreover, there is a considerable risk of neurovascular injury or circulatory compromise due to swelling. The fracture should be reduced under general anaesthesia as soon as possible, by the method described above, and then held with percutaneous crossed Kirschner wires; this obviates the necessity to hold the elbow acutely flexed. Smooth wires should be used (this lessens the risk of physeal injury) and great care should be taken not to injure the ulnar and radial nerves. Post-operative management is the same as for Type IIA.

Open reduction This is sometimes necessary for (1) a fracture which simply cannot be reduced closed; (2) an open fracture; or (3) a fracture associated with vascular damage. The fracture is exposed (preferably through two incisions, one on each side of the elbow), the haematoma is evacuated and the fracture is reduced and held by two crossed Kirschner wires.

Continuous traction Traction through a screw in the olecranon, with the arm held overhead, can be used (1) if the fracture is severely displaced and cannot be reduced by manipulation; (2) if, with the elbow flexed 100°, the pulse is obliterated and image intensification is not available to allow pinning and then straightening of the elbow; or (3) for severe open injuries or multiple injuries of the limb. Once the swelling subsides, a further attempt can be made at closed reduction. Alternatively, the child may be treated by skin traction with the elbow almost straight and the arm in a small Thomas' splint (Dunlop traction).

TREATMENT OF ANTERIORLY DISPLACED FRACTURES

This is a rare injury. However, 'posterior' fractures are sometimes inadvertently converted to 'anterior' ones by excessive traction and manipulation.

The fracture is reduced by pulling on the forearm with the elbow semi-flexed, applying thumb pressure over the front of the distal fragment and then extending the elbow fully. A posterior slab is bandaged on and retained for 3 weeks. Thereafter, the child is allowed to regain flexion gradually.

Complications

EARLY

Vascular injury The great danger of supracondylar fracture is injury to the brachial artery, which, before the introduction of percutaneous pinning, was reported as occurring in over 5% of cases. Nowadays the incidence is probably less than 1%. Peripheral ischaemia may be immediate and severe, or the pulse may fail to return after reduction. More commonly the injury is complicated by forearm oedema and a mounting *compartment syndrome* which leads to necrosis of the muscle and nerves without causing peripheral gangrene. Undue pain plus one positive sign (pain on passive extension of the fingers, a tense and tender forearm, an absent pulse, blunted sensation or reduced capillary return on pressing the finger pulp) demands urgent action. The flexed elbow must be extended and all dressings removed. If the circulation does not promptly improve, then angiography (on the operating table if it saves time) is carried out, the vessel repaired or grafted and a forearm fasciotomy performed. If angiography is not available, or would cause much delay, then Doppler imaging should be used. In extreme cases, operative exploration would be justified on clinical criteria alone.

Nerve injury The median nerve, particularly the anterior interosseous branch, may be injured. Tests for nerve function are described in Chapter 11. Fortunately loss of function is usually temporary and recovery can be expected in 6–8 weeks.

The ulnar nerve may be damaged by careless pinning. If the injury is recognized, and the pin removed, recovery will usually follow.

LATE

Malunion Malunion is common. However, backwards or sideways shifts are gradually smoothed out by modelling during growth and they seldom give rise to visible deformity of the elbow. Forwards or backwards tilt may limit flexion or extension, but consequent disability is slight.

Uncorrected sideways tilt (angulation) and rotation are much more important and may lead to varus (or rarely valgus) deformity of the elbow; this is permanent and will not improve with growth. The fracture is extra-physeal and so physeal damage should not be blamed for the deformity; usually it is faulty reduction which is responsible. Cubitus varus is disfiguring and cubitus valgus may cause late ulnar palsy. If deformity is marked, it will need correction by supracondylar osteotomy.

Elbow stiffness and myositis officans Stiffness is an ever-present risk with elbow injuries. Extension in particular may take months to return. It must not be hurried. Passive movement (which includes carrying weights) or forced movement is prohibited – this will only make matters worse and may contribute to the development of myositis ossificans. As it is, myositis ossificans is extremely rare, and should remain so if rehabilitation is properly supervised.

FRACTURES OF THE LATERAL CONDYLE

The lateral condylar (or capitellar) epiphysis begins to ossify during the first year of life and fuses with the shaft at 12–16 years. Between these ages it may be sheared off or avulsed by forceful traction.

Mechanism of injury and pathology

The child falls on the hand with the elbow extended and forced into varus. A large fragment, which includes the lateral condyle, breaks off and is pulled upon by the attached wrist extensors. The fracture line usually runs along the physis and into the trochlea; less often it continues through the lateral epiphysis and exits through the capitulotrochlear groove. In severe injuries the elbow may dislocate posterolaterally; the condyle is 'capsized' by muscle pull and remains capsized while the elbow reduces spontaneously.

The extent of this injury is often not appreciated. Because the condylar epiphysis is largely cartilaginous, the bone fragment may look deceptively small on x-ray. Displacement can be quite marked due to muscle pull. The fracture is important for two reasons: (a) it may damage the growth plate and (b) it always involves the joint. Early recognition and accurate reduction are therefore essential if a poor outcome is to be avoided.

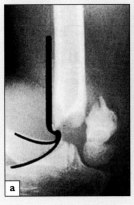
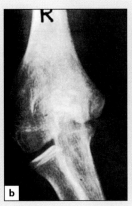
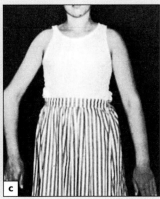

24.19 Supracondylar fractures – complications The most serious complication is arterial damage (**a**) leading to Volkmann's ischaemia. (**b, c**) Varus deformity of the right elbow following poor reduction (rotation was never corrected).

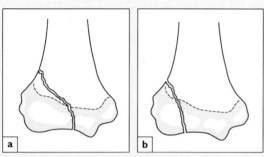

24.20 Physeal fractures of the lateral condyle (a) The commonest is a fracture starting in the metaphysis and running along the physis of the lateral condyle into the trochlea (Salter–Harris type II injury). (b) Less common is a fracture running right through the lateral condyle to reach the articular surface in the capitulotrochlear groove (Salter–Harris type IV); though uncommon, this latter injury is important because of its potential for causing growth defects.

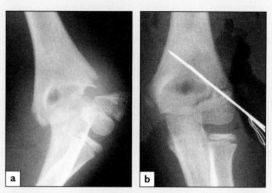

24.21 Fractured lateral condyle If displacement is more than 2mm, open reduction and internal fixation is the treatment of choice.

Clinical features

The elbow is swollen and deformed. There is tenderness over the lateral condyle. Passive flexion of the wrist (pulling on the extensors) may be painful.

X-RAY

X-ray examination must include oblique views or else the full extent of the fracture may be missed. Two types of fracture are recognized: (1) A fracture lateral to the trochlea: the humero-ulnar joint is not involved and is stable. (2) A fracture through the middle of the trochlea: this injury is more common; the elbow is unstable and it may dislocate. The fragment is often grossly displaced and capsized, and it may carry with it a triangular piece of the metaphysis. Remember that the fragment is much larger than it seems on x-ray.

Treatment

If there is no (or only minimal) displacement the arm can be splinted in a backslab with the elbow flexed 90°, the forearm neutral and the wrist extended (this position relaxes the extensor mechanism which attaches to the fragment). However, it is essential to repeat the x-ray after 5 days to make sure that the fracture has not displaced. The splint is removed after 2 weeks and exercises are encouraged.

A displaced fracture (i.e. with a gap of more than 2mm) requires accurate reduction and internal fixation. If the fragment is only moderately displaced (hinged), it may be possible to manipulate it into position by extending the elbow and pressing upon the condyle, and then fixing the fragment with percutaneous pins. If this fails, and for all widely separated fractures, open reduction and internal fixation with pins or screws is required. The arm is immobilized in a cast; cast and pins are removed after 3 or 4 weeks.

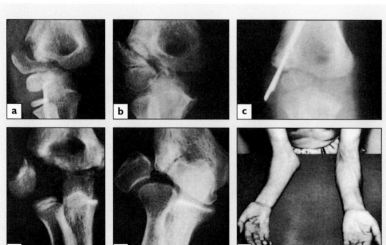

24.22 Fractured lateral condyle – complications (a, b) A large fragment of bone and cartilage is avulsed; even with reasonable reduction, union is not inevitable. (c) Open reduction with fixation is often wise. (d) Sometimes the condyle is capsized; if left unreduced non-union is inevitable (e) and a valgus elbow with delayed ulnar palsy (f) the likely sequel.

Complications

Non-union and malunion If the condyle is left capsized, non-union is inevitable; with growth the elbow becomes increasingly valgus, and ulnar nerve palsy is then likely to develop. Stiffness and pain can result. Even minor displacements sometimes lead to non-union, and even slight malunion may lead to ulnar palsy in later life; it is for these reasons that open reduction (and internal fixation) is often preferred.

Recurrent dislocation Occasionally condylar displacement results in posterolateral dislocation of the elbow. The only effective treatment is reconstruction of the bony and soft tissues on the lateral side.

FRACTURES OF THE MEDIAL CONDYLE

This is much rarer than either a fracture of the lateral condylar epipysis or a separation of the medial epicondylar apophysis.

Mechanism of injury

The injury is usually caused by a fall from a height, involving either a direct blow to the point of the elbow or a landing on the outstretched hand with the elbow forced into valgus; in the latter case it would be an avulsion injury. The fracture line runs through the physis, exiting in the trochlear notch or even further laterally, and the medial fragment may be displaced by the pull of the flexor muscle group.

Clinical features and x-ray

This is an intra-articular fracture, resulting in considerable pain and swelling. In older children the metaphyseal component is usually easily visualized on x-ray. However, in young children much of the medial condylar epiphysis is cartilaginous and therefore not visible on x-ray, so the full extent of the fracture may not be recognized; seeing only the epicondylar ossific centre in a displaced position on the x-ray may mislead the surgeon into thinking that this is only an epicondylar fracture. In doubtful cases an arthrogram may be helpful.

Treatment

Undisplaced fractures are treated by splintage; x-rays are repeated until the fracture has healed, so as to ensure that it does not become displaced.

Displaced fractures are treated by either closed reduction and percutaneous pinning or by open reduction and fixation with pins.

Post-operative management is similar to that of lateral condyle fractures.

Complications

EARLY
Ulnar nerve damage is not uncommon, but recovery is usual unless the nerve is left kinked in the joint.

LATE
Stiffness of the elbow is common and extension often limited for months; but, provided movement is not forced, it will eventually return.

Late ulnar nerve palsy may be caused by friction in the roughened bony groove.

SEPARATION OF THE MEDIAL EPICONDYLAR APOPHYSIS

Mechanism of injury and pathology

The medial epicondylar apophysis begins to ossify at the age of about 5 years and fuses to the shaft at about 16; between these ages it may be avulsed by a severe muscle or ligament strain. The child falls on the outstretched hand with the wrist and elbow extended, and the unfused epicondylar apophysis is avulsed by tension on either the wrist flexor muscles or the medial ligament of the elbow. If the elbow subluxates (even momentarily), the small apophyseal fragment may be dragged into the joint. With more severe injuries the joint dislocates laterally.

Clinical features

The diagnosis should be suspected if injury is followed by pain, swelling and bruising on the medial side of the elbow. If the joint is dislocated, deformity is of course obvious. Sensation and power in the fingers should be tested to exclude concomitant ulnar nerve damage.

X-RAY
In the anteroposterior view the medial epicondylar epiphysis may be tilted or shifted downwards; if the joint is dislocated the fragment lies distal to the lower humerus. A lateral view may show the epicondyle looking like a loose body in the joint. If in any doubt, the normal side should be x-rayed for comparison.

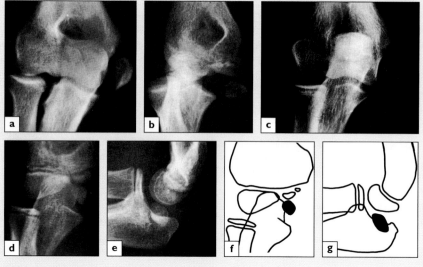

24.23 Fractured medial epicondyle (a) Avulsion of the medial epicondyle following valgus strain. (b) Avulsion associated with dislocation of the elbow; (c) after reduction.

Sometimes the epicondylar fragment is trapped in the joint (d, e); the serious nature of the injury is then liable to be missed unless the surgeon specifically looks for the trapped fragment, which is emphasized in the tracings (f, g).

Treatment

Minor displacement may be disregarded. This is an extra-articular fracture, so the elbow can be mobilized as soon as the child wishes.

If the epicondyle is trapped in the joint it must be freed. Manipulation with the elbow in valgus and the wrist hyperextended (to pull on the flexor muscles) may be successful; if this fails, the joint must be opened (the ulnar nerve must be visualized and protected) and the fragment retrieved and fixed back in position.

Displaced fractures with the fragment not trapped in the joint do not need to be operated upon: a manipulation can improve the position but open surgery and fixation does not improve the final outcome.

Complications

EARLY
Ulnar nerve damage is not uncommon. Mild symptoms usually recover spontaneously; a complete palsy suggests that the nerve may kinked in the joint and exploration should be considered.

LATE
Stiffness of the elbow is common and extension often limited for months; but, provided movement is not forced, it will eventually return.

FRACTURE-SEPARATION OF THE DISTAL HUMERAL PHYSIS

Up to the age of 7 years the distal humeral epiphysis is a solid cartilaginous segment with maturing centres of ossification. With severe injury it may separate *en bloc*. This is likely to occur with fairly severe violence; for example, in birth injuries or child abuse.

Clinical features

The child is in pain and the elbow is markedly swollen. The history may be deceptively uninformative.

X-RAY
In a very young child, in whom the bony outlines are still unformed, the x-ray may look normal. All that can be seen of the epiphysis is the pea-like ossification centre of the capitulum; its position should be compared with that of the normal side. Medial displacement of either the capitellar ossification centre or the proximal radius and ulna is very suspicious. In the older child the deformity is usually obvious.

Treatment

The injury is treated like a supracondylar fracture. If the diagnosis is uncertain, the elbow is merely splinted in flexion for 2 weeks; any resulting deformity (which is rare) can be dealt with at a later age.

FRACTURED NECK OF RADIUS

Mechanism of injury and pathology

A fall on the outstretched hand forces the elbow into valgus and pushes the radial head against the capitulum. In children the bone fractures through the neck of the radius; in adults the injury is more likely to fracture the radial head.

Clinical features

Following a fall, the child complains of pain in the elbow. There may be localized tenderness over the radial head and pain on rotating the forearm.

X-RAY

The fracture line is transverse. It is either situated immediately distal to the physis or there is true separation of the epiphysis with a triangular fragment of shaft (a Salter–Harris II injury). The proximal fragment is tilted distally, forwards and outwards. Sometimes the upper end of the ulna is also fractured.

Treatment

In chldren, up to 30° of radial head tilt and up to 3mm of transverse displacement are acceptable. The arm is rested in a collar and cuff, and exercises are commenced after a week.

Displacement of more than 30° requires reduction. With the patient's elbow extended, traction and varus force are applied; the surgeon then pushes the displaced radial fragment into position with his or her thumb. If this fails, open reduction is performed. The radial head tilt is corrected but internal fixation is unnecessarily meddlesome. The head of the radius must never be excised in children because this will interfere with the synchronous growth of radius and ulna.

Fractures that are seen a week or longer after injury should be left untreated (except for light splintage).

Following operation, the elbow is splinted in 90° of flexion for a week or two and then movements are encouraged.

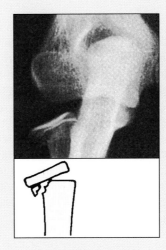

24.24 Fractured neck of radius in a child Up to 30° of tilt is acceptable. Greater degrees of angulation should be reduced; never excise the radial head in a child.

FRACTURES AND DISLOCATIONS AROUND THE ELBOW IN ADULTS

Elbow fractures in adults pose problems quite different from those in children. Fusion of the epiphyses brings a change in the mechanical properties of the bone ends, and consequently differences in the pattern of injury. Some of these fractures – especially those of the distal humerus – are high-energy injuries which are associated with vascular and nerve damage; some can be reduced and stabilized only by complex surgical techniques; and the tendency to stiffness of the elbow means that with all severe injuries the striving for anatomical perfection has to be weighed up against the realities of imperfect postoperative function.

FRACTURES OF THE DISTAL HUMERUS

The AO-ASIF Group (Müller *et al.*, 1991) have defined three types of distal humeral fracture: Type A, which is an extra-articular supracondylar fracture; Type B, an intra-articular unicondylar fracture (one condyle sheared off and the other still in continuity with the shaft); and Type C, bicondylar fractures with varying degrees of comminution.

TYPE A – SUPRACONDYLAR FRACTURES

These extra-articular fractures are rare in adults. When they do occur, they are usually displaced and unstable – probably because there is no tough periosteum to tether the fragments. In high-energy injuries there may be comminution of the distal humerus.

PULLED ELBOW

In young children the elbow may be injured by pulling on the arm, usually with the forearm pronated. It is sometimes called subluxation of the radial head; more accurately, it is a subluxation of the orbicular ligament which slips up over the head of the radius into the radiocapitellar joint.

A child aged 2 or 3 years is brought with a painful, dangling arm: there is usually a history of the child being jerked by the arm and crying out in pain. The forearm is held in pronation and extension, and any attempt to supinate it is resisted. There are no x-ray changes.

A dramatic cure is achieved by forcefully supinating and then flexing the elbow; the ligament slips back with a snap.

Treatment

Closed reduction is unlikely to be stable and Kirshner wire fixation is not strong enough to permit early mobilization. Open reduction and internal fixation is therefore the treatment of choice. With the patient prone, the distal humerus is approached through a posterior exposure and either an inverted 'V' distal reflection of the triceps tendon or an extra-articular osteotomy of the olecranon process and proximal reflexion of the triceps. A simple transverse or oblique fracture can usually be reduced and fixed with a single contoured plate and screws. Comminuted fractures may require double plates and transfixing screws.

TYPES B AND C – INTRA-ARTICULAR FRACTURES

Except in osteoporotic individuals, intra-articular condylar fractures should be regarded as high-energy injuries with soft-tissue damage. A severe blow on the point of the elbow drives the olecranon process upwards, splitting the condyles apart. Swelling is considerable, but if the bony landmarks can be felt the elbow is found to be distorted. The patient should be carefully examined for evidence of vascular or nerve injury; if there are signs of vascular insufficiency, this must be addressed as a matter of urgency.

X-RAY

The fracture extends from the lower humerus into the elbow joint; it may be difficult to tell whether one or both condyles are involved, especially with an undisplaced condylar fracture. There is often also comminution of the bone between the condyles, the extent of which is usually underestimated. Sometimes the fracture extends into the metaphysis as a T- or Y-shaped break, or else there may be multiple fragments (comminution). *The lesson is: 'Prepare for the worst before operating'.*

Treatment

These are severe injuries associated with joint damage; prolonged immobilization will certainly result in a stiff elbow. Early movement is therefore a prime objective.

Undisplaced fractures These can be treated by applying a posterior slab with the elbow flexed almost 90°; movements are commenced after 2 weeks. However, great care should be taken to avoid the dual pitfalls of underdiagnosis (displacement and comminution are not always obvious on the initial x-ray) and late displacement (always obtain check x-rays a week after injury).

Displaced Type B and C fractures If the appropriate expertise and facilities are available, open reduction and internal fixation is the treatment of choice for displaced fractures (some would say for *all* Type B and C fractures – minor displacement is easily overlooked in the early post-injury x-rays). The danger with conservative treatment is the strong tendency to stiffening of the elbow and persistent pain.

The operative approach is similar to that used for Type A fractures, but better exposure is obtained by performing an intra-articular olecranon osteotomy. The ulnar nerve should be identified and protected throughout. The fragments are reduced and held temporarily

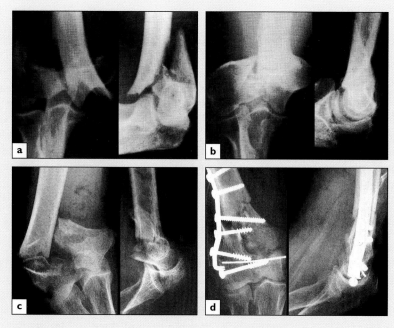

24.25 Bicondylar fractures (**a**) Before and (**b**) after treatment in a collar-and-cuff plus activity; reasonable movement was obtained by this method but a hinged brace would have been better. (**c**) Before and (**d**) after open reduction and internal fixation; the result was very good, though this is not always the case.

with Kirschner wires. A unicondylar fracture without comminution can then be fixed with screws; if the fragment is large, a contoured plate is added to prevent re-displacement. Bicondylar and comminuted fractures will require double plate and screw fixation, and sometimes also bone grafts in the gaps.

Post-operatively the elbow is held at 90° with the arm supported in a sling. Movement is encouraged but should never be forced. Fracture healing usually occurs by 12 weeks. Despite the best efforts, the patient often does not regain full extension and in the most severe cases movement may be severely restricted.

A description of this sort fails to convey the real difficulty of these operations. Unless the surgeon is more than usually skilful, the elbow may end up stiffer than if treated by activity (see below).

ALTERNATIVE METHODS OF TREATMENT
If it is anticipated that the outcome of operative treatment will be poor (either because of the degree of comminution and soft-tissue damage or because of lack of expertise and facilities) other options can be considered.

The 'bag of bones' technique The arm is held in a collar and cuff or, better, a hinged brace, with the elbow flexed above a right angle; active movements are encouraged as soon as the patient is willing. The fracture usually unites within 6–8 weeks, but exercises are continued far longer. A useful range of movement (45–90°) is often obtained.

Skeletal traction An alternative method of treating either moderately displaced or severely comminuted fractures is by skeletal traction through the olecranon (beware the ulnar nerve!); the patient remains in bed with the humerus held vertical, and elbow movements are encouraged.

Elbow replacement The elderly patient with a comminuted fracture may be best served by replacement of the elbow.

Complications

EARLY
Vascular injury Always check the circulation (repeatedly!). Vigilance is required to make the diagnosis and institute treatment as early as possible.

Nerve injury There may be damage to either the median or the ulnar nerve. It is important to examine the hand and record the findings before treatment is commenced. The nerves are particularly vulnerable during surgery.

LATE
Stiffness Comminuted fractures of the elbow always result in some degree of stiffness. However, the disabil-

ity may be reduced by encouraging an energetic exercise programme. Late operations to improve elbow movement are difficult but can be rewarding.

Heterotopic ossification Severe soft-tissue damage may lead to heterotopic ossification. Forced movement should be avoided.

FRACTURED CAPITULUM

This is an articular fracture which occurs only in adults. The patient falls on the hand, usually with the elbow straight. The anterior part of the capitulum is sheared off and displaced proximally.

Clinical features

Fullness in front of the elbow is the most notable feature. The lateral side of the elbow is tender and flexion is grossly restricted.

X-RAY
In the lateral view the capitulum (or part of it) is seen in front of the lower humerus, and the radial head no longer points directly towards it.

Treatment

Undisplaced fractures can be treated by simple splintage for 2 weeks.

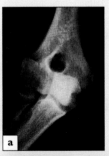
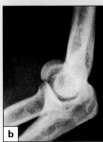
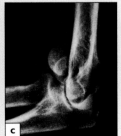

24.26 Fractured capitulum (a, b) Anteroposterior and lateral views showing proximal displacement and tilting; in (c) the capitulum has been sheared off vertically.

Displaced fractures should be either reduced or excised. Closed reduction is feasible, but prolonged immobilization may result in a stiff elbow. Operative treatment is therefore preferred. The fragment is always larger than expected. If it can be securely replaced, it is fixed in position with a small screw. If this proves too difficult, the fragment is best excised. Movements are commenced as soon as discomfort permits.

FRACTURED HEAD OF RADIUS

Radial head fractures are common in adults but are hardly ever seen in children (probably because the proximal radius is mainly cartilaginous).

Mechanism of injury

A fall on the outstretched hand with the elbow extended and the forearm pronated causes impaction of the radial head against the capitulum. The radial head may be split or broken. In addition, the articular cartilage of the capitulum may be bruised or chipped; this cannot be seen on x-ray but is an important complication. The radial head is also sometimes fractured during elbow dislocation.

Clinical features

This fracture is sometimes missed, but tenderness on pressure over the radial head and pain on pronation and supination should suggest the diagnosis.

X-RAY
Three types of fracture are identified:

Type I A vertical split in the radial head.

Type II A single fragment of the lateral portion of the head broken off and usually displaced distally.

Type III The head broken into several fragments (comminuted).

The wrist also should be x-rayed to exclude a concomitant injury of the distal radioulnar joint, which would signify damage to the interosseous membrane (acute longitudinal radioulnar dissociation).

Treatment

An undisplaced split (Type I) Worthwhile pain relief can be achieved by aspirating the haematoma and injecting local anaesthetic. The arm is held in a collar and cuff for 3 weeks; active flexion, extension and rotation are encouraged.

A single large fragment (Type II) If the fragment is displaced, it should be reduced and held with a small screw. A buried head (Herbert) screw will not impede rotation.

A comminuted fracture (Type III) This is best treated by excising the radial head. However, if there are associated forearm injuries or disruption of the distal radioulnar joint, the risk of proximal migration of the radius is considerable and the patient may develop intractable symptoms of pain and instability in the forearm; in such cases, every effort should therefore be made to reconstruct the radial head or, if it has to be excised, it must be replaced by a silicone or metal prosthesis.

Fracture-dislocation Dislocation of the elbow associated with a radial head fracture is an unstable injury. After reduction of the dislocation, it is essential to restore the radial pillar (by fixation of a displaced Type II fracture or prosthetic replacement for a Type III fracture) and to resume movement slowly and gently while the ligaments heal (see page 609).

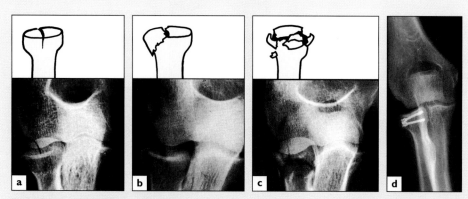

24.27 Fractured head of radius There are three main types of adult radial head fracture: (a) a chisel-like split of head, (b) a marginal fracture or (c) a comminuted fracture. Displaced marginal fractures can often be treated by (d) internal fixation.

Complications

Joint stiffness is common and may involve both the elbow and the radioulnar joints. Even with minimally displaced fractures the elbow can take several months to recover, and stiffness may occur whether the radial head has been excised or not.

Myositis ossificans is an occasional complication.

Recurrent instability of the elbow can occur if the medial collateral ligament was also injured and the radial head excised.

FRACTURE OF THE RADIAL NECK

In adults, a displaced fracture of the radial neck may need open reduction; if so, a mini-plate can be applied, making sure not to damage the articular surface.

FRACTURES OF THE OLECRANON

Two types of injury are seen: (1) a comminuted fracture which is due to a direct blow or a fall on the elbow; and (2) a clean transverse break, due to traction when the patient falls onto the hand while the triceps muscle is contracted.

The fracture enters the elbow joint and therefore also damages the articular cartilage. With transverse fractures, the triceps aponeurosis sometimes remains intact, in which case the fracture fragments stay together.

Clinical features

A graze or bruise over the elbow suggests a comminuted fracture; the triceps is intact and the elbow can be extended against gravity. With a transverse fracture there may be a palpable gap and the patient is unable to extend the elbow against resistance.

X-RAY

A properly orientated lateral view is essential to show details of the fracture, as well as the associated joint damage. The position of the radial head should be checked; it may be dislocated.

Treatment

A comminuted fracture with the triceps intact should be treated as a 'bruise'. Many of these patients are old and osteoporotic, and immobilizing the elbow will lead to stiffness. The arm is rested in a sling for a week; a further x-ray is obtained to ensure that there is no displacement and the patient is then encouraged to start active movements.

An undisplaced transverse fracture that does not separate when the elbow is x-rayed in flexion can be treated closed. The elbow is immobilized by a cast in about 60° of flexion for 2–3 weeks and then exercises are begun.

Displaced transverse fractures can be held only by splinting the arm absolutely straight – and stiffness in that position would be disastrous. Operative treatment is therefore preferred. The fracture is reduced and held by tension-band wiring. Early mobilization should be encouraged. *A very small fragment* may be excised and the triceps reattached to the ulna.

Complications

Stiffness used to be common, but with secure internal fixation and early mobilization the residual loss of movement should be minimal.

Non-union sometimes occurs after inadequate reduction and fixation of a transverse fracture. If elbow

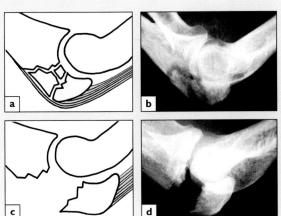
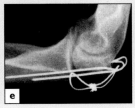
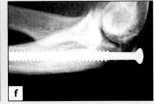
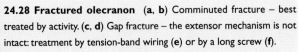

24.28 Fractured olecranon (a, b) Comminuted fracture – best treated by activity. **(c, d)** Gap fracture – the extensor mechanism is not intact: treatment by tension-band wiring **(e)** or by a long screw **(f)**.

function is good, it can be ignored; if not, rigid internal fixation and bone grafting will be needed.

Ulnar nerve symptoms can develop. These usually settle spontaneously.

Osteoarthritis is a late complication, especially if reduction is less than perfect. This can usually be treated symptomatically.

DISLOCATION OF THE ELBOW

Dislocation of the ulnohumeral joint is fairly common – more so in adults than in children. Injuries are usually classified according to the direction of displacement. However, in 90% of cases the radioulnar complex is displaced posteriorly or posterolaterally, often together with fractures of the restraining bony processes.

Mechanism of injury and pathology

The cause of posterior dislocation is usually a fall on the outstretched hand with the elbow in extension. Disruption of the capsuloligamentous structures alone can result in posterior or posterolateral dislocation. However, provided there is no associated fracture, reduction will usually be stable and recurrent dislocation unlikely. The combination of ligamentous disruption and fracture of the radial head, coronoid process or olecranon process (or, worse still, several fractures) will render the joint more unstable and, unless the fractures are reduced and fixed, liable to re-dislocation.

Once posterior dislocation has taken place, lateral shift may also occur. Soft tissue disruption is often considerable and surrounding nerves and vessels may be damaged.

Although certain common patterns of fracture-dislocation are recognized (based on the particular combination of structures involved), high-energy injuries do not follow any rules. A classic example is the so-called *side-swipe injury* which occurs, typically, when a car-driver's elbow, protruding through the window, is struck by another vehicle. The result is forwards dislocation with fractures of any or all of the bones around the elbow; soft-tissue damage (including neurovascular injury) is usually severe.

Clinical features

The patient supports his or her forearm with the elbow in slight flexion. Unless swelling is severe, the deformity is obvious. The bony landmarks (olecranon and epicondyles) may be palpable and abnormally placed. However, in severe injuries pain and swelling are so marked that examination of the elbow is impossible. Nevertheless, the hand should be examined for signs of vascular or nerve damage.

X-RAY
X-ray examination is essential (a) to confirm the presence of a dislocation and (b) to identify any associated fractures.

Treatment

UNCOMPLICATED DISLOCATION
The patient should be fully relaxed under anaesthesia. The surgeon pulls on the forearm while the elbow is slightly flexed. With one hand, sideways displacement is corrected, then the elbow is further flexed while the olecranon process is pushed forwards with the thumbs. Unless almost full flexion can be obtained, the olecranon is not in the trochlear groove.

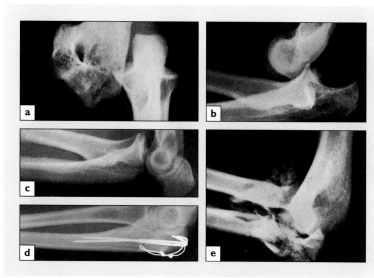

24.29 Elbow dislocations (**a, b**) The usual uncomplicated dislocation. (**c**) Forwards dislocation with fractured olecranon; this needs (**d**) reduction, with stabilization of the olecranon. (**e**) Side-swipe fracture-dislocation.

After reduction, the elbow should be put through a full range of movement to see whether it is stable. The distal nerves and circulation are checked again. In addition, an x-ray is obtained to confirm that the joint is reduced and to disclose any associated fractures.

The arm is held in a collar and cuff with the elbow flexed above 90°. After 1 week the patient gently exercises the elbow; at 3 weeks the collar and cuff are discarded. Elbow movements are allowed to return spontaneously and are never forced.

DISLOCATION WITH ASSOCIATED FRACTURES

Coronoid process Small flakes off the coronoid process need no special treatment. Large fragments are associated with instability of the ulnohumeral joint and should be fixed.

Medial epicondyle An avulsed medial epicondyle is, for practical purposes, a medial ligament disruption. If the epicondylar fragment is displaced, it must be reduced and fixed back in position. The arm and wrist are splinted with the elbow at 90°; after 3 weeks movements are begun under supervision.

Head of radius The combination of ligament disruption and a type II or III radial head fracture is an unstable injury; stability is restored only by healing or repair of the ligaments and restoration of the radial pillar – either by fracture fixation or (in the case of a comminuted fracture) by prosthetic replacement of the radial head. If there is much tissue damage, radial head replacement can be deferred for a few weeks to allow the tissues to recover.

Olecranon process In the rare forwards dislocation of the elbow, the olecranon process may fracture; a large piece of the olecranon is left behind as a separate fragment. Open reduction with internal fixation is the best treatment.

Side-swipe injuries These severe fracture-dislocations are often associated with damage to the large vessels of the arm. The priorities are repair of any vascular injury, skeletal stabilization and soft-tissue coverage. This is demanding surgery, necessitating a high level of expertise, and is best undertaken in a unit specializing in upper limb injuries.

Persistent instability In cases where the elbow remains unstable after the bone and joint anatomy has been restored, a hinged external fixator can be applied in order to maintain mobility while the tissues heal.

Complications

Complications are common; some are potentially so serious that the patient with a dislocation or a fracture-dislocation of the elbow must be observed with the closest attention.

EARLY

Vascular injury The brachial artery may be damaged. Absence of the radial pulse is a warning. If there are other signs of ischaemia, this should be treated as an emergency. Splints must be removed and the elbow should be straightened somewhat. If there is no improvement, an arteriogram is performed; the brachial artery may have to be explored.

Nerve injury The median or ulnar nerve is sometimes injured. Spontaneous recovery usually occurs after 6–8 weeks.

LATE

Stiffness Loss of 20 to 30° of extension is not uncommon after elbow dislocation. Fortunately this is usually of little functional significance. More severe degrees of stiffness can often be improved by anterior capsular release (see also page 308).

Heterotopic ossification Heterotopic bone formation may occur in the damaged soft tissues in front of the joint. In former years 'myositis ossificans' was a fairly common complication, usually associated with forceful reduction and overenthusiastic passive movement of the elbow. Nowadays it is rarely seen, but it is as well to be alert for signs such as excessive pain and tenderness, and tardy recovery of active movements. X-rays may show soft-tissue ossification as early as 4–6 weeks after injury. If the condition is suspected, exercises are stopped and the elbow is splinted in comfortable flexion until pain subsides; gentle active movements and continuous passive motion are then resumed. Anti-inflammatory drugs may help to reduce stiffness; they are also used prophylactically to reduce the risk of heterotopic bone formation.

A bone mass which markedly restricts movement and elbow function should be excised once the bone is 'mature', that is has well defined cortical margins and trabeculae.

Unreduced dislocation A dislocation may not have been diagnosed; or only the backwards displacement corrected, leaving the olecranon process still displaced sideways. Up to 3 weeks from injury, manipulative reduction is worth attempting but care is needed to avoid fracturing one of the bones. Other than this, there is no satisfactory treatment. Open reduction can be considered, but a wide soft-tissue release is required, which predisposes to yet further stiffness. Alternatively, the condition can be left, in the hope that the elbow will regain a useful range of movement. If pain is a problem, the patient can be offered an arthrodesis or an arthroplasty.

Recurrent dislocation This is rare unless there is a large coronoid fracture or radial head fracture. If recurrent elbow instability occurs, the lateral ligament and capsule can be repaired or re-attached to the lateral condyle. A cast with the elbow at 90° is worn for 4 weeks.

Osteoarthritis Secondary osteoarthritis is quite common after severe fracture-dislocations. In older patients, total elbow replacement can be considered.

ISOLATED DISLOCATION OF THE RADIAL HEAD

A true isolated dislocation of the radial head is very rare; if it is seen, search carefully for an associated fracture of the ulna (the Monteggia injury). In a child, the ulnar fracture may be difficult to detect if it is incomplete, either green-stick or plastic deformation of the shaft; it is very important to identify these incomplete fractures because even a minor deformity, if it is allowed to persist, may prevent full reduction of the radial head dislocaion.

REFERENCES AND FURTHER READING

Browner BD, Jupiter JB, Levine AM, Trafton PG (eds) (1998) *Skeletal Trauma.* WB Saunders, Philadelphia

Jupiter JB (1994) Complex fractures of the distal part of the humerus. *Journal of Bone and Joint Surgery* **76**A, 1252-1263

Modabber MR, Jupiter JB (1995) Reconstruction for post-traumatic conditions of the elbow joint. *Journal of Bone and Joint Surgery* **77**A, 1431-1446

Morrey BF (1995) Current concepts in the treatment of fractures of the radial head, the olecranon and coronoid. *Journal of Bone and Joint Surgery* **77**A, 316-327

Müller ME, Allgower M, Schneider R *et al* (1991) *Manual of Internal Fixation.* 3rd edition. Springer Verlag, Berlin, Heidelberg, New York

Neer CS II (1970) Displaced proximal humeral fractures. I. Classification and evaluation. *Journal of Bone and Joint Surgery* **52**A, 1077–1089

O'Hara LJ, Barlow JW, Clarke NMP (2000) Displaced supracondylar fractures of the humerus in children. *Journal of Bone and Joint Surgery* **82**B, 204-210

Ring D, Jupiter JB (1998) Fracture-dislocation of the elbow. *Journal of Bone and Joint Surgery* **80**A, 566-580

Rockwood CA Jr, Green DP, Bucholz RW, Heckman JD (eds) (1996) *Rockwood and Green's Fractures in Adults* 4th edition. Lippincott-Raven, Philadelphia

Wilkins KE (1984) Fractures and dislocations in the elbow region. In *Fractures in Children* vol 3 (eds Rockwood CA Jr, Wilkens KE, King RE). JB Lippincott and Co, Philadelphia.

Injuries of the forearm and wrist

FRACTURES OF THE RADIUS AND ULNA

Mechanism of injury and pathology

Fractures of the shafts of both forearm bones occur quite commonly in road accidents. A twisting force (usually a fall on the hand) produces a spiral fracture with the bones broken at different levels. A direct blow or an angulating force causes a transverse fracture of both bones at the same level. Additional rotation deformity may be produced by the pull of muscles attached to the radius: these are the biceps and supinator muscles to the upper third, the pronator teres to the middle third and the pronator quadratus to the lower third. Bleeding and swelling of the muscle compartments of the forearm may cause circulatory impairment.

Clinical features

The fracture is usually quite obvious, but the pulse must be felt and the hand examined for circulatory or neural deficit. Repeated examination is necessary in order to detect an impending compartment syndrome.

X-RAY

Both bones are broken, either transversely and at the same level or obliquely with the radial fracture usually at a higher level. In children, the fracture is often incomplete (green-stick) and only angulated. In adults, displacement may occur in any direction – shift, over-lap, tilt or twist. In low-energy injuries, the fracture tends to be transverse or oblique; in high-energy injuries, comminuted or segmental.

Treatment

CHILDREN
In children, closed treatment is usually successful because the tough periosteum tends to guide and then control the reduction. The fragments are held in a well-moulded full-length cast, from axilla to metacarpal shafts (to control rotation). The cast is applied with the elbow at 90°. If the fracture is proximal to pronator teres, the forearm is supinated; if it is distal to pronator teres, then the forearm is held in neutral. The position is checked by x-ray after a week and, if it is satisfactory, splintage is retained until both fractures are united (usually 6–8 weeks). Throughout this period hand and shoulder exercises are encouraged. The child should avoid contact sports for a few weeks to prevent re-fracture.

Occasionally an operation is required, (a) if the fracture cannot be reduced or (b) if the fragments are very unstable. Fixation with a small plate, Kirschner wires (K-wires) or flexible intramedullary nails is then needed.

ADULTS
Unless the fragments are in close apposition, reduction is difficult and re-displacement in the cast almost invariable. So predictable is this outcome that most surgeons opt for open reduction and internal fixation from the outset. The fragments are held by interfragmentary compression with

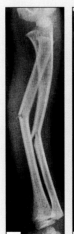
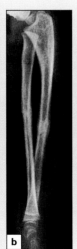
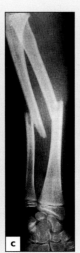
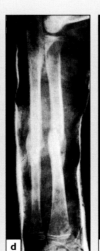
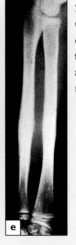

25.1 Fractured radius and ulna in children Green-stick fractures (**a**) need only correction of angulation (**b**), and plaster splintage. Complete fractures (**c**) are harder to reduce; but provided alignment is corrected and held in plaster (**d**), slight lateral shift remodels with growth (**e**).

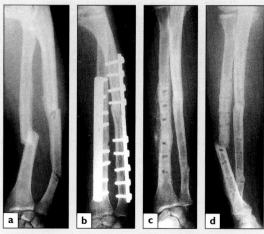

25.2 Fractured radius and ulna in adults (a, b) These fractures are usually treated by internal fixation with sturdy plates and screws. However, removal of the implants is not without risk. **(c, d)** In this case the radius fractured through one of the screw holes.

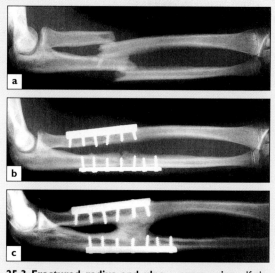

25.3 Fractured radius and ulna – cross-union If the interosseous membrane is severely damaged, even succesful plating **(a, b)** cannot guarantee that cross-union will not occur **(c)**.

plates and screws. Bone grafting is advisable if there is comminution of more than one-third of the circumference. The deep fascia is left open to prevent a build-up of pressure in the muscle compartments, and only the skin and subcutaneous tissues are sutured.

After the operation the arm is kept elevated until the swelling subsides, and during this period active exercises of the hand are encouraged. If the fracture is not comminuted and the patient is reliable, early range of movement exercises are commenced but lifting and sports are avoided. It takes 8–12 weeks for the bones to unite. With comminuted fractures or unreliable patients, immobilization in plaster is safer.

OPEN FRACTURES

Open fractures of the forearm must be managed meticulously. Antibiotics and tetanus prophylaxis are given as soon as possible; the nerves and circulation are checked. The wounds are excised and extended; the bone ends are exposed and thoroughly cleaned. The fractures are primarily fixed with compression screws and plates; bone graft, if necessary, is probably best deferred until the wounds are healed. The wound is best left open but the extensions can be closed. When there is major soft-tissue loss, the bones are better stabilized with an external fixator and the services of a plastic surgeon called in.

Complications

EARLY

Nerve injury Nerve injuries are rarely caused by the fracture, but they may be caused by the surgeon! Exposure of the radius in its proximal third risks damage to the posterior interosseous nerve where it is covered by the

superficial part of the supinator muscle. Surgical technique is particularly important here; the anterior Henry approach is safest.

Vascular injury Injury to the radial or ulnar artery seldom presents any problem, as the collateral circulation is excellent.

Compartment syndrome Fractures (and operations) of the forearm bones are always associated with swelling of the soft tissues, with the attendant risk of a compartment syndrome. The threat is even greater, and the diagnosis more difficult, if the forearm is wrapped up in plaster. A distal pulse does not exclude compartment syndrome! The byword is 'watchfulness'; if there are any signs of circulatory embarrassment, treatment must be prompt and uncompromising.

LATE

Delayed union and non-union Most fractures of the radius and ulna heal within 8–12 weeks; high-energy fractures and open fractures are less likely to unite. Delayed union of one or other bone (usually the ulna) is not uncommon; immobilization may have to be continued beyond the usual time. Non-union will require bone grafting and internal fixation

Malunion With closed reduction there is always a risk of malunion, resulting in angulation or rotational deformity of the forearm, cross-union of the fragments or shortening of one of the bones and disruption of the distal radioulnar joint. If pronation or supination is severely restricted, and there is no cross-union, mobility may be improved by excising the distal end of the ulna.

Complications of plate removal Removal of plates and screws is often regarded as a fairly innocuous procedure. Beware! Complications are common and they include damage to vessels and nerves, infection and fracture through a screw hole.

FRACTURE OF A SINGLE FOREARM BONE

Fracture of the radius alone is very rare and fracture of the ulna alone is uncommon. These injuries are usually caused by a direct blow – the 'nightstick fracture'. They are important for two reasons:

- An associated dislocation may be undiagnosed; if only one forearm bone is broken along its shaft and there is displacement, then either the proximal or the distal radioulnar joint must be dislocated. The entire forearm should always be x-rayed.
- Non-union is liable to occur unless it is realized that one bone takes just as long to consolidate as two.

Clinical features

Ulnar fractures are easily missed – even on x-ray. If there is local tenderness, a further x-ray a week or two later is wise.

X-RAY

The fracture may be anywhere in the radius or ulna. The fracture line is transverse and displacement is slight. In children, the intact bone sometimes bends without actually breaking ('plastic deformation').

Treatment

Isolated fracture of the ulna The fracture is rarely displaced; a forearm brace leaving the elbow free is usually sufficient. It takes about 8 weeks before full activity can be resumed.

Isolated fracture of the radius Radial fractures are prone to rotary displacement; to achieve reduction the forearm needs to be supinated for upper third fractures, neutral for middle third fractures and pronated for lower third fractures. The position is sometimes difficult to hold; if so, then internal fixation with a compression plate and screws is better. With rigid fixation, early movement is encouraged.

MONTEGGIA FRACTURE-DISLOCATION OF THE ULNA

The injury described by Monteggia in the early nineteenth century (without benefit of x-rays!) was a fracture of the shaft of the ulna associated with dislocation of the proximal radioulnar joint; the radiocapitellar joint is inevitably dislocated or subluxated as well. More recently the definition has been extended to embrace almost any fracture of the ulna associated with dislocation of the radiocapitellar joint, including trans-olecranon fractures in which the proximal radioulnar joint remains intact. If

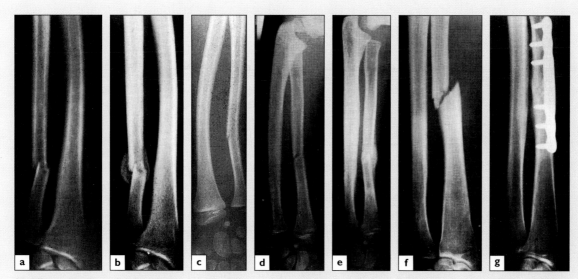

25.4 Fracture of one forearm bone *Fracture of the ulna:* A fracture of the ulna alone (**a**) usually joins satisfactorily (**b**); in children the intact radius may be bowed (**c**). *Fracture of the radius:* In a child, fracture of the radius alone (**d**) may join in plaster (**e**), but in adults a fractured radius (**f**) is better treated by plating (**g**).

the ulnar shaft fracture is angulated with the apex anterior (the commonest type) then the radial head is displaced anteriorly; if the fracture apex is posterior, the radial dislocation is posterior; and if the fracture apex is lateral then the radial head will be laterally displaced. In children, the ulnar injury may be an incomplete fracture (green-stick or plastic deformation of the shaft).

Mechanism of injury

Usually the cause is a fall on the hand; if at the moment of impact the body is twisting, its momentum may forcibly pronate the forearm. The radial head usually dislocates forwards and the upper third of the ulna fractures and bows forwards. Sometimes the causal force is hyperextension.

Clinical features

The ulnar deformity is usually obvious but the dislocated head of radius is masked by swelling. A useful clue is pain and tenderness on the lateral side of the elbow. The wrist and hand should be examined for signs of injury to the radial nerve.

X-RAY

With isolated fractures of the ulna, it is essential to obtain a true anteroposterior and true lateral view of the elbow. In the usual case, the head of the radius (which normally points directly to the capitulum) is dislocated forwards, and there is a fracture of the upper third of the ulna with forwards bowing. Backwards or lateral bowing of the ulna (which is much less common) is likely to be associated with, respectively, posterior or lateral displacement of the radial head. Trans-olecranon fractures, also, are often associated with radial head dislocation.

Treatment

The clue to successful treatment is to restore the length of the fractured ulna; only then can the dislocated joint be fully reduced and remain stable. In adults, this means an operation. The ulnar fracture must be accurately reduced, with the bone restored to full length, and then fixed with a plate and screws; bone grafts may be added for safety. The radial head usually reduces once the ulna has been fixed. Stability must be tested through a full range of flexion and extension. If the radial head does not reduce, or is not stable, open reduction should be performed.

High posterior fracture-dislocations are particularly unstable, and are sometimes associated with subluxation of the ulnohumeral joint. Check for an associated fracture of the coronoid process, which also may need fixation.

If the elbow is completely stable, then flexion/extension and rotation can be started after 10 days. If there is doubt, then the arm should be immobilized in plaster with the elbow flexed for 6 weeks.

Complications

Nerve injury Nerve injuries can be caused by over-enthusiastic manipulation of the radial dislocation or during the surgical exposure. Always check for nerve function after treatment. The lesion is usually a neurapraxia, which will recover by itself.

Malunion Unless the ulna has been perfectly reduced, the radial head remains dislocated and limits elbow flexion. In children, no treatment is advised. In adults, excision of the radial head, with or without prosthetic replacement, may be needed.

Non-union Non-union of the ulna should be treated by plating and bone grafting. If the radial head is dislocated it should be excised.

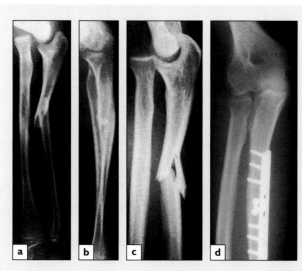

25.5 Monteggia fracture-dislocation (**a**) The ulna is fractured and the head of the radius no longer points to the capitulum. In a child, closed reduction and plaster (**b**) is usually satisfactory; in the adult (**c**) open reducation and plating (**d**) is preferred.

SPECIAL FEATURES IN CHILDREN

The general features of Monteggia fracture-dislocations are similar to those in adults. However, it is important to remember that the ulnar fracture may be incomplete (green-stick or plastic deformation); if this is not detected, and corrected, the child may end up with chronic subluxation of the radial head.

Incomplete ulnar fractures can often be reduced closed, although considerable force is needed to straighten the ulna with plastic deformation. The position of the radial head is then checked; if it is not perfect, closed reduction can be completed by flexing and supinating the elbow and pressing on the radial head. The arm is then immobilized in a cast with the elbow in flexion and supination, for 3 weeks.

Complete fractures are best treated by open reduction and fixation, as in adults.

GALEAZZI FRACTURE-DISLOCATION OF THE RADIUS

Mechanism of injury

This injury was first described in 1934 by Galeazzi. The usual cause is a fall on the hand; probably with a superimposed rotation force. The radius fractures in its lower third and the inferior radioulnar joint subluxates or dislocates.

Clinical features

The Galeazzi fracture is much more common than the Monteggia. Prominence or tenderness over the lower end of the ulna is the striking feature. It may be possible to demonstrate the instability of the radioulnar joint by 'ballotting' the distal end of the ulna (the 'piano-key sign') or by rotating the wrist. It is important also to test for an ulnar nerve lesion, which is common.

X-RAY
A transverse or short oblique fracture is seen in the lower third of the radius, with angulation or overlap. The inferior radioulnar joint is subluxated or dislocated.

Treatment

As with the Monteggia fracture, the important step is to restore the length of the fractured bone. In children, closed reduction is often successful; in adults, reduction is best achieved by open operation and compression plating of the radius. An x-ray is taken to ensure that the distal radioulnar joint is reduced. There are three possibilities:

- *The distal radioulnar joint is reduced and stable* No further action is needed. The arm is rested for a few days, then gentle active movements are encouraged. The radioulnar joint should be checked, both clinically and radiologically, during the next 6 weeks.
- *The distal radioulnar joint is reduced but unstable* The forearm should be immobilized in the position of stability (usually supination), supplemented if required by a transverse K-wire. The forearm is splinted in an above-elbow cast for 6 weeks. If there is a large ulnar styloid fragment, it should be reduced and fixed.
- *The distal radioulnar joint is irreducible* This is unusual. Open reduction is needed to remove the interposed soft tissues. The triangular fibrocartilage complex (TFCC) and dorsal capsule are then carefully repaired and the forearm immobilized in the position of stability (again, usually supination) for 6 weeks.

FRACTURES OF THE DISTAL RADIUS

The distal end of the radius is subject to six distinct types of fracture, each with its own characteristic pattern of behaviour. These are:

1. Colles' fracture – a low-energy osteoporotic fracture in postmenopausal women.

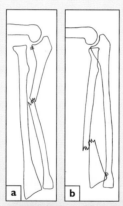

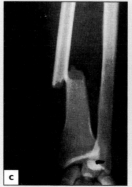

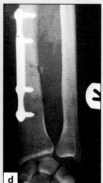

25.6 Galeazzi fracture-dislocation The diagrams show the contrast between **(a)** Monteggia and **(b)** Galeazzi fracture-dislocations. **(c, d)** Galeazzi type before and after reduction and plating.

2. Smith's fracture – similar to Colles' fracture but displaced anteriorly rather than posteriorly (hence its other name, 'reversed Colles').
3. Distal forearm fracture in children – sometimes (erroneously) called 'juvenile Colles'.
4. Radial styloid fracture – the fracture enters the wrist joint.
5. Barton's fracture – fracture-subluxation of the wrist.
6. Comminuted intra-articular fractures in young adults.

NOTE: With any of these fractures, the wrist also can suffer substantial ligamentous injury and/or distal radioulnar instability; these injuries are easily missed because the x-rays often look normal.

COLLES' FRACTURE

The injury that Abraham Colles described in 1814 is a transverse fracture of the radius just above the wrist, with dorsal displacement of the distal fragment. It is the most common of all fractures in older people, the high incidence being related to the onset of postmenopausal osteoporosis. Thus the patient is usually an older woman who gives a history of falling on her outstretched hand.

Mechanism of injury and pathological anatomy

Force is applied in the length of the forearm with the wrist in extension. The bone fractures at the corticocancellous junction and the distal fragment collapses into extension, dorsal displacement, radial tilt and shortening.

Clinical features

We can recognize this fracture (as Colles did long before radiography was invented) by the 'dinner-fork' deformity, with prominence on the back of the wrist and a depression in front. In patients with less deformity there may only be local tenderness and pain on wrist movements.

X-RAY
There is a transverse fracture of the radius at the corticocancellous junction, and often the ulnar styloid process is broken off. The radial fragment is impacted into radial and backwards tilt. Sometimes it is severely comminuted or crushed.

Treatment

UNDISPLACED FRACTURES
If the fracture is undisplaced (or only very slightly displaced), a dorsal splint is applied for a day or two until the swelling has resolved, then the cast is completed. The fracture is stable and the cast can usually be removed after 4 weeks to allow mobilization.

DISPLACED FRACTURES
Displaced fractures must be reduced under anaesthesia (haematoma block, Bier's block or axillary block). The hand is grasped and traction is applied in the length of the bone (sometimes with extension of the wrist to disimpact the fragments); the distal fragment is then pushed into place by pressing on the dorsum while manipulating the wrist into flexion, ulnar deviation and pronation. The position is then checked by x-ray. If it is satisfactory, a dorsal plaster slab is applied, extending from just below the elbow to the metacarpal necks and two-thirds of the way round the circumference of the wrist. It is held in position by a crepe bandage. *Extreme positions of flexion and ulnar deviation must be avoided*; 20° in each direction is adequate.

The arm is kept elevated for the next day or two; shoulder and finger exercises are started as soon possible. If the fingers become swollen, cyanosed or painful, there should be no hesitation in splitting the bandage.

At 7–10 days fresh x-rays are taken; redisplacement is not uncommon and is usually treated by re-reduction; unfortunately, even if manipulation is successful, re-redisplacement is common.

The fracture unites in about 6 weeks and, even in the absence of radiological proof of union, the slab may safely be discarded and exercises begun.

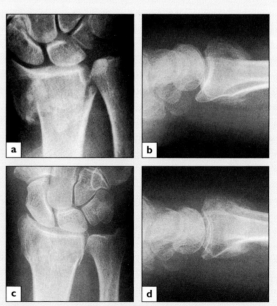

25.7 Colles' fracture (**a, b**) The typical Colles fracture is both displaced and angulated towards the dorsum and towards the radial side of the wrist. (**c, d**) Note how, after successful reduction, the radial articular surface faces correctly both distally and slightly volarwards.

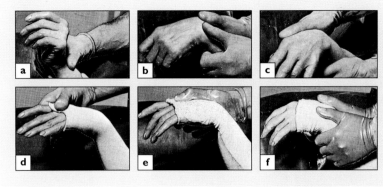

25.8 Colles' fracture – reduction and splintage
Reduction: (**a**) dis-impaction (not always necessary), (**b**) pronation and forwards shift, (**c**) ulnar deviation. *Splintage:* (**d**) Stockinette, (**e**) wet plaster slab, (**f**) slab bandaged on and reduction held till plaster sets. *Beware not to overdo the ulnar deviation and flexion.*

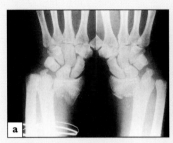
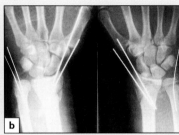

25.9 Colles' fracture – internal fixation This unfortunate patient leapt head first through a window and landed on outstretched hands. The injuries are more or less symmetrical: (**a**) severely displaced, unstable Colles' fractures. (**b**) Fixation with percutaneous K-wires gave a good result. More severely comminuted fractures in osteoporotic bone may require external fixation (see Fig. 25.16).

COMMINUTED COLLES' FRACTURES

Plaster immobilization alone may be insufficient; this can be supplemented by percutaneous K-wire fixation. The plaster and wires are removed after 5 weeks and exercises begun. In very comminuted fractures for which percutaneous wires are inadequate, external fixation is needed. Proximal pins are placed through the radius and distal pins through the shaft of the second metacarpal. Bone grafts may be added if the radius has markedly collapsed. External fixation, whilst improving the x-ray appearance, may lead to prolonged stiffness unless the ability to move is built into the fixator (see Fig. 25.16).

Complications

EARLY

The circulation in the fingers must be checked; the bandage holding the slab may need to be split or loosened.

Nerve injury is rare, but compression of the median nerve in the carpal tunnel is fairly common. If it occurs soon after injury and the symptoms are mild, they may resolve with release of the dressings and elevation. If symptoms are severe or persistent, the transverse ligament should be divided.

Reflex sympathetic dystrophy is probably quite common, but fortunately it seldom progresses to the full-blown picture of *Sudeck's atrophy*. There may be swelling and tenderness of the finger joints, a warning not to neglect the daily exercises. In about 5% of cases, by the time the plaster is removed the hand is stiff and painful and there are signs of vasomotor instability. X-rays show osteoporosis and there is increased activity on the bone scan.

TFCC injury is more common than is generally appreciated. As the distal radius displaces dorsally, the TFCC is damaged; the ulnar styloid fracture which commonly accompanies a Colles' fracture illustrates the forces which are transmitted to the TFCC, which attaches in part to it.

LATE

Malunion is common, either because reduction was not complete or because displacement within the plaster was overlooked. The appearance is ugly, and weakness and loss of rotation may persist. In most cases treatment is not necessary. Where the disability is severe and the patient relatively young, the radial deformity should be corrected by osteotomy.

Delayed union and non-union of the radius are rare, but the ulnar styloid process often joins by fibrous tissue only and remains painful and tender for several months.

Stiffness of the shoulder, elbow and fingers from neglect is a common complication. Stiffness of the wrist may follow prolonged splintage.

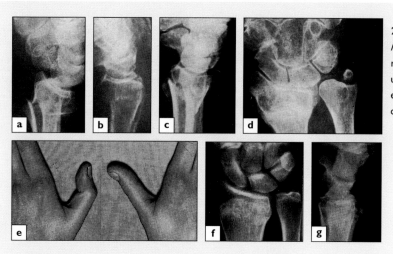

Tendon rupture (of extensor pollicis longus) occasionally occurs a few weeks after an apparently trivial undisplaced fracture of the lower radius. The patient should be warned of the possibility and told that operative treatment is available.

SMITH'S FRACTURE

Smith (a Dubliner, like Colles) described a similar fracture about 20 years later. However, in this injury the distal fragment is displaced anteriorly (which is why it is sometimes called a 'reversed Colles'). It is caused by a fall on the back of the hand.

Clinical features

The patient presents with a wrist injury, but there is no dinner-fork deformity. Instead, there is a 'garden spade' deformity.

X-RAY
There is a fracture through the distal radial metaphysis; a lateral view shows that the distal fragment is displaced and tilted anteriorly – the opposite of a Colles' fracture. The entire metaphysis can be fractured, or there can be an oblique fracture exiting at the dorsal or volar rim of the radius.

Treatment

The fracture is reduced by traction and extension of the wrist, and the forearm is immobilized in a cast for 6 weeks.

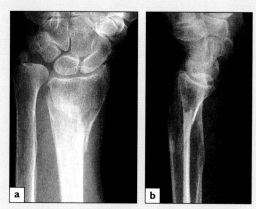

25.11 Smith's fracture (**a**, **b**) Here, in contrast to Colles' fracture, the displacement of the lower radial fragment is forwards – not backwards.

DISTAL FOREARM FRACTURES IN CHILDREN

The distal radius and ulna are among the commonest sites of childhood fractures. The break may occur through the distal radial physis or in the metaphysis of one or both bones. Metaphyseal fractures are often incomplete or green-stick.

Mechanism of injury

The usual injury is a fall on the outstretched hand with the wrist in extension; the distal fragment is forced posteriorly (this is often called a 'juvenile Colles' fracture'). However, sometimes the wrist is in flexion and the fracture is angulated anteriorly. Lesser force may do no more than buckle the metaphyseal cortex (a type of compression fracture, or torus fracture).

Clinical features

There is usually a history of a fall, though this may be passed off as one of many childhood spills. The wrist is painful, and often quite swollen; sometimes there is an obvious 'dinner-fork' deformity.

X-RAY
The precise diagnosis is made on the x-ray appearances.

Physeal fractures are almost invariably Salter–Harris type I or II, with the epiphysis shifted and tilted backwards and radially. Type V injuries are unusual; sometimes they are diagnosed in retrospect when premature epiphyseal fusion occurs.

Metaphyseal injuries may appear as mere *buckling* of the cortex (easily missed unless appropriate views are obtained), as angulated *green-stick fractures* or as *complete fractures* with displacement and shortening. If only the radius is fractured, the ulna may be bent though not fractured.

Treatment

Physeal fractures are reduced, under anaesthesia, by pressure on the distal fragment. The arm is immobilized in a full-length cast with the wrist slightly flexed and ulnar deviated, and the elbow at 90°. The cast is retained for 4 weeks. These fractures do not interfere with growth. Even if reduction is not absolutely perfect, further growth and modelling will obliterate any deformity within a year or two. Patients seen more than 2 weeks after injury are best left untreated.

Buckle fractures require no more than 2 weeks in plaster, followed by another 2 weeks of restricted activity.

Green-stick fractures are usually easy to reduce – but apt to redisplace in the cast! Some degree of angulation can be accepted: in children under 10 years of age, up to 30° and in children over ten, up 15°. If the deformity is greater, the fracture is reduced by thumb pressure and the arm is immobilized with three-point fixation in a full-length cast with the wrist and forearm in neutral and the elbow flexed 90°. The cast is changed and the fracture re-x-rayed at 2 weeks; if it has redisplaced a further manipulation can be carried out. The cast is finally discarded after 6 weeks.

Complete fractures can be embarrassingly difficult to reduce – especially if the ulna is intact. The fracture is manipulated in much the same way as a Colles' fracture; the reduction is checked by x-ray and a full-length cast is applied with the wrist neutral and the forearm supinated. After 2 weeks, a check x-ray is obtained; the cast is kept on for 6 weeks. If the fracture slips, especially if the ulna is intact, it should be stabilized with a percutaneous K-wire.

Complications

EARLY
Forearm swelling and a threatened *compartment syndrome* are prevented by avoiding overforceful or repeated manipulations, splitting the plaster, elevating the arm for the first 24–48 hours and encouraging exercises.

LATE
Malunion as a late sequel is uncommon in children under 10 years of age. Deformity of as much as 30° will straighten out with further growth and remodelling over the next 5 years. This should be carefully explained to the worried parents.

Radioulnar discrepancy Premature fusion of the radial epiphysis may result in bone length disparity and

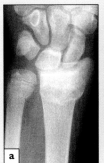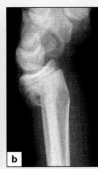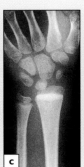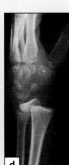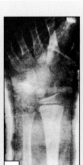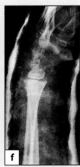

25.12 Distal forearm fractures in children (a, b) In older children the fracture is usually slightly more proximal than a true Colles', and often merely a green-stick or buckling injury. (c, d) In young children physeal fractures are usually Salter–Harris type I or II. In this case, accurate reduction has been achieved (e, f).

subluxation of the radioulnar joint. If this is troublesome, the distal end of the ulna can be excised.

Fractures of the distal radius may enter the wrist joint, causing (1) a simple osteoarticular fracture, (2) a comminuted osteoarticular fracture or (3) a fracture-subluxation of the wrist.

RADIOCARPAL FRACTURES

FRACTURED RADIAL STYLOID

This injury is caused by forced radial deviation of the wrist and may occur after a fall, or when a starting handle 'kicks back'- the so-called 'chauffeur's fracture'. The fracture line is transverse, extending laterally from the articular surface of the radius; the fragment, much more than the radial styloid, is often undisplaced. The radial styloid can also be fractured as part of the far more serious transscaphoid perilunate fracture dislocation.

Treatment If there is displacement it is reduced, and the wrist is held in ulnar deviation by a plaster slab round the outer forearm extending from below the elbow to the metacarpal necks. Imperfect reduction may lead to osteoarthritis; therefore if closed reduction is imperfect the fragment should be screwed back, or held with K-wires.

FRACTURE–SUBLUXATION (BARTON'S FRACTURE)

Volar subluxation

The true Barton's injury is a volar fracture associated with volar subluxation of the carpus. It is sometimes mistaken for a Smith's fracture, but it differs from the latter in that the fracture line runs obliquely across the volar lip of the radius into the wrist joint; the distal fragment is displaced anteriorly, carrying the carpus with it. Because the fragment is small and unsupported, the fracture is inherently unstable.

Treatment The fracture can be easily reduced, but it is just as easily redisplaced. Internal fixation, using a small anterior buttress plate, is recommended.

Dorsal subluxation

This is sometimes called a 'dorsal Barton's fracture'. Here the line of fracture runs obliquely across the dorsal lip of the radius and the carpus is carried posteriorly.

Treatment The fracture is easier to control than the volar Barton's fracture. It is reduced closed and the

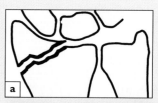
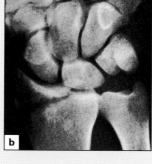

25.13 Fracture of the radial styloid process This fracture, which enters the joint, needs to be reduced accurately.

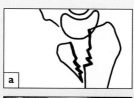
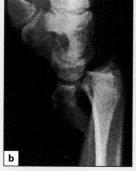
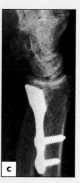

25.14 Fracture-subluxation (Barton's fracture) (a, b) The true Barton's fracture is a split of the volar edge of the distal radius with anterior (volar) subluxation of the wrist. This has been reduced and held (**c**) with a small anterior plate.

forearm is immobilized in a cast for 6 weeks. If it redisplaces, open reduction and plating is advisable.

COMMINUTED INTRA–ARTICULAR FRACTURES IN YOUNG ADULTS

In the young adult, a comminuted intra-articular fracture is a high-energy injury. A poor outcome will result unless intra-articular congruity, fracture alignment and length are restored and movements started as soon as possible. For these patients a much higher standard must be set than would be accepted for the typical osteoporotic fracture. In addition to the usual posteranterior

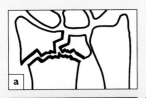
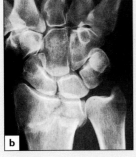
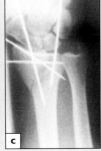

25.15 Comminuted fracture of the distal radius The 'die punch fragment' of the lunate fossa of the distal radius (**a, b**) must be perfectly reduced and fixed; here this has been achieved by closed reduction and percutaneous K-wire fixation (**c**). The wires can be used as 'joy sticks' to manipulate the fragment back before fixation.

and lateral x-rays, oblique views are useful to show the medial complex.

The simplest option is a manipulation and cast. If the anatomy is not restored, then an open reduction may be necessary. The medial complex must be anatomically reduced, which may require open reduction through dorsal and palmar approaches and a combination of wires, plates, screws, bone grafts and external fixation.

COMPLICATIONS OF RADIOCARPAL FRACTURES

EARLY

Associated injuries of the carpus Injuries of the carpus are easily overlooked while attention is focussed on the

radius. Wrist injuries must be excluded by careful clinical and x-ray examination.

Redisplacement There is a strong tendency for Barton's fracture to redisplace if it is held in a cast; hence our preference for internal fixation.

LATE

Carpal instability The patient may present years later with chronic carpal instability. The wrist injury may have been overlooked at the time.

Secondary osteoarthritis Fractures into the joint and carpal instability may eventually lead to secondary osteoarthritis. It is difficult to predict when (or even whether) this is likely to occur; symptoms develop slowly and disability is often not severe. Warning symptoms are restricted wrist movement and loss of grip strength. If pain and weakness interfere significantly with function, arthrodesis of the wrist may be need, especially if it is the dominant side which is affected.

CARPAL INJURIES

Fractures and dislocations of the carpal bones are common. They vary greatly in type and severity. *These should never be regarded as isolated injuries; the entire carpus suffers*, and sometimes, long after the fracture has healed, the patient still complains of pain and weakness in the wrist.

The commonest wrist injuries are:

1. Sprains of the capsule and ligaments.
2. Fracture of a carpal bone (usually the scaphoid).
3. Injury of the TFCC and distal radioulnar joint.
4. Dislocations of the lunate or the bones around it.
5. Subluxations and 'carpal collapse', which may be acute or chronic.

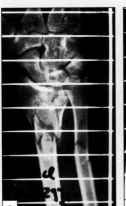
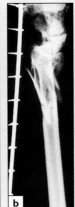
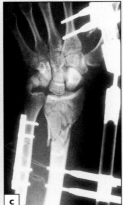
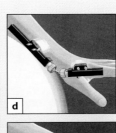
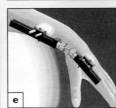

25.16 High-energy fractures of the distal forearm bones (**a, b**) Severely comminuted fractures of the distal radius and ulna may need both internal and external fixation (**c**). In this case, good reduction and fixation were achieved. Movements were started with the external fixator still in place after 2 or 3 weeks, thus reducing the risk of stiffness. (**d, e**) A Pennig fixator.

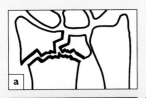

Clinical assessment

Following a fall, the patient complains of pain in the wrist. There may be swelling or well-marked deformity of the joint. Tenderness should be carefully localized; undirected prodding will confuse both the patient and the examiner. The blunt end of a pencil is helpful in testing for point tenderness. For scaphoid fractures, the 'jump spot' is in the anatomical snuffbox; for scapholunate injuries, just beyond Lister's tubercle; for lunate dislocation, in the middle of the wrist; for triquetral injuries, beyond the head of the ulna; for hamate fractures, at the base of the hypothenar eminence; for triangular fibrocartilage complex injuries, over the dorsum of the ulnocarpal joint. Movements are often limited (more by pain than by stiffness) and they may be accompanied by a palpable catch or an audible click.

Imaging

X-rays are the key to diagnosis. There are three golden rules:

- Accept only high-quality films.
- If the initial x-rays are 'normal', treat the clinical diagnosis.
- Repeat the x-ray examination 2 weeks later.

Initially three standard views are obtained: anteroposterior and lateral with the wrist neutral, and an oblique 'scaphoid' view. If these are normal and clinical features suggest a carpal injury, four further views are obtained: anteroposterior x-rays with the wrist first in maximum ulnar and then in maximum radial deviation, and lateral x-rays with the wrist in maximum flexion and extension.

The examiner should be familiar with the normal x-ray anatomy of the carpus in all the standard views, so that he or she can visualize a three-dimensional picture from the two-dimensional, overlapping images of the carpal bones.

In the anteroposterior x-rays note the shape of the carpus, whether the individual bones are clearly outlined and whether there are any abnormally large gaps suggesting disruption of the ligaments. The scaphoid may be fractured; or it may have lost its normal bean shape and look squat and foreshortened, sometimes with an inner circular density (the cortical ring sign) – features of an end-on view when the bone is hyperflexed because of damage to the restraining scapholunate ligament. The lunate is normally quadrilateral in shape, but if it is dislocated it looks triangular.

In the lateral x-ray the axes of the radius, lunate, capitate and third metacarpal are co-linear, and the scaphoid projects at an angle of about 45° to this line. With traumatic instability the linked carpal segments collapse (like the buckled carriages of a derailed train). Two patterns are recognized: dorsal intercalated

segment instability (DISI), in which the lunate is torn from the scaphoid and tilted backwards; and volar intercalated segment instability (VISI), in which the lunate is torn from the triquetrum and turns towards the palm, while the capitate assumes a complementary dorsal tilt. In addition, there may be a flake fracture off the back of a carpal bone (usually the triquetrum).

Special x-ray studies are sometimes helpful: a *carpal tunnel view* may show a fractured hook of hamate, and *motion studies* in different positions may reveal a subluxation. A *radioisotope scan* will confirm a wrist injury although it may not precisely localize it.

Magnetic resonance imaging (MRI) is sensitive and specific (especially for detecting undisclosed fractures or Kienböck's disease), but unless very fine cuts are taken it may miss TFCC and interosseous ligament tears.

Wrist arthroscopy is the best way of demonstrating TFCC or interosseous ligament tears.

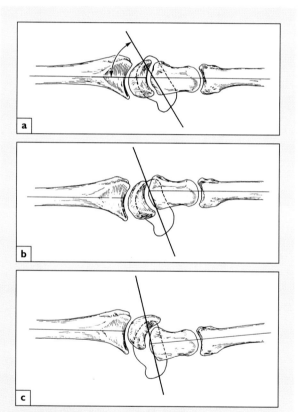

25.17 Carpal instability – x-ray patterns (a) Normal lateral view. The radius, capitate and middle metacarpal lie in a straight line and the scaphoid axis is angled at 45° to the line of the radius. (b) Dorsal intercalated segmental instability (DISI). The lunate is tilted dorsally and the scaphoid is tilted somewhat volarwards; the axes of the capitate and metacarpals now lie behind (dorsal to) that of the radius. (c) Volar intercalated segmental instability (VISI). The lunate and scaphoid are tilted somewhat volarwards and the capitate and metacarpals lie anterior (volar) to the radius.

FRACTURED SCAPHOID

Scaphoid fractures account for almost 75% of all carpal fractures although they are rare in the elderly and in children. With unstable fractures there may also be disruption of the scapholunate ligaments and dorsal rotation of the lunate.

Mechanism of injury and pathological anatomy

The scaphoid lies obliquely across the two rows of carpal bones, and is also in the line of loading between the thumb and forearm. The combination of forced carpal movement and compression, as in a fall on the dorsiflexed hand, exerts severe stress on the bone and it is liable to fracture. Most scaphoid fractures are stable; with unstable fractures the fragments may become displaced. The distal fragment, unrestrained by the scapholunate ligament, flexes and the proximal fragment tilts dorsally with the lunate (a DISI deformity); the hump-backed deformity of the scaphoid is apparent.

The blood supply of the scaphoid diminishes proximally. This accounts for the fact that 1% of distal third fractures, 20% of middle third fractures and 40% of proximal fractures result in non-union or avascular necrosis of the proximal fragment.

Clinical features

The appearance may be deceptively normal, but the astute observer can usually detect fullness in the anatomical snuffbox; precisely localized tenderness in the same place is an important diagnostic sign; the scaphoid can of course also be palpated from the front and back of the wrist and it may be tender there as well. Proximal pressure along the axis of the thumb may be painful.

X-RAY

Anteroposterior, lateral and oblique views are all essential; often a recent fracture shows only in the oblique view. Usually the fracture line is transverse, and through the narrowest part of the bone (waist), but it may be more proximally situated (proximal pole fracture). Sometimes only the tubercle of the scaphoid is fractured.

It is very important to look for subtle signs of displacement or instability: e.g. obliquity of the fracture line, opening of the fracture line, angulation of the distal fragment and foreshortening of the scaphoid image.

A few weeks after the injury the fracture may be more obvious; if union is delayed, cavitation appears on either side of the break. Old, un-united fractures

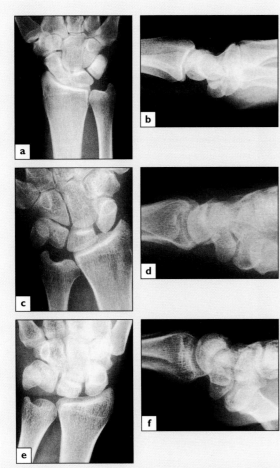

25.18 Carpal injuries (a, b) Normal appearances in anteroposterior and lateral x-rays. (c, d) Following a 'sprained wrist', this patient developed persistent pain and weakness. X-rays showed (c) scapholunate dissociation and (d) dorsal rotation of the lunate (the typical DISI pattern). (e, f) This patient, too, had a sprained wrist. The anteroposterior and lateral x-rays show foreshortening of the scaphoid and volar rotation of the lunate (VISI).

Principles of management

'Wrist sprain' should not be diagnosed unless a more serious injury has been excluded with certainty. Even with apparently trivial injuries, ligaments are sometimes torn and the patient may later develop carpal instability.

If the x-rays are normal but the clinical signs strongly suggest a carpal injury, a splint or plaster should be applied for 2 weeks, after which time the x-rays are repeated. A fracture may become more obvious after a few weeks, but a second negative x-ray still does not exclude a serious bone or ligament injury. A bone scan or MRI at this stage will confirm or exclude a fracture; however, a major ligament strain may be missed by these investigations, so it is wise to continue with immobilization until the symptoms settle or a firm diagnosis is made.

The more common lesions are dealt with below.

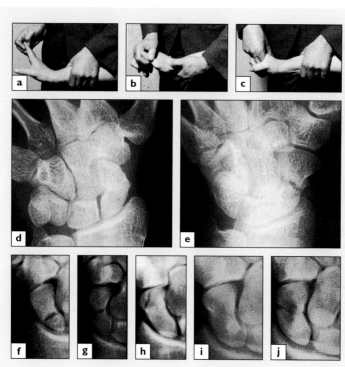

25.19 Scaphoid fractures – diagnosis *Clinical signs:* (**a**) pain on dorsiflexion, (**b**) localized tenderness, (**c**) pain on gripping. *X-ray signs:* the anteroposterior view (**d**) often fails to show the fracture; always ask for an oblique, 'scaphoid' view (**e**). Fracture may be through (**f**) the proximal pole, (**g**) the waist or (**h**) the tubercle. If the clinical features are suggestive and no fracture is seen on x-ray (**i**), a repeat film at 2 weeks (**j**) should be obtained.

have 'hard' borders, making it seem as if there is an extra carpal bone. Relative sclerosis of the proximal fragment is pathognomonic of avascular necrosis.

Treatment

Fracture of the scaphoid tubercle needs no splintage and should be treated as a wrist sprain; a crepe bandage is applied and movement is encouraged. Other scaphoid fractures are treated as follows.

Undisplaced fractures need no reduction and are treated in plaster; 90% should heal. The cast is applied from the upper forearm to just short of the metacarpophalangeal joints of the fingers, but incorporating the proximal phalanx of the thumb. The wrist is held dorsiflexed and the thumb forwards in the 'glass-holding' position. The plaster must be carefully moulded into the hollow of the hand, and is not split. It is retained (and if necessary repaired or renewed) for 6 weeks.

After 6 weeks the plaster is removed and the wrist examined clinically and radiologically. If there is no tenderness and the x-ray shows signs of healing, the wrist is left free; complete radiographic union may take several months. CT scan is the most reliable means of confirming union if in doubt.

If the scaphoid is tender, or the fracture still visible on x-ray, the cast is reapplied for a further 6 weeks. At that stage, one of two pictures may emerge:

- The wrist is painless and the fracture has healed – the cast can be discarded.

- The x-ray shows signs of delayed healing (bone resorption and cavitation around the fracture) – union can be hastened by bone grafting and internal fixation.

Displaced fractures can also be treated in plaster, but the outcome is less predictable. It is better to reduce the fracture openly and to fix it with a compression screw. This will increase the likelihood of union and reduce the time of immobilization.

Complications

Avascular necrosis The proximal fragment may die, especially with proximal pole fractures, and then at 2–3 months it appears dense on x-ray. Although revascularization and union are theoretically possible, they take years and meanwhile the wrist collapses and arthritis develops. Bone grafting, as for delayed union, may be successful, in which case the bone, though abnormal, is structurally intact. If the wrist becomes painful, the dead fragment can be excised. However, the wrist tends to collapse after this procedure; a better option would be to remove the entire proximal row of carpal bones or else to remove the scaphoid and fuse the proximal to the distal row (four-corner fusion: capitate–hamate–triquetrum–lunate).

Non-union By 3 months it may be obvious that the fracture will not unite. Bone grafting may still be attempted, especially in the younger, more vigorous type of patient, because this probably reduces the chance of later, symptomatic osteoarthritis. Two types

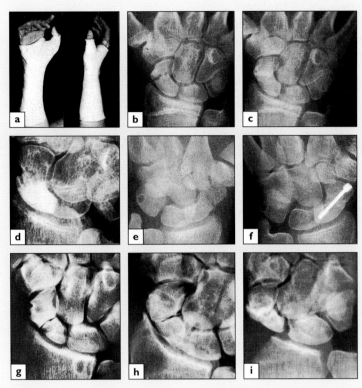

25.20 Scaphoid fractures – treatment and complications (a) Scaphoid plaster – position and extent. (b, c) Before and after treatment: in this case radiological union was visible at 10 weeks. (d) Avascular necrosis of proximal half; (e) non-union, treated successfully by (f) inserting a screw. (g) Established non-union with sclerosis; (h) non-union with localized osteoarthritic changes; (i) osteoarthritis treated by excising the radial styloid.

of graft are used. If the scaphoid has folded into a flexed 'humpback' shape, then it is approached from the front and a wedge of cortico-cancellous iliac crest graft is inserted to restore the shape of the bone. The graft is fixed with a buried screw and/or K-wires. If the scaphoid has not collapsed, the graft is inserted into a trough carved into the front of the scaphoid and again stabilized with a screw or wires. If these techniques fail to achieve union then the options are a vascularized bone graft, scaphoidectomy with proximal-to-distal-row (four-corner) fusion, proximal row carpectomy or radiocarpal arthrodesis.

In older patients, and those who are completely asymptomatic, non-union may be left untreated. Sometimes a patient is seen for the first time with a 'sprain', but x-rays show an old, un-united fracture with sclerosed edges; 3–4 weeks in plaster may suffice to make him or her comfortable once again, and no further treatment is required.

Osteoarthritis Non-union or avascular necrosis may lead to secondary osteoarthritis of the wrist. If the arthritis is localized to the distal pole, excising the radial styloid may help. As the arthritis progresses, changes appear in the scaphocapitate joint and eventually throughout the wrist. Salvage procedures include proximal row carpectomy, four-corner fusion or radiocarpal fusion.

FRACTURES OF OTHER CARPAL BONES

TRIQUETRUM

Avulsion of the dorsal ligaments is not uncommon; analgesics and splintage for a few days are all that is required. Occasionally the body is fractured; it usually heals after 4–6 weeks in plaster.

HAMATE

Fractures of the body are rare. A fracture of the hook follows a direct blow to the palm of the hand. These fractures cannot be seen on routine x-rays; a carpal tunnel view, CT or MRI is needed. The fracture does not heal readily; if symptoms are prolonged then the fragment is excised, taking care not to damage the ulnar nerve.

TRAPEZIUM

The body of the trapezium can be fractured if the shaft of the first metacarpal impacts onto it; the ridge (to which the transverse carpal ligament attaches) can be fractured by a direct blow. The latter fracture can usually be seen on a carpal tunnel view rather than standard x-rays. The body fracture may need open reduction and internal fixation if displaced; the ridge fracture usually settles with splintage for a week or two.

CAPITATE

The capitate is relatively protected within the carpus. However in severe trauma the waist can be fractured; the distal fragment can rotate, in which case open reduction and internal fixation is required.

LUNATE

Fractures of the lunate are rare and follow a hyperextension injury to the wrist. There is a real risk of non-union; undisplaced fractures should be immobilized in a cast for 6 weeks; displaced fractures should be reduced and fixed with a screw.

Repetitive microtrauma may be the cause of Kienböck's disease in a lunate which has a precarious blood supply.

ULNAR-SIDE WRIST INJURIES

The distal radioulnar joint is often injured with a radial fracture (see also Chapter 16); it can also be damaged in isolation, particularly after hyperpronation. The TFCC can be torn, the ulnar styloid avulsed or the articular surfaces of the ulnocarpal joint or distal radioulnar joint damaged.

Clinical features

There is tenderness over the distal radioulnar joint and pain on rotation of the forearm. The distal ulna may be unstable; the *piano-key sign* is elicited by holding the patient's forearm pronated and pushing sharply forwards on the head of the ulna.

Imaging and arthroscopy

A lateral x-ray in pronation and supination shows incongruity of the distal radioulnar joint. The antero-posterior view may show an avulsed ulnar styloid. Arthrography, MRI and arthroscopy may be needed to confirm the diagnosis.

Treatment

Instability usually resolves if the arm is held in supination for 6 weeks; occasionally a K-wire is needed to maintain the reduction. If the dislocation is irreducible, this may be due to trapped soft tissue, which will have to be removed. Chronic instability may require reconstructive surgery.

A TFCC tear should be repaired and the ulnocarpal capsule reefed. A displaced ulnar styloid fracture, if painful or associated with instability of the radioulnar joint, should be fixed with a small screw.

CARPAL DISLOCATIONS, SUBLUXATIONS AND INSTABILITY

The wrist functions as a system of intercalated segments or links, stabilized by the intercarpal ligaments and the scaphoid which acts as a bridge between the proximal and distal rows of the carpus. Fractures and dislocations of the carpal bones, or even simple ligament tears and sprains, may seriously disturb this system so that the links collapse into one of several well-recognized patterns (see Chapter 16).

LUNATE AND PERILUNATE DISLOCATIONS

A fall with the hand forced into dorsiflexion may tear the tough ligaments that normally bind the carpal bones. The lunate usually remains attached to the radius and the rest of the carpus is displaced backwards (*perilunate dislocation*). Usually the hand immediately snaps forwards again but, as it does so, the lunate may be levered out of position to be displaced anteriorly (*lunate dislocation*). Sometimes the scaphoid remains attached to the radius and the force of the perilunar dislocation causes it to fracture through the waist (*trans-scaphoid perilunate dislocation*).

Clinical features

The wrist is painful and swollen and is held immobile. If the carpal tunnel is compressed there may be paraesthesia or blunting of sensation in the territory of the median nerve, and weakness of palmar abduction of the thumb.

X-RAY

Most dislocations are perilunate. In the anteroposterior view the carpus is diminished in height and the bone shadows overlap abnormally. One or more of the carpal bones may be fractured (usually the scaphoid and radial styloid). If the lunate is dislocated, it has a characteristic triangular shape instead of the normal quadrilateral appearance.

In the lateral view it is easy to distinguish a lunate from a perilunate dislocation. The *dislocated lunate* is tilted forwards and is displaced in front of the radius, while the capitate and metacarpal bones are in line with the radius. With a *perilunate dislocation* the lunate is tilted only sightly and is not displaced forwards, and the capitate and metacarpals lie behind the line of the radius (DISI pattern); if there is an associated *scaphoid fracture,* the distal fragment may be flexed.

Treatment

Closed reduction The surgeon pulls strongly on the dorsiflexed hand; then, while maintaining traction, he or she slowly palmarflexes the wrist, at the same time squeezing the lunate backwards with his or her other thumb. These manoeuvres usually effect reduction; they also prevent conversion of a perilunate to a lunate dislocation. A plaster slab is applied holding the wrist neutral. Percutaneous Kirschner wires may be needed to hold the reduction.

Open reduction Reduction is imperative, and if closed reduction fails, or if a later x-ray shows that the wrist has collapsed into the familiar DISI pattern, open reduction is performed. The carpus is exposed by an anterior approach which has the advantage of decompressing the carpal tunnel. While an assistant pulls on the hand, the lunate is levered into place and kept there by a Kirschner wire which is inserted through the lunate into the capitate. If the scaphoid is fractured, this too can be reduced and fixed with a Herbert screw or Kirschner wires. Where possible, the torn soft tissues should be repaired through palmar and dorsal approaches. At the end of the procedure, the wrist is splinted in a plaster slab, which is retained for 3 weeks. Finger, elbow and shoulder exercises are practised throughout this period. The Kirschner wires are removed at 10 weeks.

This injury is frequently accompanied by severe compression of the median nerve, which should be released.

SCAPHOLUNATE DISSOCIATION

A wrist sprain may be followed by persistent pain and tenderness over the dorsum just distal to Lister's tubercle.

X-rays show an excessively large gap between the scaphoid and the lunate. The scaphoid may appear foreshortened, with a typical cortical ring sign. In the lateral view, the lunate is tilted dorsally and the scaphoid anteriorly (DISI pattern).

Treatment

Scapholunate instability causes weakness of the wrist and recurrent discomfort. If seen early (i.e less than 4

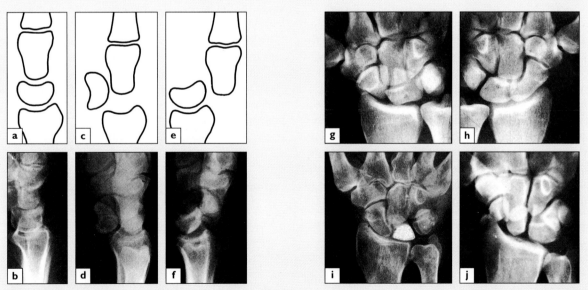

25.21 Lunate and perilunate dislocations (**a, b**) Lateral view of normal wrist; (**c, d**) lunate dislocation; (**e, f**) perilunate dislocation. (**g, h**) Anteroposterior view of both wrists with dislocated left lunate: note the triangular appearance of the lunate image. (**i**) Avascular necrosis following reduction. (**j**) Associated fracture of the scaphoid.

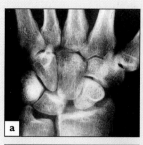

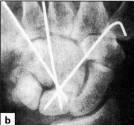

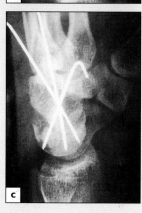

25.22 Scapholunate dissociation After a fall this patient had pain and tenderness in the anatomical snuffbox. The scaphoid is intact but (**a**) there is an obvious gap between the lunate and scaphoid. After open reduction and repair of the dorsal scapholunate ligament the scaphoid was held in position with Kirschner wires (**b, c**) until ligament healing was complete.

weeks after injury) the scapholunate ligament should be repaired directly with interosseous sutures, protected by K-wires for 6 weeks and a cast for 8–12 weeks. If seen between 4 and 24 weeks, then the ligament is unlikely to heal. Blatt's capsulodesis is helpful: a proximally based flap of dorsal capsule is attached to the back of the scaphoid to haul it back from flexion into a normal position. In chronic lesions without secondary osteoarthritis, a capsulodesis or ligament reconstruction is attempted. If there is severe symptomatic osteoarthritis then a limited intercarpal arthrodesis or radiocarpal arthrodesis is performed.

TRIQUETROLUNATE DISSOCIATION

A medial sprain followed by weakness of grip and tenderness distal to the head of the ulna should suggest disruption of the triquetrolunate ligaments.

X-rays show a noticeable gap between the triquetrum and the lunate, with a VISI carpal collapse pattern in the lateral view.

Treatment

Acute tears should be repaired with interosseous sutures, supported by temporary K-wires for 6 weeks and a cast for 8–12 weeks. In chronic injuries, a ligament substitution (e.g. a slip of extensor carpi ulnaris) or a limited intercarpal fusion may be considered.

RADIOCARPAL DISLOCATION

The most common injuries of this type involve a fracture of the anterior or posterior rim of the distal radius (Barton's fracture – see page 620). However, occasionally the ligaments which bind the carpus to the distal radius can rupture; the carpus tends to translate medially. Repair of the ligaments and temporary K-wire stabilization is needed.

MIDCARPAL DISLOCATION

The extrinsic ligaments which bind the proximal to the distal row can rupture (there are, by definition, no intrinsic ligaments between these two rows). The diagnosis is difficult but is more readily suggested in those with generalized ligament laxity and a chronic wrist problem. The patient complains of a painful, recurrent snap in the wrist; the two rows can be passively 'clunked' apart when shifted backwards and forwards. If an acute ligament rupture is diagnosed, then repair and temporary K-wire stabilization should be carried out. In a chronic lesion, fusion of the proximal row to the distal row is the most effective treatment but this operation will restrict wrist movement and may predispose to later arthritis.

REFERENCES AND FURTHER READING

Dias JJ, Thompson J, Barton NJ, Gregg PJ (1990) Suspected scaphoid fractures. *Journal of Bone and Joint Surgery* **72B**, 98–101

Herbert TJ (1990) *The Fractured Scaphoid.* Quality Medical Publishing, St Louis MO

Rockwood CA Jr, Green DP, Bucholz RW, Heckman JD (eds) (1996) *Fractures in Adults* 4th edition. Lippincott-Raven, Philadelphia

Hand injuries

Hand injuries – the commonest of all injuries – are important out of all proportion to their apparent severity, because of the need for perfect function. Nowhere else do painstaking evaluation, meticulous care and dedicated rehabilitation yield greater rewards. The outcome is often dependent upon the judgement of the doctor who first sees the patient.

Assessment

If there is skin damage the patient should be examined in a clean environment with the hand displayed on sterile drapes.

A brief but searching history is obtained; often the mechanism of injury will suggest the type and severity of the trauma. The patient's age, occupation and 'handedness' also are important.

Superficial injuries and severe fractures are obvious, but deeper injuries are often poorly disclosed. It is important in the initial examination to assess the circulation, soft tissue cover, bones, joints, nerves and tendons

X-rays should include at least three views (posteroanterior, lateral and oblique), and with finger injuries the individual digit must be x-rayed.

General principles of treatment

Most hand injuries can be dealt with under local or regional anaesthesia; a general anaesthetic is only rarely required.

The principles of treatment are as follows

* CIRCULATION If the circulation is threatened, it must be promptly restored, if necessary by direct repair or vein grafting.

* SWELLING Swelling must be controlled by elevating the hand and by early and repeated active exercises.

* SPLINTAGE Incorrect splintage is a potent cause of stiffness; it must be *appropriate* and it must be kept to a *minimum length of time*. If a finger has to be splinted, it may be possible simply to tape it to its neighbour so that both move as one; if greater security is needed, only the injured finger should be splinted. If the entire hand needs splinting, this must always be in the *position safe immobilization* – with the metacarpophalangeal joints flexed at least

70° and the interphalangeal joints almost straight. Sometimes an external splint, to be effective, would need to immobilize undamaged fingers or would need to hold the joints of the injured finger in an unfavourable position (e.g. flexion of the interphalangeal joints). If so, internal splintage is required. Wherever possible, percutaneous Kirschner wires (K-wires) are used but sometimes open reduction and fixation with screws, plates or wire loops may be necessary.

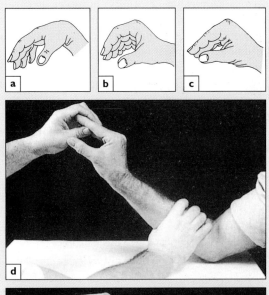

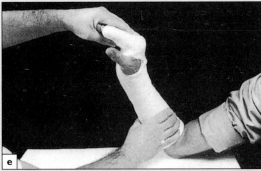

26.1 Splintage of the hand *Three positions of the hand:* (**a**) *The position of relaxation,* (**b**) *the position of function (ready for action)* and (**c**) *the position of safe immobilization, with the ligaments taut. The hand should always be splinted in the position of safe immobilization* (**d, e**), *with the knuckle joints 90° flexed, the finger joints extended and the thumb abducted. In this position the ligaments are at their longest and splintage is least likely to result in stiffness.*

- SKIN COVER Skin damage demands wound toilet followed by suture, skin grafting, local flaps, pedicled flaps and occasionally free flaps. Treatment of the skin takes precedence over treatment of the fracture.

- NERVE AND TENDON INJURY Generally, the best results will follow primary repair of tendons and nerves. Occasionally grafts are required.

METACARPAL FRACTURES

The metacarpal bones are vulnerable to blows and falls upon the hand, or the longitudinal force of the boxer's punch. Injuries are common and the bones may fracture at their *base*, in the *shaft* or through the *neck*.

Angular deformity is usually not very marked, and even if it should persist it does not interfere much with function. Rotational deformity, however, is serious. Close your hand with the distal phalanges extended, and look: the fingers converge across the palm to a point above the thenar eminence; malrotation of the metacarpal (or proximal phalanx) will cause that finger to diverge and overlap one of its neighbours. Thus, with a fractured metacarpal it is important to regain normal rotational alignment.

The fourth and fifth metacarpals are more mobile than the second and third, and therefore are better able to compensate for residual angular deformity.

Fractures of the thumb metacarpal usually occur near the base and pose special problems. They are dealt with separately below.

FRACTURES OF THE METACARPAL SHAFT

A direct blow may fracture one or several metacarpal shafts transversely, often with associated skin damage.

A twisting or punching force may cause a spiral fracture of one or more shafts. There is local pain and swelling, and sometimes a dorsal 'hump'.

Treatment

Oblique fractures or transverse fractures with slight displacement require no reduction. Splintage also is unnecessary, but a firm crepe bandage may be comforting; this should not be allowed to discourage the patient from active movements of the fingers, which should be practised assiduously.

Transverse fractures with considerable displacement are reduced by traction and pressure. Reduction can sometimes be held by a plaster slab extending from the forearm over the fingers (only the damaged ones). The slab is maintained for 3 weeks and the undamaged fingers are exercised. However, these fractures are usually quite unstable and should be fixed with percutaneous K-wires, placed either across the fracture or transversely through the neighbouring undamaged metacarpals.

Spiral fractures are liable to rotate; they should be perfectly reduced and fixed with transverse wires or lag screws and a plate.

FRACTURES OF THE METACARPAL NECK

A blow may fracture the metacarpal neck, usually of the fifth finger (the 'boxer's fracture') and occasionally one of the others. There may be local swelling, with flattening of the knuckle. X-rays show an impacted transverse fracture with volar angulation of the distal fragment.

Treatment

The main function of the *fifth and fourth fingers* is flexion ('power grip') and, as can be readily demon-

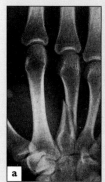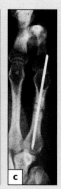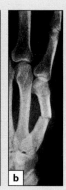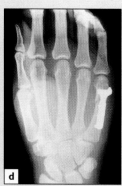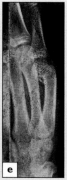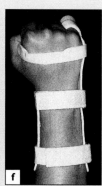

26.2 Metacarpal fractures (a) A spiral fracture of a single metacarpal (especially an 'inboard' one) is adequately held by neighbouring bones and muscles; (b) a displaced fracture (especially an 'outboard' one) can be held by a stiff K-wire (c), or better still a small plate (d), thus allowing early movement. Multiple displaced metacarpal fractures, likewise, should be plated. (e) Fracture of the fifth metacarpal neck; if splintage is used (f), only the damaged ray should be immobilized.

strated on the normal side, there is 'spare' extension available at the metacarpophalangeal joint. Therefore in these digits, a flexion deformity of about 40° can be accepted, and as long as there is no rotational deformity, a good outcome can be expected. The hand is immobilized in a gutter splint with the metacarpophalangeal joint flexed and the interphalangeal joints straight until discomfort settles – a week or two – and then the hand is mobilized. The patient is warned that the knuckle profile may be permanently lost. In *the index and middle fingers*, which function mainly in extension, no more than 20° of flexion at the fracture is acceptable.

If the fracture needs reduction, this can be done under a metacarpal block. The reduced finger is held with a gutter splint moulded at three points to support the fracture; the metacarpophalangeal joints are flexed and the interphalangeal joints are straight. Unfortunately, these fractures are usually fairly unstable because of the tone of the flexor tendons and the palmar comminution of the fracture. If there is a tendency to redisplacement, percutaneous K-wires should be used.

Complications

Malunion, with volar angulation of the distal fragment, is poorly tolerated, particularly if this affects the second and third rays. The patient may be aware of a bump in the palm from the prominent metacarpal head and the digit may take on a 'Z' appearance as the knuckle joint hyperextends to compensate for the deformity.

FRACTURES OF THE METACARPAL BASE

Excepting fractures of the thumb metacarpal, these are stable injuries which can usually be treated by ensuring that rotation is correct and then splinting the digit in a volar slab extending from the forearm to the proximal finger joint. The splint is retained for 3 weeks and exercises are then encouraged.

Displaced intra-articular fractures of the base of the fifth metacarpal may cause marked incongruity of the joint. This is a mobile joint and it may, therefore, be painful. The fracture should be reduced by traction on the little finger and then held with a percutaneous K-wire or compression screw.

FRACTURE OF THE THUMB METACARPAL

Three types of fracture are encountered: impacted fracture of the metacarpal base; Bennett's fracture-dislocation of the carpometacarpal joint; and Rolando's comminuted fracture of the base.

IMPACTED FRACTURE
A boxer may, while punching, sustain a fracture of the base of the first metacarpal. Localized swelling and tenderness are found, and x-ray shows a transverse fracture about 6mm distal to the carpometacarpal joint, with outward bowing and impaction.

Treatment If the angulation is less than 20 to 30° and the fragments impacted, the thumb is rested in a plaster of Paris cast extending from the forearm to just short of the interphalangeal thumb joint with the thumb fully abducted and extended. The cast is removed after 2–3 weeks and the thumb is mobilized.

If the angulation is greater than 30°, then the reduced thumb web span will be noticeable and so the fracture should be reduced. The surgeon pulls on the abducted thumb and, by levering the metacarpal outwards against his or her own thumb, corrects the bowing. A plaster cast is applied. If the fracture is still unstable, then a percutaneous K-wire is inserted.

BENNETT'S FRACTURE-DISLOCATION
This fracture, too, occurs at the base of the first metacarpal bone and is commonly due to punching; but the fracture is oblique, extends into the carpometacarpal joint and is unstable.

The thumb looks short and the carpometacarpal region swollen. X-rays show that a small triangular fragment has remained in contact with the medial half of the trapezium, while the remainder of the thumb has subluxated proximally.

Treatment It is widely supposed (with little evidence) that perfect reduction is essential. It should, however, be attempted and can usually be achieved by pulling on the

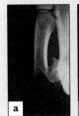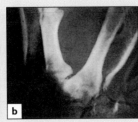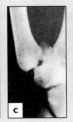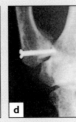

26.3 Fractures of the first metacarpal base A transverse fracture (**a**) can be reduced and held in plaster (**b**). Bennett's fracture-dislocation (**c**) is best held with a small screw (**d**) or a percutaneous K-wire.

thumb, abducting it and extending it. Reduction can then be held in one of two ways: plaster or internal fixation.

Plaster may be applied with a felt pad over the fracture, and the first metacarpal held abducted and extended (usually best achieved by *flexing* the metacarpophalangeal joint). If x-ray shows that perfect reduction is being held, the plaster is worn for 4 weeks; otherwise the method is abandoned. Plaster only works if it is applied with great skill; the pressure required to maintain a reduction can cause skin damage.

Internal fixation is usually the method of choice; it can be achieved by inserting a small screw, or by driving short lengths of K-wire through the metacarpal base (bypassing the fracture) into the carpus; the protruding ends are incorporated in a small plaster slab. After 3 weeks the slab is removed and the wires are pulled out.

ROLANDO'S FRACTURE

This is an intra-articular comminuted fracture of the base of the first metacarpal. Treatment is difficult. With a triple T or Y configuration, closed reduction and K-wiring or open reduction and mini-screw fixation can be used. With more severe comminution, external fixation is needed.

METACARPAL FRACTURES IN CHILDREN

Metacarpal fractures are less common in children than in adults. In general they also present fewer problems: the vast majority can be treated by manipulation and plaster splintage; angular deformities will almost always be remodelled with further growth. However, rotational alignment is as important as it is in adults.

Bennett's fracture is rare; but when it does occur it usually requires open reduction. This is, by definition, a Salter–Harris type III fracture-separation of the physis; it must be accurately reduced and fixed with a K-wire.

FRACTURES OF THE PHALANGES

The fingers are usually injured by direct violence, and there may be considerable swelling or open wounds. Injudicious treatment may result in a stiff finger – which, in some cases, can be worse than no finger.

FRACTURES OF THE PROXIMAL AND MIDDLE PHALANGEAL SHAFTS

The phalanx usually fractures transversely, often with forwards angulation which may damage the flexor tendon sheath. Fractures at either end of the phalanx may enter the joint; stiffness is the main threat, and if the fracture is displaced the finger may also be deformed.

Treatment

UNDISPLACED FRACTURES These can be treated by 'functional splintage'. The finger is strapped to its neighbour ('buddy strapping') and movements are encouraged from the outset. Splintage is retained for 2–3 weeks, but during this time it is wise to check the position by x-ray in case displacement has occurred.

DISPLACED FRACTURES Displaced fractures must be reduced and immobilized. The fracture is reduced by pulling on the bent finger and thumbing the phalanx straight. *It is essential to check for rotational correction* by (1) noting the convergent position of the finger when the metacarpophalangeal joint is flexed, and (2) seeing that the fingernails are all in the same plane.

If the fracture is stable after reduction, the finger can be strapped to its neighbour and movements allowed. If it is unstable, the finger must be immobilized in a malleable splint with the metacarpophalangeal joint flexed and the interphalangeal joint extended. However, fractures often slip and the finger can become stiff if it is immobilized until the fracture heals. For these reasons, it might be better to fix displaced phalangeal fractures with percutaneous wires or mini-plates and screws.

FRACTURES OF THE TERMINAL PHALANX

The terminal phalanx, small though it is, is subject to five different types of fracture.

FRACTURE OF THE TUFT

The tip of the finger may be struck by a hammer or caught in a door, and the bone shattered. The fracture is disregarded and treatment is focussed on controlling swelling and regaining movement. The painful haematoma beneath the finger nail should be drained by piercing the nail with a hot paper clip. If the nail bed is shattered and cosmesis is important, it should be meticulously repaired under magnification.

MALLET FINGER INJURY

There are three types of mallet finger:

- a tendinous avulsion;
- a small flake of bone;
- a large dorsal bone fragment, sometimes with subluxation of the joint.

After a sudden flexion injury (e.g. stubbing the finger) the terminal phalanx droops and cannot be straightened actively. One of three defects will be seen: (1) the extensor tendon is avulsed from its insertion in the base of the terminal phalanx; (2) a tiny flake of bone is pulled of with the tendon; or (3) a comparatively large fragment of bone is avulsed, sometimes resulting in subluxation of the joint.

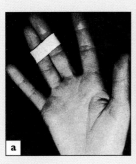
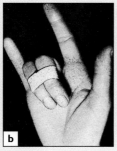
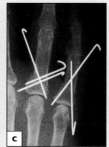

26.4 Phalangeal fractures (**a, b**) If the fracture is stable, the finger is strapped to its neighbour for splintage and movement is encouraged. (**c**) Unstable fractures should be reduced (if necessary by operation) and fixed with percutaneous wires or internal plates and screws. In all cases, movement should be started within a few days of injury or stiffness will ensue.

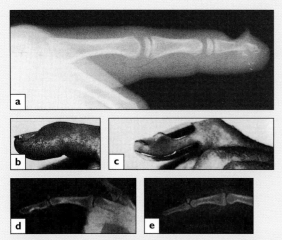

26.5 Distal phalangeal injury (**a**) Fracture of the tuft, the painful consequence of a misdirected hammer blow. (**b**) Mallet finger, treated by splintage (**c**); this is adequate when the bony fragment (if any) is small (**d**), but if the fragment is large (**e**) it is tempting (though usually unwise) to fix it.

AVULSION OF THE FLEXOR TENDON

This injury is caused by sudden hyperextension of the distal joint, typically when a football player catches his or her finger on an opponent's shirt. The ring finger is most commonly affected. The flexor digitorum profundus tendon is avulsed, either rupturing the tendon itself or taking a fragment of bone with it. If the bone fragment is small, or if only the tendon is ruptured, it can recoil into the palm. If the lesion is detected within a few days (and the diagnosis is easily missed if not thought about), then the tendon can be re-attached. If the diagnosis is much delayed, repair is likely to be unsuccessful. Tendon reconstruction is possible but very difficult, and the finger may end up stiff. Thus, for late cases, fusion of the distal joint is usually preferable.

PHYSEAL FRACTURE

The basal physis can break, usually producing a Salter–Harris II fracture. The nail may be dislocated from its fold, an injury which is easily overlooked if the finger is very swollen. The nail must be cleaned and carefully replaced into its bed.

Treatment consists of immobilizing the terminal joint in slight hyperextension by means of a special mallet-finger splint which fixes the distal joint but leaves the proximal joint free. Occasionally it may be necessary to transfix the distal joint through the pulp with a K-wire. This position is held continuously for 6–8 weeks. Treatment can be successful even if the patient presents 4 or 5 weeks after injury.

Re-attachment of the bone fragment, even when large and with a subluxated joint, is difficult and probably does not improve the outcome. Later problems are best treated by arthrodesing the distal joint.

FRACTURE OF THE SHAFT

If undisplaced, these should be ignored. If angulated, these should be reduced and held with a longitudinal K-wire through the pulp for 4 weeks. The nail is often dislocated from its fold; if so it must be carefully tucked back in and held with a suture in each corner.

JOINT INJURIES

Any finger joint may be injured by a direct blow (often the overlying skin is damaged), or by an angulation force or by the straight finger being forcibly stubbed. The affected joint is swollen, tender and too painful to move. X-rays may show that a fragment of bone has been sheared off or avulsed.

CARPOMETACARPAL DISLOCATION

The thumb is most frequently affected and clinically the injury then resembles a Bennett's fracture-dislocation; however, x-rays reveal proximal subluxation or dislocation of the first metacarpal bone without a fracture. The displacement is easily reduced by traction and hyper-pronation, but reduction is unstable and can be

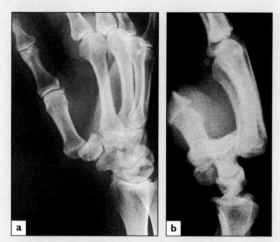

26.6 Carpometacarpal dislocation (a) Subluxation of the thumb carpometacarpal joint. (b) Complete carpometacarpal dislocation – the 'motorcyclist's injury'.

held only by one of the methods used for a Bennett's fracture-dislocation: plaster, or K-wires driven through the metacarpal into the carpus. The wire is removed after 4 weeks but a protective splint should be worn for 8 weeks because of the risk of instability.

The other carpometacarpal joints are also sometimes dislocated, typically when a motorcyclist, holding the handlebars, strikes an object and the hand is driven backwards. The hand swells up rapidly and the diagnosis is easily missed unless a true lateral x-ray is carefully examined. Closed manipulation is usually successful, although a K-wire may be needed to prevent the joint from 'spinning out' again.

METACARPOPHALANGEAL DISLOCATION

Usually the thumb is affected, sometimes the fifth finger, and rarely the other fingers. The entire finger is suddenly forced into hyperextension and the capsule and muscle insertions in front of the joint may be torn. There are two types of dislocation.

Simple dislocation The finger is extended about 75°. It is easily reduced by traction, firstly in hyperextension then

pulling the finger around. The finger is strapped to its neighbour and early mobilization is encouraged.

Complex dislocation The avulsed palmar plate sits in the joint, blocking reduction. Furthermore, the metacarpal head can be clasped between the flexor tendon and lumbrical tendon. The finger is extended only about 30° and there is usually a tell-tale dimple in the palm. Very occasionally the fracture can be reduced closed by hyperextending the metacarpophalangeal joint and flexing the interphalangeal joints to release the clasp. If this fails, open reduction is required. A dorsal approach is safest. After reduction the joint is stable and should be mobilized in a neighbour-splint.

INTERPHALANGEAL JOINT DISLOCATION

Distal joint dislocation is rare; proximal joint dislocation is more common. The dislocation is easily reduced by pulling. The joint is strapped to its neighbour for a few days and movements are begun immediately. The lateral x-ray may show a small flake of bone, representing a palmar plate avulsion; this should be ignored. The patient must be warned that it can take many months for the spindle-like swelling of the joint to settle and for full extension to recover.

CONDYLAR FRACTURE

The basal joint surface or distal joint surface of the phalanges can be fractured, usually by an angulation force. If the fragment is not displaced, it is best to disregard the fracture, strap the finger to its neighbour and concentrate on regaining movement. An x-ray after a week should be taken to ensure there is no displacement.

If the fracture is displaced, there is a risk of permanent angular deformity and loss of movement at the joint. The fracture should be anatomically reduced, either closed or by open operation and fixation with small K-wires or screws. The finger is splinted for a few days and then supervised movements are commenced.

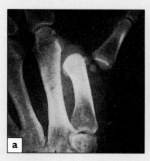
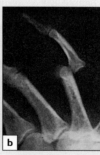
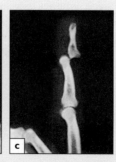

26.7 Finger dislocation
(a) Metacarpophalangeal dislocation in the thumb occasionally buttonholes and needs open reduction; (b, c) interphalangeal dislocations are easily reduced (and easily missed if not x-rayed!).

VOLAR FRACTURE–DISLOCATIONS

When the proximal interphalangeal joint dislocates, a fragment of bone may be avulsed from the base of the middle phalanx. If this fragment is large, the joint can subluxate. Surgical fixation is very difficult and can lead to permanent stiffness of the joint. The fracture can be reduced by flexing the joint to 40°. The joint is then held in a splint which allows flexion but not extension. The amount of extension block is reduced over the next 4 weeks and the splint is then discarded.

LIGAMENT INJURIES

COLLATERAL LIGAMENTS OF THE FINGERS

Partial or complete tears of the ligaments are common and usually due to forced angulation at the joint.

Mild sprains require no treatment; with more severe injuries the finger should be splinted for a week or two. Occasionally, the bone to which the ligament is attached is avulsed; if the fragment is markedly displaced (and large enough), it should be re-attached. The patient must be warned that the joint is likely to remain swollen and slightly painful for 6–12 months.

ULNAR COLLATERAL LIGAMENT OF THE THUMB METACARPOPHALANGEAL JOINT ('GAMEKEEPER'S THUMB'; 'SKIER'S THUMB')

In former years, gamekeepers who twisted the necks of little animals ran the risk of tearing the ulnar collateral ligament of the thumb metacarpophalangeal joint. Nowadays this injury is seen in skiers who fall onto the extended thumb, forcing it into hyperabduction. A small

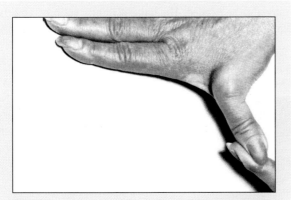

26.8 Gamekeeper's thumb The ulnar collateral ligament of the metacarpophalangeal joint is completely ruptured; immediate repair is advisable.

flake of bone may be pulled off at the same time. The resulting loss of stability may interfere markedly with prehensile (pinching) activities.

The ulnar collateral ligament inserts partly into the palmar plate. In *a partial rupture*, only the ligament proper is torn and the thumb is unstable in flexion but still more or less stable in full extension because the palmar plate is intact. In *a complete rupture*, both the ligament proper and the palmar plate are torn and the thumb is unstable in all positions. If the ligament ruptures completely (usually at its distal attachment to the base of the proximal phalanx), it will not heal unless it is repaired; this is because the distal end gets trapped in front of the adductor pollicis aponeurosis (the Stener lesion).

Clinical assessment

On examination there is tenderness and swelling precisely over the ulnar side of the thumb metacarpophalangeal joint. *An x-ray is essential, to exclude a fracture before carrying out any stress tests.* A local anaesthetic is then injected into the tissues along the inner (adductor) aspect of the joint and the thumb is stressed in abduction with the metacarpophalangeal joint flexed 30°; if there is no undue laxity (compare with the normal side) then a serious injury can be excluded. If there is significant laxity, the test is repeated with the thumb fully extended; if it now moves no more than 15° more than the normal side, then the palmar plate is still intact (i.e. it is a partial rupture); if laxity is greater than this, there is probably a complete rupture which will require operative repair.

Treatment

Partial tears can be treated by a short period (2–4 weeks) of immobilization in a cast or splint, followed by increasing movement and pinching and gripping exercises.

Complete tears need operative repair. Care should be taken during the exposure not to injure the superficial radial nerve branches. The Stener lesion is found at the proximal edge of the adductor aponeurosis. The aponeurosis is incised and retracted to expose the ligaments and capsule and the torn structures are then carefully repaired (Heyman, 1997). Post-operatively, the joint is immobilized in a thumb spica (leaving the interphalangeal joint free) for 4 weeks, followed by another 2 weeks in a removable splint.

A neglected tear leads to weakness of pinch. This is probably best treated by arthrodesis, although, in early cases without articular damage, stability may be restored by advancing the insertion of adductor pollicis to the base of the phalanx, or by using a free tendon graft, or by reinforcing the ligament with the tendon of extensor pollicis brevis.

OPEN INJURIES OF THE HAND

Over 75% of work injuries affect the hands; inadequate treatment costs the patient (and society) dear in terms of functional disability.

Clinical assessment

Open injuries comprise tidy or 'clean' cuts, lacerations, crushing and injection injuries, burns and pulp defects.

The precise *mechanism of injury* must be understood. Was the instrument sharp or blunt? Clean or dirty? The position of the fingers (flexed or extended) at the time of injury will influence the relative damage to the deep and superficial flexor tendons. A history of high pressure injection predicts major soft-tissue damage, however innocuous the wound may seem. What are the patient's occupation, hobbies and aspirations? Is he or she right-handed or left-handed?

Examination should be gentle and painstaking. *Skin damage* is important, but it should be remembered that even a tiny, clean cut may conceal nerve or tendon damage.

The circulation to the hand and each digit must be assessed. The Allen test can be applied to the hand as a whole or to an individual finger. The radial and ulnar arteries at the wrist are simultaneously compressed by the examiner while the patient clenches his or her fist for several seconds before relaxing; the hand should now be pale. The radial artery is then released; if the hand flushes it means that the radial blood-supply is intact. The test is repeated for the ulnar artery. An injured finger can be assessed in the same way. The digital arteries are occluded by pinching the base of the finger. When blood is squeezed out of the finger the pulp will become noticeably pale; one digital artery is then released and the pulp should pink up; the test is repeated for the other digital artery.

Sensation is tested in the territory of each nerve. *Two-point discrimination* may be reduced in partial injuries. In children, who are more difficult to examine, the *plastic pen* test is helpful: if a plastic pen is brushed along the skin it will tend to 'stick' due to the normal thin layer of sweat on the surface; absence of sweating (due to a nerve injury) is revealed by noting that the pen does not adhere as it should (compared to the normal side). Another observation is that the skin in the territory of a divided nerve will not *wrinkle* if immersed in water.

Tendons must be examined with similar care. Start by testing for 'passive tenodesis'. When the wrist is extended passively, the fingers automatically flex in a gentle and regular cascade; when the wrist is flexed, the fingers fall into extension. These actions rely upon the balanced tension of the opposing flexor and extensor tendons to the fingers; if a tendon is cut, the cascade will be disturbed.

Active movements are then tested for each individual tendon. Flexor digitorum profundus is tested by holding the proximal finger joint straight and instructing the patient to bend the distal joint. Flexor digitorum superficialis is tested by the examiner holding all the fingers together out straight, then releasing one and asking the patient to bend the proximal joint. Holding the fingers out straight 'immobilizes' all the deep flexors (including that of the finger being tested) which have a common muscle belly. However, in the index finger this test is not 100% reliable because the deep flexor is sometimes separate.

If a tendon is only partly divided, it will still work although it may be painful. In full-thickness skin lacerations, if there is any doubt about the integrity of the tendons, the wound should be explored.

X-rays may show fractures, foreign bodies, air or paint.

Primary treatment

PRE-OPERATIVE CARE
As usual, general measures to maintain the airway, breathing and circulation take precedence. If the hand wound is contaminated, it should be rinsed with sterile crystalloid, and antibiotics should be given as soon as possible. Prophylaxis against tetanus and gas gangrene may also be needed. The hand is lightly splinted and the wound is covered with an iodine-soaked dressing.

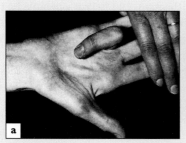 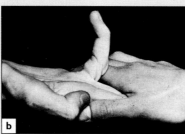

26.9 Testing superficialis To detect superficialis competence, first anchor the profundus, which is a 'mass action' muscle. (**a**) The superficialis is normal; it alone is flexing the proximal interphalangeal joint; the tip is flail. (**b**) The superficialis is not working; only by using profundus (with difficulty) can the proximal interphalangeal joint be flexed; consequently the tip is not flail.

WOUND EXPLORATION

Under general or regional anaesthesia, the wound is cleaned and explored. A pneumatic tourniquet is essential unless there is a crush injury in which muscle viability is in doubt. Skin is too precious to waste and only obviously dead skin should be excised. For adequate exposure the wound may need enlarging, but incisions must not cross a skin crease or an interdigital web. Through the enlarged wound, loose debris is picked out, dead muscle is excised and the tissues are thoroughly irrigated with isotonic crystalloid solution. A further assessment of the extent of the injury is then undertaken.

TISSUE REPAIR

Fractures are reduced and held with K-wires, unless there is some specific contraindication. *Joint capsule and ligaments* are repaired with fine sutures.

Artery and vein repair may be needed if the hand or finger is ischaemic. This done with the aid of an operating microscope. Any gap should be bridged with a vein graft.

Severed nerves are sutured under an operating microscope with the finest, non-reactive material. If the repair cannot be achieved without tension then a nerve graft (e.g. from the posterior interosseous nerve at the wrist or from the sural nerve) should be performed.

Extensor tendon repair is not as easy and the results not as reliable as some have suggested. Repair and post-operative management should be meticulous.

Flexor tendon repair is even more challenging, particularly in the region between the distal palmar crease and the flexor crease of the proximal interphalangeal joint where both the superficial and deep tendons run together in a tight sheath (Zone II or, more dramatically, 'no man's land' – see Fig. 26.11). Primary repair with fastidious post-operative supervision gives the best outcome but calls for a high level of expertise and specialized physiotherapy. If the necessary facilities are not available, then the wound should be washed out and loosely closed, and the patient transferred to a special centre. A delay of several days, with a clean wound, is unlikely to affect the outcome. The tendon repair must be strong and accurate enough to allow early mobilization (usually passive) so that the tendons can glide freely and independently from each other and the sheath. A central locked core suture is placed without handling the tendon any more than is absolutely necessary; this is supplemented by a continuous circumferential suture which strengthens the repair and smoothes it, thus making the gliding action through the sheath easier. The A2 and A4 pulleys (see Fig. 26.12) must be repaired or reconstructed, otherwise the tendons will bowstring. Cuts above the wrist (Zone V), in the palm (Zone III) or distal to the superficialis insertion (Zone I) generally have a better outcome than injuries in the carpal tunnel (Zone IV) or flexor sheath (Zone II). Division of the superficialis tendon noticeably weakens the hand and a swan-neck deformity can develop in those with lax ligaments. It should therefore always be repaired.

26.10 Hand incisions 'Permissable' incisions in hand surgery. Incisions must not cross a skin crease or an interdigital web or else scarring may cause contracture and deformity.

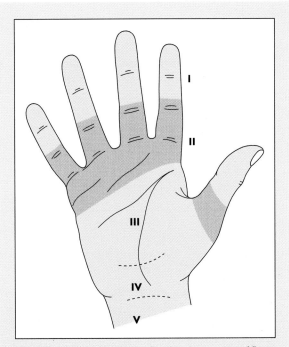

26.11 The zones of injury I – Distal to the insertion of flexor digitorum superficialis. II – Between the opening of the flexor sheath (the distal palmar crease) and the insertion of flexor superficialis. III – Between the end of the carpal tunnel and the beginning of the flexor sheath. IV – Within the carpal tunnel. V – Proximal to the carpal tunnel.

Amputation of a finger as a primary procedure should be avoided unless the damage involves many tissues and is clearly irreparable. Even when a finger has been amputated by the injury, the possibility of reattachment should be considered (see below).

Ring avulsion is a special case. When a finger is caught by a ring, the soft tissues are sheared away from the underlying skeleton. Depending on the amount of damage, skin reattachment, microvascular reconstruction or even amputation may be required.

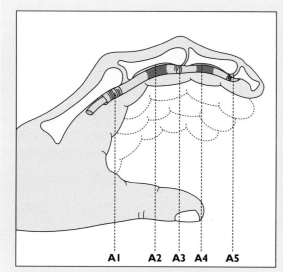

26.12 The flexor tendon sheath and pulleys Fibrous pulleys – designated A1 to A5 – hold the flexor tendons to the phalanges and prevent bowstringing during movement. A1, 3 and 5 are attached to the palmar plate near each joint; A2 and 4 have a crucial tethering effect and must always be preserved or reconstructed.

CLOSURE

The tourniquet is deflated and bipolar diathermy is used to stop bleeding. Haematoma formation leads to poor healing and tendon adhesions. Unless the wound is contaminated, the skin is closed – either by direct suture without tension or, if there is skin loss, by skin grafting. Skin grafts are conveniently taken from the inner aspect of the upper arm. If tendon or bare bone is exposed, this must be covered by a rotation or pedicled flap. Sometimes a severely mutilated finger is sacrificed and its skin used as a rotation flap to cover an adjacent area of loss.

Pulp and fingertip injuries In full thickness wounds without bone exposure, if the open area is greater than 1cm in diameter healing will be quicker with a split-skin or full-thickness graft. If bone is exposed and length of the digit is important for the individual patient, then an advancement flap or neurovascular island flap should be considered. If not, then primary cover can be achieved by shortening the bone and tailoring the skin flaps ('terminalization'). In young children, the finger tips recover extraordinarily well from injury and they should be treated with dressings rather than grafts or terminalization. Thumb length should never be sacrificed lightly.

Nail bed injuries These are often seen in association with fractures of the terminal phalanx. If appearance is important, meticulous repair of the nail bed under magnification, replacing any loss with a split thickness nail bed graft from one of the toes, will give the best cosmetic result.

DRESSING AND SPLINTAGE

The wound is covered with a single layer of paraffin gauze and ample wool roll. A light plaster slab holds the wrist and hand in the position of safe immobilization (wrist extended, metacarpophalangeal joints flexed to 90°, interphalangeal joints straight, thumb abducted).

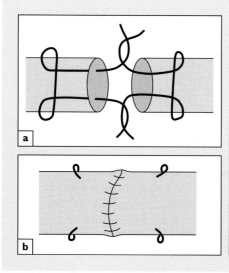

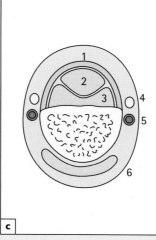

26.13 Flexor tendon repair A core suture (a) is supplemented by circumferential sutures (b). (c) The relationship of the important structures in 'no man's land': 1 – the tendon sheath; 2 – flexor digitorum profundus; 3 – flexor digitorum superficialis; 4 – digital nerve; 5 – artery; 6 – extensor tendon.

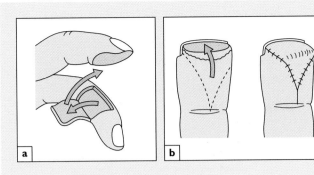

26.14 Pulp and fingertip injuries (a) Cross-finger graft for a palmar oblique fingertip injury with exposed bone. (b) V-to-Y advancement for a transverse fingertip injury with exposed bone.

This is the position in which the metacarpophalangeal and interphalangeal ligaments are fully stretched and fibrosis therefore least likely to cause contractures. *Failure to appreciate this point is the commonest cause of irrecoverable stiffness after injury.*

This position is modified in two circumstances: (1) After primary flexor tendon suture, the wrist is held in about 20° of flexion to take tension off the repair (too much wrist flexion invites wrist stiffness and carpal tunnel symptoms) but the interphalangeal joints must remain straight. (2) After extensor tendon repair, the metacarpophalangeal joints are flexed to only about 30° so that there is less tension on the repair; the wrist is extended to 30° and the interphalangeal joints remain straight.

Post-operative management

IMMEDIATE AFTERCARE
The hand is kept elevated in a roller towel or high sling. If the latter is used, the sling must be removed several times a day to exercise the elbow and shoulder. Too much elbow flexion can stop venous return and make swelling worse. Antibiotics are continued as necessary.

REHABILITATION
Movements of the hand must be commenced within a few days at most. Splintage should allow as many joints as possible to be exercised, consistent with protecting the repair. Most extensor tendon injuries are splinted for about 4 weeks. Dynamic splintage can be used, particularly for injuries at the level of the extensor retinaculum and the metacarpophalangeal joint. Various protocols are followed for flexor tendon injuries, including passive, active or elastic-band assisted flexion. Early movement promotes tendon healing and excursion. In all cases the risk of rupture is balanced against the need for early mobilization. Close supervision and attention to detail are essential.

Once the tissues have healed, the hand is increasingly used for more and more arduous and complex tasks, especially those that resemble the patient's normal job, until he or she is fit to start work; if necessary, his or her work is modified temporarily. Even if secondary surgery

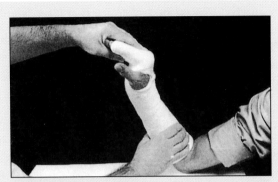

26.15 Post-operative splintage The hand is always splinted in the position of safe immobilization.

is required, tendon or nerve repair is postponed until the skin is healthy, there is no oedema and the joints have regained a normal range of passive movement.

Replantation

With modern microsurgical techniques and appropriate skill, amputated digits or hands can be replanted. An amputated part should be wrapped in sterile saline gauze, placed in a plastic bag which is itself placed in watery ice. The 'cold ischaemic time' for a finger, which contains so little muscle, is about 30 hours, but the 'warm time' is less than 6 hours. After resuscitation and attention to other potentially life-threatening injuries, the patient and the amputated part should be transferred to a centre where the appropriate surgical skills and facilities are available.

INDICATIONS The decision to replant depends on the patient's age, his or her social and professional requirements, the condition of the part (whether clean-cut, mangled, crushed or avulsed), and the warm and cold ischaemic time. Furthermore, and perhaps most importantly, it depends on whether the replanted part is likely to give better function than an amputation.

The *thumb* should be replanted whenever possible. Even if it functions only as a perfused 'post' with protective sensation, it will give useful service. *Multiple digits* also should be replanted, and *in a child even a single digit*. *Proximal amputation* (through the palm, wrist or forearm) likewise merits an attempt at replantation.

RELATIVE CONTRAINDICATIONS *Single digits* do badly if replanted. There is a high complication rate, including stiffness, non-union, poor sensation and cold intolerance; a replanted single finger is likely to be excluded from use. The exception is an amputation beyond the insertion of flexor digitorum superficialis, when a cosmetic, functioning finger tip can be retrieved. Severely *crushed, mangled or avulsed* parts may not be replantable; and parts with a *long ischaemic time* may not survive. *General medical disorders or other injuries* may engender unacceptable risks from the prolonged anaesthesia needed for replantation.

Management of burns

Generally, hand burns should be dealt with in a specialized unit. *Superficial burns* are covered with moist nonadherent dressings; the hand is elevated and finger movements are encouraged. *Partial thickness burns* can usually be allowed to heal spontaneously; the hand is dressed with an antimicrobial cream and splinted in the position of safety.

Full thickness burns will not heal. Devitalized tissue should be excised; the wound is cleaned and dressed and 2–5 days later skin-grafted. Full thickness circumferential burns may need early escharotomy to preserve the distal circulation. Skin flaps are sometimes needed in sites such as the thumb web which are prone to contracture. The hand should be splinted in the position of safety; K-wires may be needed to maintain this position.

Electric burns may cause extensive damage and thrombosis which become apparent only after several days.

Management of injection injuries

Oil, grease, solvents, hydraulic fluid or paint injected under pressure are damaging because of tension, toxicity or both. The thumb or index finger is usually involved. Substances can gain entry even through intact skin. Air or lead paint may show on x-ray. Immediate decompression and removal of the foreign substance offers the best hope, but eventually finger or partial hand amputation is often necessary.

Secondary operations

The primary treatment of hand injuries should always be carried out with an eye to any future reconstructive procedures that might be necessary. These are of three kinds:

- secondary repair or replacement of damaged structures;
- amputation of fingers;
- reconstruction of a mutilated hand.

DELAYED REPAIR

SKIN

If the skin cover has broken down or is unsuitable for surgery it is replaced by a graft or flap. As always, the skin creases must be respected. Contractures are dealt with by Z-plasty or skin replacement. When important volar surfaces are insensate, a flap of skin complete with its neurovascular supply may be transposed.

TENDONS

Primary suture may have been contraindicated by wound contamination, undue delay between injury and repair, massive skin loss or inadequate operating facilities. In these circumstances secondary repair or tendon grafting may be necessary.

In a late-presenting *injury of the profundus tendon with an intact superficialis*, advancement of a retracted tendon can cause a flexion deformity of the entire finger. Tendon grafting also is risky: the finger could become even more stiff. Unless the patient's work or hobby demands flexion of the distal joint and maximum power in the finger, fusion or tenodesis of the distal interphalangeal joint is a more reliable option.

If *both the superficialis and profundus tendons* have been divided and have retracted, a tendon graft is needed. Full passive joint movement is a pre-requisite. If the pulley system is in good condition and there are no adhesions, the tendons are excised from the flexor sheath and replaced with a tendon graft (palmaris longus, duplicated extensor digiti minimi, plantaris or a toe extensor). Rehabilitation is the same as for a primary repair. If the pulleys are damaged, the skin cover poor, the passive range of movement limited or the sheath scarred, a two-stage procedure is preferred. The tendons are excised and the pulleys reconstructed with extensor retinaculum or excised tendon. A Silastic rod is sutured to the distal stump of the profundus tendon and rehabilitation is planned to maintain a good passive range of movement. A smooth gliding surface forms around the rod. Six to eight weeks later the rod is removed through two smaller incisions and a tendon graft (palmaris longus, plantaris or a lesser toe extensor) is sutured to the proximal and distal stumps of flexor digitorum profundus. Rehabilitation is as for a primary repair.

Tenolysis is sometimes indicated. After flexor tendon repair in Zone II, a poor excursion is not infrequent because of adhesions between the tendons and the sheath. There is some active movement – indicating that the tendon is intact – but not enough for good function. The passive range of movement should be good if the tenolysis is to succeed. The tendons are painstakingly freed through small windows in the flexor sheath. Post-operatively an intensive programme of movement is essential, otherwise there will be even more scar tissue than before and the tenolysis will have made matters worse.

NERVES

Late-presenting nerve injuries must be carefully assessed. The results of repair deteriorate with time, particularly for motor nerves where the end-plate begins to fail and the muscle begins to atrophy. If several months have passed, tendon transfer may be a more reliable alternative. If nerve repair is attempted, the scar is excised and the stumps pared back until healthy nerve is found proximally and distally; a nerve graft is usually needed to avoid tension at the suture line.

JOINTS

The proximal interphalangeal joint is most prone to a flexion contracture. Active and passive exercises can be supplemented by serial static splints or dynamic splints. Surgery (capsulotomy, palmar plate and collateral ligament release) may be required but these operations themselves can invite further stiffness. Unstable or painful joints are best fused.

BONES

Malunion, especially if rotational, may require treatment. Non-union is very uncommon, but if present grafting may be required.

AMPUTATION

Indications A finger is amputated only if it remains painful or unhealed, or if it is a nuisance (i.e. if the patient cannot bend it, straighten it or feel with it), and then only if repair is impossible or uneconomic.

Technique In the finger tip, the aim is a mobile digit covered by healthy skin with normal sensation. This can be achieved by local advancement flaps or neurovascular island flaps, or by bone shortening ('terminalization'). A cross-finger flap is fairly straightforward and provides good skin cover, but sensation is limited and a flexion contracture can develop in the donor finger. The final choice depends on the patient's requirements and the surgeon's skill.

In the thumb every millimetre is worth preserving; even a stiff or deformed thumb is worth keeping.

The middle and ring fingers should not be amputated through the knuckle joint; cosmetically this is unsatisfactory and small objects will fall through the gap. If the proximal phalanx can be left, the appearance is still abnormal but function is better. The extensor tendon must never be sutured to the flexor tendon; this will act as a tether on the common belly of flexor digitorum profundus and prevent the other digits from flexing fully (the 'Quadriga effect'). If the middle phalanx is amputated distal to the flexor digitorum superficialis insertion, the profundus tendon continues to pull, but now through the lumbrical, making the proximal interphalangeal joint paradoxically extend rather than flex. This irritating anomaly is avoided by suturing the superficialis stump to the flexor sheath or by dividing the lumbrical.

For more proximal injuries, the entire finger with most of its metacarpal may be amputated; the hand is weakened but the appearance is usually satisfactory. If the middle ray is amputated through the metacarpal, the index finger may 'scissor' across it in flexion; this can be overcome by dividing the adjacent index metacarpal and transposing it to the stump of the middle metacarpal.

LATE RECONSTRUCTION

A severely mutilated hand should be dealt with by a hand expert. Certain options may be considered in exceptional cases. If all the fingers have been lost but the thumb is present, a new finger can sometimes be constructed with cortical bone, covered by a tubular flap of skin; an alternative is a neurovascular microsurgical transfer from the second toe. If the thumb has been lost, the options include pollicization (rotating a finger to oppose the other fingers), second toe transfer and osteoplastic reconstruction (a cortical bone graft surrounded by a skin flap).

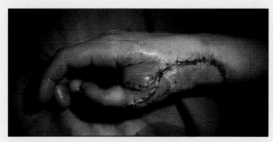

26.16 Late reconstruction The second toe has been transferred to replace the thumb, which was severed in an accident.

REFERENCES AND FURTHER READING

Heyman P (1997) Injuries to the ulnar collateral ligament of the thumb metacarpophalangeal joint. *Journal of the American Academy of Orthopaedic Surgeons* **5**, 224–229

PATHOPHYSIOLOGY OF SPINE INJURIES

STABLE AND UNSTABLE INJURIES

Spinal injuries carry a double threat: damage to the vertebral column and damage to the neural tissues. Whilst the full extent of the damage may be apparent from the moment of injury, there is always the fear that movement may cause or aggravate the neural lesion; hence the importance of establishing whether the injury is stable or unstable and treating it as unstable until proved otherwise.

A *stable injury* is one in which the vertebral components will not be displaced by normal movements; if the neural elements are undamaged, there is little or no risk of them becoming damaged.

An *unstable injury* is one in which there is a significant risk of displacement and consequent damage to the neural tissues.

In assessing spinal stability, three structural elements must be considered: the *posterior osseoligamentous complex (or posterior column)* consisting of the pedicles, facet joints, posterior bony arch, interspinous and supraspinous ligaments; the *middle column* comprising the posterior half of the vertebral body, the posterior

part of the intervertebral disc and the posterior longitudinal ligament; and the *anterior column* composed of the anterior half of the vertebral body, the anterior part of the intervertebral disc and the anterior longitudinal ligament (Denis, 1983). All fractures involving the middle column and at least one other column should be regarded as unstable. Fortunately, only 10% of spinal fractures are unstable and less than 5% are associated with cord damage.

Neurological instability refers specifically to burst fractures where a neurological deficit develops when the patient is mobilized because of bone protrusion from the vertebral body into the spinal canal.

MECHANISM OF INJURY

There are three basic mechanisms of injury: traction (avulsion), direct injury and indirect injury.

Traction injury In the lumbar spine resisted muscle effort may avulse transverse processes; in the cervical spine the seventh spinous process can be avulsed ('clay-shoveller's fracture').

Direct injury Penetrating injuries to the spine, particularly from firearms and knives, are becoming increasingly common.

Indirect injury This is the most common cause of significant spinal damage; it occurs most typically in a fall from a height when the spinal column collapses in its vertical axis, or else during violent free movements of the neck or trunk. A variety of forces may be applied to the spine (often simultaneously): axial compression, flexion, lateral compression, flexion-rotation, shear, flexion-distraction and extension.

NOTE: *Insufficiency fractures* may occur with minimal force in bone which is weakened by osteoporosis or a pathological lesion.

HEALING

Spinal injuries may damage both bone and soft tissue (ligaments, facet joint capsule and intervertebral disc). Non-union is very rare whilst malunion is very common. The bone injury will usually heal; however, if the bone structures heal in an abnormal position the

27.1 Structural elements of the spine The vertical lines show Denis' classification of the structural elements of the spine. The three elements are: the posterior complex, the middle component and the anterior column. This concept is particularly useful in assessing the stability of lumbar injuries.

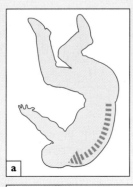

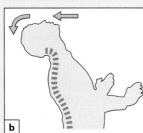

27.2 Mechanism of injury The spine is usually injured in one of two ways: (a) a fall onto the head or the back of the neck; and (b) a blow on the forehead, which forces the neck into hyperextension.

METHODS OF TEMPORARY IMMOBILIZATION

CERVICAL SPINE

In-line immobilization The head and neck are supported in the neutral position.

Quadruple immobilization A backboard, sandbags, a forehead tape and a semi-rigid collar are applied. Because children have a relatively prominent occiput, care must be taken to ensure that the neck is not flexed: padding may be required behind the shoulders.

THORACOLUMBAR SPINE

The patient should be moved without flexion or rotation of the thoracolumbar spine. A scoop stretcher and spinal board are very useful; however in the paralysed patient, there is a high risk of pressure sores – adequate padding is essential and transfer to a special bed must be undertaken as soon as possible.

If the back is to be examined, or if the patient is to be placed onto a scoop stretcher or spinal board, the *log-rolling technique* should be used.

healed soft tissues may not protect against progressive deformity. This is most likely with flexion injuries in which there is anterior wedging of the vertebral body of more than 40%. An increasing flexion deformity (kyphosis) can occur. Similarly, injuries with a predominant soft-tissue element, for example flexion-distraction with a bilateral facet dislocation and complete disruption of the posterior ligaments and disc, tend not to become stable after healing.

PRINCIPLES OF DIAGNOSIS AND MANAGEMENT

Diagnosis and management go hand in hand; inappropriate movement and examination can irretrievably change the outcome for the worse.

EARLY MANAGEMENT

The adherence to the resuscitation protocol (airway with cervical spine control, breathing, circulation and haemorrhage control) supersedes the assessment of the spinal injury. Adequate oxygenation, ventilation and circulation will minimize secondary spinal cord injury. The essential principle is that if there is the slightest possibility of a spinal injury in a trauma patient, the spine must be immobilized until the patient has been resuscitated and other life-threatening injuries have been identified and treated. Immobilization is abandoned only when spinal injury has been excluded by clinical and radiological assessment.

DIAGNOSIS

History

A high index of suspicion is essential; symptoms and signs may be minimal; the history is crucial. Every patient with a blunt injury above the clavicle, a head injury or loss of consciousness should be considered to have a cervical spine injury until proven otherwise. Every patient who is involved in a fall from a height or a high-speed deceleration accident should similarly be considered to have a thoracolumbar injury. However, lesser injuries also should arouse suspicion if they are followed by pain in the neck or back or neurological symptoms in the limbs.

Examination

NECK

The head and face are thoroughly inspected for bruises or grazes which could indicate indirect trauma to the cervical spine. The neck is inspected for deformity, bruising or penetrating injury. The patient may be supporting his or her head with their hands. The bone and soft tissues of the neck are palpated for tenderness. Of particular note are tenderness, bogginess or space between the interspinous ligaments, suggesting instability due to posterior column failure. The cervical spine is not moved as part of the examination (Look, Feel but *do not* Move) because with an unstable injury this would imperil the cord.

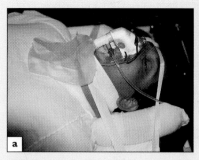
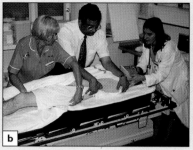
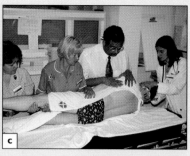

27.3 Spinal injuries – early management (a) Quadruple immobilization: the patient is on a backboard, the head is supported by sandbags and held with tape across the forehead, and a semi-rigid collar has been applied. (b, c) The log-rolling technique for exposure and examination of the back.

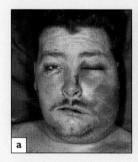
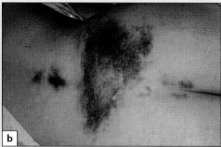

27.4 Spinal injuries – suspicious signs First appearances do matter. With severe facial bruising (a) always suspect a hyperextension injury of the neck. (b) Bruising over the lower back should raise the suspicion of a lumbar vertebral fracture.

BACK

The patient is 'log-rolled' to avoid movement of the thoracolumbar spine. The spine is inspected for deformity, penetrating injury, haematoma or bruising. The bone and soft-tissue structures are palpated, again with particular reference to the interspinous spaces. A haematoma, a gap or a step are signs of instability

SHOCK

Three types of shock may be encountered in patients with spinal injury.

Hypovolaemic shock is suggested by tachycardia, peripheral shutdown and, in later stages, hypotension.

Neurogenic shock reflects loss of the sympathetic pathways in the spinal cord; the peripheral vessels dilate causing hypotension but the heart, deprived of its sympathetic innervation, does not respond by increasing its rate. The combination of paralysis, bradycardia and hypotension suggests neurogenic shock. Over-enthusiaistic use of fluids can cause pulmonary oedema; atropine and vasopressors may be required.

Spinal shock occurs when the spinal cord fails temporarily following injury. Even parts of the cord without structural damage do not function. Below the level of the injury, the muscles are flaccid, the reflexes absent and sensation is lost. This rarely lasts for more than 48 hours and during this period it is difficult to tell whether the neurological lesion is complete or incomplete. Once the primitive reflexes return (anal wink and the bulbocavernosus reflex), spinal shock has ended; the residual motor and sensory loss reflects the true state of affairs.

NEUROLOGICAL EXAMINATION

A full neurological examination is carried out in every case; this may have to be repeated several times during the first few days. Each dermatome, myotome and reflex is tested.

Cord longitudinal column functions are assessed: corticospinal tract (posterolateral cord, ipsilateral motor power), spinothalamic tract (anterolateral cord, contralateral pain and temperature) and posterior columns (ipsilateral proprioception).

Sacral sparing should be tested for. Preservation of active great toe flexion, anal tone (on digital examination) and intact peri-anal sensation suggest a partial rather than complete lesion. Further recovery may occur.

The unconscious patient is difficult to examine; a spinal injury must be assumed until proven otherwise. Clues to the existence of a spinal cord lesion are a history of a fall or rapid deceleration, a head injury, diaphragmatic breathing, a flaccid anal sphincter, hypotension with bradycardia and a pain response above, but not below, the clavicle.

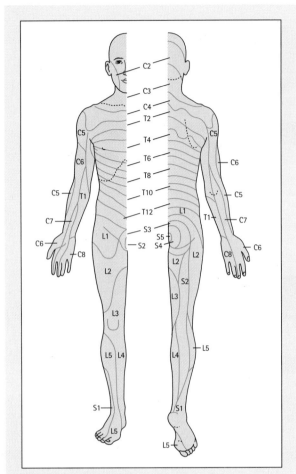

27.5 Spine injuries – neurological examination Dermatomes supplied by the spinal nerve roots.

Table 27.1 Tests for nerve root motor function

Nerve Root	Test
C5	Elbow flexion
C6	Wrist extension
C7	Wrist flexion, finger extension
C8	Finger flexion
T1	Finger abduction
L1,2	Hip abduction
L3,4	Knee extension
L5,S1	Knee flexion
L5	Great toe extension
S1	Great toe flexion

Table 27.2 Root values for tendon reflexes

Root value	Tendon reflex
C5	Biceps
C6	Brachioradialis
C7	Triceps
L3,4	Quadriceps
L5, S1	Achilles tendon

Imaging

- X-ray examination is mandatory for all accident victims complaining of pain or stiffness in the neck or back, all patients with head injuries or severe facial injuries (cervical spine), patients with rib fractures or severe seat-belt bruising (thoracic spine), and those with severe pelvic or abdominal injuries (thoracolumbar spine).
- Accident victims who are unconscious should have spine x-rays as part of the routine work-up.
- Patients with known vertebral pathology (e.g. ankylosing spondylitis) may suffer fractures after comparatively minor back injury; the spine should be x-rayed even if pain is not marked.
- Pain is often poorly localized; views should include several segments above and below the painful area.
- X-ray examination should be carried out with a minimum of movement and manipulation. No attempt should be made to obtain 'flexion-and-extension' views during the initial work-up.
- 'Difficult' areas, such as the lower cervical and upper thoracic segments which are often obscured by

shoulder and rib images, may require plain film tomography or computed tomography (CT). Odontoid fractures also are sometimes better shown on axial tomograms than on routine CT.

- In addition to anteroposterior and lateral views, open mouth views are need for the upper two cervical vertebrae and oblique views may be needed for the thoracolumbar region.
- CT is ideal for showing structural damage to individual vertebrae and displacement of bone fragments into the vertebral canal.
- Magnetic resonance imaging (MRI) is the method of choice for displaying the intervertebral discs, ligamentum flavum and neural structures.
- CT myelography, with the intrathecal introduction of contrast agent, provides information on the dimensions of the spinal canal, impingement by fracture fragments or intervertebral disc and root avulsion. This investigation has been largely replaced by MRI.
- Three-dimensional reconstruction of CT images defines certain complex fracture patterns. Spiral CT allows high-resolution sagittal reconstruction and, when available, is useful for displaying fractures of the odontoid process.
- Remember that the spine may be damaged in more than one place.
- Do not accept poor quality images.
- In difficult cases, consult with the radiologist.

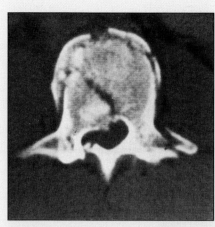

27.6 Spine injuries – x-ray diagnosis The plain x-ray showed the fracture but gave little indication of the amount of fragmentation and displacement. This CT scan revealed that one large fragment was encroaching dangerously on the spinal cord.

PRINCIPLES OF DEFINITIVE TREATMENT

The objectives of treatment are:

1. to preserve neurological function;
2. to relieve any reversible neural compression;
3. to restore alignment of the spine;
4. to stabilize the spine;
5. to rehabilitate the patient.

The *indications for urgent surgical stabilization* are (a) an unstable fracture with progressive neurological deficit and (b) an unstable fracture in a patient with multiple injuries.

PATIENTS WITH NO NEUROLOGICAL INJURY

If the spinal injury is stable, the patient is treated by supporting the spine in a position that will cause no further strain; a firm collar or lumbar brace will usually suffice, but the patient may need to rest in bed until pain and muscle spasm subside. The exception is a burst fracture of the vertebral body: a CT should be arranged which may show displaced fragments within the spinal canal; even with a fairly large retropulsed fragment, in the absence of neurological compromise surgery is not necessary. However, rehabilitation may be easier if surgery is performed. Furthermore, these patients are potentially 'neurologically unstable' and a progressive neurological deficit can develop, which is an indication for decompression and fusion. In the burst fracture without neurological compromise, the management is debatable.

The correction of *deformity* by surgery is also controversial. It is not clear that symptoms are related to minor deformity, although a kyphosis of greater than 30° is associated with back pain in the long-term. Furthermore, when there is more than 30° angulation, the posterior ligaments are likely to be relatively incompetent and the deformity may progress. Stabilization should be considered.

If the spinal injury is unstable it should be held secure until the tissues heal and the spine becomes stable. In the cervical spine this should be done as soon as possible by traction, using tongs or a halo device attached to the skull. If the halo is attached to a body cast the combination can be used as an external fixator for prolonged immobilization (see below). Alternatively (particularly in the thoracolumbar spine) internal fixation can be carried out. Dislocations and subluxations must be reduced, whether by adjusting the posture, by traction or by open operation.

PATIENTS WITH A NEUROLOGICAL INJURY

Once spinal shock has recovered, the full extent of the neurological injury is assessed.

If the spinal injury is stable (which is rare), the patient can be treated conservatively and rehabilitated as soon as possible.

With the usual unstable injury, conservative treatment can be used; this is highly demanding and is best carried out in a special unit equipped for round-the-clock nursing, 2-hourly turning routines, skin toilet, bladder care and specialized physiotherapy and occupational therapy. After a few weeks the injury stabilizes spontaneously and the patient can be got out of bed for intensive rehabilitation. This approach is most applicable to high thoracic injuries with no associated rib or sternal fractures and minimal deformity. In most other situations, early operative stabilization is preferred; it facilitates nursing, reduces the risk of spinal deformity and persistent local pain, and speeds rehabilitation.

The benefit of early surgery on neurological recovery is uncertain. However, *if neurological loss is incomplete, and especially if neurological loss is progressive,* early operative reduction or decompression and stabilization is indicated.

Intravenous methylprednisolone has been shown to improve outcome if given within 8 hours of injury. Remember, though, that short courses of high-dosage corticosteroids occasionally give rise to osteonecrosis; this is more likely if there are other, cumulative risk factors such as a background of previous corticosteroid medication or alcoholism (Solomon and Pearse, 1994) and patients should be warned about this.

TREATMENT METHODS

CERVICAL SPINE

COLLARS *Soft collars* offer very little biomechanical support to the cervical spine and their use is restricted to minor sprains for the first few days after injury. *Semi-rigid collars* limit motion quite effectively and are widely used in the acute setting. They are not adequate for very unstable injury patterns. *Four-poster braces* are more stable, applying pressure to the mandible, occiput, sternum and upper thoracic spine. They can be uncomfortable.

TONGS A pin is inserted into the outer table on each side of the skull; these are mounted on a pair of tongs and traction is applied to reduce the fracture or dislocation and to maintain the reduced position.

HALO RING At least four pins are inserted into the outer table of the skull and a ring is applied. The use of titanium pins and graphite ring allows an MRI scan to be performed. The halo ring can be used for initial traction and reduction of the fracture or dislocation, and then can be attached to a plaster vest. Proper positioning and torque-pressure of the pins is essential.

FIXATION Various operative procedures are available, depending on the level and pattern of injury. *Odontoid fractures* can be fixed with lag screws; *burst fractures* can be decompressed through an anterior approach; and *facet dislocations* can be reduced through a posterior approach. The spine can be stabilized anteriorly with plates between the vertebral bodies or posteriorly with wires between the spinous processes, or with small plates between the lateral masses.

THORACOLUMBAR SPINE

BEDS Special beds are used in the management of spinal injuries. They are designed to avoid pressure sores (with special mattresses or the facility to turn the patient frequently). Some beds allow postural reduction of fractures.

BRACE A thoracolumbar brace avoids flexion by three-point fixation. It is suitable for some burst fractures, seat-belt injuries and compression fractures.

DECOMPRESSION AND STABILIZATION The aim of surgery is to reduce the fracture, hold the reduction and decompress the neural elements. The surgical approach can be either anterior or posterior.

The anterior approach is suitable for burst fractures with significant canal impingement or as a supplement to posterior fixation in those compression fractures with considerable loss of anterior bone stock. With an anterior

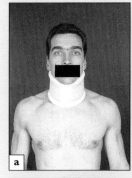
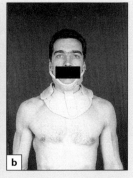
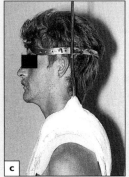

27.7 Spine injuries – treatment (a) Standard cervical collar. (b) More rigid variety. (c) Halo-body cast.

approach, the spine is exposed through a transthoracic, transdiaphragmatic or transperitoneal approach depending on the level of the fracture. The vertebral body is removed so that the spinal canal is decompressed; a bone graft (rib, fibula or iliac crest) is then inserted and special plates are applied between the intact vertebral bodies above and below the injured level.

The posterior approach is more suitable for flexion-compression injuries, seat belt injuries and fracture-dislocations. Some burst fractures can also be reduced indirectly from a posterior approach using implants that apply distraction to the fracture. Hook and rod systems provide fixation between intact vertebrae several segments above and below the injury. The advent of *segmental spinal instrumentation*, with the fixation device attached to the spinal column through pedicle screws, allows secure fixation of a much shorter implant, reaching only one or two segments away from the injury. These devices also allow correction of the deformity by distraction and extension. Bone graft is required so that a biological fusion can supplement the implants.

CERVICAL SPINE INJURIES

The patient will usually give a history of a fall from a height, a diving accident or a vehicle accident in which the neck is forcibly moved. In a patient unconscious from a head injury, a fractured cervical spine should be assumed (and acted upon) until proved otherwise.

An abnormal position of the neck is suggestive, and careful palpation may elicit tenderness. Movement is best postponed until the neck has been x-rayed. Pain or paraesthesia in the limbs is significant, and the patient should be examined for evidence of spinal cord or nerve root damage.

Imaging

Plain x-rays must be of high quality and should be inspected methodically.

- In the anteroposterior view the lateral outlines should be intact, and the spinous processes and tracheal shadow in the midline. An open-mouth view is necessary to show C1 and C2 (for odontoid and lateral mass fractures).
- The lateral view must include all seven cervical vertebrae and the upper half of T1, otherwise a serious injury at the cervicothoracic junction will be missed. If the cervicothoracic junction cannot be seen, then the lateral view should be repeated while the patient's shoulders are pulled down. If this fails, then a 'swimmer's view' is obtained. If this, too, fails, then tomography or a CT scan is required.
- The smooth lordotic curve should be followed, tracing four parallel lines formed by the front of the vertebral bodies, the back of the bodies, the posterior borders of the lateral masses and the bases of the spinous processes; any irregularity suggests a fracture or displacement. Forwards shift of the vertebral body by 25% suggests a unilateral facet dislocation and by 50% a bilateral facet dislocation.
- The distance between the odontoid peg and the back of the anterior arch of the atlas should be no more than 3mm in adults and 4.5mm in children.

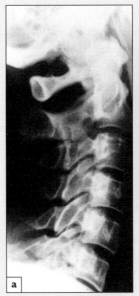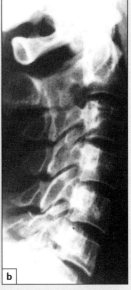

27.9 Cervical spine injuries – x-ray diagnosis (a) Following a traffic accident this patient had a painful neck and consulted her doctor three times; on each occasion she was told 'the x-rays are normal'. But count the vertebrae! There are only six in this film. If the C7–T1 junction cannot be seen, then a shoulder pull-down, swimmer's view or CT scan is required. (b) When a shoulder pull-down view was made to show the entire cervical spine, a dislocation of C6 on C7 could be seen at the very bottom of the film.

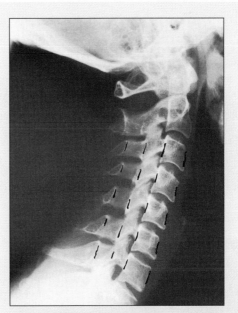

27.10 Cervical spine – normal x-ray In the lateral projection, four parallel lines can be traced unbroken from C1 to C7. They are formed by: (1) the anterior surfaces of the vertebral bodies; (2) the posterior surfaces of the bodies; (3) the posterior borders of the lateral masses; and (4) the bases of the spinous processes.

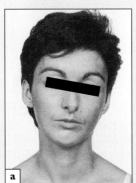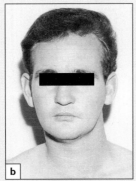

27.8 Cervical spine injuries – clinical signs Skew neck is a common finding after neck 'sprains'. The woman shown in (a) had suffered a 'whiplash injury'; the man in (b), who has a similar postural deformity, gave a history of a fall some weeks before and was found to have a fractured odontoid process.

- Compare the shape of each vertebral body with that of the others; note particularly any loss of height, fragmentation or backwards displacement of the posterior border of the vertebral body.
- Examine the soft-tissue shadows. The retropharyngeal space may contain a haematoma; the prevertebral soft tissue shadow should be less than 5mm in thickness above the level of the trachea and less than one vertebral body's width in thickness below. The interspinous space may be widened after ligament rupture.

Diagnostic pitfalls in children

Children are often distressed and difficult to examine; more than usual reliance may be placed on the x-rays. It is well to recall some common pitfalls.

An increased atlanto-dental interval (up to 4.5mm) may be quite normal; this is because the skeleton is incompletely ossified and the ligaments relatively lax during childhood. There may also be apparent subluxation of C2 on C3 (*pseudosubluxation*).

An increased retropharyngeal space can be brought about by forced expiration during crying.

Growth plates and synchondroses can be mistaken for *fractures*. The normal synchondrosis at the base of the dens has usually fused by the age of 6 years, but it can be mistaken for an undisplaced fracture; the spinous process growth plates also resemble fractures; and the growth plate at the tip of the odontoid can be tasken for a fracture in older children.

SCIWORA is an acronym for Spinal Cord Injury Without Obvious Radiographic Abnormality. Normal radiographs in children do not exclude the possibility of spinal cord injury.

UPPER CERVICAL SPINE

OCCIPITO–ATLANTAL DISLOCATION

This is usually fatal; occasionally a patient survives a subluxation without neurological deficit. The diagnosis is made on the lateral cervical radiograph: the tip of the odontoid should be no more than 5mm in vertical alignment and 1mm in horizontal alignment from the basion (anterior rim of the foramen magnum). Greater distances are allowable in children. The injury is managed initially by halo ring immobilization *without* traction, followed by posterior fusion of the occiput to the upper cervical spine.

C1 FRACTURE

Sudden severe load on the top of the head may cause a 'bursting' force which fractures the ring of the atlas (Jefferson's fracture). There is no encroachment on the neural canal and, usually, no neurological damage. The fracture is seen on the open mouth view (if the lateral masses are spread away from the odontoid peg) and the lateral view. A CT scan is particularly helpful in defining

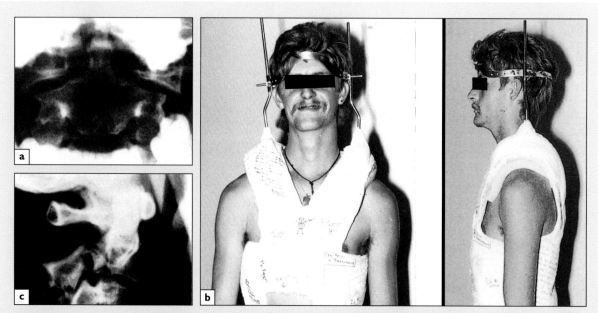

27.11 Fractures of C1 and C2 – neural arches (a) Fractures of C1 with disruption of the arch (Jefferson fracture). The open-mouth view shows spreading of the lateral masses; the spine is unstable, and a halo-body cast (b) may be indicated. (c) Fracture of the pedicle or lateral pillar of C2 is usually due to an extension injury ('hangman's fracture').

the fracture. If it is undisplaced, the injury is stable and the patient wears a semi-rigid collar or halo-vest until the fracture unites. If there is sideways spreading of the lateral masses (more than 7mm on the open-mouth view), the transverse ligament has ruptured; this injury is unstable and should be treated by a halo-vest for several weeks. If there is persisting instability on x-ray, a posterior C1/2 arthrodesis is considered.

A hyperextension injury can fracture either the anterior or posterior arch of the atlas. These are usually relatively stable and are managed with a halo-vest or semi-rigid collar until union occurs.

Fractures of the atlas are associated with injury elsewhere in the cervical spine in up to 50% of cases; odontoid fractures and 'hangman's fractures' in particular should be excluded.

ODONTOID FRACTURE (C2)

Odontoid fractures are uncommon. They usually occur as flexion injuries in young adults after high-velocity accidents or severe falls. However, they also occur in elderly, osteoporotic people as a result of low-energy trauma in which the neck is forced into hyperextension, e.g. a fall onto the face or forehead.

A displaced fracture is really a fracture-dislocation of the atlanto-axial joint in which the atlas is shifted forwards or backwards, taking the odontoid process with it. Cord damage is seen in about a quarter of patients; at this level about a third of the internal diameter of the atlas is free space, a third filled with the odontoid and a third with the cord. Thus there is space available for displacement without neurological injury.

Classification

Odontoid fractures have been classified by Anderson and D'Alonzo as follows:

- *Type I* – An avulsion fracture of the tip of the odontoid process due to traction by the alar ligaments. The fracture is stable and unites without difficulty.
- *Type II* – A fracture at the junction of the odontoid process and the body of the axis. This is the most common (and potentially the most dangerous) type. The fracture is unstable and prone to non-union.
- *Type III* – A fracture through the body of the axis. The fracture is stable and almost always unites with immobilization.

Clinical features

The history is usually that of a severe neck strain followed by pain and stiffness due to muscle spasm. Diagnosis is not as easy as it sounds; odontoid fractures are often associated with other, more obvious injuries which command immediate attention. In some cases the clinical features are mild and continue to be overlooked for weeks on end. Neurological symptoms occur in about 20% of cases.

Imaging

Plain x-rays usually show the fracture, although the extent of the injury is not always obvious – e.g. there may be an associated fracture of the atlas. X-ray

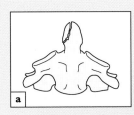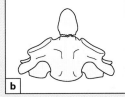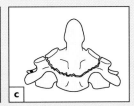

27.12 Odontoid fractures – classification (a) Type I – fracture through the tip of the odontoid process. (b) Type II – fracture at the junction of the odontoid process and the body. (c) Type III – fracture through the body of the axis. (Anderson and D'Alonzo, 1974).

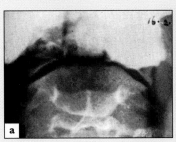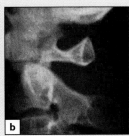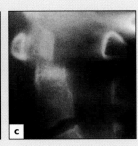

27.13 Odontoid fractures – x-ray (a, b) Fractured base of odontoid peg, permitting forwards shift of the atlas and skull. (c) X-ray tomography may show the lesion more clearly.

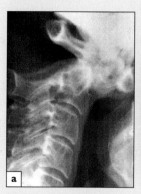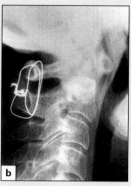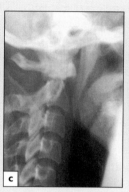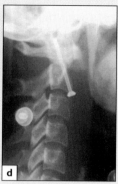

27.14 Odontoid fractures – treatment (a) A severely displaced odontoid fracture. (b) In this case the fracture was reduced by skull traction and held by fixing the spinous process of C1 to that of C2. (c, d) An alternative method of fixation.

tomography is helpful but MRI has the advantage that it may reveal rupture of the transverse ligament; this can cause instability in the absence of a fracture.

Treatment

Type I fractures need no more than immobilization in a rigid collar until discomfort subsides.

Type II fractures are often unstable and prone to non-union, especially if displaced more than 5mm. Undisplaced fractures can be held by fitting a halo-vest. Displaced fractures need to be reduced by traction and are then held by operative screw fixation or by halo-cast immobilization with x-ray monitoring to check for stability.

Type III fractures, if undisplaced, are treated in a halo-vest for 8–12 weeks. If displaced, the fracture must first be reduced by halo traction, which will allow positioning in either flexion or extension, depending on whether the displacement is forwards or backwards; the neck is then immobilized in a halo-vest for 8–12 weeks.

FRACTURED PEDICLE(S) OF C2 (HANGMAN'S FRACTURE)

In the true judicial hangman's fracture, the pedicles of the axis are fractured and the C1/2 disc is torn; the mechanism is extension with distraction. In civilian injuries, the mechanism is more complex, with varying degrees of extension, compression and flexion. This is one cause of death in motor vehicle accidents when the forehead strikes the dashboard. Neurological damage, however, is unusual because the fracture of the posterior arch tends to decompress the spinal cord. Nevertheless the fracture is potentially unstable.

Undisplaced fractures which are shown to be stable on supervised flexion–extension views are treated in a semi-rigid collar or halo-vest until united. Displaced fractures may need reduction; however, because the mechanism of

injury usually involves distraction, traction must be avoided. After reduction, the neck is held in a halo-vest until union has occurred. Fusion is sometimes required for persistent instability. Occasionally, the hangman's fracture is associated with a C2/3 facet dislocation; open reduction and stabilization is required.

LOWER CERVICAL SPINE

Fractures of the lower cervical spine, from C3 to C7, tend to produce characteristic fracture patterns, depending on the mechanism of injury: flexion, axial compression, flexion–rotation or hyperextension.

WEDGE COMPRESSION FRACTURE

A pure flexion injury results in a wedge-compression fracture of the vertebral body. The middle and posterior elements remain intact and the injury is stable. All that is needed is a comfortable collar.

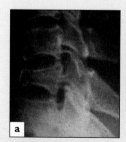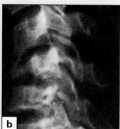

27.15 Compression fractures of the cervical spine A true wedge-compression fracture (a) is stable because the middle and posterior elements remain intact. (b) At first glance this also looks like a simple compression fracture, but it isn't! The middle column is broken and the vertebral body is driven backwards; the fracture is unstable and the cord is threatened. This needs CT or MRI to show the true state of affairs.

A note of warning: The x-ray should be carefully examined to exclude damage to the middle column and posterior displacement of the vertebral body fragment, that is features of a burst fracture which is potentially dangerous. If there is the least doubt, CT or MRI is required.

POSTERIOR LIGAMENT INJURY

Sudden flexion of the mid-cervical spine can result in damage to the posterior ligament complex (the interspinous ligament, facet capsule and supraspinous ligament). The upper vertebra tilts forwards on the one below, opening up the interspinous space posteriorly.

The patient complains of pain and there may be localized tenderness posteriorly. *X-ray* may reveal a slightly increased gap between the adjacent spines; however, if the neck is held in extension this sign can be missed, so it is always advisable to obtain a lateral view with the neck in the neutral position. A flexion view would, of course, show the widened interspinous space more clearly, *but flexion should not be permitted in the early post-traumatic period.*

The assessment of stability is essential in these injuries. If the angulation of the vertebral body with its neighbour exceeds 11°, if there is anterior translation of one vertebral body upon the other of more than 3.5mm or if the facets are fractured or displaced, then the injury is unstable and it should be treated as a subluxation or dislocation. If it is certain that the injury is stable, a semi-rigid collar for 6 weeks is adequate; if the injury is unstable then posterior fixation and fusion is advisable.

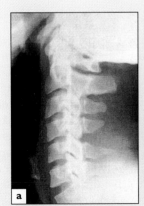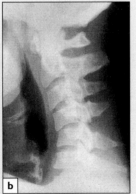

27.16 Cervical spine – posterior ligament injury (a) The film taken in extension shows no displacement of the vertebral bodies, but there is an unduly large gap between the spinous processes of C4 and 5. (b) With the neck slightly flexed the subluxation is obvious. *NB: flexion–extension views are potentially dangerous and should be used only in specific situations under direct supervision of an experienced surgeon.*

BURST FRACTURE

These severe injuries are due to axial compression of the cervical spine, usually in diving or athletic accidents. Persistent neurological injury is common.

Plain x-rays show a comminuted fracture of the vertebral body; the films should be carefully examined for evidence of middle column damage and posterior displacement (even very slight displacement) of the body fragment. Traction must be applied immediately and *CT or MRI* should be performed to look for retropulsion of large fragments into the spinal canal.

If there is no neurological deficit, the injury is treated by immobilization in a halo-vest. If there is any neurological deficit, then urgent anterior decompression is considered; immobilization for 6–8 weeks is, of course, also needed.

'TEAR-DROP FRACTURE'

With combined axial compression and flexion, an antero-inferior fragment of the vertebral body is sheared off; this fragment, the eponymous 'tear-drop', may look benign but there is a very real danger that the middle column and posterior elements may also be damaged, making it a very unstable injury (see Fig. 27.17).

X-ray may show that the greater part of the vertebral body is displaced posteriorly. However, evaluation by *CT or MRI* is much better: if there is middle or posterior column damage, the injury should be managed by anterior or posterior stabilization. If there are signs of cord impingement, decompression and stabilization will be needed.

FLEXION–ROTATION INJURIES

UNILATERAL FACET DISLOCATION

This also is a flexion-rotation injury but only one apophyseal joint is dislocated. There may be an associated fracture of the facet. On the lateral x-ray the vertebral body appears to be partially displaced (less than one-half of its width); on the anteroposterior x-ray the alignment of the spinous processes is disrupted. Cord damage is unusual and the injury is stable.

The dislocation is reduced by skull traction, starting with 5kg and then increasing, under x-ray control, up to about one-third of body weight. When the facet is seen to be perched, a gentle extension and rotaton manoeuvre can achieve full reduction. The traction is then reduced to maintain the reduction. The patient should be awake during reduction and any neurological symptoms mean that further attempts at closed reduction should be stopped.

If closed reduction with traction fails, a manipulation can be performed if the operator is experienced;

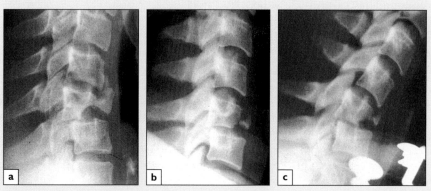

27.17 Tear-drop fracture (**a**) This comminuted vertebral body fracture has produced a large anterior fragment and obvious posterior displacement of the posterior fragment. (**b**) In this case the anterior 'tear-drop' was noted but the severity of the injury was underestimated; careful examination shows that the main body fragment is displaced slightly posteriorly. The patient was treated in a collar; 3 weeks later (**c**) the fracture had collapsed and the large body fragment was now very obviously tilted and displaced posteriorly. By then he was complaining of tingling and weakness in the right arm. Beware the innocent tear-drop!

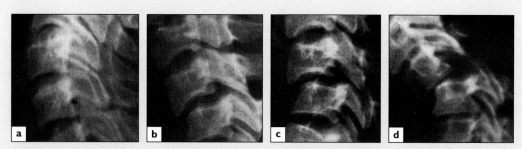

27.18 Cervical subluxation and dislocation In (**a**) the cervical spine looks normal, but the film in flexion (**b**) shows forwards subluxation – the posterior ligaments are torn. (**c**) Fracture-dislocation with moderate forwards shift signifying a unilateral facet dislocation. (**d**) Fracture-dislocation with displacement of both facets and marked forwards shift.

otherwise open reduction and internal fixation are advisable. Patients left with an unreduced unilateral facet dislocation are liable to develop neck pain and nerve root symptoms.

After reduction, the injury is usually stable if there is no fracture. The neck is immobilized in a halo-vest for 6–8 weeks. If there is an associated facet fracture or recurrent dislocation in the external fixator, then posterior fusion should be considered.

BILATERAL FACET DISLOCATION OR FRACTURE-DISLOCATION
These injuries result from severe flexion and rotation; the articular facets ride forwards over the facets below. One or both of the articular masses is fractured or there may be a pure dislocation ('jumped facets'). The posterior ligaments are ruptured and the spine is unstable. Usually there is cord damage. The lateral radiograph shows forwards displacement of a vertebra on the one below of greater than one-half its width.

The displacement must be reduced as a matter of urgency. Skull traction is used, starting with 5kg and increasing it step-wise by similar amounts up to 30kg; intravenous muscle relaxants and a bolster beneath the shoulders may help. If x-rays show that the dislocation had been reduced, traction is diminished to about 5kg and maintained for 6 weeks; thereafter the patient wears a collar for another 6 weeks. More convenient for the patient is to immobilize the neck in a halo-vest for 12 weeks. A third method is to carry out a posterior fusion as soon as reduction has been achieved; the patient is allowed up in a cervical brace which is worn for 6–8 weeks.

If reduction with traction fails, then a posterior open reduction and fusion will be required.

After reduction, the spine should be imaged urgently by myelography, CT or MRI as extruded disc fragments are not uncommon and may further compromise the spinal cord. An anterior decompression would be required.

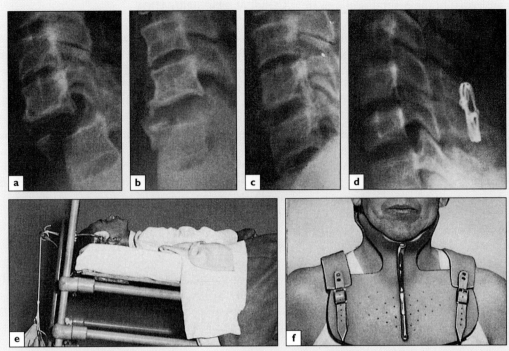

27.19 Treatment of fracture-dislocation (**a**, **b**, **c**) Stages in the reduction of a fracture-dislocation by skull traction; (**d**) subsequent wiring to ensure stability. (**e**) The patient was kept on skull traction until the wound had healed. A polythene collar as in (**f**) was then applied.

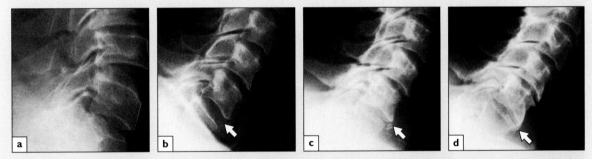

27.20 Hyperextension injuries (**a**) The anterior longitudinal ligament has been torn; in the neutral position the gap will close and reduction will be stable, but a collar or brace will be needed until the soft tissues are healed. (**b**) X-ray in this case showed a barely visible flake of bone anteriorly at the C6/7 disc space. (**c**) 1 month later the traction fracture at C6/7 was more obvious, as was the disc lesion at C5/6. (**d**) A year later C6/7 has fused anteriorly; the patient still has neck pain due to the C5/6 disc degeneration.

HYPEREXTENSION INJURY

Hyperextension strains of soft-tissue structures are common and may be caused by comparatively mild acceleration forces. Bone and joint disruptions, however, are rare.

The more severe injuries are suggested by the history and the presence of facial bruising or lacerations. The posterior bone elements are compressed and may fracture; the anterior structures fail in tension, with tearing of the anterior longitudinal ligament or an avulsion fracture of the anterosuperior or anteroinferior edge of the vertebral body, opening up of the anterior part of the disc space, fracture of the back of the vertebral body and/or damage to the intervertebral disc. In patients with pre-existing cervical spondylosis, the cord can be pinched between the bony spurs or disc and the posterior ligamentum flavum; oedema and haematomyelia may cause an acute central cord syndrome (quadriplegia, sacral sparing and more upper limb than lower limb deficit, a flaccid upper limb paralysis and spastic lower limb paralysis).

These injuries are stable in the neutral position, in which they should be held by a collar for 6–8 weeks. Healing may lead to spontaneous fusion between adjacent vertebral bodies.

DOUBLE INJURIES

With high-energy trauma the cervical spine may be injured at more than one level. Discovery of the most obvious lesion is no reason to drop one's guard. Two salutary examples are shown in Figures 27.21 and 27.22.

AVULSION INJURY OF THE SPINOUS PROCESS

Fracture of the C7 spinous process may occur with severe voluntary contraction of the muscles at the back of the neck; it is known as the *clay-shoveller's fracture*. The injury is painful but harmless. No treatment is required; as soon as symptoms permit, neck exercises are encouraged.

CERVICAL DISC HERNIATION

Acute post-traumatic disc herniation may cause severe pain radiating to one or both upper limbs, and neurological symptoms and signs ranging from mild paraesthesia to weakness, loss of a reflex and blunted sensation. Rarely a patient presents with full-blown paresis. The diagnosis is confirmed by MRI or CT-myelography.

Sudden paresis will need immediate surgical decompression. With lesser symptoms and signs, one can afford to wait a few days for improvement; if this does not occur, then anterior discectomy and interbody fusion will be needed.

NEURAPRAXIA OF THE CERVICAL CORD

Accidents causing sudden, severe axial loading with the neck in hyperflexion or hyperextension are occasionally followed by transient pain, paraesthesia and weakness in the arms or legs, all in the absence of any

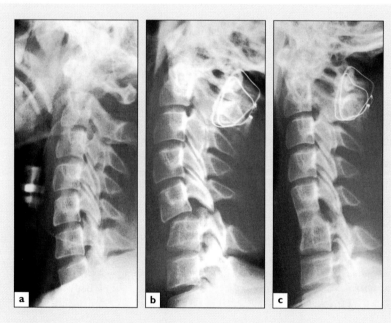

27.21 Double cervical injuries (a) This patient with a neck injury was suspected of having an odontoid fracture. This was confirmed and a posterior stablization was performed. Only when the brace was removed and he started flexing his neck did the x-ray show an obvious subluxation lower down (b). This was treated by anterior fusion (c).

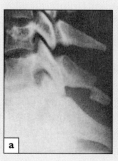
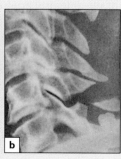
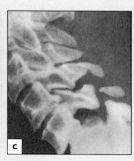

27.22 Avulsions (a) The clay-shoveller's fracture. Jerking the neck backwards has resulted in avulsion of one of the spinous processes – a benign injury. (b) This patient might be thought to have a similar fracture, but a subsequent flexion film (c) shows the serious nature of the injury – a severe fracture-dislocation.

x-ray or MRI abnormality. Symptoms may last for as little as a few minutes or as long as 2 or 3 days. The condition has been called neurapraxia of the cervical cord and is ascribed to pinching of the cord by the bony edges of the mobile spinal canal and/or local compression by infolding of the posterior longitudinal ligament or the ligamentum flavum (Thomas *et al.*, 1999). Congenital narrowing of the spinal canal may be a predisposing factor.

Treatment consists of reassurance (after full neurological investigation) and graded exercises to improve strength in the neck muscles.

SPRAINED NECK (WHIPLASH INJURY)

Soft-tissue sprains (or wrenching injuries) of the neck are so common after car accidents that they now constitute a veritable epidemic; and the imaginative term *whiplash injury* has served effectively to enhance public apprehension at its occurrence. It usually follows a rear-end collision in which the occupant's body is thrown forwards and the head jerked backwards with hyperextension of the lower cervical spine; however, it can also occur with flexion and rotation injuries. Women are affected more often than men, perhaps because their neck muscles are more gracile. There is disagreement about the exact pathology but it is likely that the anterior longitudinal ligament and the capsular fibres of the facet joints are strained; in some cases the intervertebral discs also may be damaged. There is no tidy correlation between the amount of damage to the vehicle and the severity of complaints.

Clinical features

Often the victim is unaware of any abnormality immediately after the collision. Pain and stiffness of the neck usually appear with the next 12 to 48 hours, or occasionally only several days later. Pain sometimes radiates to the shoulders or interscapular area and may be accompanied by other, more ill-defined, symptoms such as headache, dizziness, blurring of vision, paraesthesia in the arms, temporomandibular discomfort and tinnitus. Neck muscles are tender and movements often restricted (see Fig. 27.8). Other physical signs – including neurological defects – are uncommon.

X-ray examination may show straightening out of the normal cervical lordosis, a sign of muscle spasm; in other respects the appearances are usually normal. In some cases, however, there are features of long-standing intervertebral disc herniation or degenerative changes in the uncovertebral joints; it may be that these patients suffer more, and for longer spells, than others. *MRI* may show disc abnormalities but there is doubt as to whether these are more common than in the population at large.

Table 27.3 Proposed grading of whiplash-associated injuries

Grade	Clinical pattern
0	No neck symptoms or signs
1	Neck pain, stiffness and tenderness
	No physical signs
2	Neck symptoms and musculoskeletal signs
3	Neck symptoms and neurological signs
4	Neck symptoms and fracture or dislocation

For purposes of comparison, the severity grading system proposed by the Quebec Task Force on Whiplash-Associated Disorders is useful (Table 27.3).

Differential diagnosis

The diagnosis of sprained neck is reached largely by a process of exclusion, that is the inability to demonstrate any other credible explanation for the patient's symptoms. X-rays should be carefully scrutinized to avoid missing a *vertebral fracture* or a mid-cervical *subluxation*. The presence of neurological signs such as muscle weakness and wasting, a depressed reflex or definite loss of sensibility should suggest *an acute disc lesion* and is an indication for MRI.

Seat-belt injuries often accompany neck sprains. They do not always cause bruising of the chest, but they can produce pressure or traction injuries of the *suprascapular nerve* or the *brachial plexus*, either of which may cause symptoms resembling those of a whiplash injury. The examining doctor should be familiar with the clinical features of these conditions.

Treatment

Collars are more likely to hinder than help recovery. Simple pain-relieving measures, including analgesic medication, may be needed during the first few weeks. However, the emphasis should be on graded exercises, beginning with isometric muscle contractions and postural adjustments, then going on gradually to active movements and lastly movements against resistance. The range of movement in each direction is slowly increased without subjecting the patient to unnecessary pain. Many patients find osteopathy and chiropractic treatment to be helpful.

Progress and outcome

The natural history of whiplash injury is extremely variable, and this is reflected in the widely divergent statistics appearing in the medical literature. Some patients become asymptomatic within a few weeks; others complain of pain, restriction of movement and significant loss of function for the rest of their lives. In most cases symptoms diminish after about 3 months and go on improving over the next year or two. Some investigators have suggested that there is little chance of further improvement after the first year and that a significant number of patients (estimates range from 10 to 40%) will continue to suffer discomfort for many years (literature review by Bannister and Gargan, 1993). Negative prognostic indicators are increasing age, severity of symptoms at the outset, prolonged duration of symptoms and the presence of pre-existing intervertebral disc degeneration. Unfortunately most of these studies have been flawed from the outset because they are based on selected groups of patients (usually those who attended a hospital after the accident) and little is known of the natural progress in the thousands of people who experience similar injuries and either do not develop symptoms or do not report them.

Chronic whiplash–associated disorder

Those patients who, in the absence of any objective clinical or imaging signs, continue almost indefinitely to complain of pain, restriction of movement, loss of function, psychological changes and inability to work constitute a sizeable problem in terms of medical resources, compensation claims, legal costs and – not least – personal suffering. Opinions on the causes of these long-term difficulties differ widely from one investigator to another. The subject is well reviewed in the *Current Concepts* monograph edited by Gunzburg and Szpalski (1997). The significance of peer copying (amoung both patients and doctors!) and the role of cultural and psychosocial factors and emphasized in several recent publications (Livingston, 1999).

THORACIC SPINE INJURIES

Most thoracic spine injuries result from hyperflexion; fractures are usually wedge-compressions but fracture-dislocations also occur. The rib cage tends to protect all but the lower two or three segments from injury patterns that commonly occur in the flexible cervical and lumbar areas, and most thoracic spine fractures are mechanically stable. However, the spinal canal in this area is relatively narrow so cord damage is not uncommon and when it does occur it is usually complete (Bohlman, 1985).

Plain radiographs, whilst showing the lower thoracic spine quite clearly, may be difficult to interpret for the upper thoracic spine because the scapula and shoulders get in the way. Tomography or MRI may be needed; CT is helpful if cord impingement is suspected.

Treatment

Stable fracture patterns (less than about 30° of kyphosis) without neurological injury are managed symptomatically. If angulation is more marked, bracing or posterior fusion are indicated to avoid an increasing kyphosis.

If there is complete paraplegia with no improvement after 48 hours, conservative management is adequate; the patient can be rested in bed for 5–6 weeks, then gradually mobilized in a brace. With severe bony injury, however, increasing kyphosis may occur and internal fixation should be considered.

If the paraplegia is partial, there is the potential for further recovery; decompression and stabilization are carried out through a transthoracic approach.

THORACIC DISC HERNIATION

Intervertebral discs can be damaged at any level. In the thoracic spine this is particularly significant because there is little spare space around the spinal cord. Pain may be localized to the back or may radi-

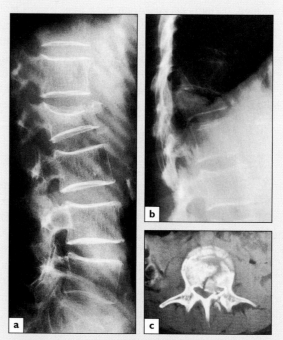

27.23 Thoracic vertebral fractures (a) Compression fractures are relatively common in elderly, osteoporotic people. Note the absence of transverse trabeculae and sharply pencilled cortices, classic signs of postmenopausal osteoporosis. (b) This severe compression fracture (really a type of burst fracture) was due to a fall from a horse. The posterior part of the vertebral body is shattered and pushed backwards into the spinal canal; this is shown more clearly in the CT scan (c). The injury was treated by internal fixation and grafting (same case as Fig. 27.28).

ate around the chest wall or towards the groin; it may be accompanied by paraesthesia. On examination there may be an ataxic gait, weakness or paralysis of the lower limbs, hypertonic leg reflexes and upgoing plantar reflexes. The diagnosis is confirmed by CT myelography or MRI.

Treatment requires an anterior transthoracic discectomy. Posterior laminotomy and decompresson are contraindicated because the cord can be damaged by the retraction needed to expose the disc.

THORACOLUMBAR AND LUMBAR INJURIES

The thoracolumbar junction is particularly prone to injury because of the transition between the relatively fixed thoracic spine and the relatively mobile lumbar spine. Forces applied to the thoracolumbar and lumbar spine cause typical injury patterns, which (following Denis) are classified as *minor* (fractures of the vertebral processes and pars interarticularis) and *major* (compression, burst, fracture-dislocation and jack-knife injuries). Here, as in the cervical spine, it is important to establish whether the fracture is stable or unstable.

The *anteroposterior x-ray* may show loss of height or splaying of the intervertebral body with a crush fracture. Widening of the distance between the pedicles at one level, or an increased distance between two adjacent spinous processes, is associated with posterior column damage. The *lateral view* is examined for alignment, bone outline, structural integrity, disc space defects and soft-tissue shadows abnormalities. *Supplementary views* may be required to show the pedicles, the pars interarticularis, facet joints or intervertebral foramena. *CT* is invaluable for demonstrating posterior displacement of vertebral body fragments and encroachment on the spinal canal. *MRI* also may be necessary in the assessment of neurological damage.

'MINOR INJURIES'

FRACTURES OF THE TRANSVERSE PROCESSES

The transverse processes can be avulsed with sudden muscular activity. Isolated injuries need no more than symptomatic treatment. More ominous than usual is a fracture of the transverse process of L5; this should alert one to the possibility of a vertical shear injury of the pelvis.

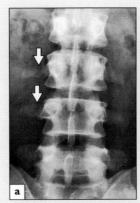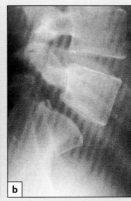

27.24 Thoracolumbar injuries – minor fractures (a) Fracture of the transverse processes on the right at L3 and L4 (arrows). As usual with undisplaced fractures, they are difficult to see. (**b**) Fracture of the pars interarticularis at L5.

EXTENSION INJURIES

Extension of the thoracolumbar spine can cause fractures of the spinous processes, facets, laminae and pars interarticularis. There may be an avulsion flake of the antero-inferior corner of the vertebral body. These injuries are usually stable and respond to symptomatic treatment. A particular example of an extension injury is seen when a weight-lifter, gymnast, cricketer or athlete has a sudden onset of back pain. The injury is often inappropriately ascribed to a disc prolapse, whereas in fact it is due to a stress fracture of the pars interarticularis (*traumatic spondylolysis*). This is best seen in the oblique x-rays, but a thin fracture line is easily missed; a week or two later, an isotope bone scan may show a 'hot' spot. Bilateral fractures occasionally lead to spondylolisthesis. The fracture usually heals spontaneously, provided the patient is prepared to forego his or, more often, her athletic passion for several months.

MAJOR INJURIES

COMPRESSION INJURY

This is by far the most common vertebral fracture and is due to spinal flexion. In osteoporotic patients, fracture may occur with minimal trauma. The posterior ligaments usually remain intact, although they may be damaged by distraction. CT shows that the posterior part of the vertebral body (middle column) is unbroken. Pain is usually quite marked but the fracture is stable. Neurological injury is extremely rare.

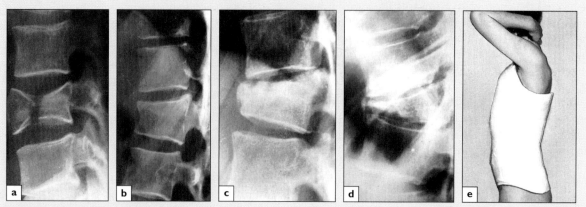

27.25 Thoracolumbar compression fractures (**a**) Central compression fracture with intact posterior half of vertebral body. (**b**) Anterior wedge fracture with 20% loss of height. (**c**) Wedge fracture with 50% loss of height. (**d**) Severe wedge fracture with more than 50% loss of height. Stable injuries and lesser degrees of wedging can be treated by bracing or (**e**) a plaster jacket.

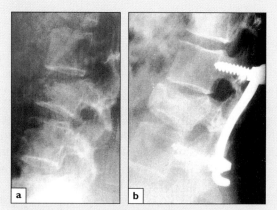

27.26 Wedge-compression fracture (**a**) Left alone, the deformity in this case would almost certainly have increased. (**b**) Posterior fixation has prevented further collapse.

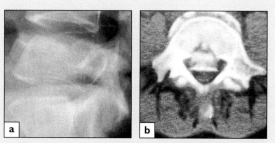

27.27 Lumbar burst fracture Severe compression may shatter the middle column and cause retropulsion of the vertebral body (**a**). The extent of spinal canal encroachment is best shown by CT (**b**).

The patient is kept in bed for a week or two until pain subsides and is then mobilized. For minimal wedging, no support is needed. For those with greater wedging (say 10–40°) a thoracolumbar brace is helpful. At 3 months, flexion–extension views are taken out of the brace; if there is no instability, the brace is gradually discarded.

If loss of vertebral height is greater that 40%, it is likely that the posterior ligaments have been damaged by distraction and will be unable to resist further collapse and deformity. Although conservative treatment with a brace or plaster jacket is feasible, surgical correction and internal fixation is preferable.

BURST INJURY

Severe axial compression may 'explode' the vertebral body, causing failure of both the anterior and the middle columns. The posterior column is usually, but not always, undamaged. The posterior part of the vertebral body is shattered and fragments of bone and disc may be displaced into the spinal canal. The injury is usually unstable.

Anteroposterior x-rays may show spreading of the vertebral body with an increase of the interpedicular distance. Posterior displacement of bone into the spinal canal (retropulsion) is difficult to see on the plain lateral radiograph; a CT is required.

If there is minimal retropulsion of bone, no neurological damage and minimal anterior wedging, the patient is kept in bed until the acute symptoms settle and is then mobilized in a thoracolumbar brace which is discarded at about 12 weeks.

Even if CT shows that there is considerable compromise of the spinal canal, provided there are no neurological symptoms or signs non-operative treatment is still appropriate; the fragments sometimes remodel. However, the patient must be rested in bed for at least 3–6 weeks before being mobilized in a brace. The fractures are neurologically 'unstable', and so any symptoms such as tingling, weakness or alteration of bladder or bowel function must be reported immediately; anterior decompression and stabilization may then be needed.

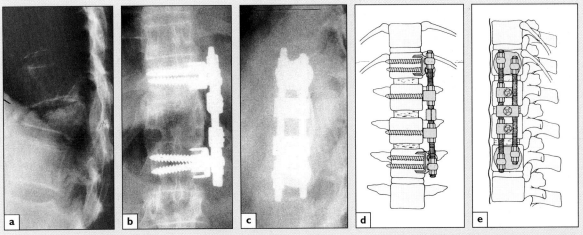

27.28 Burst fracture – treatment (a) Burst fracture in a 44-year-old man who fell from his horse; 3 months later he developed paraesthesia in both legs. (**b–e**) Internal fixation and grafting through a transthoracic transdiaphragmatic approach provided total stability (the Kaneda method).

JACK–KNIFE INJURY

Combined flexion and distraction may cause the mid-lumbar spine to 'jack-knife' around an axis that is placed anterior to the vertebral column. This is seen most typically in *lap seat-belt injuries*, where the body is thrown forwards against the restraining strap. There is little or no crushing of the vertebral body, but the posterior and middle columns fail in distraction; thus these fractures are unstable in flexion.

The tear passes transversely through the bones or the ligament structures, or both. The most perfect example of tensile failure is the injury described by Chance in 1948, in which the split runs through the spinous process, the transverse processes, pedicles and the vertebral body. Neurological damage is uncommon, though the injury is (by definition) unstable. X-rays may show horizontal fractures in the pedicles or transverse processes, and in the anteroposterior view the apparent height of the vertebral body may be increased. In the lateral view there may be opening up of the disc space posteriorly.

The Chance fracture (being an 'all bone' injury) heals rapidly and requires 3 months in a plaster jacket or well-fitting brace. Flexion–extension lateral views should then be taken to ensure that there is no unstable deformity.

Severe ligamentous injuries are less predictable and posterior spinal fusion is advisable.

FRACTURE–DISLOCATION

Segmental displacement may occur with various combinations of flexion, compression, rotation and shear. All three columns are disrupted and the spine is grossly unstable. These are the most dangerous injuries

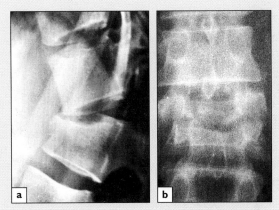

27.29 Jack-knife injuries (**a**) Whereas flexion usually crushes the vertebral body and leaves the posterior ligaments intact, the jack-knife injury disrupts the posterior ligaments causing only slight anterior compression. (**b**) The rare Chance fracture.

and are often associated with neurological damage to the lowermost part of the cord or the cauda equina.

The injury most commonly occurs at the thoracolumbar junction. X-rays may show fractures through the vertebral body, pedicles, articular processes and laminae; there may be varying degrees of subluxation or even bilateral facet dislocation. Often there are associated fractures of transverse processes or ribs. CT is helpful in demonstrating the degree of spinal canal occlusion.

Most fracture-dislocations will benefit from early surgery. *In fracture-dislocation with paraplegia*, surgery will facilitate nursing, shorten the hospital stay, help the patient's rehabilitation and reduce the chance of painful deformity. *In fracture-dislocation with a partial*

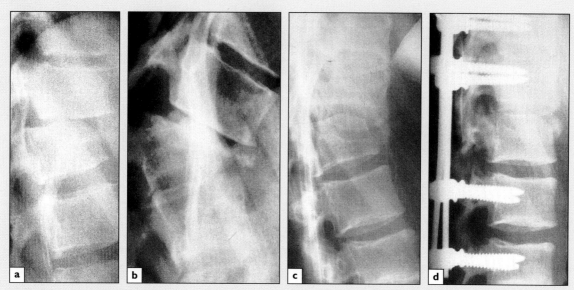

27.30 Thoracolumbar fracture-dislocation (a) Fracture-dislocation at T11/12 in a 32-year-old woman who was a passenger in a truck that overturned. She was completely paraplegic and operation was not thought worthwhile. (b) 4 weeks later the deformity has increased, leaving her with a marked gibbus. (c, d) A similar injury in a 17-year-old man, treated by open reduction and internal fixation.

neurological deficit, surgical stabilization and decompression should give the best neurological outcome. This may require a combined posterior and anterior approach. *In fracture-dislocation without neurological deficit*, surgical stabilization will prevent neurological complications and allow earlier rehabilitation.

When specialized surgery cannot be performed and safe transfer is impractical, these injuries can be managed non-operatively with postural reduction, bed rest and bracing.

NEURAL INJURIES

In spinal injuries the displaced structures may damage the cord or the nerve roots, or both; cervical lesions may cause quadriplegia, and thoracolumbar lesions paraplegia. The damage may be partial or complete. Three varieties of lesion occur: neurapraxia, cord transection and root transection.

NEURAPRAXIA

Motor paralysis (flaccid), burning paraesthesia, sensory loss and visceral paralysis below the level of the cord lesion may be complete, but within minutes or a few hours recovery begins and soon becomes full. The condition is most likely to occur in patients who, for some reason other than injury, have a small-diameter anteroposterior canal; there is, however, no radiological evidence of recent bony damage.

CORD TRANSECTION

Motor paralysis, sensory loss and visceral paralysis occur below the level of the cord lesion; as with cord concussion, the motor paralysis is at first flaccid. This is a temporary condition known as cord shock, but the injury is anatomical and irreparable.

After a time, however, the cord below the level of transection recovers from the shock and acts as an independent structure; that is, it manifests reflex activity. Within 48 hours the primitive anal wink and bulbocavernosus reflexes recover and the plantar responses become extensor. The flaccid paralysis becomes spastic, with increased tone, increased tendon reflexes and clonus; flexor spasms and contractures may develop but sensation never returns.

ROOT TRANSECTION

Motor paralysis, sensory loss and visceral paralysis occur in the distribution of the damaged roots. Root transection, however, differs from cord transection in two ways: recovery may occur and residual motor paralysis remains permanently flaccid.

Anatomical levels

CERVICAL SPINE
With cervical spine injuries the segmental level of cord transection nearly corresponds to the level of bony damage. Not more than one or two additional roots are likely to be transected. High cervical cord

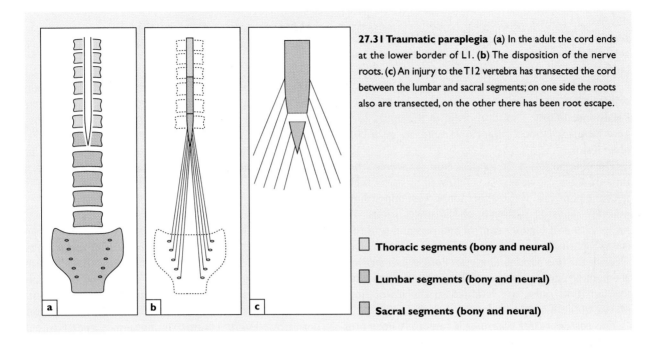

27.31 Traumatic paraplegia (a) In the adult the cord ends at the lower border of L1. (b) The disposition of the nerve roots. (c) An injury to the T12 vertebra has transected the cord between the lumbar and sacral segments; on one side the roots also are transected, on the other there has been root escape.

- ☐ Thoracic segments (bony and neural)
- ☐ Lumbar segments (bony and neural)
- ☐ Sacral segments (bony and neural)

transection is fatal because all the respiratory muscles are paralysed. At the level of the C5 vertebra, cord transection isolates the lower cervical cord (with paralysis of the upper limbs), the thoracic cord (with paralysis of the trunk) and the lumbar and sacral cord (with paralysis of the lower limbs and viscera). With injury below the C5 vertebra, the upper limbs are partially spared and characteristic deformities result.

BETWEEN T1 AND T10 VERTEBRAE

The first lumbar cord segment in the adult is at the level of the T10 vertebra. Consequently, cord transection at that level spares the thoracic cord but isolates the entire lumbar and sacral cord, with paralysis of the lower limbs and viscera. The lower thoracic roots may also be transected but are of relatively little importance.

BELOW T10 VERTEBRA

The cord forms a slight bulge (the conus medullaris) between the T10 and L1 vertebrae, and tapers to an end at the interspace between the L1 and L2 vertebrae. The L2 to S4 nerve roots arise from the conus medullaris and stream downwards in a bunch (the cauda equina) to emerge at successive levels of the lumbosacral spine. Therefore, spinal injuries above the T10 vertebra cause cord transection, those between the T10 and L1 vertebrae cause cord and nerve root lesions, and those below the L1 vertebra only root lesions.

The *sacral roots* innervate:

- sensation in the 'saddle' area (S3, S4), a strip down the back of the thigh and leg (S2) and the outer two-thirds of the sole (S1);
- motor power to the muscles controlling the ankle and foot;

- the anal and penile reflexes, plantar responses and ankle jerks;
- control of micturition and bowels.

The *lumbar roots* innervate:

- sensation to the groins and entire lower limb other than that portion supplied by the sacral segment;
- motor power to the muscles controlling the hip and knee;
- the cremasteric reflexes and knee jerks.

It is essential, when the bony injury is at the thoracolumbar junction, to distinguish between cord transection with root escape and cord transection with root transection. A patient with root escape is much better off than one with cord and root transection.

Diagnosis

Clinical examination of the back nearly always shows the signs of an unstable fracture; however, a 'burst' fracture with paraplegia is stable. The nature and level of the bone lesion are demonstrated by x-ray, and that of the neural lesion by CT or MRI.

Neurological examination should be painstaking. Without detailed information, accurate diagnosis and prognosis are impossible; rectal examination is mandatory.

COMPLETE CORD LESIONS

Complete paralysis and anaesthesia below the level of injury suggest cord transection. During the stage of spinal shock when the anal reflex is absent (seldom longer than the first 24 hours) the diagnosis cannot be absolutely certain; if the anal reflex returns and the neural deficit persists, the cord lesion is complete. Any complete lesion lasting more than 72 hours will not recover.

INCOMPLETE CORD LESIONS

Persistence of any sensation distal to the injury (perianal pinprick is most important) suggests an incomplete lesion.

The commonest is the *central cord syndrome* where the initial flaccid weakness is followed by lower motor neurone paralysis of the upper limbs with upper motor neurone (spastic) paralysis of the lower limbs, and preservation of bladder control and perianal sensation (sacral sparing).

With the less common *anterior cord syndrome* there is complete paralysis and anaesthesia but deep pressure and position sense are retained in the lower limbs (dorsal column sparing).

The *posterior cord syndrome* is rare; only deep pressure and proprioception are lost.

The *Brown–Séquard syndrome* (due to cord hemisection) is usually associated with penetrating thoracic injuries. There is loss of motor power on the side of the injury and loss of pain and temperature sensation on the opposite side. Most of these patients improve and regain bowel and bladder function and some walking ability.

High root lesions sometimes cause confusion. Below the T10 vertebra, discrepancies between neurological and skeletal levels are due to transection of roots descending from cord segments higher than the vertebral lesion.

Frankel grading

A well-established method of recording the functional deficit after an incomplete spinal cord injury was that described by Frankel:

Grade A = Absent motor and sensory function.
Grade B = Sensation present, motor power absent.
Grade C = Sensation present, motor power present but not useful.
Grade D = Sensation present, motor power present and useful (grade 4 or 5).
Grade E = Normal motor and sensory function.

Frankel observed that 60% of patients with partial cord lesions (Grades B, C or D) improved (spontaneously) by one grade regardless of the treatment type.

MANAGEMENT OF TRAUMATIC PARAPLEGIA AND QUADRIPLEGIA

With *partial paralysis*, decompression and stabilization offer the best chance of further recovery. With *complete paralysis* it is the overall management that is important, especially the early management.

The patient must be transported with great care to prevent further damage, and preferably taken to a spinal centre. The strategy is outlined below.

SKIN

Within a few hours anaesthetic skin may develop large pressure sores; this can be prevented by meticulous nursing. Immediate fixation of the spine enables these essential nursing procedures to be carried out much more easily and without discomfort to the patient. Creases in the sheets and crumbs in the bed are not permitted. Every 2 hours the patient is gently rolled onto his or her side and the back is carefully washed (without rubbing), dried and powdered. After a few weeks the skin becomes a little more tolerant and the patient can turn him or herself. Later the patient should be taught how to relieve skin pressure intermittently during periods of sitting. If sores have been allowed to develop, they may never heal without excision and skin grafting.

BLADDER AND BOWEL

For the first 24 hours the bladder distends only slowly, but, if the distension is allowed to progress, overflow incontinence occurs and infection is probable. In special centres it is usual to manage the patient from the outset by intermittent catheterization under sterile conditions. If early transfer to a paraplegia centre is not possible, continuous drainage through a fine Silastic catheter is advised. The catheter drains in a closed manner into a disposable bag, and is changed twice weekly to prevent blockage. When infection supervenes, antibiotics are given.

Bladder training is begun as early as possible. Although retention is complete to begin with, partial recovery may lead to either an automatic bladder which works reflexly or an expressible bladder which is emptied by manual suprapubic pressure.

A few patients are left with a high residual urine after emptying the bladder. They need special investigations, including cystography and cystometry; transurethral resection of the bladder neck or sphincterotomy may be indicated but should not be performed until at least 3 months of bladder training have been completed.

The bowel is more easily trained, with the help of enemas, aperients and abdominal exercises.

MUSCLES AND JOINTS

The paralysed muscles, if not treated, may develop severe flexion contractures. These are usually preventable by moving the joints passively through their full range twice daily. Later, splints may be necessary.

With lesions below the cervical cord, the patient should be up within 3 months; standing and walking are valuable in preventing contractures.

Calipers are usually necessary to keep the knees straight and the feet plantigrade. The calipers are removed at intervals during the day while the patient lies prone, and while he or she is having physiotherapy. The upper limbs must be trained until they develop sufficient power to enable the patient to use crutches and a wheelchair.

If flexion contractures have been allowed to develop, tenotomies may be necessary. Painful flexor spasms are rare unless skin or bladder infection occurs. They can sometimes be relieved by tenotomies, neurectomies, rhizotomies or the intrathecal injection of alcohol.

Heterotopic ossification is a common and disturbing complication; it is more likely to occur with high lesions and complete lesions. It may restrict or abolish movement, especially at the hip. It is doubtful whether ossification can be prevented, but once the new bone is mature it can safely be excised.

TENDON TRANSFERS

Some function can be regained in the upper limb by the use of tendon transfers. The aim with patients who have a low cervical cord injury is to use the limited number of functioning muscles in the arm to provide a primitive pinch mechanism (normally powered by C8 or T1 which, being below the level of injury, are lost). One must establish which muscles are working, which are not and which are available for transfer.

- *If only deltoid and biceps are working (C5, C6)* then a posterior-deltoid to triceps transfer using interposition tendon grafts will replace the lost C7 function of elbow extension; this will enable the patient to propel or push him or herself out of a wheelchair or walk with crutches.
- *If brachioradialis (C6) is working*, this can be transferred to become a wrist extensor (since its prime function as an elbow flexor is duplicated by biceps). A primitive thumb pinch can be achieved by the Moberg procedure in which the thumb interphalangeal joint is fused and the basal joint of the thumb is tenodesed with a loop of the redundant flexor pollicis longus. On active extension of the wrist, the basal joint of the thumb is passively flexed.
- *If extensor carpi radialis longus and brevis (C7) are both available*, one of them can be transferred into the flexor pollicis longus to provide active thumb flexion (normally supplied by C8).

MORALE

The morale of a paraplegic patient is liable to reach a low ebb, and the restoration of his or her self-confidence is an important part of treatment. Constant enthusiasm and encouragement by doctors, physiotherapists and nurses are essential. Their scrupulous attention to his or her comfort and toilet are of primary importance; the unpleasant smells associated with skin or urinary infection must be prevented. The earlier the patient gets up the better, and he or she must be trained for a new job as quickly as possible.

REFERENCES AND FURTHER READING

Advanced Trauma Life Support (1997). American College of Surgeons

Anderson LD, D'Alonzo RT (1974) Fractures of the odontoid process of the axis. *Journal of Bone and Joint Surgery* 56A, 1663-1674

Bannister G, Gargan M (1993) Prognosis of whiplash injuries: A review of the literature. *Spine* 7, 557–569

Bohlman HH (1985) Treatment of fractures and dislocations of the thoracic and lumbar spine – current concepts review. *Journal of Bone and Joint Surgery* 67A, 165-169

Chance CQ (1948) Note on a type of flexion fracture of the spine. *British Journal of Radiology* 21, 452-453

Denis F (1983) The three column spine and its significance in the classification of acute thoracolumbar spinal injuries. *Spine* 8, 817-831

Gargan MF, Bannister GC (1990) Long-term prognosis of soft-tissue injuries of the neck. *Journal of Bone and Joint Surgery* 72B, 901-903

Gunzburg R, Szpalski M (1997) *Whiplash Injuries. Current concepts in prevention, diagnosis and treatment of the cervical whiplash syndrome.* Lippincott-Raven, Philadelphia

Livingston M (1999) Common whiplash injury: A modern epidemic. Charles C Thomas, Springfield Il

Slucky AV, Eismont FJ (1994) Treatment of acute injury of the cervical spine. *Journal of Bone and Joint Surgery* 76A, 1882-1895

Solomon L, Pearse MF (1994) Osteonecrosis following low-dose short-course corticosteroids. *Journal of Orthopaedic Rheumatology* 7, 203-205

Spitzer WO, Skovron ML, Salmi LR *et al* (1995) Scientific monograph of the Quebec Task Force on whiplash-associated disorders: redefining whiplash and its management. *Spine* 20 (suppl.), 8

Thomas BE, McCullen GM, Yuan HA (1999) Cervical spine injuries in football players. *Journal of the American Academy of Orthopaedic Surgeons* 7, 338-347

Fractures of the pelvis account for less than 5% of all skeletal injuries, but they are particularly important because of the high incidence of associated soft-tissue injuries and the risks of severe blood loss, shock, sepsis and adult respiratory distress syndrome (ARDS). Like other serious injuries, they demand a combined approach by experts in various fields.

About two-thirds of all pelvic fractures occur in road accidents involving pedestrians; over 10% of these patients will have associated visceral injuries, and in this group the mortality rate is probably in excess of 10%.

Surgical anatomy

The pelvic ring is made up of the two innominate bones and the sacrum, articulating in front at the symphysis pubis (the anterior or pubic bridge) and posteriorly at the sacroiliac joints (the posterior or sacroiliac bridge). This basin-like structure transmits weight from the trunk to the lower limbs and provides protection for the pelvic viscera, vessels and nerves.

The stability of the pelvic ring depends upon the rigidity of the bony parts and the integrity of the strong ligaments that bind the three segments together across the symphysis pubis and the sacroiliac joints. The strongest and most important of the tethering ligaments are the sacroiliac and iliolumbar ligaments; these are supplemented by the sacrotuberous and sacrospinous ligaments and the ligaments of the symphysis pubis.

As long as the bony ring and the ligaments are intact, load-bearing is unimpaired.

The major branches of the common iliac arteries arise within the pelvis between the level of the sacroiliac joint and the greater sciatic notch. With their accompanying veins they are particularly vulnerable in fractures through the posterior part of the pelvic ring. The nerves of the lumbar and sacral plexuses, likewise, are at risk with posterior pelvic injuries.

The bladder lies behind the symphysis pubis. The trigone is held in position by the lateral ligaments of the bladder and, in the male, by the prostate. The prostate lies between the bladder and the pelvic floor. It is held laterally by the medial fibres of the levator ani, whilst anteriorly it is firmly attached to the pubic bones by the puboprostatic ligament. In the female the trigone is attached also to the cervix and the anterior vaginal fornix. The urethra is held by both the pelvic floor muscles and the pubourethral ligament. Consequently in females the urethra is much more mobile and less prone to injury.

In severe pelvic injuries the membranous urethra is damaged when the prostate is forced backwards whilst the urethra remains static. When the puboprostatic ligament is torn, the prostate and base of the bladder can become grossly dislocated from the membranous urethra.

The pelvic colon, with its mesentery, is a mobile structure and therefore not readily injured. However, the rectum and anal canal are more firmly tethered to the urogenital structures and the muscular floor of the pelvis and are therefore vulnerable in pelvic fractures.

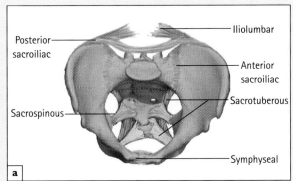
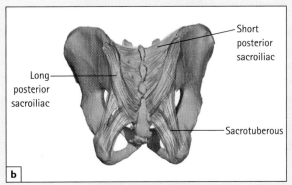

28.1 Ligaments supporting the pelvis Some ligaments run transversely and will resist rotational forces which separate the two halves (the posterior sacroiliac and iliolumbar ligaments can be thought of as a posterior tension band), whilst those that are oriented longitudinally tend to resist vertical shear.

Pelvic instability

If the pelvis can withstand weight-bearing loads without displacement, it is stable; this situation exists only if the bony and key ligamentous structures are intact.

An anterior force applied to both halves of the pelvis forces apart the symphysis pubis. If a diastasis occurs because of capsular rupture, the extent of separation is checked by the anterior sacroiliac and sacrospinous ligaments. Should these restraints fail through the application of a still greater force, the pelvis opens like a book until the posterior iliac spines abut; because the more vertically oriented long posterior sacroiliac and sacro-tuberous ligaments remain intact, the pelvis still resists vertical shear but it is rotationally unstable. If, however, the posterior sacroiliac and sacrotuberous ligaments are damaged, then the pelvis is not only rotationally and vertically unstable, but there is also posterior translation of the injured half of the pelvis. Vertical instability is therefore ominous as it suggests complete loss of the major ligamentous support posteriorly.

It should be remembered that some fracture patterns can cause instability which mimics that of ligamentous disruption; e.g. fractures of both pubic rami may behave like symphyseal disruptions, and fractures of the iliac wing combined with ipsilateral pubic rami fractures are unstable to vertical shear.

Clinical assessment

Fracture of the pelvis should be suspected in every patient with serious abdominal or lower limb injuries. There may be a history of a road accident or a fall from a height or crush injury. Often the patient complains of severe pain and feels as if he or she has fallen apart, and there may be swelling or bruising of the lower abdomen, the thighs, the perineum, the scrotum or the vulva. All these areas should be rapidly inspected, looking for evidence of extravasation of urine. *However, the first priority, always, is to assess the patient's general condition and look for signs of blood loss. It may be necessary to start resuscitation before the examination is completed.*

The abdomen should be carefully palpated. Signs of irritation suggest the possibility of intraperitoneal bleeding. The pelvic ring can be gently compressed from side to side and back to front. Tenderness over the sacroiliac region is particularly important and may signify disruption of the posterior bridge.

A rectal examination is then carried out in every case. The coccyx and sacrum can be felt and tested for tenderness. If the prostate can be felt, which is often difficult due to pain and swelling, its position should be gauged; an abnormally high prostate suggests a urethral injury.

Enquire when the patient passed urine last and look for bleeding at the external meatus. An inability to void and blood at the external meatus are the classic

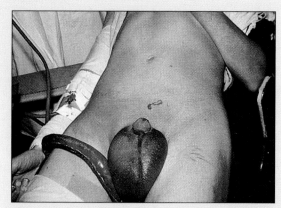

28.2 Fractures of the pelvis This young man crashed on his motorcycle and was brought into the Accident and Emergency Department with a fractured femur. His perineum and scrotum were swollen and bruised, he was unable to pass urine and a streak of blood appeared at the external meatus. X-rays confirmed that he had a fractured pelvis.

features of a ruptured urethra. However, the absence of blood at the meatus does not exclude a urethral injury, because the external sphincter may be in spasm, halting the passage of blood from the site of injury. Thus every patient who has a pelvic fracture must be considered to be at risk.

The patient can be encouraged to void; if he or she is able to do so, either the urethra is intact or there is only minimal damage which will not be made worse by the passage of urine. *No attempt should be made to pass a catheter, as this could convert a partial to a complete tear of the urethra.* If a urethral injury is suspected, it can be diagnosed more accurately and more safely by retrograde urethrography.

A ruptured bladder should be suspected in patients who do not void or in whom a bladder is not palpable after adequate fluid replacement. This palpation is often difficult because of abdominal wall haematoma. The physical findings initially can be minimal, with normal bowel sounds, as extravasation of sterile urine produces little peritoneal irritation. Only a very small proportion of patients with a ruptured bladder are hypotensive, so if a patient is hypotensive another cause must be sought.

Neurological examination is important; there may be damage to the lumbar or sacral plexus.

If the patient is unconscious, the same routine is followed. However, early x-ray examination is essential in these cases.

Imaging of the pelvis

During the initial survey of every severely injured patient, a plain anteroposterior x-ray of the pelvis should be obtained at the same time as the chest x-ray. In most cases this film will give sufficient information to make a preliminary diagnosis of pelvic fracture. The exact nature of the injury can be clarified by more detailed radiography once it is certain that the patient can tolerate an extended period of positioning and repositioning on the x-ray table. Five views are necessary: anteroposterior, an inlet view (tube cephalad to the pelvis and tilted 30° downwards), an outlet view (tube caudad to the pelvis and tilted 40° upwards), and right and left oblique views.

If any serious injury is suspected, a computed tomography (CT) scan at the appropriate level is extremely helpful (some would say essential). This is particularly true for posterior pelvic ring disruptions and for complex acetabular fractures, which cannot be properly evaluated on plain x-rays.

Three-dimensional CT re-formation of the pelvic image gives the most accurate picture of the injury; however, with practice almost as much information can be gleaned from a good set of plain radiographs and standard CT images.

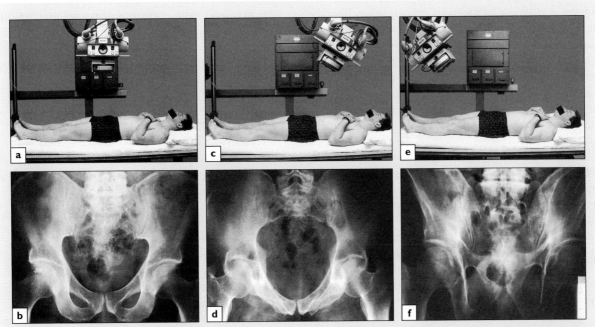

28.3 Pelvic fractures – x-ray diagnosis (1) (a, b) The anteroposterior view is usually taken during the initial assessment of the multiply-injured patient as part of a 'trauma series'. It is useful in quickly diagnosing gross disruptions or fractures. The x-ray should be read systematically: Is the picture well centred? Look for asymmetry in the pubic symphysis, the pubic rami, the iliac blades, the sacroiliac joints and the sacral foramina. If the patient's condition permits, at least two additional views should be obtained: (c, d) an *inlet* view with the tube titled 30° downwards and (e, f) an *outlet* view with the tube titled 40° upwards.

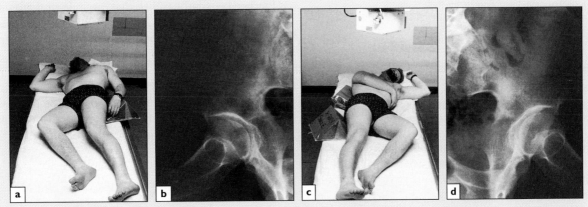

28.4 Pelvic fractures – x-ray diagnosis (2) Oblique views are helpful for defining the ilium and acetabulum on each side. (a, b) the *right oblique* view; and (c,d) the *left oblique* view. These can be omitted if facilities for CT are available.

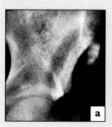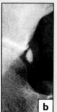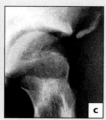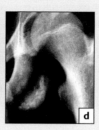

28.5 Avulsion injuries These all result from powerful muscle action. (**a**) Avulsion of sartorius attachment; this should not be confused with (**b**) an os acetabuli, which is well-defined on all sides. (**c**) Avulsion of rectus origin. (**d**) Avulsion of hamstring origin – the clinical condition is much less alarming than the x-ray.

Imaging of the urinary tract

If there is evidence of upper abdominal injury, and the patient has haematuria, an intravenous urogram is performed to exclude renal injury. This will also show whether there is any ureteric or major bladder damage. In a case of urethral rupture, the base of the bladder may be riding high (dislocated prostate) or there may be a tear-drop deformity of the bladder owing to compression by blood and extravasated urine (prostate-in-situ).

When a urethral injury is considered likely, a urethrogram should be undertaken using 25–30ml of water-soluble contrast agent with a suitable aseptic technique. A film must be taken during injection of the contrast agent to ensure that the urethra is fully distended. This technique will confirm a urethral tear and will show whether it is complete or incomplete.

In a patient with possible rupture of the bladder (so long as there is no evidence of a urethral injury) a cystogram should be performed.

Types of injury

Injuries of the pelvis fall into four groups: (1) isolated fractures with an intact pelvic ring; (2) fractures with a broken ring – these may be stable or unstable; (3) fractures of the acetabulum – although these are ring fractures, involvement of the joint raises special problems and therefore they are considered separately; and (4) sacrococcygeal fractures.

ISOLATED FRACTURES

AVULSION FRACTURES

A piece of bone is pulled off by violent muscle contraction; this is usually seen in sportsmen and athletes. The anterior superior iliac spine can be pulled off by sartorins, the anterior inferior iliac spine by rectus femoris, the pubis by adductor longus, and part of the ischium by the hamstrings. All are essentially muscle injuries, needing only rest for a few days and reassurance.

Pain may take months to disappear and, because there is often no history of impact injury, biopsy of the callus may lead to an erroneous diagnosis of a tumour. Rarely, avulsion of the ischial apophysis by the hamstrings may lead to persistent symptoms, in which case open reduction and internal fixation is indicated (Wootton *et al.*, 1990).

DIRECT FRACTURES

A direct blow to the pelvis, usually after a fall from a height, may fracture the ischium or the iliac blade. Bed rest until pain subsides is usually all that is needed.

STRESS FRACTURES

Fractures of the pubic rami are fairly common (and often quite painless) in severely osteoporotic or osteomalacic patients. More difficult to diagnose are stress fractures around the sacroiliac joints; this is an uncommon cause of 'sacroiliac' pain in elderly osteoporotic individuals. Obscure stress fractures are best demonstrated by radioisotope scans.

FRACTURES OF THE PELVIC RING

It has been cogently argued that, because of the rigidity of the pelvis, a break at one point in the ring must be accompanied by disruption at a second point; exceptions are fractures due to direct blows (including fractures of the acetabular floor), or ring fractures in children, whose symphysis and sacroiliac joints are springy. Often, however, the second break is not visible – either because it reduces immediately or because the sacroiliac joints are only partially disrupted.

Mechanisms of injury

The basic mechanisms of pelvic ring injury are anteroposterior compression (APC), lateral compression (LC), vertical shear (VS) and combinations of these.

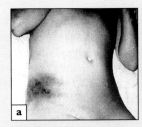
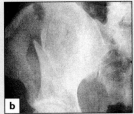

28.6 Fractured iliac blade (**a**) The bruise suggests the site of the fracture. (**b**) The fracture looks alarming and is certainly painful but, if the remainder of the bony pelvis is intact, it poses no serious threat to the patient.

ANTEROPOSTERIOR COMPRESSION This injury is usually caused by a frontal collision between a pedestrian and a car. The pubic rami are fractured or the innominate bones are sprung apart and externally rotated, with disruption of the symphysis – the so-called 'open book' injury. The anterior sacroiliac ligaments are partially torn, or there may be a fracture of the posterior part of the ilium.

LATERAL COMPRESSION Side-to-side compression of the pelvis causes the ring to buckle and break. This is usually due to a side-on impact in a road accident or a fall from a height. Anteriorly the pubic rami on one or both sides are fractured, and posteriorly there is a severe sacroiliac strain or a fracture of the sacrum or ilium, either on the same side as the fractured pubic rami or on the opposite side of the pelvis. If the sacroiliac injury is much displaced, the pelvis is unstable.

VERTICAL SHEAR The innominate bone on one side is displaced vertically, fracturing the pubic rami and disrupting the sacroiliac region on the same side. This occurs typically when someone falls from a height onto one leg. These are usually severe, unstable injuries with gross tearing of the soft tissues and retroperitoneal haemorrhage.

COMBINATION INJURIES In severe pelvic injuries there may be a combination of the above.

Stable and unstable fractures

Stability in a pelvic injury can often be deduced from the fracture pattern and displacement. Because the mechanisms which cause these injuries are fairly consistent, typical patterns are defined which make it possible to deduce the mechanism of injury, the type of ligament damage and the degree of pelvic instability. Occasionally the decision on stability cannot be made until the patient is examined under anaesthesia.

Several classifications are in use. The one presented here is based on that of Young and Burgess (1986; 1987).

ANTEROPOSTERIOR COMPRESSION INJURIES
The 'open book' pattern appears as either diastasis of the pubic symphysis or fracture(s) of the pubic rami; as the pelvis is sprung open, the sacroiliac elements also are strained. This general pattern is subclassified according to the severity of the injury.

In *APC-I injuries* there may be only slight (less than 2cm) diastasis of the symphysis; however, although invisible on x-ray, there will almost certainly be some strain of the anterior sacroiliac ligaments. The pelvic ring is stable.

In *APC-II injuries* diastasis is more marked and the anterior sacroiliac ligaments (often also the sacrotuberous and sacrospinous ligaments) are torn. CT may show slight separation of the sacroiliac joint on one side. If the posterior sacroiliac ligaments are intact, the pelvic ring is still stable.

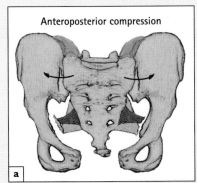
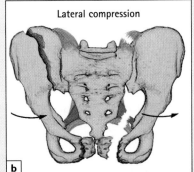
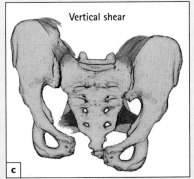

28.7 Types of pelvic ring fracture The three important types of injury are shown. (**a**) Anteroposterior compression with lateral rotation may cause the 'open book' injury, the hallmark of which is diastasis of the pubic symphysis. Widening of the anterior portion of the sacroiliac joint is best seen on an inlet view. (**b**) Lateral compression causing the ring to buckle and break; the pubic rami are fractured, sometimes on both sides. Posteriorly the iliac blade may break or the sacrum is crushed. (**c**) Vertical shear, with disruption of both the sacroiliac and symphyseal regions on one side.

In *APC-III injuries* the anterior and posterior sacroiliac ligaments are torn. CT shows a shift or separation of the sacroiliac joint; the one hemipelvis is effectively disconnected from the other anteriorly and from the sacrum posteriorly. The ring is unstable.

LATERAL COMPRESSION INJURIES

The hallmark of this injury is a transverse fracture of the pubic ramus (or rami), often best seen on an inlet view x-ray. There may also be a compression fracture of the sacrum. In its simplest form this would be classified as a *LC-I injury*. The ring is stable.

The *LC-II injury* is more severe; in addition to the anterior fracture, there may be a fracture of the iliac wing on the side of impact. However, the ring remains stable.

The *LC-III injury* is worse still. As the victim is run over, the lateral compression force on one iliac wing results in an opening anteroposterior force on the opposite ilium, causing injury patterns typical for that mechanism.

VERTICAL SHEAR INJURIES

The hemipelvis is displaced in a cranial direction, and often posteriorly as well, producing a typically asymmetrical appearance of the pelvis. As with APC-III injuries, the hemipelvis is totally disconnected and the pelvic ring is unstable.

COMBINATION INJURIES

Combination patterns do occur but, in the main, the above classification defines the most common types of injury. The LC-II pattern is linked to abdominal, head and chest injuries; all the unstable patterns carry a high risk of severe haemorrhage and are life-threatening (Dalal *et al.*, 1989).

Clinical features

In fractures which do not affect the pelvic ring, as well as stable ring fractures, the patient is not severely shocked but has pain on attempting to walk. There is localized tenderness but seldom any damage to pelvic viscera (the exception is a severe LC-II injury). Plain x-rays reveal the fractures.

In unstable injuries of the pelvic ring the patient is severely shocked, in great pain and unable to stand. He or she may also be unable to pass urine and there may be blood at the external meatus. Tenderness is widespread, and attempting to move one or both blades of the ilium is very painful. If the patient permits it, pulling or pushing may reveal the vertical instability (Olson and Pollack, 1996). One leg may be partly anaesthetic because of sciatic nerve injury.

These are extremely serious injuries, carrying a high risk of associated visceral damage, intra-abdominal and retroperitoneal haemorrhage, shock, sepsis and ARDS; the mortality rate is considerable.

IMAGING

This may show fractures of the pubic rami, ipsilateral or contralateral fractures of the posterior elements, separation of the symphysis, disruption of the sacroiliac joint or combinations of these injuries. The films are often difficult to interpret and CT scans are much the best way of visualizing the nature of the injury.

Management

EARLY MANAGEMENT

Treatment should not await full and detailed diagnosis. It is vital to keep a sense of priorities and to act on any information that is already available while moving along to the next diagnostic hurdle. 'Management' in this context is a combination of assessment and treatment.

Six questions must be asked and the answers acted upon as they emerge:

- Is there a clear airway?
- Are the lungs adequately ventilated?
- Is the patient losing blood?
- Is there an intra-abdominal injury?
- Is there a bladder or urethral injury?
- Is the pelvic fracture stable or unstable?

With any severely injured patient, the first step is to make sure that the airway is clear and ventilation is unimpaired. Resuscitation must be started immediately and active bleeding controlled. The patient is rapidly examined for multiple injuries and, if necessary, painful fractures are splinted. A single anteroposterior x-ray of the pelvis is obtained.

A more careful examination is then carried out, paying attention to the pelvis, the abdomen, the perineum and the rectum. The urethral meatus is inspected for signs of bleeding. The lower limbs are examined for signs of nerve injury.

If the patient's general condition is stable, further x-rays can then be obtained. If a urethral tear is suspected, a urethrogram is gently performed. The findings up to that stage may dictate the need for an intravenous urogram.

By now the examining doctor will have a good idea of the patient's general condition, the extent of the pelvic injury, the presence or absence of visceral injury and the likelihood of continued intra-abdominal or retroperitoneal bleeding. Ideally, a team of experts will be on hand to deal with the individual problems or undertake further investigations.

MANAGEMENT OF SEVERE BLEEDING

The general treatment of shock is described in Chapter 22. If there is an unstable fracture of the pelvis, haemorrhage will be reduced by rapidly applying an external fixator (Evers *et al.*, 1989).

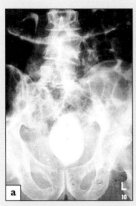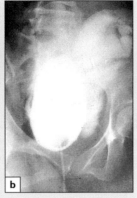

28.8 Pelvic fractures and bladder injury (a) Intravenous urogram outlining the bladder and showing the typical globular appearance due to compression by blood and extravasated urine. There is also marked gastric dilation suggesting retroperitoneal bleeding. (b) Cystogram showing extravasation of radio-opaque material. This patient had a ruptured bladder.

The diagnosis of persistent bleeding is often difficult, and even when it seems clear that continuing shock is due to haemorrhage, it is not easy to determine the source of the bleeding. Patients with suspicious abdominal signs should be further investigated by peritoneal aspiration or lavage. If there is a positive diagnostic tap, the abdomen should be explored in an attempt to find and deal with the source of bleeding. However, if there is a large retroperitoneal haematoma, it should not be evacuated as this may release the tamponade effect and lead to uncontrollable haemorrhage. Pressure packing can be applied to compress the vessels around the sacrum and sacroiliac joints.

If there is no evidence of intra-abdominal bleeding and laparotomy is not contemplated, but the patient shows signs of continuing blood loss, then angiography should be performed with a view to carrying out embolization.

MANAGEMENT OF THE URETHRA AND BLADDER

Urological injury occurs in about 10% of patients with pelvic ring fractures. As these patients are often seriously ill from other injuries, a urinary catheter may be required to monitor urinary output, and therefore the urologist is placed under pressure to make a rapid diagnosis of urethral damage.

There is no place for passing a diagnostic catheter as this will most probably convert any partial tear to a complete tear. For an incomplete tear, the insertion of a suprapubic catheter as a formal procedure is all that is required. Around half of all incomplete tears will heal and require little long-term management.

The treatment of a complete urethral tear is controversial. Primary realignment of the urethra may be achieved by performing suprapubic cystostomy, evacuating the pelvic haematoma and then threading a catheter across the injury to drain the bladder. If the bladder is floating high it is repositioned and held down by a sling suture passed through the lower anterior part of the prostatic capsule, through the perineum on either side of the bulbar urethra and anchored to the thighs by elastic bands. An alternative – and much simpler – approach is to perform the cystostomy as soon as possible, making no attempt to drain the pelvis or dissect the urethra, and to deal with the resulting stricture 4–6 months later. The latter method is contraindicated if there is severe prostatic dislocation or severe tears of the rectum or bladder neck. With both methods there is a significant incidence of late stricture formation, incontinence and impotence.

TREATMENT OF THE FRACTURE

For patients with very severe injuries, early external fixation is one of the most effective ways of reducing haemorrhage and counteracting shock (Evers *et al.*, 1989; Poka and Libby, 1996). If there are no life-threatening complications, definitive treatment is as follows.

Isolated fractures and minimally displaced fractures need only bed rest, possibly combined with lower limb traction. Within 4–6 weeks the patient is usually comfortable and may then be allowed up using crutches.

Open-book injuries, provided the anterior gap is less than 2cm and it is certain that there are no displaced posterior injuries, can usually be treated satisfactorily by bed rest; a posterior sling or an elastic girdle helps to 'close the book'.

In more severe injuries, the most efficient way of maintaining reduction is by external fixation with pins in both iliac blades connected by an anterior bar; 'closing the book' may also reduce the amount of bleeding. Placing the pins is made easier if two temporary Kirschner wires are first inserted, hugging the medial and lateral surfaces of each iliac blade, and then directing the fixing pins between them. Internal fixation by

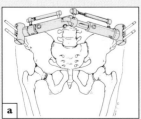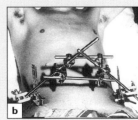

28.9 Pelvic fractures – external fixation Displaced fractures can often be reduced and held by external fixation.

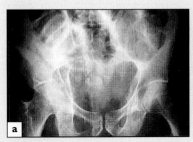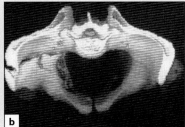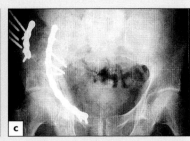

28.10 Pelvic fractures – internal fixation (**a, b**) X-ray examination and CT, together with reconstructed three-dimensional images, enabled appropriate pre-operative planning and (**c**) stable internal fixation with plates and screws. (Courtesy of Mr RN Brueton and Dr RL Guy.)

attaching a plate across the symphysis should be performed: (1) during the first few days after injury only if the patient needs a laparotomy; and (2) later on if the gap cannot be closed by less radical methods.

Fractures of the iliac blade can often be treated with bed rest. However, if displacement is marked, or if there is an associated anterior ring fracture or symphysis separation, then open reduction and internal fixation with plates and screws will need to be considered (e.g. in displaced LC-II injuries causing a leg length discrepancy greater than 1.5cm). It is also possible to reduce and hold some of these fractures by external fixation.

APC-III and VS injuries are the most dangerous and the most difficult to treat. It may be possible to reduce some or all of the vertical displacement by skeletal traction combined with an external fixator; even so, the patient needs to remain in bed for at least 10 weeks. This prolonged recumbency is not without risk. As these injuries represent loss of both anterior and posterior support, both areas will need to be stabilized. Two techniques are used: (a) anterior external fixation and posterior stabilization using screws across the sacroiliac joint, or (b) plating anteriorly and screws posteriorly. The operation is hazardous (the dangers include massive haemorrhage and infection) and should be attempted only by surgeons with considerable experience in this field. Persisting with skeletal traction and external fixation is probably safer, though the malposition is likely to leave a legacy of posterior pain. It should be emphasized that more than 60% of pelvic fractures need no fixation.

Open pelvic fractures are managed by external fixation. A diversion colostomy may be necessary.

Secondary complications

Sciatic nerve injury It is essential to test for sciatic nerve function both before and after treating the pelvic fracture. If the nerve is injured it is usually a neurapraxia and one can afford to wait several weeks for recovery. Occasionally, though, nerve exploration is necessary.

Urogenital problems Urethral injuries sometimes result in *stricture, incontinence* or *impotence* and may require prolonged treatment.

Persistent sacroiliac pain Unstable pelvic fractures are often associated with partial or complete sacroiliac joint disruption, and this can lead to persistent pain at the back of the pelvis. Occasionally arthrodesis of the sacroiliac joint is needed.

FRACTURES OF THE ACETABULUM

Fractures of the acetabulum occur when the head of the femur is driven into the pelvis. This is caused either by a blow on the side (as in a fall from a height) or by a blow on the front of the knee, usually in a dashboard injury when the femur also may be fractured.

Acetabular fractures combine the complexities of pelvic fractures (notably the frequency of associated soft-tissue injury) with those of joint disruption (namely, articular cartilage damage, malcongruent loading and secondary osteoarthritis).

Patterns of fracture

Several classifications of acetabular fractures are currently popular (Letournel, 1981; Müller *et al.,* 1991; Tile, 1995). All use similar anatomical descriptions, but Tile's universal classification has much to commend it for simplicity.

The fractures are divided into four major types; though they are distinguished on anatomical grounds, it is important to recognize that they also differ in their ease of reduction, their stability after reduction and their long-term prognosis.

ACETABULAR WALL FRACTURES
Fractures of the anterior or posterior part of the acetabular rim affect the depth of the socket and may lead to hip instability unless they are properly reduced and fixed.

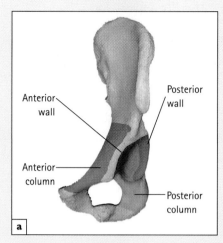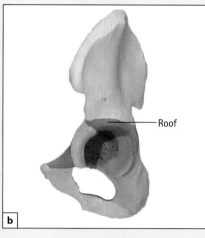

28.11 Acetabular fractures
Fractures occur through the wall (rim) or supporting columns. Of particular importance is the roof (superior dome) which carries a high proportion of the load in walking.

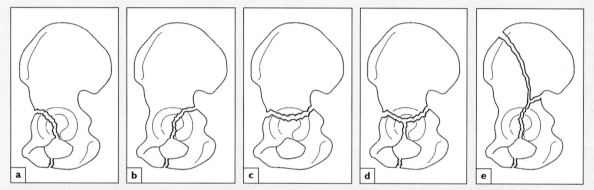

28.12 Tile's classification of acetabular fractures There are four types of injury: (**a**, **b**) a simple fracture involving either the anterior or the posterior wall or column; (**c**) a transverse or (**d**) a T-type fracture involving two columns; (**e**) the both-column fracture, resulting in a 'floating' acetabulum with no part of the socket attached to the ilium (compare this with the transverse or T-type fractures).

COLUMN FRACTURES

The *anterior column* extends from the pubic symphysis, along the superior pubic ramus, across the acetabulum to the anterior part of the ilium. On the x-ray it is shown in profile by the iliopectineal line in the oblique view. Anterior column fractures are uncommon, do not involve the weight-bearing area and have a good prognosis.

The *posterior column* extends from the ischium, across the posterior aspect of the acetabular socket to the sciatic notch and the posterior part of the innominate bone. In an iliac oblique x-ray it is seen in profile as the ilioischial line. A posterior column fracture usually runs upwards from the obturator foramen into the sciatic notch, separating the posterior ischiopubic column of bone and breaking the weight-bearing part of the acetabulum. It is usually associated with a posterior dislocation of the hip and may injure the sciatic nerve. Treatment is more urgent and usually involves internal fixation to obtain a stable joint.

TRANSVERSE FRACTURE

This fracture runs transversely through the acetabulum, involving both the anterior and posterior columns, and separating the iliac portion above from the pubic and ischial portions below. A vertical split into the obturator foramen may coexist, resulting in a T-fracture. Note that in both transverse and T-type fractures, a portion of the acetabulum remains attached to the ilium. These fractures are usually difficult to reduce and to hold reduced.

COMPLEX FRACTURES

Many acetabular fractures are complex injuries which damage either the anterior or the posterior columns (or both) as well as the roof or the walls of the acetabulum. Of particular note, and sometimes a cause of confusion, is the *'both-column fracture'* – this is really a variant of the T-fracture in that the two columns are involved but the transverse part of the 'T' lies just *above* the acetabulum; effectively, no portion of the acetabulum remains connected to the

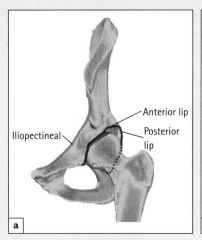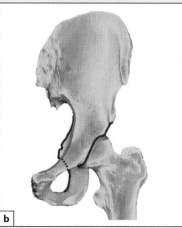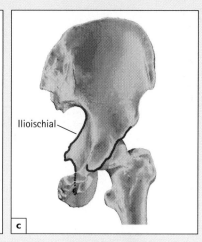

28.13 Imaging the pelvis for acetabular fractures Although CT scans have become the standard in assessing acetabular fractures, plain x-rays have much to offer. The obturator oblique (**a**), standard anteroposterior (**b**) and iliac oblique (**c**) views will allow the trained eye to picture the structures involved in the injury. The iliopectineal line represents a profile of the anterior column whereas the ilioischial line defines the posterior column. The margins of the anterior and posterior walls are usually seen in all three views.

rest of the pelvis. Understandably, the confusion arises when the term 'both-column' is used to refer to a transverse fracture – perhaps the term 'high T' would have been better!

Complex fracture patterns share the following features: (1) the injury is severe; (2) the joint surface is disrupted; (3) they usually need operative reduction and internal fixation; and (4) the end result is likely to be less than perfect, unless surgical restoration has been exact.

Clinical features

There has usually been a severe injury, either a traffic accident or a fall from a height. Associated fractures are not uncommon and, because they may be more obvious, are liable to divert attention from the more urgent pelvic injuries. Whenever a fractured femur, a severe knee injury or a fractured calcaneum is diagnosed, the hips also should be x-rayed.

The patient may be severely shocked, and the complications associated with all pelvic fractures should be sought. Rectal examination is essential. There may be bruising around the hip and the limb may lie in internal rotation (if the hip is dislocated). No attempt should be made to move the hip.

Careful neurological examination is important, testing the function of the sciatic, femoral, obturator and pudendal nerves.

IMAGING
At least four *x-ray views* should be obtained in every case: a standard anteroposterior view, the pelvic inlet view and two 45° oblique views. Each view shows a different profile of the acetabulum; with practice the various landmarks (iliopectineal line, ilioischial line and the boundaries of the anterior and posterior walls) can

be identified, thus providing a fairly good mental picture of the fracture type, the degree of comminution and the amount of displacement. *CT scans* and *three-dimensional re-formations* are added refinements, and are particularly helpful if surgical reconstruction is planned.

Treatment

EMERGENCY TREATMENT
The first priority is to counteract shock and reduce a dislocation. Traction is then applied to the distal femur (10kg will suffice) and during the next 3–4 days the patient's general condition is brought under control. Occasionally, additional lateral traction through the greater trochanter is needed for central hip dislocations. Definitive treatment of the fracture is delayed until the patient is fit and operation facilities are optimal.

NON-OPERATIVE TREATMENT
In recent years opinion has moved in favour of operative treatment for displaced acetabular fractures. However, conservative treatment is still preferable in certain well-defined situations: (1) acetabular fractures with minimal displacement (in the weight-bearing zone, less than 3mm); (2) displaced fractures that do not involve the superomedial weight-bearing segment (roof) of the acetabulum – usually distal anterior column and distal transverse fractures; (3) a both-column fracture that retains the ball and socket congruence of the hip by virtue of the fracture line lying in the coronal plane and displacement being limited by an intact labrum; (4) fractures in elderly patients, where closed reduction seems feasible; (5) patients with 'medical' contraindications to operative treatment (including local sepsis). Comminution in itself is not a

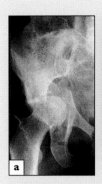
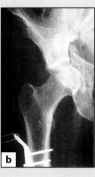
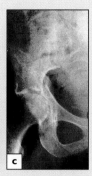

28.14 Fractured acetabulum – conservative treatment This severely displaced acetabular fracture (**a**) was almost completely reduced by (**b**) longitudinal and lateral traction. (**c**) The fracture healed and the patient regained a congruent joint with a fairly good range of movement.

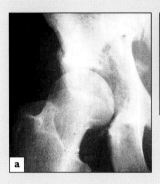
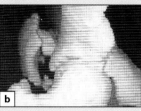
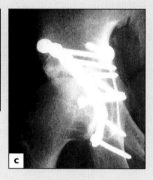

28.15 Fractured acetabulum – internal fixation (**a**) X-ray and (**b**) three-dimensional CT before reduction, showing a large posterior fragment which needed accurate repositioning and internal fixation (**c**). (Courtesy of Mr RN Brueton and Dr RL Guy.)

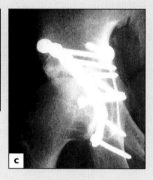

contraindication to operative treatment, provided adequate facilities and expertise are available.

Matta and Merritt (1988) have listed certain criteria which should be met if conservative treatment is expected to succeed: (1) when traction is released, the hip should remain congruent; (2) the weight-bearing portion of the acetabular roof should be intact; and (3) associated fractures of the posterior wall should be excluded by CT. Non-operative treatment is more suitable for patients aged over 50 years than for adolescents and young adults (Matta and Merritt, 1988).

If there are medical contraindications to operative treatment, closed reduction under general anaesthesia is attempted. In all patients treated conservatively, longitudinal traction, if necessary supplemented by lateral traction, is maintained for 6–8 weeks; this will unload the articular cartilage and will help to prevent further displacement of the fracture. During this period, hip movement and exercises are encouraged. The patient is then allowed up, using crutches with minimal weight-bearing for a further 6 weeks.

OPERATIVE TREATMENT

Operative treatment is indicated for all unstable hips and fractures resulting in significant distortion of the ball and socket congruence, as well as for associated fractures of the femoral head and/or retained bone fragments in the joint. The hip may be dislocated centrally, anteriorly or posteriorly. If a stable closed reduction cannot be achieved, or if the joint re-dislocates, then immediate open reduction and stabilization should be performed. In other cases operation is usually deferred for 4 or 5 days.

Matta and Merritt (1988) have made the important point that open reduction is an operation on the pelvis and not merely the acetabular socket. Adequate exposure is essential, if possible through a single approach which is selected according to the type of fracture. The posterior Kocher–Langenbach exposure allows good access to the posterior wall and column but may have to be combined with a trochanteric osteotomy to gain adequate sight in transverse fractures. The anterior ilioinguinal approach is suited for anterior wall and column fractures. Both exposures are usually needed in T-type and both-column fractures – this is a considerable undertaking, encouraging some surgeons to adopt the singular triradiate or extended iliofemoral approaches instead. The fracture (or fractures) are fixed with lag screws or special buttressing plates which can be shaped in the operating theatre. It is useful to monitor somatosensory-evoked potentials during the operation, in order to avoid damaging the sciatic nerve (separate electrodes are required for medial and lateral popliteal branches).

Prophylactic antibiotics are used, and post-operatively hip movements are started as soon as possible. Some prophylaxis against heterotopic ossification is often used, usually indomethacin. The patient is allowed up, partial weight-bearing with crutches, after 7 days. Exercises are continued for 3–6 months; it may take a year or longer for full function to return.

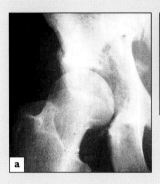

Complications

Operative treatment should aim for a perfect anatomical reduction and is best undertaken in centres which specialize in this form of treatment.

Iliofemoral venous thrombosis is fairly common and potentially serious. It is doubtful, however, whether routine prophylactic anticoagulation is warranted (Montgomery, 1996).

Sciatic nerve injury may occur either at the time of fracture or during the subsequent operation. Unless the nerve is seen to be unharmed during the operation, there can be no certainty about the prognosis. Intraoperative somatosensory monitoring is advocated as a means of preventing serious nerve damage. For an established lesion, it is worth waiting for 6 weeks to see if there is any sign of recovery. If there is none, the nerve should be explored in order to establish the diagnosis and ensure that the nerve is not being compressed.

Hereterotopic bone formation is common after severe soft-tissue injury and extended surgical dissections. In cases where this is anticipated, prophylactic indomethacin is useful.

Avascular necrosis of the femoral head may occur even if the hip is not fully dislocated. The condition is probably overdiagnosed because of erroneous interpretation of the x-ray appearances following impacted marginal fractures of the acetabulum (Gruen *et al.*, 1988).

Loss of joint movement and secondary osteoarthritis are common sequelae after displaced acetabular fractures involving the weight-bearing portion of the joint. This may, ultimately, require joint replacement. However, the operation should be deferred until the fractures have consolidated; the acetabular implant is bound to work loose if there is any movement of the innominate segments.

INJURIES TO THE SACRUM AND COCCYX

A blow from behind, or a fall onto the 'tail', may fracture the sacrum or coccyx, or sprain the joint between them. Women seem to be affected more commonly than men.

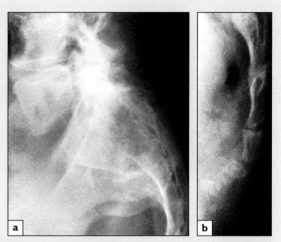

28.16 Sacrococcygeal fractures (a) Fractured sacrum; (b) fractured coccyx.

Bruising is considerable and tenderness is elicited when the sacrum or coccyx is palpated from behind or per rectum. Sensation may be lost over the distribution of sacral nerves.

X-rays may show: (1) a transverse fracture of the sacrum, in rare cases with the lower fragment pushed forwards; (2) a fractured coccyx, sometimes with the lower fragment angulated forwards; or (3) a normal appearance if the injury was a sprain of the sacrococcygeal joint.

Treatment If the fracture is displaced, reduction is worth attempting. The lower fragment may be pushed backwards by a finger in the rectum. The reduction is stable, which is fortunate. The patient is allowed to resume normal activity, but is advised to use a rubber-ring cushion when sitting. Occasionally, sacral fractures are associated with urinary problems, necessitating sacral laminectomy.

Persistent pain, especially on sitting, is common after coccygeal injuries. If the pain is not relieved by the use of a cushion or by the injection of local anaesthetic into the tender area, excision of the coccyx may be considered.

REFERENCES AND FURTHER READING

Dalal SA, Burgess AR, Siegel JH *et al* (1989) Pelvic fracture in multiple trauma. *J Trauma* **29**, 981-1000

Evers BM, Cryer HM, Miller SB (1989) Pelvic fracture haemorrhage. Priorities in management. *Archives of Surgery* **124**, 422-424

Gruen GS, Mears DC, Tauxe WN (1988) Distinguishing avascular necrosis from segmental impaction of the femoral head following an acetabular fracture. *Journal of Orthopaedic Trauma* **2**, 5-9

Letournel E (1981) *Fractures of the Acetabulum.* Springer, Berlin

Matta JM, Merritt PO (1988) Displaced acetabular fractures. *Clinical Orthopaedics and Related Research* **230**, 83-97

Montgomery KD, Geerts WH, Potter HG, Helfet DL (1996) Thromboembolic complications in patients with pelvic trauma. *Clinical Orthopaedics and Related Research* **329**, 68-87

Mostafavi HR, Tornetta P 3rd (1996) Radiologic evaluation of the pelvis. *Clinical Orthopaedics and Related Research* **329**, 6-14

Müller ME, Allgower M, Schneider R, Willeneger H (1991) *Manual of Internal Fixation* 3rd edition. Springer Verlag, Berlin, Heidelberg and New York

Olson SA, Pollak AN (1996) Assessment of pelvic ring stability after injury. Indications for surgical stabilisation. *Clinical Orthopaedics and Related Research* **329**, 15-27

Poka A, Libby EP (1996) Indications and techniques for external fixation of the pelvis. *Clinical Orthopaedics and Related Research* **329**, 54-9

Tile M (1995) *Fractures of the Pelvis and Acetabulum* 2nd edition. Williams and Wilkins, Baltimore

Wootton JR, Cross MJ, Holt KWG (1990) Avulsion of the ischial apophysis. *Journal of Bone and Joint Surgery* **72B**, 625-627

Young JWR, Burgess AR, Brumback RJ, Poka A (1986) Lateral compression fractures of the pelvis: the importance of plain radiographs in the diagnosis and surgical management. *Skeletal Radiology* **15**, 103-109

Young JWR, Burgess AR (1987) *Radiologic Management of Pelvic Ring Fractures: Systematic radiographic diagnosis.* Urban and Schwarzenberg, Baltimore

DISLOCATION OF THE HIP

With the rise in the number of road accidents, dislocation of the hip has become more common. Often small fragments of bone are chipped off as the joint dislocates; if there is a major fragment, or comminution, it is regarded as a fracture-dislocation.

The injuries are classified according to the direction of dislocation: *posterior* (by far the commonest variety), *anterior* and *central* (a comminuted or displaced fracture of the acetabulum).

POSTERIOR DISLOCATION

Mechanism of injury

Four out of five traumatic hip dislocations are posterior. Usually this occurs in a road accident when someone seated in a truck or car is thrown forwards, striking the knee against the dashboard. The femur is thrust upwards and the femoral head is forced out of its socket; often a piece of bone at the back of the acetabulum (the posterior wall of the socket) is sheared off, making it a fracture-dislocation.

Clinical features

In a straightforward case the diagnosis is easy: the leg is short and lies adducted, internally rotated and slightly flexed. However, if one of the long bones is fractured – usually the femur – the injury can easily be missed. The golden rule is to x-ray the pelvis in every case of severe injury, and, with femoral fractures, to insist on x-rays that include the hip and the knee. The lower limb should be examined for signs of sciatic nerve injury.

X-RAY

In the anteroposterior film the femoral head is seen out of its socket and above the acetabulum. A segment of acetabular rim or femoral head may have been broken off and displaced; oblique films are useful in demonstrating the size of the fragment. If any fracture is seen, other bony fragments (which may need removal) must be suspected. A computed tomography (CT) scan is the best way of demonstrating an acetabular fracture or any bony fragment.

Thompson and Epstein (1951) suggested a classification which is helpful in planning treatment. Type I is a dislocation with no more than minor chip fractures. Type II is a dislocation with a single large fracture of the posterior acetabular wall. In type III the posterior wall is comminuted. Type IV has an associated fracture of the acetabular floor, and type V an associated fracture of the femoral head, (which can be further subdivided acording to Pipkin's (1957) classification.

Treatment

The dislocation must be reduced as soon as possible under general anaesthesia. In the vast majority of cases this is

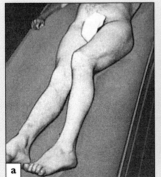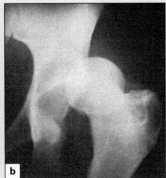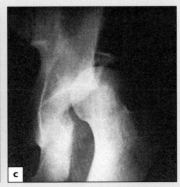

29.1 Posterior dislocation of the hip (a, b) Uncomplicated posterior dislocation; reduction is usually straightforward, but it is important to be sure that no loose bony fragments remain in the joint. **(c)** Associated acetabular fracture which may need open reduction and fixation.

performed closed. An assistant steadies the pelvis; the surgeon starts by applying traction in the line of the femur as it lies (usually in adduction and internal rotation), and then gradually flexes the patient's hip and knee to 90°, maintaining traction throughout. At 90° of hip flexion, traction is increased and sometimes a little rotation (both internal or external) is required to accomplish reduction. A satisfying 'clunk' terminates the manoeuvre. X-rays are essential to confirm reduction and to exclude a fracture. If there is the slightest suspicion that bone fragments have been trapped inside the joint, CT is needed.

Reduction is usually stable in type I injuries, but the hip has been severely injured and needs to be rested. The simplest way is to apply traction and maintain it for 3 weeks. Movement and exercises are begun as soon as pain allows. At the end of 3 weeks the patient is allowed to walk with crutches.

If the post-reduction x-rays or CT scan show the presence of intra-articular fragments, they should be removed and the joint washed out through a posterior approach. This is usually postponed until the patient's condition has stabilized.

Type II fracture-dislocations are often treated by immediate open reduction and anatomical fixation of the detached fragment, the rationale being that many large posterior wall fragments either do not reduce well or remain a cause of instability even after reduction. However, if the patient's general condition is suspect, or the necessary surgical skills are not available, the hip is reduced closed, as described above. Traction can be applied until conditions are appropriate for surgery – open reduction and internal fixation will remedy the source of instability, return congruity to the joint and remove any trapped bone fragments. In all type II cases, traction is maintained for 6 weeks.

Type III injuries are treated closed, but there may be retained fragments and these should be removed by open operation; traction is maintained for 6 weeks. Fixation of a comminuted posterior wall is sometimes impossible – if persistent instability is present, referral to a specialist centre, where reconstruction using a segment of iliac crest could be undertaken, is advisable.

Type IV and V injuries are treated initially by closed reduction. The bone fragment may automatically fall into place; this can be confirmed by CT. If the fragment remains unreduced, operative treatment is indicated: a small fragment can simply be removed, but a large fragment should be replaced; the joint is opened, the femoral head dislocated and the fragment fixed in position with a countersunk screw. Post-operatively, traction is maintained for 4 weeks and full weight-bearing is deferred for 12 weeks.

Complications

EARLY

Sciatic nerve injury The sciatic nerve is damaged in 10–20% of cases, but fortunately it usually recovers. If, after reducing the dislocation, a sciatic nerve lesion and an unreduced acetabular fracture are diagnosed, the nerve should be explored and the fragment correctly replaced (and screwed in position). Recovery often takes months and in the meantime the limb must be protected from injury and the ankle splinted to overcome the foot drop.

Vascular injury Occasionally the superior gluteal artery is torn and bleeding may be profuse. If this is suspected, an arteriogram should be performed. The torn vessel may need to be ligated.

Associated fractured femoral shaft When this occurs at the same time as hip dislocation, the dislocation is often missed. It should be a rule that with every femoral shaft fracture the buttock and trochanter are palpated, and the hip clearly seen on x-ray. Even if this precaution has been omitted, a dislocation should be suspected whenever the proximal fragment of a transverse shaft fracture is seen to be adducted. Reduction of the dislocation is much more difficult, but a gentle closed manipulation should still be attempted. If this fails, open reduction should be performed, and at the same time the femur can be fixed with an intramedullary nail.

LATE

Avascular necrosis The blood supply of the femoral head is seriously impaired in at least 10% of traumatic hip dislocations; if reduction is delayed by more than a few hours, the figure rises to 40%. Avascular necrosis shows on x-ray as increased density of the femoral head; but this change is not seen for at least 6 weeks, and sometimes very much longer (up to 2 years), depending on the rate of bone repair. In the early weeks, radioscintigraphy may reveal signs of bone ischaemia. If the femoral head shows signs of fragmentation, an operation may be needed. If there is a small necrotic segment, realignment osteotomy is the method of choice. Otherwise, in younger patients, the choice is between femoral head replacement with a bipolar prosthesis or hip arthrodesis (never an easy procedure). In patients over the age of 50 years a total hip replacement is better.

Myositis ossificans This is an uncommon complication, probably related to the severity of the injury. Being difficult to predict, it is difficult to prevent. But movements should never be forced and in severe injuries the period of rest and non-weight-bearing may need to be prolonged.

Unreduced dislocation After a few weeks an untreated dislocation can seldom be reduced by closed manipulation and open reduction is needed. The incidence of stiffness or avascular necrosis is considerably increased and the patient may later need reconstructive surgery.

Osteoarthritis Secondary osteoarthritis is not uncommon and is due to (1) cartilage damage at the time of

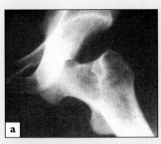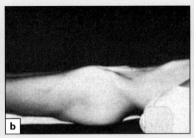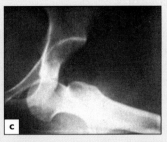

29.2 Anterior hip dislocations (**a, b**) The usual appearance of an anterior dislocation: the hip is only slightly abducted and the head shows clinically as a prominent lump (**c**). Occasionally an anterior dislocation is in wide abduction.

the dislocation, (2) the presence of retained fragments in the joint or (3) ischaemic necrosis of the femoral head. In young patients treatment presents a difficult problem (see Chapter 5).

ANTERIOR DISLOCATION

Anterior dislocation is rare compared with posterior. The usual cause is a road accident or air crash – even a posteriorly directed force on an abducted and externally rotated hip will cause the neck to impinge on the acetabular rim and lever the femoral head out in front. The femoral head will then lie superiorly (type I) or inferiorly (type II). Dislocation of one or even both hips may occur when a weight falls onto the back of a miner or building labourer who is working with his legs wide apart, knees straight and back bent forwards.

Clinical features

The leg lies externally rotated, abducted and slightly flexed. It is not short, because the attachment of rectus femoris prevents the head from displacing upwards. Occasionally the leg is abducted almost to a right angle. Seen from the side, the anterior bulge of the dislocated head is unmistakable, especially when the head has moved anteriorly and superiorly. The prominent head is easy to feel, either anteriorly (superior type) or in the groin (inferior type). Hip movements are impossible.

X-RAY

In the anteroposterior view the dislocation is usually obvious, but occasionally the head is almost directly in front of its normal position; any doubt is resolved by a lateral film.

Treatment and complications

The manoeuvres employed are similar to those used to reduce a posterior dislocation, except that while the hip is gently flexed upwards, it should be kept adducted; an assistant then helps by applying lateral traction to the thigh. Reduction is usually heard and felt. The subsequent treatment is similar to that employed for posterior dislocation.

In some superior dislocations there may be pressure on the femoral neurovascular bundle. Avascular necrosis occurs in less than 10% of cases.

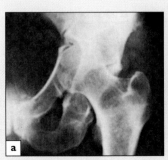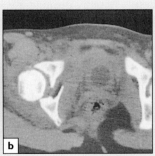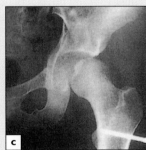

29.3 Central dislocation (**a**) The plain x-ray gives a good picture of the displacement, but (**b**) a CT scan shows the pelvic injury more clearly. (**c**) Skeletal traction, which often needs both longitudinal and lateral vectors, is an effective method of reduction.

CENTRAL DISLOCATION

A fall on the side, or a blow over the greater trochanter, may force the femoral head medially through the floor of the acetabulum (see also Chapter 28). Although this is called 'central dislocation', it is really a fracture of the acetabulum. The condition is dealt with on page 674.

FRACTURES OF THE FEMORAL NECK

The femoral neck is the commonest site of fractures in the elderly. The vast majority of patients are Caucasian women in their seventh and eighth decades, and the association with osteoporosis is so manifest that the incidence of femoral neck fractures has been used as a measure of age-related osteoporosis in population studies. Other *risk factors* include bone-losing or bone-weakening disorders such as osteomalacia, diabetes, stroke (disuse), alcoholism and chronic debilitating disease. In addition, old people often have weak muscles and poor balance, resulting in an increased tendency to fall. By contrast, people whose bone mass is above the population average seldom suffer hip fractures; this is reflected in the low incidence among negroid populations and in patients with osteoarthritis of the hip.

The association of femoral neck fracture with post-menopausal bone loss has stimulated renewed interest in screening for osteoporosis and prophylactic measures in the 'at-risk' population (see Chapter 7).

Mechanism of injury

The fracture usually results from a fall directly onto the greater trochanter. In very osteoporotic people, less force is required – perhaps no more than catching a toe in the carpet and twisting the hip into external rotation. Some patients have evidence of a preceding stress fracture of the femoral neck.

In younger individuals, the usual cause is a fall from a height or a blow sustained in a road accident; these patients often have multiple injuries and in 20% there is an associated fracture of the femoral shaft.

Pathological anatomy and classification

The most useful classification is that of Garden, which is based on the amount of displacement apparent in the pre-reduction x-rays (Garden, 1961). Once fractured, the head and neck become displaced in progressively severe stages. *Stage I* is an incomplete impacted fracture, including the so-called abduction fracture in which the femoral head is tilted into valgus in relation

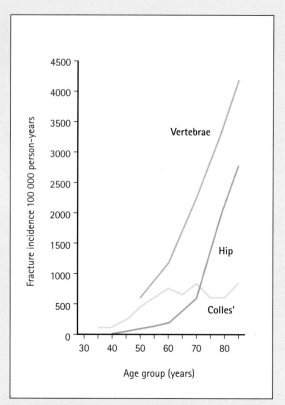

29.4 Incidence of 'osteoporotic' fractures The incidence of 'osteoporotic' fractures in women rises sharply from the menopause onwards.

to the neck. *Stage II* is a complete but undisplaced fracture. *Stage III* is a complete fracture with moderate displacement. And *Stage IV* is a severely displaced fracture. This is essentially a radiographic classification; the distinctive x-ray features are described below.

Garden I and II fractures, which are only slightly displaced, have a much better prognosis for union and for viability of the femoral head than the more severely displaced Garden III and IV fractures. This has an important influence on the choice of treatment for the various stages. However, there is little room for complacency with any of these fractures; left untreated, a comparatively benign-looking stage I fracture may rapidly disintegrate to stage IV.

Healing of femoral neck fractures is bedevilled by two problems: the threat of bone ischaemia and tardy union. The femoral head obtains its blood supply from three sources: (1) intramedullary vessels in the femoral neck; (2) ascending cervical branches of the medial and lateral circumflex anastomosis, which run within the capsular retinaculum before entering the bone at the edge of the femoral head; and (3) the vessels of the ligamentum teres. The intramedullary supply is always interrupted by the fracture; the retinacular vessels, also, may be kinked or torn if the fracture is displaced. In elderly people, the remaining supply in the ligamentum teres is at best fairly meagre and, in 20% of cases,

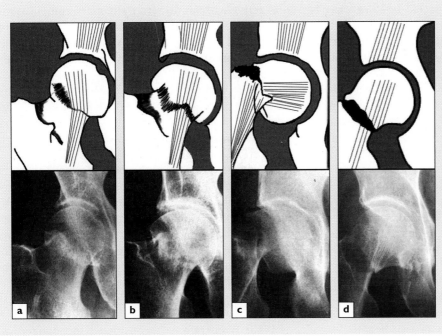

29.5 Garden's classification of femoral neck fractures
(a) *Stage I*: incomplete (so-called abducted or impacted) – the femoral head in this case is in slight valgus. (b) *Stage II*: complete without displacement. (c) *Stage III*: complete with partial displacement – the fragments are still connected by the posterior retinacular attachment; the femoral head trabeculae are no longer in line with those of the innominate bone. (d) *Stage IV*: complete with full displacement – the proximal fragment is free and lies correctly in the acetabulum so that the trabeculae appear normally aligned with those of the innominate.

non-existent. Hence the high incidence of avascular necrosis in displaced femoral neck fractures.

Transcervical fractures are, by definition, intracapsular. They have a poor capacity for healing because (1) by tearing the capsular vessels the injury deprives the head of its main blood supply; (2) intra-articular bone has only a flimsy periosteum and no contact with soft tissues which could promote callus formation; and (3) synovial fluid prevents clotting of the fracture haematoma. Accurate apposition and impaction of bone fragments are therefore of more importance than usual. There is evidence that aspirating a haemarthrosis increases the blood flow in the femoral head by relieving tension in the capsule (Harper *et al.*, 1991).

Clinical features

There is usually a history of a fall, followed by pain in the hip. If the fracture is displaced, the patient lies with the limb in lateral rotation and the leg looks short.

Beware, though: not all hip fractures are so obvious. With an impacted fracture the patient may still be able to walk; and debilitated or mentally handicapped patients may not complain at all – even with bilateral fractures.

Young adults with severe injuries of the lower limbs – whether they complain of hip pain or not – should always be examined for an associated femoral neck fracture.

X-RAY
Two questions must be answered: is there a fracture, and is it displaced? Usually the break is obvious, but an impacted fracture can be missed by the unwary. Displacement is judged by the abnormal shape of the bone outlines and the degree of mismatch of the trabec-

ular lines in the femoral head and neck and the supra-acetabular (innominate) part of the pelvis. This assessment is important because impacted or undisplaced fractures do well after internal fixation, whereas displaced fractures have a high rate of non-union and avascular necrosis.

In *Garden I fractures* the femoral head is in its normal position or tilted into valgus and impacted on the femoral neck stump. The medial cortex may be intact. The femoral head stress trabeculae are normally aligned with the innominate trabeculae.

In *Garden II fractures* the femoral head is normally placed and the fracture line may be difficult to discern.

In *Garden III fractures* the anteroposterior x-ray shows that the femoral head is tilted out of position and the trabecular markings are not in line with those of the innominate bone; this is because the proximal fragment retains some contact with the neck stump and is pushed out of alignment.

In *Garden IV fractures* the femoral head trabeculae are normally aligned with those of the innominate bone; the reason is that the proximal fragment has lost contact with the femoral neck and lies in its normal position in the acetabular socket.

Diagnosis

There are four situations in which a femoral neck fracture may be missed, sometimes with dire consequences.

1 Stress fractures The elderly patient with unexplained pain in the hip should be considered to have a stress fracture until proved otherwise. The x-ray is usually normal, but a bone scan will show the 'hot' lesion.

2 Undisplaced fractures Impacted fractures may be extremely difficult to discern on plain x-ray. If there is a fracture it will show up on magnetic resonance imaging (MRI), or a bone scan after a few days.

3 Painless fractures A bed-ridden patient may develop a 'silent' fracture. Even a fit patient occasionally walks about without pain if the fracture is impacted. If the context suggests an injury, investigate – whether the patient complains or not.

4 Multiple fractures The patient with a femoral shaft fracture may also have a hip fracture, which is easily missed unless the pelvis is x-rayed.

Treatment

Initial treatment consists of pain-relieving measures and simple splintage of the limb. If operation is delayed, a femoral nerve block may be helpful.

Operative treatment is almost mandatory. Displaced fractures will not unite without internal fixation, and in any case old people should be got up and active without delay if pulmonary complications and bed sores are to be prevented. Impacted fractures can be left to unite, but there is always a risk that they may become displaced, even while lying in bed, so fixation is safer.

The one indication for non-operative management of an impacted Garden I fracture is an 'old' injury where the diagnosis is made only after the patient has been walking about for several weeks without deleterious effect on the fracture position.

When should the operation be performed? In young patients operation is urgent: interruption of the blood supply will produce irreversible cellular changes after 12 hours and the way to prevent this is to obtain accurate reduction and internal fixation as soon as possible. In older patients also the longer the delay the greater is the likelihood of complications; however, here speed is tempered by the need for adequate preparation, especially in the very elderly, who are often ill and debilitated.

What if operation is considered too dangerous? Lying in bed on traction may be even more dangerous, and leaving the fracture untreated too painful; the patient least fit for operation may need it most.

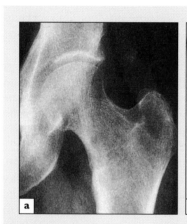
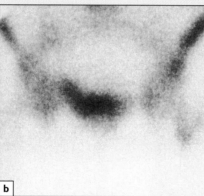

29.6 Fracture of the femoral neck – diagnosis (a) An elderly woman tripped on the pavement and complained of pain in the left hip. The plain x-ray showed no abnormality. 2 weeks later she was still in pain; (b) a bone scan showed a 'hot' area medially at the base of the femoral neck, suggesting a stress fracture. Prophylactic fixation was performed.

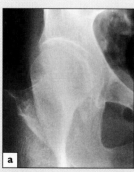
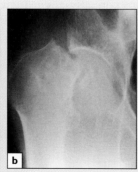
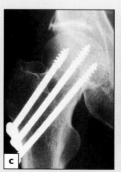
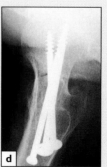

29.7 Femoral neck injuries – treatment (a) This fracture was thought to be securely impacted, but (b) a few days later it displaced completely. A pity it had not been fixed – the operation would have been easier and the prognosis better. (c, d) In this case the fracture was fixed with three cannulated screws; alignment is perfect in both anteroposterior and lateral views.

Internal fixation Notwithstanding the advances in joint replacement, for most patients the principles of treatment are as of old: accurate reduction, secure internal fixation and early activity. Displaced fractures must first be reduced: with the patient under anaesthesia, the fracture is disimpacted by applying traction with the hip held in 45° of flexion and slight abduction; the limb is then slowly brought into extension and finally internally rotated; as traction is released, the fracture re-impacts in the reduced position.

The reduction is assessed by x-ray. The femoral head should be positioned correctly so that the stress trabeculae are aligned close to their normal position in both anteroposterior and lateral views, as shown in Fig 29.8 (Garden, 1974). To fix an imperfectly reduced fracture is to invite failure. If a stage III or IV fracture cannot be reduced closed, and the patient is under 60 years of age, open reduction through an anterolateral approach is advisable. However, in older patients (and certainly in those over 70 years of age) this is seldom justified; if two careful attempts at closed reduction fail, prosthetic replacement is preferable.

Once the fracture is reduced, it is held with cannulated screws or a sliding screw and side-plate which attaches to the femoral shaft. A lateral incision is used to expose the upper femur. Guide-wires, inserted under fluoroscopic control, are used to ensure correct placement of the fixing device. Usually two cannulated screws

will suffice; they should lie parallel and extend to within 5mm of the subchondral bone plate; in the lateral view they must be central in the head and neck and in the anteroposterior view the distal screw ideally should lie against the inferior cortex of the neck (Olerud *et al.*, 1991). If there is marked posterior comminution, a third screw may be needed as a buttress for the calcar femorale. If a sliding screw is used, the femoral neck will first have to be reamed; a temporary guide-wire should always be introduced before reaming so as to prevent the femoral head from rotating with the reamer and tearing the remaining soft-tissue attachments. Once the sliding screw is fixed, the guide-wire is replaced by a single screw to reduce the risk of femoral head rotation during fracture healing.

From the first day the patient should sit up in bed or in a chair. She is taught breathing exercises, and encouraged to help herself and to begin walking (with crutches or a walker) as soon as possible. To delay weight-bearing may be theoretically appropriate but is rarely practicable.

Prosthetic replacement Some argue that the prognosis for stage III and IV fractures is so unpredictable that prosthetic replacement is always preferable. This underestimates the morbidity associated with replacement. Our policy is therefore to attempt reduction and fixation in all patients aged under 75 years of age and to reserve replacement for (1) the very old and the very

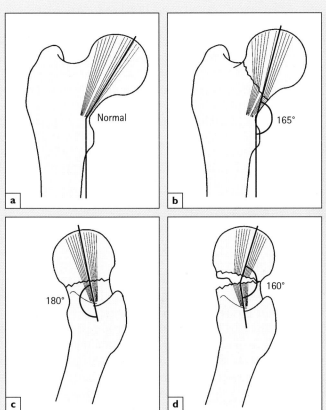

29.8 Garden's index for assessing reduction in subcapital fractures On the anteroposterior x-ray (**a, b**), the medial femoral shaft and the axis of trabecular markings over the medial aspect of the femoral neck lie at an angle of 160°; an acceptable reduction is deemed to lie between 155° and 180°. On the lateral view (**c, d**), the trabecular markings would be in line (i.e. 180°) if the fracture was perfectly reduced; an acceptable reduction is within 20° of this ideal. Garden (1974) noted that there was a higher association with complications such as avascular necrosis, non-union and osteoarthritis if the quality of reduction was outside these acceptable limits.

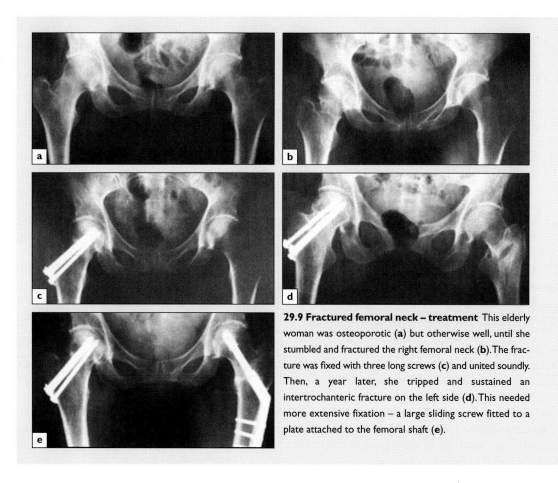

29.9 Fractured femoral neck – treatment This elderly woman was osteoporotic (**a**) but otherwise well, until she stumbled and fractured the right femoral neck (**b**). The fracture was fixed with three long screws (**c**) and united soundly. Then, a year later, she tripped and sustained an intertrochanteric fracture on the left side (**d**). This needed more extensive fixation – a large sliding screw fitted to a plate attached to the femoral shaft (**e**).

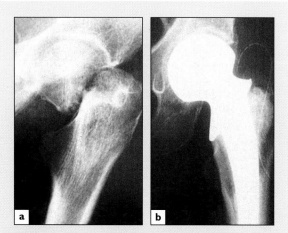

29.10 Fracture of the femoral neck – treatment (**a**) In a very old patient with a severely displaced fracture, prosthetic replacement (**b**) may be quicker and less traumatic than fixation and may also permit earlier rehabilitation.

frail, (2) patients in whom closed reduction fails, and (3) pathological fractures. The least traumatic replacement is an uncemented femoral prosthesis or a bipolar prosthesis inserted through a posterior approach. Stability and durability rely on a good interference fit;

careful pre-operative planning and operative technique are essential. Patients who, despite their age, are still very active may do better with a cemented prosthesis.

Total hip replacement may be preferable (1) if treatment has been delayed for some weeks and acetabular damage is suspected, or (2) in patients with metastatic disease or Paget's disease.

Post-operatively, breathing exercises and early mobilization are important. Speed of recovery depends largely on how active the patient was before the fracture; after 2–4 months, further improvement is unlikely.

Complications

General complications These patients, most of whom are elderly, are prone to general complications such as deep vein thrombosis, pulmonary embolism, pneumonia and bed sores; not to mention disorders that might have been present before the fracture and which lead to death in a substantial proportion of cases. In some centres anticoagulants are used routinely.

Notwithstanding the advances in perioperative care, the mortality rate in elderly patients may be as high as 20% at 4 months after injury. Among the survivors over 80 years of age, about half fail to resume independent walking.

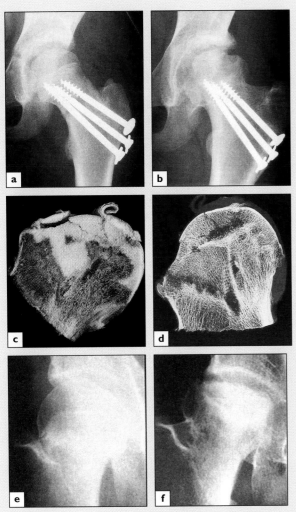

29.11 Fracture of the femoral neck – avascular necrosis (a) The post-reduction x-ray may look splendid but the blood supply is compromised and 6 months later (b) there is obvious necrosis of the femoral head. (c) Section across the excised femoral head, showing the large necrotic segment and splitting of the articular cartilage. (d) Fine detail x-ray of the same. (e, f) Even an impacted fracture, if it is displaced in valgus, can lead to avascular necrosis.

Avascular necrosis Necrosis of the femoral head occurs in about 30% of patients with displaced fractures and 10% of those with undisplaced fractures. There is no way of diagnosing this at the time of fracture. A few weeks later, a nanocolloid scan may show diminished vascularity. X-ray changes may not become apparent for months or even years. Whether the fracture unites or not, collapse of the femoral head will cause pain and progressive loss of function.

In patients over 45 years of age, treatment is by total joint replacement. In younger patients, the choice of treatment is controversial. Core decompression has no place in traumatic osteonecrosis. Realignment/rotational osteotomy is suitable for those with a relatively small necrotic segment. Arthrodesis is often mentioned in armchair discussions, but in practice it is seldom carried out. Provided the risks are carefully explained, including the likelihood of at least one revision procedure, joint replacement (hemi- or total) may be justifiable even in this group.

Non-union More than 30% of all femoral neck fractures fail to unite, and the risk is particularly high in those that are severely displaced. There are many causes: poor blood supply, imperfect reduction, inadequate fixation, and the tardy healing that is characteristic of intra-articular fractures. The bone at the fracture site is ground away, the fragments fall apart and the nail or screw cuts out of the bone or is extruded laterally. The patient complains of pain, shortening of the limb and difficulty with walking. The x-ray shows the sorry outcome.

The method of treatment depends on the cause of the non-union and the age of the patient. In the relatively young, three procedures are available. (1) If the fracture is unduly vertical but the head is alive, subtrochanteric osteotomy with nail-plate fixation changes the fracture line to a more horizontal angle. (2) If the reduction or fixation was faulty and there are no signs of necrosis, it is reasonable to remove the screws, reduce the fracture, insert fresh screws correctly and also to apply a bone graft across the fracture, either a segment of fibula or a muscle pedicle graft. (3) If the head is avascular but the joint unaffected, prosthetic replacement may be suitable; if the joint is damaged or arthritic, total replacement is indicated.

In elderly patients, only two procedures should be considered. (1) If pain is considerable, then the femoral head, no matter whether it is avascular or not, is best removed; if the patient is reasonably fit, total joint replacement is performed. (2) If the patient is old and infirm and pain not unbearable, a raised heel and a stout stick or elbow crutch are often sufficient.

Osteoarthritis Avascular necrosis or femoral head collapse may lead, after several years, to secondary osteoarthritis of the hip. If there is marked loss of joint movement and widespread damage to the articular surface, total joint replacement will be needed.

Combined fractures of the neck and shaft

Young patients with high-energy fractures of both the femoral neck and the ipsilateral femoral shaft present a special problem. Both fractures must be fixed, and there are several ways of doing this. The aesthetically most pleasing is also the most difficult: fixation of the shaft fracture using an intramedullary nail with two locking screws at the upper end. Inserting the screws correctly in both the nail and the femoral head can be a formidable task. Most surgeons prefer to reduce the femoral neck fracture, hold it temporarily with Kirschner wires while reducing and nailing the shaft fracture, then replacing the Kirschner wires with two or three cannulated screws inserted around the nail. The easiest of all – and probably the method of choice for the novice – is to reduce and pin the femoral neck fracture in the usual way and then fix the shaft fracture with a plate and screws.

INTERTROCHANTERIC FRACTURES

Intertrochanteric fractures are, by definition, extracapsular. As with femoral neck fractures, they are common in elderly, osteoporotic people; most of the patients are women in the eigth decade. However, in contrast to intracapsular fractures, extracapsular trochanteric fractures unite quite easily and seldom cause avascular necrosis.

Mechanism of injury

The fracture is caused either by a fall directly onto the greater trochanter or by an indirect twisting injury. The crack runs up between the lesser and greater trochanter and the proximal fragment tends to displace in varus. There may be comminution of the posteromedial cortex.

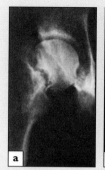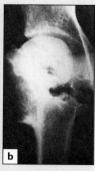

29.12 Fractures of the femoral neck – non-union In this relatively young patient non-union has been treated successfully by intertrochanteric osteotomy.

Pathological anatomy

Intertrochanteric fractures are divided into *stable* and *unstable* varieties. In essence, unstable fractures are those where there is poor contact between the fracture fragments, as in four-part intertrochanteric types, or where the fracture pattern is such that weight-bearing forces tend to displace the fracture further, as in reverse oblique types. Instability may also arise if the postero-medial cortex is shattered, displacing a large fragment that includes the lesser trochanter; these are particularly difficult to hold with internal fixation. Bone quality also influences post-fixation stability and hence the risk of implant failure.

A more detailed classification is described by Kyle *et al.* (1994); four basic patterns are separated, reflecting increasing instability as well as the difficulty of reduction and fixation (see Fig 29.13).

Clinical features

The patient is usually old and unfit. Following a fall she is unable to stand. The leg is shorter and more externally rotated than with a cervical fracture (because the fracture is extracapsular) and the patient cannot lift her leg.

X-RAY
Undisplaced, stable fractures may show no more than a thin crack along the intertrochanteric line; indeed, there is often doubt as to whether the bone is fractured and the diagnosis may have to be confirmed by scintigraphy or MRI.

More often the fracture is displaced and there may be considerable comminution. If the lesser trochanter is separated and the medial cortex fragmented, internal fixation may not be stable and weight-bearing should be delayed.

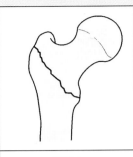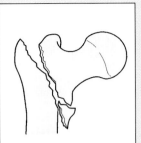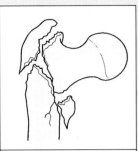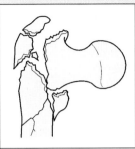

TYPE 1	TYPE 2	TYPE 3	TYPE 4
Undisplaced	Displaced	Displaced	Severely comminuted
Uncomminuted	Minimal comminution	Greater trochanter fracture	Subtrochanter extension
	Lesser trochanter fracture	Comminuted	(Also reverse oblique)
	Varus	Varus	

29.13 Intertrochanteric fractures – classification Types 1 to 4 are arranged in increasing degrees of instability and complexity. Types 1 and 2 account for the majority (nearly 60%). The reverse oblique type of intertrochanteric fracture represents a subgroup of Type 4; it causes similar difficulties with fixation.

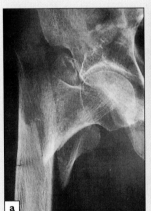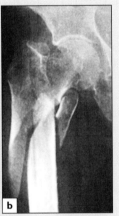

29.14 Intertrochanteric features Two contrasting types of intertrochanteric fracture. (a) Type 2 fracture: the fracture runs obliquely downwards from the lateral to medial cortex, in this case associated with a lesser trochanter fracture and resulting in a typical varus deformity. This is an unstable fracture. (b) Type 4 'reverse oblique' fracture: here the fracture line runs downwards from medial to lateral cortex, to give an even more unstable geometry.

Treatment

Intertrochanteric fractures are almost always treated by early internal fixation – not because they fail to unite with conservative treatment (they unite quite readily), but (a) to obtain the best possible position and (b) to get the patient up and walking as soon as possible and thereby reduce the complications associated with prolonged recumbency.

Minimally displaced fractures are reduced by slight traction and internal rotation; the position is checked by x-ray and the fracture is fixed with an angled device – preferably a sliding nail or screw – that grips the femoral head and neck and is fixed to the shaft with screws, yet allows the bone fragments to impact during weight-bearing. Positioning of the screw is important if it is to be prevented from cutting out of the osteoporotic bone. It should pass up the femoral neck at a high angle (closer to 150° than the usual 'anatomical' 135°) towards the centre of the femoral head; the tip should rest about 5mm from the subchondral bone plate. The side-plate should be long enough to accommodate at least four screws below the fracture line. A small lesser trochanteric fragment may be 'caught' with additional screws.

With the less common 'reversed oblique' fracture (where the fracture line runs downwards obliquely from medial to lateral cortex) there is a tendency for the distal fragment to shift medially under the proximal fragment as the hip screw slides in the barrel; in these cases a 95° device or an intramedullary device with a hip screw gives more stable fixation.

If closed reduction fails to achieve a satisfactory position, open reduction and manipulation of the fragments will be necessary. A large posteromedial fragment (often including the lesser trochanter) may need additional fixation. The addition of bone grafts may hasten union of the medial cortex.

In those cases where anatomical reduction proves impossible, a valgus osteotomy may be needed to allow the proximal fragment to sit securely on the femoral shaft (Dimon and Hughston, 1967).

Post-operatively, exercises are started on the day after operation and the patient is allowed up and partial weight-bearing as soon as possible.

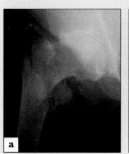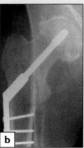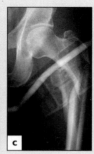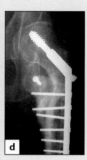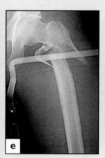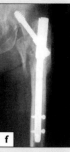

29.15 Intertrochanteric fractures – treatment Anatomic reduction is the ideal; but stable fixation is equally important. Types 1 and 2 fractures (**a, b**) can usually be held in good position with a compression screw and plate. If this is not possible, an osteotomy of the lateral cortex (**c ,d**) will allow a screw to be inserted up the femoral neck and into the head of the femur; this can be used as a lever to reduce the fracture so that the medial spike of the proximal fragment engages securely into the femoral canal; fixation is completed with a side plate. Reverse oblique fractures (**e, f**) are inherently unstable even after perfect reduction; here one can use an intramedullary device with a locking screw that engages the femoral head. (Courtesy of Mr M Manning and Mr JS Albert.)

Complications

EARLY
Early complications are the same as with femoral neck fractures, reflecting the fact that most of these patients are in poor health.

LATE
Failed fixation Screws may cut out of the osteoporotic bone if reduction is poor or if the fixation device is incorrectly positioned. If union is delayed, the implant itself may break. In either event, reduction and fixation may have to be re-done.

Malunion Varus and external rotation deformities are common. Fortunately they are seldom severe and rarely interfere with function.

Non-union Intertrochanteric fractures seldom fail to unite. If healing is delayed (say beyond 6 months) the fracture probably will not join and further operation is advisable; the fragments are repositioned (usually in some valgus), the fixation device is applied more securely and bone grafts are packed around the fracture.

Pathological fractures

Pertrochanteric fractures may be due to metastatic disease or myeloma. Unless patients are terminally ill, fracture fixation is essential in order to ensure an acceptable quality of life for their remaining years. In addition to internal fixation, methylmethacrylate cement may be packed in the defect to improve stability.

If there is involvement of the femoral neck, bone replacement with a cemented prosthesis may be preferable.

PROXIMAL FEMORAL FRACTURES IN CHILDREN

Hip fractures rarely occur in children but when they do they are potentially very serious.

The fracture is usually due to high velocity trauma; for example, falling from a height or a car accident. Pathological fractures sometimes occur through a bone cyst or benign tumour. In children under 2 years of age, the possibility of child abuse should be considered.

There is a high risk of complications, such as avascular necrosis, premature physeal closure and coxa vara.

At birth the proximal end of the femur is entirely cartilaginous and for several years, as ossification proceeds, the area between the capital epiphysis and greater trochanter is unusually vulnerable to trauma. Moreover, between the ages of 4 and 8 years the ligamentum teres contributes very little to the blood supply of the epiphysis; hence its susceptibility to post-traumatic ischaemia.

Classification

The most useful classification is that of Delbet, which is based on the level of the fracture (Hughes and Beaty, 1994). *Type I* is a fracture-separation of the epiphysis; sometimes the epiphyseal fragment is dislocated from the acetabulum. *Type II* is a transcervical fracture of the femoral neck; this is the commonest variety, accounting for almost half of the injuries. *Type III* is a basal (cervico-trochanteric) fracture, the second most common injury. *Type IV* is an intertrochanteric fracture.

Clinical features

Diagnosis can be difficult, especially in infants in whom the epiphysis is not easily defined on x-ray. Type I fractures are easily mistaken for hip dislocation. Ultrasonography, MRI and arthrography may help. In older children the diagnosis is usually obvious on plain x-ray examination.

It is important to establish whether the fracture is displaced or undisplaced; the former carries a much higher risk of complications. Type IV fractures are the least likely to give rise to complications.

Treatment

These fractures should be treated as a matter of urgency, and certainly within 24 hours of injury. Initially the hip is supported or splinted while investigations are carried out. Early aspiration of the intracapsular haematoma is advocated by some authors as a means of reducing the risk of epiphyseal ischaemia; however, the benefits are uncertain and the matter is controversial (Hughes and Beaty, 1994).

Undisplaced fractures may be treated by immobilization in a plaster spica for 6–8 weeks. However, fracture position is not always maintained and there is a considerable risk of late displacement and malunion or non-union.

Displaced type IV fractures also can be treated non-operatively: closed reduction, traction and spica immobilization. Careful follow-up is essential; if position is lost, operative fixation will be needed.

Type I, II and III fractures are treated by closed reduction and then internal fixation with smooth pins or cannulated screws. 'Closed reduction' means one gentle manipulation; if this fails, open reduction is performed. In small children, operative fixation is supplemented by a spica cast for 6–12 weeks.

Complications

Avascular necrosis of the femoral head This is the most common (and most feared) complication; it occurs in about 30% of all cases. Important risk factors are (1) an age of more than 10 years; (2) a high velocity injury; (3) a type I or II fracture; and (4) displacement. The child complains of pain and loss of movement; x-ray changes usually appear within 3 months of injury. Treatment is problematic. Non-weight-bearing, or 'containment splintage' in abduction and internal rotation, is sometimes advocated but there is little evidence that this makes any difference. The outcome depends largely on the size of the necrotic area; unfortunately most patients end up with intrusive pain and marked restriction of movement. Arthrodesis may be advisable, as a late salvage procedure.

Coxa vara Femoral neck deformity may result from malunion, avascular necrosis or premature physeal closure. If the deformity is mild, remodelling may take care of it. If the neck-shaft angle is less than 110°, subtrochanteric valgus osteotomy will probably be needed.

Diminished growth Physeal damage may result in retarded femoral growth. Limb length equalization may later be needed.

ISOLATED FRACTURES OF THE TROCHANTERS

In adolescents, the *lesser trochanter* apophysis may be avulsed by the pull of the psoas muscle; the injury nearly always occurs during hurdling. Less commonly, part of the *greater trochanter* is avulsed by the abductor muscles. With either injury the patient needs to rest in bed for

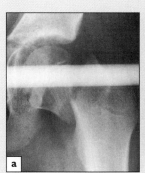
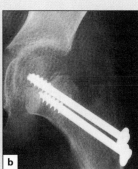
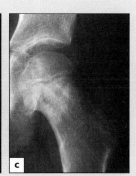
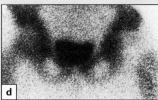

29.16 Femoral neck fractures in children (a) Fracture of the femoral neck in a child is particularly worrying because, even with perfect fixation (b), there is often ischaemia of the femoral head. The fracture united and the screws were removed (c), but the radioisotope scan shows no activity in the left femoral head (d), i.e. ischaemic necrosis.

only 2–3 days and may then get up using crutches. As soon as he or she can balance on the affected leg, crutches may be discarded, but the patient is unlikely to resume athletic activities until the following season. Functional recovery is usually good.

Occasionally the greater trochanter is fractured by a direct blow. A large, separated fragment should be fixed back in position with cancellous screws. Full weight-bearing is prohibited for 6–8 weeks.

SUBTROCHANTERIC FRACTURES

Subtrochanteric fractures may occur at any age if the injury is severe enough; but most occur with relatively trivial injury, in elderly patients with osteoporosis, osteomalacia, Paget's disease or a secondary deposit. Blood loss is greater than with femoral neck or trochanteric fractures. The head and neck are abducted and externally rotated by the gluteal muscles, and flexed by the psoas.

Fracture healing is slow and, if an angled screw-plate is used, the implant may fail before the fracture unites.

Clinical features

The leg lies externally rotated and short, and the thigh is markedly swollen. Movement is excruciatingly painful.

X-RAY
The fracture is through or below the lesser trochanter. It may be transverse, oblique or spiral, and is frequently comminuted. The upper fragment is flexed and appears deceptively short; the shaft is adducted and is displaced proximally.

Three important features should be looked for, as the presence of any one will influence treatment: (1) an unusually long fracture line extending proximally towards the greater trochanter and piriformis fossa; (2) a large, displaced fragment which includes the lesser trochanter; and (3) lytic lesions in the femur.

Treatment

Open reduction and internal fixation is the treatment of choice. For fractures at the level of the lesser trochanter, a compression (dynamic) hip screw and plate is satisfactory. A large medial fragment including part of the lesser trochanter may need separate reduction and fixation to ensure stability.

Intramedullary nails are equally good for stabilizing the fracture. If the break is below the lesser trochanter, a standard locking nail will suffice; if the fracture extends proximally, the locking screws will need to grip the femoral head. If the medial cortex is comminuted or deficient, bone grafts should be added. For a pathological fracture, a full-length nail should be used as there may be tumour deposits in the distal part of the femur. Intramedullary nailing is unsuitable for fractures which extend into the piriformis fossa, because of the high risk of fixation failure; a 95° angled-plate is safer.

Post-operatively the patient is allowed partial weightbearing (with crutches) until union is secure.

Complications

Malunion, usually in varus and external rotation, is fairly common and, if marked, may need operative correction.

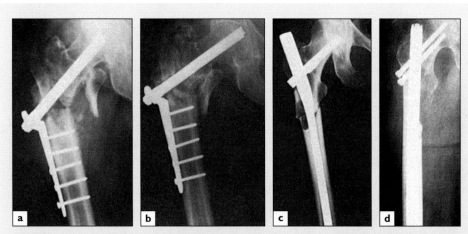

29.17 Subtrochanteric fractures (**a, b**) Fixation with a pin and plate often fails if the important posteromedial fragment is not reduced and fixed. Intramedullary fixation (**c**) is better; but if a posteromedial fragment is present it may need fixation to the shaft with cerclage wires. (**d**) Subtrochanteric fractures are not uncommonly through secondary deposits; there may be lesions also more distally, so it is best to use very secure fixation of the entire femoral shaft.

Non-union occurs in about 5% of cases; this will require operative correction of any deformity, renewed fixation and bone grafting.

FEMORAL SHAFT FRACTURES

The femoral shaft is well padded with powerful muscles – an advantage in protecting the bone from all but the most powerful forces, but a disadvantage in that fractures are often severely displaced by muscle pull, making reduction difficult.

Mechanism of injury

This is essentially a fracture of young adults and usually results from a high-energy injury. Diaphyseal fractures in elderly patients should be considered 'pathological' until proved otherwise. In children under 4 years of age the possibility of physical abuse must be kept in mind.

A spiral fracture is usually caused by a fall in which the foot is anchored while a twisting force is transmitted to the femur. *Transverse* and *oblique fractures* are more often due to angulation or direct violence and are therefore particularly common in road accidents. With severe violence (often a combination of direct and indirect forces) the fracture may be *comminuted,* or the bone may be broken in more than one place (*segmental fracture).*

Pathological anatomy

Most fractures of the femoral shaft have some degree of comminution, although it is not always apparent on x-ray; it is a reflection of the amount of force involved in these injuries. Small bone fragments, or a single large 'butterfly' fragment, may separate at the fracture line, but they usually remain attached to the adjacent soft tissue and retain their blood supply. With more extensive comminution there is no point of firm contact between proximal and distal fragments and the fracture is completely unstable. This is the basis of a helpful classification by Winquist *et al.* (1984).

Displacement is determined by the pull of muscles attached to each fragment. In proximal shaft fractures, the proximal fragment flexes, abducts and externally rotates because of gluteus medius and iliopsoas; the distal fragment is frequently adducted. In mid-shaft fractures, the proximal fragment abducts less but flexion and external rotation by iliopsoas persists. In lower third fractures, the proximal fragment adducts and the distal fragment is flexed by the gastrocnemius.

The soft tissues are always injured, and bleeding from the perforators of the profunda femoris may be severe. Over a litre may be lost into the tissues.

Clinical features

There is swelling and deformity of the limb, and any attempt to move the limb is painful. The effects of blood loss and other injuries, some of which can be life-threatening, may dominate the clinical picture. It is important to exclude neurovascular problems and other lower limb or pelvic fractures. The combination of femoral shaft and tibial shaft fractures on the same side, producing a 'floating knee', signals a high risk of multisystem injury in the patient.

X-RAY

It may be difficult to obtain adequate views in the Accident and Emergency Room setting, especially views that provide reliable information on proximal or distal fracture extensions or joint involvement; these can be postponed until better facilities and easier patient positioning are possible. *But never forget to x-ray the hip*

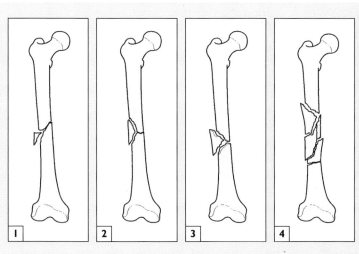

29.18 Femoral shaft fractures – classification
Winquist's classification reflects the observation that the degrees of soft-tissue damage and fracture instability increase with increasing grades of comminution. In *Type 1* there is only a tiny cortical fragment. In *Type 2* the 'butterfly fragment' is larger but there is still at least 50% cortical contact between the main fragments. In *Type 3* the butterfly fragment involves more than 50% of the bone width. *Type 4* is essentially a segmental fracture.

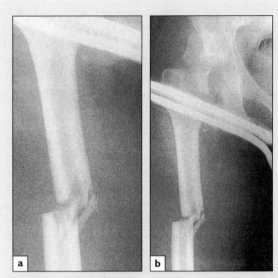

29.19 Femoral shaft fractures – diagnosis (a) The upper fragment of this femur is adducted, which should alert the surgeon to the possibility of (b) an associated hip dislocation. With this combination of injuries the dislocation is frequently missed; the safest plan is to *x-ray the pelvis with every fracture of the femoral shaft.*

and knee as well. A baseline chest x-ray is useful as there is a risk of adult respiratory distress syndrome (ARDS) in those with multiple injuries.

The fracture pattern should be carefully noted; it will form a guide to treatment.

Emergency treatment

At the site of the accident, shock should be treated and the fracture splinted before the patient is moved. The injured limb may be tied to the other leg or to any convenient splint. For transport a Thomas' splint is ideal: the leg is pulled straight and threaded through the ring of the splint; the shod foot is tied to the cross-piece so as to maintain traction, and the limb and splint are firmly bandaged together. This temporary stabilization helps to control pain, reduces bleeding and makes transfer easier. Once the patient is in hospital, skin traction can be changed to skeletal traction if operative treatment is to be delayed or if non-operative treatment is planned.

Definitive treatment

Femoral shaft fractures are usually caused by high-energy trauma and patients have an increased potential for developing fat embolism, ARDS and multi-organ failure. The medical staff should be alert to the early signs of these complications. Blood volume should be restored and maintained and a definitive plan of action instituted as soon as the patient's condition has been assessed.

The risk of systemic complications can be significantly reduced by early stabilization of the fracture. The most effective way of achieving this is by locked intramedullary nailing; however, the method is highly dependent on operator skill and experience and the availability of special equipment and facilities for intra-operative image intensification. Alternative methods can be used, but the indications, strengths and limitations of the various approaches need to be known.

TRACTION AND BRACING

Traction can reduce and hold most fractures in reasonable alignment, except those in the upper third of the femur. Joint mobility can be ensured by active exercises. The chief drawback is the length of time spent in bed (10–14 weeks for adults) with the attendant problems of maintaining fracture alignment to the end and reducing patient morbidity and frustration. Some of these difficulties are overcome by reducing the time in traction and then changing to a plaster spica or – in the case of lower third fractures – functional bracing; this is acceptable once the fracture is 'sticky', usually around 6–8 weeks.

The main indications for traction are (1) fractures in children; (2) contraindications to anaesthesia; and (3) lack of suitable skill or facilities for internal fixation. It is a poor choice for elderly patients, for pathological fractures and for those with multiple injuries.

The various methods of traction are described in Chapter 23. For children, *skin traction* without a splint is usually all that is needed. Infants under 12 kg in weight are most easily managed by suspending the lower limbs from overhead pulleys ('gallows traction'), but no more than 2 kg weight should be used and the feet must be checked frequently for circulatory problems. Older children are better suited to *Russell's traction* (see page 550). Fracture union occurs within 2–4 weeks (depending on the age of the child) and at that stage a *hip spica* is applied and the child is allowed up. Consolidation is usually complete by 6–12 weeks.

Adults (and older adolescents) require *skeletal* traction through a pin or a tightly strung Kirschner wire behind the tibial tubercle. Traction (8–10kg for an adult) is applied over pulleys at the foot of the bed. The limb is usually supported on a *Thomas' splint* and a flexion piece allows movement at the knee. However, a splint is not essential; indeed, *skeletal traction without a splint* (Perkins' traction) has the advantages of producing less distortion of the fracture and allowing freer movement in bed. Exercises are begun as soon as possible. Once the fracture is sticky (at about 8 weeks in adults) traction can be discontinued and the patient allowed up and partial weight-bearing in a *cast or brace*. For fractures in the upper half of the femur, a plaster spica is the safest but it will almost certainly prolong the period of knee stiffness. For fractures in the lower half of the femur, cast-bracing is suitable.

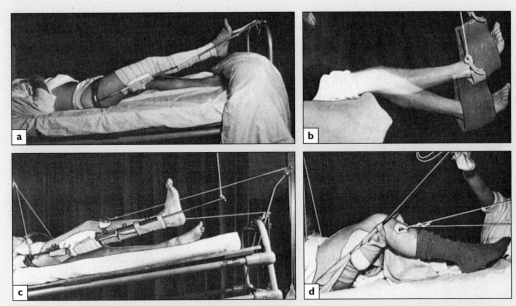

29.20 Femoral shaft fractures – treatment by traction (**a**) *Fixed traction on a Thomas' splint:* the splint is tied to the foot of the bed which is elevated. This method should be used only rarely because the knee may stiffen; (**b**) this was the range in such a case when the fracture had united. (**c, d**) *Balanced traction:* one way to minimize stiffness is to use skeletal balanced traction; the lower slings can be removed to permit knee flexion while traction is still maintained.

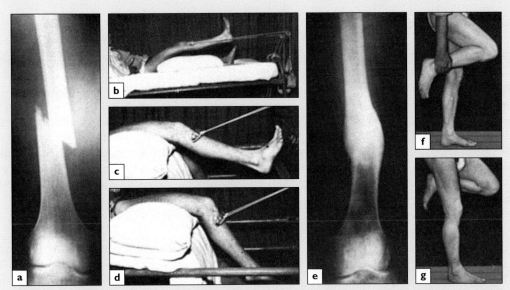

29.21 Femoral shaft fractures – traction Even in the adult, traction without a splint can be satisfactory, but skeletal traction is essential. The patient with this rather unstable fracture (**a**) can lift his leg and exercise his knee (**b, c, d**). At no time was the leg splinted, but clearly the fracture has consolidated (**e**), and the knee range (**f**) is only slightly less than that of the uninjured left leg (**g**).

This type of protection is needed until the fracture has consolidated (16–24 weeks).

OPEN REDUCTION AND PLATING

Plating is a comparatively easy way of obtaining accurate reduction and firm fixation. The method was popular at one time but went out of favour because of the high complication rate, including implant failure. The main indications today are (1) the combination of shaft and femoral neck fractures and (2) a shaft fracture with an associated vascular injury.

The least destructive technique is 'indirect reduction' using a femoral distractor. A single stout plate is then applied to the lateral surface of the femur with at least

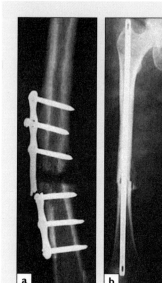
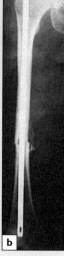
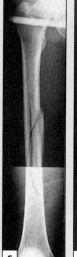
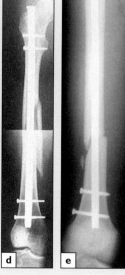

29.22 Femoral shaft fractures – internal fixation (a) This plate is absurdly inadequate to hold a fractured femur; longer and stronger plates can be used, but most surgeons nowadays prefer (b) intramedullary nailing. Proximal and distal locking (c, d) should be standard – not only to control length but also to resist rotation. With this modification, intramedullary nailing has become the treatment of choice also for distal third fractures (e).

five screws in each of the main fragments; bone grafts are added on the medial aspect across the fracture. Severely comminuted fractures are simply bridged by a plate of suitable length.

INTRAMEDULLARY NAILING

Intramedullary nailing is the method of choice for most femoral shaft fractures. However, it should not be attempted unless the appropriate facilities and expertise are available. The basic implant system consists of an intramedullary nail (in a range of sizes) which is perforated near each end so that locking screws can be inserted transversely at the proximal and distal ends; this controls rotation and ensures stability even for subtrochanteric and distal third fractures.

The operation is performed with the patient on his or her back or side and skeletal traction still in place. The fracture is then reduced under x-ray control; if closed reduction cannot be achieved, the fracture is exposed through a limited incision and reduced with the aid of a distracting device. The tip of the greater trochanter is identified through a gluteal muscle-splitting incision; slightly behind and medial to this is the piriform fossa, where the nail will be introduced. The cortex is perforated with a sharp 'bayonet' and then, under fluoroscopic control, a guide rod is passed down the femur crossing the fracture. If closed reduction cannot be achieved and repeated attempts to persuade a guide-wire across the fracture site fail, a small exposure to achieve reduction is permissable. Flexible reamers are used to widen the medullary canal. A pre-bent nail of suitable length and width (usually 1.5mm smaller than the widest reamer used) is chosen; this is passed over the guide rod (or a second, stiffer, guide rod) and driven home under fluoroscopic control.

Stability is improved by using interlocking screws; all locking holes in the nail should be used. Often there is enough shared stability between the nail and fracture ends to allow some weight-bearing early on. The fracture usually heals within 20 weeks and complication rates are low; sometimes malunion (more likely malrotation) or delayed union (from leaving the fracture site over-distracted) occurs.

Slim nails which can be inserted without reaming are now available; these have helped to shorten operation times. The results of these unreamed nails are promising in the early reports, but they are as yet unproved as being significantly better than the older type.

Open medullary nailing is a feasible alternative where facilities for closed nailing are lacking. A limited lateral exposure of the femur is made; the fracture is reduced and a guide-wire is passed between the main proximal and distal fragments; a small exposure to achieve reduction does not significantly affect the risk of complications or fracture healing.

EXTERNAL FIXATION

This method of femoral shaft fracture stabilization was previously reserved for open fractures. Newer designs of fixator half-pins and fixator bodies have improved the outcome from this technique – union rates of over 90% have been reported (DeBastiani *et al.*, 1984). Like closed intramedullary nailing, it has the advantage of not exposing the fracture site and small amounts of axial movement can be fed to the bone by allowing a telescoping action to occur in the fixator body. As the callus increases in volume and quality, the fixator can be adjusted to increase stress transfer to the fracture site, thus promoting quicker consolidation. However, there are still problems with pin-site infection, pin loosening and (if the half-pins are applied close to joints) limitation of movement due to interference with sliding structures.

The main indications for external fixation are (1) the treatment of severe open injuries; (2) management of patients with multiple injuries where there is a need to reduce operating time; and (3) dealing with severe bone loss by the technique of bone transport. External fixation is also useful for (4) treating femoral fractures in adolescents.

Post-operatively, the limb is left free and exercises are begun as soon as possible. Knee movement is more rapidly regained with a continuous passive motion (CPM) machine.

After a week or 10 days the patient is allowed up, partial weight-bearing on crutches. Full weight-bearing is usually achieved 4–6 weeks later, but comminuted fractures should be protected for longer than this.

Open fractures

Open femoral fractures should be carefully assessed for (1) skin loss; (2) wound contamination; (3) muscle ischaemia; and (4) injury to vessels and nerves.

The immediate treatment is similar to that of closed fractures; in addition, the patient is started on intravenous antibiotics. Wound cleansing and debridement should be carried out with as little delay as possible. If there is tissue death or obvious contamination, the wound should be extended and dead tissue carefully excised.

Thereafter, the major decision is how to stabilize the fracture. This will depend on the degree of contamination, the length of time from injury to operation and the amount of soft-tissue damage. If there is no obvious contamination, open fractures of all grades up to IIIA (Gustilo classification) can be treated as for a closed injury; immediate intramedullary nailing produces union rates as good as those in closed fractures of a comparable nature but with an incidence of infection of 3–5%. More severe injuries should be left open and the fracture stabilized by *external fixation*.

Complex injuries

Fractures associated with vascular injury Warning signs of an associated vascular injury are (1) excessive bleeding or haematoma formation; and (2) paraesthesia, pallor or pulselessness in the leg and foot. Doppler examination may be helpful, but do not accept 'arterial spasm' as a cause of absent pulses; arteriography will show the level of the injury which may be an intimal tear. The fracture should be stabilized as quickly as possible – preferably by nailing, or else by plating or external fixation if these methods are quicker – and the vascular repair or bypass is then carried out. Ischaemia should not be allowed to persist beyond 6 hours.

Fracture associated with knee injury Femoral fractures are frequently accompanied by injury to the ligaments of the knee. With attention focused on the femur, the knee injury is easily overlooked, only to re-emerge as a

persistent complaint weeks or months later. As soon as the fracture has been stabilized, the knee should be carefully examined and any associated abnormality treated.

'Floating knee' Ipsilateral fractures of the femur and tibia may leave the knee joint 'floating'. This is a very serious fracture pattern and other injuries are frequently present. Both fractures will need immediate stabilization – it is usual to fix the femur first.

Combined neck and shaft fractures This is dealt with on page 690. The most important thing is diagnosis: always examine the hip and obtain an x-ray of the pelvis. Both sites must be stabilized, first the femoral neck and then the femur.

Multiple injuries Resuscitation and attention to head and chest injuries take priority. Thereafter, long-bone fractures should be stabilized as soon as possible. Reaming is best avoided in patients with chest injuries; venous emboli may increase the risk of ARDS.

Pathological fractures Fractures through metastatic lesions should be fixed by intramedullary nailing. Provided the patient is fit enough to tolerate the operation, a short life expectancy is not a contraindication. 'Prophylactic fixation' is also indicated if a lytic lesion is (a) greater than half the diameter of the bone; (b) longer than 3cm on any view or (c) painful, irrespective of its size (see Fig. 23.50).

Paget's disease may present a problem. The bone is likely to be very hard and to bleed excessively. If the femur is bowed, it may have to be osteotomized to allow the nail to be inserted fully.

Periprosthetic fractures Femoral shaft fractures around a hip implant are uncommon; they may happen during primary hip surgery when reaming or preparing the medullary canal, or when forcing in an over-sized uncemented prosthesis, or during revision surgery as when extracting cement or whilst attempting to dislocate the hip if the soft-tissue release has been insufficient. Sometimes the fracture occurs much later, and there are usually x-ray signs of osteolysis or implant loosening suggesting a reason for bone weakness.

If the prosthesis is worn or loose, it should be removed and replaced by one with a long stem, thereby treating both problems. If the primary implant is neither loose nor worn, plate fixation of the fracture with structural allografts bridging the fracture offers a suitable solution.

Complications

All the complications described in Chapter 23, with the exception of visceral injury and avascular necrosis, are encountered in femoral shaft fractures. The more common ones are as follows.

Shock 1–2 litres of blood can be lost even with a closed fracture, and shock may be severe. Prevention is better than cure; most patients will require a transfusion.

Fat embolism and ARDS Fracture through a large marrow-filled cavity almost inevitably results in small showers of fat emboli being swept to the lungs. This can usually be accommodated without serious consequences, but in some cases (and especially in those with multiple injuries and severe shock, or in patients with associated chest injuries) it results in progressive respiratory distress and multi-organ failure (ARDS). Blood gases should be measured soon after admission, and any suspicious signs such as shortness of breath, restlessness or a rise in temperature or pulse rate should prompt a search for petechial haemorrhages over the upper body, axillae and conjunctivae. Treatment is supportive, with the emphasis on preventing hypoxia and maintaining blood volume.

Thromboembolism Prolonged traction in bed predisposes to thrombosis. Movement and exercise are important in preventing this, but should be supplemented by foot compression devices or prophylactic doses of anticoagulants. If thigh or pelvis thrombosis is suspected, special investigations should be carried out as soon as possible (see page 257); if the diagnosis confirmed, full anticoagulant treatment is started forthwith.

Infection In open injuries, and following internal fixation, there is always a risk of infection. Prophylactic antibiotics, and careful attention to the principles of fracture surgery, should keep the incidence below 2%. If the bone does become infected, the patient should be treated as for an acute osteomyelitis. The presence of pus or a sequestrum calls for operative treatment; the wound is explored, all dead and infected tissue is removed and the fracture (if it has not been fixed) is stabilized by fitting an external fixator. If a medullary nail is already in place and fixation is stable, the nail should be left there; even worse than an infected fracture is an infected unstable fracture! However, if the fracture is unstable, the nail should be replaced by one with a larger diameter, or else by an external fixator.

The long-term management of chronic osteomyelitis is discussed in Chapter 2.

LATE
Delayed union and non-union It is said that a fractured femur should unite in 100 days, plus or minus 20. If union is delayed beyond this time, an exchange nailing is performed using a slightly larger nail; in addition the fracture may need bone grafting.

Malunion Fractures treated by traction and bracing often develop some deformity; no more than 15° of angulation should be accepted. Even if the initial reduction was satisfactory, until the x-ray shows solid union the fracture is too insecure to permit weight-bearing; the bone will bend and what previously seemed a satisfactory reduction may end up with lateral or anterior bowing.

Malunion is much less likely in those treated with static interlocked nails; yet it does still occur – especially malrotation – and this can be prevented only by meticulous intra-operative and post-operative assessment followed, where necessary, by immediate correction. Shortening is seldom a major problem; if it occurs, it can usually be accommodated by building up the shoe.

Joint stiffness The knee is often affected after a femoral shaft fracture. The joint may be injured at the same time, or it stiffens due to soft-tissue adhesions during treatment; hence the importance of repeated evaluation and early physiotherapy.

Refracture and implant failure Fractures which heal with abundant callus are unlikely to recur. By contrast, in those treated by internal fixation, callus formation is often slow and meagre. With delayed union or non-union, the integrity of the femur may be almost wholly dependent on the implant and sooner or later it will fail. If a comminuted fracture is plated, bone grafts should be added and weight-bearing delayed so as to protect the plate from reaching its fatigue limit too soon. Intramedullary nails are less prone to break. However, sometimes they do, especially with a slow-healing fracture of the lower third and a static locked nail; the break usually occurs through the screw hole closest to the fracture. Treatment consists of replacing the nail and adding bone grafts.

FEMORAL SHAFT FRACTURES IN CHILDREN

Mechanism

Fractures of the femur are quite common in older children and are usually due to *direct violence* (e.g. a road accident) or a *fall* from a height. However, in children under 2 years of age the commonest cause is child abuse; if there are several fractures in different stages of healing, this is very suspicious. *Pathological fractures* are common in generalized disorders such as spina bifida and osteogenesis imperfecta, and with local bone lesions (e.g. a benign cyst or tumour).

Treatment

The principles of treatment are discussed above. It should be emphasized that in young children open treatment is rarely necessary. The choice of closed method depends largely on the age and weight of the child.

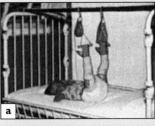
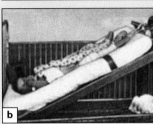
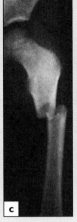
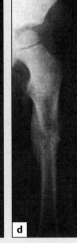
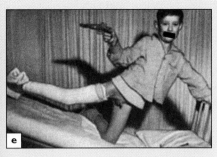

29.23 Femoral shaft fractures in children
(**a–d**) Traction without a splint is certainly adequate in children, and skin traction is sufficient. (**e**) In this case the fracture has clearly united!

Infants need no more than 1–2 weeks in balanced traction, followed by a spica cast for another 3–4 weeks. Angulation of up to 30° can be accepted, as the bone remodels quite remarkably with growth.

Children between 2 and 10 years of age can be treated either with balanced traction (Russell's traction – see above) for 2–3 weeks followed by a spica cast for another 4 weeks, or by early reduction and a spica cast from the outset. Shortening of 1–2cm and angulation of up to 20° are acceptable.

Teenagers require somewhat longer (4–6 weeks) in balanced traction, and those aged over 15 years (or even younger adolescents if they are large and muscular) may need skeletal traction. Once the fracture feels firm, traction is exchanged for either a spica cast (in the case of upper third and mid-shaft fractures) or a cast-brace (for lower third fractures), which is retained for a further 6 weeks. The position should be checked every few weeks; the limit of acceptable angulation in this age group is 15° in the anteroposterior x-ray and 25° in the lateral.

If a satisfactory reduction cannot be achieved by traction, internal or external fixation is justified. This applies particularly to older children and those with multiple injuries. Three methods are illustrated in Fig. 29.24.

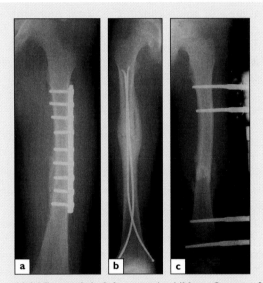

29.24 Femoral shaft fractures in children Operative fixation is occasionally needed for fractures in older children and in those with multiple injuries. This can be achieved by using (**a**) a plate and screws, (**b**) flexible intramedullary nails or (**c**) external fixation. (Courtesy of Mr JC Dorgan and Mr NK Garg)

Complications

Shortening Overlapping and comminution of the bone fragments may shorten the femur. However, anything up to 1.5cm is quite acceptable; indeed, some surgeons regard this as an advantage because there is a tendency for the fractured bone to 'overgrow'. Unfortunately, the effect on growth is unpredictable.

Malunion Angulation can usually be tolerated within the limits mentioned above. However, the fact that bone modelling is excellent in children is no excuse for casual management; bone may be forgiving but parents are not. Rotational malunion is not corrected by growth or remodelling.

SUPRACONDYLAR FRACTURES OF THE FEMUR

Supracondylar fractures of the femur are seen (a) in young adults, usually as a result of high-energy trauma, and (b) in elderly, osteoporotic individuals.

Mechanism and pathological anatomy

Direct violence is the usual cause. The fracture line is just above the condyles, but may extend between them. In the worst cases the fracture is severely comminuted.

When the lower fragment is intact it may be markedly displaced by the pull of gastrocnemius, thus risking injury to the popliteal artery.

Clinical features

The knee is swollen and deformed; movement is too painful to be attempted. The tibial pulses should always be palpated.

X-RAY

The fracture is just above the femoral condyles and is transverse or comminuted. The distal fragment is often tilted backwards. *The entire femur should be x-rayed so as not to miss a proximal fracture or dislocated hip.*

Treatment

NON-OPERATIVE

If the fracture is only slightly displaced and extra-articular, or if it reduces easily with the knee in flexion, it can be treated quite satisfactorily by traction through the proximal tibia; the limb is cradled on a Thomas' splint with a knee flexion piece, and movements are encouraged. If the distal fragment is displaced by gastrocnemius pull, a second pin above the knee, and vertical traction, will correct this. At 4–6 weeks, when the fracture is beginning to unite, traction can be replaced by a cast-brace and the patient allowed up and partially weight-bearing with crutches. Non-operative treatment is most likely to be considered if the patient is young and has not suffered multiple injuries.

OPERATIVE

If closed reduction fails, open reduction and internal fixation with an angled compression device, though difficult, may be successful. This does not necessarily lead to earlier mobilization because the bone is often osteoporotic and the patient may be old and frail, but nursing in bed is easier and knee movements can be started sooner. Unprotected weight-bearing is not permitted until the fracture has consolidated (usually around 12 weeks).

Locked intramedullary nails which are introduced retrograde through the intercondylar notch are also used for these fractures. They provide adequate stability, even in the presence of osteoporotic bone, but (as with compression plates) unprotected weight-bearing is best avoided until union is assured.

Complications

EARLY

Arterial damage There is a small but definite risk of arterial damage and distal ischaemia. Careful assessment of the leg and peripheral pulses is essential, even if the x-ray shows only minimal displacement.

LATE

Joint stiffness Knee stiffness is almost inevitable. A long period of exercise is necessary but full movement is rarely regained.

Non-union Knee stiffness increases the likelihood of non-union. This combination is difficult to treat and, unless great care is exercised, the ultimate range of movement at the knee may be less than that at the fracture.

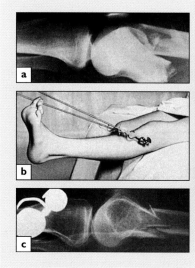
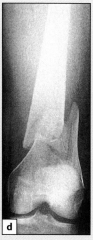
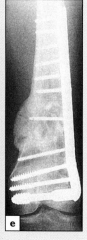

29.25 Supracondylar fractures (a, b, c) These fractures can sometimes be treated successfully by traction through the upper tibia; if there is much posterior displacement (endangering the popliteal vessels) it may be corrected by vertical traction through a second pin above the knee. **(d, e)** If the bone is not too osteoporotic, internal fixation with a dynamic condylar screw and plate is a good alternative.

FEMORAL CONDYLE FRACTURES

Mechanism of injury

Condylar fractures are often associated with supra-condylar fractures where a distal extension into the knee joint may cause one or both condyles to be split apart. They can also occur in isolation; a direct injury or a fall from a height may drive the tibia upwards into the intercondylar fossa.

Pathological anatomy

Because of the overlap in mechanism and pattern of injury, condylar and supracondylar fractures are often classified together (Müller *et al.*, 1991). Thus, one can define three groups of fractures: (A) purely extra-articular, supracondylar fractures; (B) intra-articular fracture of one condyle – usually the lateral; and (C) intra-articular bicondylar fractures, which are effectively also 'supracondylar'.

Clinical features

The knee is swollen and may be deformed. There is a tender, 'doughy' feel characteristic of a haemarthrosis. The joint is too painful to move, but the foot should be examined to exclude nerve and arterial damage.

X-RAY

One femoral condyle may be fractured obliquely and shifted upwards, or both condyles may be split apart so that the fracture line is T-shaped or Y-shaped. Beware: a coronal plane fracture of the posterior part of the condyle (the Hoffa fracture) is easily missed unless good lateral and oblique views are obtained.

Treatment

Closed reduction is sometimes successful; indeed, the fracture may not necessarily be severely displaced and the position may be almost acceptable. Skeletal traction is applied through the proximal tibia and the fracture is 'reduced' by manual compression. Traction is maintained for 4–6 weeks and is then exchanged for a cast-brace which is worn until the fracture is firmly united.

Open reduction is indicated if closed methods fail to bring the condylar fragments together. It may also be the preferred method of primary treatment in a young, fit patient who is anxious to be up and mobile as soon as possible. The fracture is exposed through a lateral or medial incision; a good view of the knee joint helps to ensure accurate reduction and anatom-

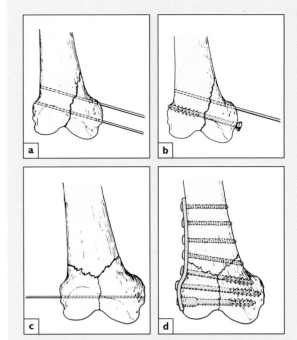

29.26 Femoral condyle fractures – treatment (**a**) A single condylar fracture can be reduced open and held with Kirschner wires preparatory to (**b**) inserting compression screws. (**c**) T- or Y-shaped fractures are best fixed with a dynamic condylar screw and plate (**d**).

ical restoration of the articular surface. The fragments are fixed with cannulated screws, a blade-plate or a dynamic condylar screw and plate (the size of the fragments will determine the choice). Provided fixation is secure, the patient can begin knee exercises and be got out of bed within a day or two, but very little weight should be taken through the leg until the fracture is consolidated.

FRACTURE-SEPARATION OF THE DISTAL FEMORAL EPIPHYSIS

In the childhood or adolescent equivalent of a supracondylar fracture, the lower femoral epiphysis may be displaced (1) to one side (usually laterally) by forced angulation of the straight knee or (2) forwards by a hyperextension injury. Although not nearly as common as physeal fractures at the elbow or ankle, this injury is important because of its potential for causing abnormal growth and deformity of the knee.

The fracture is usually a Salter–Harris type 2 lesion – i.e. physeal separation with a large triangular metaphyseal bone fragment. Although this type of fracture usually has a good prognosis, asymmetrical growth arrest is not uncommon and the child may end up with a valgus or varus deformity. All grades of injury, but

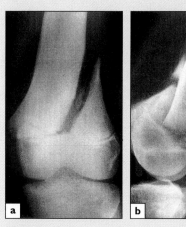

29.27 Fracture-separation of epiphysis These fractures are not difficult to reduce and can usually be held adequately in plaster, but they must be watched carefully for several weeks.

displacement of the epiphysis, the popliteal artery may be obstructed by the lower femur.

especially Salter–Harris types 3 and 4, may result in femoral shortening. Nearly 70% of the femur's length is derived from the distal physis, so early arrest can present a major problem.

Clinical features

The knee is swollen and perhaps deformed. The pulses in the foot should be palpated because, with forwards

Treatment

The fracture can usually be perfectly reduced manually, but further x-ray checks will be needed over the next few weeks to ensure that reduction is maintained. Occasionally open reduction is needed; a flap of periosteum may be trapped in the fracture line. Salter–Harris types 3 and 4 should be accurately reduced and fixed. If there is a tendency to redisplacement, the fragments may be stabilized with percutaneous Kirschner wires or lag screws driven across the metaphyseal spike. The limb is immobilized in plaster and the patient is allowed partial weight-bearing on crutches. The cast can be removed after 6–8 weeks and physiotherapy started.

Complications

EARLY
Vascular injury There is danger of gangrene unless the hyperextension injury is reduced without delay.

LATE
Physeal arrest Damage to the physis is not uncommon and residual deformity may require corrective osteotomy at the end of the growth period. Shortening, if it is marked, can be treated by femoral lengthening.

REFERENCES

Barnes R, Brown JT, Garden RS, Nicol EA (1976) Subcapital fractures of the femur. A prospective review. *Journal of Bone and Joint Surgery* 58B, 2-24

Cooper C (1989) Osteoporosis - an epidemiological perspective: a review. *Journal of the Royal Society of Medicine* 82, 753-757

DeBastiani G, Aldegheri R, Renzi Brivio L (1984) The treatment of fractures with a dynamic axial fixator. *Journal of Bone and Joint Surgery* 66B, 538-545

Dimon JH, Hughston JC (1967) Unstable intertrochanteric fractures of the hip. *Journal of Bone and Joint Surgery* 49A, 440-450

Garden RS (1961) Low-angle fixation in fractures of the femoral neck. *Journal of Bone and Joint Surgery* 43B, 647-663

Garden RS (1974) Reduction and fixation of subcapital fractures of the femur. *Orthoptic Clinics of North America* 5, 683-712

Gustilo RB, Merkow RL, Templeman D (1990) The management of open fractures. *Journal of Bone and Joint Surgery* 72A, 299-304

Harper WM, Barnes MR, Gregg PJ (1991) Femoral head blood flow in femoral neck fracture. *Journal of Bone and Joint Surgery* 73B, 73-75

Hughes LO, Beaty JA (1994) Fractures of the head and neck of femur in children. *Journal of Bone and Joint Surgery* 76A, 283-293

Kyle RF, Cabanela ME, Russell TA *et al* (1994) Fracture of the proximal part of the femur. *Journal of Bone and Joint Surgery* 76A, 924-950

Müller ME, Allgower M, Schneider R, Willeneger H (1991) *Manual of Internal Fixation* 3rd edition. Springer, Berlin, pp598-600

Olerud C, Rehnberg L, Hellquist E (1991) Internal fixation of femoral neck fractures. *Journal of Bone and Joint Surgery* 73B, 16-19

Pipkin G (1957) Treatment of grade IV fracture dislocation of the hip. *Journal of Bone and Joint Surgery* 39, 1027-1042

Thompson VP, Epstein HC (1951) Traumatic dislocation of the hip. *Journal of Bone and Joint Surgery* 33A, 746-778

Winquist RA, Hansen ST Jr, Clawson DK (1984) Closed intramedullary nailing of femoral fractures: a report of five hundred and twenty cases. *Journal of Bone and Joint Surgery* 66A, 529-539

ACUTE KNEE LIGAMENT INJURIES

The bony structure of the knee joint is inherently unstable; were it not for the strong capsule, intra- and extra-articular ligaments and controlling muscles, the knee would not be able to function effectively as a mechanism for support, balance and thrust.

Valgus stresses are resisted by the fascia lata, pes anserinus, superficial and deep layers of the medial collateral ligament (MCL) and the tough posteromedial part of the capsule. In full extension all these structures, as well as the anterior cruciate ligament (ACL), act together to prevent both valgus and rotation. At 30° of flexion, the MCL is the main stabilizer.

The main checks to varus angulation are the iliotibial tract and the lateral collateral ligament (LCL). The LCL is taut in full extension; as the knee is flexed the ligament relaxes, but the popliteus tendon comes into play and provides stability in flexion.

The cruciate ligaments provide both anteroposterior and rotary stability; they also help to resist excessive valgus and varus angulation. Both cruciate ligaments have a layered structure and some fibres of each ligament are taut in all positions of the knee. Anterior displacement of the tibia (the anterior drawer sign) is resisted by both the anteromedial part of the ACL and the posteromedial part of the capsule. Posterior displacement is prevented by the posterior cruciate ligament (PCL).

Injuries of the knee ligaments are common, particularly in sporting pursuits but also in road accidents where they may be associated with fractures or dislocations. They vary in severity from a simple sprain to complete rupture. It is important to recognize that these injuries are seldom 'unidirectional'; they often involve more than one structure and it is therefore useful to refer to them in functional terms (e.g. anteromedial instability) as well as anatomical terms (e.g. torn MCL and ACL).

Mechanism of injury and pathological anatomy

Most ligament injuries occur while the knee is bent, i.e. when the capsule and ligaments are relaxed and the femur is allowed to rotate on the tibia. The damaging force may be a straight thrust (e.g. a dashboard injury forcing the tibia backwards) or, more commonly, a combined rotation and thrust as in a football tackle. The medial structures are most often affected but if the injury has a twist in addition to a valgus force, the ACL also may be damaged. This twisting force in a weight-bearing knee often tears the medial meniscus, causing a well-recognized triad of MCL, ACL and medial meniscal injury. A knee with a solitary MCL injury, if sufficiently severe, can be shown to 'open' on the medial side when the knee is flexed to 30° and a valgus stress is applied, but if this is still detectable when the knee is extended, then it is likely the capsule and ACL are also damaged.

Forces that push the tibia into varus will damage the lateral structures, but these forces are relatively uncommon; as with medial injuries, the cruciate ligaments are at risk if there is a twisting component, and a clinically detectable opening on varus stressing in an extended knee suggests that there is also capsular and cruciate damage.

Cruciate ligament injuries occur singly or in combination with damage to other structures. The ACL is the more commonly affected. Solitary cruciate ligament injuries result in instability in the sagittal plane, i.e. the tibia can be pushed backwards or pulled forwards in relation to the femur. If there is damage to a collateral ligament or the capsule as well, then the direction of instability is often oblique and there may be a problem in controlling rotation.

Oblique plane and rotatory instabilities are complex; in essence, one of the cruciate ligaments is ruptured and there is also laxity in one of the areas of the knee joint capsule. This causes movement of the tibia on the femur, usually around an axis of remaining intact capsule or supporting ligament. Thus, in the more common anterolateral instability, where the ACL, lateral capsule and LCL are injured, the lateral plateau of the tibia can be made to sublux anteriorly when the tibia is rotated internally. If this is done with the knee fully extended whilst maintaining a valgus force, and the knee is then gradually flexed, a palpable reduction of this subluxation is felt at 20–30°. This is the basis of the *pivot shift test*; it is thought the tibia rotates around the axis of an intact MCL.

The common rotatory instability patterns are summarized in Table 30.1, showing the likely ligaments involved and the clinical tests for assessment.

Clinical features

The patient gives a history of a twisting or wrenching injury and may even claim to have heard a 'pop' as the tissues snapped. The knee is painful and (usually) swollen – and, in contrast to the story in meniscal injury, the swelling appears almost immediately.

Table 30.1 Rotary instabilities of the knee

Type of instability	Test	Positive result	Likely structures damaged
Anterolateral rotatory instability	Anterior drawer test but with the foot internally rotated 30°	The tibia subluxes forwards	ACL
			LCL
	The pivot shift manoeuvre	The tibia can be felt to sublux and reduce	Lateral aspect of knee capsule
Anteromedial rotatory instability	Anterior drawer test but with the foot externally rotated 15°	The tibia subluxes forwards	ACL
			MCL
			Medial aspect of knee capsule (posterior oblique ligament)
Posterolateral rotatory instability	Reverse (external rotation) pivot shift manoeuvre	The tibia subluxes forwards	PCL
	Pick up the foot by grasping the medial forefoot	The knee hyperextends and tibia externally rotates	Arcuate complex (LCL, arcuate ligament and popliteus)

Tenderness is most acute over the torn ligament, and stressing one or other side of the joint may produce excruciating pain. The knee may be too painful to permit deep palpation or much movement.

For all the apparent consistency, the findings can be somewhat perverse: thus, with a complete tear the patient may have little or no pain, whereas with a partial tear the knee is painful. Swelling also is worse with partial tears, because haemorrhage remains confined within the joint; with complete tears the ruptured capsule permits leakage and diffusion. With a partial tear attempted movement is always painful; the abnormal movement of a complete tear is often painless or prevented by spasm.

Abrasions suggest the site of impact, but bruising is more important and indicates the site of damage. The doughy feel of a haemarthrosis distinguishes ligament injuries from the fluctuant feel of the synovial effusion of a meniscus injury. Tenderness localizes the lesion, but the sharply defined tender spot of a partial tear (usually medial and 2.5cm above the joint line) contrasts with the diffuse tenderness of a complete one. The entire limb should be examined for other injuries and for vascular or nerve damage.

The most important aspect of the examination is to test for ligamentous stability. Partial tears permit no abnormal movement, but the attempt causes pain. Complete tears permit abnormal movement which sometimes is painless. To distinguish between the two is critical because their treatment is different; so, *if there is doubt, examination under anaesthesia is mandatory.*

Sideways tilting (varus/valgus) is examined, first with the knee at 30° of flexion and then with the knee straight. Movement is compared with the normal side. If the knee angulates only in slight flexion, there is probably an isolated tear of the collateral ligaments; if it angulates in full extension, there is almost certainly rupture of the capsule and cruciate ligaments as well as the collateral ligament.

Anteroposterior stability is assessed first by placing the knees at 90° with the feet resting on the couch and looking from the side for posterior sag of the proximal tibia; when present, this is a reliable sign of posterior cruciate instability. Next, the drawer test is carried out in the usual way; a positive drawer sign is diagnostic of a tear, but a negative test does not exclude one. The Lachman test is more reliable; anteroposterior glide is tested with the knee flexed 15–20°.

Rotational stability can usually be tested only under anaesthesia.

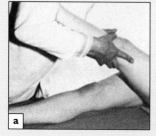
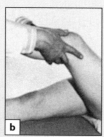
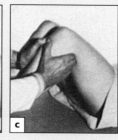

30.1 Knee ligaments – examination Grips used in examination for abnormal movements. **(a)** Sideways tilting with the knee straight, and **(b)** with the knee flexed tests the collateral ligaments; **(c)** anteroposterior glide (this should also be tested with the knee flexed to 20°) tests the anterior cruciate ligament.

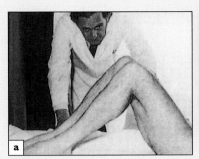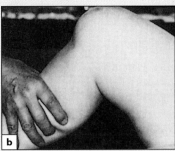

30.2 Posterior cruciate ligaments (a) Viewed from the side, any backwards displacement of the upper tibia is plainly visible and can be confirmed by (b) pushing the tibia backwards.

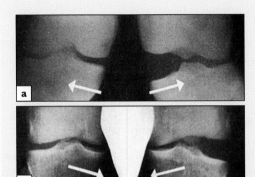

30.3 Stress x-rays Stress films show: **(a)** complete tear of medial ligament, left knee; **(b)** complete tear of lateral ligament. In both, the anterior cruciate also was torn.

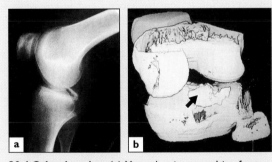

30.4 Other imaging **(a)** X-ray showing an avulsion fracture at the insertion of the posterior cruciate ligament. **(b)** Three-dimensional CT reconstruction. The fragment, and its bed, are clearly defined.

Imaging

Plain x-rays may show that the ligament has avulsed a small piece of bone – the medial ligament usually from the femur, the lateral ligament from the fibula, the anterior cruciate ligament from the tibial spine and the posterior cruciate from the back of the upper tibia.

Stress films (if necessary under anaesthesia) demonstrate if the joint hinges open on one side.

Magnetic resonance imaging (MRI) is sometimes needed to distinguish partial from complete ligament tears. This may also reveal 'bone bruising', a hitherto poorly recognized source of pain.

Three-dimensional computed tomography (CT) reconstruction may help to define osteo-articular fractures prior to internal fixation.

Arthroscopy

With severe tears of the collateral ligaments and capsule, arthroscopy should not be attempted; fluid extravasation will hamper diagnosis and may complicate further procedures. The main indication for arthroscopy is in suspected 'isolated' cruciate ligament tears, and in lesser sprains to exclude other internal injuries such as meniscal tears, which (if present) can be dealt with then and there.

Treatment

SPRAINS AND PARTIAL TEARS
The intact fibres splint the torn ones and spontaneous healing will occur. The hazard is adhesions, so active exercise is prescribed from the start, facilitated by aspirating a tense effusion, applying ice-packs to the knee and, sometimes, by injecting local anaesthetic into the tender area. Weight-bearing is permitted but the knee is protected from rotation or angulation strains by a heavily padded bandage or a functional brace. A complete plaster cast is unnecessary and disadvantageous; it inhibits movement and prevents weekly reassessment – an important precaution if the occasional error is to be avoided. With a dedicated exercise programme, the patient can usually return to sports training by 6–8 weeks.

COMPLETE TEARS
Isolated tears of the MCL, i.e. where the knee is stable in full extension, usually heal well enough to permit near-normal function. Operative repair is unnecessary (Sandberg *et al.*, 1987). A long cast-brace is worn for 6 weeks and thereafter graded exercises are encouraged.

Isolated tears of the LCL are rare. If the diagnosis is certain, these can be treated conservatively as for MCL tears.

Isolated tears of the ACL should, in theory, be treated by early operative reconstruction. Indeed, such are the pressures on professional sportsmen that this is often demanded. Operation may also be indicated for non-professionals if the tibial spine is avulsed; the bone fragment, with the attached ACL, is replaced and fixed under arthroscopic control and the knee is immobilized for 6 weeks. In all other cases it is more prudent to follow the conservative regime described above; the cast-brace is worn only until symptoms subside and thereafter movement and muscle-strengthening exercises are encouraged. About half of these patients regain sufficiently good function not to need further treatment. The remainder complain of varying degrees of instability; late assessment will identify those who are likely to benefit from ligament reconstruction.

Isolated tears of the PCL are treated conservatively. Most patients end up with little or no loss of function. However, a few experience instability walking up stairs and some are sufficiently disabled to warrant late reconstruction.

Combined injuries Acute knee ligament injuries resulting in significant loss of function usually involve more than one structure. With combined ACL and collateral ligament injury, reconstruction of the ACL often obviates the need for collateral ligament treatment; however, early operation carries the risk of post-operative joint fibrosis, so it is wiser to start treatment with joint support and physiotherapy in order to restore a good range of movement before following on with ACL reconstruction. A similar approach is adopted for combined injuries involving the PCL, but here all damaged structures will need to be repaired.

Complications

Adhesions If the knee with a partial ligament tear is not actively exercised, torn fibres stick to intact fibres and to bone. The knee 'gives way' with catches of pain; localized tenderness is present, and pain occurs on medial or lateral rotation. The obvious confusion with a torn meniscus can be resolved by the grinding test (page 460), or by manipulation and injection under anaesthesia, which is often curative. If there is still doubt about the possibility of a torn meniscus, MRI or arthroscopy is indicated.

Ossification in the ligament (Pellegrini–Stieda's disease) Occasionally an abduction injury is followed by ossification near the upper attachment of the medial ligament. This is usually discovered as a chance finding in x-rays of the knee.

Instability The knee may continue to give way. The instability tends to get worse and predisposes to osteoarthritis. This important subject is discussed under a separate heading below.

CHRONIC LIGAMENTOUS INSTABILITY

Instability ('giving way') of the knee may be obvious soon after the acute injury has healed, or it may only become apparent much later. It is usually progressive (a meniscectomy is likely to make it worse) but, except in people engaged in strenuous sport, dancing or certain work activities, the disability is often tolerated without complaint. In more severe and long-standing cases, osteoarthritis may eventually supervene.

Functional pathology

Unstable tibiofemoral relationships may result in abnormal sideways tilt (varus or valgus), excessive glide (forwards, backwards or even in an oblique direction), unnatural rotation (internal or external) or combinations of these.

Seldom is only one ligament at fault. Stability is normally maintained by both primary and secondary stabilizers (not to mention the dynamic forces of surrounding muscles). In different positions, different structures come into play as primary stabilizers. Therefore, when testing for *medial and lateral stability*, valgus and varus stresses should be applied with the knee first in full extension and then in 30° of flexion.

Abnormal translation or rotation of the tibia on the femur is even more complex. A positive anterior drawer sign is the result of a torn ACL, but a solitary cruciate injury is unusual. More commonly there *is anterolateral rotatory instability* where, in addition to a torn ACL, the lateral capsule and lateral collateral ligament are torn or 'stretched'. In this instance, not only will the anterior drawer test be positive, but the lateral tibial condyle can be made to sublux forwards as the tibia rotates abnormally around an axis through the medial condyles; this is the basis of the *pivot shift phenomenon* (Losee *et al.*, 1978; Galway and MacIntosh, 1980).

A positive posterior drawer sign means that the posterior cruciate ligament is torn. Soon after injury, however, this sign is difficult to elicit unless the LCL, arcuate ligament and popliteus tendon also are torn. Chronic deficiency of these 3 structures (sometimes referred to as the arcuate complex) and the PCL causes a type of *posterolateral rotatory instability* which is the counterpart of the pivot shift phenomenon. Complete tears of all the posterior structures also allow the knee to hyperextend.

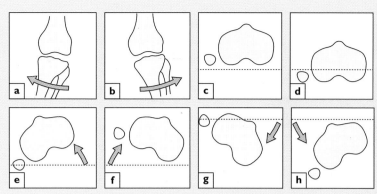

30.5 Types of instability *Straight subluxations*: **(a)** tilting into varus, **(b)** into valgus; **(c)** forwards shift, **(d)** backwards. *Rotatory subluxations*: **(e)** anteromedial instability; **(f)** anterolateral instability; **(g)** posteromedial instability (rare); **(f)** posterolateral instability.

Clinical features

The patient complains of a feeling of insecurity and of giving way. With collateral ligament instability the cause is obvious even to the patient, but with anterolateral rotatory instability the symptoms are more subtle – the knee suddenly gives way as he or she pivots on the affected side (effectively causing a pivot shift to occur). Trickey (1987) noted how patients describe this jerking sensation by grinding the knuckles of clenched fists upon each other. The explanation is that, with the knee just short of full extension, the lateral tibial condyle slips forwards (subluxes); then, as the knee is flexed, the iliotibial band pulls the condyle back into the reduced position with a 'clunk'. For a sportsman, 'cutting' is particularly troublesome. Locking is not a feature of instability and should always suggest an associated meniscal tear.

In the less common posterior cruciate insufficiency, symptoms are mild unless the arcuate ligament complex also is torn or stretched; instability is sometimes felt only on climbing stairs.

The joint looks normal apart from slight wasting; there is rarely any tenderness but excessive movement in one or more directions can usually be demonstrated. Comparison with the normal knee is essential. A useful routine is to examine the knee first for dynamic instability, then for hyperextension, then for increased tilting into varus or valgus (at 0° and 30° knee flexion), then for increased gliding by the drawer tests at 90° and the more specific Lachman test (*see below*), and finally to perform special tests for rotational instability.

Start by watching the patient walk and noting knee posture and movement in the stance phase. Then ask the patient to stand on one leg – those with severe instabilities may not be able to achieve this task, whereas others who do may demonstrate the problem.

Hyperextension is tested with the patient supine and the knee straight; with the patient relaxed, lift each heel in turn. Repeat the test, but this time grasping the medial forefoot – if the tibia sags posteriorly and externally rotates, this suggests both posterior

cruciate and posterolateral capsule are torn (*posterolateral rotatory instability*).

To test stability in the coronal plane, grasp the patient's thigh with one hand and his or her leg with the other and stress the knee in valgus and varus; perform the test first with the knee straight and then flexed at 30°. If the limb is too large for your hands, tuck the leg between your body and your upper arm while your hands support the knee and control the varus and valgus stress.

Next, place the knees at 90° with the feet flat on the couch and the heels lined up; the quadriceps should be relaxed. Looking from the side, note if there is any posterior sag of the upper tibia by checking the levels of the tibial tuberosities on each leg – a posterior sag is a sure sign of posterior cruciate laxity. Then ask the patient to slide the foot slowly down the couch; as the quadriceps contracts, the sag is pulled up and the proximal tibia shifts forwards (Daniel *et al.*, 1988).

Again with the knees flexed at 90° and both feet resting on the couch (it is useful to sit across the couch to prevent the feet sliding forwards), grasp the upper tibia in both hands and, making sure the hamstrings are relaxed, test for anterior and posterior laxity (the drawer signs). A more reliable test for anterior cruciate laxity is to examine for anteroposterior displacement with the knee flexed to 20° (the Lachman test). Hold the calf with one hand and the thigh with the other, and try to displace the joint backwards and forwards. Surgeons with small hands may find it easier to do the Lachman test with the patient prone (Feagin and Cooke, 1989).

Rotational stability can be tested in several ways:

Modified drawer test The anterior drawer test is performed with the tibia in 30° of internal rotation; if positive, it suggests anterolateral rotatory instability. Likewise, a positive drawer sign with the knee in external rotation (about 15°) suggests anteromedial rotatory instability.

Jerk test This is a demonstration of the pivot shift phenomenon. The examiner supports the knee in 90°

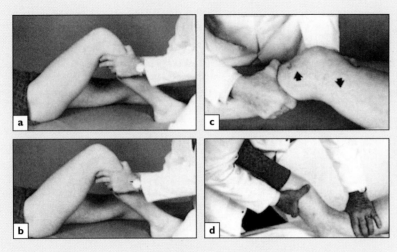

30.6 Testing for cruciate ligament tears
(**a, b**) Testing at 90° may reveal a positive drawer sign but (**c**) Lachman's test is more sensitive. (**d**) For those surgeons with small hands, it is best performed with the patient prone.

of flexion with the tibia internally rotated (the reduced position); the knee is then gradually extended while a valgus stress is applied. In a positive test, as the knee reaches 20 or 30°, there is a sudden jerk as the lateral tibial condyle slips forwards *(anterolateral rotatory subluxation)*. A modification of the classic jerk test may be used to diagnose *posterolateral rotatory instabilty*: the tibia is held in external rotation and a valgus stress is applied to the knee; a characteristic 'clunk' as the knee is extended signals the change from a subluxed to a reduced position (the reverse pivot shift).

MacIntosh test The test originally described by MacIntosh is quite difficult and is often more reliably performed with the patient anaesthetized. Starting with the knee fully extended (and supporting the foot and knee in a way similar to the jerk test), the knee is gradually flexed; as the joint begins to flex, the lateral tibial condyle subluxes anteriorly but as flexion increases (again around 20 or 30°) there is a sudden 'jump' as the condyle slips back to its reduced position.

Imaging

MRI is a reliable method of diagnosing both cruciate ligament and meniscal injuries, providing almost 100% sensitivity and over 90% accuracy.

Arthroscopy

Arthroscopy is indicated if: (1) the diagnosis, or the extent of the ligament injury, remains in doubt; (2) other lesions, such as meniscal tears or cartilage damage, are suspected; or (3) surgical treatment is anticipated. Partial meniscectomy and removal of loose cartilage tags can be performed at the same time.

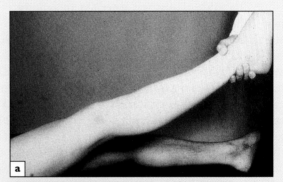

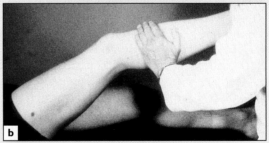

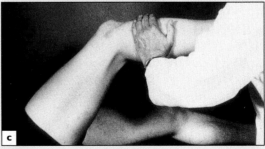

30.7 Cruciate ligament tears – MacIntosh's test (**a**) The leg is lifted with the knee straight. (**b**) The fibula is pushed forwards – if the anterior cruciate is torn the lateral tibial condyle is now subluxed forwards. (**c**) It is held forwards while the knee is flexed; at 30–40° the condyle reduces with a jerk. This may be painful and an alternative method is to lift the straight leg by holding it with both hands just above the ankle, rotating the leg inwards, then flexing the knee – the jerk is often visible and usually painless.

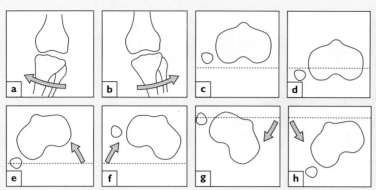

30.5 Types of instability *Straight subluxations*: **(a)** tilting into varus, **(b)** into valgus; **(c)** forwards shift, **(d)** backwards. *Rotatory subluxations*: **(e)** anteromedial instability; **(f)** anterolateral instability; **(g)** posteromedial instability (rare); **(f)** posterolateral instability.

Clinical features

The patient complains of a feeling of insecurity and of giving way. With collateral ligament instability the cause is obvious even to the patient, but with anterolateral rotatory instability the symptoms are more subtle – the knee suddenly gives way as he or she pivots on the affected side (effectively causing a pivot shift to occur). Trickey (1987) noted how patients describe this jerking sensation by grinding the knuckles of clenched fists upon each other. The explanation is that, with the knee just short of full extension, the lateral tibial condyle slips forwards (subluxes); then, as the knee is flexed, the iliotibial band pulls the condyle back into the reduced position with a 'clunk'. For a sportsman, 'cutting' is particularly troublesome. Locking is not a feature of instability and should always suggest an associated meniscal tear.

In the less common posterior cruciate insufficiency, symptoms are mild unless the arcuate ligament complex also is torn or stretched; instability is sometimes felt only on climbing stairs.

The joint looks normal apart from slight wasting; there is rarely any tenderness but excessive movement in one or more directions can usually be demonstrated. Comparison with the normal knee is essential. A useful routine is to examine the knee first for dynamic instability, then for hyperextension, then for increased tilting into varus or valgus (at 0° and 30° knee flexion), then for increased gliding by the drawer tests at 90° and the more specific Lachman test (*see below*), and finally to perform special tests for rotational instability.

Start by watching the patient walk and noting knee posture and movement in the stance phase. Then ask the patient to stand on one leg – those with severe instabilities may not be able to achieve this task, whereas others who do may demonstrate the problem.

Hyperextension is tested with the patient supine and the knee straight; with the patient relaxed, lift each heel in turn. Repeat the test, but this time grasping the medial forefoot – if the tibia sags posteriorly and externally rotates, this suggests both posterior cruciate and posterolateral capsule are torn (*posterolateral rotatory instability*).

To test stability in the coronal plane, grasp the patient's thigh with one hand and his or her leg with the other and stress the knee in valgus and varus; perform the test first with the knee straight and then flexed at 30°. If the limb is too large for your hands, tuck the leg between your body and your upper arm while your hands support the knee and control the varus and valgus stress.

Next, place the knees at 90° with the feet flat on the couch and the heels lined up; the quadriceps should be relaxed. Looking from the side, note if there is any posterior sag of the upper tibia by checking the levels of the tibial tuberosities on each leg – a posterior sag is a sure sign of posterior cruciate laxity. Then ask the patient to slide the foot slowly down the couch; as the quadriceps contracts, the sag is pulled up and the proximal tibia shifts forwards (Daniel *et al.*, 1988).

Again with the knees flexed at 90° and both feet resting on the couch (it is useful to sit across the couch to prevent the feet sliding forwards), grasp the upper tibia in both hands and, making sure the hamstrings are relaxed, test for anterior and posterior laxity (the drawer signs). A more reliable test for anterior cruciate laxity is to examine for anteroposterior displacement with the knee flexed to 20° (the Lachman test). Hold the calf with one hand and the thigh with the other, and try to displace the joint backwards and forwards. Surgeons with small hands may find it easier to do the Lachman test with the patient prone (Feagin and Cooke, 1989).

Rotational stability can be tested in several ways:

Modified drawer test The anterior drawer test is performed with the tibia in 30° of internal rotation; if positive, it suggests anterolateral rotatory instability. Likewise, a positive drawer sign with the knee in external rotation (about 15°) suggests anteromedial rotatory instability.

Jerk test This is a demonstration of the pivot shift phenomenon. The examiner supports the knee in 90°

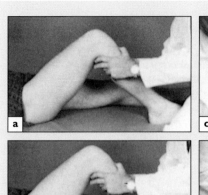
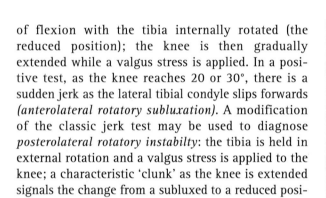
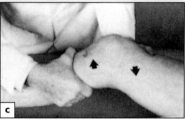

30.6 Testing for cruciate ligament tears (**a, b**) Testing at 90° may reveal a positive drawer sign but (**c**) Lachman's test is more sensitive. (**d**) For those surgeons with small hands, it is best performed with the patient prone.

of flexion with the tibia internally rotated (the reduced position); the knee is then gradually extended while a valgus stress is applied. In a positive test, as the knee reaches 20 or 30°, there is a sudden jerk as the lateral tibial condyle slips forwards *(anterolateral rotatory subluxation)*. A modification of the classic jerk test may be used to diagnose *posterolateral rotatory instabilty*: the tibia is held in external rotation and a valgus stress is applied to the knee; a characteristic 'clunk' as the knee is extended signals the change from a subluxed to a reduced position (the reverse pivot shift).

MacIntosh test The test originally described by MacIntosh is quite difficult and is often more reliably performed with the patient anaesthetized. Starting with the knee fully extended (and supporting the foot and knee in a way similar to the jerk test), the knee is gradually flexed; as the joint begins to flex, the lateral tibial condyle subluxes anteriorly but as flexion increases (again around 20 or 30°) there is a sudden 'jump' as the condyle slips back to its reduced position.

Imaging

MRI is a reliable method of diagnosing both cruciate ligament and meniscal injuries, providing almost 100% sensitivity and over 90% accuracy.

Arthroscopy

Arthroscopy is indicated if: (1) the diagnosis, or the extent of the ligament injury, remains in doubt; (2) other lesions, such as meniscal tears or cartilage damage, are suspected; or (3) surgical treatment is anticipated. Partial meniscectomy and removal of loose cartilage tags can be performed at the same time.

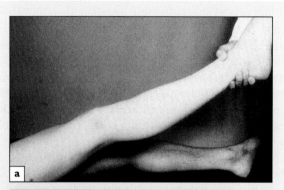
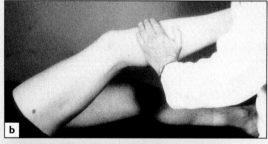
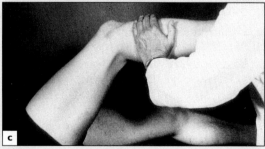

30.7 Cruciate ligament tears – MacIntosh's test (**a**) The leg is lifted with the knee straight. (**b**) The fibula is pushed forwards – if the anterior cruciate is torn the lateral tibial condyle is now subluxed forwards. (**c**) It is held forwards while the knee is flexed; at 30–40° the condyle reduces with a jerk. This may be painful and an alternative method is to lift the straight leg by holding it with both hands just above the ankle, rotating the leg inwards, then flexing the knee – the jerk is often visible and usually painless.

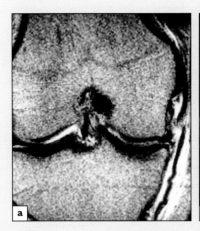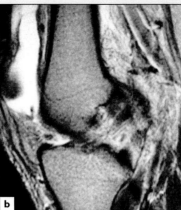

30.8 Torn knee ligaments – MRI (a) Coronal T2-weighted image showing a medial collateral ligament tear with surrounding oedema and joint effusion. (b) Sagittal T2-weighted image showing an intra-substance tear of the anterior cruciate ligament with a large joint effusion.

Treatment

Most patients with chronic instability have reasonably good function and will not require an operation. The first approach should always be a supervised, disciplined and progressively vigorous exercise programme to strengthen the quadriceps and the hamstrings. At the end of 6 months the patient is re-evaluated.

The indications for operation are: (1) recurrent locking, with MRI or arthroscopic confirmation of a meniscal tear (arthroscopic meniscectomy alone may alleviate the patient's symptoms, though this may later lead to increased instability); (2) intolerable symptoms of giving way; (3) suboptimal function in a sportsman or others with similarly demanding occupations (even in this group, some patients will accept the use of a knee-brace for specific activities that are known to cause trouble); and (4) adolescents with ligament injuries (the long-term effects of chronic instability in this group are more marked).

There is still much controversy about the need for surgery in partial tears of the ACL. The decision should be made on the basis of symptoms and functional capacity rather than the appearance of the ligament. Young adults with chronic anterior cruciate insufficiency and proved partial tears show diminished activity and run the risk of developing secondary problems such as meniscal lesions, cartilage damage, increasing instability and (eventually) secondary osteoarthritis (Fruensgaard and Johannsen, 1989). With careful follow-up and reassessment, those most at risk can usually be identified and advised to undergo reconstructive surgery.

OPERATIVE TREATMENT

Medial collateral ligament insufficiency seldom causes much disability unless there is an associated anterior cruciate tear. However, if valgus instability is marked, and particularly if it is progressive, ligament reconstruction, by advancing the proximal or distal end of the ligament, restoring the tension of the posteromedial capsule and reinforcing the medial structures with the semimembranosus tendon, is justified.

Isolated lateral instability is uncommon and symptoms are rarely troublesome enough to warrant surgery. If operative reconstruction is attempted, it should follow the lines described above.

Isolated PCL insufficiency rarely causes any loss of function. Conservative treatment (mainly quadriceps strengthening exercises) will usually suffice.

Isolated ACL insufficiency is uncommon and can usually be managed by physiotherapy. Splints or braces may be used to speed the return to weight-bearing. Patients seeking to resume competitive sport may need something more; reconstructive surgery involves replacing the torn ACL with an autologous graft, usually a strip of patellar tendon with bone attachments at either end.

Combined injuries Anterolateral and anteromedial rotatory instabilities are the commonest reasons for reconstructive surgery. When the ACL is damaged together with either the MCL or LCL, reconstruction of the ACL alone often suffices. The torn ACL is replaced by an autograft (usually from the patellar tendon but sometimes from hamstring tendons) or by an allograft. The ideal synthetic graft has yet to be developed. Post-operative care will depend on the fixation of the new ligament; in many cases a short period of splintage can be followed by regular physiotherapy to avoid joint stiffness and improve muscle control. Many patients return to sports within 6 months.

The treatment of combined injuries in which the PCL is involved is changing; until recently, it was thought that most of these patients had good function and therefore did not need reconstructive surgery. Newer studies have shown that there is an increased risk of osteoarthritis (especially of the medial compartment) and this is seen as an indication for PCL reconstruction in patients who have more than 10–15mm of posterior tibial translation in the drawer test. Unlike injuries involving the ACL, combination injuries involving the PCL require all damaged structures to be repaired.

FRACTURED TIBIAL INTERCONDYLAR EMINENCE OR SPINE

Severe valgus or varus stress, or twisting injuries, may severely strain the knee ligaments and cause a fracture of the intercondylar eminence or tibial spine. This is, in fact, a type of traction injury, the adolescent variant of a cruciate ligament tear. It is said to be most common after bicycle accidents.

Pathological anatomy

The detached bone fragment (usually the anterior part of the intercondylar eminence) may remain almost undisplaced, held in position by the soft tissues; it may be partially displaced, the anterior end lifted away on a posterior hinge; or it may be completely detached and displaced. Because its articular surface is covered with cartilage – invisible on x-ray – the image seen on x-ray is smaller than the actual fragment.

Clinical features

The patient – usually an older child or adolescent – presents with a swollen, immobile knee. The joint feels tense, tender and 'doughy' and aspiration will reveal a haemarthrosis. Examination under anaesthesia may show that extension is blocked. There may also be associated ligament injuries; always test for varus and valgus stability and cruciate laxity.

X-RAY
The fracture is not always obvious and a small posterior fragment may be missed unless the x-rays are carefully examined. The fragment – often including part of the intercondylar eminence – may be undisplaced, tilted upwards or completely detached.

If a collateral ligament injury is suspected, stress x-rays should be performed under general anaesthesia.

Treatment

Under anaesthesia the joint is aspirated and gently manipulated into full extension. Often the fragment falls back into position and the x-ray shows that the fracture is reduced. If the fragment is only very slightly elevated but the knee able to extend fully, the position can be accepted. If there is a block to full extension, or if the bone fragment remains significantly displaced, operative reduction is essential. The fragment – often larger than suspected – is restored to its bed and anchored by sutures. Small screws can be used if the physis has closed.

After either closed or open reduction, a long plaster cylinder is applied with the knee almost straight; it is worn for 6 weeks and then movements are encouraged.

The outcome is usually good and full movement is regained within 3 months; although there may be some residual laxity on examination, this rarely causes symptoms.

Complications

Unreduced fracture The diagnosis may be missed or the fragment may be left unreduced. This should be suspected if the knee fails to regain full extension within 4 months of injury; the diagnosis can be confirmed by x-ray or CT. Treatment is difficult: if the prominent fragment is excised, there may be some loss of cruciate function, although this need not necessarily cause disability; if the ligament has not contracted, it may be possible to excavate the fragment and embed it more deeply.

Associated ligament injury Persistent instability suggests an associated collateral ligament injury. Stress x-rays will help with the diagnosis.

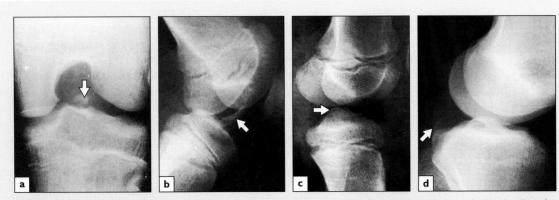

30.9 Tibial spine fracture (a, b) This young man injured his knee while playing football; x-rays showed a large, displaced avulsion fracture of the tibial spine. **(c)** An undisplaced tibial spine fracture. **(d)** Posterior fractures, with avulsion of the posterior cruciate ligament, are often missed.

DISLOCATION OF THE KNEE

The knee can be dislocated only by considerable violence, as in a road accident. The cruciate ligaments and one or both lateral ligaments are torn.

Clinical features

There is severe bruising, swelling and gross deformity. The circulation in the foot must be examined because the popliteal artery may be torn or obstructed. Distal sensation and movement should be tested to exclude nerve injury.

X-RAY

In addition to the dislocation, the films occasionally reveal a fracture of the tibial spine (cruciate ligament avulsion). If there is any doubt about the circulation, an arteriogram should be obtained.

Treatment

Reduction under anaesthesia is urgent; this is usually achieved by pulling directly in the line of the leg, but hyperextension must be avoided because of the danger to the popliteal vessels. If reduction is achieved, the limb is rested on a back-splint with the knee in 15° of flexion; the circulation is checked repeatedly during the next week. Because of swelling, a plaster cylinder is dangerous. If the joint is unstable, an anterior external fixator can be applied.

Occasionally closed reduction fails because the torn medial ligament lies between the femur and the tibial condyles; open reduction must then be performed, the ligament is sutured back into place and the capsule is repaired. Similarly, if there is an open wound, or vascular damage which needs operation, the opportunity is taken to repair the ligaments and capsule. Otherwise, these structures are left undisturbed.

When swelling has subsided, a cast is applied and is worn for 12 weeks. Quadriceps muscle exercises are practised from the start. Weight-bearing in the plaster is permitted as soon as the patient can lift his or her leg. Knee movements are regained when the plaster is removed.

Complications

EARLY
Arterial damage Popliteal artery damage is common and needs immediate repair.

Nerve injury The lateral popliteal nerve may be injured, but fortunately it usually recovers by itself.

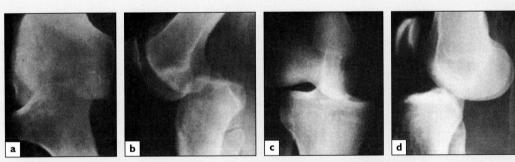

30.10 Dislocations of the knee (**a, b**) Posterolateral dislocation; (**c, d**) anteromedial dislocation.

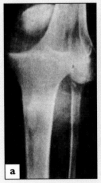 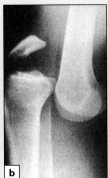 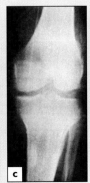 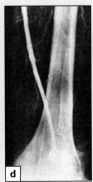

30.11 Knee dislocation and vascular trauma (**a, b**) This patient was admitted with a dislocated knee. After reduction (**c**) the x-ray looked satisfactory, but the circulation did not. (**d**) An arteriogram showed vascular cut-off just above the knee; had this not been recognized and treated, amputation might have been necessary.

LATE

Joint instability Anteroposterior glide or a lateral wobble often remains but, provided the quadriceps muscle is sufficiently powerful, the disability is not severe.

Stiffness Loss of movement, due to prolonged immobilization, is a common problem and may be even more troublesome than instability.

ACUTE INJURIES OF THE EXTENSOR APPARATUS

Disruption of the extensor apparatus may occur in the quadriceps tendon, at the attachment of the quadriceps tendon to the proximal surface of the patella, through the patella and retinacular expansions, at the junction of the patella and the patellar ligament, in the patellar ligament or at the insertion of the patellar ligament to the tibial tubercle. *(Note: The patellar ligament is often called the patellar tendon.)*

In all but direct fractures of the patella, the mechanism of injury is the same: sudden resisted extension of the knee or (essentially the same thing) sudden passive flexion of the knee while the quadriceps is contracting. The patient gives a history of stumbling on a stair, catching the foot while running or kicking hard at a muddy football.

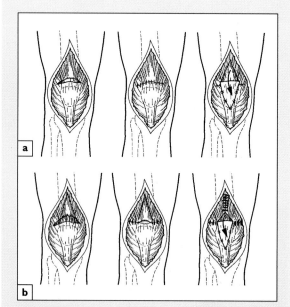

30.12 Repairing ruptures of the quadriceps tendon
(a) Acute ruptures can usually be sutured and reinforced with a partial thickness flap of the quadriceps tendon (Scuderi). When the patient presents late (b), the retracted ends may have to be bridged by a full thickness V-shaped flap (Codivilla).

The lesion tends to occur at progressively higher levels with increasing age: adolescents suffer avulsion fractures of the tibial tubercle; young adult sportsmen tear the patellar ligament, middle-aged adults fracture their patellae; and older people (as well as those whose tissues are weakened by chronic illness or corticosteroid medication) suffer acute tears of the quadriceps tendon.

RUPTURE OF THE QUADRICEPS TENDON

The patient is usually elderly, may have a history of diabetes or rheumatoid disease, or may have been treated with corticosteroids. Occasionally acute rupture is seen in a young athlete. The typical injury is followed by tearing pain and giving way of the knee. There is bruising and local tenderness; sometimes a gap can be felt proximal to the patella. Active knee extension is either impossible (suggesting a complete rupture) or weak (partial rupture). The diagnosis can be confirmed by MRI.

Treatment

Partial tears Non-operative treatment will suffice: a plaster cylinder is applied for 6 weeks, followed by physiotherapy which concentrates on restoring knee flexion and quadriceps strength.

Complete tears Early operation is needed, or else the ruptured fibres will retract and repair will be more difficult. End-to-end suturing can be reinforced by turning down a partial thickness triangular flap of quadriceps tendon proximal to the repair (Scuderi). If the tendon has been avulsed from the proximal pole of the patella, it should be re-attached to a trough created at that site using pull-through sutures. Post-operatively the knee is held in extension in a cast for 6 weeks; this is followed by physiotherapy.

'Chronic' ruptures (usually the result of delayed presentations or missed diagnoses) are difficult to repair because the ends have retracted. The gap can often be made smaller by closing the medial and lateral ends, and the remaining central gap is then covered by a full thickness V-flap turned down from the proximal quadriceps tendon (Codivilla). A pull-out or cerclage wire protects the repair.

The results of acute repairs are good, with most patients regaining full power, a good range of movement and little or no extensor lag. Late repairs are less predictable.

RUPTURE OF THE PATELLAR LIGAMENT

This is an uncommon injury; it is usually seen in young athletes and the tear is almost always at the proximal or distal attachment of the ligament. There may be a previous history of 'tendinitis' and local injection of corticosteroid.

The patient gives a history of sudden pain on forced extension of the knee, followed by bruising, swelling and tenderness at the lower edge of the patella or more distally.

X-rays may show a high-riding patella and a telltale flake of bone torn from the proximal or distal attachment of the ligament.

MRI will help to distinguish a partial from a complete tear.

Treatment

Partial tears can be treated by applying a plaster cylinder. *Complete tears* need operative repair or re-attachment to bone. Tension on the suture line can be lessened by inserting a temporary pull-out wire to draw the patella downwards towards the tibial tuberosity. Post-operatively the knee is immobilized in extension for 6 weeks.

Late cases are difficult to manage because of proximal retraction of the patella. A two-stage operation may be needed: first to release the contracted tissues and apply traction directly to the patella, then at a later stage to repair the patellar ligament and reinforce it with fascia lata. Here, again, a tension-relieving pull-out wire is helpful. Post-operatively a long leg cast is used to hold the knee in extension for 6 weeks; this is followed by a further period in a knee brace until the knee feels absolutely stable.

Early repair of acute ruptures gives excellent results. Late repairs are less successful and the patient may be left with a permanent extension lag.

FRACTURES OF THE TIBIAL TUBERCLE

Fracture or avulsion of the tibial tubercle usually occurs as a sports injury in young people. If the knee is suddenly forced into flexion while the quadriceps is contracting, a fragment of the tubercle – or sometimes the entire apophysis – may be wrenched from the bone. The diagnosis is suggested by the history. The area over the tubercle is swollen and tender; active extension causes pain.

The lateral x-ray shows the fracture. Sometimes the patella is abnormally high, having lost part of its distal attachment.

An incomplete fracture can be treated by applying a long-leg cast with the knee in extension for 6 weeks. Complete separation requires open reduction and fixation with pins or cancellous screws; a cast is applied for 6 weeks.

Osgood–Schlatter's disease Repetitive strain on the patellar ligament may give rise to a painful, tender swelling over the tibial tubercle. The condition is fairly common in adolescents who are keen on sport. Treatment consists of restricting sports activities until the symptoms subside (see page 478).

FRACTURED PATELLA

The patella is a sesamoid bone in continuity with the quadriceps tendon and the patellar ligament (also called the patellar tendon). There are additional insertions from the vastus medialis and lateralis into the medial and lateral edges of the patella. The extensor 'strap' is completed by the medial and lateral extensor retinacula (or quadriceps expansions) which bypass the patella and insert into the proximal tibia.

The mechanical function of the patella is to hold the entire extensor 'strap' away from the centre of rotation of the knee, thereby lengthening the anterior lever arm and increasing the efficiency of the quadriceps.

The key to the management of patellar fractures is the state of the entire extensor mechanism. If the extensor retinacula are intact, active knee extension is still possible even if the patella itself is fractured.

Mechanism of injury and pathological anatomy

The patella may be fractured, either by a direct force that cracks the bone like a tile under the blow of a hammer or by an indirect traction force that pulls the bone apart (and often tears the extensor expansions as well).

Direct injury – usually a fall onto the knee or a blow against the dashboard of a car – causes either an undisplaced crack or else a comminuted ('stellate') fracture without severe damage to the extensor expansions.

Indirect injury occurs, typically, when someone catches his or her foot against a solid obstacle and, to avoid falling, contracts the quadriceps muscle forcefully. This is a transverse fracture with a gap between the fragments.

Clinical features

Following one of the typical injuries, the knee becomes swollen and painful. There may be an abrasion or bruising over the front of the joint. The patella is tender and sometimes a gap can be felt.

Active knee extension should be tested. If the patient can lift the straight leg, the quadriceps mechanism is still intact. If this manoeuvre is too painful, active extension can be tested with the patient lying on his or her side.

If there is an effusion, aspiration may reveal the presence of blood and fat droplets.

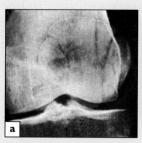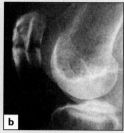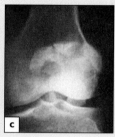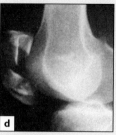

30.13 Fractured patella – stellate (**a, b**) A fracture with little or no displacement can be treated conservatively by a posterior slab of plaster which is removed several times a day for gentle active exercises. (**c, d**) With severe comminution, patellectomy is arguably the best treatment, although some surgeons would consider preserving as many useful fragments as possible.

X-RAY

The x-ray may show one or more fine fracture lines without displacement, multiple fracture lines with irregular displacement or a transverse fracture with a gap between the fragments. Comparative x-rays of the opposite knee may help to distinguish normal from abnormal appearances in undisplaced fractures.

Patellar fractures are classified as transverse, longitudinal, polar or comminuted (stellate). Any of these may be either undisplaced or displaced. Separation of the fragments is significant if it is sufficient to create a step on the articular surface of the patella or, in the case of a transverse fracture, if the gap is more than 3mm.

A fracture line running obliquely across the superolateral corner of the patella should not be confused with the smooth, regular line of a (normal) bipartite patella. Check the opposite knee; bipartite patella is often bilateral.

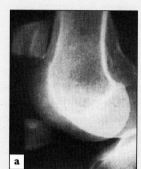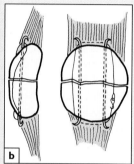

30.14 Fractured patella – transverse The separated fragments (**a**) are transfixed by Kirschner wires; malleable wire is then looped around the protruding ends of the Kirschner wires and tightened over the front of the patella (**b**).

Treatment

UNDISPLACED OR MINIMALLY DISPLACED FRACTURES

If there is a haemarthrosis it is aspirated. The extensor mechanism is intact and treatment is mainly protective. A plaster cylinder holding the knee straight is worn for 3–4 weeks, and during this time quadriceps exercises are practised every day.

COMMINUTED (STELLATE) FRACTURE

The extensor expansions are intact and the patient may be able to lift the leg. However, the undersurface of the patella is irregular and there is a serious risk of damage to the patellofemoral joint. For this reason some people advocate patellectomy, whatever the degree of displacement. To others it seems reasonable to preserve the patella if the fragments are not severely displaced (or to remove only those fragments that obviously distort the articular surface); a back-

slab is applied but removed several times daily for exercises to mould the fragments into position and to maintain mobility.

DISPLACED TRANSVERSE FRACTURE

The lateral expansions are torn and the entire extensor mechanism is disrupted. Operation is essential.

Through a longitudinal incision the fragments are reduced and transfixed with two stiff Kirschner wires; flexible wire is then looped tightly around the protruding Kirschner wires and over the front of the patella. The tears in the extensor expansions are then repaired. A plaster backslab is worn until active extension of the knee is regained; the backslab may be removed every day to permit active knee-flexion exercises.

Small residual irregularities of the articular surface may be smoothed away by active use. If severe symptoms and signs develop later, the patella can then be excised; the knee recovers more quickly than it does after immediate post-traumatic patellectomy.

Outcome

Patients usually regain good function but, depending on the severity of the injury, there is a significant incidence of late patellofemoral osteoarthritis.

DISLOCATION OF THE PATELLA

Because the knee is normally angled in slight valgus, there is a natural tendency for the patella to pull towards the lateral side when the quadriceps muscle contracts. Lateral deviation of the patella during knee extension is prevented by a number of factors: the patella is seated in the intercondylar groove, which has a high lateral 'embankment'; the force of extensor muscle contraction pulls it firmly into the groove; and the extensor retinacula and patellofemoral ligaments guide it centrally as it tracks along the intercondylar runway. The most important static 'checkrein' on the medial side is the medial patellofemoral ligament, a more or less distinct structure extending from the superomedial border of the patella towards the medial femoral condyle deep to vastus medialis (Conlan *et al.*, 1993). Additional restraint is provided by the medial patellomeniscal and patellotibial ligaments and the associated medial retinacular fibres. In the normal knee, considerable force is required to wrench the patella out of its track. However, if the intercondylar groove is unusually shallow, or the patella seated higher than usual or the ligaments abnormally lax, dislocation is not that difficult.

Mechanism of injury

While the knee is flexed and the quadriceps muscle relaxed, the patella may be forced laterally by direct violence; this is rare. More often traumatic dislocation is due to indirect force: sudden, severe contraction of the quadriceps muscle while the knee is stretched in valgus and external rotation. Typically this occurs in field sports when a runner dodges to one side. The patella dislocates laterally and the medial patellofemoral ligament and retinacular fibres may be torn.

Predisposing factors are anatomical variations such as genu valgum, tibial torsion, high-riding patella (patella alta) and a shallow intercondylar groove, as well as patellar hypermobility due to generalized ligamentous laxity or localized muscle weakness.

Clinical features

In a 'first-time' dislocation the patient may experience a tearing sensation and a feeling that the knee has gone 'out of joint'; when running, he or she may collapse and fall to the ground. Often the patella springs back into position spontaneously; however, if it remains unreduced there is an obvious (if somewhat misleading) deformity: the displaced patella, seated on the lateral side of the knee, is not easily noticed but the uncovered medial femoral condyle is unduly prominent and may be mistaken for the patella; neither active nor passive movement is possible. In the rare intra-articular (downwards) dislocation the patella is stuck between the condyles and there is a marked prominence on the front of the knee.

If the dislocation has reduced spontaneously, the knee may be swollen and there may be bruising and tenderness on the medial side. If there is fluid in the joint, aspiration may show that it is blood-stained; the presence of fat droplets suggests a concurrent osteochondral fracture.

With recurrent dislocation the symptoms and signs are much less marked, though still unpleasant. After spontaneous reduction the knee looks normal, but the apprehension test is positive.

IMAGING

Anteroposterior, lateral and tangential ('skyline') *x-ray views* are needed. In an unreduced dislocation, the patella is seen to be laterally displaced and tilted or rotated. In 5% of cases there is an associated osteochondral fracture.

MRI may reveal a soft-tissue lesion (e.g. disruption of the medial patellofemoral ligament) as well as articular cartilage and/or bone damage.

Treatment

In most cases the patella can be pushed back into place without much difficulty and anaesthesia is not always

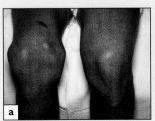
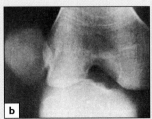
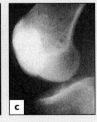

30.15 Dislocation of the patella (**a**) The right patella has dislocated laterally; the flattened appearance is typical. (**b**, **c**) Anteroposterior and lateral films of traumatic dislocation of the patella.

necessary; the exception is an intra-articular (intercondylar) dislocation which may need open reduction.

If there are no signs of soft tissue rupture – i.e. there is minimal swelling, no bruising and little tenderness – cast splintage alone will usually suffice. The knee is aspirated and then immobilized in almost full extension; a small pad along the lateral edge of the patella may help to keep the medial soft tissues relaxed. The cast is retained for 2 or 3 weeks and the patient then undergoes a long period (2–3 months) of quadriceps strengthening exercises.

The same approach has been advocated for more severe forms of dislocation. However, if there is much bruising, swelling and tenderness medially, the patellofemoral ligaments and retinacular tissues are probably torn and immediate operative repair will reduce the likelihood of later recurrent dislocation.

OPERATIVE TREATMENT

The area is approached through a medial incision. If the patellofemoral ligament is avulsed from the femur, it is reattached with suitable anchors. Midsubstance tears of the ligaments are sutured directly. At the same time, if the lateral retinaculum is tight it is released. Osteochondral fragments are removed – unless they are single, large and amenable to re-attachment. Post-operatively a padded cylinder cast is applied with the knee in extension; this can be renewed when the swelling has subsided and is retained for 6 weeks, during which time weight-bearing is permitted. After removal of the cast, quadriceps exercises are encouraged.

Complications

Recurrent dislocation The main 'complication' is recurrent dislocation. Patients treated non-operatively for a first-time dislocation have a 15–20% chance of suffering further dislocations. This depends also on whether there are other predisposing abnormalities, and prevention consists of dealing with all these conditions (the subjects of recurrent dislocation, subluxation, chronic patellar instability and patellar mal-tracking are dealt with in Chapter 20).

OSTEOCHONDRAL INJURIES

Osteochondral fractures and osteochondritis dissecans are similar injuries of the articular cartilage and subchondral bone. The knee joint is a common site for both conditions. The lesion is usually located on one of the femoral condyles, the intercondylar groove or the medial facet of the patella, and is thought to be due to the patella striking the opposed articular surface.

OSTEOCHONDRAL FRACTURES

The patient gives a history of patellar dislocation or a blow to the front of the knee. The joint is swollen and aspiration yields blood-stained fluid mixed with fat globules.

Standard anteroposterior and lateral x-rays seldom show the abnormality; if the diagnosis is suspected, tunnel and patellar skyline views are needed, and even then the fracture may be hard to see because the damaged area consists largely of articular cartilage. MRI or arthroscopy will be more helpful.

Treatment Small fragments should be removed as they may cause symptoms. Larger fragments, and especially those from load-bearing areas, can be reattached with smooth pins or screws (counter-sunk Herbert or small fragment screws). Post-operatively a long leg cast is applied for 6 weeks before movement is allowed.

Sometimes a large area of cartilage damage, or even a crater, is discovered on the anterior intercondylar surface. In the past it was felt that little could be done about this, except trimming of any ragged parts. More recently, cartilage transplantation into these defects has shown promising results.

OSTEOCHONDRITIS DISSECANS

Teenagers and young adults who complain of intermittent pain in the knee are sometimes found to have developed a small segment of osteochondral necrosis, usually on the lateral aspect of the medial femoral condyle. This is probably a traumatic lesion, caused by repetitive contact with the overlying patella or an adjacent ridge on the tibial plateau. The condition is described in Chapter 6.

TIBIAL PLATEAU FRACTURES

Mechanism of injury

Fractures of the tibial plateau are caused by a varus or valgus force combined with axial loading (a pure valgus force is more likely to rupture the ligaments). This is sometimes the result of a car striking a pedestrian (hence the term 'bumper fracture'); more often it is due to a fall from a height in which the knee is forced into valgus or varus. The tibial condyle is crushed or split by the opposing femoral condyle, which remains intact.

Pathological anatomy

The fracture pattern and degree of displacement depend on the type and direction of force as well as the quality of the bone at the upper end of the tibia. The most useful classification is that of Schatzker (1987).

Type 1 – vertical split of the lateral condyle This is a fracture through dense bone, usually in younger people. It may be virtually undisplaced, or the wedge-shaped condylar fragment may be pushed inferiorly and tilted; the damaged lateral meniscus may be trapped in the crevice.

Type 2 – vertical split of the lateral condyle combined with depression of the adjacent load-bearing part of the condyle The wedge fragment, which varies in size from a small piece of the condylar rim to a substantial part of the condyle, is displaced laterally; the joint is widened and, if the fracture is not reduced, may later develop a valgus deformity.

Type 3 – depression of the articular surface with an intact condylar rim This injury, which is the commonest type of plateau fracture, occurs in older people who are somewhat osteoporotic. It is usually due to low-energy trauma. The joint is usually stable and may tolerate early movement.

Type 4 – fracture of the medial tibial condyle Two types of fracture are seen: (a) a depressed, crush fracture of osteoporotic bone in an elderly person (a low-energy lesion), and (b) a high-energy fracture resulting in a condylar split which runs obliquely from the intercondylar eminence to the medial cortex. The momentary varus angulation may be severe enough to cause a rupture of the lateral collateral ligament and a traction injury of the peroneal nerve. The severity of these injuries should not be underestimated.

Type 5 – fracture of both condyles Both condyles are split and the tibial shaft is wedged between them.

Type 6 – combined condylar and subcondylar fractures This is a high-energy injury which may result in severe comminution. The tibial shaft is effectively disconnected from the tibial condyles.

Clinical features

The knee is swollen and may be deformed. Bruising is usually extensive and the tissues feel 'doughy' because of haemarthrosis. Gentle examination (or examination under anaesthesia) may suggest medial or lateral instability. The leg and foot should be carefully examined for signs of vascular or neurological injury. Traction injury of the peroneal or tibial nerves is not uncommon and it is important to establish whether this is present at the time of admission and before operation.

X-RAY
Anteroposterior, lateral and oblique x-rays will usually show the fracture, but the amount of comminution or

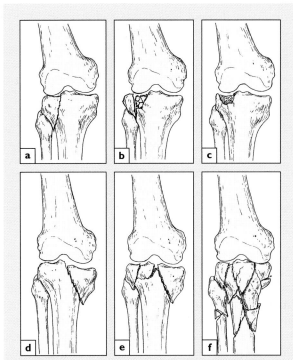

30.16 Tibial plateau fractures (**a**) Type 1 – simple split of the lateral condyle. (**b**) Type 2 – a split of the lateral condyle with a more central area of depression. (**c**) Type 3 – depression of the lateral condyle with an intact rim. (**d**) Type 4 – a fracture of the medial condyle. (**e**) Type 5 – fractures of both condyles, but with the central portion of the metaphysis still connected to the tibial shaft. (**f**) Type 6 – combined condylar and subcondylar fractures; effectively a disconnection of the shaft from the metaphysis.

plateau depression may not be appreciated without tomography. With CT, reconstruction of axial images can provide sagittal and coronal views. It is important not to miss the posterior condylar component in high-energy condylar fractures because this may require separate posteromedial or posterolateral exposure for internal fixation. Stress views (under anaesthesia) are sometimes helpful in assessing the degree of joint instability. With a crushed lateral condyle the medial ligament is often intact, but with a crushed medial condyle the lateral ligament is often torn.

Treatment

Treatment by traction is simple and often produces a well-functioning knee, but residual angulation is not uncommon (Apley, 1979). On the other hand, obsessional surgery to restore the shattered surface may produce a good x-ray appearance – and a stiff knee, especially if the operation is followed by prolonged immobilization.

Type 1 fractures Undisplaced type 1 fractures can be treated conservatively. The haemarthrosis is aspirated and a compression bandage is applied. The limb is rested on a continuous passive motion (CPM) machine and knee movements are begun. As soon as the acute pain and swelling have subsided (usually within a week), a hinged cast-brace is fitted and the patient is allowed up; however, weight-bearing is not allowed for another 3 weeks. Thereafter, partial weight-bearing is permitted but full weight-bearing is delayed until the fracture has healed (usually around 8 weeks).

Displaced fractures should be treated by open reduction and internal fixation. The condylar surface is examined and trapped fragments are released or removed. One should aim for a perfect reduction; two lag screws are usually sufficient for fixation.

Type 2 fractures If depression is slight (less than 5mm) and the knee is not unstable, or if the patient is old and frail or osteoporotic, the fracture is treated closed with the aim of regaining mobility and function rather than anatomical restitution. After aspiration and compression bandaging, skeletal traction is applied via a threaded pin passed through the tibia 7cm below the fracture. An attempt is made to squeeze the condyle into shape; the knee is then flexed and extended several times to 'mould' the upper tibia on the opposing femoral condyle. The leg is cradled on pillows and, with 5kg traction in place, active exercises are carried out every day. Alternatively, the knee can be treated from the outset on a CPM machine, increasing the range of movement progressively; after a week of this treatment the machine is removed and active exercises are begun. As soon as the fracture is 'sticky' (usually at 3–4 weeks), the traction pin is removed, a hinged cast-brace is applied and the patient is allowed up on crutches. Full weight-bearing is deferred for another 6 weeks.

In younger patients, and more so in those with a central depression of more than 5 mm, open reduction with elevation of the plateau and internal fixation with a buttress plate is preferred. A midline incision offers good exposure; with the additional help of a limited transverse arthrotomy beneath the lateral meniscus, the interior of the joint can be seen well enough to provide a check on the quality of reduction. Bone graft is needed to support the elevated fragments. The fracture can be fixed with a buttress plate, though occasionally cannulated screws will do if care is taken to place at least two beneath the subchondral bone and a third at the apex of the lateral wedge fragment (anti-glide function). Postoperatively the knee is treated on a CPM machine; after a few days active exercises are begun and at 2 weeks the patient is allowed up in a cast-brace which is retained until the fracture has united.

Type 3 fractures The principles of treatment are similar to those applying to type 2 fractures. However, the fact that the lateral rim of the condyle is intact means that the knee is usually stable and a satisfactory outcome is more predictable. The depressed fragments usually need to be elevated through a window in the metaphysis; reduction should be checked by x-ray or arthroscopy. The elevated fragments are supported with bone grafts and the whole segment is fixed in position with screws or a buttress plate. Post-operatively, exercises are begun as soon as possible and 2 weeks later the patient is allowed up in a cast-brace which is retained until the fracture has united.

Type 4 fractures Osteoporotic *crush fractures* of the medial plateau are difficult to reduce; in the long term the patient is likely to be left with some degree of varus

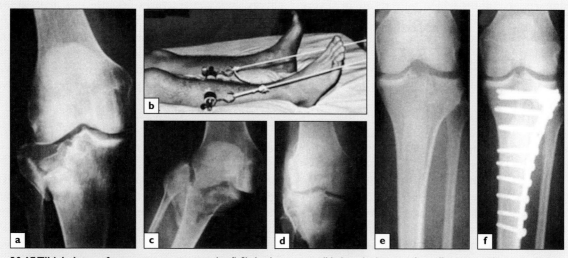

30.17 Tibial plateau fractures – treatment (**a–d**) Skeletal traction well below the knee is often effective in reducing these fractures, especially when combined with early movements. However, some residual angulation is common, though if mild this may not be clinically important. (**e, f**) The alternative is internal fixation, which certainly produced a satisfying x-ray.

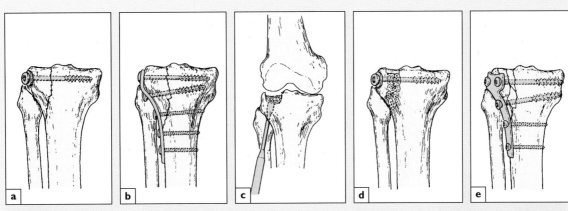

30.18 Tibial plateau fractures – fixation (**a**) One or two lag screws may be sufficient for a simple split (type 1), though (**b**) a buttress plate and screws is more secure. (**c**) Depression of more than 5mm in a type 2 fracture can be treated by elevation from below and (**d**) supported by bone grafts and fixation. (**e**) Type 3 fractures require a combination of both techniques – direct reduction, elevation of depressed areas, bone grafting and buttress plate fixation.

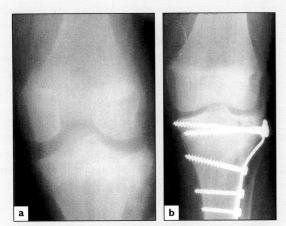

30.19 Tibial plateau fractures – fixation (**a**) A tomograph showed significant depression and some lateral displacement. (**b**) Open reduction and internal fixation was performed.

deformity. The principles of treatment are the same as for crush fractures of the lateral plateau.

Medial condylar *split fractures* usually occur in younger people and are caused by high-energy trauma. Before attempting reduction it is wise to test for lateral ligament damage which may need repair. The fracture itself is often more complex than is appreciated at first sight; there may be a second, posterior split in the coronal plane which cannot be fixed through the standard anterior approach. Good lateral x-rays or CT are needed to define the fracture pattern. If the fracture is undisplaced it can be treated closed, as for an undisplaced type 1 fracture. Displaced fractures will need open reduction and internal fixation; if necessary, the lateral ligament can be repaired at the same time.

Type 5 and 6 fractures These are severe injuries that carry the added risk of a compartment syndrome. A simple bicondylar fracture in an elderly patient can often be reduced by traction and the patient is then treated as for a type 2 injury – some residual angulation may follow. More complex fractures with comminution, especially in younger adults, are better managed operatively. The danger is that the wide exposure necessary to gain access to both condyles may strip the supporting soft tissues, thus increasing the risk of wound breakdown and delayed union or non-union. Double buttress plates should be avoided; an effective alternative is screw fixation with a ring external fixator.

PRINCIPLES OF REDUCTION AND FIXATION
Distraction is used to achieve as much reduction as possible without exposing the fracture. This can be done by applying bone distractors across the knee joint or by traction on a traction table. Many of the fragments which have soft-tissue attachments will reduce spontaneously.

If direct reduction is needed, the operation should be carefully planned. High-quality imaging is needed to define the fracture pattern accurately. The difficulty of fixing plateau fractures should not be underestimated; operative treatment should be undertaken only if the full range of implants and the necessary expertise are available.

The standard approach is through a longitudinal parapatellar incision. The aim is to preserve the meniscus while fully exposing the fractured plateau; this is best done by entering the joint through a transverse capsular incision beneath the meniscus. If exposure of both medial and lateral compartments is needed, the patellar tendon is divided in a Z-fashion.

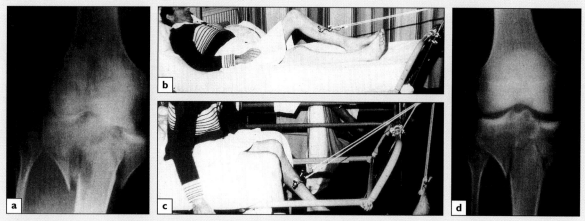

30.20 Complex plateau fractures – non-operative treatment (a) Even in this complex bicondylar fracture, non-operative treatment with (b, c) a low traction pin and early movements is possible. (d) The x-ray 10 days later shows very good reduction and the end result was excellent.

A single large fragment may be repositioned and held with cancellous screws and washers; a buttress plate is added for security. Comminuted, depressed fractures must be elevated by pushing the fragmented mass upwards from below; the osteoarticular surface is then supported by packing the subchondral area with cortico-cancellous grafts (obtained from the iliac crest) and held in place by applying a suitably contoured buttress plate and screws to the side of the bone. Unless it is torn, the meniscus should be preserved and sutured back in place when the capsule is repaired.

Displaced fractures with splits in both the sagittal and the coronal plane (triplane fractures) may be impossible to reduce and fix through the anterior approach; a second, posteromedial or posterolateral approach is the answer.

Extensive exposure and manipulation of highly comminuted fractures can sometimes be self-defeating. These injuries may be better treated by percutaneous manipulation of the fragments (under traction) and circular-frame external fixation.

Stability is all-important; no matter which method is used, fixation must be secure enough to permit early joint movement. There is little point in ending up with a pleasing x-ray and a stiff knee.

Post-operatively the limb is elevated and splinted until swelling subsides; movements are begun as soon as possible and active exercises are encouraged. At the end of 6 weeks the patient can usually be allowed up partial weight-bearing with crutches; full weight-bearing is resumed when healing is complete, usually after 12–16 weeks.

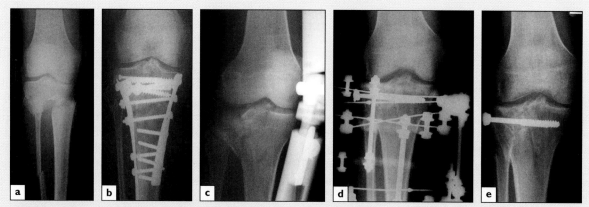

30.21 Complex plateau fractures – fixation In high energy fractures (a, b), double plating may give a satisfying x-ray appearance, but in this case the wound broke down leading to infection. A safer approach is to use indirect reduction techniques: an external fixator is temporarily placed across the joint (c) which helps control the soft-tissue swelling and enables easy access to monitor for compartment syndrome. Later, depressed fragments are elevated and defects bone-grafted, and definitive fixation in the form of lag screws and a circular external fixator (d) applied; this allows early movement of the knee joint. This fracture took 14 weeks to heal (e).

Complications

EARLY
Compartment syndrome With closed types 5 and 6 fractures there is considerable bleeding and swelling of the leg – and a risk of developing a compartment syndrome. The leg and foot should be examined repeatedly for suggestive signs.

LATE
Joint stiffness With severely comminuted fractures, and after complex operations, there is a considerable risk of developing a stiff knee. This is prevented by avoiding prolonged immobilization and encouraging movement as early as possible.

Deformity Some residual valgus or varus deformity is quite common – either because the fracture was incompletely reduced or because, although adequately reduced, the fracture became redisplaced during treatment. Fortunately, moderate deformity is compatible with good function, although constant overloading of one compartment may predispose to osteoarthritis in later life.

Osteoarthritis If, at the end of treatment, there is marked depression of the plateau, deformity of the knee or ligamentous instability, secondary osteoarthritis is likely to develop after 5 or 10 years. This may eventually require reconstructive surgery.

FRACTURE-SEPARATION OF THE PROXIMAL TIBIAL EPIPHYSIS

This uncommon injury is usually caused by a severe hyperextension and valgus strain. The epiphysis displaces forwards and laterally, often taking a small fragment of the metaphysis with it (a Salter-Harris type 2 injury). There is a risk of popliteal artery damage where the vessel is stretched across the step at the back of the tibia.

Clinical features

The knee is tensely swollen and extremely tender. If the epiphysis is displaced, there may be a valgus or hyperextension deformity. All movements are resisted.

X-RAY
Salter–Harris types 1 and 2 injuries may be undisplaced and difficult to define on x-ray; a few small bone fragments near the epiphysis may be the only clue. In the more serious injuries the entire upper tibial epiphysis may be tilted forwards or sideways.

Treatment

Under anaesthesia, closed manipulative reduction can usually be achieved. The direction of tilt may suggest the mechanism of injury; the fragment can be reduced by gentle traction in a direction opposite to that of the fracturing force. Fixation using smooth Kirschner wires or screws may be needed if the fracture is unstable. Occasionally, when the entire tibial epiphysis cannot be accurately reduced by closed manipulation, it is repositioned at operation and held by a screw. The rare Salter–Harris 3 or 4 fractures also may need open reduction and fixation.

Following reduction, whether closed or open, a long-leg cast is applied. For the usual hyperextension injury the knee is held flexed at 30°; for the less common flexion and varus injuries the knee is kept straight. The cast is worn for 6–8 weeks, with partial weight-bearing from the outset. Knee movement quickly returns when the cast is removed.

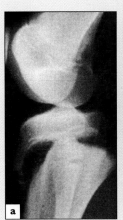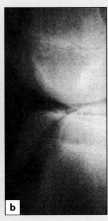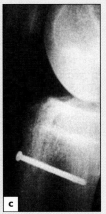

30.22 Fracture-separation of proximal tibial epiphysis (**a**) This hyperextension type of fracture needs urgent reduction because the popliteal vessels are endangered. (**b**) A flexion type of fracture-separation, but essentially a Salter–Harris type 4 pattern; in this case reduction was held with internal fixation (**c**).

Complications

Epiphyseal fractures in young children sometimes result in angular deformity of the proximal tibia. This may later require operative correction. With the higher grades of injury there is a risk of complete growth arrest at the proximal tibia. If the predicted leg length discrepancy is greater than 2.5cm, tibial lengthening (or epiphysiodesis of the opposite limb) may be needed.

FRACTURE OF THE PROXIMAL END OF THE FIBULA

Fracture of the proximal end of the fibula may be caused by either direct injury or an indirect twisting injury of the lower limb. *Beware: an isolated fracture of the proximal fibula is rare; it may be merely the most visible part of a more extensive rotational injury of the leg involving a serious fracture or ligament injury of the ankle (the Maisonneuve fracture). Always x-ray the ankle!*

The fracture itself is of little moment and it requires no treatment. However, associated injuries are frequent and they may result in prolonged disability.

Complications

Associated injuries Associated lesions, which should be looked for in every case, are: (1) the ankle injury mentioned above; (2) peroneal nerve injury and (3) collateral ligament injury. An occasional late complication is (4) peroneal nerve entrapment. Each of these conditions requires specific treatment.

DISLOCATION OF THE PROXIMAL TIBIOFIBULAR JOINT

A blow or twisting injury may cause subluxation or dislocation of the proximal tibiofibular joint. Isolated injuries are rare; they usually occur in parachuting or similar activities. Occasionally the condition is habitual and associated with generalized ligamentous laxity.

The fibular head displaces upwards, anterolaterally or posteromedially. There is usually pain and local tenderness; the abnormal contour over the lateral aspect of the knee is best seen when the two knees are flexed to 90° on the examination couch. Always check for peroneal nerve injury.

X-RAY

In the normal anteroposterior x-ray of the knee the fibular head overlaps the lateral tibial condyle; in a dislocation the fibular head stands clear of the tibia, and in the lateral view the fibular head is displaced anteriorly.

Treatment Manual reduction is carried out by flexing the knee to 90° (to relax the lateral collateral ligament) and pressing upon the fibular head; a plaster cylinder is applied for 4 weeks. Recurrent subluxation may call for excision of the fibular head.

FRACTURES OF THE TIBIA AND FIBULA

Because of its subcutaneous position, the tibia is more commonly fractured, and more commonly sustains an open fracture, than any other long bone.

Mechanism of injury

A twisting force causes a spiral fracture of both leg bones at different levels; an angulatory force produces transverse or short oblique fractures, usually at the same level.

Indirect injury is usually low energy; with a spiral or long oblique fracture one of the bone fragments may pierce the skin from within.

Direct injury crushes or splits the skin over the fracture; this is usually a high-energy lesion and the most common cause is a motorcycle accident.

Pathological anatomy

The behaviour of these injuries – and therefore the choice of treatment – depends on the following factors.

(a) The state of the soft tissues The risk of complications and the progress to fracture healing are directly related to the amount and type of soft-tissue damage. Closed fractures are best classified according to Tscherne's (1984) method (Table 30.2). For open injuries, Gustilo's grading (Table 30.3) is more useful (Gustilo *et al.*, 1990). The incidence of tissue breakdown and/or infection ranges from 1% for Gustilo type I to 30% for type IIIC.

Table 30.2 Tscherne's classification of skin lesions in closed fractures

IC1	No skin lesion
IC2	No skin laceration but contusion
IC3	Circumscribed degloving
IC4	Extensive, closed degloving
IC5	Necrosis from contusion

Table 30.3 Gustilo's classification of open fractures

Grade	Wound	Soft-tissue injury	Bone injury
I	Less than 1cm long	Minimal	Simple low-energy fractures
II	Greater than 1cm long	Moderate, some muscle damage	Moderate comminution
IIIA	Usually greater than 1cm long	Severe deep contusion; ± compartment syndrome	High-energy fracture patterns; comminuted but soft-tissue cover possible
IIIB	Usually greater than 10cm long	Severe loss of soft-tissue cover	Requires soft-tissue reconstruction for cover
IIIC	Usually greater than 10cm long	As IIIB, with need for vascular repair	Requires soft-tissue reconstruction for cover

(b) The severity of the bone injury High-energy fractures are more damaging and take longer to heal than low-energy fractures; this is regardless of whether the fracture is open or closed. Low-energy breaks are typically closed or Gustilo I or II, and spiral. High-energy fractures are usually caused by direct trauma and tend to be open (Gustilo IIIB or IIIC), transverse or comminuted.

(c) Stability of the fracture Will it displace if weight-bearing is allowed? Long oblique fractures tend to shorten; those with a butterfly fragment tend to angulate towards the butterfly; severely comminuted fractures are the least stable of all, and the most likely to need mechanical fixation.

Clinical features

The limb should be carefully examined for signs of soft-tissue damage: bruising, severe swelling, crushing or tenting of the skin, an open wound, circulatory changes, weak or absent pulses, diminution or loss of sensation and inability to move the toes. Any deformity should be noted but no attempt is made to move the fracture. *Always be on the alert for signs of an impending compartment syndrome.*

X-RAY

The entire length of both the tibia and fibula, as well as the knee and ankle joints, must be seen. The type of fracture, its level and the degree of angulation and displacement are recorded. Rotational deformity can be gauged by comparing the width of the tibio-fibular interspace above and below the fracture.

Spiral fractures without comminution are low-energy injuries. Transverse, short oblique and comminuted fractures, especially if displaced, are usually high-energy injuries.

Management

The main objectives are: (1) to limit soft-tissue damage and preserve skin cover; (2) to prevent – or at least recognize – compartment swelling; (3) to obtain and hold fracture alignment; (4) to start early weight-bearing (loading promotes healing); and (5) to start joint movements as soon as possible.

The first step is to gain a clear idea of the character of the injury – what some have called the 'fracture personality'. Uncomminuted, spiral fractures with minimal soft-tissue damage (including open injuries up to Gustilo II) are likely to heal with a minimum of trouble; they can be treated conservatively unless there is a definite indication for surgery (see below). Fractures associated with severe soft-tissue damage (whether open or closed) need much more careful attention if complications are to be avoided (BOA, BAPS Working Party Report, 1993).

LOW-ENERGY FRACTURES

Conservative management Most low-energy fractures, including Gustilo I and II injuries after attention to the wounds, can be treated by non-operative methods.

If the fracture is *undisplaced or minimally displaced* a full-length cast from upper thigh to metatarsal necks is applied with the knee slightly flexed and the ankle at a right angle. Displacement of the fibular fracture is unimportant and can be ignored.

If the fracture is *displaced,* it is reduced under general anaesthesia with x-ray control. Apposition need not be complete but alignment must be near-perfect (no more than 7° of angulation) and rotation absolutely perfect. A full-length cast is applied as for undisplaced fractures (note, however, that if placing the ankle at 0° causes the fracture to displace, a few degrees of equinus would be acceptable). The position is checked by x-ray; minor degrees of angulation can still be corrected by making a transverse cut in the plaster and wedging it into a better position.

The limb is elevated and the patient is kept under observation for 48–72 hours. If there is excessive swelling, the cast is split. Patients are usually allowed up (and home) on the second or third day, bearing minimal weight with the aid of crutches. The immediate application of plaster may be unwise if skin viability is doubtful, in which case a few days on skeletal traction is useful as a preliminary measure.

After 2 weeks the position is checked by x-ray. The cast is retained (or renewed if it becomes loose) until

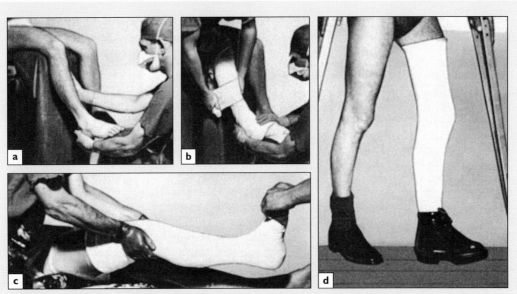

30.23 Fractured tibia and fibula – closed treatment (1) Reduction is facilitated by bending the knee over the end of the table, with the normal leg alongside for comparison (**a**). The surgeon holds the position while an assistant applies plaster from the knee downwards (**b**). When the plaster has set, the leg is lifted and the above-knee plaster completed (**c**); note that the foot is plantigrade, the knee slightly bent, and the plaster moulded round the patella. A rockered boot is fitted for walking (**d**).

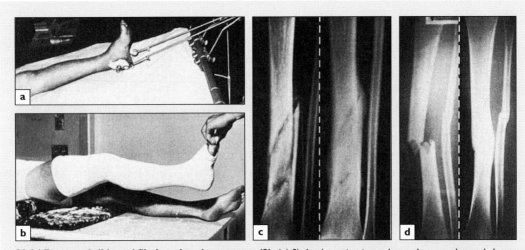

30.24 Fractured tibia and fibula – closed treatment (2) (**a**) Skeletal traction is used to reduce overlap, and also as provisional treatment when skin viability is doubtful. Plaster is applied 10–14 days later (**b**), using the technique shown in Figure 30.23, except that the skeletal pin is retained until the plaster has set. Examples of spiral and transverse fractures treated in this way are shown in (**c**) and (**d**).

the fracture unites, which is around 8 weeks in children but seldom under 16 weeks in adults.

With stable fractures the full-length cast may be changed after 4–6 weeks to a *functional below-knee cast or brace* which is carefully moulded to bear upon the upper tibia and patellar tendon. This liberates the knee and allows full weight-bearing (Sarmiento *et al.*,

1989). A snug fit is important and the fastening straps will need to be tightened as the swelling subsides.

From the start, the patient is taught to exercise the muscles of the foot, ankle and knee. When he or she gets up, an overboot with a rocker sole is fitted and the patient is taught to walk correctly. When the plaster is removed, a crepe bandage is applied and the patient is told that he or she may either elevate and exercise the limb or walk correctly on it, but it must not be allowed dangle idly.

Indications for skeletal fixation In hospitals where experience and facilities for operative skeletal fixation are lacking, non-operative treatment is not only feasible but positively desirable. However, it should be recognized that, although the period of hospitalization is shorter than with operative treatment, subsequent follow-up is more demanding and prolonged. Conservative treatment also carries a higher risk of delayed union and malunion (Hooper *et al.,* 1991). Thus, if non-operative treatment is employed and follow-up x-rays show unsatisfactory fracture alignment which cannot be corrected by wedging, or frank non-union, the plaster should be abandoned and the fracture reduced and fixed. Indeed, many surgeons would hold that unstable fractures are better treated by skeletal fixation from the outset.

Closed intramedullary nailing This is the method of choice for internal fixation. The fracture is reduced under x-ray control and image intensification. The proximal end of the tibia is exposed; a guide-wire is passed down the medullary canal and the canal is reamed. A nail of appropriate size and shape is then introduced from the proximal end across the fracture site. Transverse locking screws are inserted at the proximal and distal ends. Post-operatively, partial weight-bearing is started as soon as possible, progressing to full weight-bearing when this is comfortable.

For diaphyseal fractures, union can be expected in over 95% of cases. However, the method is less suitable for fractures near the bone ends.

Plate fixation Plating is best for metaphyseal fractures that are unsuitable for nailing. It is also sometimes used for unstable low-energy fractures in children. Disadvantages are (a) the need to expose the fracture site; (b) stripping of soft tissues around the fracture; (c) an increased risk of introducing infection; and (d) less secure fixation and delayed weight-bearing. After 6–8 weeks of partial weight-bearing the patient still has to wear a protective cast until union is complete.

External fixation This is an excellent alternative to closed nailing; it avoids exposure of the fracture site and it allows further adjustments to be made if this should be needed. Partial weight-bearing is permitted and the external fixator can be replaced by a functional brace once there are signs of union (although, with modern fixators, this is usually unnecessary because fracture loading can be controlled and adjusted in the fixator).

HIGH-ENERGY FRACTURES
Initially, the most important consideration is the viability of the damaged soft tissues and underlying bone.

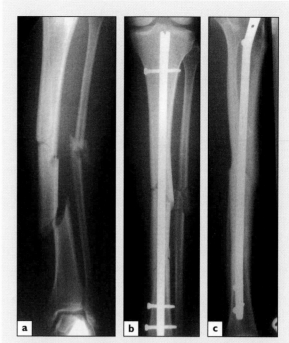

30.25 Fractured tibia and fibula – intramedullary nailing
Closed intramedullary nailing is now the preferred treatment for unstable tibial fractures. This series of x-rays shows the fracture before and after nailing. Active movements and partial weight-bearing were started soon after operation.

Tissues around the fracture should be disturbed as little as possible and open operations should be avoided unless there is already an open wound.

Transverse fractures are usually stable after reduction; they can be treated 'closed', provided a careful watch is kept for symptoms and signs of complications (excessive pain, swelling, tightness or sensory change).

Comminuted and segmental fractures, those associated with bone loss, and indeed any high-energy fracture which is inherently unstable, require early surgical stabilization. For open fractures, external fixation is the method of choice. For closed fractures, external fixation and closed nailing are equally suitable; in both cases the tissues around the fracture are left undisturbed.

In cases of bone loss, small defects can be treated by delayed bone grafting; larger defects will need either bone transport or compression-distraction with an external fixator (see page 263).

OPEN FRACTURES
A suitable mantra for the treatment of open tibial fractures is:

* antibiotics;
* debridement;
* stabilization;
* soft-tissue cover;
* rehabilitation.

Antibiotics are started immediately. A second generation cephalosporin is suitable for Gustilo grades I–IIIA wounds, but more severe grades benefit from Gram-negative cover as well (an aminoglycoside like gentamicin is often used). If the wound resulted from an agricultural accident, anaerobic cover with metronidazole should be added. The period of antibiotic use in open tibial fractures is variable, but most surgeons would continue treatment for a full therapeutic course, which is 3–5 days.

The wound should be photographed on first inspection in the Emergency Department using a Polaroid-type camera, and then covered with a sterile dressing. Any further assessment is left to be done in the operating theatre.

Adequate debridement is possible only if the original wound is extended. However, excise as little skin as possible and discuss wound extensions with a plastic surgeon if there appears to be a need for local or free skin flaps. *Ideally treatment should be conducted from the onset by a partnership of orthopaedic and plastic surgeons.* All dead and foreign material is removed; this includes bone without any significant soft-tissue attachments. Tissue of doubtful viability may be left for a second look in 48 hours. The wound and the fracture site are then washed out with large quantities of normal saline – more than 10 litres in severe injuries.

Swabs are taken for bacterial culture; if necessary, a more appropriate antibiotic is substituted during the post-operative period. Remember, though, that infecting organisms may be different from those cultured at operation and it is wise to obtain further swab samples if infection should occur.

Gustilo grade I injuries can be closed primarily and then treated as for closed injuries. More severe wounds are left open and re-examined within the next 48 hours; if necessary, a further debridement is carried out. In general one should aim to have the wound closed within the first 3 or 4 days; this usually involves split skin grafting or flap cover (free flaps, fasciocutaneous flaps or local muscle flaps).

It is important to stabilize the fracture. For Gustilo I, II and IIIA injuries, locked intramedullary nailing is permissible. In specialized units, grade IIIB fracutures also have been treated successfully by locked nailing (Keating *et al.*, 2000); however, in units which do not have much experience in handling the more severe grades of open fracture, it is wiser to apply an external fixator, leaving the wound free to be inspected and treated as necessary.

Post-operative management

Swelling is common after tibial fractures; even after skeletal fixation the soft tissues continue to swell for several days. The limb should be elevated and frequent checks made for signs of compartment syndrome (see below).

After the nailing of a transverse or short oblique fracture, weight-bearing can be started within a few days, progressing to full weight when this is comfortable. If the fracture is comminuted or segmental, almost all the load is taken by the nail, and therefore only partial weight-bearing is permitted until some callus is seen on x-ray.

With plate fixation, additional support with a cast is needed if partial weight-bearing is to start soon after surgery; otherwise weight-bearing is delayed for 6 weeks. Unlike fractures treated with intramedullary nails, callus formation is not seen as rapidly and as such it is a poor indicator for increasing the amount of weight-bearing.

Patients with fractures stabilized with external fixators can usually partially weight-bear early unless there is major bone loss. The effect of controlled dynamization provided by some external fixators allows the stimulus of weight-bearing without risk of loss of length or alignment. Weight-bearing through the fractured tibia is increased when callus is visible on x-ray; the device is later fully dynamized to allow some collapse to occur when the callus bridge consolidates. This does away with the need for exchanging the external fixator for a functional brace. However, if the pin sites are in poor condition or there is loosening, functional bracing is helpful.

Early complications

VASCULAR INJURY Fractures of the proximal half of the tibia may damage the popliteal artery. This is an emergency of the first order, requiring exploration and repair.

COMPARTMENT SYNDROME Tibial fractures – both open and closed – and intramedullary nailing are the commonest causes of compartment syndrome in the leg. The combination of tissue oedema and bleeding (oozing) causes swelling in the muscle compartments and this may precipitate ischaemia. Additional *risk factors* are young patients, severe injury, long delay to treatment, haemorrhagic shock, difficult and prolonged operation and the use of traction during operation.

The diagnosis is usually suspected on clinical grounds. Warning symptoms are increasing pain, a feeling of tightness or 'bursting' in the leg and numbness in the leg or foot. These complaints should always be taken seriously and followed by careful and repeated examination for pain provoked by muscle stretching and for loss of sensibility and/or muscle strength.

Heightened awareness is all! The diagnosis can be confirmed by measuring the compartment pressures in the leg. Indeed, so important is the need for early diagnosis that some surgeons now advocate the use of continuous compartment pressure monitoring for *all* tibial fractures (McQueen *et al.*, 1996). This deals admirably with patients who are unconscious or uncooperative, and those with multiple injuries. It also serves as an 'early warning system' in less problematic cases. A split-tip 20-gauge catheter is introduced

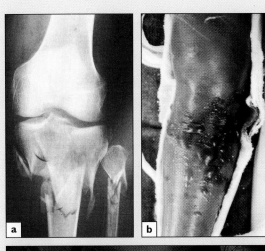

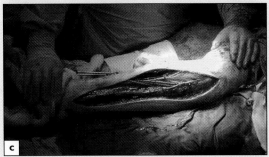

30.26 Compartment syndrome (**a**) With a fracture at this level the surgeon should be constantly on the alert for symptoms and signs of a compartment syndrome. This patient was treated in plaster. Pain become intense and when the plaster was split (which should have been done immediately after its application), the leg was swollen and blistered (**b**). Tibial compartment decompression (**c**) requires fasciotomies of *all* the compartments in the leg.

of the fibula to the lateral malleolus, and the fascia is split along the length of each compartment taking care not to damage the peroneal nerves. A second, similar incision is made posterior to the medial crest of the tibia; the fascial covering of the superficial posterior compartment is split; the muscle bulk of the superficial compartment is then retracted posteriorly, thus exposing the fascial envelope of the deep posterior compartment, which is likewise split down its entire length. Segmental arteries which perforate the fascia from the posterior tibial artery should be preserved for possible use in local skin flaps. The incisions are left open, a well-padded dressing is applied and the leg is splinted with the ankle in the neutral position. The fracture (if it has not already been nailed) is treated as a grade III open injury requiring an external fixator and delayed wound closure or skin grafting.

Outcome Compartment decompression within 6 hours of the onset of symptoms (or critical pressure measurement) should result in full recovery. Delayed decompression carries the risk of permanent dysfunction, the extent of which varies from mild sensory and motor loss to severe muscle and nerve damage, joint contractures and trophic changes in the foot.

INFECTION Open fractures are always at risk; even a small perforation should be treated with respect and debridement carried out before the wound is closed.

If the diagnosis is suspected, wound swabs and blood samples should be taken and antibiotic treatment started forthwith, using a 'best guess' intravenous preparation; once the laboratory results are obtained, a more suitable antibiotic may be substituted.

With established infection, skeletal fixation should not be abandoned if the system is stable; infection control and fracture union are more likely if fixation is secure. However, if there is a loose implant it should be removed and replaced by external fixation.

Late complications

MALUNION Slight shortening (up to 1.5cm) is usually of little consequence, but rotation and angulation deformity, apart from being unsightly, can be disabling because the knee and ankle no longer move in the same plane.

Angulation should be prevented at all stages; anything more than 7° in either plane is unacceptable. Angulation in the sagittal plane, especially if accompanied by a stiff equinus ankle, produces a marked increase in sheer forces at the fracture site during walking; this may result in either refracture or non-union.

Varus or valgus angulation will alter the axis of loading through the knee or ankle, causing increased stress in some part of the joint. This is often cited as a cause of secondary osteoarthritis; however, while this may be true for angular deformities close to the joint,

into the anterior compartment of the leg and the pressure is measured close to the level of the fracture (Heckman *et al.*, 1994). A differential pressure (ΔP) – the difference between diastolic pressure and compartment pressure – of less than 30mmHg (4.00kPa) is regarded as critical and an indication for compartment decompression. Ideally the pressure should be measured in all four compartments but this is often impractical; however, if the clinical features suggest a compartment syndrome and the anterior compartment pressure is normal or borderline, pressures should be measured in the other compartments.

Fasciotomy and decompression Once the diagnosis is made, decompression should be carried out with the minimum delay – *and that means all four compartments at the first operation.* This is best and most safely accomplished through two incisions, one anterolateral and one posteromedial (see Fig. 30.27). The anterolateral incision is made over the intermuscular septum between the anterior and lateral compartments extending from the neck

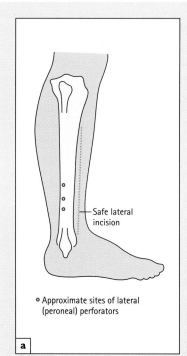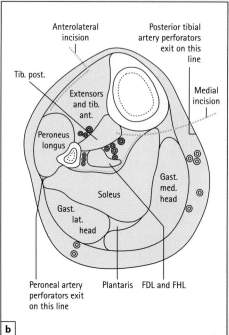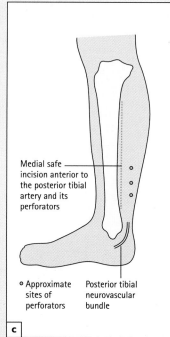

30.27 Fasciotomies for compartment decompression (a) The first incision is usually anterolateral, giving access to the anterior and lateral compartments. *But this is not enough.* The superficial and deep posterior compartments also must be opened; their position is shown in (b), a cross section of the leg. This requires a second incision (b, c), which is made a finger's breadth behind the posteromedial border of the tibia; care must be taken not to damage the deep perforators of the posterior tibial artery. Note that the two incisions should be placed at least 7cm apart so as to ensure a sufficient skin bridge without risk of sloughing.

long-term studies have failed to show that it applies to moderate deformities in the middle third of the bone (Merchant and Dietz, 1989).

Rotational alignment should be near-perfect (as compared with the opposite leg). This may be difficult to achieve with closed methods, but it should be possible with locked intramedullary nailing.

Late deformity, if marked, should be corrected by tibial osteotomy.

DELAYED UNION High-energy fractures are slow to unite and liable to non-union or fatigue failure if a nail has been used. This has prompted the use of 'prophylactic' bone grafting as soon as the soft tissues have healed (Watson, 1994). An alternative is exchange nailing of the tibia at around 12 weeks if there are no signs of callus on x-ray; the first nail is removed, the canal reamed and a larger nail inserted. If the fibula has united before the tibia, it should be osteotomized so as to allow better apposition and compression of the tibial fragments.

NON-UNION This may follow bone loss or deep infection, but a common cause is faulty treatment. Either the risks and consequences of delayed union have not been recognized, or splintage has been discontinued too soon, or the patient with a recently united fracture has walked with a stiff equinus ankle.

Hypertrophic non-union can be treated by intramedullary nailing (or exchange nailing) or compression plating. Atrophic non-union needs bone grafting in addition. If the fibula has united, a small segment should be excised so as to permit compression of the tibial fragments. Intractable cases will respond to nothing except radical Ilizarov techniques.

JOINT STIFFNESS Prolonged cast immobilization is liable to cause stiffness of the ankle and foot, which may persist for 12 months or longer in spite of active exercises. This can be avoided by changing to a functional brace as soon as it is safe to do so, usually by 4–6 weeks.

OSTEOPOROSIS Osteoporosis of the distal fragment is so common with all forms of treatment as to be regarded as a 'normal' consequence of tibial fractures. Axial loading of the tibia is important and weight-bearing should be re-established as soon as possible. After prolonged external fixation, special care should be taken to prevent a distal stress fracture.

ALGODYSTROPHY With distal third fractures, algodystrophy is not uncommon. Exercises should be encouraged throughout the period of treatment. The management of established algodystrophy is discussed on page 226.

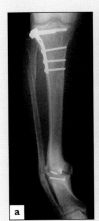
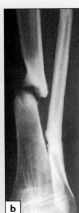
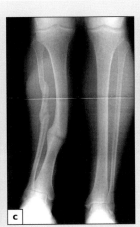
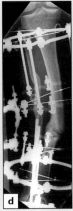
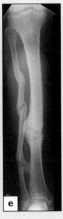

30.28 Fractured tibia and fibula – late complications (a) *Hypertrophic non-union*: the exuberant callus formation and frustrated healing process are typical. (b) *Atrophic non-union*: there is very little sign of biological activity at the fracture site (c) *Malunion*: treated, in this case, by gradual correction in an Ilizarov fixator (d, e).

FRACTURE OF THE TIBIA ALONE

A direct injury, such as a kick or a blow with a club, may cause a transverse or slightly oblique fracture of the tibia alone at the site of impact. Children sometimes suffer a spiral fracture after a twisting injury, but this is rare in adults.

Local bruising and swelling are usually evident, but knee and ankle movements are possible. The child with a spiral fracture may be able to stand on the leg, and, as the fracture may be almost invisible in an antero-posterior film, unless two views are taken the injury can be missed; a few days later an angry mother brings the child with a lump which proves to be callus. Transverse and slightly oblique fractures are easily seen on x-ray but displacement is slight.

Treatment

If the fracture is displaced, reduction should be attempted. An above-knee plaster is applied as with a fracture of both bones; first a split plaster and then, when swelling has subsided, a complete one. A fracture of the tibia alone takes just as long to unite as if both bones were broken, so at least 12 weeks is needed for consolidation and sometimes much more. The child with a spiral fracture, however, can be safely released after 6 weeks; and with a mid-shaft transverse fracture the surgeon may (if he or she is a skilled plasterer and reduction is perfect) replace the above-knee plaster by a short plaster gaiter.

Complications

Delayed union Isolated tibial fractures, especially in the lower third, may be slow to join and the temptation is to discard splintage too soon. Even slight displacement may delay union, so open reduction with internal fixation is

often preferred. If healing seems to be at a standstill, union can sometimes be hastened by excising 2.5cm of the fibula, which allows the tibial fragments to impact.

FRACTURE OF THE FIBULA ALONE

Isolated spiral fractures should be regarded with suspicion: they are often associated with other injuries and it is wise to obtain x-rays of the ankle and knee.

A transverse or short oblique fracture may be due to a direct blow. There is local tenderness, but the patient is able to stand and to move the knee and ankle. Pain can usually be controlled by analgesic medication and the patient will need no more than an elastic bandage, from knee to toes, for 2–3 weeks. In the occasional case where pain is more severe, a below-knee walking cast may be necessary.

Pathological fractures sometimes occur in patients with osteomyelitis or bone tumours. Treatment is that of the underlying condition.

FATIGUE FRACTURES

Repetitive stress may cause a fatigue fracture of the tibia (usually in the upper half of the bone) or the fibula (most often in the lower third). This is seen in army recruits, runners and ballet dancers, who complain of pain in the leg. There is local tenderness and slight swelling. The condition may be mistaken for a chronic compartment syndrome.

X-RAY For the first 4 weeks there may be nothing abnormal about the x-ray, but a bone scan shows increased activity. After some weeks periosteal new bone may be seen, with a small transverse defect in the

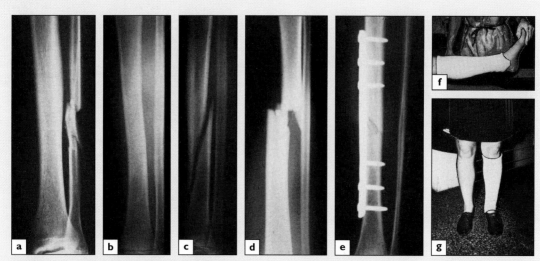

30.29 Fracture of one bone only (a) Fracture of the fibula alone. (b, c) In this child's leg the spiral fracture of the tibia shows only in one view. (d) Transverse fracture of the tibia alone in the adult: it has been plated (e) and is now so stable that a plaster gaiter (f, g) is the only protection needed. Nowadays, an intramedullary nail would be the preferred method of fixation.

cortex. There is a danger that these appearances may be mistaken for those of an osteosarcoma, with tragic consequences. If the diagnosis of stress fracture is kept in mind, such mistakes are unlikely.

TREATMENT The patient is told to avoid the stressful activity. Usually after 8–10 weeks the symptoms settle down. A short leg gaiter can be applied for comfort during weight-bearing.

REFERENCES AND FURTHER READING

Apley AG (1979) Fractures of the tibial plateau. *Orthopedic Clinics of North America* 10, 61-74

BOA/BAPS Working Party Report on Severe Tibial Injuries (1993) The early management of severe tibial fractures: the need for combined plastic and orthopaedic management. British Orthopaedic Association, London

Conlan T, Garth WP Jr, Lemons JE (1993) Evaluation of the medial soft-tissue restraints of the extensor mechanism of the knee. *Journal of Bone and Joint Surgery* 75A, 682-693

Daniel DM, Stone ML, Barnett P, Sachs R (1988) Use of the quadriceps active test to diagnose posterior cruciate ligament disruption and measure posterior laxity of the knee. *Journal of Bone and Joint Surgery* 70A, 386-391

Feagin JA, Cooke TDV (1989) Prone examination for anterior cruciate ligament insufficiency. *Journal of Bone and Joint Surgery* 71B, 863

Fruensgaard S, Johannsen HV (1989) Incomplete ruptures of the anterior cruciate ligament. *Journal of Bone and Joint Surgery* 71B, 526-530

Galway HR, MacIntosh DL (1980) The lateral pivot shift: a symptom and sign of anterior cruciate ligament insufficiency. *Clinical Orthopaedics and Related Research* 147, 45-50

Gustilo RB, Merkow RL, Templeman D (1990) The management of open fractures. *Journal of Bone and Joint Surgery* 72A, 299-304

Heckman MM, Whitesides TE Jr, Grewe SR, Rooks MD (1994) Compartment pressure in association with closed tibial fractures. The relationship between tissue pressure, compartment and the distance from the site of the fracture. *Journal of Bone and Joint Surgery* 76A, 1285-1292

Hooper GJ, Keddell RC, Penny ID (1991) Conservative management or closed nailing for tibial shaft fractures. A randomised prospective trial. *Journal of Bone and Joint Surgery* 73B, 83-85

Keating JK, Blachut PA, O'Brien PJ, Court-Brown CM, (2000) Reamed nailing of Gustilo grade-IIIB tibial fractures. *Journal of Bone and Joint Surgery* 82B, 1113-1116

Losee RE, Johnson TR, Southwick WD (1978) Anterior subluxation of the lateral tibial plateau. A diagnostic test and operative repair. *Journal of Bone and Joint Surgery* 60A, 1015-1030

McQueen MM, Christie J, Court-Brown CM (1996) Acute compartment syndrome in tibial diaphyseal fractures. *Journal of Bone and Joint Surgery* 78B, 95-98

Merchant TC, Dietz FR (1989) Long-term follow-up after fractures of the tibial and fibular shafts. *Journal of Bone and Joint Surgery* 71A, 599-606

Sandberg R, Balkfors B, Nilsson B, Westlin N (1987) Operative versus non-operative treatment of recent injuries to the ligaments of the knee: a prospective randomized study. *Journal of Bone and Joint Surgery* 69A, 1120-1126

Sarmiento A, Gersten LM, Sobol PA *et al* (1989) Tibial shaft fractures treated with functional braces. *Journal of Bone and Joint Surgery* 71B, 602-609

Schatzker J (1987) Fractures of the tibial plateau. In *The Rationale of Operative Fracture Care* (eds Schatzker J, Tile M). Springer, Berlin, pp279-296

Trickey EL (1987) Soft tissue injuries of the knee – clinical evaluation. *Current Orthopaedics* 1, 135-139

Tscherne H (1984) The management of open fractures. In *Fractures with Soft Tissue Injuries* (eds Tscherne H, Gotzen L). Springer, Berlin, pp10-32

Watson JT (1994) Treatment of unstable fractures of the shaft of the tibia. *Journal of Bone and Joint Surgery* 76A, 1575-1584

31 Injuries of the ankle and foot

The ankle is a close-fitting hinge of which the two parts interlock like a mortise (the box formed by the distal ends of the tibia and fibula) and tenon (the upwards projecting talus). The mortise bones are held together as a syndesmosis by the distal (inferior) tibiofibular and interosseous ligaments, and the talus is prevented from slipping out of the mortise by the medial and lateral collateral ligaments and joint capsule. The ankle moves only in one plane (flexion/extension); sideways movement is prevented by the malleolar buttresses and the collateral ligaments. If the talus is forced to tilt or rotate, something must give: the ligaments, the malleoli or both. Whenever a fracture of the malleolus is seen, it is important to ask 'What is the associated ligament injury?'

ANKLE LIGAMENT INJURIES

Although ankle ligament injuries are often associated with sporting activities they are, if anything, even more common in pedestrians and country walkers who stumble on stairways, pavements and potholes.

A sudden twist of the ankle momentarily tenses the structures around the joint. This may amount to no more than a painful wrenching of the soft tissues – what is commonly called a *sprained ankle*. If more severe force is applied, the ligaments may be strained to the point of rupture. With a *partial tear*, most of the ligament remains intact and, once it has healed, it is able to support the weight of the body. With a *complete tear*, the ligament may still heal but it never regains its original form and the joint will probably be unstable.

Functional anatomy

The lateral collateral ligaments consist of the anterior talofibular, the posterior talofibular and (between them) the calcaneofibular ligaments. The anterior talofibular ligament runs almost horizontally from the anterior edge of the lateral malleolus to the neck of the talus; it is relaxed in dorsiflexion and tense in plantarflexion. The calcaneofibular ligament stretches from the tip of the lateral malleolus to the posterolateral part of the calcaneum; thus it helps also to stabilize the subtalar joint. Maximum tension is produced

by inversion and dorsiflexion of the ankle. The posterior talofibular ligament runs from the posterior border of the lateral malleolus to the posterior part of the talus.

The medial collateral (deltoid) ligament consists of superficial and deep portions. The superficial fibres spread like a fan from the medial malleolus as far anteriorly as the navicular and inferiorly to the calcaneum and talus. Its chief function is to resist eversion of the hindfoot. The deep portion is intra-articular, running directly from the medial malleolus to the medial surface of the talus. Its principal effect is to prevent external rotation of the talus. The combined action of restraining eversion and external rotation makes the deltoid ligament the major stabilizer of the ankle.

The distal tibiofibular joint is held by four ligaments: anterior, posterior, inferior transverse and the interosseous 'ligament', which is really a thickened part of the interosseous membrane. This strong ligament complex still permits some movement at the tibiofibular joint during flexion and extension of the ankle.

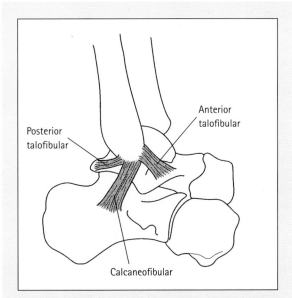

31.1 Lateral ligaments of the ankle The three main ligaments on the lateral side of the ankle are the anterior talofibular ligament, the posterior talofibular ligament and, between them, the calcaneofibular ligament. With isolated tears of the anterior talofibular ligament, lateral stability is largely preserved but the ankle feels insecure because of the resulting anteroposterior instability. (The talocalcaneal ligaments are not shown.)

INJURIES OF THE LATERAL LIGAMENTS

Over 90% of ankle ligament injuries involve the lateral complex – usually the anterior talofibular, or both this and the calcaneofibular ligament; only in the most severe injuries is the posterior talofibular ligament torn.

Mechanism of injury and pathology

The common 'twisted ankle' is due to unbalanced loading with the ankle inverted and plantarflexed. First the anterior talofibular and then the calcaneofibular ligament is strained; sometimes the talocalcaneal ligaments also are injured. If fibres are torn there is bleeding into the soft tissues. In some cases the peroneal tendons are injured.

Clinical features

A history of a twisting injury followed by pain and swelling could suggest anything from a minor sprain to a fracture. If the patient is able to walk, and bruising only faint and slow to appear, it is probably a sprain; if bruising is marked and the patient unable to put any weight on the foot, this suggests a more severe injury. Tenderness is maximal just distal and slightly anterior to the lateral malleolus. The slightest attempt at passive inversion of the ankle is extremely painful. It is impossible to test for abnormal mobility without using local or general anaesthesia.

With all ankle injuries it is essential to examine the entire leg and foot; undisplaced fractures of the fibula or the tarsal bones are easily missed and injuries of the distal tibiofibular joint and the peroneal tendon sheath cause features that mimic those of a ligament strain.

X-RAY

Anteroposterior, lateral and 'mortise' (30° oblique) views of the ankle should be obtained in all but the mildest cases; 45° oblique views are also sometimes helpful. Localized soft-tissue swelling and, in some cases, a small avulsion fracture of the tip of the lateral malleolus or the anterolateral surface of the talus are the only corroborative signs of lateral ligament injury. However, it is important to exclude other injuries, such as an undisplaced fibular fracture or diastasis of the tibiofibular syndesmosis. If tenderness extends onto the foot, or if swelling is so severe that the area cannot be properly examined, additional x-rays of the foot are essential.

Stress x-rays to demonstrate instability are unnecessary in the acute case unless operative repair is being considered; local or general anaesthesia will be needed.

MRI

Acute lateral ligament tears can be demonstrated by magnetic resonance imaging (MRI). However, the investigation is rarely justified unless primary repair is considered essential.

Treatment

PARTIAL TEAR

Sprains and strains should be treated by activity. An elastic bandage is applied and active exercises are begun immediately and persevered with until full movement is regained. Ultrasound may hasten recovery. The patient is not allowed to dangle the leg and the bandage is worn until swelling has disappeared. Weight may be taken as soon as the patient will walk, but he or she must be taught to walk correctly with the normal heel-toe gait. A common cause of prolonged pain is repeated stress due to unstable footwear or weak muscles.

COMPLETE TEAR

Operative repair of acutely ruptured ligaments may be advisable in top class athletes and dancers. In most patients, however, the injury can be treated by cast immobilization, extending from just below the knee to the toes, with the foot plantigrade. If there is swelling, the cast is split and replaced when the swelling has subsided. After 6 weeks the cast can be replaced by a removable brace and physiotherapy is begun. The ligament takes about 10 weeks to heal; at that stage the splint is discarded and the patient is encouraged to return gradually to normal activity.

Outcome

In most cases the ligament heals and the symptoms gradually settle down, although some patients go on complaining of pain on stressing the ankle. There may also be residual weakness of the peroneal tendons. The most serious complication is recurrent or chronic instability of the ankle.

RECURRENT LATERAL INSTABILITY

Clinical features

The patient gives a history of a 'sprained ankle', which never quite seems to recover and is followed by recurrent 'giving way' or a feeling of instability when walking on uneven surfaces. This is said to occur in about 20% of cases after acute lateral collateral ligament tears (Colville, 1994).

The ankle looks normal and passive movements are full. However, stress tests for abnormal lateral ligament laxity may show either excessive talar tilting in the sagittal plane or anterior displacement (an anterior drawer sign) in the coronal plane. In the chronic phase

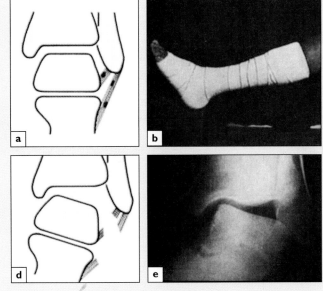

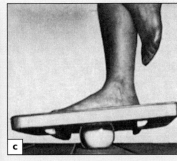

31.2 Ankle sprains The commonest injury is a partial tear of the lateral ligament (**a**). In treatment a crepe bandage (**b**) is more efficient than adhesive strapping. The balancing (wobble) board (**c**) is a useful method of strengthening the muscles and improving proprioception. A complete tear of the lateral ligament (**d**) may cause recurrent giving way; a strain film reveals talar tilt (**e**).

these tests are painless and can be performed either manually or with the use of special mechanical stress devices. Both ankles are tested, so as to allow comparison of the abnormal with the normal side.

The talar tilt test With the ankle held in the neutral position, the examiner stabilizes the tibia by grasping the leg with one hand above the ankle; his or her other hand is then used to force the heel into maximum inversion. The range of movement can be estimated clinically and compared with that of the normal ankle. The exact degree of talar tilt can also be measured by x-rays, which should be taken with the ankles in 30° of internal rotation (mortise views); 15° of talar tilt (or 5° more than in the normal ankle) is regarded as abnormal. Inversion laxity suggests injury to both the calcaneofibular and the anterior talofibular ligament.

The anterior drawer test The patient's knee is held in full flexion and the ankle in 10° of plantarflexion. The lower leg is stabilized with one hand while the other hand forces the patient's heel forwards under the tibia. In a positive test the talus can be felt sliding forwards and backwards. The position of the talus is verified by lateral x-rays; anterior displacement of 10mm (or 5mm more than on the normal side) indicates abnormal laxity of the anterior talofibular ligament. *NOTE*: With an isolated tear of the anterior talofibular ligament, the anterior drawer test may be positive in the absence of abnormal talar tilt.

Treatment

Recurrent 'giving way' can usually be prevented by raising the outer side of the heel and extending it

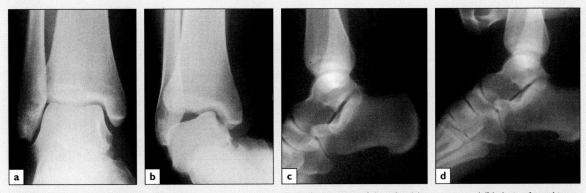

31.3 Tests for ankle instability *The talar tilt test:* stress x-rays show the position of the talus (**a**) in repose and (**b**) during forced inversion; 15° of tilt (or more than 5° worse than the normal side) is diagnostic. *The anterior drawer test:* the heel is pulled forwards under the tibia in an attempt to displace the talus anteriorly. Lateral x-rays show the position (**c**) in repose and (**d**) during anterior traction; note the amount of talar displacement compared with that on the normal side.

laterally. Ankle exercises to strengthen the peroneal muscles are helpful, and a light brace can be worn during stressful activities. If, in spite of these measures, the patient continues to experience instability during everyday activities, reconstruction of the lateral ligament should be considered.

Various operations are described; they fall mainly into two groups: (a) those which aim to repair or tighten the ligaments, and (b) those which are designed to construct a 'checkrein' against the unstable movement. The *Brostrom–Karlsson operation* is an example of the first type: the anterior talo-fibular and calcaneofibular ligaments are exposed and repaired, usually by an overlapping (or 'double-breasting' technique) (Karlsson *et al.*, 1989). In the second type of operation a substitute ligament is constructed by using peroneus brevis to act as a tenodesis and prevent sudden movements into varus (Chrisman and Snook, 1969).

Post-operatively the ankle is immobilized in eversion for 2 weeks; a below-knee cast is then applied for another 4 weeks, during which time the patient can bear weight. Thereafter, a removable brace is worn and exercises are encouraged. The brace can usually be discarded after 3 months but it may need to be used from time to time for sports activities.

DELTOID LIGAMENT TEARS

Rupture of the deltoid ligament is usually associated with either a fracture of the distal end of the fibula or tearing of the distal tibiofibular ligaments (or both). The effect is to destabilize the talus and allow it to move into eversion and external rotation. The diagnosis is made by x-ray: there is widening of the medial joint space in the mortise view; sometimes the talus is tilted, and diastasis of the tibiofibular joint may be obvious.

Treatment Provided the medial joint space is completely reduced, the ligament will heal. The fibular fracture or diastasis must be accurately reduced, if necessary by open operation and internal fixation. Occasionally the medial joint space cannot be reduced; it should then be explored in order to free any soft tissue trapped in the joint. A below-knee cast is applied with the foot plantigrade and is retained for 8 weeks.

DISLOCATION OF THE PERONEAL TENDONS

Acute dislocation of the peroneal tendons may accompany – or may be mistaken for – a lateral ligament strain. Tell-tale signs on x-ray are an oblique fracture of the lateral malleolus (the so-called 'rim fracture') or a small flake of bone lying lateral to the lateral malleolus (avulsion of the retinaculum). Treatment in a below-knee cast for 6 weeks will succeed in over half the cases; the remainder will complain of residual symptoms.

Recurrent subluxation or dislocation is unmistakable, for the patient can demonstrate that the peroneal tendons dislocate forwards over the fibula during dorsiflexion and eversion. Treatment is operative and is based on the observation that the attachment of the retinaculum to the periosteum on the front of the fibula has come adrift, creating a pouch into which the tendons displace. Using non-absorbable sutures through drill holes in the bone, the normal anatomy is recreated (Das De and Balasubramaniam, 1985).

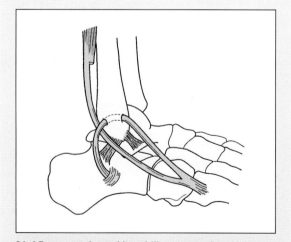

31.4 Recurrent lateral instability – operative treatment
One way of augmenting the lateral ligament is to re-route part of the peroneus brevis tendon so that is acts as a checkrein (tenodesis; the Chrisman-Snook operation).

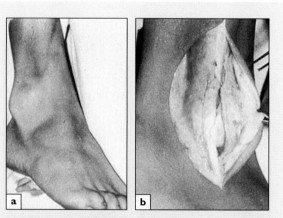

31.5 Dislocation of peroneal tendons (**a**) On movement of the ankle, the peroneal tendons slip forwards over the lateral malleolus. (**b**) The anterior part of the retinaculum is being reconstructed.

TEARS OF THE INFERIOR TIBIOFIBULAR LIGAMENTS

The inferior tibiofibular ligaments may be torn, allowing partial or complete separation of the tibiofibular joint (diastasis). *Complete diastasis,* with tearing of both the anterior and posterior fibres, follows a severe abduction strain. *Partial diastasis,* with tearing of only the anterior fibres, is due to an external rotation force. These injuries may occur in isolation, but they are usually associated with fractures of the malleoli or rupture of the collateral ligaments.

Clinical features

Following a twisting injury, the patient complains of pain in the front of the ankle. There is swelling and marked tenderness directly over the inferior tibiofibular joint. A 'squeeze test' has been described by Hopkinson *et al.* (1990); when the leg is firmly compressed some way above the ankle, the patient experiences pain over the syndesmosis. Be sure, though, to exclude a fracture before carrying out the test.

X-RAY
With a partial tear the fibula usually lies in its normal position and the x-ray looks normal. With a complete tear the tibiofibular joint is separated and the ankle mortise is widened; sometimes this becomes apparent only when the ankle is stressed in abduction. There may be associated fractures of the distal tibia or fibula, or an isolated fracture more proximally in the fibula.

Treatment

Partial tears can be treated by strapping the ankle firmly for 2–3 weeks. Thereafter exercises are encouraged.

Complete tears are best managed by internal fixation with a transverse screw just above the joint. This must be done as soon as possible so that the tibiofibular space does not become clogged with organizing haematoma and fibrous tissue. If the patient is seen late and the ankle is painful and unstable, open clearance of the syndesmosis and transverse screw fixation may be warranted. The ankle is immobilized in plaster for 8 weeks; 4 weeks later the screw is removed. However, some degree of instability usually persists.

FRACTURES OF THE ANKLE

Fractures and fracture-dislocations of the ankle are common. One such injury was described by Percival Pott in 1768, and the group as a whole was for a long time referred to as Pott's fracture.

The most obvious injury is a fracture of one or both malleoli; often, though, the 'invisible' part of the injury – rupture of one or more ligaments – is just as serious.

Mechanism of injury

The patient stumbles and falls. Usually the foot is anchored to the ground while the body lunges forwards. The ankle is twisted and the talus tilts and/or rotates forcibly in the mortise, causing a low-energy fracture of one or both malleoli, with or without associated injuries of the ligaments. If a malleolus is pushed off, it usually fractures obliquely; if it is pulled off, it fractures transversely. The precise fracture pattern is determined by (a) the position of the foot and (b) the direction of force at the moment of injury. The foot may be either pronated or supinated and the force upon the talus is towards adduction, abduction or external rotation, or a combination of these.

Pathological anatomy

There is no completely satisfactory classification of ankle fractures. *Lauge-Hansen* grouped these injuries according to the likely position of the foot and the direction of force at the moment of fracture. This is useful as a guide to the method of reduction (reverse the pathological force); it also gives a pointer to the associated ligament injuries. However, some people find this classification overly complicated. For a detailed description the reader is referred to the original paper by Lauge-Hansen (1950).

A simpler (perhaps too simple) classification is that of *Danis and Weber* (Müller *et al.*, 1991), which focuses on the fibular fracture (Fig. 31.6). Type A is a transverse fracture of the fibula below the tibiofibular syndesmosis, perhaps associated with an oblique or vertical fracture of the medial malleolus; this is almost certainly an adduction (or adduction and internal rotation) injury. Type B is an oblique fracture of the fibula in the sagittal plane (and therefore better seen in the lateral x-ray) at the level of the syndesmosis; often there is also an avulsion injury on the medial side (a torn deltoid ligament or fracture of the medial malleolus). This is probably an external rotation injury and it may be associated with a tear of the anterior tibiofibular ligament. Type C is a more severe injury, above the level of the syndesmosis – which means that the tibiofibular ligament and part of the interosseous membrane must have been torn. This is due to severe abduction or a combination of abduction and external rotation. Associated injuries are an avulsion fracture of the medial malleolus (or rupture of the medial collateral ligament), a posterior malleolar fracture and diastasis of the tibiofibular joint.

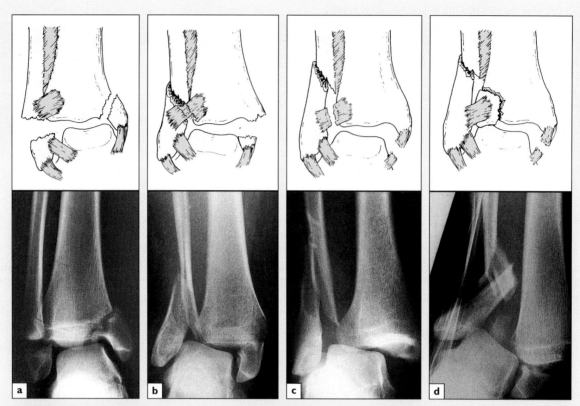

31.6 Ankle fractures – classification The Danis–Weber classification is based on the level of the fibular fracture. (**a**) *Type A* – a fibular fracture below the syndesmosis and an oblique fracture of the medial malleolus (caused by forced supination and adduction of the foot). (**b**) *Type B* – a fracture at the syndesmosis, often associated with disruption of the anterior fibres of the tibiofibular ligament and fracture of the posterior and/or medial malleolus, or disruption of the medial ligament (caused by forced supination and external rotation). (**c**) *Type C* – a fibular fracture above the syndesmosis; the tibiofibular ligament must be torn, or else (**d**) the ligament avulses a small piece of the tibia. Here, again, there must also be disruption on the medial side of the joint – either a medial malleolar fracture or rupture of the deltoid ligament.

Clinical features

Ankle fractures are seen in skiers, footballers and climbers; an older group includes women with post-menopausal osteoporosis.

A history of a severe twisting injury, followed by intense pain and inability to stand on the leg suggests something more serious than a simple 'sprain'. The ankle is swollen and deformity may be obvious. The site of tenderness is important; if both the medial and the lateral sides are tender, a double injury (bony or ligamentous) must be suspected.

X-RAY

At least three views are needed: anteroposterior, lateral and a 30° oblique 'mortise' view. The level of the fibular fracture is often best seen in the lateral view; diastasis may not be appreciated without the mortise view. Further x-rays may be needed to exclude a proximal fibular fracture.

From a careful study of the x-rays it should be possible to reconstruct the mechanism of injury.

Treatment

The four guiding principles are:

- don't delay;
- treat the entire injury, not only the fracture;
- reduce accurately;
- check and maintain reduction.

Swelling is usually rapid and severe. If the injury is not dealt with within a few hours, definitive treatment may have to be deferred for several days while the leg is elevated so that the swelling can subside; this can be hastened by using a foot pump (which also reduces the risk of deep vein thrombosis).

Fractures are visible on x-ray; ligaments are not. Always look for clues to the invisible ligament injury – widening of the tibiofibular space, asymmetry of the talotibial space, widening of the medial joint space or tilting of the talus – before deciding on a course of action.

Like other intra-articular injuries, ankle fractures must be accurately reduced and held if later mechani-

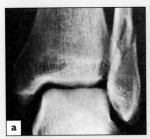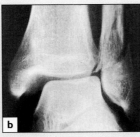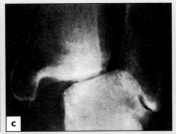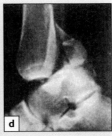

31.7 Ankle fractures – stable or unstable? (**a**) *Stable fracture*: in this Danis–Weber Type B fracture the tibiofibular syndesmosis has held; the surfaces of the tibia and talus are precisely parallel and the width of the joint space is regular both superiorly and medially. (**b**) *Slight subluxation*: the syndesmosis is intact but the talus has moved laterally with the distal fibular fragment; the medial joint space is too wide, signifying a deltoid ligament rupture. It is vital, after reduction of the fibular fracture, to check that the medial joint space is normal; if it isn't, the ligament has probably been trapped in the joint and it must be freed so as to allow perfect re-positioning of the talus. (**c**) *Fracture-dislocation*: in this high fibular fracture the syndesmosis has given way, the medial collateral ligament has been torn and the talus is displaced and tilted. The fibula must be fixed to full length and the tibiofibular joint secured before the ankle can be stabilized. (**d**) *Posterior fracture-dislocation*: if the posterior margin of the tibia is fractured, the talus may be displaced upwards. The fragment must be replaced and fixed securely.

cal dysfunction is to be prevented. Persistent displacement of the talus, or a step in the articular surface, leads to increased stress and predisposes to secondary osteoarthritis.

In assessing the accuracy of reduction, four objectives must be met: (1) the fibula must be restored to its full length; (2) the talus must sit squarely in the mortise, with the talar and tibial articular surfaces parallel; (3) the medial joint space must be restored to its normal width, that is the same width as the tibiotalar space (about 4mm); and (4) oblique x-rays must show that there is no tibiofibular diastasis.

Ankle fractures are often unstable. Whatever the method of reduction and fixation, the position must be checked by x-ray during the period of healing.

UNDISPLACED FRACTURES

The first step is to decide whether the injury is stable or unstable. An isolated, *undisplaced Danis–Weber type A fracture* is stable and will need minimal splintage: a firm bandage or plaster slab is applied mainly for comfort until the fracture heals.

Undisplaced type B fractures are potentially unstable only if the tibiofibular ligament is torn or avulsed, or if there is a significant medial-sided injury. X-rays will show if the syndesmosis or mortise is intact; if it is, a below-knee cast is applied with the ankle in the neutral (anatomical) position. The plaster may need to be split and, if so, it must be completed or replaced when swelling has subsided. A check x-ray is taken at 2 weeks to confirm that the fracture remains undisplaced. An overboot is fitted and the patient is taught to walk correctly as soon as possible. The cast can usually be discarded after 6–8 weeks. Ankle and foot movements are regained by active exercises when the plaster is removed. As with any lower limb fracture, the leg must not be allowed to dangle idly – it must be exercised and elevated.

Undisplaced type C fractures are deceivingly innocent-looking but are often accompanied by disruption of the medial joint structures as well as the tibiofibular syndesmosis and interosseous membrane. These defects may become apparent only when the fracture displaces in a cast; arguably, therefore, type C fractures are better fixed from the outset.

DISPLACED FRACTURES

Reduction of these joint disruptions is a prerequisite to all further treatment; knowledge of the causal mechanism (and this is where the Lauge-Hansen classification is useful) helps to guide the method of closed reduction. Although internal fixation is usually performed to stabilize the reduction, not all such fractures require surgery.

Displaced Weber type A fractures The medial malleolar fracture is nearly vertical and after closed reduction it often remains unstable; internal fixation of the malleolar fragment with one or two screws directed almost parallel to the ankle joint is advisable. A perfect reduction should be aimed for, with accurate restoration of the tibial articular surface. Loose bone fragments are removed. The lateral malleolar fracture, unless it is already perfectly reduced and stable, should be fixed with a plate and screws or tension-band wiring. Postoperatively a 'walking cast' is applied for 6 weeks.

Displaced Weber type B fractures The most common fracture pattern is a spiral fracture of the fibula and an oblique fracture of the medial malleolus. The causal mechanism is external rotation of the ankle when the foot is caught in a supinated position. Closed reduction therefore needs traction (to disimpact the fracture) and then internal rotation of the foot. If closed reduction succeeds, a cast is applied, following the same routine as for undisplaced fractures. Failure of closed reduction (sometimes a torn medial ligament is caught between

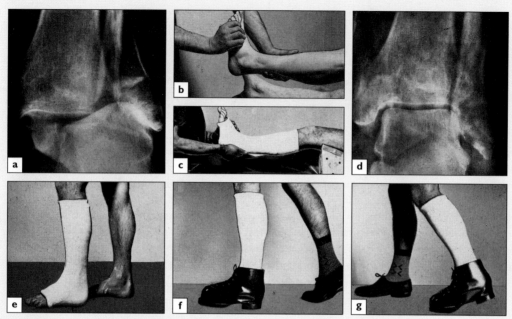

31.8 Ankle fractures – closed treatment A supination–external rotation fracture (**a**) is reduced by traction followed by internal rotation (**b**); a below-knee plaster is applied, moulded and held till it has set (**c**). Reduction is checked by x-ray (**d**). The plaster must be plantigrade (**e**); a 'rocker boot' permits an almost normal gait (**f, g**).

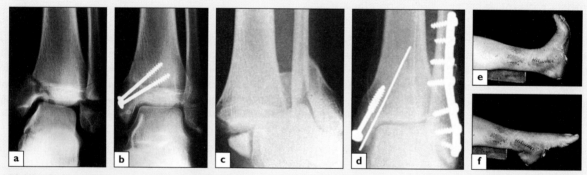

31.9 Ankle fractures – open treatment (1) (**a, b**) Danis–Weber type A fractures can often be treated conservatively, but if the medial malleolar fragment involves a large segment of the articular surface, it is best treated by accurate open reduction and internal fixation with one or two screws. (**c, d**) An unstable fracture-dislocation such as this almost always needs open reduction and internal fixation. The fibula should be restored to full length and fixed securely; in this case the medial malleolus also needed internal fixation; (**e**) and (**f**) show the range of ankle movement a few days after operation and before a 'walking plaster' was applied.

the talus and medial malleolus) or late redisplacement calls for operative treatment.

Type B fractures may also be caused by abduction; often the lateral aspect of the fibula is comminuted and the fracture line more horizontal. Despite accurate reduction (the ankle is adducted and the foot supinated), these injuries are unstable and often poorly controlled in a cast; internal fixation is therefore preferred.

Displaced Weber type C fractures The fibular fracture is well above the syndesmosis and frequently there are associated medial and posterior malleolar fragments. An isolated type C fibular fracture should raise strong

suspicions of major ligament damage to the syndesmosis and medial side of the joint. Almost all type C fractures are unstable and will need open reduction and internal fixation. The first step is to reduce the fibula, restoring its length and alignment; the fracture is then stabilized using a plate and screws. If there is a medial fracture, this also is fixed. The syndesmosis is then checked, using a hook to pull the fibula laterally. If the joint opens out, it means that the ligaments are torn; the syndesmosis is stabilized by inserting a transverse screw across from the fibula into the tibia (the ankle should be held in 10° of dorsiflexion when the screw is inserted).

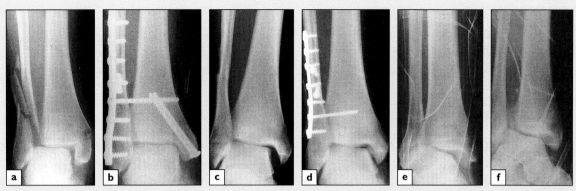

31.10 Ankle fractures with diastasis – open treatment (2) (a) In this type B fracture there is partial disruption of the distal tibiofibular syndesmosis. Treatment (b) required medial and lateral fixation as well as a tibiofibular screw. (c) A type C fracture must, inevitably, disrupt the tibiofibular ligament; in this case the medial malleolus was intact but the deltoid ligament was torn (look at the wider-than-normal medial joint space). (d) By fixing the fibular fracture and using a tibiofibular screw, the ankle was completely reduced and it was therefore unnecessary to explore the deltoid ligament. (e) This patient presented 5 days after his injury; he, too, had a diastasis with disruption of the deltoid ligament (f). In this case the tibiofibular joint as well as the deltoid ligament had to be explored before the ankle could be reduced.

Delayed treatment Fracture-subluxations more than a week old may prove difficult to reduce because of clot organization in the syndesmosis. Granulation tissue should be removed from the syndesmosis and transverse tibiofibular fixation secured.

Post-operative management After open reduction and fixation of ankle fractures, movements should be regained before applying a below-knee plaster cast. The patient is then allowed partial weight-bearing with crutches; the cast is retained until the fractures have consolidated (anything from 6 to 12 weeks).

If a transverse tibiofibular screw has been inserted, the patient should be recalled to have this removed after 3 months.

OPEN FRACTURES

Open fractures of the ankle pose special problems. If the fracture is not reduced and stabilized at an early stage, it may prove impossible to restore the anatomy. For this reason unstable injuries should be treated by internal fixation even in the presence of an open wound, provided the soft tissues are not too severely damaged and the wound is not contaminated. If internal fixation seems too risky, an external fixator can be used. Treatment in other respects follows the principles outlined in Chapter 23.

Complications

EARLY

Vascular injury With a severe fracture-subluxation the pulses may be obliterated. The ankle should be immediately reduced and held in a splint until definitive treatment has been initiated.

Wound breakdown and infection Diabetic patients are at greater than usual risk of developing wound-edge necrosis and deep infection. In dealing with displaced fractures, these risks should be carefully weighed against the disadvantages of conservative treatment; casts may also cause skin problems if not well padded and are less effective in preventing malunion.

LATE

Incomplete reduction Incomplete reduction is common and, unless the talus fits the mortise accurately, degenerative changes may occur. This can sometimes be prevented by a corrective osteotomy.

Non-union The medial malleolus occasionally fails to unite because a flap of periosteum is interposed between it and the tibia. It should be prevented by operative reduction and screw fixation.

Joint stiffness Swelling and stiffness of the ankle are usually the result of neglect in treatment of the soft tissues. The patient must walk correctly in plaster and, when the plaster is removed, he or she must, until circulatory control is regained, wear a crepe bandage and elevate the leg whenever it is not being used actively. Physiotherapy is also helpful.

Algodystrophy often follows fractures of the ankle. The patient complains of pain in the foot; there may be swelling and diffuse tenderness, with gradual development of trophic changes and severe osteoporosis. Management is discussed on page 226.

Osteoarthritis Malunion and/or incomplete reduction may lead to secondary osteoarthritis of the ankle. If symptoms becomes severe, arthrodesis may be necessary.

PILON FRACTURES

Unlike the twisting injuries which cause the common ankle fractures, this injury to the ankle joint occurs when a large force drives the talus upwards against the tibial plafond, like a pestle (pilon) being struck into a mortar. There is considerable damage to the articular cartilage and the subchondral bone may be broken into several pieces; in severe cases, the comminution extends some way up the shaft of the tibia.

Clinical features

There may be little swelling initially but this rapidly changes and fracture blisters are common. The ankle may be deformed or even dislocated; prompt reduction is mandatory.

X-RAYS

This is a comminuted fracture of the distal end of the tibia, extending into the ankle joint. The fracture may be classified according to the amount of displacement and comminution (Rüedi and Allgöwer, 1979), though this will usually require accurate definition by computed tomography (CT). Rüedi *type 1* is an intra-articular fracture with little or no displacement of the fragments; in *type 2* there is more severe disruption of the articular surface but without very marked comminution; and *type 3* is a severely comminuted fracture with displacement of the fragments and gross articular irregularity (see Fig. 31.11). In severe injuries, accurate definition of the fragments is impossible without CT, and preferably three-dimensional CT reconstruction.

Treatment

Control of soft-tissue swelling is a priority; this is best achieved either by elevation and calcaneal traction or by applying an external fixator across the ankle joint. It may take 2–3 weeks before the soft tissues improve, by which time surgery may be considered if the fracture is displaced. Unfortunately most are, and reduction and fixation will be needed.

Once the skin has recovered, an open reduction and fixation with plates and screws (usually with bone grafting) may be possible. However, the more severe injuries (types 2 and 3) do not readily tolerate large surgical exposures for plating and wound breakdown and infection rates of 18–37% are reported (Teeny and Diss, 1993). Better results have followed wider use of indirect reduction techniques (e.g. applying a femoral distractor across the ankle joint to obtain as much reduction as possible through ligamentotaxis) and plating through limited exposures. Recently, these injuries have also been successfully treated by using a combination of indirect reduction methods and small screws to hold the articular fragments; bone grafts are often added to defects in the metaphysis and a circular fixator is then applied to stabilize the tibial plafond on the shaft.

The soft-tissue swelling following these injuries is substantial. After fixation, elevation and early movement help to reduce the oedema; arteriovenous impulse devices applied to the sole of the foot are also helpful.

Pilon fractures usually take 12–16 weeks to heal. Post-operatively, physiotherapy is focused on joint movement and reduction of swelling. During the early weeks weight-bearing is forbidden because of the risk of displacement. If the fracture is treated with a circular external fixator, partial weight-bearing is

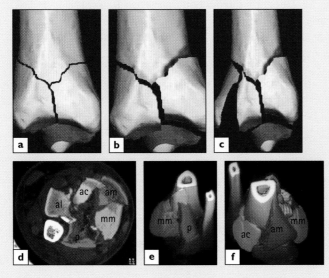

31.11 Pilon fractures – imaging These are either (**a**) undisplaced (type 1), (**b**) minimally displaced (type 2) or (**c**) markedly displaced (type 3).

CT (**d**) shows that there are usually five major tibial fragments: anterolateral (al), anterocentral (ac), anteromedial (am), the medial malleolus (mm) and the posterior fragment (p). These elements are better defined by three-dimensional CT reconstruction (**e, f**).

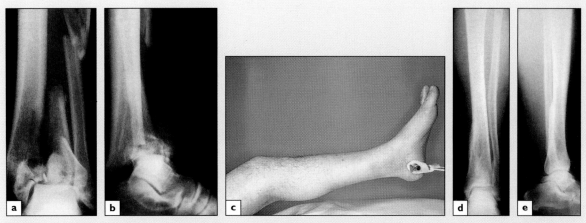

31.12 Pilon fracture – conservative treatment This complex fracture (**a**, **b**) was treated by (**c**) traction and movements. By 12 weeks the fracture had healed in good position. X-rays at one year are shown in (**d**) and (**e**).

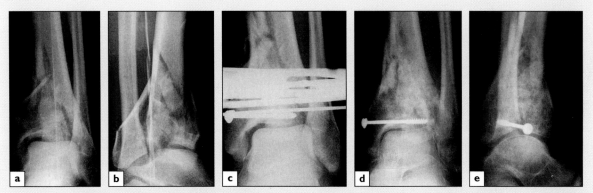

31.13 Pilon fractures – operative treatment High energy pilon fractures (**a**, **b**) carry a risk of wound breakdown and infection if treated by wide open reduction and plating. Indirect reduction techniques (ligamentotaxis and percutaneous manipulation of fragments) with minimal internal fixation are better tolerated. This may be combined with circular external fixation and tensioned wires (**c**); reduction is maintained until union occurs (**d**, **e**) – in this case it took 14 weeks.

permitted after 6 weeks, by which time sufficient healing between the articular fragments will have occurred to make the risk of displacement minimal. Plated fractures need protection from weight-bearing for longer.

Outcome

The methods outlined above have reduced the incidence of major complications such as infection and non-union; however, long-term outcome studies are still awaited. Although bony union may be achieved, the fate of the joint is decided by the degree of cartilage injury – the 'invisible' factor on x-rays. Secondary osteoarthritis is still a frequent late complication.

ANKLE FRACTURES IN CHILDREN

Physeal injuries are quite common in children and almost a third of these occur around the ankle.

Mechanism of injury

The foot is fixed to the ground or trapped in a crevice and the leg twists to one or the other side. The tibial (or fibular) physis is wrenched apart, usually resulting in a *Salter–Harris type 1 or 2 fracture*. With severe external rotation or abduction the fibula may also fracture more proximally. The tibial metaphyseal spike may come off posteriorly, laterally or posteromedially;

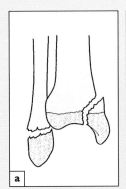
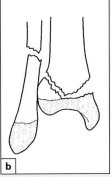
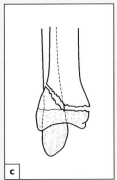
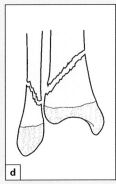

31.14 Physeal injuries of the distal tibia The classification suggested by Dias and Tachdjian (1978) has the merit of pointing to the required reduction manoeuvre – the reverse of the causal mechanism. (**a**) *Supination–inversion*: the fibular fracture is usually an avulsion (Salter–Harris type 1) whereas the medial malleolar fracture can be variable; (**b**) *Pronation–eversion–external rotation*: the fibular fracture is often high and transverse; (**c**) *Supination–plantarflexion*: a fracture of the distal tibia only (Salter–Harris type 1 or 2) with posterior displacement, (**d**) *Supination–external rotation*: an oblique fibular fracture coupled with a fracture of the distal tibia.

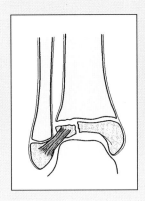

31.15 Tillaux fracture Diagram illustrating the elements of this unusual injury.

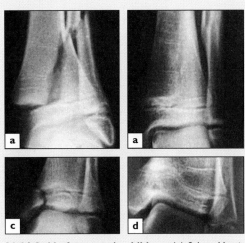

31.16 Ankle fractures in children (**a**) Salter–Harris type 2 injury; after reduction (**b**) growth has proceeded normally. (**c**) Salter–Harris type 3 injury; (**d**) the medial side of the physis has fused prematurely, resulting in distorted growth.

its position is determined by the mechanism of injury and suggests the method of reduction. With adduction injuries the tip of the fibula may be avulsed.

Type 3 and 4 fractures are uncommon. They are due to a supination–adduction force. The epiphysis is split vertically and one piece of the epiphysis (usually the medial part) may be displaced.

Two unusual injuries of the growing ankle are the Tillaux fracture and the notorious triplane fracture. The *Tillaux fracture* is an avulsion of a fragment of tibia by the anterior tibiofibular ligament; in the child or adolescent this fragment is the lateral part of the epiphysis and the injury is therefore a Salter–Harris type 3 fracture.

The *triplane fracture* occurs on the medial side of the tibia and is a combination of Salter–Harris types 2 and 3 injuries. Fracture lines appear in the coronal, sagittal and transverse planes. Injury to the physis may result in either asymmetrical growth or arrested growth.

Clinical features

Following a sprain the ankle is painful, swollen, bruised and acutely tender. There may be an obvious deformity, but sometimes the injury looks deceptively mild.

X-RAY

Undisplaced physeal fractures – especially those in the distal fibula – are easily missed. Even a hint of physeal widening should be regarded with great suspicion and the child x-rayed again after a week. In an infant the state of the physis can sometimes only be guessed at, but a few weeks after injury there may be extensive periosteal new-bone formation.

In triplane fractures the tibial epiphysis may be split in one plane and the metaphysis in another, thus making it difficult to see both fractures in the same x-ray. CT scans are particularly helpful in these and other type 3 injuries.

Treatment

Salter–Harris type 1 and 2 injuries are treated closed. If it is displaced, the fracture is gently reduced under general anaesthesia; the limb is immobilized in a full-length cast for 3 weeks and then in a below-knee walking cast for a further 3 weeks. Occasionally, surgery is needed to extract a periosteal flap which prevents an adequate reduction.

Type 3 or 4 fractures, if undisplaced, can be treated in the same manner, but the ankle must be x-rayed again after 5 days to ensure that the fragments have not slipped. Displaced fractures can sometimes be reduced closed by reversing the forces that produced the injury. However, unless reduction is near-perfect, the fracture should be reduced open and fixed with interfragmentary screws which are inserted parallel to

the physis. Post-operatively the leg is immobilized in a below-knee cast for 6 weeks.

Tillaux fractures are treated in the same way as type 3 fractures. Triplane fractures, if undisplaced, can be managed closed but require vigilant monitoring for late displacement. Displaced fractures must be reduced and fixed.

Complications

Malunion Imperfect reduction may result in angular deformity of the ankle – usually valgus. In children under 10 years old, mild deformities may be accommodated by further growth and modelling. In older children the deformity should be corrected by a supra-malleolar closing-wedge osteotomy.

Asymmetrical growth Fractures through the epiphysis (Salter–Harris type 3 or 4) may result in localized fusion of the physis. The bony bridge is usually in the medial half of the growth plate; the lateral half goes on growing and the distal tibia gradually veers into varus. MRI or CT is helpful in showing precisely where

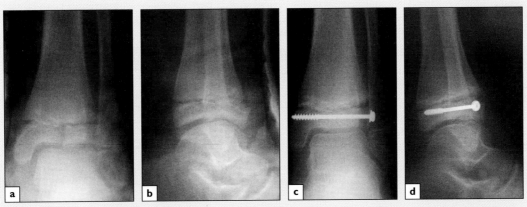

31.17 The Tillaux fracture (**a, b**) This avulsion fracture of the lateral part of the physis was reduced and fixed percutaneously (**c, d**).

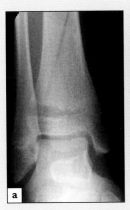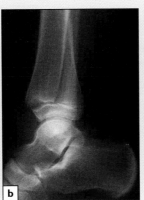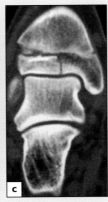

31.18 The triplane fracture The three fracture planes may not be seen in a single x-ray, but can be visualized from a combination of images. In this case the epiphyseal fracture is clearly seen only in the coronal plane CT scan (**c**).

physeal arrest has occurred. If the bony bridge is small (less than 30% of the physeal width) it can be excised and replaced by a pad of fat in the hope that physeal growth may be restored. If more than half of the physis is involved, or the child is near the end of the growth period, a supramalleolar closing-wedge osteotomy is indicated.

Shortening Early physeal closure occurs in about 20% of children with distal tibial injuries. Fortunately the resulting limb length discrepancy is usually mild. If it promises to be more than 2cm and the child is young enough, proximal tibial epiphysiodesis in the opposite limb may restore equality. If the discrepancy is marked, or the child near the end of the growth period, leg lengthening is indicated.

PRINCIPLES IN MANAGING INJURIES OF THE FOOT

Injuries of the foot are apt to be followed by residual symptoms and loss of function which seem out of proportion to the initial trauma. Severe injuries affect the foot as a whole, whatever the particular bone which might be fractured. A global approach is therefore essential in dealing with these injuries, the objective being a return to full weight-bearing without pain.

CLINICAL ASSESSMENT The entire foot should be examined systematically, no matter that the injury may appear to be localized to one spot. Multiple fractures, or combinations of fractures and dislocations, are easily missed. The circulation and nerve supply must be carefully assessed; a well-reduced fracture is a useless achievement if the foot becomes ischaemic or insensitive.

Fractures and dislocations may cause tenting of the skin; this is always a bad sign because there is a risk of skin necrosis if reduction is delayed.

IMAGING Imaging routinely begins with anteroposterior, lateral and oblique x-rays of the foot. Special projections are called for if a fracture of the talus or calcaneum, or fracture-dislocation of the mid-tarsal joints, is suspected. CT is especially useful for evaluating fractures of the calcaneum, and MRI is helpful in diagnosing osteo-chondral fractures of the talus. *Familiarity with the talo-calcaneal anatomy is essential if fractures of the hindfoot are to be properly diagnosed.*

TREATMENT Swelling is always a problem. Not only does it make clinical examination difficult, but more importantly it may lead to definitive treatment being delayed and sometimes the optimal moment is lost; fractures and dislocations are more difficult to reduce in a swollen foot. Work quickly; splint the foot, keep it elevated and apply ice-packs; make the diagnosis and institute treatment as soon as possible.

If the foot has to be immobilized, exercise those joints that can be left free. Start weight-bearing as soon as the patient will tolerate it, provided this will not jeopardize the reduction. If a removable splint will fit the purpose, use it so that non-weight-bearing exercises can be started as soon as possible. Prolonged immobilization predisposes to osteoporosis and reflex sympathetic dystrophy.

INJURIES OF THE TALUS

Talar fractures and dislocations are relatively uncommon. They usually involve considerable violence – car accidents in which the occupants are thrown against the

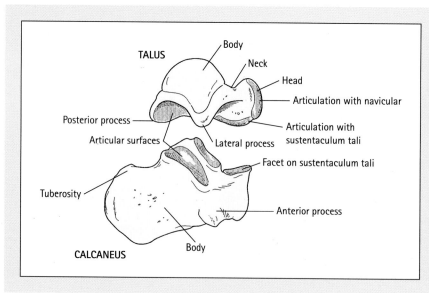

31.19 The talus and calcaneus The main features of these two bones, and their relationship to each other, are shown here.

resistant frame of the vehicle, falls from a height or severe wrenching of the ankle. The injuries include fractures of the head, the neck, the body, or the bony processes of the talus, dislocations of the talus or the joints around the talus, osteochondral fractures of the superior articular surface and a variety of chip or avulsion fractures.

The significance of the more serious injuries is enhanced by two important facts: (a) the talus is a major weight-bearing structure (the superior articular surface carries a greater load per unit area than any other bone in the body), and (b) it has a vulnerable blood supply and is a relatively common site for post-traumatic ischaemic necrosis.

Blood vessels enter the bone from the anterior tibial, posterior tibial and peroneal arteries, as well as anastomotic vessels from the surrounding capsule and ligaments. The head of the talus is richly supplied by intraosseous vessels. However, the body of the talus is supplied mainly by vessels which enter the talar neck from the tarsal canal and then run from anterior to posterior. In fractures of the talar neck these vessels are divided; if the fracture is displaced, the extraosseous plexus too may be damaged and the body of the talus becomes ischaemic.

Mechanism of injury

Fracture of the talar neck is produced by violent hyperextension of the ankle. The neck of the talus is forced against the anterior edge of the tibia, which acts like a cleaver. If the force continues, the fracture is displaced and the surrounding joints may subluxate or dislocate.

Fracture of the body is usually a compression injury due to a fall from a height. Avulsion fractures are associated with ligament strains around the ankle.

Clinical features

The patient has usually been involved in a motor vehicle accident or has fallen from a height. The foot and ankle are painful and swollen; if the fracture is displaced, there may be an obvious deformity, or the skin may be tented or split. Tenting is a dangerous sign; if the fracture or dislocation is not promptly reduced, the skin may slough and become infected. The pulses should be checked and compared with those in the opposite foot.

X-RAY

Anteroposterior, lateral and oblique views are essential; additional views may be needed to exclude associated injuries of the ankle and foot. Both malleoli, the ankle mortise, the talus and all the adjacent tarsal bones should be clearly visualized. Undisplaced fractures are not always easy to see, and sometimes even severely displaced fractures are missed because of unfamiliarity with the normal appearance in various x-ray projections. CT is particularly helpful with fractures of the body of the talus.

Fractures of the head of the talus are rare. They usually involve the talonavicular joint.

Fractures of the neck of the talus are classified as:

- Type I – undisplaced;
- Type II – displaced (however little) and associated with subluxation or dislocation of the subtalar joint;
- Type III – displaced, with dislocation of the body of the talus from the ankle joint (Hawkins, 1970).

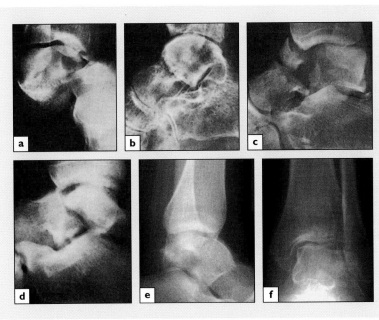

31.20 Injuries of the talus – x-rays (a) Talocalcaneal fracture-dislocation. (b) Undisplaced fracture of the talar neck. (c) Type III fracture of the neck. (d) Displaced fracture of the body of the talus. (e) This fracture of the body was thought to be well reduced; however, in the AP view (f) one can see two overlapping outlines, indicating that the fragments are malrotated.

Fractures of the body of the talus are uncommon. They are often displaced and they may cause distortion of the talocalcaneal joint. Rotational malalignment of the fragments is difficult to diagnose on plain x-ray examination; the deformity is best visualized by three-dimensional CT reconstruction.

Fractures of the lateral and posterior processes are usually associated with ankle ligament strains. It is sometimes difficult to distinguish between a fracture of the posterior process and a normal os trigonum. A simple rule is 'if it's not causing symptoms it doesn't really matter'.

Osteochondral fractures following acute trauma usually occur on the lateral part of the dome of the talus. The diagnosis is often missed when the patient is first seen and may come to light only after CT or MRI.

Treatment

The general principles set out on page 746 should be observed.

UNDISPLACED FRACTURES

A split below-knee plaster is applied and, when the swelling has subsided, is replaced by a complete cast with the foot plantarflexed. Weight-bearing is not permitted for the first 4 weeks; thereafter, the plaster is removed, the fracture position is checked by x-ray, a new cast is applied and weight-bearing is gradually introduced. Further plaster changes will allow the foot to be brought up, slowly, to plantigrade. At 8 weeks the cast is discarded and function is regained by normal use.

DISPLACED FRACTURES OF THE NECK

Even the slightest displacement makes it a type II fracture, which needs to be reduced. If the skin is tight, reduction becomes urgent because of the risk of skin necrosis. Reduction must be *perfect*, (a) in order to ensure that the subtalar joint is mechanically sound, and (b) to lessen the chance – or at any rate lessen the effects – of avascular necrosis.

With *type II fractures*, closed manipulation under general anaesthesia can be tried first. Traction is applied with the ankle in plantarflexion; the foot is then steered into inversion or eversion to correct the displacement shown on x-ray. The reduction is checked by x-ray; nothing short of 'anatomic' is acceptable. A below-knee cast is applied (with the foot still in equinus) and this is retained, non-weight-bearing, for 4 weeks. Cast changes after that will allow the foot to be gradually brought up to plantigrade; however, weightbearing is not permitted until there is evidence of union (8–12 weeks).

If closed reduction fails, open reduction is essential; indeed, some would say that *all* type II fractures should be managed by open reduction and internal fixation without attempting closed treatment. Through an anteromedial incision the fracture is exposed and manipulated into position; wider access can be obtained by osteotomizing the medial malleolus. The position is checked by x-ray and the fracture is then fixed with two Kirschner wires or a lag screw. Post-operatively a below-knee cast is applied; weightbearing is not permitted until there are signs of union (8–12 weeks).

Type III fracture-dislocations need urgent open reduction and internal fixation. A posteromedial approach is used; the medial malleolus is pre-drilled for an AO malleolar screw and osteotomized and retracted distally without injuring the deltoid ligament. This wide exposure is essential to permit removal of small fragments from the ankle joint and perfect reduction of the displaced talar body under direct vision; even then, it is difficult! The position is checked by x-ray and the fracture is then fixed with Kirschner wires or a lag screw. If there is the slightest doubt about the condition of the skin, the wound is left open and delayed primary closure carried out 5 days later. Post-operatively the foot is splinted and elevated until the swelling subsides; a below-knee cast is then applied, following the same routine as for type II injuries.

DISPLACED FRACTURES OF THE BODY

Fractures through the body of the talus are usually displaced or comminuted and involve the ankle and/or the talocalcaneal joint; occasionally the fragments are completely dislocated.

Minimal displacement can be accepted; a below-knee non-weight-bearing cast is applied for 6–8 weeks; this is then replaced by a weight-bearing cast for another 4 weeks.

Horizontal fractures that do not involve the ankle or subtalar joint are treated by closed reduction and cast immobilization (as above).

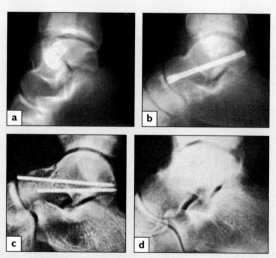

31.21 Fractures of the talus – treatment (a) This displaced fracture of the body was reduced and fixed with a countersunk screw (b), giving a perfect result. Fractures of the neck, even if well reduced, (c) are still at risk of developing ischaemic necrosis (d).

Displaced fractures with dislocation of the adjacent joints should be accurately reduced. In almost all cases open reduction and internal fixation will be needed. A step-cut osteotomy of the medial malleolus is useful for adequate exposure of the talus; the malleolus is pre-drilled before the osteotomy and fixed back in position after the talar fracture has been dealt with. The prognosis for these fractures is poor: there is a considerable incidence of malunion, joint incongruity, avascular necrosis and secondary osteoarthritis of the ankle or talocalcaneal joint.

DISPLACED FRACTURES OF THE HEAD

The main problem is injury to the talonavicular joint. If the fragments are large enough, open reduction and internal fixation with small countersunk screws is the recommended treatment. If there is much comminution, it may be better simply to excise the smaller fragments. Post-operative immobilization is the same as for other talar fractures.

FRACTURES OF THE TALAR PROCESSES

If the fragment is large enough, open reduction and fixation with Kirschner wires or small screws is advisable. Tiny fragments, if they become symptomatic, can be excised.

OSTEOCHONDRAL FRACTURES

These small surface fractures of the dome of the talus usually occur with severe ankle sprains or subtalar dislocations. Most acute lesions can be treated by cast immobilization for 4–6 weeks. Occasionally a displaced fragment is large enough to warrant operative replacement and internal fixation with a countersunk mini-fragment screw or Herbert screw. More often it is very small and, if it is separated from its bed, it is best excised: the exposed bone is then drilled to encourage repair by fibrocartilage.

OPEN FRACTURES

Fractures of the talus are often associated with burst skin wounds. In some cases the fracture becomes 'open' when stretched or tented skin starts sloughing. There is a high risk of infection in these wounds and prophylactic antibiotics are advisable.

The injury is treated as an emergency. Under general anaesthesia, the wound is cleaned and debrided and all necrotic tissue is removed. The fracture is then dealt with as for closed injuries, except that the wound is left open and closed by delayed primary suture or skin grafting 5–7 days later when swelling has subsided and it is certain that there is no infection.

Sometimes, in open injuries, the talus is completely detached and lying in the wound. After adequate debridement and cleansing, the talus should be replaced in the mortise and stabilized, if necessary with crossed Kirschner wires.

Complications

Malunion The importance of accurate reduction has been stressed. Malunion may lead to distortion of the joint surface, limitation of movement and pain on weightbearing. If early follow-up x-rays show redisplacement of the fragments, a further attempt at reduction is justified. Persistent malunion predisposes to osteoarthritis.

Avascular necrosis Avascular necrosis of the body of the talus occurs in displaced fractures of the talar neck. The incidence varies with the severity of displacement: in type I fractures it is less than 10%; in type II about 30–40%; and in type III more than 90%. The earliest x-ray sign (often present by the sixth week) is apparent increased density of the avascular segment; in reality it is the rest of the tarsus that has become slightly porotic with disuse, but the avascular portion remains unaffected and therefore looks more 'dense'. The opposite is also true: if the dome of the talus becomes osteoporotic, this means that it has a blood supply and it will not develop osteonecrosis. This is the basis of Hawkins' sign, which should be looked for 6–8 weeks after injury.

If osteonecrosis does occur, the body of the talus will eventually become densely sclerotic due to reactive new bone formation.

Despite necrosis, the fracture may heal, so treatment should not be interrupted by this event; if anything, weight-bearing should be delayed in the hope that the bone is not unduly flattened. Function may yet be reasonable. However, if the talus becomes flattened or fragmented, or pain and disability are marked, the ankle may need to be arthrodesed.

Secondary osteoarthritis Osteoarthritis of the ankle and/or subtalar joints occurs some years after injury in over 50% of patients with talar neck fractures. There are several causes: articular damage due to the initial trauma; malunion and distortion of the articular surface; and avascular necrosis of the talus. Pain and stiffness can usually be managed by judicious analgesic medication and orthotic adjustments. Operative treatment should be avoided if possible; fusion of one joint is likely to hasten the appearance of symptoms in the other.

FRACTURES OF THE CALCANEUM

The calcaneum is the most commonly fractured tarsal bone, and in 5–10% of cases both heels are injured simultaneously. Crush injuries, although they always heal in the biological sense, are likely to be followed by long-term disability.

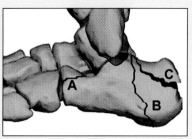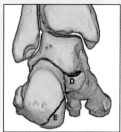

31.22 Extra-articular fractures of the calcaneum
Fractures may occur through (**A**) the anterior process, (**B**) the body, (**C**) the tuberosity, (**D**) the sustentaculum tali or (**E**) the medial tubercle. Treatment is closed unless the fragment is large and badly displaced, in which case it will need to be fixed back in position.

Mechanism of injury

In most cases the patient falls from a height, often from a ladder, onto one or both heels. The calcaneum is driven up against the talus and is split or crushed. Over 20% of these patients suffer associated injuries of the spine, pelvis or hip.

Avulsion fractures sometimes follow traction injuries of the tendo Achillis or the ankle ligaments

Occasionally the bone is shattered by a direct blow.

Pathological anatomy

Based largely on the work of Palmer (1948) and Essex-Lopresti (1952), it has been customary to divide calcaneal fractures into *extra-articular fractures* (those involving the various calcaneal processes or the body posterior to the talocalcaneal joint) and *intra-articular fractures* (those that split the talocalcaneal articular facet).

EXTRA-ARTICULAR FRACTURES
These account for 25% of calcaneal injuries. They usually follow fairly simple patterns, with shearing or avulsion of the anterior process, the sustentaculum tali, the tuberosity or the inferomedial process. Fractures of the posterior (extra-articular) part of the body are caused by compression. Extra-articular fractures are usually easy to manage and have a good prognosis.

INTRA-ARTICULAR FRACTURES
These injuries are much more complex and unpredictable in their outcome. They are best understood by imagining the impact of the talus cleaving the bone from above to produce a *primary fracture line* that runs obliquely across the posterior articular facet and the body from posteromedial to anterolateral. Where it splits the posterior articular facet depends upon the position of the foot at impact; if the heel is in valgus (abducted), the fracture is in the lateral part of the facet; if the heel is in varus (adducted), the fracture is more medial.

This may occasionally be the entire extent of the injury, that is a two-part fracture with a larger posterolateral segment and a slightly smaller antero-medial segment. Much more frequently a *secondary fracture line* appears in the posterolateral segment, thus converting it into a three-part fracture. This secondary fracture usually propagates in one of two ways, often referred to as 'tongue-type' and 'joint depression' fractures (Essex-Lopresti, 1952). In the 'tongue-type' fracture, the crack runs posteriorly from the crucial angle (Gissane's angle) to the tuberosity, creating what looks like a large 'tongue' of bone in the lateral x-ray (in fact the superolateral part of the body of the talus, including much of the articular facet). In the 'joint depression' fracture, the secondary crack curves round behind the articular facet, thus isolating a small fragment consisting of the thalamic portion of the calcaneum with the lateral part of the articular facet. In both types, the lateral x-ray shows what looks like tilting or depression of the thalamic part of the calcaneum; in reality (as shown by CT) the lateral joint fragment swivels posterolaterally, the body of the calcaneum is driven upwards and laterally (as well as often tilting into varus) and the medial sustentacular fragment maintains its relationship to the talus. The lateral joint fragment may sometimes be trapped within the body of the calcaneum and can only be reduced if the lateral wall of the body is osteotomized so as to gain access to it (Eastwood *et al.*, 1993b). The upwards displacement of the body of the calcaneum produces one of the classic x-ray signs of a 'depressed' fracture: flattening of the angle subtended by the posterior articular surface and the upper surface of the body posterior to the joint (Böhler's angle).

The advent of CT, and the trend towards operative reduction and fixation of depressed calcaneal fractures, have sharpened our understanding of these complex injuries. In most cases there are more than three fragments, with considerable variability in the pattern of displacement (Eastwood *et al.*, 1993a; Langdon *et al.*, 1994). The fracture often extends across the anterior facet into the calcaneocuboid joint; the lateral wall of the calcaneum may be comminuted and the posterior articular facet is sometimes split sagitally into three or more pieces. Lateral displacement of the body causes the heel to be widened and the tip of the fibula may impinge on the lateral wall, compressing the peroneal tendons.

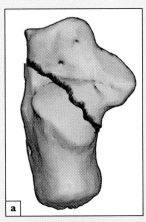
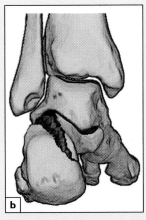
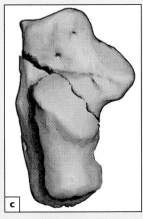
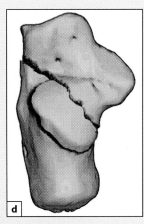

31.23 Intra-articular fractures of the calcaneum The primary fracture line (**a, b**) is created by the impact of the talus on the calcaneum – it runs from posteromedial to anterolateral. Secondary fracture lines may create 'tongue' (**c**) or 'joint depression' (**d**) variants to the fracture pattern.

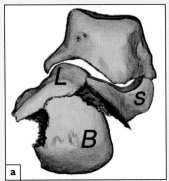
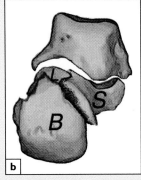
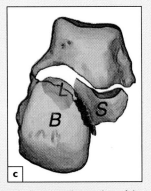

31.24 Intra-articular fractures of the calcaneum CT scans have allowed a better understanding of the fracture anatomy. A coronal CT scan enables the identification of three major fragments in most intra-articular fractures: the lateral joint fragment (L), the sustentaculum tali (S) and the body fragment (B). In type 1 fractures (**a**), the lateral joint fragment is in valgus whereas the body is in varus. In type 2 fractures (**b**), the sustentaculum tali is in varus and the lateral joint fragment is elevated in relation to it. In type 3 fractures (**c**) the lateral joint fragment is impacted and buried within the body fragment (Eastwood et al., 1993).

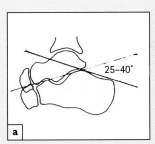
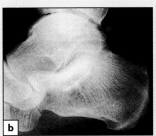
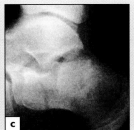
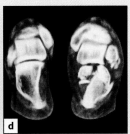

31.25 Fracture of the calcaneum – imaging (**a, b**) Measurement of Böhler's angle and the x-ray appearance in a normal foot. (**c**) Flattening of Böhler's angle in a fractured calcaneum. (**d**) The CT scan in this case shows how the articular fragments have been split apart.

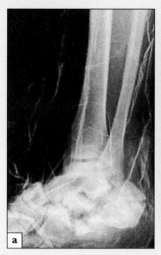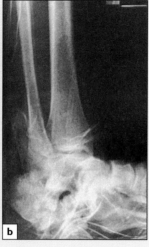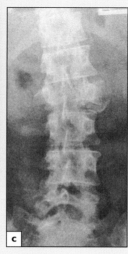

31.26 Calcaneal fractures – imaging Bilateral calcaneal fractures (**a**, **b**) are caused by a fall on the heels from a height or by an explosion from below. In either case the spine also may be fractured, as it was (**c**) in this patient. With bilateral heel fractures, always x-ray the spine.

Clinical features

Unless the patient is unconscious, he or she will give a history of a fall from a height; in elderly osteoporotic people even a comparatively minor injury may fracture the calcaneum.

The foot is painful and swollen and a large bruise appears on the lateral aspect of the heel. The heel may look broad and squat. The surrounding tissues are thick and tender, and the normal concavity below the lateral malleolus is lacking. The subtalar joint cannot be moved but ankle movement is possible.

Always check for signs of a compartment syndrome of the foot (intense pain, very extensive bruising and diminished sensibility).

X-RAY

Plain x-rays should include lateral, oblique and axial views. Extra-articular fractures are usually fairly obvious. Intra-articular fractures, also, can often be identified in the plain films and if there is displacement of the fragments the lateral view may show flattening of the tuber-joint angle (Böhler's angle).

For accurate definition of intra-articular fractures, CT is essential. Coronal sections will show the fracture 'geometry' clearly enough to permit accurate diagnosis of most intra-articular fractures (Lowrie *et al.*, 1988; Crosby and Fitzgibbons, 1993).

With severe injuries – and especially with bilateral fractures – it is essential to x-ray the knees, the spine and the pelvis as well.

Treatment

For all except the most minor injuries, the patient is admitted to hospital so that the leg and foot can be elevated and treated with ice packs until the swelling subsides. This also gives time to obtain the necessary x-rays and CT scans.

EXTRA-ARTICULAR FRACTURES

The byword for the management of extra-articular fractures is 'mobility and function are more important than anatomical repositioning'. The vast majority are treated non-operatively: compression bandaging, ice packs and elevation until the swelling subsides; exercises as soon as pain permits; no weight-bearing for 4 weeks, followed by partial weight-bearing for another 4 weeks. Variations from this routine relate to specific injuries.

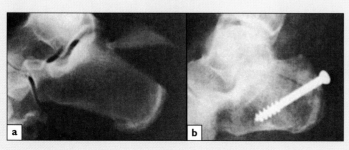

31.27 Extra-articular calcaneal fractures – treatment (**a**) Avulsion fracture of posterosuperior corner (**b**) fixed by a screw.

Fractures of the anterior process Most of these are avulsion fractures and many are mistaken for an ankle sprain. Oblique x-rays will show the fracture, which almost always involves the calcaneocuboid joint. If there is a very large displaced fragment, internal fixation may be needed; this is followed by the usual 'closed' routine.

Fractures of the tuberosity These are usually due to avulsion by the tendo Achillis; clinical signs are similar to those of a torn Achilles tendon. If the fragment is displaced, it should be reduced and fixed with cancellous screws; the foot is then immobilized in slight equinus to relieve tension on the tendo Achillis; weight-bearing can be permitted after 4 weeks.

Fractures of the body If it is certain that the subtalar joint is not involved, the prognosis is good and the fracture can be treated by the usual 'closed' routine. However, if there is much sideways displacement and widening of the heel, closed reduction by manual compression should be attempted. Weight-bearing is avoided for 6–8 weeks; however, cast immobilization is unnecessary except if both heels are fractured or if the patient simply cannot manage a one-legged gait with crutches (e.g. those who are elderly or frail).

INTRA-ARTICULAR FRACTURES

Undisplaced fractures are treated in much the same way as extra-articular fractures: compression bandaging, ice-packs and elevation followed by exercises and non-weight-bearing for 6–8 weeks. As long as vertical stress is avoided, the fracture will not become displaced; cast immobilization is therefore unnecessary and it may even be harmful in that it increases the risk of stiffness and reflex sympathetic dystrophy. In a small series of well-documented cases assessed by CT, Crosby and Fitzgibbons (1993) reported good or excellent results in 90% of patients with undisplaced intra-articular fractures.

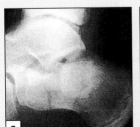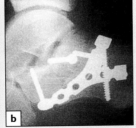

31.28 Fracture of the calcaneum – operative treatment (a) In this displaced fracture of the calcaneum, Böhler's angle is completely flattened. (b) After open reduction and internal fixation, the normal anatomy is restored. (Courtesy of Mr RM Atkins).

Displaced intra-articular fractures are best treated by open reduction and internal fixation as soon as the swelling subsides. CT has greatly facilitated this approach; the medial and lateral fragments can be clearly defined and, with suitable drawings or models, the surgical procedure can be carefully planned and rehearsed.

The operation is usually performed through a single, wide lateral approach; access to the posterior facet and medial fragment is achieved by taking down the lateral aspect of the calcaneum, performing the reduction and then rebuilding this wall. The various fragments are held with interfragmentary screws – bone grafts are sometimes added to fill in defects. The anterior part of the calcaneum and the calcaneocuboid joint also need attention; the fragments are similarly reduced and fixed. Finally a contoured plate is placed on the lateral aspect of the calcaneum to buttress the entire assembly. The wound is then closed and drained. This is specialized surgery which should not be attempted by the novice.

Post-operatively the foot is lightly splinted and elevated. Exercises are begun as soon as pain subsides and after 2–3 weeks the patient can be allowed up non-weight-bearing on crutches. Partial weight-bearing is permitted only when the fracture has healed (seldom before 8 weeks) and full weight-bearing about 4 weeks after that. Restoration of function may take 6–12 months.

Outcome

Extra-articular fractures and undisplaced intra-articular fractures, if properly treated, usually have a good result. However, the patient should be warned that it may take 6–12 months before full function is regained, and in about 10% of cases there will be residual symptoms which might preclude a return to their previous job if this involved walking on uneven surfaces or balancing on ladders.

The outcome for *displaced intra-articular fractures* is much less predictable. The results of operative treatment are heavily dependent on the severity of the fracture and the experience of the surgeon (Buckley and Meek, 1992; Sanders and Gregory, 1995). In expert hands, this is now the method of choice; good results can be achieved in over 70% of cases. However, it is not an enterprise for the tyro and unless the appropriate skills and facilities are available the patient should be referred to a specializing centre.

Closed treatment, though it may be the only alternative, has a bad reputation. Crosby and Fitzgibbons (1993), in a follow-up of 30 patients who had undergone closed treatment, found that 50% of those with uncomplicated displaced intra-articular fractures were contemplating having an arthrodesis within 4 years of injury; only two out of 10 patients had a 'good' result. Those with comminuted fractures fared even worse: all of them were assessed as having a poor result.

Complications

EARLY

Swelling and blistering Intense swelling and blistering may jeopardize operative treatment. The limb should be elevated with the minimum of delay.

Compartment syndrome About 10% of patients develop intense pressure symptoms. The risk of a full-blown compartment syndrome can be minimized by starting treatment early. If operative decompression is done, this will delay any definitive procedure for the fracture.

LATE

Malunion Closed treatment of displaced fractures, or injudicious weight-bearing after open reduction, may result in malunion. *The heel is broad and squat*, and the patient has a problem fitting shoes. Usually the foot is in valgus and walking may be impaired.

Peroneal tendon impingement Lateral displacement of the body of the calcaneum may cause painful compression of the peroneal tendons against the lateral malleolus. Treatment consists of operative paring down of protuberant bone on the lateral wall of the calcaneum.

Insufficiency of the tendo Achillis The loss of heel height may result in diminished tendo Achillis action. If this interferes markedly with walking, subtalar arthrodesis with insertion of a bone block may alleviate the problem.

Talocalcaneal stiffness and osteoarthritis Displaced intra-articular fractures may lead to joint stiffness and, eventually, osteoarthritis. This can usually be managed conservatively but persistent or severe pain may necessitate subtalar arthrodesis. If the calcaneocuboid joint is also involved, a triple arthrodesis is better.

MID-TARSAL INJURIES

Injuries in this area vary from minor sprains, often incorrectly labelled as 'ankle' sprains, to severe fracture-dislocations which can threaten the survival of the foot. The mechanism differs accordingly, from benign twisting injuries to crushing forces which produce severe soft-tissue damage; bleeding into the fascial compartments of the foot may cause a typical compartment syndrome.

Isolated injuries of the navicular, cuneiform or cuboid bones are rare. Fractures in this region should be assumed to be 'combination' fractures or fracture-subluxations until proved otherwise.

Pathological anatomy

The most useful classification is that of Main and Jowett (1975), which is based on the mechanism of injury.

Medial stress injuries are caused by violent inversion of the foot and vary in severity from sprains of the mid-tarsal joint to subluxation or fracture-subluxation of the talonavicular or mid-tarsal joints.

Longitudinal stress injuries are the most common. They are caused by a severe longitudinal force with the foot in plantarflexion. The navicular is compressed between the cuneiforms and the talus, resulting in fracture of the navicular and subluxation of the mid-tarsal joint.

Lateral stress injuries are usually due to falls in which the foot is forced into valgus. Injuries include fractures and fracture-subluxations of the cuboid and the anterior end of the calcaneum as well as avulsion injuries on the medial side of the foot.

Plantar stress injuries result from falls in which the foot is twisted and trapped under the body; they usually present as dorsal avulsion injuries or fracture-subluxation of the calcaneocuboid joint.

Crush injuries usually cause open comminuted fractures of the mid-tarsal region.

Clinical features

The foot is bruised and swollen. Tenderness is usually diffuse across the mid-foot. A medial mid-tarsal dislocation looks like an 'acute clubfoot' and a lateral dislocation produces a valgus deformity; with longitudinal stress injuries there is often no obvious deformity. Any attempt at movement is painful. It is important to exclude distal ischaemia or a compartment syndrome.

X-RAY

Multiple views are necessary to determine the extent of the injury; be sure that *all* the tarsal bones are clearly shown. Tarsometatarsal dislocation may be missed if the forefoot falls back into place; fractures of the tarsal bones or bases of the metatarsals should alert the surgeon to this possibility.

Treatment

Ligamentous strains The foot may be bandaged until acute pain subsides. Thereafter, movement is encouraged.

Undisplaced fractures The foot is elevated to counteract swelling. After 3 or 4 days a below-knee cast is applied and the patient is allowed up on crutches with limited weight-bearing. The plaster is retained for 4–6 weeks.

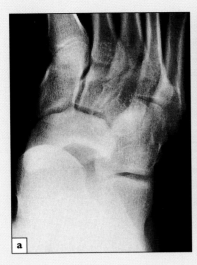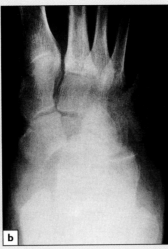

31.29 Tarso-metatarsal injuries X-rays of two patients showing (**a**) talonavicular dislocation and (**b**) a longitudinal compression fracture of the navicular.

Displaced fractures An isolated navicular or cuboid fracture is sometimes displaced and, if so, may need open reduction and screw fixation.

Fracture-dislocation These are severe injuries. Under general anaesthesia, the dislocation can usually be reduced by closed manipulation but holding it is a problem. If there is the least tendency to redisplacement, percutaneous Kirschner wires are run across the joints to fix them in position. The foot is immobilized in a below-knee cast for 6–8 weeks. Exercises are then begun and should be practised assiduously; it may be 6–8 months before function is regained.

If accurate reduction cannot be achieved by closed manipulation, then open reduction and screw fixation is necessary; the importance of anatomical reduction cannot be over-emphasized. However, missed fractures are a lost cause and open reduction will seldom improve the situation in those who present late (more than 3 weeks after injury).

Comminuted fractures Severely comminuted fractures defy accurate reduction. Attention should be paid to the soft tissues; there is a risk of ischaemia. The foot is splinted in the best possible position and elevated until swelling subsides. Early arthrodesis, with restoration of the longitudinal arch, is advisable.

Outcome

A major problem with mid-tarsal injuries is the frequency with which fractures and dislocations are missed at the first examination, resulting in under-treatment and a poor outcome. Even with accurate reduction of mid-tarsal fracture-dislocations, post-traumatic osteoarthritis may develop and about 50% of patients fail to regain normal function. If symptoms are persistent and intrusive, arthrodesis may be indicated.

TARSO-METATARSAL INJURIES

The five tarso-metatarsal joints form a structural complex which is held intact partly by the interdigitating joints and partly by the strong ligaments which bind the metatarsal bones to each other and to the tarsal bones of the mid-foot.

Sprains are quite common but dislocation is rare; twisting and crushing injuries are the usual causes.

Tarso-metatarsal dislocation or fracture-dislocation should always be suspected in patients with pain and swelling of the foot after high-velocity car accidents. Only with severe injury is there an obvious deformity.

X-rays may be difficult to interpret; something looks wrong, but it is often difficult to tell what; multiple views may be needed and comparison with the normal foot is helpful. Concentrate on the second and fourth metatarsals: the medial edge of the second should be in line with the medial edge of the second cuneiform, and the medial edge of the fourth should line up with the medial side of the cuboid. If a fracture-dislocation is suspected (the displacement may reduce spontaneously and not be immediately detectable), stress views may reveal the abnormality.

Treatment

The method of treatment depends on the severity of the injury. Undisplaced sprains require cast immobilization for 4–6 weeks. Subluxation or dislocation calls for accurate reduction. This can often be achieved by traction and manipulation under anaesthesia; the position is then held with percutaneous Kirschner wires or screws and cast immobilization. The cast is changed after a few days when swelling has subsided; the new cast is retained, non-weight-

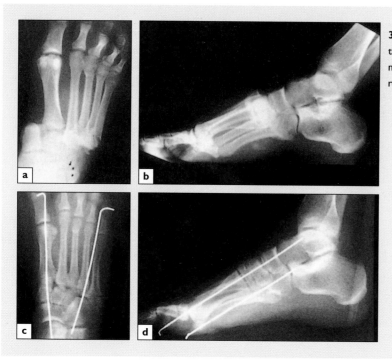

31.30 Tarso-metatarsal injuries (**a, b**) X-ray of the foot showing fracture-dislocation of the tarso-metatarsal joints. This injury was treated by open reduction and fixation with Kirschner wires (**c, d**).

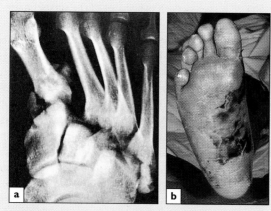

31.31 Tarso-metatarsal injuries – complications (**a**) A severe injury such as this inevitably causes bleeding into the soft tissues of the foot. (**b**) This patient developed a compartment syndrome and threatened Volkmann's ischaemia. Prompt incision and decompression of the plantar compartment prevented a disaster.

bearing, for 6–8 weeks. The Kirschner wires are then removed and rehabilitation exercises begun.

If closed reduction fails, open reduction is essential. The key to success is the second tarso-metatarsal joint. Through a longitudinal incision, the base of the second metatarsal is exposed and the joint manipulated into position. Reduction of the remaining parts of the tarso-metatarsal articulation will not be too difficult. The bones are fixed with percutaneous Kirschner wires or screws and the foot is immobilized as described above. If stability cannot be achieved, external fixation may be needed.

Complications

Compartment syndrome A tensely swollen foot may hide a serious compartment syndrome which could result in ischaemic contractures. If this is suspected, intracompartmental pressures should be measured (see page 563). Treatment should be prompt and effective: through a medial longitudinal incision, all the compartments can be reached and decompressed; the wound is left open until swelling subsides and the skin can be closed without tension.

INJURIES OF THE METATARSAL BONES

Metatarsal fractures are relatively common and are of four types: crush fractures due to a direct blow, a spiral fracture of the shaft due to a twisting injury, avulsion fractures due to ligament strains and insufficiency fractures due to repetitive stress.

Clinical features

In acute injuries pain, swelling and bruising of the foot are usually quite marked; with stress fractures, the symptoms and signs are more insidious.

X-rays should include routine anteroposterior, lateral and oblique views of the entire foot; multiple injuries are not uncommon. Undisplaced fractures may be difficult to detect and stress fractures usually show nothing at all until several weeks later.

Treatment

Treatment will depend on the type of fracture, the site of injury and the degree of displacement.

UNDISPLACED AND MINIMALLY DISPLACED FRACTURES

These can be treated by immobilization in a below-knee cast, non-weight-bearing, for 3 weeks, followed by a further 3 weeks in a weight-bearing cast or splint. At the end of that period, exercise is very important and the patient is encouraged to resume normal activity.

If this method is adopted, it is wise to keep the patient under observation for the first 48 hours to ensure that swelling and soft-tissue damage are not severe.

An alternative approach is to aim for early movement and functional activity. The foot is splinted and elevated and active movements are started immediately. As soon as the swelling has subsided, firm strapping is applied, the patient is given an oversized boot and walking is encouraged. Slight malunion rarely results in disability once mobility has been regained.

DISPLACED FRACTURES

Displaced fractures can usually be treated closed. The foot is elevated until swelling subsides. The fracture is then reduced by traction under anaesthesia and the leg immobilized in a cast – non-weight-bearing – for 4 weeks. At the end of that period weight-bearing is permitted but the cast is retained for a further 2 weeks or until the fracture has healed.

What if closed reduction fails? For the second to fifth metatarsals, displacement in the coronal plane can be accepted and closed treatment, as above, is satisfactory. However, for the first metatarsal and for all fractures with significant displacement in the sagittal plane (i.e. depression or elevation of the displaced fragment) open reduction and internal fixation with crossed Kirschner wires is advisable. A below-knee cast is applied and weight-bearing is avoided for 3 weeks; this is then replaced by a weight-bearing cast for another 4 weeks, at which time the Kirschner wires are removed.

Fractures of the metatarsal neck have a tendency to displace, or redisplace, with closed immobilization. It is therefore important to check the position repeatedly if closed treatment is used. If the fracture is unstable, it may be possible to maintain the position by percutaneous Kirschner wire fixation. However, if this is unsuccessful, open reduction and internal fixation with an intramedullary Kirschner wire is advisable. The wire is removed after 3 weeks; cast immobilization is retained for 4–6 weeks.

TRACTION INJURY

Forced inversion of the foot (the 'pot-hole injury') may cause avulsion of the base of the fifth metatarsal. Pain due to a sprained ankle may overshadow pain in the foot. Examination will disclose a point of tenderness directly over the prominence at the base of the fifth metatarsal bone.

X-ray shows a transverse fracture near the tip of the metatarsal base; the small fragment is usually only slightly displaced. Occasionally a normal peroneal ossicle in this area may be mistaken for a fracture; x-ray of the other foot will show a symmetrical opacity.

If pain is severe, the foot should be rested and elevated for a few days. Thereafter, activity is encouraged and the patient walks as normally as possible in an ordinary shoe. Full painless function is rapidly regained.

If the fragment is markedly separated, a painful non-union occasionally ensues. This can be treated by fixation with an interfragmentary screw.

STRESS INJURY (MARCH FRACTURE)

In a young adult (often a military recruit or a nurse) the foot may become painful and slightly swollen after overuse. A tender lump is palpable just distal to the mid-shaft of a metatarsal bone. Usually the second metatarsal is affected, especially if it is much longer than an 'atavistic' first metatarsal. The x-ray appearance may at first be normal but a radioisotope scan will show an area of intense activity in the bone. Later a hairline crack may be visible and later still a mass of callus is seen.

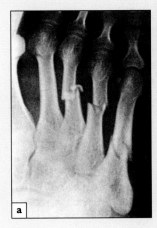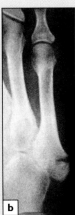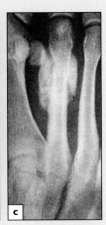

31.32 Metatarsal injuries (a) Transverse fractures of three metatarsal shafts. (b) Avulsion fracture of the base of the fifth metatarsal – the pot-hole injury, or Robert Jones fracture. (c) Florid callus in a stress fracture of the second metatarsal.

Unaccountable pain in elderly osteoporotic people may be due to the same lesion; x-ray diagnosis is more difficult because callus is minimal and there may be no more than a fine linear periosteal reaction along the metatarsal.

Metatarsal pain after Keller's operation also may be due to stress fractures of the adjacent metatarsals, a consequence of redistributed stresses in the foot.

No displacement occurs and neither reduction nor splintage is necessary. The forefoot may be supported with an elastic bandage and normal walking is encouraged.

INJURIES OF THE METATARSOPHALANGEAL JOINTS

Sprains and dislocations of the metatarsophalangeal joints are common in dancers and athletes. A simple sprain requires no more than light splinting; strapping the toe to its neighbour for a week or two is the easiest way. If the toe is dislocated, it should be reduced by traction and manipulation; the foot is then protected in a short walking cast for a few weeks.

FRACTURED TOES

A heavy object falling on the toes may fracture phalanges. If the skin is broken it must be covered with a sterile dressing. The fracture is disregarded and the patient encouraged to walk in a suitably mutilated boot. If pain is marked, the toe may be splinted by strapping it to its neighbour for 2–3 weeks.

FRACTURED SESAMOIDS

One of the sesamoids (usually the medial) may fracture from either a direct injury (landing from a height on the ball of the foot) or sudden traction; chronic, repetitive stress is more often seen in dancers and runners.

The patient complains of pain directly over the sesamoid. There is a tender spot in the same area and sometimes pain can be exacerbated by passively hyperextending the big toe. X-rays will usually show the fracture (which must be distinguished from a smooth-edged bipartite sesamoid).

Treatment is often unnecessary, though a local injection of lignocaine helps for pain. If discomfort is marked, the foot can be immobilized in a short-leg walking cast for 2–3 weeks. Occasionally, intractable symptoms call for excision of the offending ossicle; care should be taken not to disrupt the flexor attachment to the proximal phalanx as this may result in valgus, varus or cock-up deformity of the great toe.

REFERENCES AND FURTHER READING

Broström L (1966) Sprained ankles. Surgical treatment of 'chronic' ligament ruptures. *Acta Chirurgie Scandinavica* 132, 551-565

Buckley RE, Meek RN (1992) Comparison of open versus closed reduction of intra-articular calcaneal fractures: a matched cohort in workmen. *Journal of Orthopaedic Trauma* 6, 216-222

Chrisman OD, Snook GA (1969) Reconstruction of lateral ligament tears of the ankle: an experimental study and clinical evaluation of seven patients treated by a new modification of the Elmslie procedure. *Journal of Bone and Joint Surgery* 51A, 904-912

Colville MR (1994) Reconstruction of the lateral ankle ligaments. *Journal of Bone and Joint Surgery* 76A, 1092-1102

Crosby LA, Fitzgibbons T (1993) Intra-articular calcaneal fractures: Results of closed treatment. *Clinical Orthopaedics* 290, 46-54

Das De S, Balasubramaniam P (1985) A repair operation for recurrent dislocation of the peroneal tendons. *Journal of Bone and Joint Surgery* 67B, 585-587

Dias LS, Tachdjian MO (1978) Physeal injuries of the ankle in children. *Clinical Orthopaedics* 136, 230

Eastwood DM, Gregg PJ, Atkins RM (1993a) Intra-articular fractures of the calcaneum. Part 1: Pathological anatomy and classification. *Journal of Bone and Joint Surgery* 75B, 183-188

Eastwood DM, Langkamer VG, Atkins RM (1993b) Intra-articular fractures of the calcaneum. Part 2: Open reduction and internal fixation by the extended lateral transcalcaneal approach. *Journal of Bone and Joint Surgery* 75B, 189-195

Essex-Lopresti P (1952) The mechanism, reduction technique and results in fractures of the os calcis. *British Journal of Surgery* 39, 395-419

Hawkins LG (1970) Fractures of the neck of the talus. *Journal of Bone and Joint Surgery* 52A, 991-1002

Hopkinson WJ, St Pierre P, Ryan JB *et al* (1990) Syndesmosis sprains of the ankle. *Foot Ankle* 10, 325

Karlsson J, Bergsten T, Lansinger O *et al* (1989). Surgical treatment of chronic lateral instability of the ankle joint. A new procedure. American Journal of Sports Medicine 17, 268-274

Langdon IJ, Kerr PS, Atkins RM (1994) Fractures of the calcaneum: the anterolateral fragment. *Journal of Bone and Joint Surgery* 76B, 303-305

Lauge-Hansen N (1950) Fractures of the ankle. II. Combined experimental–surgical and experimental–roentgenologic investigations. *Archives of Surgery* 60, 957-985

Lowrie IG, Finlay DB, Brenkel IJ, Gregg PJ (1988) Computerised tomographic assessment of the subtalar joint in calcaneal fractures. *Journal of Bone and Joint Surgery* 70B, 247-250

Main BJ, Jowett RL (1975) Injuries of the midtarsal joint. *Journal of Bone and Joint Surgery* 57B, 89-97

Müller ME, Allgöwer M, Schneider R, Willeneger H (1991) *Manual of Internal Fixation* 3rd edition. Springer, Berlin, pp598-600

Palmer I (1948) The mechanism and treatment of fractures of the calcaneus. *Journal of Bone and Joint Surgery* 30A, 2-8

Rüedi TP, Allgöwer M (1979) The operative treatment of intra-articular fractures of the lower end of the tibia. *Clinical Orthopaedics* 138, 105-110

Sanders R, Gregory P (1995) Operative treatment of intra-articular fractures of the calcaneus. *Orthopaedic Clinics of North America* 26, 203-214

Teeny SM, Wiss DA (1993) Open reduction and internal fixation of tibial plafond fractures. *Clinical Orthopaedics* 292, 108-117

Vander Griend R, Michelson JD, Bone LB (1996) Fractures of the ankle and distal part of the tibia. *Journal of Bone and Joint Surgery* 78A, 1772-1783

Page numbers in **bold** refer to major discussions and can include aetiology/pathology/diagnosis/clinical features/imaging and treatment.

Page numbers in *italics* refer to pages on which figures/tables appear.

vs denotes differential diagnosis or comparisons.

A

Abbreviated Injury Scale (AIS) 538
abdominal injuries **529–530**, 547
abduction 8, 278, 408
abscess 27
 Brodie's 32
 cold (tuberculosis) 44, 387, 388, *389*
 epidural 212
 hand infections 350
 horse-shoe 352
 psoas 65, *389*
 subperiosteal 28
absorptiometry 114
accessory nerve, spinal *240*, 297
accidents
 management at scene **521–523**
 management in hospital **523–525**
 see also trauma
acetabulum 446, *675*
 dysplasia 80, **416–418**, *417*
 fractures **674–678**, *675*
  treatment 676–677, *677*
 lateral indentation *120*
 protrusio acetabuli (otto pelvis) 84, *419*, **419**
Achilles tendon *see* tendo Achilles
achondroplasia *141*, **141–142**, 145
acid–base balance 111
acrocephalosyndactyly 150
acromegaly 130
acromioclavicular joint *585*
 dislocations 586
 injuries *585*, **585–586**, *586*
 osteoarthritis *298*, **298**
 rheumatoid arthritis 293
 sprains 585, 586
acromion, fractures 585
acromioplasty 284–285
acrosyndactyly 337
acrylic cement 273
actinomycosis 47
action potentials 24, 229
acute phase proteins 21
adamantinoma *193*, **193**

adduction 8, 278, 408
adductor longus train 440
adhesions, knee 708
adhesive capulitis *287*, **287–289**
adolescents
 flat foot 492–493
 hallux valgus 500
 idiopathic scoliosis 378–381
 kyphosis *see* Scheuermann's disease
adrenal corticosteroids 110, 130
adrenocortical dysfunction **130–131**
Adson's test 251, 358
adult respiratory distress syndrome (ARDS) *535*, **535**, 696, 700
age
 bone changes **111–112**
 fracture type *545*
 intervertebral disc changes 390
 osteoarthritis and 77–78
airway
 problems after trauma **525**
 protection/maintenance after accidents 521–522, 523, 525, 532, 533
Aitkin's classification 421, *421*
Albers-Schönberg disease *147*, **147–148**
Albright's syndrome 174
alcohol abuse
 osteonecrosis after 92, 95, *96*, 97
 osteoporosis 119
 radial nerve injuries 241
algodystrophy *see* reflex sympathetic dystrophy (RSD)
alkaline phosphatase, serum levels 114, 127
alkaptonuria 74, *74*, **159**
Allen test 636
allografts, bone 261
alpha-fetoprotein (AFP) 136
ambulances 523
amelia 162
amniocentesis 136
amputations **267–271**, *268*
 complications **270–271**
 fingers 638, 641
 indications and types 267
 other sites 269–270
 principle of method 268–269
 prostheses *270*, **270**
 sites of election 267–269, *268*
 Syme's 163, *269*, **269–270**
 tumours 172
amyloidosis 58, 67
amyotrophic lateral sclerosis **221**
anaemia, hypochromic 21
anaesthesia 12
analgesic arthropathy 84
anatomical snuffbox 330

aneurysm, popliteal 478
aneurysmal bone cyst *180*, **180–181**
ankle **485–517**
 amputations above 269–270
 anatomy **515–516**, 733
 clonus 12
 dislocation of peroneal tendons 736, *736*
 examination *485*, **485–488**
  imaging *487*, **487–488**
 fracture-dislocations *739*
 fractures **737–741**
  children **743–746**, *744*
  displaced 739–741
  open 741
  pilon 742, **742–743**, *743*
  treatment 738–741, *740*, 741
  undisplaced 739
 'giving way' **734–736**
 injuries **733–759**
 instability **734–736**, *737*
  tests *735*, **735**
 ligament(s) **515–516**, 733, *733*
  lateral 733, *733*, 734
  medial collateral (deltoid) 733, 736
 ligament injuries **733–737**
  deltoid tears 736
  lateral ligament *733*, 734
  tears 733, 734
 movements 486, *486*, 516
 osteoarthritis 507, *507*, 750
 rheumatoid arthritis **505**, *506*
 sprains 733, 734–736, *735*, 754
 stability 487
 stiffness 730, 741
 symptoms and signs 485–487
 tuberculous arthritis **504**, *505*
 'twisted' 734
 see also foot; talus; tendo Achilles
ankylosing hyperostosis 61
ankylosing spondylitis **58–61**
 cervical spine **368**
 clinical features *59*, **59–60**
 deformities 60, *60*, 61
 differential diagnosis 55, 422
 irritable hip *vs* 422
ankylosis 8
 juvenile chronic arthritis 67
annulus fibrosus 402
anterior cord syndrome 664
anterior cruciate ligament *see* cruciate ligaments
anterior drawer sign 705
anterior drawer test 735, *735*
anterior interosseous nerve
 compression 248
 lesions *243*

anterior interosseous nerve syndrome 248
antibiotics
  acute haematogenous osteomyelitis 31
  acute suppurative arthritis 40
  brucellosis 46
  chronic osteomyelitis 38
  hand infections 350
  open fractures 559
  postoperative infection prevention 36
anticoagulation 258
aorta, ruptured 527, *527*
Apert's syndrome 150
Apley's test 453
apprehension test 8
  at knee *453*, 463, *463*, 581
  at shoulder 289, 589
arachnodactyly 151
arachnoid 530
arachnoiditis 393–394
arm
  cerebral palsy 210–211
  transverse absence 317
  transverse deficiency 162
  see also elbow; forearm; humerus;
    limb; shoulder; wrist
Arnold and Hilgartner classification 88
arthritis
  acute suppurative 30, 32, *39*, **39–41**
  chronic erosive, HA crystal deposition
    75, *75*
  degenerative *see* osteoarthritis
  enteropathic 63, **64–65**
  gonococcal **41**, 63
  haemorrhagic 45
  hypertrophic 79
  juvenile chronic *see* juvenile chronic
    arthritis (JCA)
  neuropathic, elbow **308**
  Paget's 128, *128*
  psoriatic *see* psoriatic arthritis
  pyogenic *see* pyogenic arthritis
  reactive **61–63**
  septic *see* septic arthritis
  subacute 45
  tuberculous 42–46, *43*, *45*
arthritis mutilans 64, *64*, 341
arthrocentesis 21
arthrodesis 8, *86*, **266**, *266*
  elbow **312**
  hip 266, 436, 443, *443*, *444*
  interphalangeal (foot) 503
  knee 86, 481, *481*
  metatarsophalangeal joint 502
  osteoarthritis 86
  poliomyelitis *220*
  rheumatoid arthritis 58
  shoulder 238, **299**, *300*
arthrography 16, *17*
  shoulder 279, 283
arthrogryposis 337
arthrogryposis multiplex congenita
  221–222, *222*, 318
arthroplasty *86*, **266–267**, *267*
  elbow **311–312**
  knee *see* knee, replacement
  osteoarthritis 86

revision 37
  shoulder *299*, **299**
  see also joint replacement
arthroscopy **23–24**
  complications 24
  elbow **311**
  hip 24, 408–409
  indications 23
  knee 23, 454, *455*, 479, 707, 710
  osteoarthritis 82
  shoulder 23, 280, **298**
  technique 23
  wrist 24, 317, 323
arthrotomy **265**
ascorbic acid deficiency **124–125**, *125*
aspirin 258
ataxia 204, 205
  Friedreich's **211**, 224
athetosis 205
atlantoaxial joint
  instability 368
  rotatory displacement 360–361
  subluxation *368*
atlanto-dental interval 650
atlanto-occipital dislocation 650
atlanto-occipital erosion 368
atlas, fracture 651
autoantibodies 51, 67
autografts 260–261
avascular necrosis *see* osteonecrosis
axillary nerve *240*
  injuries **240–241**, 588
axon(s) 201, 229
  degeneration/regeneration 230
  diffuse injury 533
axonotmesis 230, *231*

B

Babinski sign 12
back *see* spine
backache/back pain 371
  chronic 400, *401*
  chronic back pain syndrome **401**
  persistent postoperative 393
  in pregnancy 131
  recurrent 395
  segmental instability 394
  sudden acute 400
  transient after activity 400
  see also low back pain
back strain 400
'bag of bones' technique 605
Baker's cyst 83, 477
Bankart lesion/procedure 289, 290
Barlow's test *410*, 410–411
Barton's fracture 616, 620, *620*
baseball pitcher's elbow 311
basilar impression 361
Batson's plexus 403
battered baby syndrome *577*
  see also child abuse
Baumann's angle 596, *597*
Becker's muscular dystrophy 228
Beck's triad 526

bed sores 571
Bennett's fracture-dislocation *631*,
  631–632, 634
biceps jerk 12
biceps tendinitis 286, *286*
biceps tendon lesions **285–287**, 293
  distal, avulsion **311**
  rupture 286, *286*
biochemical tests 21
biopsy
  bone 22–23, 114–115, **168–169**
  muscle 204
  synovial 55
bisphosphonates 117, 129
bites 353
bladder 667
  injuries 673, *673*
  ruptured 668
  training after paraplegia 664
bleeding
  into joints 40, 87, 88
  therapeutic anticoagulation causing
    258
  see also haemorrhage
bleeding disorders
  swelling of knee 475
  see also haemophilia
blisters, fracture 566
blood loss, accidents 523, *524*, 528–529
blood supply
  femoral head *423*, 447, 684
  spine 403
blood tests 21
blood vessel tumours **198**
blood volume 528
Blount's disease *457*, 457–458
body proportions 136, *136*
Böhler's angle 750, *751*, *753*
bone 105, **105–112**
  age-related changes **111–112**
  amputation complications 271
  biopsy 22–23, 114–115, **168–169**
  cells **105–106**
  composition **105–106**
  cyst *15*, **178–180**, *179*, *182*, 593
    aneurysmal *180*, **180–181**
    solitary (unicameral) 178, *179*
  cyst-like lesions *182*
  deformities 10
    correction **263**, *264*
  density 15
    measurement/scan 113, *113*, 114
    osteoarthritis risk factor 81
  destruction, suppurative arthritis 41
  disappearing **183**
  electrical stimulation 111
  examination 6, 14
  fixation *260*, **260**
  formation 28–29, 153, 260, 445
    see also ossification
  functions 105
  grafts 172, **260–261**, *261*, 612
  growth 106–108, 112, *112*
    acute suppurative arthritis 41
    alterations 32, 578
    developmental disorders *139*

hydatid disease 48, *48*
induction 111
infection 22, 170
  see also osteomyelitis
ischaemic necrosis 28, *91*, 423
  see also osteonecrosis
lengthening 262, *263*
loss 115, 117
  after fractures 572
  postmenopausal *see* osteoporosis
lumps 10, *10*
mass and strength 112
mechanical stress 111
mineral exchange **108–111**
remodelling/modelling **106–108**, *107*, 423
  fracture repair 543, *543*
remodelling unit 107
resorption 107, 112
shape 14
structure 106, *107*
subchondral, osteoarthritis 80
surgery **259–265**
transport 263, *263*
tumours *see* bone tumours
turnover **108–111**, 126
types 106, 539
'vacant areas' 15, *15*
wormian 153
woven 543
x-ray examination 14–15
bone cements
  acrylic **273**
  bioactive 261
bone marrow, osteonecrosis pathogenesis 92, *92*
bone marrow oedema syndrome *100*, **100**, **439–440**, *440*
bone morphogenetic protein (BMP) 111
bone-seeking isotopes 20
bone tumours **167–200**, 577
  benign **173–183**
  classification *167*
  differential diagnosis 169–170
  imaging 17, 18, *19*, 168
  metastatic 15, 167, **193–195**, *194*, *576*, 577
  primary malignant **184–193**
  see also tumours; *specific tumours*
Boston brace 379, *379*
Bouchard's nodes 83
boutonnière deformity 339–341, *340*, *346*, 348, 356
bow legs 455–457, *456*, *457*
bowstring sign 373, *373*
boxer's fracture 630–631
brachial artery injuries 598, 609
brachial neuritis, acute 225, *225*
brachial plexus 236, *236*
brachial plexus injuries **236–238**, *237*
  palsy, obstetrical **238–239**, *239*
bracing, functional 551–553, *552*
  femoral shaft fractures 696, *697*
Brailsford's disease 512
brain 530
brain injuries 530–531, *531*

contusions 533
brain stem 530
breast cancer 577
breathing, management after accidents 521–522, 523, 533
Bristow-Laterjet operation 290
brittle bones *see* osteogenesis imperfecta
Brodie's abscess 32
Brostrom-Karlsson operation 736
Brown-Séquard syndrome 212, *212*, 664
brown tumours *123*
brucellosis **46**
buckle fractures 619
'buddy strapping' 632, *633*
bunion 499
  tailor's 504
burns **533–534**
  hands 640
bursitis
  hip **440–441**
  iliopsoas 441
  infrapatellar 477, *477*
  olecranon *311*, **311**
  prepatellar 477
  trochanteric **440**
  ulnar 306
burst fractures 648, 653, 660, *660*, *661*

C

café-au-lait spots 155, *156*, 174, *199*
Caffey's disease *34*, **34**
Caisson disease 98
calcaneal bone lesions 511
calcaneal fractures *750*, **750–754**, *752*, *753*
  displaced 753
  extra-articular 750, *750*, 752–753
  intra-articular 750, *751*, 753
calcaneal pitch 497, *497*
calcaneofibular ligament 733
calcaneus *746*
calcification
  calcium hydroxyapatite deposition 74
  joints/discs 73
  knee **479**
  rotator cuff **285–286**
  supraspinatus tendon *14*, 285, *286*
calcitonin 110, 117, 128
calcitriol 109
calcium 107, 108, **108–109**, 114
calcium hydroxyapatite deposition disorders **74–75**
calcium pyrophosphate deposition disease **72–74**
  chronic arthropathy 73–74
  differential diagnosis 56
  elbow 308, *308*
calipers 665
callosities 485
callotasis (callus distraction) 262, *262*
callus 169, 541, *542*, 543
  foot 514–515
  formation 542–543
Calve's disease *183*

camptodactyly 337, *337*
Camurati's disease (Engelmann's disease) *148*, **148**
cancellous (trabecular) bone 106, 539
cancer *see* tumours; *specific tumours*
candidiasis 47
candle bones 148, *149*
capillaries, endoneurial 230
capitate bone, fractures 626
capitulum of humerus, fractures *605*, 605–606
carbon fibre implants **273**
carcinomatosis 119
cardiac failure, high-output 128
cardiac tamponade 523–524, 526, 529
cardiogenic shock 529
carpal bones/joints 319–320, *320*, 330
  chronic instability *321*, 321–323, *322*, 572
  dislocations/subluxations **626–628**, *627*
  fractures **625–626**
  fusions 317
  injuries **621–623**, *622*, *623*
  instability 621, *622*
  see also mid-carpal joints; radio-carpal joint
carpal tunnel 247, 330
carpal tunnel syndrome 83, 131, 247, *247*, **247–248**, 330, 348
carpometacarpal joints 355
  dislocation 633–634, *634*
  osteoarthritis 327
carrying angle, forearm 596
cartilage 77
  breakdown/weakness 41, 78, 79
  disorders *139*
  osteoarthritis aetiology/pathology 78, 79
  transplants 86
cartilage-capped exostosis **178**, *179*
cast splintage 551, *552*, 566
Catterall classification 423, *424*
cauda equina 663
  compression 392
causalgia 226, **226–227**, *227*
cellulitis 30
cement *see* bone cements
central cord syndrome 664
ceramic implants **272–273**
cerebellar function, assessment 12
cerebral palsy **205–211**
  clinical features 206–207, *207*
  early diagnosis 205–206, *206*
  hand 342, *342*
  management 208–211
  regional survey 209–211
cerebrospinal fluid (CSF) 530
cervical collar *363*, 648, *648*
cervical ribs 251, *251*
  see also thoracic outlet syndrome
cervical spine
  acute disc prolapse *362*, **362–363**, *363*, 656
  anatomy 369
  ankylosing spondylitis 368

anomalies in children 361, *361*
avulsion injury (spinous process) 656
cord compression 212
double injuries 656, *656*
examination *357*, 357–359, *358*
  imaging 358–359, *359*, *649*
facet dislocation 653–654, *654*, *655*
facet fracture-dislocation 654, *654*
flexion–rotation injuries 653–654
fractures
  burst 648, 653
  C1 *650*, 650–651
  C2 (odontoid) 648, *651*, 651–652, *656*
  'tear-drop' 653, *654*
  wedge compression *652*, 652–653
hyperextension injury 651, *655*,
    655–656
immobilization 644
infections 363
injuries **648–650**
lower, injuries **652–657**
movements *358*, 369
myelopathy **365–366**
nerve root transection 662–663
neurapraxia of cord 656–657
posterior ligament injury 653, *653*
protection after accidents 521–522,
    523, 525
pyogenic infection 366–367, *367*
rheumatoid arthritis 367–368, *368*
stenosis 365–366
tuberculosis 367
tumours 363, 364
unstable injuries 647
upper, injuries **650–652**
vertebral fusion in Klippel-Feil
    syndrome *161*, 161
see also neck; spine
cervical spondylosis 251, 363–365, *364*
cervical-vertebral synostosis 361, *361*
Chance fracture 661, *661*
Charcot–Marie–Tooth disease 223
Charcot's disease 84, *89*, 89–90, 475
Charcot's joints 222, 508
Charnley hip replacement *445*
chauffeur's fracture 620
cheilectomy 502
chemonucleolysis 393
chemotherapy, tumours 172–173
chest
  expansion 60
  injuries 547
    management **525–528**
  stove-in (flail) 526–527
  sucking wounds 526
Chiari's pelvic osteotomy *417*
child abuse *577*, 595, *602*
children
  acute haematogenous osteomyelitis 28,
    29, 31
  acute suppurative arthritis 39
  bow legs and knock knees 455–457,
    456, *457*
  cervical spine injuries 650
  developmental dysplasia of hip 414, *414*
  dislocation of patella 462–465, *463*

examination 13
flat foot 492–493
fractures
  ankle **743–746**, *744*
  distal forearm **618–620**, *619*
  elbow **596–603**
  femoral shaft **700–701**, *701*
  humerus 593, *593*, 595
  metacarpal 632
  proximal femoral **692–693**, *693*
  radius and ulna 611
genetic disorder diagnosis 136–137
hypopituitarism 129
limp *411*
multifocal non-suppurative
    osteomyelitis 33
neck deformities 360–361
pyogenic arthritis of hip 430, *430*
rickets 119
shoulder dislocation 591
cholecalciferol 109
chondroblastoma *177*, **177**
chondrocalcinosis 72, *72*, 74
chondrocytes 77
chondrodiatasis 262, *263*
chondrodysplasia (dysostosis), metaphy-
    seal *143*, **143**
chondrodysplasia punctata **146–147**
chondrolysis 430
chondroma (enchondroma) *176*,
    176–177, 184
  periosteal **177**
chondromalacia 79
  patella *455*, **465–467**, *466*
  sesamoid 513, *514*
chondromyxoid fibroma **177–178**, *178*
chondro-osteodystrophies **138–151**
  see also skeletal dysplasia
chondroplasty 467
chondrosarcoma *184*, **184–185**, *185*,
    576
chordoma **192–193**
chorionic villus sampling 136
Christmas disease 86
chromosome disorders 133–134, *139*, 160
chronic pain syndrome 227
  back pain **401**
circulation, management after accidents
    522, 523–524, 533·
circumduction 8
clavicle
  condensing osteitis 297
  congenital pseudarthrosis **296**
  disorders **295–298**
  fractures *583*, **583–584**
  pseudarthrosis 164, *164*
claw hand 7, 242, 342, *342*
claw toes 221, 224, *496*, 502, *503*, **503**
'clay-shoveller's fracture' 643, 656, *656*
cleft hand 337
cleidocranial dysplasia **149–150**, *150*,
    296
clergyman's knee 477
clinodactyly 337
club foot *488*, **488–491**, *489*, *490*
  correction 263

club hand 317–318, 336–337, *337*
coagulopathies 92, 96
Cobb's angle 377, *377*
coccyx injuries **678**
cock-up deformity 504
Codman's triangle 185, *186*
coin test *388*
cold ischaemic time 639
Coleman's block test 497, *497*
collagen 151
  type I 105, 153
  type II 77
collateral ligaments, of fingers, injuries
    635
collateral ligaments, of knee 705
  calcific deposits 462, 479
  injuries 705
  lateral 483
  medial 483
    calcification 479
    insufficiency 711
    partial tear 460
  reconstruction 479
  tears 460, 707–708
  tests 451, *452*
Colles' fracture 319, 615, *616*, **616–618**,
    617
  comminuted 617
  complications 617–618, *618*
  juvenile 616, **618–620**, *619*
  reversed (Smith's fracture) 616, *618*, 618
coma 524, 531, 533
common peroneal nerve lesions 245
compact (cortical) bone 106
compartment syndrome 87, **252**,
    563–564, *564*
  acute/chronic 246, 252
  after osteotomy 260
  foot 752, 754, 756
  fractures associated 563–564
    radius/ulna 612
    supracondylar 599
    tibia and fibula 728–729, *729*
    tibial plateau 723
  management 564, 729, *730*
complex regional pain syndrome *see*
    reflex sympathetic dystrophy (RSD)
compound palmar ganglion 329–330,
    330
computed tomography (CT) 17–18, *18*
  applications 17
  bone tumours 17, 168
  brain injuries 531–532, *532*
  CT-guided procedures 17
  neck 359
  osteonecrosis 95
  pelvis 669
  quantitative 114
  spiral 646
condylar fracture, phalangeal 634
congenital malformations/deformities
    138, *139*, **160–165**
  cervical vertebrae **161**
  clasped thumb 337
  elbow **304**
  foot **488–491**

hands 336–338, *337*
hip *see* developmental dysplasia of hip (DDH)
limb 162–165
scapula 161
shoulder 295–296
thoracospinal 162
vertebral 160–161
wrist *317*, 317–318
see also skeletal dysplasia; *specific anomalies*
congenital trigger thumb 338
conjunctivitis, Reiter's syndrome 62, *62*
connective tissue 77
connective tissue disorders 9, **67**, *139*, **151–156**
Conradi's disease 146–147, *147*
constriction bands, hand 338
contractures 10, 202
    after fractures 572
    cerebral palsy 208
    hand *338*, 338–339, *339*, *339*
    in paraplegia 665
    skin (hand) 338, *338*
    superficial palmar fascia 338–339
    see also individual contractures
coracoacromial ligament *280*, 300
coracoid process, fractures 584
cord shock 662
corns 485, 514–515
cortical function, assessment 12
corticosteroids
    osteonecrosis after 92, 95, 97
    rheumatoid arthritis 56
    secondary osteoporosis after 118
    side-effects *57*
Cotrel-Dubousset system 379
counselling 137
coxa vara 163, **419–421**, 430, 446
    acquired *420*, 420–421
    congenital 420, *420*
cranial nerves
    compression, Paget's disease 127
    third 530
craniodiaphyseal dysplasia **148**
craniofacial dysplasia **150**
craniometaphyseal dysplasia **147**
C-reactive protein 21
crepitus 7
crescent sign 94, 435
cretinism 131, 145
cricothyrotomy 525
Crohn's disease, arthritis 64–65
crossed sciatic tension 373, 391
crossover syndrome 328–329
cruciate ligaments 483, 705
    examination *707*
    injuries 705
    insufficiency 711
    reconstruction 479
    tears 460, 708, *710*, 711
    tests 451, *452*, 709–710, *710*
crush injury 267, 536–537, 750
    mid-tarsal 754
crush syndrome **536–537**
crutch palsy 230, 241

crystal deposition disorders **69–75**
    calcium hydroxyapatite deposition **74–75**
    see also calcium pyrophosphate deposition disease; gout
cubital tunnel syndrome 248–249
cubitus valgus 304–305, *305*
cubitus varus 305, *305*
cuff tear arthropathy 295
Cushing's disease/syndrome 118, 131
cyst(s)
    Baker's 83, 477
    bone *see* bone, cyst
    ganglion 329, *330*, 462
    meniscus *461*, 461–462, *462*, 477
    popliteal 477, 477–478
    subarticular, osteoarthritis 79, 80, *80*
cytokines 110–111

D

dactylitis 97
Danis–Weber classification 737, *738*, *739*
dead arm syndrome 289
debridement, open fractures 559
decompression sickness 98
deep peroneal nerve lesions 245
deep vein thrombosis (DVT) 257, 258
deformities 4, *5*, 9–10, 202
    assessment 203
    fixed 9, 10
    postural/structural 10
    see also specific deformities/joints/diseases
deltoid muscle
    power, examination 279
    wasting 241, 292
demyelination 223
de Quervain's disease 328, *328*
dermatitis, pustular, feet 62, *63*
dermatomes *203*, 232, *232*, *646*
developmental disorders
    classification 138, *139*
    see also congenital malformations; genetic disorders; skeletal dysplasia
developmental dysplasia of hip (DDH) *18*, **409–416**
    aetiology/pathogenesis 409–410
    clinical features *410*, 410–412, *411*
    imaging *411*, 411–412, *412*
    management 412–415, *413*, *414*, *415*
        reduction *413*, 413–414
    unilateral dislocation 415
diabetes mellitus
    ankle fractures 741
    foot **507–509**, *508*, *509*
    neuropathy 224, 508
diagnosis, orthopaedic 3–25
diagnostic imaging 13–21
diaphragm, ruptured 527
diaphyseal aclasis (hereditary multiple exostosis) **139–141**, *140*, 178
diaphyseal dysplasias **147–148**, *148*
diastematomyelia 214
diastrophic dysplasia **149**

diffuse idiopathic skeletal hyperostosis (DISH) 85, *85*, 365
digital anomalies 165
    see also fingers; toe(s)
digital nerve compression, foot 252
dihydroxycholecalciferol (DHCC) 109
'dinner-fork' deformity 616, 619
diplegia 205, 207
disc *see* intervertebral disc
discitis 386, *387*
discogenic disease, chronic 213
discography 16, *17*, 374
dislocation 10, 581
    acromioclavicular joint 586
    carpal bones/joints **626–628**, *627*
    carpometacarpal joints 633–634, *634*
    cervical spine 653–654, *654*, *655*
    elbow *see* elbow
    habitual (voluntary) 581
    hip *see* hip
    interphalangeal joint 634, *634*
    knee *713*, 713–714
    lunate 626–627
    metacarpophalangeal joints 634, *634*
    mid-carpal joints 628
    occipito-atlantal 650
    radiocarpal 628
    recurrent 572, 581, 589
    shoulder *see* shoulder
    sternoclavicular **586–587**, *587*
    thumb 633–634
    ulnohumeral joint 608
    wrist **626–628**, *627*
    see also fracture-dislocation
disseminated intravascular coagulation (DIC) **536**
distraction histogenesis **261–264**
dorsal intercalated segment instability (DISI) 321, 622, 623
dorsal root ganglia 229
'double crush' phenomenon/syndrome 231, 246, 251
Down's syndrome *160*, 160
drainage
    acute haematogenous infections 31
    acute suppurative arthritis 40–41
    hand infections 350
drawer test 289, 451, 487, 706
    modified 709
drop foot 204, *245*
drop wrist 7, 319
drugs, osteonecrosis induced by 92, 95, 97
dual-energy X-ray absorptiometry (DEXA) 114, 116
Duchenne muscular dystrophy *227*, **227–228**
Dunn's operation 429, *429*
Dupuytren's contracture 338–339, *343*, **343–344**, *344*
Dupuytren's disease 287
dwarfism 141, *142*, 143
dyschondroplasia 14, **143–144**, *144*
dyschondrosteosis 143
dysmorphism 136
dysplasia *see* skeletal dysplasia

dysplasia epiphysealis hemimelica **146**, *147*
dysraphism 160, 214, *214*, *215*
dystonia 204, *204*, 206
dystrophia myotonica 228
Dywer method 379–380

E

eburnation 79
ectromelia 162
Ehlers–Danlos syndrome 152, *152*
elbow **303–312**
  acquired deformities **304–305**
  anatomy 312, 596
  arthrodesis 312
  arthroplasty *307*, **311–312**
  arthroscopy 311
  congenital disorders **304**
  dislocation 304, *608*, **608–610**
    recurrent 609–610
  epiphyses at 596, 599
  examination *303*, **303–304**, *304*
  flail *309*
  fracture-dislocations 606
  fractures in adults **603–610**
    bicondylar 604, *604*
    capitulum *605*, 605–606
    distal humerus **603–605**
    intra-articular 604
    medial epicondyle 609
    olecranon *607*, **607–608**, 609
    supracondylar 603–604
  fractures in children **596–603**
    lateral condyle **599–601**, *600*
    medial condyle 601, *602*
    supracondylar **596–599**, *597*, *598*
  gout and pseudogout 308
  loose bodies 306, *309*
  medial epicondylar apophysis separa-
    tion **601–602**
  movements 304, *304*, 312
  neuropathic arthritis 308
  operations/surgery **311–312**
  osteoarthritis 308, *309*, 610
  osteochondritis dissecans **305–306**,
    306
  overuse/repetitive strain syndromes
    310, **310–311**
  pain 303
  poliomyelitis 219
  pulled 305, 603
  recurrent instability **309–310**
  replacement *307*
  rheumatoid arthritis **306–308**, *307*, 311
  stability 303, 312, 596
  stiffness 303, **308–309**, 599, 601, 602,
    605, 607, 609
  symptoms and signs 303–304
  tennis 249, 310, *310*
  tuberculosis *306*, **306**
elderly
  femoral neck fractures 686, 688, 690
  kyphosis **385–386**
electrical burns 533–534, 640

electrodiagnosis *24*, 24–25, 204
electromyography (EMG) 25, 204, 233
'elephantiasis' *156*
elongation–derotation–flexion (EDF)
  plaster cast 381
embolism
  fat 92, **535–536**, *536*, 700
  hand 354
emphysema, surgical 528
'empty glenoid' sign 589
enchondroma (chondroma) *176*,
  176–177, 184
enchondromatosis **143–144**
endocrine disorders **129–131**
endoneurium 230
endosteal membrane 106
Engelmann's disease *148*, **148**
enteropathic arthritis 63, **64–65**
enthesopathy 59
entrapment syndromes *see* nerve
  compression syndromes
eosinophilic granuloma **182–183**, *183*
epicondylitis
  lateral (tennis elbow) 249, 310, *310*
  medial 311
epidural abscess 212
epidural anaesthesia 258
epineurium 230
epiphyseal arrest 264
epiphyseal growth plate *see* physes
epiphyseal ring sign *125*
epiphyseodesis 264
epiphyses
  dysplasias involving **144–147**, *147*
  in renal osteodystrophy *125*
  stippled **146–147**
epiphysiolysis 426
equinus of foot 210
Erb's palsy 239, *239*
erythrocyte sedimentation rate (ESR)
  21
Ewing's sarcoma *190*, **190**
examination, physical 5–12
  movement assessment 6–9, *7*
  neurological *see* neurological assessment
  paediatric 13
  special situations 13
excision arthroplasty 266
exercise, after fractures **557–558**, *558*
exostosis
  cartilage-capped **178**, *179*
  hereditary multiple (diaphyseal aclasis)
    139–141, *140*, *178*
  ivory **176**
exsanguination 256, 350
extension 8
extensor pollicis longus, ruptured 339,
  571, 618
extensor retinaculum 328
extensor tendons
  hands 335, **355–356**, 637
    rupture 348
  wrist 329
external fixation **555–557**, *556*
extradural haematoma *532*, 533

F

facet joints
  abnormalities 394
  arthrography 374
  dislocations, cervical 648
  displacement 390
  dysfunction **394–396**
  injections 396
facetography 16
facioscapulohumeral dystrophy 228
family history 5, 81, 137
fasciotomy 564, 729, *730*
fat embolism 92, 700
fat embolism syndrome **535–536**, *536*
fat pad, painful under heel 512
'fat pad sign' 596
fatty tumours **195–196**, *196*
felon 351, *351*
femoral anteversion **418–419**, *419*
femoral epiphysis
  distal, fracture-separation **703–704**,
    704
  slipped capital 422, **426–430**, *427*
femoral head 447
  blood supply *423*, 447, 684
  osteonecrosis 91, 97, *159*, 422,
    436–439, 678
    after femoral neck fractures 689, *689*
    after hip dislocation 682
    differential diagnosis 468
    proximal femoral fractures 693
    staging and treatment 438–439, *439*
    see also osteonecrosis; Perthes'
    disease
femoral neck 447
  fractures 92, 117, 128, **684–690**, 690
    complications 688–690, *689*, *690*
    impacted 685, 686
    mechanism and classification
      684–685
    metastatic bone tumours 195
    osteoporotic *684*
    stress 575, **685–686**
    treatment, 688 *686*, **686–688**, *687*
  persistent fetal alignment 419
femoral neck-shaft angle 446
femoral nerve injuries **244**
femoral shaft, fractures 682, 690, *695*,
  695–697
  children **700–701**, *701*
  complex 699
  open 699
  pathological 699, 700
  periprosthetic 699
  refracture 700
femoral stretch test 373, *373*
femur
  amputations 269
  congenital short (deficiency) 162–163
  dysplasia 162–163, *163*
  fractures
    condyle *703*, **703**
    intertrochanteric **690–692**, *691*, *692*
    pathological *576*, 577, 692
    proximal, in children **692–693**, *693*

subtrochanteric *694*, **694–695**
supracondylar **701–702**, *702*
trochanters 690, 693–694
see also femoral neck; femoral shaft
infections 418
proximal femoral focal deficiency
421, **421**
'shepherd's crook' *174*
shortening 264
fetal imaging 136
fibrillation 77, 79
fibrodysplasia ossificans progressiva
155, **155**
fibroma **196**
chondromyxoid **177–178**, *178*
non-ossifying *173*, **173–174**
fibromatosis **196**
fibrosarcoma **196–197**
of bone *189*, **189**
fibrous ankylosis 8
fibrous cortical defects *173*, **173–174**
fibrous dysplasia *174*, **174–175**, *175*
fibrous tumours **196–197**
fibula
congenital absence 164
fractures **731**, *732*
proximal **724**
tibia fracture with **724–730**
finger pulp
infections 351, *351*
injuries 638, *639*
fingers
amputation 638, 641
boutonnière deformity 339–341, *340*,
346, 348, 356
clawing *11*
cold ischaemic time 639
collateral ligament injuries 635
congenital anomalies 165
dropped 339, *340*
fractures 630–631, **632–633**, *633*
see also phalangeal fractures
mallet *see* mallet finger
movements, muscles 355
osteoarthritis 348–349
polyarthritis 85
replantation 639–640
rheumatoid arthritis 348
ring avulsion 638
spider 151, *152*
swan-neck deformity *340*, 341, *341*,
346, 348
terminalization 638, 641
tourniquet 256
trigger *344*, **344–345**
see also hand(s)
fingertip injuries 638, *639*
Finkelstein's test 328
fishmonger's infection 353–354
fixation
bone *260*, **260**
delayed union 566
external **555–557**, *556*
internal *see* internal fixation
open fractures 560, *560*
flaccidity 11

flail chest 526–527
flail elbow *309*
flat foot **491–495**, *492*, *493*
adults 494–495, *495*
children/adolescents 492–493
flexible/rigid 492, *493*, 494
peroneal spastic 493–494
flexion 8
flexor digitorum profundus tendon 636
avulsion 633
repair 637, 640
flexor digitorum superficialis *636*, 636,
640
flexor tendinitis, wrist 329
flexor tendons
avulsion in finger 633
hands 335, 636, 637
rupture 348
repair 637–638, *638*
tendon sheath and pulleys *638*
wrist 329
flexor tenosynovitis 348
hand 352
fluid replacement, after accidents
523–524, 529, 533
fluoride 111, 117
fluorine 125
fluorosis **125–126**
foot **485–517**
amputations at/in 270
anatomy **516**
congenital deformities **488–491**, 516
diabetic **507–509**, *508*, *509*
digital nerve compression 252
drop 204, *245*
examination *485*, **485–488**
imaging *487*, 487–488
flat *see* flat foot
gout *506*, **506**
high-arched (pes cavus) *495*, **495–498**,
496, *498*
injuries **746–759**
management **746**
instability 221
painful **511–514**
paralysed **510–511**, *511*
poliomyelitis 221
positions 516
pronated *see* pes valgus
pustular dermatitis 62, *63*
rheumatoid arthritis 505, *506*
skin disorders **514–515**
spina bifida 217–218
symptoms and signs 485–487
valgus/varus deformity 221
weight-bearing X-rays 497, *497*
see also ankle; forefoot; midfoot
footprints *516*
forearm
carrying angle 596
distal, fractures *621*
children **618–620**, *619*
fractures 319
injuries **611–620**
poliomyelitis 219
see also radius; ulna

forefoot
deformities 489, 490
pain 512–514, *514*
rheumatoid arthritis 505, *506*
foreign body granuloma 515
Forestier's disease (ankylosing hyperostosis) 61, *396*
fracture blisters 566
'fracture disease' 551
fracture-dislocation
ankle *739*
Bennett's **631**, 631–632, 634
cervical spine 654, *654*
elbow 606
Galeazzi, of radius 320, **615**, *615*, *615*,
615
hip 682
humerus 592–593
mid-tarsal injuries 755
Monteggia, of ulna *546*, 610, **613–615**,
614, *615*
shoulder 588, *589*
talocalcaneal *747*
thoracolumbar spine 661–662, *662*
volar 635
fractures
angulation 546, 547
avascular necrosis 570, **570–571**
buckle 619
causes/mechanisms *539*, **539–540**
classification 540, *541*, 547, 724, 725
clinical features **544–547**
closed (simple) 539, 547, *724*
complications **562–563**
treatment **547–558**
comminuted 540
complete/incomplete 540, *540*
complications *562*, **562–574**
early *562*, **562–566**
late **566–574**
compression 540
consolidation 543, **544**
displacement **540–541**, *541*, 547,
548, 579
examination 545–547
fixation *see* fixation
greenstick 540, *540*, 611, 619
healing **541–543**, *542*, *543*, 547
holding reduction 549, **549–557**
imaging 545–546, *546*
implant failure 555
infections 36, 560, *560*, **564–565**, *565*,
567, *576*
juvenile chronic arthritis 67
malunion **569–570**, *570*, 574
manipulation 547, 548, *548*
metaphyseal 574
non-union *544*, **544**, 555, 568,
568–569, *569*
atrophic *544*, 568, 731
hypertrophic *544*, 568, 731
open (compound) 539, *725*
classification/severity 558
complications 563
infections 560, *560*
post-traumatic osteomyelitis 34–35

treatment **558–561**, *559*
osteoarthritis risk factor 81
osteogenesis imperfecta 153, 155
Paget's disease 128, *576*
pathological *see* pathological fractures
physeal *578*, 578–580
postmenopausal osteoporosis and 116, *116*
principles **539–582**
reduction 547, *548*, 548–549
repair *543*, 543–544
shape 547
stabilization 549, 560, *560*
stress (fatigue) *see* stress fractures
traction *see* traction
traumatic 539
treatment 561
  closed fractures **547–558**
  in metastatic bone tumours 195
  open fractures **558–561**, *559*
  quartet 547, *547*, 549, 551
  see also fixation; traction
types **540**
union 543–544
  delayed 566–568, *567*
see also specific bones
Freiberg's disease 101, *101*, 513, 574
Friedreich's ataxia 211, 224
Fröhlich's adiposogenital syndrome 129, *130*
Froment's sign 242
frozen shoulder *287*, **287–289**
fulcrum test 289
functional disability 5, 82
fungal infections **46–48**, 354

G

gait 203–204, 406, 485
  abnormal 12, 204, 207, 209
  cerebral palsy 206–207
  in-toe **418–419**, *419*
  phases of walking 485–486, *486*
Galeazzi fracture-dislocation, of radius 320, *615*, **615**, *615*, **615**
gallium-67 20
gamekeeper's thumb 635, *635*
gamma-globulins, plasma 21
ganglion, compound palmar 329–330, *330*
ganglion cysts 329, *330*, 462
Garden's classification 684, 685, *685*
'garden spade' deformity 618
Garré's sclerosing osteomyelitis **32–33**
gas gangrene 270, *565*, 565–566
Gaucher's disease 31, 40, **98–99**, *99*, 158–159, *159*
gene, therapy 138
genes 133
  mapping 135
  mutations 137
  single gene disorders 133–134
genetic disorders **133–165**
  autosomal dominant 134, *135*
  autosomal recessive 134, *135*

chromosome disorders 133–134, *139*
  management 137–138
  single gene disorders 133–134
  X-linked 134, *135*
genetic heterogeneity 134
genetic markers 134–135
gentamicin-impregnated beads 38
genu recurvatum 220, 458, 723
genu valgum *456*, 458, 483
genu varum 458
giant-cell sarcoma 182
giant-cell tumour *181*, 181–182, *182*
  of tendon sheath *197*, **197**
gibbus 371, 382
gigantism 130, *130*
Gla protein (osteocalcin) 105, 114
Glasgow coma scale 524, *524*, 531, 537
glenohumeral joint disorders **292–295**
glenoid fractures 584
glomus tumour 198
glucocorticoids 130, 131
gluteus medius tendinitis 440
glycosaminoglycans 156, *157*
golfer's elbow 311
gonadal hormone insufficiency 118
goniometer 7
gonococcal arthritis 41, 63
Gorham's disease **183**
gout **69–71**, *71*
  ankle and foot *506*, **506**
  differential diagnosis 40, 55–56, 63, 73, *73*, 85, 170
  elbow **308**
  hand 342
  primary/secondary 69–70
Gowers' sign 227
grafts
  bone *see* bone
  nerve 235, 238
  skin, hand injuries 638
granulation tissue 27, 423
granuloma
  eosinophilic **182–183**, *183*
  foreign body 515
growth defects/disturbance
  after fractures 571
  ankle fractures 745
  juvenile chronic arthritis 67
growth hormone, deficiency 130
gunshot injuries *561*, **561–562**
'gun-stock' deformity 305, *305*
Gustilo's classification 558, *725*
Guyon's canal 242, 249

H

haemangioma 143, *183*, **183**, 198
haemarthrosis
  after fractures 564
  post-traumatic, knee 475
haematoma 169, *169*, 541
haemochromatosis **73–74**, *74*
haemophilia 40, 86, *87*, 87–88, *88*
  arthritis of knee **475**
haemophilic arthropathy **86–88**, *87*, *88*

haemorrhage
  head injuries 532
  pelvic ring injuries 672–673
  trauma causing 522, 523–524, *524*
  see also bleeding
haemothorax 526, 528
hallux rigidus **501–502**, *502*
hallux valgus **498–501**, *499*, *500*, *501*
  adolescents 500
halo rings 648, *648*
hamartoma 198
hamate, fracture 625
hammer toe 502, **503**, *504*
hamstring, lengthening 209, *210*
hand(s) **333–356**, 353, *353*
  acquired deformities **338–343**
  acute infections **349–354**, *350*, *351*
    deep fascial space 352
    fungal 354
    septic arthritis 353, *353*
  applied anatomy **354–356**
  bone lesions 342
  burns 640
  claw 7, 242, 342, *342*
  congenital anomalies **336–338**, *337*
  contractures 338, 338–339
  differentiation failure 337–338
  duplication 338
  examination **333–336**, *334*, *335*
  formation failure 336–337
  functions 354–355
  grip strength *334*, 335
  immobilization position *350*, 355
  incisions 637, *637*
  injuries 342, **629–641**
    joints **633–635**
    ligament **635**
    treatment 629–630
  joint disorders 341–342
  joints 355
  movements 333, 335, *335*, 639
  muscles and tendons 355–356
  nerves 356
  neuromuscular disorders 342–343
  open injuries **636**, **636–641**
    assessment 636, *636*
    delayed repair 640–641
    injection (oil/solvents) 640
    late reconstruction 641, *641*
    zones 637, *637*
  osteoarthritis 83, *84*, **348–349**
  over-/undergrowth 338
  poliomyelitis 219
  positions 355, 629, *629*
  rehabilitation 639, 640
  rheumatoid arthritis *345*, **345–348**, *346*, *347*
  splintage 629, *629*, 638–639, *639*
  symptoms and signs 333, 335
  tendon lesions 339–341
  vascular disorders **354**
  weakness 346
  see also fingers; thumb
Hand-Schüller-Christian disease 183, *183*
hangman's fracture *650*, 652
Harrington system 379, *380*

Harrison's sulcus 119
Haversian system/canals 106
head
  examination after trauma 531
  injuries 530–533, *532*
Heberden's nodes 83, *84*
heel pain 511–512
height 136
hemiplegia 205
heparin 258, 259
hepatitis B 257
hereditary motor and sensory neuropathy *11*, 223–224
hereditary multiple exostosis (diaphyseal aclasis) 139–141, *140, 178*
hereditary neuropathies *223*, 223–225
heroin addicts 31
herpes zoster 224–225, *225*
Herring's lateral pillar classification 424, *425*
heterozygous, definition 134
high-density polyethylene (HDPE) implants 272
'high ulnar paradox' 242
Hilgrenreiner's epiphyseal angle 420, *420*
Hill-Sachs lesion 289
hindfoot, rheumatoid arthritis 505, *506*
hip 405–448
  acetabular dysplasia 416–418, *417*
  adduction deformity 209, *209*
  amputation at 269
  applied anatomy 446–447
  arthrodesis 266, 436, 443, *443, 444*
  arthroscopy 24, 408–409
  biomechanics/forces 447, *447*
  bursitis 440–441
  congenital dislocation *see* developmental dysplasia of hip (DDH)
  development 410
  diagnostic calendar of disorders 409, *409*
  dislocation
    acquired 418–419
    anterior 683, *683*
    central *683*, 684
    children 414–415
    persistent in adults *415*, 415–416, *416*
    persistent traumatic 418
    posterior *681*, 681–684
  dysplasia *see* developmental dysplasia of hip (DDH)
  examination 405–406
    imaging *16*, 408, *409*
  exposure (surgical) 441
  flexion deformity 209, 407
  fracture
    thromboembolism 257
    see also acetabulum; femoral neck
  fracture-dislocations 682
  infections 418
  injuries 681–704
  instability 409
  internal rotation deformity 209
  irritable **422**
  ligaments 447
  movement 407–408, *408*

loss 678
nerve supply 447
normal *16*
operations/surgery **441–446**
osteoarthritis *16, 82, 83, 409, 434,* **434–436,** *435, 436,* 442, 678
pain 422, *440*
poliomyelitis 220
pyogenic arthritis 418, *430,* 430–431, *431*
replacement 16, *16,* 415, *416,* 443–446, *445*
  after fractures 687–688
  complications 445–446
  loosening 445–446, *446*
  sciatic palsy after 244–245
  thromboembolism 257
rheumatoid arthritis *433,* 433–434, *434*
septic arthritis 65
slipped femoral epiphysis 422, 426–430, *427*
snapping 441
spina bifida 217
subluxation 209, 416–418, *417*
  congenital *417*
symptoms and signs 405–406, *406*
tendinitis **440–441**
transient osteoporosis (marrow oedema) *100,* 100, **439–440,** *440*
tuberculosis *431,* 431–433, *432*
Hippocratic method 587
histamine test 237
histiocytoma, malignant fibrous *189,* 189–190
histocytosis-X 182
history-taking 3, 167
HIV-1 infection, septic arthritis 41
HLA antigens 21, 133
HLA-B27 59, 62, 63, 65
Homans' sign 258
homocystinuria 151, *159*
homozygous, definition 134
hormonal therapy 195
hormone replacement therapy (HRT) 116–117, 118
hormones
  effect on bone 110
  imbalance 426
housemaid's knee 477
Howship's lacunae 106
humerus
  distal, fractures **603–605**
  distal physis, fracture-separation 602
  fracture-dislocations 592–593
  head, avascular necrosis 593
  neck, fractures 592
  proximal, fractures **591–593,** *592*
    in children 593, *593*
  shaft, fractures **593–595,** *594*
Hunter's syndrome 156, 157, *157*
Hurler's syndrome 157, *157*
hyaline cartilage 77
hydatid disease *48,* 48
hydrocephalus 214, 215
hydroxyapatite 105, **273**
hydroxyapatite composites 261, **273**

hydroxymethylene diphosphonate, ⁹⁹ᵐTc-labelled 20
hydroxyproline 114, 126
hyperaesthesia 12
hypercalcaemia 123, 128, 195
hypercortisonism 118, *118,* 131
hyperextension injury
  cervical spine 651, *655,* 655–656
  knee 220, 458, 723
hyperkyphosis 9, 61, 371, 382
hyperlordosis 9, 371
hypermobility 9, *9*
hyperostosis
  infantile cortical (Caffey's disease) *34,* 34
  sternoclavicular *297,* **297–298**
  sterno-costo-clavicular **34**
hyperparathyroidism **122–124**
  primary 123, *123*
  secondary 121, 124
hyperpituitarism 130
hyperthyroidism 118–119
hypertrophic reaction 82
hyperuricaemia 69
  congenital **159**
hypervitaminosis **125**
hypoaesthesia 12
hypochondroplasia *142,* 142–143, 145
hypophosphataemia 122, *122*
hypophosphataemic rickets/osteomalacia 121–122
hypopituitarism **129–130**
hypothermia, avoidance after accidents 524
hypothyroidism 131
hypovolaemic shock 528–529, 645

iliac blade, fracture *671, 674*
iliofemoral venous thrombosis 678
iliopsoas bursitis 441
iliopsoas function, assessment 406
Ilizarov method 38, 164, **261–264,** 265, *490, 491*
imaging
  diagnostic 13–21
  tumours 168
  see also individual conditions/diseases; individual techniques
immobilization, osteoporosis associated 119
immune response, rheumatoid arthritis 51–52
immunocompromised patients 31
impact injuries 92, 101
impingement sign 282
impingement syndrome **280–285**
impingement test 282
implants
  failure 271, 272, 555
  materials **271–273**
  tumour management 172
in-breeding 134
indium-111-labelled leucocytes 21

infantile cortical hyperostosis (Caffey's disease) *34*, **34**
infantile idiopathic scoliosis 381, *381*
infants
  acute haematogenous osteomyelitis 28, 29
  acute suppurative arthritis 39
  examination 13
  infection(s) 27–49
    acute pyogenic 27, 35
    chronic 27
    fractures 560, *560*, 564–565, *565*, 567, *576*
    fungal (mycotic) **46–48**, 354
    Gram-negative 31
    internal fixation complication 553, 555
    metastatic 32
    postoperative 35–36
    prevention in surgery 256–257
    rheumatoid arthritis 58
    treatment principles 27, 349–351
    see also osteomyelitis; *specific infections/bones*
  inflammation
    acute haematogenous osteomyelitis 28
    fracture healing 541, *542*
    rheumatoid arthritis 51
inflammatory arthritis 16
inflammatory arthropathies 85
inflammatory bowel disease, arthritis 64–65
infraclavicular lesions 236
inheritance 134, *135*
injuries *see* trauma
Injury Severity Scale (ISS) 538
insect bites *353*
insulin-like growth factor I 110
intercarpal joints, chronic instability *321*, 321–323
interdigital nerve compression 514
interfragmentary screws 553, *554*
interleukin-1 (IL-1) 110
internal fixation 36, **553–557**
  complications 555, *555*
  types 553–555, *554*
interphalangeal joints 355
  dislocation 634, *634*
  osteoarthritis 348–349
  replacement 347
  rheumatoid arthritis 348
intersection syndrome 328–329
intertrochanteric fractures **690–692**, *691*, *692*
intertrochanteric realignment osteotomy 436, 441–442
intervertebral disc *390*, 402
  age-related changes 390
  anatomy 402
  bulging 391, *391*
  cervical spine 369
  degeneration 390–394, *391*, 395
  disorders 390–403, *391*
  operative removal 393
  prolapse (herniation/rupture) 213, **390–394**
    cervical *362*, **362–363**, *363*, 656

differential diagnosis 392–393
    lumbar *372*
    pain 391
    thoracic 658–659
    treatment 393
intervertebral disc space, narrowing 394, 395
intervertebral foramina 402
intracranial pressure 530
intramedullary nails *554*, 555
  femoral shaft fractures 697
  tibial fractures *727*
intrauterine surgery 138
intrinsic hand muscles 355
  paralysis 342
  shortening 339
intrinsic-minus hand 342–343
intrinsic-plus hand 339, 342, 355
iodides, contrast media 16
iridocyclitis, chronic 65, 67
ischaemia 564
  bone *91*, 423
    see also osteonecrosis
  muscle 564, 572, *572*
  transient, nerve injuries 230
  Volkmann's *see* Volkmann's ischaemic contracture
isotopes, bone-seeking 20
ivory exostosis **176**

J

jack-knife injury 661, *661*
javelin throwers' elbow 311
Jefferson's fracture *650*, 650–651
jerk test 709–710
Johannson-Larson's disease *102*
joint(s)
  amputation complications 271
  bleeding into, haemophilia 40, 87, *87*, 88
  contractures, correction **263**
  debridement, osteoarthritis 86
  deformities *see individual joints/deformities*
  density 15
  destruction 10, 52
  disorders, hand 341–342
  dysplasia 80
  examination 6, 15–16
  excision *58*
  flail 219
  haemophilic arthropathy 88
  hypermobility 9, *9*, 151, 152, 153
  infections *see* arthritis, acute suppurative
  injuries *580*, **580–581**
    hand **633–635**, 641
  instability 4, 572
  irritable 8, 40
  laxity 9, *151*, **151**
  loading 77, 78, 79
  position 6
  posture sense, testing 12
  realignment **265–266**, *266*
  reconstruction, skeletal dysplasia 138
  rheumatoid arthritis 52, *58*

rupture 58
  shape 15
  sprain *see* sprains
  stiffness *see* stiffness
  surgery **265–267**
  swelling 21, 81
  see also individual joints
joint capsule
  herniation 83
  osteoarthritis 79, 80
'joint mouse' 469, *469*
joint replacement
  internal fixation 36–37
  osteoarthritis 86
  rheumatoid arthritis *58*
  thromboembolism 257
  see also arthroplasty; *specific joints*
juvenile chronic arthritis (JCA) **65–67**, *66*
  hands 341
  irritable hip *vs* 422
juvenile Colles' fracture 616, **618–620**, *619*

K

Kaneda method *661*
Kashin-Beck disease 83
keratoderma blenorrhagicum 62, *63*
Kienbock's disease 101, *101*, **323–324**, *324*, 626
Kirner's deformity 337
Klinefelter's syndrome **160**
Klippel-Feil syndrome *161*, **161**
  cervical spine 361, *361*
  shoulder 296, *296*
Klumpke's palsy 239
knee **449–517**
  adhesions 708
  amputation at/below 269
  anatomy **482–483**, 705
  arthrodesis 481, *481*
  arthroplasty *see* knee, replacement
  arthroscopy 23, 454, *455*, 479, 707, 710
  bursitis 477
  calcification around 479
  Charcot's disease 475
  chronic ligamentous instability **462**
  deformities **455–458**
    flexion 209, 220
  diagnostic calendar 454
  dislocation *713*, **713–714**
  examination *449*, **449–454**
    imaging 453–454, 707, *707*
  extensor apparatus ruptures *478*, 478–479
  'floating' 699
  giving way 449, 460, 469, 708
  haemophilic arthritis **475**
  hyperextension 220, 458, 723
  injuries **705–724**
    extensor apparatus **714–715**
    femoral shaft fractures 699
    imaging 707, *707*
  instability 220, 706, 708
    chronic **708–711**

rotatory *706, 708, 709*
  types *709*
intra-articular fluid 450
knock knees 455–457, *456*
lax ligaments 458
ligament injuries **705–708**
  tears 706, 707–708
ligaments
  examination *706, 706–707*
  ossification 708
  reconstruction 479
  see also collateral ligaments; cruciate
    ligaments
locking 449, 459, 460, 468
loose bodies 459, 467, **468–469**, *469*
movements *450, 451, 451, 483*
operations/surgery **479–483**
ossification around **479**
osteoarthritis *82*, **472–473**, *473*, 723
osteochondritis dissecans 101–102,
  467–468, *468*
osteonecrosis *474*, **474**
osteotomy *480*, 480–481
pain 449, 465, *466*
poliomyelitis 220
realignment osteotomy 471, 473
replacement 472, 473, *481*, 481–482
  thromboembolism 257
rheumatoid arthritis *471*, **471–472**,
  472, 476
septic arthritis 476
spina bifida 217
sprains 707
stability 705, 708
  testing *451, 452*, 706, 709–710
stiffness 700, 702, 714, 723
swellings **475–478**, *476*
symptoms and signs **449–451**
synovial chondromatosis **469**
synovial disorders 476
tenderness 706
traumatic synovitis 476
tuberculosis *470*, **470–471**
tumours 462
knock knees 455–457, *456*
Kocher's method 587–588
Köhler's disease 101, *101*, 512, *513*
Kugelberg–Welander disease **221**
Kussmaul's sign 526
kyphos 371, 382, *383*
kyphosis 9, *9*, 371, **382–383**, *383*
  adolescent *see* Scheuermann's disease
  congenital 383
  elderly **385–386**
  osteoporotic 385–386
  postural 382–383, *384*
  senile *386*
  spina bifida 217
  structural 383

L

Lachman test 451, *452, 453*, 709
lamellar bone 106
laminectomy, partial 393

Larsen's syndrome **152–153**
lateral cutaneous nerve of thigh,
  compression 252
lateral plantar nerve, entrapment 512
Lauge-Hansen classification 737
laxity, joint/ligaments 9, *151*, **151**,
  458, 572
leg
  amputations 267–268, 269–270
  bow 455–457, *456, 457*
  cerebral palsy 209
  compression syndromes **252**
  intermittent pneumatic compression
    258
  length 376, 406–407
    equalization **264–265**
    inequality 264
    real *vs* apparent 407, *407*
  lengthening 265, *265*
  muscle power 372
  short, scoliosis 375, *375*
  shortening 407, *407*
  see also limb; *individual bones/joints;
    individual ligaments*
Legg-Calvé-Perthes disease *see* Perthes'
  disease
leontiasis 148
leprosy 224, *224*
Leri's disease **148**, *149*
Lesch–Nyhan syndrome 159
Letterer–Siwe disease 183
leucocytosis 21
Lhermitte's sign 368
ligament(s)
  ossification 586
  pelvis *667*
  rupture 580, 581
  strains 580–581
  see also individual ligaments
ligament injuries
  ankle *see* ankle
  cervical spine 653, *653*
  hands **635**
  knee **705–708**
limb
  anomalies **162–165**
  compression, crush injury 536
  deformities, treatment *211*
  elevation 557
  examination, after head injuries 531
  lengthening 262, *262, 263*
  reconstruction **261–264**
  replantation **267**, *268*
  trauma, thromboembolism 257
limb buds 162
limb girdle dystrophy 228
limb-sparing surgery 172
limp, children *411*
lipid storage disorders *183*
lipoma **195–196**, *196*
liposarcoma **196**, *196*
'locked back' 394
locking 4
log-rolling technique 644, 645, *645*
loose bodies 15, 83
  elbow **306**, *309*

knee 459, 467, **468–469**, *469*
Lorain syndrome 129
lordosis 9, 371
low back pain 390, 391, 400
  causes and differential diagnosis 60–61
  diagnostic approach **400–401**
  see also backache/back pain
lower limb *see* foot; leg; limb
lower motor neurone lesions 202, 212,
  218, 510
lumbar backache *see* low back pain
lumbar lordosis *384*
lumbar spine
  burst fractures 660, *660*
  cord lesions 212
  disc prolapse 390, 391–392, *392*
  imaging 374, *374*
  injuries *645*, **659**
  nerve root transection 663, *663*
  scoliosis *378*
  stenosis 399, *399*
  see also spine; thoracolumbar spine
lumbosacral nerve root compression 61
lumbosacral plexus injuries **244**
lumps 167
  bony 10, *10*
lunate
  dislocation 626–627, *627*
  fractures 626
luno-triquetral ballotment 322
luno-triquetral dissociation 323
luno-triquetral joint test 316
luxatio erecta 587, **590–591**
lymphadenopathy, rheumatoid arthritis 52

M

MacIntosh test 710, *710*
McMurray's test 452, *460*
macrodactyly 338
Madelung's deformity 318, *318*
maduromycosis 47, *47*
Maffucci's syndrome 143, **144**
magnesium 109
magnetic resonance imaging (MRI) 17,
  18–19, *19*
  acute haematogenous infections 30
  bone tumours 18, 168
  knee *454*, 454, *711*
  neck 359, *359*
  osteonecrosis *94*, 95, 435
  short tau inversion recovery (STIR) 18
  shoulder 280
major histocompatibility complex (MHC)
  133
malabsorption, intestinal 121
malignant fibrous histiocytoma *189*,
  189–190
malleolus fractures 737
  'rim' 736
mallet finger 339, *340*, 356
  types and treatment 632–633, *633*
mallet toes 502, **504**, *504*
Mannerfelt lesion 348
marble bones *147*, **147–148**

march fracture 757
Marfan's syndrome **151–152**, *152*
marrow oedema syndrome *100*, **100**, **439–440**, *440*
Meary's angle 497
mechanical stress 78, *78*, 81, 111
median nerve 312, 356
    compression *247*, **247–248**, 352, 627
    see also carpal tunnel syndrome
    injuries **242–244**, *243*, 599
melorheostosis 148, *149*
meninges 530
meningocele *214*
meniscectomy *461*
meniscus 458
    anatomy 483
    cysts *461*, **461–462**, *462*, 477
    degeneration 461
    discoid lateral 461, *461*
    lesions **458–462**
    medial, tears 458–461, *459*
    prolapsed torn 462
    repair 461, *461*
    tears *455*, 458–461, *459*, 462
menopause, osteoporosis *see* post-menopausal osteoporosis
meralgia paraesthetica 252
metabolic bone disease 22, 113–115
metabolic disorders **112–132**, *139*, **156–159**
    in CPPD crystal deposition 72, 73
metabolism, response to trauma **534**
metacarpal fractures *630*, **630–632**
    base fractures 631, *631*
    children 632
    neck fractures 630–631
    shaft fractures 630
metacarpophalangeal joints 355
    dislocation 634, *634*
    osteoarthritis 349
    rheumatoid arthritis 347
    ulnar collateral ligament rupture 635
metal implants **271–272**
metaphyseal chondrodysplasia (dysostosis) *143*, **143**
metaphyseal dysplasia (Pyle's disease) **147**
metaphyses
    dysplasias involving **138–144**
    infections 28, *29*
metastatic bone tumours *15*, 167, **193–195**, *194*, 576, 577
metatarsal bones 499
    fractures 757
    injuries **756–758**, *757*
    stress fracture 513–514, 757
metatarsalgia 512–513
metatarsophalangeal joint
    arthrodesis 502
    hallux valgus 499
    injuries **758**
    painful 513
    rigidity 501
metatarsus adductus 491, *491*
metatarsus primus varus 499
methylprednisolone, intravenous 647
metrizamide 16, 17

microdiscectomy 393
microsurgery **267**, *268*, 639
mid-carpal joints 319–320, *320*
    dislocation 628
    instability 322, 323
midfoot
    deformities 497–498
    pain 512, *513*
mid-palmar space, infection 352
mid-tarsal injuries **754–755**
    fracture-dislocation 755
mid-tarsal joint 486
Milwaukee brace 379, *379*
Milwaukee shoulder 75, *295*, **295**
mineralocorticoids 130
Moberg pick-up test 233
mononeuropathy 222, 223
Monteggia fracture-dislocation *546*, 610, **613–615**, *614*, *615*
morphine 522
Morquio–Brailsford syndrome *157*, 157–158
Morton's metatarsalgia 514
motor action potential 24
motor nerve conduction 24
motor neuron disease **221**
motor neuron disorders **221**
motor neurons 229
motor power *see* muscle, power
movement assessment 6–9, *7*
    see also individual joints
Mseleni joint disease 83–84
mucopolysaccharidoses **156–158**, *157*
Müller's classification, fractures 540, *541*
multiple epiphyseal dysplasia 84, **144–145**, *145*
multiple exostosis 139, 178
multiple myeloma 119, *191*, **191–192**, *576*
multisystem organ failure (MSOF) **537**
muscle **201–202**, *202*
    amputation complications 271
    biopsy 204
    bleeding into 87
    charting 215
    contraction 25, 202
    contractures *see* contractures
    fibres 201–202
    hand 355–356
    imbalance 10, 418
    ischaemia 564, 572, *572*
    nerve root supply *203*
    power 11, 203
        grading/testing 11, *11*, 233
    tumours **199**
    wasting 44, 202
    weakness 4, 11, 202
        after fractures 572
        poliomyelitis 219
        rheumatoid arthritis 52, 57–58, 346
muscle flap, transfer 38
muscle transfer, brachial plexus injuries 238
muscular atrophy, peroneal 223, *223*
muscular dystrophies **227–228**
mycobacterial infections

    hand 353–354
    see also tuberculosis
mycoses **46–48**, *47*, 354
    deep 47–48, 354
    superficial 47
myelin 230
myelography 16–17, *17*, 359, 374, 646
    lumbar 392
myeloma 119, *191*, **191–192**, *576*
myelomeningocele *214*
myelopathy, cervical **365–366**
myocardial contusion 527, 529
myositis, streptococcal necrotizing 30
myositis ossificans 571, *571*
    after hip dislocation 682
    differential diagnosis 169
    elbow injuries 599, 609
myositis ossificans progressiva *155*, **155**
myotonia congenita 228
myotonic disorders **228**
myxoedema 131

N

nail bed injuries 638
nail-fold infections 351, *351*
nail-fold lesions *346*
nailing, fracture fixation 594–595
nail–patella syndrome *150*, **150**
navicular, accessory 493
neck **357–369**
    anatomy **369**
    congenital short *161*, **161**
    deformities in children **360–361**
    examination *357*, **357–359**, *358*
    pain 357, 363
    skew *649*
    soft-tissue strain 362
    sprained (whiplash injury) *649*, *657*, **657–658**
    wry 360, *362*
    see also cervical spine
Neer's classification 591
Neisseria gonorrhoea 41
nerve(s) *201*, **201**
    acute compression 230
    amputation complications 271
    bleeding into 87
    conduction 24, 237
    entrapment *see* nerve compression syndromes
    grafting 235, 238
    hands 356
    structure and function *229*, **229–230**
    supply
        hip 447
        spine 403
    transfer 235, 238
    tumours **198–199**, 393
nerve compression syndromes **246–252**, 512
    after fractures 563, **571–572**
    cervical spondylosis 364
    foot 512
    see also individual nerves

nerve injuries
  fracture complications 562–563, *563*
  hands 641
  shoulder dislocation 588
  spinal 647
  traction causing 550
  see also peripheral nerve injuries
nerve roots *203*, 402–403
  cervical spine 369
  lumbar 663
  motor function assessment *646*
  tendon reflexes *646*
  transection 662–664
nerve sheath tumours
  benign **198**
  malignant **199**
nervous system 201
neuralgic amyotrophy 225, *225*, 362
neural tube defects 214
neurapraxia 230, *231*, 588
  cervical cord 656–657
  thoracolumbar cord 662
neurilemmoma 198
neurofibroma **198–199**
neurofibromatosis **155–156**, *156*,
    198–199, *199*
  scoliosis *382*, **382**
neurogenic shock 529, 645
neurological assessment 10–12, *11*
  hands 335–336
  spinal injuries 645–646, *646*
'neurological pain' (tarsal tunnel
    syndrome) 252, 514
neuroma **198**, 231, 271
neuromuscular disorders **201–228**
  clinical assessment **202–204**
  hand 342–343
  imaging 204, *204*
  scoliosis **382**
neurons 201, 229
neuropathic joint disease (Charcot's
    disease) 84, *89*, **89–90**, 508
neuropathies
  hereditary *223*, **223–225**
  peripheral **222–225**
neurosarcoma (malignant schwannoma)
    199
neurotmesis 230–231, *231*, 595
night splints 66
'nightstick' fracture 613
non-Hodgkin's lymphoma *19*,
    190–191, *191*
non-steroidal anti-inflammatory drugs
    (NSAIDs) 56, 61
nucleus pulposus 402
numbness 5
nutritional supplementation, after
    trauma 534

O
obesity, osteoarthritis risk factor 81
obstetrical palsy **238–239**, *239*
ochronosis 74, 159, *396*
odontoid anomalies 361

odontoid fractures 648, 651, *651–652*, *656*
oedema, prevention after fractures 557
oestrogen 110, 116–117
  deficiency/insufficiency 118
olecranon
  bursitis *311*, **311**
  fractures *607*, **607–608**, *609*
Ollier's disease **143–144**
onychogryposis 515
orthopaedic operations *see* surgery
Ortolani's test 410, *410*
Osgood–Schlatter's disease 102, *102*,
    170, **478–479**, 715
ossification
  ankylosing spondylitis 59
  around knee **479**
  endochondral 106, 176
  heterotopic 445, 605, 609, 665, 678
  ligaments 586
  membranous 107
  posterior longitudinal ligament *365*, **365**
  quadriceps tendon *14*
osteitis condensans ilii 131, *401*
osteitis deformans *see* Paget's disease
osteitis fibrosa 113
osteoarthritis **77–90**
  acromioclavicular joint *298*, **298**
  aetiology 77–78, *78*, 434
  after fractures 574
  ankle *507*, **507**, 750
  clinical features *81*, 81–82
  in CPPD crystal deposition 73
  deformities *81*, 82
  differential diagnosis 56, 84–85, *85*, 89
  elbow 308, *309*, 610
  hands and fingers 83, *84*, 341–342,
    348–349
  hip *16*, 82, *83*, 409, 434, **434–436**,
    435, *436*, 442, 678
  knee *82*, **472–473**, *473*, 723
  management 85–86
  natural history and complications
    82–83
  negative association with osteoporosis
    81
  non-progressive *78*
  in Paget's disease 128
  pathogenesis 78–79, *79*
  pathology 79, *79–80*, *435*
  prevalence 80
  primary 434
  progressive *78*
  rapidly destructive 84, *84*
  risk factors 80–81, *434*
  secondary 56, *83*, 434
    ankle 750
    hip 678, **682–683**, 690
    knee 723
    radiocarpal fractures 621
    wrist 625
  shoulder *294*, **294–295**, 586
  spinal 390, 395, *395*
  variants and sites 83–84, *435*
  wrist **326–328**, *327*
  x-ray features 16
osteoblastoma **176**

osteoblasts 105
osteocalcin (Gla protein) 105, 114
osteochondral fractures **718**, 748, *749*
osteochondral injuries **718**
osteochondritis (osteochondrosis) *101*,
    101–102, *102*
  vertebral 101, *383*, **383–385**
osteochondritis dissecans 101–102, 718
  elbow **305–306**, *306*
  knee *455*, **467–468**, *468*
  talus **506–507**, *507*
osteochondroma *10*, **178**, *179*
osteochrondroses 92
osteoclast-activating factor (OAF) 110
osteoclasts **105–106**
osteoconduction 260, *261*
osteocytes 105
osteogenesis 260
osteogenesis imperfecta *14*, **153–155**,
    154, *155*
  clinical variants 153, *154*
osteoid osteoma **175**, *175*
  giant (osteoblastoma) 176
osteoinduction 260, *261*
osteolysis **183**, 446
osteoma
  compact (ivory exostosis) **176**
  osteoid *see* osteoid osteoma
osteomalacia 113, **119–122**, *120*, *121*
osteomyelitis
  acute haematogenous **27–32**, *28*, *29*, 40
  chronic 32, 37, **37–38**
  clavicle 298
  differential diagnosis 170, 384
  Garré's sclerosing **32–33**
  multifocal non-suppurative **33–34**, *34*
    subacute recurrent 33–34
  postoperative **35–37**
  post-traumatic **34–35**
  pyogenic, spine *386*, **386–387**
  subacute haematogenous 32, *33*
osteonecrosis **91–103**, **436–439**
  aetiology/pathogenesis *91*, 91–92, *92*,
    435, 438
  after slipped femoral epiphysis 430
  atraumatic, of talus **507**
  bone marrow oedema *vs* 100
  clinical features 93, 435
  conditions associated *91*, **97–100**
  in congenital hip dislocation 415
  differential diagnosis 84–85, *85*
  dysbaric 98
  fracture complications 570, **570–571**
  imaging and diagnosis 93–95, *94*, *435*,
    435–436
  knee *474*, **474**
  non-traumatic 437, 507
  pathology and natural history 92–93,
    93, 438
  prevention and treatment 96, **96–97**,
    439
  radiation necrosis 99, **99–100**
  segmental 91
  shoulder 295, *295*
  talus fractures 750
  traumatic/post-traumatic 92, 95, 437

see also femoral head
osteonectin 105
osteopathia striata **148,** *149*
osteopenia 65, 115
osteopetrosis (marble bones) *147,* **147–148**
osteopetrosis congenita 148
osteopetrosis tarda 147
osteophytes 15, 79, 80, 364
osteopoikilosis **148,** *149*
osteoporosis 113, **115–119**
   after fractures 573, *573,* 730
   clinical assessment 113–115
   diabetics 508
   femoral neck fractures *684*
   generalized 115
   involutional (senile) 117
   kyphosis 385–386
   negative association with osteoarthritis 81
   osteomalacia comparison *121*
   postmenopausal 112, 115, *115, 116,* **116–117,** 385–386
   primary 115–117
   regional 29–30, 115
   regional migratory 100
   secondary *118,* 118–119
   senile 386
   tibial fractures and 730
   transient 100, *400,* **439–440**
osteosarcoma **185–187,** *186, 187*
   diagnosis and staging 185–186
   differential diagnosis 574
   in Paget's disease 128
   treatment 186–187
   variants 187–189
osteotomy **259–260**
   around joints 265–266
   Chiari's pelvic *417*
   intertrochanteric 436, 441–442
   knee *480,* 480–481
     realignment 471, 473
   osteoarthritis 86, *86*
   periacetabular *418*
   Salter 414, *414*
   spinal *60*
   supracondylar 471
   wedge 259, *259*
otto pelvis (protrusio acetabuli) 84, *419,* **419**
overbone 512
overuse injuries *see* repetitive strain syndromes
oxygenation, management after accidents 523, 525, 532

P

Paget's arthritis 128, *128*
Paget's disease *14, 126,* **126–129,** *127, 449, 576*
   deformities 126, *126*
   femoral shaft fracture 699
   sarcoma *188,* 188–189
pain 3–4, **225–227**
   acute/chronic 226
   autonomic 4
   back *see* backache/back pain
   bone tumours 167, 195
   complex regional pain syndrome *226,* 226–227
   elbow 303
   foot **511–514**
   grading and severity 3
   heel **511–512**
   hip 422, *440*
   knee 449, 465, *466*
   location 3, *4*
   metastatic bone tumours 193
   neck 357, 363
   osteoarthritis 81
   osteosarcoma 185
   perception 225–226
   referred 3–4, 277
   sacroiliac 674
   shoulder 277, *288*
   spine 371
painful arc syndrome 281–282, *282*
palmar aponeurosis 355
palsy 205
Pancoast's syndrome 251
Panner's disease 101
Papineau technique 38
paraesthesia 202
paralysis 203
   care of joints/limbs 235
   foot **510–511,** *511*
   intrinsic hand muscles 342
   poliomyelitis 218
paraplegia 658, 661
   traumatic *663,* **664–665**
parathyroid hormone (PTH) 109, 110, 114, 122–124
   see also hyperparathyroidism
paresis, adult spastic (stroke) 211
paronychia 351, *351*
parosteal osteosarcoma 187–188, *188*
pars interarticularis 397
   stress fracture 659
'passive tenodesis' 636
past medical history 5, 137
patella 482
   anatomy 715
   dislocation *717,* **717–718**
     non-traumatic 465, 717
     recurrent 717
   examination *453*
   fracture **715–717,** *716*
   instability *463,* 463–465, *464*
   in knee replacement 482
   realignment 464, *464,* 467
   recurrent dislocation 460, **462–465,** *463*
   recurrent subluxation 465
   tendon rupture above/below 478
   tracking 466
patellar friction test *453*
patellar hollow test *450*
patellar ligament (tendon) 482, 714
   distal elevation 467
   rupture 714–715
patellar pain syndrome **465–467**
patellar tap *450*
patella 'tendinopathy' 479
patellectomy 465, 467, 473
patellofemoral joint 453, 465, 482
   osteoarthritis 473
patellofemoral overload syndrome **465–467,** *466*
pathological fractures 167, 193, 540, **575–577,** *576*
   causes *575*
   femoral shaft 699, 700
   femur *576,* 577, 692
   humerus, in children 593
   spine 577
Pavlik harness 412, *413*
pectoral girdle **277–301**
   see also shoulder
pedobarography 488
Pellegrini–Stieda's disease 479, 708
pelvic ring 667
   compression injuries 670–671, *671–672*
   fractures **670–674,** *671*
     management 672–674
     'open-book' 671, 673
pelvis
   anatomy 667
   cerebral palsy 211
   fractures **670**
   imaging 668–779, *669*
   injuries **667–679**
     avulsion 670, *670*
   instability 668
   ligaments *667*
   otto (protrusio acetabuli) 84, *419,* **419**
   'trefoil' *120*
periacetabular osteotomy *418*
periarthritis, acute/subacute 74–75
perilunate dislocation 626–627, *627*
perineurium 230
periosteal chondroma **177**
periosteal membrane 106
periosteal osteosarcoma 188
periosteum, x-ray *15*
peripheral nerve compression *see* nerve compression syndromes
peripheral nerve injuries **229–254**
   acute and chronic types 232
   assessment 25, 232–233, *234*
   classification **231–232**
   clinical features **232–233**
   delayed repair 234–235
   electromyography 25, 233
   foot paralysis 510
   grades 231, *231*
   hand 342
   iatrogenic 252–253
   pathology **230–231**
   primary repair/suture 233–234, *234*
   prognosis **235–236**
   regional survey **236–246**
   repair (pathology) 230–231, *231*
   treatment **233–235**
peripheral nerves 201
   exploration after injury 233
peripheral neuropathy **222–225,** 246
   diabetic 224, 508

peritendinitis crepitans 328–329
Perkin's timetable 544
peroneal muscular atrophy *11*, 223, *223*
peroneal nerve lesions 245, **245–246**, 260
peroneal spastic flat foot 493–494
peroneal tendons
    dislocation 736, *736*
    impingement 754
Perthes' disease **422–426**, *424*, *425*
    differential diagnosis 97, 145, 422, 424
    osteoarthritis risk factor 80
    prognosis and management 424–426,
        426
pes cavus *495*, **495–498**, *496*, *498*
pes planus **491–495**
pes valgus 210, **491–495**
    congenital convex 492
pes varus 210
phalangeal fractures **632–633**, *633*
    proximal/middle shafts 632
    terminal 632–633
Phalen's test 248
phantom limb 271
phocomelia 162
phosphate 114, 121
phosphorus 108, 109
physeal injuries *578*, **578–580**, *579*, 743
    fractures 619, 633
    wrist 319
physes (growth plates) 106, 141
    growth abnormalities **138–144**
physical examination *see* examination,
        physical
physiotherapy
    cerebral palsy 208
    cervical spondylosis 364
    osteoarthritis 85–86
    segmental instability 396
piano-key sign 320, 325, 626
pigmented villonodular synovitis *197*,
        197, 476
pilon fractures *742*, **742–743**, *743*
Pirogoff's amputation 270
piso-triquetral joint test 316
pituitary dysfunction **129–130**
pivot shift phenomenon 708
pivot shift test 322, 705
plantar fasciitis 511–512
plantar reflex 12
plantar venous compression, intermit-
        tent 258
plantar warts 515
plant thorn injuries 349
Plaster of Paris casts 551
plaster sores 566
'plastic pen test' 232
plates, internal fixation 554, *554*
platyspondyly 157, *157*
plica syndrome **469–470**
pneumothorax 521–522, 528
    tension 522, 525–526, *526*, 528, 529
policeman's heel *512*
poliomyelitis *218*, **218–221**, 219, *220*
    scoliosis *382*
polyarthritis 55, 73, 85
polydactyly 338

polymyalgia rheumatica 56
polyneuropathy 222, *223*
popliteal aneurysm 478
popliteal cyst *477*, **477–478**
position sense, testing 12
posterior cord syndrome 664
posterior interosseous nerve 312
    compression **249**
posterior interosseous syndrome 249
posterior ligament injury, cervical spine
        653, *653*
posterior longitudinal ligament, ossifica-
        tion *365*, **365**
postganglionic lesions, brachial plexus
        236, 237
postmenopausal osteoporosis 112, 115,
        115, *116*, **116–117**, 385–386
    fractures 116, *116*
postoperative infections 35–36
posture *7*, 203–204
    ankylosing spondylitis 59–60
    cerebral palsy 206
    deformity 10
    neurological disorders 10–11
'pot-hole' injury 757
Pott's fracture 737
Pott's paraplegia 388
preganglionic lesions, brachial plexus
        236, 237
pregnancy 100, **131**
prenatal diagnosis **135–136**
pressure sores 551, 566, *566*, 664
pronation 8
pronator syndrome 248
prostaglandins 111
prostheses
    after amputation *270*, **270**
    for hallux rigidus 502
    hip *444*
    see also implants
proteoglycans 77, 105, 156
protrusio acetabuli (otto pelvis) 84,
        419, **419**
proximal femoral focal deficiency *421*,
        421
pseudarthrosis 544
    clavicle 164, *164*
    congenital *14*
    in neurofibromatosis 156
    tibia 164, *164*
pseudoachondroplasia 145, **149**
pseudo-boutonnière deformity *340*
pseudoclaudication 400
pseudogout 40, 70, 72, 73, *73*
    elbow **308**
pseudoparesis 39
psoas abscess 65, *389*
psoriatic arthritis **63–64**, *64*
    differential diagnosis 85
    hands 341
pubic rami, fractures 670
pulmonary contusion 527, 528
pulmonary embolism 257, 258, 259
pupils, examination 531
pus 30
pustulosis, palmo-plantar 297, 298

Putti–Platt operation 290
pyknodysostosis **148**
Pyle's disease **147**
pyogenic arthritis 45, 418
    hip 418, *430*, **430–431**, *431*
pyridinium compounds 114
pyrophosphate 111
pyrophosphate arthropathy, chronic 72,
        72, *73*
pyrophosphate crystal deposition 70, *71*

Q

quadriceps muscle
    contracture 465
    paralysis 219
quadriceps reflex 392
quadriceps tendon
    heterotopic ossification *14*
    rupture 714, *714*
Quadriga effect 641
quadriplegia **664–665**
quadruple immobilization, spine 644, *645*

R

radial club hand 317–318, 336, *337*
radial dysplasia *317*
radial head *see* radius, head
radial nerve 356
    compression **249**
    injuries *241*, **241–242**, 595
    palsy 595
radial styloid fracture 616, 620, *620*
radial tunnel syndrome 249
radiation necrosis *99*, **99–100**
radiculopathy 363
radio-carpal joint 319–320, *320*
    chronic instability 321–323
    dislocation 628
    fractures *620*, **620–621**
        comminuted intra-articular 620–621,
            621
        fracture-subluxation 620, *620*
    osteoarthritis 326–327
    translocation 322
radioculography 392
radiography
    acute haematogenous infections 29–30
    ankle and foot 487, *487*
    ankylosing spondylitis 60
    bone tumours 168
    brain injuries 531, *532*
    chronic osteomyelitis 37
    contrast media 16–17, *17*
    fractures 545–546, *546*
    gout 70, *71*
    hip 408, *409*
    intraoperative 255
    neck 358–359, *359*
    osteonecrosis *94*, **94–95**, 435, *435*
    osteoporosis *113*, 113–114
    plain film **13–16**
    rheumatoid arthritis *54*, 55

rule of twos 545–546
shoulder 279, *279*, 283
stress X-rays 487, *707*
tuberculosis 44, *45*
radionuclide compounds 20
radionuclide imaging (radioscintigraphy)
    20, 20–21
  acute haematogenous infections 30, *30*
  bone tumours 168
  chronic osteomyelitis 37
  knee 453–454
  metastatic bone tumours 194, *194*
  osteonecrosis *94*
radiotherapy 173, 195
radio-ulnar joint
  discrepancy 619–620
  distal 319, *319*
    injuries 626
    instability 320
    osteoarthritis 327, *327*
radius
  absence/hypoplasia 162
  distal
    comminuted fracture 620–621, *621*
    fractures **615–616**
  dorsal malunion 323
  fracture-dislocation, Galeazzi 320,
      615, **615**
  head
    fractures *606*, 606–607, 609
    isolated dislocation 610
    subluxation/dislocation 305, *305*,
      603
  isolated fracture *613*, **613**
  longitudinal deficiency 317–318, 336,
      337
  longitudinal instability 320
  neck fractures **602–603**, *603*, 607
  shaft fractures **611–613**, *612*, 613, *613*
  styloid process 330
Ranvier, nodes of 230
Raynaud's disease/phenomenon 251, 354
reactive arthritis **61–63**
  see also Reiter's disease/syndrome
rectal examination 530, 668
reflexes 12, 201, 229, *646*
reflex sympathetic dystrophy (RSD) 100,
    226, 226–227, 479, 573
  after Colles' fracture 617
  post-traumatic 226, *573*, 573–574
rehabilitation
  disc prolapse 393
  hands, after infections 350–351
Reiter's disease/syndrome **61–63**, *63*
  differential diagnosis 46, 55, 61, 70, 73
renal failure 121, 124, *124*
renal osteodystrophy *124*, **124**
renal tubular defects 122
reperfusion injury 536
repetitive strain syndromes
  elbow *310*, 310–311
  wrist 329
replantation of digits 639–640
respiration, paradoxical 526–527
reticulum-cell sarcoma **190–191**, *191*
Revised Trauma Score (RTS) 537–538

rhabdomyoma 199
rhabdomyosarcoma **199**
rheumatic disorders **51–67**, 131
rheumatic fever 40
rheumatism, acute 30
rheumatoid arthritis **51–58**
  ankle and foot **505**, *506*
  blood tests 21
  cause 51–52
  cervical spine **367–368**, *368*
  clinical features 52–54, *53*, *54*
  complications 57–58
  deformities 52, 53, *53*, *54*, *55*, 57
    treatment/prevention *57*
  diagnosis and investigations 55, 55–56
  differential diagnosis 55–56, 70
  elbow **306–308**, *307*, 311
  finger deformities 348
  hands 341, *345*, **345–348**, *346*, *347*
  hip *433*, **433–434**, *434*
  knee *471*, **471–472**, *472*, 476
  metacarpophalangeal deformities 347
  monarticular 45
  pathology 52
  prognosis 58
  shoulder 293–294, *294*
  tenosynovitis and tendon rupture 348
  thumb 347
  treatment 56–57
  wrist *315*, 319, **324–326**, *325*, *326*
rheumatoid factor (RF) 21, 51–52
rheumatoid nodule 52, 53, 306, *307*
  hands 345
rib-cage excursion 372
rib fractures **527–528**, *528*
rib hump 380
rickets **119–122**, *120*
'rickety rosary' 119
rigidity 11
Risser's sign 377
rocker-bottom deformity 489, *492*
rod and sublaminar wiring (Luque) 379
Rolando's fracture 632
Romberg's sign 12
Roos's test 251
rotation, external/internal 8
rotator cuff *280*, 300
  open repair 285, *285*
rotator cuff disorders **280–289**
rotator cuff lesions 75, 251, *283*
  calcification **285–286**
  differential diagnosis 363, 364
  disruption/tears 282–283, 588
  osteoarthritis 83
  progression (wear/tear/repair) 281, *281*
rotator cuff syndrome 280, 586
round-cell tumour 190

S

sacral agenesis *161*
sacral injuries **678**
sacral nerve roots 663
sacral sparing 645
sacrococcygeal fractures 678 *678*

sacroiliac joints
  ankylosing spondylitis 59, 60
  fusion *60*
sacroiliac pain 674
sacroiliitis 63, 65
Salter and Harris classification 578–579,
    619, *744*
Salter and Thompson classification 424
Salter osteotomy 414, *414*
sarcoidosis 56
sarcoma 170, 172
  giant cell **182**
  in Paget's disease 128
Saturday-night palsy 230, 241
scalp wounds 532
scaphoid 330, 623
  avascular necrosis 624
  fractures 545, **623–625**, *624*, *625*
scapho-lunate advanced collapse
    (SLAC) 328
scapho-lunate joint 316
  dissociation 321, 323, 627–628, *628*
  incompetence 322
scapula
  congenital elevation **295–296**
  disorders **295–298**
  elevation **161–162**
  fractures *584*, **584–585**
  grating **297**
  instability **296–297**
  undescended **161–162**
  winging *239*, *277*, **296**, 296–297
scapulohumeral rhythm 278, *278*
scapulothoracic dissociation **585**
scars 6, *6*
Scheuermann's disease 101, *383*,
    383–385, *384*, *385*
  thoracolumbar 385, *385*
Schmorl's nodes 384, *385*
Schwann cells 230
Schwann cell tumours 155
Schwannoma, malignant **199**
sciatica 59, 371, 392, 393, 400
sciatic nerve injuries **244–245**, *245*,
    674, 678, 682
sciatic palsy 244–245
scleroderma, hand 341
scoliosis 9, 10, **374–377**, *375*
  adolescent idiopathic 378–381
  angle of curvature 377, *377*
  cerebral palsy 208, 211
  clinical features 375–376
  congenital (osteopathic) **381–382**
  idiopathic **377–381**, *378*
  imaging 377
  infantile idiopathic 381, *381*
  juvenile idiopathic 381
  Marfan's syndrome *152*
  neurofibromatosis 156, *382*, **382**
  neuropathic and myopathic 382
  non-idiopathic 382, *382*
  poliomyelitis 219, *382*
  postural 375, *375*
  sciatic 375, 391
  spina bifida *216*, 217
  structural (fixed) 375–377, *376*, *380*

thoracic 375–376
treatment 378–381, *380*
scratch test, shoulder *288*
screws, internal fixation 553, *554,*
    554–555
scurvy **124–125,** *125*
seat-belt injuries 657, 661
segmental instability **394–396,** *395*
semimembranosus bursa 477, *477*
sensation, cerebral palsy 207
sensibility, changes 5, 12
    testing 12
sensory loss 222
sensory nerve action potential (SNAP) 24
sensory nerve conduction, assessment
    24–25
sensory neurons 229
sensory neuropathies 25
sensory pathways 12
septicaemia 31
septic arthritis **41,** 65, 73
    hands 353, *353*
    knee 476
    sternoclavicular joint **297**
septic shock 529
seronegative arthropathies 21, 61
    ankle and foot **506**
    juvenile chronic arthritis 66
seronegative inflammatory polyarthritis
    55
serratus anterior palsy/weakness 239, 297
sesamoiditis 513
sesamoids, fracture **758**
Sever's disease 102, *102,* 511, *512*
Sharrard's operation 217, *217*
Shenton's line *409,* 416
Shimizu's classification 95
shingles (herpes zoster) 224–225, *225*
shock **528–529,** 645
shoulder **277–301, 583–591**
    anatomy **299–300**
    arthrodesis 238, 299, *300*
    arthroplasty *299,* **299**
    arthroscopy 23, 280, **298**
    atraumatic dislocation/subluxation **292**
    disarticulation 269
    dislocations **587–591**
        anterior 587–589, *588*
        children 591
        inferior *590,* 590–591
        posterior 589–590, *590*
    examination *277,* **277–280**
        imaging *279,* 279–280
    exercises 251, *251*
    fracture-dislocation 588, *589*
    fractures **583–591**
    frozen (adhesive capsulitis) *287,*
        287–289
    injuries 547, **583–591**
    instability 277, **289–292**
        anterior **289–290,** *290*
        multidirectional 291, *292*
        posterior *291,* **291**
    Klippel–Feil syndrome 296, *296*
    Milwaukee 75, *295,* **295**
    movements *277,* 278–279, *279,* 300

operations/surgery **298–299**
osteoarthritis *294,* **294–295,** 586
osteonecrosis 295, *295*
painful *288*
poliomyelitis 219
rheumatoid arthritis **293–294,** *294*
Sprengel's deformity 296, *296*
stability 300
stiffness 277, 288, 584, 588–589, 593
subluxation 289, 291, 292, *292*
    recurrent 289, 589, *589*
symptoms 277
tuberculosis 292, *293*
see also individual joints/bones
shoulder–hand syndrome 226, 226–227
sickle-cell crisis 30–31, 97
sickle-cell disease 31, **97–98,** *98*
side-swipe injury 608, *609*
Silastic implants 272
silicon compound implants **272**
Simmonds' test 509, *510*
Sinding–Johansson-Larsen's disease 479
sinography 16
skeletal dysplasia 136, 138, **138–151**
    combined/mixed **148–151**
    with diaphyseal changes **147–148**
    with epiphyseal changes **144–147**
    with physeal/metaphyseal changes
        138–144, *139*
skeletal maturity, assessment 377, *377*
skier's thumb 635
skin
    abrasion, cast splintage causing 551
    amputation complications 270–271
    appearance 6
    contractures, hand *338,* 338–339
    grafts, hand injuries 638
    hand 355
    preparation for surgery 256
    tags 338
skin disorders, foot and ankle **514–515**
skull
    fractures 531, 532
    Paget's disease 127, *127*
SLAP lesions 287
slipped capital femoral epiphysis 422,
    426–430, *427*
Smith-Petersen approach 441
Smith's fracture 616, *618,* **618**
social history 5
soft tissue
    contracture 10
    density 14
    haematoma 169
    x-ray examination 13–14, *14*
soft-tissue tumours **195–199**
    see also specific tumours
soleus muscle, tears 509, *510*
somatomedin C 110
somatosensory evoked potentials
    (SEPs) 24
Soutter's muscle slide 217, *217,* 220
spasmodic torticollis *369,* **369**
spasticity 11
spastic paresis, hand 342
Speed's test 286

spina bifida **214–218,** *216*
spinal accessory nerve 240
    injuries **239–240,** 297
spinal bifida 215–218
spinal bifida cystica 214, 215
spinal bifida occulta 214
spinal canal 402
    narrowing *see* spinal stenosis
    thoracic 658
spinal cord 211–212, 402
    complete/incomplete lesions 663–664
    compression 58, 61, 212
    injuries 547, 645, 662
        without radiographic abnormality 650
    lesions **211–213,** *213*
    neurapraxia
        cervical 656–657
        thoracolumbar 662
    neurological assessment 645
    tethering 217
    transection, thoracolumbar 662
    tumours 213
spinal muscular atrophy **221**
spinal shock 212, 645
spinal stenosis 213, 391, *399,*
    399–400, *400*
    cervical **365–366**
    osteoarthritis 83
    Paget's disease 128
spine **371–403**
    applied anatomy **401–403,** *402, 643*
    bamboo *60*
    blood supply 403
    cerebral palsy 211
    compression injuries 659–660
    deformities **374–386**
        spina bifida 217
        see also scoliosis
    developmental abnormalities 138
    examination **371–374,** *372*
        imaging 374, *374*
    forward shift 397
    fractures 643
        ankylosing spondylitis 61
        burst 648, 653, 660, *660, 661*
        pathological compression 577
        wedge *660*
    fusion 396
    immobilization, temporary 644
    infections **386–389**
    injuries 212, **643–665,** *645*
        assessment 644–646, *646*
        definitive treatment **647**
        diagnosis and management **644–646**
        healing 643–644
        mechanisms 643, *644*
        neurological injuries 647
        pathophysiology **643–644**
        stable/unstable 643, 647
    movements 371–372, 394, 402
    nerve supply 403
    osteoarthritis 390
    osteotomy *60*
    pain 371
        see also backache/back pain
    spina bifida 217

stabilization, in bone tumours 195
stiffness 371
support 396
symptoms and signs 371–374
traction injuries 643
tuberculosis 44, **387–389**, *388, 401*
see also cervical spine; lumbar spine;
    thoracolumbar spine; vertebrae
spirochaetal infections **41–42**
splenomegaly 52
splintage
  at accident scene 522–523
  acute haematogenous osteomyelitis 31
  acute suppurative arthritis 40
  cast 551, *552*
  cerebral palsy 208
  complications 551
  delayed union 566
  developmental dysplasia of hip
      412–413, 413, 414
  fractures 541, 547
  hand 629, *629*, 638–639, *639*
  hand infections 350
  tuberculosis 45
spondylitis
  ankylosing *see* ankylosing spondylitis
  enteropathic arthritis 65
  psoriatic arthritis 63
  tuberculous 384
spondyloepiphyseal dysplasia **145–146,**
    146, 384
spondylolisthesis *397*, **397–399**, *398*
  osteoarthritis 83
spondylolysis, traumatic 659
spondylometaphyseal dysplasia 148–149
spondylosis 395, *396*
  cervical 251, **363–365**, *364*
sporotrichosis 354
sports
  meniscal tears 459, *459*
  osteoarthritis risk factor 81
  quadriceps tendon rupture 714
  tibial tubercle fracture 715
spotted bones **148**, *149*
sprains 580
  acromioclavicular joint 585, 586
  ankle 733, **734–736**, *735*, 754
  knee 707
  neck (whiplash) *649*, 657, **657–658**
  tarso-metatarsal 755
  wrist 621, 623
Sprengel's deformity **161–162**, 296, *296*
staphylococcal infections 28, 31
stature 136
  short 136, 141
  surgery to increase 265
steal syndromes, Paget's disease 127
Stener lesion 635
stenosing tenovaginitis, digital *344,*
    344–345
stereognosis 12
sternal fracture 528, *528*
sternoclavicular joint *587*
  dislocations **586–587**, *587*
  hyperostosis *297*, **297–298**
  septic arthritis **297**

sternomastoid muscle 360
stiffness 4, 8–9
  after fractures 561, 573
  cast splintage causing 551
  generalized/localized 4
  juvenile chronic arthritis 65
  morning 4, 52
  osteoarthritis 81
  post-traumatic, elbow 308–309
  rheumatoid arthritis 52
  see also individual joints
Still's disease 65
Stimson's technique 587
Stokes–Gritti operation 269
storage disorders *139, 183*
straight leg raising test 373, *373*, 394
strains, ligament 580–581
streptococcal necrotizing myositis 30
stress fractures (fatigue fractures) *169,*
    540, **574–575**, *575*
  causes 574
  differential diagnosis 169, 574
  femoral neck 575, 685–686
  metatarsals 513–514, 757
  pars interarticularis 659
  tibia **731–732**
stress injuries, mid-tarsal 754
striped bones **148**, *149*
stroke 211
students' elbow 311, *311*
subacromial bursa 293
subdural haematoma 533
subluxation 581
  see also individual joints
subtalar joint 486
Sudeck's atrophy *226*, **226–227**, *573,*
    573–574
sulphan blue 38
sulphur colloid, ⁹⁹ᵐTc-labelled 20
'sunburst effect' 185, *186*
superficial palmar fascia contracture
    338–339
superficial peroneal nerve lesions 246
supination 8
suppuration 28
supraclavicular nerve lesions 236
supracondylar fractures
  elbow **596–599**, *597, 598*, 603–604
  femur **701–702**, *702*
suprascapular nerve **240**
  compression **249–250**
supraspinatus tendinitis **280–285**, 285
  tests 282
supraspinatus tendon
  calcification *14*, 285, *286*
  tears *283*
surgery (orthopaedic) **255–274**
  amputations **267–271**
  ankylosing spondylitis 61
  'bloodless field' 255–256
  bone **259–265**
  cerebral palsy 208–209
  chronic osteomyelitis 38
  elbow 311–312
  equipment and magnification 255
  hip 441–446

iatrogenic peripheral nerve injuries
    252–253
  joints **265–267**
  knee **479–483**
  microsurgery and limb replantation
    267, *268*
  Paget's disease 129
  postoperative infections 35–37
  preparation **255–257**
  protective gowns/gloves 256, 257
  tumours 171–172
swan-neck deformity *340*, 341, *341,*
    346, 348
sway-back *384*
swellings 4, *6*
  around wrist **329–330**, *330*
Syme's amputation 163, *269*, 269–270
sympathetic nerve supply 230
symphalangism, hereditary 337
symptoms **3–5**
synchondroses 650
syndactyly 337, *337*
syndesmophytes *60*
synostosis **164–165**
  cervical-vertebral 361, *361*
  congenital, elbow 304
  radio-ulnar (post-traumatic) 309
synovectomy 471
  elbow 307
  hands 346
synovial biopsy 55
synovial chondromatosis **469**, 476
synovial fluid, analysis 21–22, *22*
synovial sarcoma *197*, **197–198**
synovial tumours **197–198**
synovioma, malignant *197*, **197–198**
synovitis
  acute 21, 73
    see also pseudogout
  ankylosing spondylitis 59
  chronic 21, 52
  knee 476
  rheumatoid arthritis 52, *53, 54*, 55
  tibialis posterior 495
  transient 45
  traumatic, knee 476
syphilis 41, 42, *42*, 213
  tabes dorsalis 89, 213
syringomyelia 213
systemic lupus erythematosus (SLE) 67,
    341

T

tabes dorsalis 89, 213
tailor's bunion 504
talar tilt test 735, *735*
talipes calcaneovalgus 491, *491*
talipes equinovarus *488*, 488–491,
    489, 490
talocalcaneal fracture-dislocation *747*
talocalcaneal stiffness 754
talus *746*
  atraumatic osteonecrosis 507
  congenital vertical 492

fractures 747, *747*, *750*
injuries **746–749**
osteochondritis dissecans **506–507**, *507*
tarsal coalition 493–494, *494*
tarsal tunnel syndrome 252, 514
tarso-metatarsal injuries *755*,
   755–756, *756*
technetium-99m 20
telopeptides 114
temperature recognition test 12
tenderness, examination for 6, *7*, 10
tendinitis 571
  biceps 286, *286*
  gluteus medius 440
  hip **440–441**
  supraspinatus *see* supraspinatus
    tendinitis
  tendo Achilles 509
tendo Achilles *510*
  disorders **509–510**
  insufficiency 754
  lengthening *210*
  peritendinitis 509
  rupture 509–510
  tight 493
tendon reflexes 12, *646*
tendons
  avulsion injuries 169–170
  hand 355–356, 636
  lesions
    after fractures 571
    hands 339–341
  repair in hands 637
    delayed 640–641
  rheumatoid arthritis 52
tendon sheath 351, 355
  giant-cell tumour *197*, **197**
  infection, hands 351–352
  xanthoma 197
tendon transfers 235
  brachial plexus injuries 238
  paraplegia management 665
  poliomyelitis *220*
tennis elbow 249, 310, *310*
tenolysis 640–641
tenosynovitis
  extensor 328–329
  hand 348
  pyogenic 352
  rheumatoid arthritis 293, 348
  shoulder 293
  suppurative 351–352
  tuberculous 353
  wrist **328–329**
tenovaginitis, stenosing, hand *344*,
  344–345
tensor fascia femoris 447
Terry Thomas sign 322
tetanus 534–535, 558
thenar space, abscess 352
Thomas' test 408, 434
thoracic nerve, long, injuries *239*, **239**
thoracic outlet syndrome 247, *250*,
  250–251
  differential diagnosis 364
thoracic spine

cord lesions 212
disc herniation 658–659
fractures 658, *658*
injuries **658–659**
nerve roots 663
scoliosis 375–376, *378*
see also spine; thoracolumbar spine
thoracolumbar spine
  anomalies **162**
  compression fractures 660, *660*
  cord lesions 662
  extension injuries 659
  fracture-dislocation 661–662, *662*
  fractures 659, *659*
    burst *660*, *661*
  immobilization 644
  injuries 648, **659**
threshold tests, nerve injury 233
thromboembolism 257, 700
  treatment 259
thromboprophylaxis **257–259**
thrombosis, intravascular 92
thumb
  congenitally clasped 337, 344
  congenital trigger 338
  dislocation 633–634
  gamekeeper's 635, *635*
  metacarpal fracture *631*, 631–632
  movements 335
  replantation 639–640
  rheumatoid arthritis 347
  trigger, infantile 344
  ulnar collateral ligament 635
  W-thumb *340*
thumb-in-palm deformity 210–211, 342
thyroid dysfunction **131**
thyroxine 110, 118
tibia
  bent *14*
  congenital absence 163
  congenital anomalies 156, 164, *164*
  distal, physeal injuries 743–744, *744*
  dysplasia 156
  external torsion 210
  fractures **731**, *732*
    fibula fracture with **724–730**
    stress (fatigue) **731–732**
    tibial spine 460, *712*, **712**
    tibial tubercle 715
    see also tibial plateau fractures
  proximal epiphysis, fracture-separation
    723, **723–724**
  pseudarthrosis 164, *164*
  sabre *14*
tibial intercondylar eminence fracture 712
tibialis posterior synovitis 495
tibialis posterior tendon
  rupture 495
  tenosynovitis *506*
tibial nerve injuries **246**
tibial plateau fractures **718–723**, *719*,
  720–721
  crush fracture 720
  fixation *721*, 721–722, *722*
tibial spine fracture 460, *712*, **712**
tibial tubercle

apophysitis 478–479
  fractures 715
tibiofemoral joint 453, 482
tibiofibular joint 733
  proximal, dislocation 724
tibiofibular ligaments, anterior, tears 737
Tile's classification, acetabular fractures
  674, *675*
Tillaux fracture 744, *744*, *745*
tinea infections 354
Tinel's sign 12, 198, *231*, 233, 248
tingling 5
tissue typing 21
toe(s) 486
  claw *see* claw toes
  deformities **502–504**
  fifth, deformities 504
  fracture **758**
  gout *506*, **506**
  hammer 502, **503**, *504*
  mallet 502, **504**, *504*
  overlapping 504, *504*
toenail disorders *515*, **515**
tomography 17
  see also computed tomography (CT)
tone 11, 202
'too-many-toes' sign 485, *485*
tophi 69, 70, 71, *71*, 72
torticollis *360*, 360–361
  spasmodic *369*, **369**
tourniquet 522
tourniquet cuff 255–256
tourniquet pressure 256
  peripheral nerve injuries 253
tourniquet time 256
trabecular (cancellous) bone 106, 539
traction 549, *549*, *550*
  brachial plexus injuries due to 236
  cervical disc prolapse 363
  complications 550, 566
  continuous 549, *549*, *550*
  delayed union 566
  dislocation of hip 414
  elbow fractures 605
  femoral shaft fractures 696, *697*
  methods/types 549–550, *550*
traction apophysitis (pulling osteochondritis) 102, *102*, 511
transforming growth factors 110
transverse absence, upper limb 317
trapezio-metacarpal joint, osteoarthritis
  327, *327*
trapezium, fracture 625–626
trauma
  acute suppurative arthritis *vs* 40
  assessment (primary/secondary
    surveys) 523–525
  complications **534–536**
  fractures *see* fractures
  'golden hour' 521, 523
  gunshot injuries *561*, **561–562**
  management **521–538**
    at accident scene **521–523**, *522*
    in hospital **523–525**
  metabolic response **534**
  mortality rates 521, *521*

osteoarthritis risk factor 81
osteonecrosis 92, 95
scoring methods **537–538**
slipped capital femoral epiphysis 427
Trauma Score-Injury Severity Score 538
Trendelenburg sign 405, *405*
Trendelenburg's test 405, *406*
Trethowan's sign 427
Trevor's disease (dysplasia epiphysealis
    hemimelica) 146, *147*
triage 537
triangular fibrocartilage 316
triangular fibrocartilage complex
    (TFCC) 319
  disorders 320–321
  injuries after fractures 615, 617
triplane fracture 744, *744, 745*
triqueotrolunate dissociation 628
triquetrum, fracture 625
trisomy 21 (Down's syndrome) *160*, **160**
trochanteric bursitis **440**
trochanters, fractures 690, 693–694
trophic ulcers *245*
Tscherne's classification *724*
tuberculosis **42–46**, *44, 46*
  ankle and foot **504**, *505*
  arthritis 42–46, *43, 45*
  cervical spine **367**
  clinical features 44
  diagnosis 44–45
  elbow *306*, **306**
  hip *45*, 422, *431*, **431–433**, *432*
  knee *470*, **470–471**
  pathology 42–44, *43*
  shoulder 292, *293*
  spine 44, **387–389**, *388, 401*
  synovitis, hip 422
  tenosynovitis (hand) 353
  treatment 389
  wrist **324**, *325*
tumours **167–200**
  benign 171
  bone *see* bone tumours
  clinical presentation 167–168
  excision 171–172, *172*
  malignant 171
  management 171–173, *173*
  soft-tissue **195–199**
  staging 170–171, *173*
  see also individual tumours
Turner's syndrome **160**
two-point discrimination test 12, 233, 636

U

ulcerative colitis, arthritis 64–65
ulcers, diabetic foot 508, *508, 509*
ulna
  fracture-dislocation (Monteggia) *546*,
    610, **613–615**, *614, 615*
  hypoplasia/absence 162
  incomplete fractures 615
  isolated fracture 613, *613*
  longitudinal deficiency 318, 336–337
  longitudinal instability 320

shaft, fractures **611–613**, *612*, 613
ulnar artery, thrombosis 354
ulnar club hand 336–337
ulnar drift 345, *345, 346*
ulnar dysplasia, distal 318, *318*
ulnar nerve 312, 356
  compression **248–249**
  entrapment 242
  injuries 242, *243*, 599, 602
  palsy 304–305, *305*, 601
ulnar neuritis 242
ulnar neuropathy 247
ulno-carpal impaction syndrome 321, *321*
ulnohumeral joint, dislocation 608
ultrasound
  acute haematogenous infections 30
  applications 19–20
  developmental dysplasia of hip 411, 412
  diagnostic 19–20
  principle 19
upper limb *see* arm; hand; wrist
upper motor neurone lesions 202, 212, 510
urate crystals 69, 70, *71*
urethral injuries 530, 667, 668, 673
urethritis 62, *62*
uricosuric drugs 70–71
urinary problems, spina bifida 216
urinary retention/incontinence 371
urinary tract, imaging 670

V

'vacuum sign' 395
valgus deformity 9, 221
  cubitus 304–305, *305*
  foot 221
  knee *9*, 449, 482
Van Nes operation 163
varus deformity 9, 221
  cubitus 305, *305*
  foot 221
  knee *9*, 449
vascular disorders, hands **354**
vascular injuries 588
  fracture complications 562, *562, 563*,
    699
vascular sinusoids 91
vasculitis 52, 58
venous insufficiency, chronic 257, 258
vertebrae
  anatomy 401–402
  codfish (biconcave) *120*
  congenital anomalies **160–161**, 381, 383
  metastases *576*
  osteochondritis *383*, **383–385**
  rotation in structural scoliosis 375
  transverse process fractures 659, *659*
  tumours 393
  see also spine
vertebral body 402
  fracture *18*, 647
  osteoporosis 113
  syndesmophytes and fusion *60*
vertebral disease, spinal cord lesions 213
vibration test 12

vibration white finger 354
vitamin A hypervitaminosis 125
vitamin C deficiency **124–125**, *125*
vitamin D 109, *109*, 114
  deficiency 109, 121
  hypervitaminosis 125
  metabolites and deficiency 109, 121
volar fracture-dislocation 635
volar intercalated segment instability
    (VISI) 321, 622
Volkmann canals 28, 106
Volkmann's ischaemia *563*
Volkmann's ischaemic contracture 339,
    496, 563–564, 572, *572*
von Recklinghausen's disease 155,
    198–199, *199*
Von Rosen's splint 412, *413*

W

wake-up test 380
wallerian degeneration 230, 231
wall test 372
warfarin 258, 259
warts, plantar 515
Watson–Jones approach 441
Watson's test 322
weakness *see* muscle, weakness
Weaver Dunn procedure 586
Werdnig–Hoffman disease **221**
whiplash-associated disorder, chronic 658
whiplash injuries 649, 657, **657–658**
whitlow, herpetic 351, *351*
Wilkin's classification 596
Wilson's sign 467
wires, internal fixation 553–554, *554*
Wolff's law 111, *111*
wounds
  cleansing/excision 559, 637
  closure, open fractures 559–560
  infections, burns 533
woven bone 106
Wright's test 251, 358
wrist **315–331**
  acquired deformities 210, **319**
  anatomy 319–320, **330**
  arthroscopy 24, 317, 323
  articulations 319–320
  avascular necrosis 624
  chronic instability 319–320
  congenital/childhood deformities *317*,
    317–318
  dislocations/subluxations **626–628**, *627*
  drop *7*, 319
  examination *315*, 315–317, *316*
    imaging 316–317
  extensor/flexor tendons 329
  fractures 572
  injuries **621–623**
    ulnar-side **626**
  movements 315–316, *316, 317*, 330
  occupational pain disorders 329
  osteoarthritis **326–328**, *327*
  physeal injury 319
  poliomyelitis 219

rheumatoid arthritis *315*, 319,
 324–326, *325*, *326*
sprains 621, 623
stability 330
swellings around **329–330**, *330*
symptoms and signs 315–316
tenosynovitis/tenovaginitis **328–329**
tuberculosis **324**, *325*

X
xanthine oxidase 69
xanthoma, tendon sheath 197
xenografts 261
x-rays *see* radiography

Y
yaws 42
Z
Z-collapse 345
Zielke method 379–380, *380*
Z-plasties 338, 343